Rook's
Dermatology
Handbook

Rook's Dermatology Handbook

EDITED BY

Christopher E. M. Griffiths, OBE, MD, FMedSci

Foundation Professor of Dermatology
The Dermatology Centre
Salford Royal NHS Foundation Trust
The University of Manchester
Manchester, UK

Tanya O. Bleiker, FRCP

Consultant Dermatologist
Department of Dermatology
University Hospitals of Derby and Burton
Derby, UK

Daniel Creamer, MD, FRCP

Consultant Dermatologist
Department of Dermatology
King's College Hospital
London, UK

John R. Ingram, MA, MSc, DM(Oxon), FRCP(Derm), FAcadMEd

BJD Editor-in-Chief
Clinical Reader and Consultant Dermatologist
Division of Infection and Immunity
Cardiff University
Cardiff, UK

Rosalind C. Simpson, PhD, MRCP(Derm)

Associate Professor and Consultant Dermatologist
Centre of Evidence Based Dermatology
University of Nottingham
Nottingham, UK

WILEY Blackwell

Registered Offices
John Wiley & Sons, Inc., 111 River Street, Hoboken, NJ 07030, USA
John Wiley & Sons Ltd, The Atrium, Southern Gate, Chichester, West Sussex, PO19 8SQ, UK

Editorial Office
9600 Garsington Road, Oxford, OX4 2DQ, UK

For details of our global editorial offices, customer services, and more information about Wiley products visit us at www.wiley.com.

Wiley also publishes its books in a variety of electronic formats and by print-on-demand. Some content that appears in standard print versions of this book may not be available in other formats.

Library of Congress Cataloging-in-Publication Data

Names: Griffiths, C. (Christopher), editor. | Bleiker, Tanya, 1969- editor.
    | Creamer, Daniel, editor. | Ingram, John R., editor. | Simpson,
    Rosalind C., editor.
Title: Rook's dermatology handbook / edited by Christopher E. M. Griffiths,
    Tanya O. Bleiker, Daniel Creamer, John R. Ingram, Rosalind C. Simpson.
Other titles: Dermatology handbook
Description: Hoboken, NJ : Wiley-Blackwell, 2020. | Includes index.
Identifiers: LCCN 2020024268 (print) | LCCN 2020024269 (ebook) | ISBN
    9781119428190 (paperback) | ISBN 9781119428350 (adobe pdf) | ISBN
    9781119428374 (epub)
Subjects: MESH: Skin Diseases
Classification: LCC RL74 (print) | LCC RL74 (ebook) | NLM WR 140 | DDC
    616.5–dc23
LC record available at https://lccn.loc.gov/2020024268
LC ebook record available at https://lccn.loc.gov/2020024269

Cover Design: Wiley
Cover Images: Skin surface, SEM © Science Photo Library / Getty Images, Inc., Blue Blue blur bokeh spring fresh romantic background © Vijay kumar / Getty Images

Set in 8.5/10.5 pt Utopia by Straive, Pondicherry, India

Printed in Singapore
M WEP236471 311023

Contents

Acknowledgements

This handbook has been compiled from *Rook's Textbook of Dermatology*, Ninth Edition, edited by Christopher Griffiths, Jonathan Barker, Tanya O. Bleiker Robert Chalmers and Daniel Creamer. © 2016 John Wiley & Sons, Ltd. Published 2016 by John Wiley & Sons, Ltd. The Editors thank all of the chapter authors from the Rook parent book for their original contributions. Where necessary, the original material has been rewritten to suit a different readership.

Thanks also to John Ingram's colleagues in Cardiff for supplying additional images: Drs Mabs Chowdhury, Manju Kalavala, Colin Long, Richard Motley, Catherine Roberts, Rachel Abbott and Ru Katugampola, and Professors Andrew Finlay and Vincent Piguet.

Preface

Rook's Textbook of Dermatology is a four volume behometh of information, arguably THE dermatological reference. First published in 1968 Rook has evolved from the visionary text produced by Arthur Rook, Darrell Wilkinson and John Ebling and is now in its 9th edition. Indubitably this is indispensable as a detailed reference on dermatology but is neither a pocket book for ready access in clinic nor a skin disease "101" for trainees, non-dermatologists and hard pressed consultants. The Rook editors had discussed the relative merits of a "Rook Handbook" for several years and eventually decided, by popular demand, that the time had come for the talking to stop and work to begin on such a book.

Rook's Dermatology Handbook is a 1000 page, fully illustrated guide to facilitate the rapid diagnosis of skin diseases and provide ready access to key relevant facts about them. The format comprises epidemiology, pathophysiology, clinical features, differential diagnosis, investigations and management. The basic science is kept to a minimum, there are no photomicrographs of histology and management is top line only. The reader would be expected to turn to more detailed references for in-depth information. We have pared down the text from Rook's textbook, retained many of its high-quality images and introduced new tables and new sections, including dermatological vocabulary and differential diagnosis of common clinical presentations such as blisters, hair loss and erythroderma. Three of the editors of the textbook – Chris Griffiths, Tanya O. Bleiker and Daniel Creamer – have been joined in the venture by two next generation clinicians, John Ingram and Rosalind Simpson. We are delighted with the book but the proof will come from how it performs in the clinic as an aid to the diagnosis, understanding and management of dermatological disease. We are indebted to all of the authors from the Rook 9th edition who freely gave us permission to recycle and synopsise their chapters.

The book would not have seen the light of day without the unstinting support and expertise of Claire Bonnett, Jenny Seward and Nick Morgan of Wiley, and Production team.

Chris Griffiths
Tanya O. Bleiker
Daniel Creamer
John Ingram
Rosalind Simpson

Glossary

Alopecia	Decreased density or thickness of hairs
Artefact	Induced by exogenous injury, sometimes self-inflicted
Callus	Reactive hyperkeratosis, usually due to friction and/or pressure, leading to enhanced skin markings
Comedone (open and closed)	*Open:* dilated hair infundibulum with oxidised (black) keratinous debris ('blackhead')
	Closed: expansion of hair infundibulum by keratinous debris, usually with no connection to skin surface ('whitehead')
Dysaesthesia	Inappropriate sensations, e.g. paraesthesias
Exanthem	Acute widespread eruption, usually due to a viral infection or drug reaction
Fissure	Linear disruption of stratum corneum; may extend into the dermis
Infarct	Ischaemia of tissue due to arterial occlusion
Induration	Deep thickening of the skin can result from oedema, inflammation, or infiltration
Keratoderma	Thickening of the stratum corneum and/or epidermis of the palms and soles, often inherited
Keratosis	Focal thickening of the epidermis, especially the stratum corneum
Kerion	Boggy plaque, due to infection, that often contains pustules
Lichenification	Accentuation of skin markings, often due to rubbing
Poikiloderma	Simultaneous presence of atrophy, telangiectasia and hypo- and hyperpigmentation
Prurigo	Papules or nodules due to scratching or picking
Purpura	Haemorrhage into the skin due to pathological processes, primarily of blood vessels
Stria	Linear atrophy along tension lines; initially can be red to purple in colour
Telangiectasia	Permanently dilated capillaries and venules which are visible to the naked eye

Abbreviations

ACTH	adrenocorticotropic hormone	HLA	human leukocyte antigen
AE	atopic eczema	HPV	human papilloma virus
AGEP	acute generalised exanthematous pustulosis	HSV	herpes simplex virus
AIDS	acquired immune deficiency syndrome	IF	immunofluorescence
AK	actinic keratoses	IFN	interferon
ALP	alkaline phosphatase	IgE	immunoglobulin E
ALT	alanine aminotransferase	IL	interleukin
ANA	antinuclear antibody	IMF	immunofluorescence
ANCA	antineutrophil cytoplasmic antibodies	IV	intravenous
ASOT	antistreptolysin O titre	KC	keratinocyte carcinoma
AST	aspartate aminotransferase	LDH	lactate dehydrogenase
ATP	adenosine triphosphate	LE	lupus erythematosus
BCC	basal cell carcinoma	LFT	liver function test
BCG	bacille Calmette–Guérin	LP	lichen planus
BP	blood pressure	MHC	major histocompatibility complex
BSA	body surface area	MM	Investigations malignant melanoma
CBT	cognitive behavioural therapy	MMR	mumps measles rubella vaccination
CMV	cytomegalovirus	MRI	magnetic resonance imaging
CNS	central nervous system	MRSA	meticillin-resistant Staphylococcus aureus
CREST	calcinosis, Raynaud phenomenon, oesophageal dysmotility, sclerodactyly and telangiectasia	NSAID	non-steroidal anti-inflammatory drug
		PAS	periodic acid–Schiff
CRP	C-reactive protein	PASI	Psoriasis Area Severity Index
CT	computerised tomography	PCR	polymerase chain reaction
CTCL	cutaneous T-cell lymphoma	PUVA	psoralen and ultraviolet A
CVI	chronic venous insufficiency	PVL	Panton–Valentine leukocidin
CXR	chest X-ray	PXE	pseudoxanthoma elasticum
DEJ	dermal–epidermal junction	RAS	Recurrent aphous stomatitis
DLE	discoid lupus erythematosus	RNA	ribo nucleic acid
DLQI	Dermatology Life Quality Index	QoL	quality of life
DNA	deoxyribonucleic acid	SCC	squamous cell carcinoma
EBV	Epstein–Barr virus	Sinus	Tract leading from a deeper focus to the skin surface
EGFR	epidermal growth factor receptor	SLE	systemic lupus erythematosus
ELISA	enzyme-linked immunosorbent assay	SPF	sun protection factor
ENA	extractable nuclear antigen	TCR	T-cell receptor
ESR	erythrocyte sedimentation rate	TFT	thyroid function test
FBC	full blood count	TNF	tumour necrosis factor
5-FU	5-fluorouracil	TPMT	thiopurine methyltransferase
G6PD	glucose-6-phosphate dehydrogenase	U&E	urea and electrolytes
GvHD	graft-versus-host disease	UV	ultraviolet
H&E	haematoxylin and eosin	UVR	ultraviolet radiation
Hb	haemaglobin	VZV	varicella-zoster virus
HHV	human herpesvirus	WCC	white cell count
HIV	human immunodeficiency virus	WHO	World Health Organization

Introduction

Human skin consists of a stratified, cellular epidermis and an underlying dermis of connective tissue, separated by a dermal–epidermal basement membrane (Figure 1.1). Beneath the dermis is a layer of subcutaneous fat, which is separated from the rest of the body by a vestigial layer of striated muscle.

The skin performs a number of functions, including:

- Providing a physiological barrier against the external environment.
- Maintaining fluid balance by restricting water loss through the skin.

- Forming an innate immune defence against bacteria, fungi and viruses through keratinocyte-derived endogenous antibiotics, defensins and cathelicidins. Langerhans cells have a primary role in epidermal immune surveillance.
- Supporting thermoregulation: vasodilatation or vasoconstriction of the blood vessels in the deep and superficial plexuses helps to regulate body temperature. Eccrine sweat glands, found at all skin sites, also play a role in heat control.
- Providing insulation and trauma protection: subcutaneous fat limits excessive heat loss and shields internal structures from physical trauma.

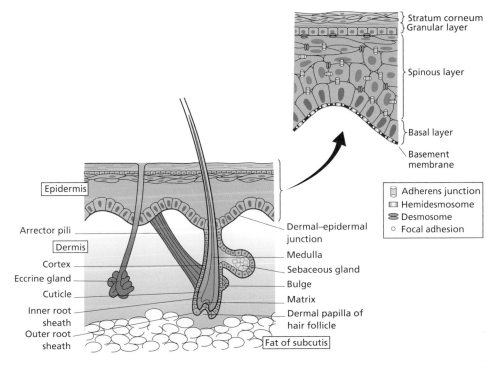

Figure 1.1 The skin and its appendages.

Rook's Dermatology Handbook, First Edition. Edited by Christopher E. M. Griffiths, Tanya O. Bleiker, Daniel Creamer, John R. Ingram and Rosalind C. Simpson.
© 2022 John Wiley & Sons Ltd. Published 2022 by John Wiley & Sons Ltd.

ROOK'S DERMATOLOGY HANDBOOK

Fat also has an endocrine function, releasing the hormone leptin, which acts on the hypothalamus to regulate hunger and energy metabolism.
- Vitamin D production.
- Performing a psychosocial function: the appearance of human skin and its associated structures, especially scalp hair, has a major impact on self-image and thus on interpersonal relationships.
- Protection from ultraviolet (UV) radiation through production of melanin from melanocytes. Variation in response to sunlight has historically been   divided into six categories according to the Fitzpatrick classification (Table 1.1). It is acknowledged that whilst these 'skin types' describe response to UV exposure, they do not adequately encompass the wide variation of tones seen in skin of colour.

History taking

Clinical assessment of a patient presenting with a skin disorder follows the standard approach of history-taking and physical examination. Investigations may be needed to supplement information obtained at the consultation.

Although a dermatological diagnosis might be swiftly apparent, it is essential to take a full history before examining the skin. The history of the presenting complaint will yield the story of the symptoms and the clinical features of the dermatosis (Box 1.1). Further questions will give details about any associated clinical problems and the patient's background medical history (Table 1.2). The act of questioning (and listening to the answers) contributes to a consultation's therapeutic function.

Table 1.1 Fitzpatrick classification of skin types

Skin type	Skin colour on sun-protected site	Sunburn risk	Tanning ability	Skin cancer risk
I	White	++++	±	High
II	White	+++	+	High
III	White	++	++	Moderate
IV	Olive	+	+++	Moderate
V	Brown	±	++++	Low
VI	Black/dark brown	±	++++	Low

Box 1.1 History of the presenting complaint

Essential points in the history: rashes

- Location: Where did the rash start, where did it spread to?
- Temporal: When did it start, does it come and go, if so, how long does it last?
- Exacerbating factors: What makes it worse?
- Alleviating factors: Physical factors, diet, treatment?
- What are the predominant symptoms: itch, pain, disfigurement?
- Occupational factors: Does it get worse at work? Does it improve away from work?
- Open questions: Do you have any thoughts as to what has caused this? What concerns you most about this problem?

Essential points in the history: lesions

- Where is the lesion? Is it single or multiple?
- Was there any trauma before it arose?
- Temporal: How long has it taken to develop to this size? Is it still growing or is it resolving?
- Symptoms: Is it tender, painful or itchy? Are there any exacerbating factors? Has it bled?
- Past history: Have you had anything similar before?
- Sun exposure: How much sun exposure have you had, including living/ working abroad and use of sun beds? Any history of blistering sun burns?

Table 1.2 Background medical history

Further history	Rationale	Example
General medical history	Systemic diseases may have cutaneous features	Dermatomyositis and other connective tissue disorders
Medication history	Certain dermatoses are induced by drugs	Drug-induced exanthem
Allergy history	Certain dermatoses are caused by an allergy to a food or drug or contact allergen	Oral allergy syndrome
Family history	Certain dermatoses are inherited	Basal cell carcinoma syndrome (Gorlin syndrome)
Occupational history	The trigger for a dermatosis may be found only at the patient's workplace	Allergic contact dermatitis in a hairdresser
Leisure history	Certain dermatoses are related to leisure activities	Allergic contact dermatitis to plants in gardening
Travel history	Certain dermatoses are more commonly encountered abroad	Leishmaniasis
Social history	Certain dermatoses are associated with lifestyle habits	Palmo-plantar pustulosis is associated with smoking
Ethnicity	Certain disorders are more prevalent in particular ethnic groups	Sarcoidosis and lupus erythematosus occur more frequently in patients with black skin
Quality of life	Effects of dermatosis on work, relationships, activities etc. can be quantified	Dermatology Life Quality Index

Clinical examination

As in any medical consultation, examination follows history-taking and the correct assessment of skin signs is only achieved in the context of a patient's symptoms. Effective interpretation of cutaneous clinical features relies on the principle that most skin diseases have characteristic lesions with a predilection for certain body sites. An understanding of these disease-specific patterns is intrinsic to diagnosis in dermatology, an assertion which is especially true in the appraisal of a rash.

The patient should always be examined in a good light, preferably daylight, and with magnification of lesions if necessary. A mobile light on a flexible stand can be helpful in illuminating areas that are in the shade from overhead lights, such as the mouth and the flexures. Ideally, the entire skin should be examined in every patient, including the scalp and nails. Full skin examination may also reveal suspicious skin lesions that the patient was not aware of, for example lesions on the back.

Examination of a lesion

When assessing a solitary skin lesion there are a number of features relating to its morphology which direct the physician to a diagnosis. All skin lesions can be assigned to one of the descriptive entities defined in Table 1.3 (illustrated in Figure 1.2). Recognition of the lesion type is the basis of clinical examination in dermatology. Thereafter a more detailed appreciation of the lesion's properties will enhance the assessment. Use of the 5Ss is helpful in describing, and thus identifying, a lesion: **S**ite, **S**ize, **S**ymmetry, **S**hape and **S**urface.

Table 1.3 Descriptive terms for cutaneous lesions (adapted from Nast et al. 2016)

Term	Definition	Example
Bulla (Figure 2a)	A circumscribed lesion >1 cm in diameter that contains liquid (clear, serous or haemorrhagic)	Bullous pemphigoid
Macule (Figure 2b)	A flat, circumscribed, non-palpable lesion that differs in colour from the surrounding skin	Junctional naevus
Nodule (Figure 2c)	An elevated, solid, palpable lesion >1 cm usually located primarily in the dermis and/or subcutis	Squamous cell carcinoma
Papule (Figure 2d)	An elevated, solid, palpable lesion that is ≤1 cm in diameter	Intradermal naevus
Patch (Figure 2e)	A flat circumscribed area of discoloration, >1 cm	Vitiligo
Plaque (Figure 2f)	A circumscribed, palpable lesion >1 cm in diameter; most plaques are elevated	Psoriatic plaque
Pustule (Figure 2g)	A circumscribed lesion that contains pus	Palmoplantar pustulosis
Vesicle	A circumscribed lesion ≤1 cm in diameter that contains liquid (not pus)	Herpes simplex
Weal	A transient elevation of the skin due to dermal oedema	Urticaria
Scale (Figure 2h)	A visible accumulation of keratin, forming a flat plate or flake	Psoriasis
Crust	Dried serum, blood or pus on the surface of the skin	Impetigo
Erosion	Loss of either a portion of the epidermis or the entire epidermis	Pemphigus vulgaris
Excoriation	A loss of the epidermis and a portion of the dermis due to scratching or an exogenous injury	Scratching from any cause
Ulcer	Full-thickness loss of the epidermis plus at least a portion of the dermis	Venous leg ulcer

Source: Adapted from A. Nast et al. The 2016 International League of Dermatological Societies' revised glossary for the description of cutaneous lesions. British Journal of Dermatology, 2016, 174, pp. 1351–1358. John Wiley & Sons Ltd on behalf of the British Association of Dermatologists.

Examination of a rash

In the initial assessment of a rash the type of primary lesion, from which the dermatosis is constituted, needs to be identified. Thereafter the configuration of lesional skin on the skin's surface will point to the diagnosis, a deductive process termed pattern recognition. The description of a rash should comment on the morphology of individual lesions, including colour and shape (Table 1.4), as well as information on body sites of involvement and distribution pattern (Table 1.5) (illustrated in Figure 1.3). Palpation of lesional skin imparts additional information about texture, skin thickness, tenderness and temperature.

Medical photographs

Medical photography is a useful tool to record the current state of a dermatosis and to permit serial comparisons over time to assess change. Patient consent and secure image storage are important considerations.

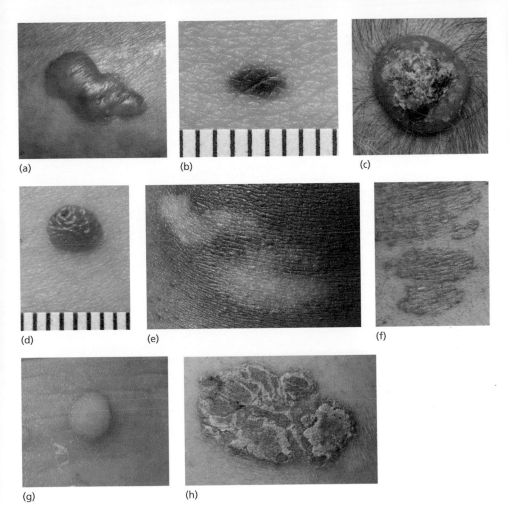

Figure 1.2 Types of cutaneous lesion: (a) bulla: bullous pemphigoid; (b) macule: junctional naevus; (c) nodule: squamous cell carcinoma; (d) papule: intradermal naevus; (e) patch: vitiligo; (f) plaque: psoriasis; (g) pustule: palmoplantar pustulosis; (h) scale: psoriasis. (Source: Reproduced with permission of Cardiff and Vale University Health Board.)

Bedside tests
Dermoscopy
(Syn. Dermatoscopy)

A dermatoscope (Syn. Dermoscope) provides polarised light and magnification to aid examination of the skin. The dermatoscope lens is applied to the skin surface with a film of oil on the lesion to enhance examination of subcorneal structures. Analysis of the colours and appearances of structural elements, such as the pigment network, is especially useful in the diagnosis of pigmented lesions. The images may be viewed directly, photographed or recorded digitally for subsequent or sequential analysis. Dermatoscopes can also be useful in distinguishing haemangiomas, angiokeratomas, pigmented basal cell carcinomas and seborrhoeic keratoses. Additional uses include the identification of scabies mites and other parasitic infections. Trichoscopy is use of a dermatoscope for hair and scalp lesions, and aids diagnostic accuracy in scalp disorders.

Table 1.4 Shapes of cutaneous lesions (adapted from Nast et al. 2016)

Term	Definition	Example
Acuminate	Elevated lesion with a sharp point	Cutaneous horn
Annular (Figure 3a)	Shape of a ring (clear centrally)	Tinea corporis
Arciform, arcuate	A segment of a ring; arch-like	Erythema annulare centrifugum
Digitate	Finger-shaped	Digitate dermatosis, a form of parapsoriasis
Discoid; nummular (Figure 3b)	Circular or coin-shaped	Nummular eczema
Linear	Lesional skin forming a band or line	Lichen striatus
Papillomatous	Lesion with multiple surface projections	Epidermal naevus
Pedunculated	Papule or nodule attached by a thinner stalk	Skin tag
Polymorphic	Variable sizes and shapes as well as types of lesions	Acne vulgaris
Polycyclic	Coalescence of several rings	Subacute cutaneous lupus erythematosus
Reticulate (Figure 3e)	Net-like or lacy pattern	Mucosal lichen planus
Serpiginous (Figure 3c)	Wavy pattern, reminiscent of a snake	Cutaneous larva migrans
Targetoid	Lesion composed of concentric rings	Erythema multiforme
Umbilicated	Lesion with a small surface depression	Molluscum contagiosum
Verruciform	Lesion with multiple projections resembling a wart	Viral wart

Source: Adapted from A. Nast et al. The 2016 International League of Dermatological Societies' revised glossary for the description of cutaneous lesions. British Journal of Dermatology, 2016, 174, pp. 1351–1358. John Wiley & Sons Ltd on behalf of the British Association of Dermatologists.

A dermatoscope can also be used in the assessment of nail fold capillaries in connective tissue diseases (e.g. dermatomyositis).

Skin swabs (bacterial/viral)

In a suspected bacterial infection skin swabs for bacteriology should be sent to confirm the organism and provide antibiotic sensitivities to guide antibiotic selection.

Detection of viral skin infection, for example herpes simplex, requires a specific viral swab for viral culture. Increasingly polymerase chain reaction (PCR) amplification of viral DNA/RNA can provide a diagnosis within hours.

Mycological sample collection

Skin. Scraping samples of surface scale from an active margin are taken with a disposable scalpel blade or banana-shaped scalpel. The scrapings should be transported in folded paper, which keeps the specimen dry, thus preventing overgrowth of bacterial contaminants.

Hairs. If tinea capitis is suspected, the hairs should be plucked with the roots intact; cut hairs are unsuitable. Brush samples from the scalp are excellent for culture, but with this technique microscopy is not possible.

Table 1.5 Distribution patterns of cutaneous lesions (adapted from Nast et al. 2016)

Term	Definition	Example
Acral	Lesions involving distal extremities (e.g. ears, nose, fingers and toes)	Acrocyanosis
Asymmetrical	Distribution pattern which lacks symmetry along an axis (e.g. the midline)	Lichen striatus
Blaschkoid; along Blaschko lines	Lesions occurring on embryonic growth lines (Blaschko lines)	Incontinentia pigmenti
Dermatomal (zosteriform)	Lesions confined to one or more dermatome (a segment of skin innervated by a single spinal nerve)	Shingles (herpes zoster)
Disseminated	Lesions distributed randomly over most of the body surface area	Viral exanthem
Exposed skin	Areas exposed to external agents (e.g. airborne allergens, irritants, sunlight)	Airborne allergic contact dermatitis
Extensor sites	Areas overlying muscles and tendons involved in extension (e.g. dorsal forearm, elbow, posterior upper arm)	Psoriasis
Flexural sites	Areas overlying muscle and tendons involved in flexion of joints (e.g. antecubital fossa)	Atopic dermatitis
Follicular	Lesions located within or around hair follicles	Keratosis pilaris
Generalised/ widespread	Distributed over most of the body surface area (see above)	Viral exanthem
Intertriginous	Present in major body folds (axillae, submammary folds, inguinal creases, natal cleft)	Flexural psoriasis
Kobnerised (displaying Kobner phenomenon)	Lesions arranged in a distribution which reflects physical stimuli (e.g. scratching, sunburn)	Lichen planus
Palmo-plantar	Involving palmar and plantar skin	Palmo-plantar pustulosis
Periorificial (e.g. perioral, periorbital)	Involving the skin around orifices	Peri-oral dermatitis
Seborrhoeic	Involving areas with the highest density of sebaceous glands (e.g. scalp, face, upper trunk)	Seborrhoeic dermatitis
Sporotrichoid (Figure 3d)	Lesions occurring along lymphatic vessels, usually of arm or leg	*Mycobacterium marinum* infection
Symmetrical	Lesions occurring with symmetry along an axis, commonly the midline	Psoriasis

Source: Adapted from A. Nast et al. The 2016 International League of Dermatological Societies' revised glossary for the description of cutaneous lesions. British Journal of Dermatology, 2016, 174, pp. 1351–1358. John Wiley & Sons Ltd on behalf of the British Association of Dermatologists.

ROOK'S DERMATOLOGY HANDBOOK

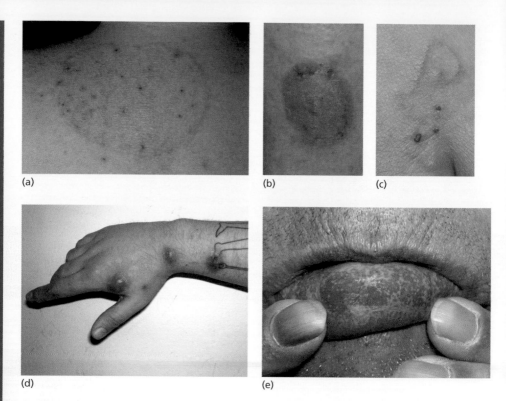

Figure 1.3 Shapes and distribution patterns of skin lesions: (a) annular: tinea cruris; (b) discoid (round): nummular eczema; (c) serpiginous: cutaneous larva migrans; (d) sporotrichoid: Mycobacterium marinum infection; (e) reticulate: lichen planus on the lower lip. (Source: (a), (b) and (c) reproduced with permission of Cardiff and Vale University Health Board.)

Nails. Isolation of the pathogen from nail material is more difficult than in other samples. The full thickness of the nail should be sampled. Debris from under the nail is a fruitful source of material.

Wood's light

This is a source of UV light from which visible light has been excluded by a Wood's (nickel oxide) filter. Variations in epidermal pigmentation are more apparent under Wood's light than under visible light, whereas variations in dermal pigment are less apparent. For example, Wood's light accentuates the epidermal depigmentation of vitiligo, whereas the pallor from localised dermal vasoconstriction in naevus anaemicus disappears under Wood's lamp. Some organisms produce chemicals that fluoresce under Wood's lamp, including *Corynebacterium minutissimum*, the bacterium responsible for erythrasma

(Figure 1.4). Wood's light examination is a useful tool in the diagnosis of superficial mycoses, particularly infections due to *Microsporum* species which fluoresce green (Table 1.6).

Specific investigations
Biopsy

A biopsy of lesional skin provides essential information on the dermatopathology of almost all skin disorders. Sections from a paraffin-embedded biopsy specimen are usually stained with haematoxylin and eosin (H&E) for standard histopathological reporting. Special stains can be used to detect the presence of microorganisms (e.g. dermatophytes), the distribution of particular components of the skin (e.g. elastin) and the deposition of pathological substances (e.g. amyloid). Antibody deposition in the skin in immunobullous diseases is assessed

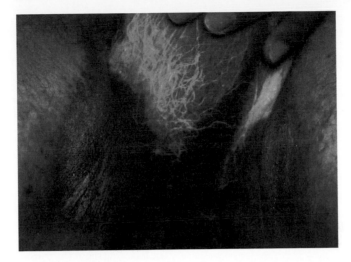

Figure 1.4 Wood's light illumination of erythrasma of the groins. The fluorescence in erythrasma is coral pink.

Table 1.6 Colour under Wood's light linked to clinical examples (adapted from Nast et al. 2016)

Colour under Wood's light	Clinical example(s)
Blue-green to yellow-green	Tinea capitis due to *Microsporum* spp.
Coral pink	Erythrasma
Red	Urine in some forms of porphyria
White	Well-developed lesions of vitiligo
Yellow to yellow-green	Pityriasis (tinea) versicolor

Source: Adapted from A. Nast et al. The 2016 International League of Dermatological Societies' revised glossary for the description of cutaneous lesions. British Journal of Dermatology, 2016, 174, pp. 1351–1358. John Wiley & Sons Ltd on behalf of the British Association of Dermatologists.

by direct immunofluorescence. Skin biopsies are processed specifically for this purpose; the immunofluorescence laboratory technique is performed on frozen sections.

Several different types of biopsy can be performed under local anaesthetic. Punch biopsies provide a small full thickness sample of skin, shave biopsies provide information on superficial skin layers and incisional biopsies may be used to sample a full-thickness section of a larger skin lesion or rash.

Patch tests

Patch tests are typically used to detect contact allergy of the delayed hypersensitivity type. Multiple chemicals are applied to the patient's back to assess for an eczematous reaction. Patch tests are usually read at 2 days and 4 days (see Chapter 69). A patch test technique can be used to detect contact urticaria when the results are read at 15–30 min.

Prick tests

Prick testing investigates immediate type I hypersensitivity reactions. A small quantity of the test solution is placed on the skin and a prick is made through it with a sharp needle. The size of the weal and flare is measured after 15 min and compared with an adjacent control solution.

2 Introduction to dermatological therapeutics

Treatment modalities for skin disease comprise:

- Topical treatment
- Dressings (not discussed further in this book)
- Local injection
- Systemic agents (Chapter 82)
- Phototherapy
- Surgical removal of tissue
- Physical destruction of tissue such as with cryotherapy, cautery/diathermy, hyfrecation, and laser.

Topical treatment

There are different 'vehicles' (Box 2.1) that can be used to apply topical medication or emollients to the skin. As a rule, acutely inflamed skin is best treated with bland preparations that are least likely to irritate. Moist or exudative eruptions are conventionally treated with lotions or creams, whilst dry skin responds well to ointments.

Prescribing topical treatment

The following should be considered when making a prescription for a topical treatment:

Prescription requirements: In general, a prescription of topical agent should comprise drug name, vehicle (cream or ointment), quantity to be dispensed, frequency, site of application and duration of treatment.

Frequency: Emollients should be applied frequently enough to maintain their physical effect, which may mean several applications per day. Active preparations are usually applied once or twice daily. Twice-daily application of topical corticosteroids is only marginally more effective than once-daily application.

Box 2.1 Different types of vehicle

Ointments: Semi-solid vehicles composed of lipid, such as white soft paraffin BP (petrolatum). Contain fewer preservatives than other vehicles. Occlusive and emollient properties.

Creams: Semi-solid emulsions containing both lipid and water. Emollient, lubricant and mildly occlusive.

Pastes: Semi-solid preparations containing a high proportion of finely powdered material such as zinc oxide or starch. Occlusive, protective and hydrating.

Lotions: Liquid formulations, usually simple suspensions or solutions of medication in water, alcohol or other liquids. Suitable for treating the scalp and other hairy areas of skin.

Gels: Thickened lotions. Suitable for treating the scalp and other hairy areas of skin.

Powders: Occasionally used to deliver drugs such as antifungal agents applied to the feet.

Paints: Liquid preparations which are usually applied with a brush to the skin or mucous membranes.

Dressings: Impregnated dressings, e.g. bandages containing ichthammol or zinc oxide, or tapes containing topical steroid.

Rook's Dermatology Handbook, First Edition. Edited by Christopher E. M. Griffiths, Tanya O. Bleiker, Daniel Creamer, John R. Ingram and Rosalind C. Simpson.
© 2022 John Wiley & Sons Ltd. Published 2022 by John Wiley & Sons Ltd.

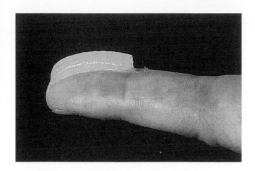

Figure 2.1 The fingertip unit: from the distal crease of the forefinger to the ventral aspect of the fingertip

Quantity: The quantity of active topical agent (such as topical corticosteroids) needed for effective treatment should be explained to the patient. 'Fingertip units' are a useful guide for topical corticosteroid application (see Figure 2.1 and Table 2.1). Emollients should be applied more liberally.

Timing of application: Leave a suitable amount of time between emollient and active agent. This avoids dilution of the active medication and prevents spread over areas of skin where it is not required.

Potential hazards: Localised irritant or allergic reactions are the most frequent adverse effects (see Chapter 69). All topically applied drugs are absorbed to some degree, but systemic side effects are relatively rare. Absorption varies considerably depending on the region of skin being treated (absorption greatest from the genital area and least from the soles and palms). Occlusion greatly enhances drug penetration. Inflammation of the skin significantly increases drug absorption, especially in erythrodermic patients. Bath oils tend to make the bath slippery; paraffin-based ointments are flammable, which is a particular risk in smokers.

Table 2.2 lists frequently used topical treatments, but is not intended to provide an exhaustive list.

Topical corticosteroids

Topical corticosteroids (TCS) are the mainstay of treatment in eczematous dermatoses and are used either regularly or occasionally in the management of most inflammatory skin diseases. TCS vary in potency from mild to very potent (Table 2.3). Classification of potency is important to predict response and possible adverse effects. Penetration of TCS is increased by occlusion using polythene film, dressings, gloves or bandages. This improves beneficial effects but also increases the potential for adverse effects.

Side effects

Significant side effects are rare, especially with short term use. The most common side effects are localised to application sites: skin atrophy, striae, erythema, telangiectasia and purpura; atrophic changes can become irreversible with long-term use of potent preparations. Areas most vulnerable to atrophy are those where the skin is already relatively thin, e.g. flexures and face.

Other local side effects are development of contact allergy, exacerbation of infection and if used on the face acneiform eruptions (see Chapter 40). It is advisable to avoid the use of topical corticosteroids in the presence of active viral infection, including herpes simplex, viral warts or molluscum contagiosum.

It is recommended that patients should use no more than 50 g of a superpotent steroid or 100 g of a potent steroid preparation per week and that prolonged usage at this high rate should be avoided to minimise the risk of systemic absorption leading to Cushing syndrome and hypothalamic-pituitary-adrenal axis suppression.

Rebound worsening of disease may occur when topical corticosteroids are withdrawn, particularly in psoriasis. This is most likely after withdrawal of potent or very potent corticosteroids.

'Steroid phobia' describes the fear of using topical corticosteroids which is out of proportion to the likelihood of side effects developing.

Topical calcineurin inhibitors

Topical calcineurin inhibitors (TCIs) have been developed for topical treatment of atopic eczema and have numerous additional applications. TCIs (e.g. tacrolimus and pimecrolimus) exhibit their anti-inflammatory effect by inhibition of calcineurin, which suppresses lymphocyte activation. They do not induce cutaneous atrophy. Theoretically, the local immunosuppression related to these

ROOK'S DERMATOLOGY HANDBOOK

Table 2.1 Fingertip units required for a single treatment of various regions in children and adults (the unit is measured using an adult finger)

Age	Face and neck	One upper limb	One lower limb	Trunk (including buttocks)	Whole body
3–6 months	1	1	1.5	2.5	8.5
1–2 years	1.5	1.5	2	5	13.5
3–5 years	1.5	2	3	6.5	18
6–10 years	2	2.5	4.5	8.5	24.5
Adult	2.5	4.5	7.6	13.5	40

Source: Finlay AY, Edwards PH, Harding KG. 'Fingertip Unit' in dermatology. Lancet, 1989, 11, 155 and Long CC, Mills CM, Finlay AY. A practical guide to topical therapy in children. Br J Dermatol 1998, 138, 293–296.

Table 2.2 Different types of topical treatments and their main uses

Type of agent	Common example(s)	Indication
Antimicrobial agents	Alcohols: isopropyl alcohol, ethanol and *n*-propanol Benzalkonium chloride Chlorhexidine, iodine Antibiotics	Alcohols can be used for skin cleansing Present in antiseptic creams Used as a skin cleanser prior to surgery Topical antibiotics are frequently used in the treatment of superficial infections, acne vulgaris and rosacea
Antifungal agents	Allylamines (e.g. terbinafine), imidazoles (e.g. clotrimazole), morpholines (e.g. amorolfine) and polyenes (e.g. nystatin)	Treatment of mild dermatophyte and yeast infections
Antiparasitic agents	Pyrethroids (e.g. permethrin), malathion, dimeticone, Ivermectin	Treatment of lice infestations and scabies
Antiperspirants	Aluminium chloride	Hyperhidrosis of the axillae, palms and soles
Antiviral agents	Aciclovir, podophyllin, cidofovir	Treatment of herpes simplex virus types I and II, treatment of genital warts
Astringents	Aqueous solutions of potassium permanganate, aluminium acetate, and silver nitrate	Used to reduce exudation by precipitation of protein. These also have antiseptic properties.
Calcineurin inhibitors	Tacrolimus, pimecrolimus	Licensed for treatment of atopic eczema, especially in facial and flexural areas Also used in multiple other inflammatory dermatoses
Corticosteroids	Topical: see Table 2.3 Intralesional, e.g. triamcinolone	Topical: mainstay of treatment in eczematous dermatoses and other inflammatory dermatoses Intralesional: recalcitrant dermatoses, e.g. alopecia areata, keloid scars, lichen simplex, nodular prurigo
Cytotoxic and antineoplastic agents	5-fluorouracil, diclofenac, ingenol mebutate, imiquimod	Actinic keratosis, Bowen disease, superficial BCC, viral warts (refer to individual drug regarding indication)
Depigmenting agents	Hydroquinone, azelaic acid	Melasma
Emollients	White soft paraffin	Used to protect, lubricate and moisturise dry skin Also use instead of soap ('soap substitute') on inflamed skin
Keratolytic agents Miscellaneous agents	Salicylic acid, urea Brimonidine Capsaicin Dithranol Nicotinamide/nicotinic acid	To treat hyperkeratosis Rosacea Neuralgia, nodular prurigo, other localised intractable itch Psoriasis Acne vulgaris

ROOK'S DERMATOLOGY HANDBOOK

Table 2.2 (Continued)

Type of agent	Common example(s)	Indication
Retinoids	Retinoic acid (tretinoin), isotretinoin, adapalene Bexarotene	Acne Early plaque stage mycosis fungoides
Sensitising agents	Dinitrocholorobenzene, diphencyprone	Treatment of alopecia areata and warts
Soothing agents	Menthol, calamine	To help soothe itching and discomfort
Special dermatological formulations ('specials')	Examples: Coal tar solution BP 5% w/w in betamethasone valerate 0.025% w/w ointment 100 g Salicylic acid 5% w/w/propylene glycol 47.5% w/w in Dermovate® cream 100 g Reflectant (Dundee) sunscreens (available in coffee, coral pink, beige) 50 g	For moderate-severe psoriasis of trunk and limbs when other treatments such as vitamin D analogues have been ineffective For use on palmoplantar skin for hyperkeratotic eczema, palmopustular pustulosis and psoriasis not responding to Clobetasol propionate and emollients alone To treat photosensitivity disorders where the patient is sensitive to visible light, e.g. solar urticaria and porphyrias
Tars	Coal tar	Psoriasis
Vitamin D analogues	Calcipotriol, calcitriol, maxacalcitol, tacalcitol	Psoriasis

Table 2.3 Potency of some common topical corticosteroids as per *British National Formulary*

Topical corticosteroid potency	Examples
Very potent	Clobetasol propionate Diflucortone valerate 0.3%
Potent	Beclometasone dipropionate 0.025% Betamethasone valerate 0.1% Fluocinolone acetonide 0.025% Hydrocortisone 17-butyrate Mometasone furoate 0.1% Fluticasone propionate
Moderate	Betamethasone valerate 0.025% Clobetasone butyrate Fludroxycortide 0.0125% Fluocinolone acetonide 0.00625% Alclometasone dipropionate 0.05%
Mild	Hydrocortisone 1% Hydrocortisone 2.5% Fluocinolone acetonide 0.0025%

compounds could increase the risks of infections and cutaneous neoplasia. In practice these risks have not proved problematic and the risk of neoplasia remains hypothetical. It is recommended that TCIs are used at night-time and advice on sun protection should be given. Patients often experience a burning sensation in the early stages of TCI use. These preparations should be built up slowly to minimise such side effects.

Intralesional steroids

Intralesional steroids have a wide range of indications, e.g. inflammatory acne cysts, lichen planus, lichen simplex, chondrodermatitis and alopecia areata. Aqueous suspensions of triamcinolone acetonide (10 and 40 mg/mL) are available and can be diluted with saline or lidocaine. Triamcinolone acetonide 10 mg/mL is sufficient for all conditions except keloids, for which the more potent preparation is usually required to achieve the desired degree of collagen resorption. The amount injected normally ranges from 0.1 to 0.5 mL of 10 mg/mL solution. The injection should be given using a 27–30-gauge needle deep in the dermis when possible to minimise the risk of collagen atrophy. Serious adverse effects may result from inadvertent intravascular injection. This is especially important when injecting lesions around the forehead, where accidental intra-arterial injection and retrograde flow of a bolus of particles may result in retinal artery occlusion and blindness.

Phototherapy

Modern phototherapy uses specific wavelengths typically within the ultraviolet (UV) part of the electromagnetic spectrum. The following are used to treat a variety of skin diseases:

- *UVB phototherapy (narrow-band UVB, 311–313 nm)*: The most commonly used phototherapy and the phototherapy of first choice for most indications.
- *Photochemotherapy (psoralen and UVA (PUVA), 315–400 nm)*: Used mainly for UVB phototherapy treatment failures and in specific conditions, e.g. palmoplantar pustulosis, pustular psoriasis and pityriasis rubra pilaris. Psoralen can be administered either topically or orally. 8-methoxypsoralen (8-MOP) and 5-methoxypsoralen (5-MOP) are the most

commonly used psoralens for oral use. Psoralen can be applied topically in a variety of ways: a bath solution for whole-body treatment and soak, paint, or cream or gel for hands and feet, scalp and other localised areas.

- *UVA-1 phototherapy (340–400 nm)*: Useful for the treatment of sclerotic skin conditions, e.g. morphoea, and for atopic eczema.
- *Extracorporeal photochemotherapy (photopheresis)*: Indicated for severe forms of cutaneous T-cell lymphoma, Sézary syndrome and graft-versus-host disease.

The main short-term hazard of UV therapy is burning of the skin and the primary long-term concern is skin cancer risk. Systemic PUVA is associated with a dose-related increased risk of squamous cell carcinoma (SCC). No evidence of increased risk of skin cancer has yet been shown for UVB or UVA-1 phototherapy. To avoid adverse events, careful patient selection, education and assessment of skin cancer risk are important. In addition, accurate dosimetry and UV lamp maintenance are required. Patient and staff safety are of paramount importance and ensured by the establishment of good clinical governance pathways. Staff who conduct dosimetry should wear goggles, face shields, appropriate clothing and sunscreen (SPF > 30) if they have to enter the cabinet with the lamps on. When UV cabinets are being used, the lamps should be switched off before opening or entering the cabinet. See Box 2.2 for patient safety measures.

Photodynamic therapy

Topical photodynamic therapy (PDT) is widely used for the treatment of superficial non-melanoma skin cancer and dysplasia, and has been shown to be at least as effective as non-surgical standard comparators such as topical fluorouracil and cryotherapy. The main indications for topical PDT are actinic keratoses, intraepithelial carcinoma and superficial basal cell carcinoma (BCC).

PDT has three key components: photosensitising agents which are taken up by precancerous/cancerous cells, light and oxygen. Together, these result in photochemical activation leading to oxidative stress, inflammation and cell death. Licensed pro-drugs in current use are 5-aminolaevulinic acid (ALA)

Box 2.2 Patient safety during phototherapy or PUVA

Eye protection

- Patients must wear UV-blocking goggles while receiving treatment.
- Individuals receiving oral PUVA must wear UVA-blocking glasses for 12 h following ingestion of psoralen (longer if risk factors for cataract development are present).
- Patients should be provided with a list of approved UV-protective eyewear and have their own glasses checked.

Prevention of burning

- Minimal erythema dose/minimal phototoxic dose testing allows more accurate determination of starting dose than that based on skin type.
- Accurate dosimetry: The irradiance of cabinets should be regularly checked by a medical physicist using an appropriately calibrated radiometer.
- Patient education: Factors that can lead to inadvertent burning should be discussed with each patient.
- Obese patients may require a modified treatment protocol, i.e. a lower starting dose, as areas such as the breasts, buttocks and abdomen are closer to the lamps.
- Use of correct UV source: In cabinets that have combined UVB and UVA lamps it is essential that the correct tubes are selected for treatment.
- Lamp maintenance: Cabins should be kept clean and lamps should be inspected regularly. Tubes should be replaced when their output falls to a predetermined threshold as agreed with the local medical physicist. If a number of tubes need to be changed at the same time, the new tubes should be spaced out and not replaced side by side to minimise the risk of burning due to uneven irradiance from the cabinet. The irradiance should be rechecked once lamp replacement has been completed.
- Psoralen dosage: It is important to ensure that the patient has taken the correct number of tablets at the correct time prior to skin irradiation.

Reducing skin cancer risk

- Male patients should wear appropriate clothing to protect the genitalia.
- The face (if not involved by the dermatosis being treated) should be shielded with a visor to avoid unnecessary UV exposure.
- For some indications, whole-body treatment may not be required (e.g. for polymorphic light eruption desensitisation, treatment limited to the photoexposed skin may be sufficient). Treatment planning should take such factors into account to reduce overall UV exposure load.
- Maximum lifetime dose of systemic PUVA should not exceed 1000–1500 J/cm^2 or 150–200 exposures. Exposure over this amount should trigger skin cancer screening review.
- Narrowband UVB has not as yet been proven to increase skin cancer risk, but if >500 lifetime treatments are received, skin cancer screening review should be triggered.

---

and methyl aminolevulinate (MAL). Following the application of pro-drugs to a skin lesion and uptake, protoporphyrin IX (PpIX) accumulates in the target tissue. PpIX is a potent photosensitiser that can be activated by light of the appropriate wavelengths. Photochemical activation of PpIX by red light at 630–635 nm penetrates tissue to a depth of 6–7 mm.

PDT is a particularly good treatment choice for multiple and/or large low-risk (and therefore generally thin) lesions, diffuse field change at sites where healing may be problematic, such as the lower leg, or where cosmetic outcome is important. It is contraindicated for disease with metastatic potential such as invasive SCC or melanoma. Topical PDT is not advisable for thick tumours such as thick nodular BCC or for morphoeic BCC. Patients with porphyria or xeroderma pigmentosum should not be treated with PDT. Tumours at high-risk sites such as the midface should also not be considered for topical PDT unless a more conventional surgical approach is contraindicated.

Destruction of tissue

Cryotherapy

Liquid nitrogen cryotherapy (–195°C) is an effective method of treating a wide range of skin lesions, e.g. viral warts, actinic keratoses, seborrhoeic keratoses and superficial BCCs <20mm diameter.

The extent of tissue injury is determined by the rate of freezing, the coldest temperature reached, freeze time and rate of thawing. Maximum damage is produced by rapid freezing and slow thawing. Repeating the freeze–thaw cycle produces much greater tissue damage than a single freeze because the greater conductivity of the previously frozen skin and the already impaired circulation both allow a greater and faster depth of cold penetration.

Liquid nitrogen can be applied using cotton-wool swabs dipped into the liquid of an unsealed vacuum flask. Alternatively, a liquid nitrogen spray from a pressurised container is easier to direct accurately, faster and more convenient.

Side effects are pain during procedure, tissue swelling, blister formation, slow healing, hypopigmentation and temporary post-inflammatory hyperpigmentation. Nerve damage resulting in paraesthesiae occasionally occurs, although this usually resolves within a matter of months.

Electrocautery

Cautery is the application of heat to living tissue. In electrocautery the metal element or burner is heated by the passage of electricity and the hot element is applied to the skin or lesion to be treated. Heat causes tissue coagulation and if excessive will lead to unsightly hypertrophic scarring. Electrocautery units vary in size from small disposable pen size units that are popular for eyelid surgery to portable battery- and mains-powered units.

Electrocautery may be used on its own or in combination with curettage to destroy a wide range of superficial skin lesions. It can also be used for haemostasis after simple shave excisions. No electricity passes through the patient and so electrocautery is completely safe in patients with implanted cardiac devices. Care must be taken due to fire risk of liquids, vapours, gases and dry cotton gauze.

Electrosurgery

Electrosurgery, also known as radiosurgery, radiofrequency surgery or surgical diathermy, creates heat in tissues by the passage of high-frequency alternating current. It has largely replaced electrocautery in clinical practice.

There are two ways of delivering electrosurgical current to the skin (monopolar and bipolar), two types of electrical contact with the patient (monoterminal and biterminal), two different types of electrosurgical generator (ground (earth) referenced and isolated machines) and a number of distinct electrosurgical techniques, including electrosection, fulguration, electrodessication and electrocoagulation. Local guidance should be followed regarding use of this technique in patients with pacemaker and implantable cardiac devices.

Surgical removal of tissue

Local anaesthesia

Dermatological surgical procedures are performed under local anaesthesia. Local anaesthetics (via either topical application or subcutaneous injections) work by blocking the sodium channels that facilitate nerve impulses in tissues. Direct infiltration just beneath the dermis is the most efficient way of delivering the local anaesthetic as close to the nerves as possible.

There are different classes of local anaesthetic: esters, e.g. benzocaine (derivatives of para-aminobenzoic acid, PABA), and amides, e.g. lidocaine (non-PABA based). The latter class carry a lower risk of producing allergic reactions.

Methods of administration of local anaesthetic are the following:

- Topical: Generally inadequate for incisional surgery, but reduces discomfort associated with needle puncture. Particularly useful in young children.
- Injection into area to be treated.
- Nerve blocks (regional anaesthesia): Local anaesthetic agents are injected adjacent to larger nerves, resulting in anaesthesia of large areas supplied by that nerve.
- Tumescent anaesthesia: Involves subcutaneous infiltration of large volumes of tumescent fluid containing lidocaine (0.05% or 0.1%),

Table 2.4 Maximum recommended local anaesthetic doses in adults

Drug	Concentration (mg/ml)	Maximum dose (mg/kg)	Maximum volume (ml)								
			35 kg	40 kg	45 kg	50 kg	60 kg	70 kg	80 kg	90 kg	100 kg
Lidocaine **1%**	10 mg/ml	3 mg/kg	10.5	12	13.5	15	18	20ml (200mg)			
Lidocaine **1%** *with* Adrenaline *(1:200000)*	10 mg/ml	7 mg/kg	24.5	28	31.5	35	42	49	50ml (500mg)		
Lidocaine **2%** *with* Adrenaline *(1:200000)*	20 mg/ml		12.25	14	15.75	17.5	21	24.5	25ml (500mg)		
Prilocaine **1%**	10 mg/ml	**6 mg/kg**	21	24	27	30	36	40ml (400mg)			

When lidocaine 2% is used, the maximum volume should be halved. Source: Data from Nottingham University Hospitals guidelines

saline and adrenaline. It is used for dermatological surgical procedures involving large areas of skin.

*Lidocaine is t*he most frequently used local anaesthetic. It is rapid acting and relatively free from toxicity and sensitivity. Preparations available are lidocaine alone or lidocaine combined with adrenaline. The effects of combining with adrenaline are to prolong the duration of anaesthesia, reduce associated bleeding and increase the intensity of the nerve blockade. Care should be given to areas where there are end arteries when using adrenaline.

The maximum safe adult dose is 3 mg/kg for plain lidocaine and 7 mg/kg for lidocaine with adrenaline. These maximum doses should be halved when used in the elderly and in children. See Table 2.4 for the maximum recommended local anaesthetic doses in adults.

Local anaesthetics are generally well tolerated. When used appropriately and according to maximum dose limits there is minimal chance of side effects. Local side effects include temporary stinging, burning and bruising secondary to the injection.

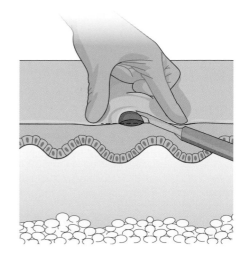

Figure 2.2 Shave excision of a superficial lesion redraw

Shave excision

Shave excision is a simple and rapid method for removing benign superficial lesions (Figure 2.2). The technique can also be used for obtaining tissue samples from protuberant nodular skin tumours (but not for suspected melanoma). Following the shave procedure, haemostasis should be obtained using cautery, electrodessication or a chemical haemostatic agent. On average, such wounds take 2–3 weeks to heal, leaving a scar of a similar size to the removed lesion.

Curettage

Curettage can be used to treat benign lesions as well as small Bowen disease, BCC and in certain specific situations small low-risk SCC. The technique relies on the principle that the curetted material is more fragile than normal skin, e.g. BCC, or there is a natural cleavage plane, e.g. seborrhoeic keratosis, between the lesion and the surrounding skin. Disposable ring curettes range in size from 2 to 7 mm and contain a sharp (cutting) edge on one side, enabling a clean plane of cleavage (Figure 2.3). Haemostasis is achieved using either a chemical haemostatic agent cautery or electrosurgery/electrocautery.

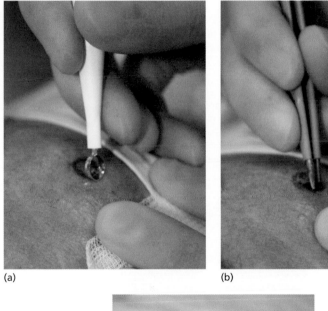

(a)

(b)

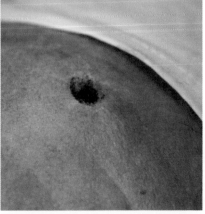

(c)

Figure 2.3 Ring curette. (a) Curettage of a small nodular BCC on the forehead using a ring curette. (b) Haemostasis with bipolar diathermy. (c) Wound bed post treatment.

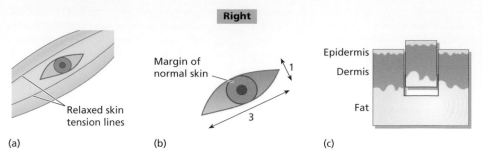

Figure 2.4 Principles of elliptical excision. The ellipse is designed to follow skin-crease lines (a) and should be approximately three times as long as it is wide (b). Ensure that an appropriate margin of normal skin is also excised (b). The blade should be held at 90° to the skin when cutting the ellipse so that the wound has vertical sides down to fat (c). (Source: From Lawrence CM, An Introduction to Dermatological Surgery, 2nd edn. Mosby, St Louis, 2002.)

Excision biopsy

The elliptical excision biopsy is used for tumour or lesion removal (Figure 2.4). The entire thickness of skin down to the fat is excised, which provides the dermatopathologist with an optimal amount of tissue to provide accurate histological assessment. An appropriate margin according to suspected diagnosis should be taken.

Part 1
Infections and Infestations

Viral infections

3

A virus particle, or virion, consists of a length of nucleic acid, either RNA or DNA, within a protein shell, the capsid. A simple classification of viruses that cause illness involving the skin in humans is given in Table 3.1.

Table 3.1 Classification of viruses causing human skin disease

Nucleic acid	Family	Genus	Species/disease
DNA-ds	*Poxviridae*	*Orthopoxvirus*	Variola
			Vaccinia
			Monkeypox
			Cowpox
		Parapoxvirus	Orf
			Pseudocowpox
		Yatapoxvirus	Tanapox
		Molluscipox	Molluscum contagiosum
	Herpesviridae	*Simplex virus*	Herpes simplex 1 and 2
			Cercopithacine herpesvirus (herpes B virus)
		Varicellovirus	Varicella zoster
		Cytomelagovirus	Cytomegalovirus
		Roseolovirus	Human herpesvirus 6
			Human herpesvirus 7
		Lymphocryptovirus	Epstein–Barr
		Rhadinovirus	Human herpesvirus 8
	Polyomaviridae	*Polyomavirus*	Merkel cell carcinoma virus (Chapter 83)
			Human polyomavirus 6
			Human polyomavirus 7
			Human polyomavirus 10
	Papillomaviridae	α *Papillomavirus*	Warts, mucosal intraepithelial neoplasia and squamous cell carcinoma
		β *Papillomavirus*	Epidermodysplasia verruciformis, skin cancer
		γ *Papillomavirus*	Cutaneous warts
		μ *Papillomavirus*	Palmar and plantar warts
		ν *Papillomavirus*	Cutaneous warts, skin cancer

(Continued)

Rook's Dermatology Handbook, First Edition. Edited by Christopher E. M. Griffiths, Tanya O. Bleiker, Daniel Creamer, John R. Ingram and Rosalind C. Simpson.
© 2022 John Wiley & Sons Ltd. Published 2022 by John Wiley & Sons Ltd.

Table 3.1 (Continued)

Nucleic acid	Family	Genus	Species/disease
DNA-ds*	*Hepadnaviridae*	*Orthohepadnavirus*	Hepatitis B
DNA-ss	*Parvoviridae*	*Erythroparvovirus*	Human parvovirus (B19)/ erythroparvovirus
			Parvovirus 4 and 5
		Bocaparvovirus	HBoV-1
RNA-ss (+)	*Retroviridae*	*Deltaretrovirus* *Lentiviruses*	HTLV-1, HTLV-2 HIV-1, HIV-2
	Togaviridae	*Rubivirus* *Alphavirus*	Rubella Ross River, Sinbis, Chikungunya, O'Nyong-Nyong, Mayaro, Barmah Forest, equine encephalitis viruses
	Flaviviridae	*Hepacivirus* *Flavivirus*	Hepatitis C Dengue Yellow fever
	Hepeviridae *Picornaviridae*	*Hepevirus* *Aphthovirus* *Enterovirus* *Hepatovirus* *Parechovirus*	Hepatitis E Foot and mouth disease Enterovirus A–J, rhinovirus A–C Hepatitis A Human parechovirus
RNA-ss (−)	*Rhabdoviridae*	*Lyssavirus* *Vesiculovirus*	Rabies Vesicular stomatitis virus
	Filoviridae	*Ebolavirus* *Marburgvirus*	Ebola disease Marburg disease
	Paramyxoviridae	*Morbillivirus* *Respirovirus* *Rubulavirus* *Pneumovirus*	Measles Parainfluenza Mumps Respiratory syncytial virus
	Orthomyxoviridae	*Influenzavirus A–C*	Influenza
	Arenaviridae	*Arenavirus*	Lassa fever, Lujo virus haemorrhagic fever, Junin virus, Argentinian haemorrhagic fever, Mapucho virus, Chapare virus, Bolivian haemorrhagic fever, Guanarito virus, Venezuelan haemorrhagic fever, Sabia virus, Latino virus, Bolivian haemorrhagic fever, whitewater arroyo virus
	Bunyaviridae	*Nairovirus* *Orthobunyavirus* *Phlebovirus*	Crimean–Congo haemorrhagic fever Bunyamwera Bwama fever virus Oropouche virus Rift valley fever

ds, double stranded; ds*, incomplete ds; ss, single stranded; ss (+), single stranded (plus strand); ss (−), single stranded (minus strand).

EXANTHEMS OF VIRAL INFECTIONS

A widespread rash, or exanthem, may be a manifestation of viral infections that cause a viraemia. (Table 3.2) Those commonly affecting neonates and infants are covered in chapters 63 and 64.)

Table 3.2 Viral exanthems

Type of rash	Pathogen associated
Macular	Rubella (Chapter 63) Echovirus (esp. 2, 4, 6, 9, 11, 16, 18, 19, 23, 25, 32) Coxsackie A (esp. 4, 5, 6, 9, 10, 16) and B (esp. 5, 3) Epstein–Barr virus (infectious mononucleosis) Human herpesvirus 6 (roseola) (Chapter 64) Human herpesvirus 7
Maculopapular	Togaviruses Echovirus (esp. 6, 9) Measles (Chapter 64) Human parvovirus (B19) (erythema infectiosum) (Chapter 64)
Maculopapular-vesicular	Coxsackie A (occasional 5, 9, 10, 16) Echovirus (occasional 4, 9, 11) Ebola, Marburg
Maculopapular-petechial	Togavirus (esp. Chikungunya) and bunyavirus haemorrhagic fevers (including Lassa)
Urticarial	Coxsackie A9 (occasional) Hepatitis B (occasional)
Vesicular	Herpes simplex virus Hand, foot and mouth disease (coxsackie 16, 4, 5) (Chapter 64) Vesicular stomatitis virus
Vesiculopapular Papulovesiculopustular	Varicella-zoster Vaccinia Variola Cowpox
Papulovesicular	Orf Milker's nodule
Papular	Molluscum contagiosum (Chapter 64) Warts Gianotti–Crosti syndrome (Chapter 64)

POXVIRUS INFECTIONS

The poxviruses are double-stranded DNA viruses (Table 3.3). Spread is mainly by direct-contact inoculation.

Table 3.3 Human poxvirus infections

Genus	Species/disease	Epidemiology	Clinical features
Orthopoxvirus	Cowpox	Natural reservoir rodents, also cows and zoo animals	5–7 days after contact Inflammatory vesicles which crust and heal with scarring on hands, arms and face Malaise, myalgia, lymphadenitis, lymphangitis, low grade fever Resolves in 2–4 weeks
Parapoxvirus	Orf (ecthyma contagiosum)	Contact with sheep and goats particularly during breeding season	Single lesion 5–6 days after contact 2–3 cm haemorrhagic pustule or bulla on hands or forearms (Figure 3.1) Lymphadenitis/lymphangitis, mild fever Heals after 3–6 weeks Erythema multiforme (EM) occurs in 10% of cases 2–3 weeks post infection (Figure 3.2) Immune after first episode but second infections do occur
	Pseudocowpox (Milker's nodule)	Workers with close contact with animals harbouring the virus e.g. farmers, milkers and veterinary personnel Farmers, milkers and veterinary personnel	5–14 days after contact Small papule mainly on hands and forearms enlarges to reddish-blue, firm nodule/vesicle often with ring of erythema Normally well Occasional EM Resolves in 4–6 weeks
Molluscipoxvirus	Molluscum contagiosum	See Chapter 64	

EM, erythema multiforme.

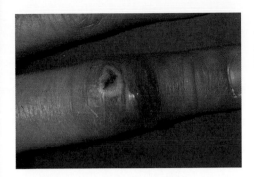

Figure 3.1 Orf. (Source: Courtesy of Addenbrooke's Hospital, Cambridge, UK.)

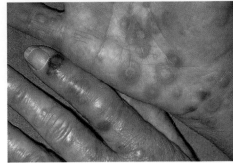

Figure 3.2 Orf on the dorsum of the left index finger with secondary, targetoid, lesions of erythema multiforme (Source: Courtesy of Dr A.S. Highet, York District Hospital, UK.)

HERPESVIRUS INFECTIONS

The herpesvirus group are enveloped DNA viruses. After primary infection, they can remain latent within the host. Eight members of the group can infect humans (Table 3.4).

Table 3.4 Herpesviruses causing disease in humans

Virus	Disease
HSV-1, HSV-2	Primary herpetic gingivostomatitis, recurrent oro-facial and cutaneous herpes, primary and recurrent Genital Herpes, neonatal herpes (Chapter 63), inoculation herpes simplex
VZV	Primary infection: varicella (chickenpox) Reactivation: zoster (shingles)
CMV	Dermal erythropoiesis ('blueberry muffin' baby) (Chapter 63) Primary CMV mononucleosis
HHV-6	Roseola infantum (Chapter 64)
HHV-7	
EBV	Infectious mononucleosis Other associated diseases: Gianotti–Crosti syndrome (Chapter 64), Lipschütz ulcers (painful genital) and rarely the severe haemophagocytic syndrome (haemophagocytic lymphohistiocytosis) Oral hairy leucoplakia (reactivation of EBV with immunodeficiency due to HIV infection) EBV-associated lymphomas, e.g. Burkitt
HHV-8	HHV-8 associated Kaposi sarcoma (Chapter 77)

CMV, cytomegalovirus; EBV, Epstein–Barr virus; HHV-6, human herpesvirus type 6; HHV-7, human herpesvirus type 7; HHV-8, human herpesvirus type 8; HSV-1, herpes simplex virus, type 1; HSV-2, herpes simplex virus, type 2; VZV, varicella-zoster virus.

Primary herpetic gingivostomatitis

(Syn. Herpes labialis, cold sore)
Primary infection with herpes simplex virus (HSV) is usually minimal or subclinical but may rarely produce a painful vesicular stomatitis.

Epidemiology
Primary type 1 infections occur mainly in children; usually minimal and often subclinical. In the developing world, over 90% of children have antibody by the age of 5 years. In more temperate areas and higher socioeconomic groups the incidence is lower in children and rises with age.

Pathophysiology
Usually HSV-1 less frequently HSV-2 Acquired by direct contact with, or droplets from, infected secretions entering via skin or mucous membrane.

Intraepidermal vesicles are formed by the combination of intra- and intercellular oedema. The dermis, and later the epidermis, are infiltrated with polymorphonuclear leukocytes.

Clinical features
Following a 5-day incubation period the stomatitis begins with fever, malaise, restlessness and excessive dribbling. The gums are swollen, inflamed and bleed easily, drinking is painful and breath foul smelling. Vesicles present as white plaques on the tongue, pharynx, palate and buccal mucous membranes which develop into ulcers with a yellowish pseudomembrane. Regional lymph nodes are enlarged and tender. Pharyngitis may occur in 10% of cases. Disseminated or systemic infection may occur in the immunodeficient and in neonates not protected by maternally acquired antibody. Encephalitis, untreated, has a high mortality and a high incidence of disability in survivors. After 3–5 days, the fever subsides and recovery occurs within 2 weeks.

Differential diagnosis
Streptococcal infections, diphtheria, candidiasis, aphthosis and coxsackie infections including herpangina, Behçet syndrome and Stevens–Johnson syndrome.

Investigations
Culture of vesicle fluid requires 1–5 days. For a more rapid diagnosis immunofluorescence, electron microscopy and PCR.

Management
Mild uncomplicated infection may not require treatment. Anaesthetic mouthwashes may help to relieve pain. For more severe infections, oral or intravenous acyclovir. Treatment does not affect the establishment of virus latency nor rates of recurrence.

Recurrent oro-facial and cutaneous herpes

(Syn. Herpes labialis, cold sore)
Reactivation of latent HSV can cause asymptomatic shedding or recurrent disease in 30–50% of people.

Pathophysiology
The virus remains latent in the ganglia of sensory nerves innervating the primary infection site. Recurrences may be triggered by minor trauma, infections and UV radiation. Menstruation and stress also blamed. Trauma may be endogenous (autoinoculation), e.g. to the finger in nail biters.

Clinical features
Itching or burning 1–2 hours prior to the development of small closely grouped vesicles on an inflamed base, predominantly around the mouth (Figure 3.3) (herpes labialis, cold sore), but can be

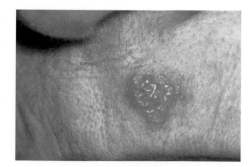

Figure 3.3 Herpes labialis. Typical recurrent lesion above the upper lip. (Source: Courtesy of Dr A.S. Highet, York District Hospital, UK.)

anywhere on the body. Lesions usually become pustular and crusted before healing in 7–10 days without scarring. Recurrences tend to be in the same region, but not always on the identical site.

Constitutional symptoms, cranial nerve palsies and neuralgic pain are rarely associated with episodes of recurrence. Eczema herpeticum can be associated with recurrent as well as primary HSV. In the immunocompromised, persistent ulcerative or verruciform lesions may occur. If recurrent herpes simplex involves the eye, keratoconjunctivitis, dendritic ulcers, disciform or hypopyon keratitis and iridocyclitis may occur. Other associations with HSV reactivation include recurrent erythema multiforme (Chapter 19), Bell palsy, recurrent lymphocytic meningitis and encephalitis.

Inoculation herpes simplex: Skin lesions develop 5–7 days after inoculation (Figure 3.4). Inoculation of the fingertips results in a 'herpetic whitlow', in which painful deep vesicles coalesce to give a honeycombed appearance or a large bulla. The regional nodes are enlarged but fever and constitutional symptoms are usually mild. Facial contact during rugby can result in HSV virus infection, commonly called 'scrumpox'.

Management
Recurrent herpes labialis may need no treatment. Sunscreen may prevent or reduce intensity of episodes. An ophthalmological opinion required if eye involvement.

First-line treatment is with topical acyclovir or penciclovir. If recurrences are frequent, long-term prophylactic oral acyclovir for 4–6 months may reduce frequency.

In the immunocompromised patient intravenous aciclovir or penciclovir for active infection or post-exposure prevention with intravenous or oral acyclovir.

Primary genital herpes

Epidemiology
Genital herpes is usually transmitted sexually. Seropositivity is low in children, but about a third of young adults are seropositive for type 2 and this rises to up to half the population by later life. In children with genital herpes (HSV-1 or HSV-2), sexual abuse must be considered.

Pathophysiology
HSV-2 the most common type in this area, although HSV-1 is increasing.

Clinical features
Penile ulceration from herpetic infection (Figure 3.5) is the most frequent type of genital ulceration seen in genito-urinary medical clinics in the UK. They are sore and painful. In men who have sex with men, herpes simplex is common in the perianal area and may extend into the rectum. In females, similar lesions occur on the external genitalia and mucosae of the vulva, vagina and cervix. Pain and dysuria are common. Infection of the cervix may progress to a severe ulcerative cervicitis. Genital lesions can last for 2–3 weeks if untreated. In HIV infection, ulceration of the primary infection

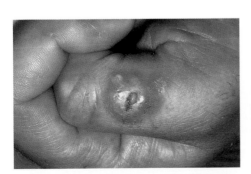

Figure 3.4 Herpes simplex. Inoculation lesion on the thumb of a dermatologist. (Source: Courtesy of Dr A.S. Highet, York District Hospital, UK.)

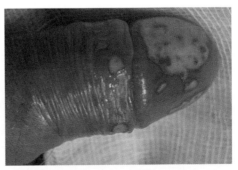

Figure 3.5 Genital Herpes. Confluent lesions resulting in large erosions. (Source: Courtesy of Addenbrooke's Hospital, Cambridge, UK.)

may become chronic, thickened and verrucous, causing diagnostic confusion with neoplasia.

Radiculoneuropathy is seen occasionally in women, and especially in perianal disease in homosexual men. There may be sacral paraesthesia, urinary retention, constipation and, in men, impotence. Recovery takes a few days to a few weeks.

Headache and meningism is common in primary genital herpes simplex with full recovery. Encephalitis is a rare complication.

Recurrent genital herpes after primary infection with establishment of latent infection is fairly common, occurring two to six times per year with clusters of small vesicles. Frequent recurrences are more likely in HSV-2 (95%) than with HSV-1(50%) infection. Reactivation episodes are of shorter duration than the initial infection.

Investigations

See Investigation of primary herpetic gingivostomatitis herpes.

Management

An infected individual may reduce the risk of spread by regular use of condoms and by avoiding sexual contact during an episode.

Oral aciclovir, valaciclovir or famciclovir in primary and recurrent infection. Prophylaxis should be considered for frequent recurrences or for associated erythema multiforme.

Varicella

(Syn. Chickenpox)
Primary infection with varicella zoster virus (VZV).

Epidemiology

Over half of primary infections occur before the age of 5 and 85% before puberty.

Pathophysiology

The virus is transmitted by droplet infection from the nasopharynx. A brief first viraemic stage, when the virus can disseminate to other organs, is followed by a second viraemia coinciding with the onset of the rash. Patients are infectious to others from about 2 days before to 5 days after the onset of the rash and 60–100% of non-immune individuals will contract the infection if exposed to someone in the infectious stage of chickenpox or zoster. Vesicle fluid in either disease contains a large amount of virus and may be a route of droplet infection. Completely dry scabs are not infectious.

Histologically, multinucleate giant cells with up to 15 nuclei are produced mainly by cell fusion. Intracellular and intercellular oedema forms the vesicle, the roof of which consists of the upper Malpighian and horny layers. A mild inflammatory reaction in the dermis later extends to the epidermis. In fatal cases of varicella, similar cytological changes with areas of focal necrosis are found in the liver, kidney and other organs.

Clinical features

The incubation period is 14–17 days. 1–2 days prodrome of fever and malaise is followed by the development of papules, which rapidly become vesicles (Figure 3.6). Vesicles appear in three to five crops over 2–4 days with a centripetal distribution. Characteristically lesions are at different stages in each site. Lesions may be few or profuse. Vesicles are common in the mouth, especially on the palate; occasionally seen on the conjunctiva and genitalia. After about 4 days, no new crops of lesions appear and existing vesicles dry and crust.

Haemorrhagic varicella, with extensive haemorrhagic vesicles, high fever and severe constitutional symptoms, is mainly seen in immunocompromised patients.

Infection in pregnancy, especially during the second trimester, carries a 2% risk of the rare congenital varicella syndrome. Maternal primary infection at the time of delivery can result in very severe infection of the baby, with a

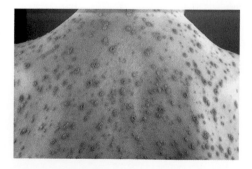

Figure 3.6 Varicella. (Source: Courtesy of York District Hospital, UK.)

mortality of about 30%. Chickenpox in a neonate when the mother is immune to VZV is usually mild due to maternal antibodies.

Complications are rare in otherwise healthy children. Varicella in immunocompromised people may be severe and progressive with a mortality of 7–10%. Features associated with a progressive varicella include haemorrhagic varicella, pneumonitis, hepatitis, encephalitis and acute retinal necrosis syndrome.

Varicella confers lasting immunity and second attacks are uncommon in immunologically healthy subjects.

Investigations
In most cases, the diagnosis of varicella is clinical. The quickest way to confirm diagnosis is by PCR of vesicle fluid or a scraping taken from the base of a blister.

Management
Prevention is possible with pre-exposure vaccination (live attenuated vaccine), post-exposure immunoglobulin (zoster immune globulin (ZIG) administered within 10 days of contact) and antiviral prophylaxis (only effective in immunocompetent).

ZIG should be given to neonates whose mothers develop varicella within the period from 7 days before to 7 days after delivery. ZIG is also indicated for healthy neonates in contact with active chickenpox or zoster and for immunocompromised children and adults (e.g. organ transplant recipients) and non-immune patients exposed to VZV who have taken oral steroids for at least 14 days within the previous 3 months. It should also be given to exposed non-immune pregnant women.

Treatment of varicella in a healthy child is symptomatic. Primary varicella infection during pregnancy should be treated with intravenous acyclovir. An antiviral is indicated for varicella in adults and for severe varicella or zoster infections at any age in the immunocompromised. Started within the first 1 or 2 days.

Zoster

(Syn. Shingles)
Zoster (zoster = a girdle) is a segmental eruption due to reactivation of latent VZV from dorsal root ganglia. Zoster patients are infectious, both from virus in the lesions and, in some instances, the nasopharynx. In susceptible contacts of zoster, chickenpox can occur.

Epidemiology
Uncommon in childhood and young adult life. The incidence rises with age, at 80 years the incidence is approximately 10 cases per 1000 patient-years.

Pathophysiology
Factors determining the site of an eruption of zoster are often unclear, may be pressure on or trauma to nerve roots, by neoplastic deposits, radiotherapy, surgery, or often trivial trauma.

Clinical features
The first manifestation is pain, which may be severe, accompanied by fever, headache, malaise and tenderness localised to areas of one or more dorsal roots. The thoracic (53%), cervical (usually C2, 3 or 4, 20%), trigeminal, including ophthalmic (15%) and lumbosacral (11%) dermatomes are most commonly involved at all ages; ophthalmic zoster increases in old age. Occasionally, the pain is not followed by the eruption ('zoster sine eruptione').

The time between the start of the pain and the onset of the eruption averages 1.4 days in trigeminal zoster and 3.2 days in thoracic disease. Closely grouped red papules, rapidly becoming vesicular and then pustular, develop in a continuous or interrupted band in the area of one, occasionally two, and, rarely, more contiguous dermatome with a striking cut-off at the mid line (Figure 3.7). Mucous membranes within the affected dermatomes are also involved. New vesicles continue to appear for several days. In 16% of patients, vesicles develop beyond the dermatome within a few days of the local eruption; more common in the elderly and the course of zoster unchanged. In the elderly and undernourished, the local eruption often becomes necrotic and heal with scarring. The lymph nodes draining the affected area are enlarged and tender. In uncomplicated cases recovery is complete in 2–3 weeks in children and young adults, and 3–4 weeks in older patients. Recurrent shingles can occur, either affecting the same dermatome or at a different site.

Maternal zoster in pregnancy is not associated with intrauterine infection.

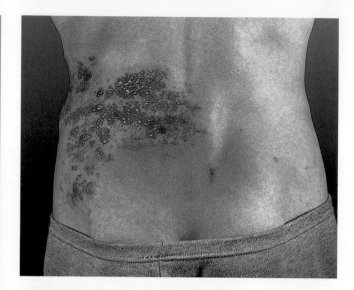

Figure 3.7 Zoster of the trunk. (Source: Courtesy of York District Hospital, UK.)

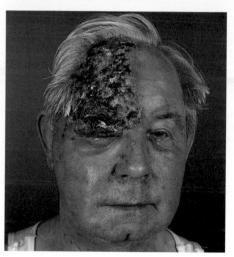

Figure 3.8 Ophthalmic zoster. (Source: Courtesy of York District Hospital, UK.)

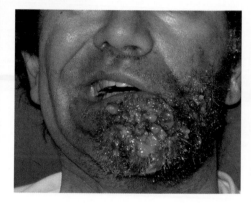

Figure 3.9 Herpes zoster oticus showing unilateral zoster with facial palsy (Ramsay Hunt syndrome).

Trigeminal nerve zoster: In ophthalmic nerve zoster (Figure 3.8), the eye is affected in two-thirds of cases, especially when vesicles on the side of the nose indicate involvement of the nasociliary nerve (Hutchinson sign). Ocular complications include uveitis, keratitis, conjunctivitis, conjunctival oedema, ocular muscle palsies, proptosis, scleritis, retinal vascular occlusion, ulceration, scarring and even necrosis of the lid. Involvement of the ciliary ganglia may give rise to Argyll–Robertson pupil.

Motor involvement occurs in 5% of cases, commoner in older patients and in those with malignancy, and in cranial compared with spinal nerve involvement. The motor weakness usually follows the pain and the eruption, by a few days to a few weeks. Complete recovery is expected in 55% and significant improvement in a further 30%. Herpes zoster oticus accounts for about 10% of cases of facial palsy, Ramsay Hunt syndrome (Figure 3.9) with full recovery only in about 20% of untreated cases. Zoster of the anogenital area may be associated with disturbances of defecation or urination.

Post-herpetic neuralgia is the commonest and most intractable sequel of zoster. Defined as persistence or recurrence of pain more than a month after the onset of zoster. It occurs in about 30% of patients over 40 and is most frequent when the trigeminal nerve is involved. It is more likely to develop if there was prolonged dermatomal pain prior to the eruption, if the acute pain of zoster was severe and if the rash was prolonged. The pain has two main forms: a continuous burning pain with hyperaesthesia and a spasmodic shooting type. Allodynia, pain caused by normally innocuous stimuli, is often the most distressing symptom and occurs in 90% of people with post-herpetic neuralgia. The neuralgia varies from inconvenient to profoundly disabling.

In patients with impaired immunity (particularly lymphoma), the incidence and severity of zoster are increased, and it is frequently complicated by disseminated cutaneous disease and systemic involvement, usually pneumonia, hepatitis or encephalitis. Anti-tumour necrosis factor (TNF)-α therapy is estimated to increase the risk of zoster threefold. In HIV, zoster is 10 times more common than in the normal population and may become disseminated and chronic.

Investigations

Diagnosis of typical zoster is clinical. Confirmation can be made by culture or PCR.

Management

Shingles is a self-limiting infection. Analgesia and treatment of secondary infection often required.

Prevention: Vaccination can help to reduce the occurrence or severity of zoster and the risk of post-herpetic neuralgia. The zoster vaccine is the same as the varicella vaccine but at a higher virus titre and is given as a single dose. Vaccination is recommended where available (over 60 years in the USA and at age 70 in the UK). Contraindicated in patients with severe immune deficiency. In those for whom immunosuppressive treatment is being considered, vaccination can be administered at least 2 weeks prior to commencing immunosuppression. The vaccine can be considered in those receiving immune suppression at a lower level (prednisolone ≤20 mg/day, azathioprine ≤3 mg/kg/day,

methotrexate 0.4 mg/kg/day). The vaccine is contraindicated in patients receiving biological therapies but may be given after 3–6 months following discontinuation of the immune suppression.

Treatment with rest and analgesics are sufficient for mild attacks of zoster in the young.

An antiviral is indicated for painful zoster infections in adults and at any age in facial zoster and in the immunocompromised. Treatment should be started within the first 1 or 2 days, prevents progression of the eruption, reduces the systemic complications of varicella and zoster and lessens zoster pain during treatment. Many believe that aciclovir or famciclovir started early in shingles can reduce the chance and the duration of post-herpetic neuralgia, especially in the older patient.

For post-herpetic neuralgia amitriptyline, nortriptyline, sodium valproate, gabapentin or pregabalin.

Infectious mononucleosis

(Syn. Glandular fever)
An acute febrile illness caused by Epstein-Barr virus (EBV).

Epidemiology

In early childhood, the virus is spread by contact with saliva on fingers or fomites. In more developed communities, early childhood infection is less frequent and primary infection occurs most commonly in early adult life, normally through kissing. Most primary infection, especially in childhood, is asymptomatic or mild, but when it is delayed to adolescence or adulthood, clinically obvious infectious mononucleosis is more frequent.

Clinical features

The incubation period from contact to symptoms is 1 to 2 months. It is characterised by fever, sore throat and lymphadenopathy with a variable degree of malaise and fatigue. Enlargement of the spleen in half of those acutely infected. Petechiae at the junction of the hard and soft palate are a distinctive feature of the disease and usually appear on the second or third day of fever.

A macular or maculopapular exanthem occurs in about 10% of cases, between days 4 and 6 on the trunk and upper arms first, and a few days later to face and forearms. Skin lesions fade after a few days to a week. The acute disease clears within a month, but cervical lymphadenopathy may take 3 months to settle. There may be relapsing episodes of malaise, fatigue, fever and lymphadenopathy, but no recurrent skin eruption.

If ampicillin or amoxicillin is taken during the course of the illness, an extensive maculopapular or morbilliform eruption develops in over 90% of cases, 7–10 days after the start of treatment most marked on extensor surfaces and pressure areas.

Complication with thrombocytopenic purpura is common but counts below 100 000/μL are rare. Splenic rupture and encephalitis are life-threatening complications.

Differential diagnosis

An acute mononucleosis-like disease can occur in infection with CMV, HHV-6, primary HIV and toxoplasma.

Investigations

In acute disease, lymphocytosis with at least 10% atypical cells on blood film. Abnormalities in liver function tests with jaundice in about 4%. The heterophile antibody test (e.g. monospot test) is positive in 90% of patients after 1–2 weeks, so not useful in the early stages. False negatives common in childhood. False positives can occur in other infectious diseases, lymphomas and leukaemias.

Antibodies to viral antigens can be detected in early infection (early antigen and viral capsid antigen) and after acute infection (antibodies to the EBV nuclear antigen A).

Management

General supportive measures only.

Eczema herpeticum

(Syn. Kaposi varicelliform eruption)
A widespread cutaneous infection with a virus which normally causes localised or mild vesicular eruptions, occurring in a patient with pre-existing skin disease.

Pathophysiology

The usual causative virus is HSV-1. HSV-2, VZV, coxsackie A6 and A16 (eczema coxsackium)

and vaccinia (eczema vaccinatum) are all associated with a similar eruption. Atopic eczema is the commonest predisposing condition. Other susceptible, less common dermatoses include Darier disease, pemphigus foliaceous and benign familial pemphigus.

Patients who develop eczema herpeticum are usually immunocompetent. An association with systemic or topical steroid treatment has not been consistently found. Topical tacrolimus and pimecrolimus, and systemic immunosuppression have been associated.

Clinical features (Figure 3.10)

A history of herpes labialis is not often seen. With known contact with HSV infection the incubation period is about 10 days.

Vesicles, which become pustular, erupt in crops, confined to abnormal skin but often widely disseminated and may generalise. They may be haemorrhagic and the face may become grossly oedematous. The skin is painful and generally erythematous. The vesicles rupture, leaving small superficial erosions which weep and crust. New crops of vesicles may appear for 5–7 days. Fever develops 2–3 days after the onset of the eruption and constitutional symptoms may be severe. Regional lymph nodes enlarged. The fever subsides after 4 or 5 days and the pustules become crusted and slowly heal without significant scarring. Rarely, there may be progression to potentially fatal systemic infection. Recurrences of eczema herpeticum occur but are rare and generally milder than the initial episode.

Investigations

Blister fluid or a surface swab should be analysed for HSV

Management

Oral aciclovir, valaciclovir or famciclovir. Bacterial infection and the underlying eczema or other dermatosis should be treated in the usual way. If aciclovir is being withheld, more cautious use of steroid therapy is advised until the viral lesions have healed. If antiviral therapy is given, the use of topical steroids does not appear to lead to a longer disease course. Severe cases should receive intravenous aciclovir. Frequently recurrent disease requires prophylactic aciclovir or valaciclovir.

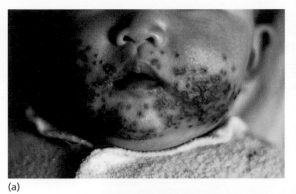
(a)

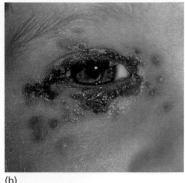
(b)

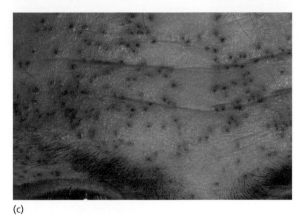
(c)

Figure 3.10 Eczema herpeticum: (a) perioral; (b) Periocular; (c) forehead. (Source: Part (c) courtesy of Addenbrooke's Hospital, Cambridge, UK.)

HUMAN PAPILLOMAVIRUS INFECTIONS

The human papillomavirus (HPV) is a small DNA virus that can infect and cause disease at any site in stratified squamous epithelium, either keratinising (skin) or non-keratinising (mucosa). Over 150 types have been recognised and characterised.

The clinical problems are broadly divided into benign (cutaneous warts, ano-genital warts, oral warts and laryngeal warts) and premalignant or malignant (intraepithelial neoplasia and squamous cell cancers of the anogenital area and upper respiratory tract).

Cutaneous warts

(Syn. common wart: verruca vulgaris; plane wart: verruca plana)

Epidemiology
2–30% of school-age children and young adults have warts. More common and persistent in conditions of immune compromise.

Pathophysiology
Common warts (excluding plantar warts) are due mainly to HPV-2, but also to the closely related types 27 and 57, and types 1 and 4. Plantar warts are caused by HPV-1, -2, -4, -27 or -57. Mosaic warts are commonly caused by HPV-2. Plane warts are due mainly to HPV-3 and -10.

Warts are spread by direct or indirect contact. Impairment of the epithelial barrier function, by trauma (including mild abrasions), maceration or both, greatly predisposes to inoculation of the virus, as in the following examples:

- Plantar warts commonly acquired from swimming pool or shower room floors: rough surfaces abrade moistened keratin from infected feet and help to inoculate virus into the softened skin of others.

- Common hand warts may spread widely round the nails in those who bite their nails or periungual skin, or habitually sucked fingers.
- Shaving may spread wart infection over the beard area.
- Occupational handlers of meat, fish and poultry have high incidences of hand warts, attributed to cutaneous injury and prolonged contact with wet flesh and water.

Histologically viral warts show acanthosis and hyperkeratosis, usually with the characteristic feature of koilocytosis of upper keratinocytes. In most warts there is also papillomatosis.

Clinical features

Warts on the skin may present in a number of different morphological forms, dependent on virus type, body site, immunological status of the patient and environmental influences.

Common warts (Figure 3.11): Firm papules with a rough horny surface 1 mm to 1 cm in diameter on the backs of the hands and fingers, and in children on the knees; may occur anywhere. New warts may form at sites of trauma, though this Koebner-like isomorphic phenomenon is less than in plane warts. Usually symptomless but may be tender on the palmar aspects of the fingers, when fissured or when growing beneath the nail plate. Common warts account for only 1% or 2% of warts on or around the genitalia in adults; in the male, they are almost always confined to the shaft of the penis. In children, HPVs causing common warts may account for up to two-thirds of ano-genital warts.

Periungual warts (Figure 3.12): Warts around the nails, especially at the nail folds or beneath the nail, can disturb nail growth. Nail biting may increase the risk of infection at this site.

Plantar warts: First appear as a small shining 'sago-grain' papule, but soon assume the typical appearance of a sharply defined rounded lesion, with a rough keratotic surface surrounded by a smooth collar of thickened horn. If gently pared with a scalpel, the abrupt separation between the wart tissue and the protective horny ring becomes more obvious, as the epithelial ridges of the plantar skin are not continued over the surface of the wart. If the paring is

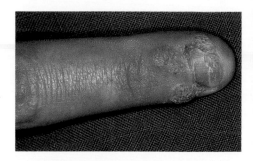

Figure 3.12 Periungual warts in a nail-biter. (Source: Courtesy of York District Hospital, UK.)

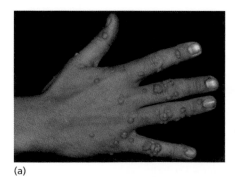

(a)

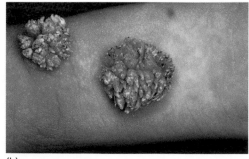

(b)

Figure 3.11 Common warts: (a) hand (Source: Courtesy of Addenbrooke's Hospital, Cambridge, UK.); (b) dorsum of the finger, filiform warts. (Source: Courtesy of Dr A.S. Highet, York District Hospital, UK.)

continued, small bleeding points, the tips of the elongated dermal papillae, are evident.

Most plantar warts are beneath pressure points, the heel or the metatarsal heads. Mosaic warts are so described from the appearance presented by a plaque of closely grouped small warts (Figure 3.13). The angular outlines of the tightly compressed individual warts are seen when the surface is pared.

Plane warts (flat warts) (Figure 3.14a): Smooth, flat or slightly elevated and are skin coloured or greyish yellow but may be pigmented. Round or polygonal in shape and vary in size from 1 to 5 mm or more in diameter. The face, backs of hands and shins common sites; number ranges from two or three to many hundreds. Contiguous warts may coalesce and a linear arrangement in scratch marks is a characteristic feature (Figure 3.14b).

Filiform and digitate warts (Figure 3.15): Occur commonly in the male, on the face and neck, irregularly distributed and often clustered.

Butchers' warts: Occupational handlers of meat, poultry or fish have a high incidence of hand warts where the skin is in prolonged contact with moist animal flesh. Lesions affect the hands,

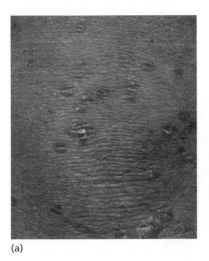

Figure 3.13 Mosaic plantar wart. (Source: Courtesy of Addenbrooke's Hospital, Cambridge, UK.)

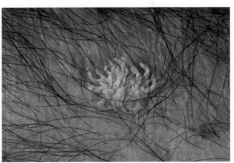

Figure 3.15 Filiform wart on the forearm. (Source: Courtesy of Addenbrooke's Hospital, Cambridge, UK.)

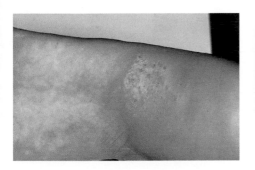

(a)

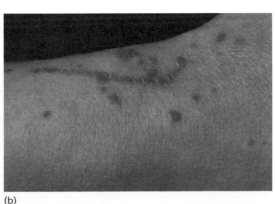

(b)

Figure 3.14 Plane warts: (a) warts on the knee; (b) warts on the arm with spread into a scratch. (Source: Courtesy of Addenbrooke's Hospital, Cambridge, UK.)

are often larger than common warts and have a high risk of recurrence even after successful treatment. HPV-2 is frequently found in butchers' warts, but HPV-7 is present in a third to a half of lesions.

Human papillomavirus in immune compromise: Long-term immune compromise, whether primary, acquired (HIV, leprosy, lymphoma) or iatrogenic (transplant recipients), can be associated with extensive evidence of HPV infection of the skin and mucosal surfaces. Warts may be extensive (Figure 3.16). Patients have an increased risk of head and neck and ano-genital squamous neoplasia.

Cutaneous squamous cell carcinoma without immunosuppression: Squamous cell carcinoma or Bowen disease of the fingertip and nail bed has been associated with high-risk genital HPVs, especially when in association with genital HPV disease.

Differential diagnosis

Hand warts: epidermal naevus, Bowen disease, actinic keratosis and callus.
Plantar warts: corns and calluses, punctate keratoderma of genetic origin.

Investigations

Clinical diagnosis of warts is often sufficient, but atypical, subclinical or dysplastic lesions may need laboratory confirmation of HPV infection. Dermoscopy can help to distinguish a plantar wart from a corn or a callosity. In warts, the plantar ridges of the epidermis are seen to be pushed apart and the mosaic and papillomatous features, sometimes with dark pinpoints of thrombosed capillaries, are visible. A callus or corn has a more amorphous appearance, and the central keratotic 'seed' may be seen.

Management

Many warts are asymptomatic and will resolve spontaneously. Spontaneous regression occurs sooner in children than in adults. In primary school-aged children, about half will clear within a year. About 65% of warts disappear spontaneously within 2 years and 95% within 4 years. Mosaic warts tend to be especially persistent. Simple measures can be advised to limit the spread of the infection, e.g. 'verruca socks' or pool-side sandals at communal bathing areas and by stopping nail biting.

First line: Removal of surface keratin with a pumice stone, emery board or foot file followed by topical 12–26% salicylic acid, with or without lactic acid, daily for 3 months; occlusion can improve the response rate.

Other topical treatments include 10% glutaraldehyde, 2–3% formalin in water, duct tape occlusion, 5% cream of 5-fluorouracil (5-FU), caustics (e.g. monochloroacetic acid, trichloroacetic acid). Retinoic acid may be tried in plane warts.

Second line: Cryotherapy until a 1-mm rim of frozen tissue around the wart then stop or maintain for 5–30 s depending on the size and site of the wart. A second freeze cycle will

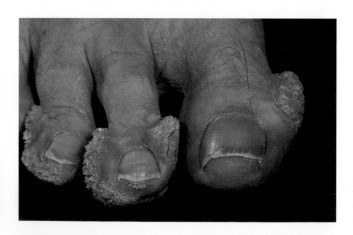

Figure 3.16 Extensive plantar warts in a renal transplant recipient. (Source: Courtesy of Addenbrooke's Hospital, Cambridge, UK.)

improve the cure rate in plantar warts. Cryotherapy may also lead to clearance by stimulating the development of an immune response. Treatment repeated every 3 weeks.

Other treatments include the pulsed dye laser, carbon dioxide laser, surgical excision or curettage and photodynamic therapy.

Ano-genital warts and HPV-associated intraepithelial and invasive neoplasias of genitalia and mucosae

See Chapter 61.

Epidermodysplasia verruciformis

A rare inherited disorder in which there is widespread and persistent infection with HPV.

Usually autosomal recessive. There are at least 20 HPV types characteristic of epidermodysplasia verruciformis (EV). HPV-5 and -8 are the main types associated with malignancy.

Clinically there is a characteristic combination of plane warts, pityriasis versicolor-like lesions and reddish plaques. The warts usually develop rapidly in childhood and are most numerous on the face and neck, and the backs of the hands and feet. Dysplastic and malignant changes occur most often on exposed skin. Squamous cell carcinoma develops in one or more lesions in about 20–30% of reported cases. Patients must be advised on sun protection and skin surveillance.

Acquired epidermodysplasia verruciformis

Long-term immunosuppressed individuals may develop lesions very like those in EV, with small erythematous non-warty plaques and squamous cell carcinomas especially on sun-exposed areas (Figure 3.17). Those at risk are organ and bone marrow transplant recipients, patients receiving long-term immunosuppression for inflammatory disease and those with disorders of immune compromise such as primary immunodeficiencies, lymphoma and HIV/AIDS. In

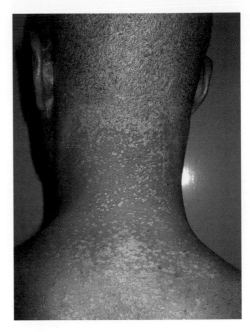

Figure 3.17 Acquired epidermodysplasia verruciformis. Widespread flat hyper- and hypopigmented lesions affecting the neck. (Source: Courtesy of Dr K.W. Shum, Derby Hospitals NHS Trust, UK.)

acquired EV, the risk of malignant progression seems to be lower than in congenital EV, but surveillance for malignancy is advised. For HIV-associated EV, antiretroviral therapy does not lead to a decrease in the skin lesions.

VIRAL INSECT-BORNE AND HAEMORRHAGIC FEVERS

Viral haemorrhagic fevers (VHFs) are caused by viruses from four different families: Arenaviridae (Lassa fever, Junin and Machupo), Bunyaviridae (Crimean-Congo haemorrhagic fever, Rift Valley fever, Hantaan haemorrhagic fevers), Filoviridae (Ebola and Marburg) and Flaviviridae (yellow fever, dengue, Omsk haemorrhagic fever, Kyasanur forest disease) (Table 3.5). Most of these viruses cause zoonotic infections, the human being an accidental host, but person-to-person transmission also occurs.

Table 3.5 Examples of VHF

Virus	Disease	Epidemiology	Clinical features
Arenaviruses			
Lassa virus	Lassa fever	West Africa Natural host: Multimammate rat	Incubation period 7–18 days Fever, nausea, abdominal pain, cough, pharyngitis, pleural effusion, pericardial effusion, swelling of the head or face, or asymptomatic Quarter of survivors have deafness Mortality rate 2–4% (10–20% for hospitalised patients)
Filoviruses			
Marburg virus	Marburg haemorrhagic fever	Very similar diseases Africa, sporadic outbreaks Natural host: fruit bats Transmission: • handling infected animals • person to person (body fluids may remain infectious for as long as 80 days)	Incubation period 1–2 weeks Generalisation phase (days 1–5): sudden headache, high fever and myalgia, often followed by a measles-like rash; petechial or purpuric if severe Second/ early organ phase (days 5–13): diarrhoea, dehydration, hepatitis, haemorrhages and renal damage Third phase (days 8–17): convalescent or late organ stage, severe blood loss, shock and death
Ebola virus	Ebola haemorrhagic fever		
Flaviviruses			
Dengue virus	Dengue fever (break bone fever)	Africa, Central and South America, the Indian subcontinent, Australia and Oceania, South-East Asia Mosquito vector	Incubation period 3–14 days Asymptomatic, acute self-limiting febrile illness or haemorrhagic fever with 1–10% mortality Rash develops on third/fourth day of the fever in half patients Maculopapular or scarlatiniform

The VHFs are all severe, multisystem diseases in which vascular damage and haemorrhage are frequent and prominent features. The mortality is high. They are seen mainly in tropical areas where they are endemic, but with increasing global travel cases are now not uncommonly seen outside these areas. Suspected cases of VHF should be isolated. Handling of specimens for testing must only be carried out at the highest level of biological containment and therefore be discussed with the microbiologist before any material is taken.

OTHER CUTANEOUS PROBLEMS ASSOCIATED WITH VIRAL INFECTIONS

Several patterns of cutaneous reaction are associated with viral (and other) infections. These include asymmetrical periflexural exanthem of childhood, erythema nodosum (see Chapter 51), erythema multiforme (see Chapter 19), Gianotti–Crosti syndrome (see Chapter 64), Kikuchi–Fujimoto disease (see Chapter 23), papular-pruritic gloves and socks syndrome, pityriasis rosea, polyarteritis nodosa (see Chapter 54) and TORCH syndrome.

Papular-pruritic gloves and socks syndrome

Papular-pruritic gloves and socks syndrome presents as an acute acral dermatosis.

Epidemiology
Mainly young adults. Less commonly in children.

Pathophysiology
Predominantly parvovirus B19 infection. In children, EBV or CMV may be associated.

Clinical features
The hands, wrists, feet and ankles are intensely pruritic with macular and papular erythema and oedema. There may be purpura and rarely petechiae. Often with a distinct cut-off at wrists and ankles. Frequently accompanied by oral inflammation with petechiae, vesicopustules and ulceration. Malaise and fever can follow a few days after the onset of the eruption and there may be lymphadenopathy.

Settles within 1–2 weeks but in children may last a month. Skin clearance usually involves desquamation.

Pityriasis rosea

An acute self-limiting disease characterised by a distinctive skin eruption and minimal constitutional symptoms.

Epidemiology
Estimated annual incidence 170/100 000. In temperate climates, there may be a seasonal variation. Occurs between ages of 10 and 35 years, slight female preponderance.

Pathophysiology
The cause is uncertain, generally felt to be of viral aetiology. Involvement of two herpesviruses, HHV-6 and HHV-7, has been suggested. Other possible viral triggers include HHV-8, HSV-2, hepatitis C and H1N1 influenza.

The herald patch and secondary lesions show similar histological features, but these are not diagnostic.

Clinical features
Prodromal symptoms are usually absent. The first manifestation of the disease is the herald patch, which is larger and more conspicuous than the lesions of the later eruption and usually situated on the thigh or upper arm, trunk or neck; may be absent or undetected in 20% of cases (Figure 3.18). It is a sharply defined, erythematous, round or oval plaque 2–5 cm in size, with fine scale. After an interval of 5 to 15 days the general eruption begins to appear in crops at 2–3-day intervals, over 7–10 days. The eruption consists of discrete, dull pink oval lesions with fine scale. The centre tends to clear and assumes a wrinkled, atrophic appearance with a marginal collarette of scale. The long axes of the lesions characteristically follow the lines of cleavage parallel to the ribs in a Christmas tree pattern on the upper chest and back. The lesions are usually confined to the trunk, base of the neck and upper third of the arms and legs but involvement of the face and scalp is quite common, especially in children. There may be pruritus and mild constitutional symptoms.

Lesions fade after 3–6 weeks. There may be temporary hyper- or hypopigmentation, but usually the lesions vanish without trace. Second attacks occur in about 2% of cases after an interval of a few months or many years.

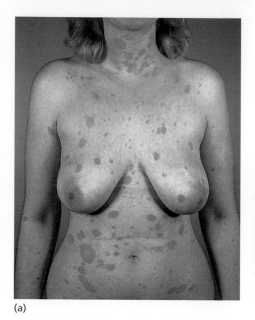

(a)

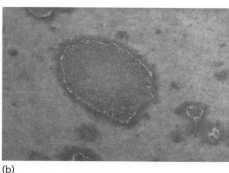

(b)

Figure 3.18 Pityriasis rosea (a) with herald patch on the right of the abdomen, shown in close-up in (b). (Source: Courtesy of York District Hospital, UK.)

Differential diagnosis

Pityriasis rosea-like drug reaction, seborrhoeic dermatitis, secondary syphilis, guttate psoriasis, pityriasis lichenoides, pityriasis versicolor.

Investigations

Diagnosis is usually made on clinical grounds; skin biopsy may be helpful if diagnostic uncertainty.

Management

The common asymptomatic and self-limiting cases require no treatment. If itch is troublesome, or the appearance distressing, a moderate potency topical steroid or UVB can be helpful.

Asymmetric periflexural exanthem of childhood

Most common in young children aged 1–5 years. The eruption starts asymmetrically, affecting the axilla, groin or trunk, and then spreads centrifugally. There are small papules or macules, which can be slightly itchy. There may be associated lymphadenopathy and a low-grade fever. After 2–4 weeks the rash fades with desquamation. Evidence of concurrent parainfluenza, adenovirus, parvovirus B19 or HHV-7 infections have been reported.

COVID-19

Infection with the severe acute respiratory syndrome-coronavirus-2 (SARS-CoV-2) is the cause of the COVID-19 pandemic resulting in worldwide health, societal and economic disruption.

Epidemiology

The disease was first identified in December 2019 in Wuhan, China and rapidly spread across the globe leading the World Health Organization to declare the outbreak a Public Health Emergency of International Concern in January 2020 and a pandemic in March 2020. As of August 2021, approximately 209 million cases of COVID-19 have been confirmed, with more than 4.3 million deaths. Cutaneous manifestations occur in up to 20% of COVID-19 patients.

Pathophysiology

The SARS-CoV-2 virus gains access to alveolar epithelial cells via respiratory droplet transmission. It may also be spread from contact with contaminated surfaces. The virus triggers a vigorous immune response to produce an inflammatory cytokine storm which causes pneumonia, acute respiratory distress syndrome, coagulation dysfunction and multi-organ failure.

Clinical features

The incubation period for SARS-CoV-2 is 2 to 14 days, median 5 days. The clinical features of COVID-19 are highly variable ranging from none, to mild flu-like symptoms, to life-threatening type 1 respiratory failure. Early features of COVID-19 include fever, cough, loss of taste and anosmia (loss of sense of smell). Up to 15% of patients develop dyspnoea and hypoxia, and 5% will progress to respiratory failure or multi-organ failure.

Cutaneous manifestations of COVID-19 are, in general, only a minor feature of the disorder. A maculo papular viral exanthem is the commonest dermatosis. Urticaria can occur in the early phase of the disease, or prior to the onset of systemic symptoms (Figure 3.19). A pruritic papulo-vesicular rash on the trunk is a rare manifestation, as is livedo reticularis. Erythema multiforme and aphthous ulcers have been described. Of particular interest is the development of perniosis on fingers and toes ('Covid toes') as a complication of COVID-19. It is more commonly seen in younger patients (Figure 3.20). A coagulopathy and endothelial dysfunction ('thromboinflammation') underlies the susceptibility to pulmonary embolism, a common and serious complication of patients with severe COVID-19. Inflammatory thrombosis can occur in other vessels, this process appears to be the cause of red-blue, tender nodules on the digits (chilblains or perniosis).

Investigations

Infection with SARS-CoV-2 is confirmed with reverse transcription polymerase chain reaction (RT-PCR) performed on a nasopharyngeal swab. This test detects the presence of SARS-CoV-2 viral RNA.

Management

Approximately 80% of COVID-19 patients have mild disease, but up to 20% of patients will require hospitalisation for supportive treatment with oxygen therapy. Fluid replacement is important in the management of severe COVID-19. Prophylactic anticoagulation is given to most hospitalised patients; those with a proven thrombosis receive treatment doses of anticoagulation. Active intervention recommendations highlight the benefit of systemic corticosteroid (usually dexamethasone) for severely affected patients. Other immunomodulatory therapies are being trialled, as are a variety of anti-viral drugs. Methods used to mitigate the spread of SARS-CoV-2 include social distancing, face masks, frequent hand hygiene and self-isolation for symptomatic individuals or people exposed to COVID-19. Vaccination programmes are ongoing. The cutaneous complications of COVID-19 can usually be managed with symptomatic therapy.

PART 1: INFECTIONS AND INFESTATIONS

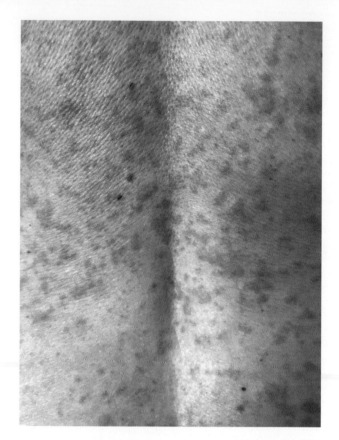

Figure 3.19 Urticarial eruption on trunk in a patient with SARS-CoV-2. Source: Galván Casas, C., et.al. (2020). Classification of the cutaneous manifestations of COVID-19: a rapid prospective nationwide consensus study in Spain with 375 cases. The British journal of dermatology, 183(1), 71–77. https://doi.org/10.1111/bjd.19163

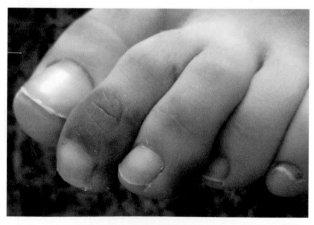

Figure 3.20 Perniosis of left second toe in a patient with SARS-CoV-2. Source: Galván Casas, C., et.al. (2020). Classification of the cutaneous manifestations of COVID-19: a rapid prospective nationwide consensus study in Spain with 375 cases. The British journal of dermatology, 183(1), 71–77. https://doi.org/10.1111/bjd.19163

Bacterial infections and sexually transmitted bacterial diseases

4

GRAM-POSITIVE BACTERIA

STAPHYLOCOCCUS AUREUS

The Gram-positive cocci bacterium *Staphylococcus aureus* is the main pathogenic species that causes skin infections (Box 4.1).

Up to 10–20% of the general population are persistent carriers of *S. aureus*, and this is higher in patients with atopic eczema and with HIV infection. Skin infections with *S. aureus* are more common in patients with breaks in the skin such as scratches, wounds, and ulcers, those who have other skin infections such as tinea pedis and herpesvirus or those with an underlying inflammatory skin disease such as atopic eczema. More than one family/group member may be affected. Other risk factors include contact sports, travel abroad, contact with animals, previous history of MRSA, immunosuppression, men who have sex with men, healthcare workers, renal/liver disease, prosthetic implants and intravenous lines.

Meticillin-resistant Staphylococcus aureus (MRSA)

The widespread use of broad-spectrum antibiotics is thought to have contributed to the increasing incidence of antibiotic-resistant strains, including MRSA. The risk factors identified for patients developing MRSA infection include previous antibiotic use, contact with a healthcare worker or nursing home resident, residence in a long-term care facility, admission to an intensive care unit, intravenous drug use, indwelling devices, haemo- or peritoneal dialysis, nasogastric or other invasive tubes,

---

Box 4.1 Involvement of *S. aureus* in cutaneous disease

Direct infection of skin and adjacent tissues

- Impetigo
- Ecthyma
- Folliculitis
- Furunculosis
- Carbuncle
- Sycosis
- Occasionally in cellulitis
- Others

Secondary infection

- Eczema, infestations, ulcers, etc.

Cutaneous disease due to effect of bacterial toxin

- Staphylococcal scalded skin syndrome
- Toxic shock syndrome
- Staphylococcal scarlatina
- Recurrent toxin-mediated perineal erythema

Rook's Dermatology Handbook, First Edition. Edited by Christopher E. M. Griffiths, Tanya O. Bleiker, Daniel Creamer, John R. Ingram and Rosalind C. Simpson.
© 2022 John Wiley & Sons Ltd. Published 2022 by John Wiley & Sons Ltd.

Box 4.2 Involvement of streptococci (mostly group A) in cutaneous disease

Direct infections of skin or subcutaneous tissue

- Impetigo
- Ecthyma
- Erysipelas
- Cellulitis
- Vulvovaginitis
- Perianal infection
- Streptococcal ulcers
- Blistering distal dactylitis
- Necrotising fasciitis
- Others

Secondary infection

- Eczema, infestations, ulcers, etc.

Tissue damage from circulating toxin

- Scarlet fever
- Toxic-shock-like syndrome
- Recurrent toxin-mediated perineal erythema

Skin lesions attributed to allergic hypersensitivity to streptococcal antigens

- Erythema nodosum (Chapter 51)
- Vasculitis (Chapter 54)

Skin disease provoked or influenced by streptococcal infection (mechanism uncertain)

- Psoriasis, especially guttate forms (Chapter 10)
- Kawasaki disease (Chapter 54)

---

immunosuppression and surgical procedures. Refer to local guidelines for the treatment of MRSA infections.

Community-acquired Meticillin-resistant Staphylococcus aureus (CA-MRSA)

CA-MRSA infections have become common recently. The majority of the infections present as abscesses or folliculitis. The staphylococci are genetically distinct from those acquired in the hospital setting and often carry the Panton–Valentine leukocidin (PVL) virulence gene, although there is now much cross-over in the strains isolated from patients in hospital.

PVL is a toxin that destroys white blood cells and is a virulence factor in some strains of *S. aureus*. Risk factors for PVL infections include overcrowding/close contact, poor hygiene and skin breaks. High-risk groups include healthcare/care home/nursery workers, military personnel, contact sports (rugby, judo, wrestling) athletes and food handlers.

STREPTOCOCCI

Gram-positive catalase-negative cocci, which are nearly all facultative anaerobes. Streptococcal bacteria are classified into group α, β or γ according to their ability to haemolyse red blood cells:

- Alpha-haemolytic streptococci include:
  S. viridans (mainly present in the mouth and leads to dental caries, gingival infections and endocarditis following dental extraction)
  S. pneumonia (causes community-acquired pneumonia, sinusitis, otitis media, conjunctivitis, osteomyelitis, endocarditis, cellulitis, meningitis).
- β-haemolytic species include Lancefield groups A–H:
  S. pyogenes (group A, Box 4.2)
  S. agalactiae (group B, mainly in neonates and the elderly, including pneumonia and meningitis).

The major streptococcal pathogens in humans belong to group A streptococcus (GAS), collectively referred to as *Streptococcus pyogenes*. 5–15% of the population are colonise by the bacteria, usually in the respiratory tract, causing disease when the balance between host immunity (immunosuppression) and bacterial factors (virulence) is altered.

GAS is highly transmissible, passing from person to person through direct skin contact, respiratory droplets and nasal discharge. Streptococci residing in the perianal skin and under fingernails are more frequently spread in conditions of overcrowding and poor hygiene. There is usually a history of skin trauma, abrasion, wounds or underlying skin disease for *S. pyogenes* to cause a cutaneous infection.

SKIN DISEASE DUE TO STAPHYLOCOCCAL AND STREPTOCOCCAL INFECTION

Impetigo

A contagious, superficial pyogenic infection of the skin. Two main clinical forms: non-bullous and bullous impetigo.

Epidemiology
Non-bullous impetigo is frequent worldwide. Large outbreaks often occur, with summer peaks. Preschool and young school age children are most often affected. In adults, males predominate. Overcrowding, poor hygiene and existing skin disease, especially scabies, predispose to infection.
Bullous impetigo is usually sporadic, most frequent in the summer months.

Pathophysiology
Non-bullous impetigo may be caused by both *S. aureus* and streptococcal bacteria. Bullous impetigo is a superficial cutaneous infection with *S. aureus* which produces an exfoliative toxin (ET) that selectively digests one of the intracellular adhesion molecules, desmoglein 1, resulting in superficial blisters. Histology from bullous impetigo classically demonstrates an epidermal split just below the stratum granulosum.

Clinical features
In non-bullous impetigo, the initial lesion is a thin-walled vesicle on an erythematous base which ruptures so rapidly that it is seldom seen. The exudate dries to form yellowish brown crusts (Figure 4.1), which are usually thicker and 'dirtier' in the streptococcal form (Figure 4.2). Lesions enlarge and coalesce. The crusts eventually dry and separate to leave erythema, which fades without scarring. In severe cases, there may be regional adenitis with fever and other constitutional symptoms. The face,

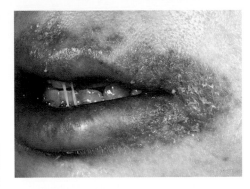

Figure 4.1 Staphylococcal impetigo. (Source: Courtesy of King's College Hospital Dermatology Department, London, UK.)

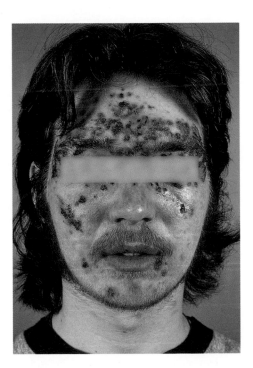

Figure 4.2 Streptococcal (group A) pyoderma.

especially around the nose and mouth, and the limbs are most commonly affected. Involvement of the scalp is frequent in tinea capitis, and lesions may occur anywhere on the body, especially in children with atopic eczema or scabies. There is a tendency to spontaneous cure in

2–3 weeks but a prolonged course is common, particularly in the presence of underlying parasitic infestations or eczema, or in hot and humid climates. In heavily pigmented skin, the lesions may be followed by temporary hypopigmentation or hyperpigmentation.

In bullous impetigo, the bullae are less rapidly ruptured and become much larger; a diameter of 1–2 cm is common but may be bigger, and persist for 2 or 3 days (Figure 4.3); some may become erosive (Figure 4.4). Regional adenitis is rare.

Infective complications are uncommon in the absence of systemic disease or malnutrition. Streptococcal impetigo accounts for the majority of cases of poststreptococcal acute glomerulonephritis.

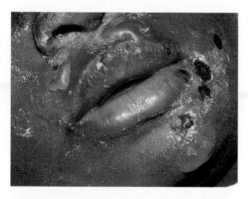

Figure 4.3 Bullous impetigo. (Source: Courtesy of King's College Hospital Dermatology Department, London, UK.)

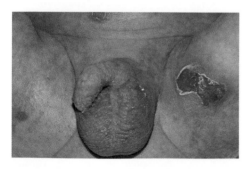

Figure 4.4 Erosive bullous impetigo in a neonate. (Source: Courtesy of King's College Hospital Dermatology Department, London, UK.)

Differential diagnosis

Immunobullous diseases, localised staphylococcal scalded skin syndrome (SSSS), contact dermatitis (irritant or allergic) and herpes simplex infections.

Investigations

Microbiological skin swabs taken from affected skin.

Management

Impetigo is usually self-limiting and resolves within days to weeks with the appropriate use of topical cleansers and antibiotics. Spread to close contacts is common and relapse is more frequently seen in individuals with underlying skin diseases and in staphylococcal carriers.

General measures: Wash affected skin daily with disinfectants, e.g. chlorhexidine, povidone–iodine or sodium hypochlorite. Handwashing for patient and close contacts.

Localised disease: Topical antibiotics for 5 7 days, e.g. mupirocin, fusidic acid, or 2% clindamycin cream.

Widespread or bullous disease or local lymphadenopathy: Systemic antibiotics for 1 week. First-line antibiotics include flucloxacillin (dicloxacillin), cephalexin, co-amoxiclav, cloxacillin and clindamycin. Second-line antibiotics include macrolides such as erythromycin and clarithromycin (macrolide resistance can be quite high) and co-trimoxazole. Third-line antibiotics include trimethoprim and tetracyclines.

Ecthyma

A pyogenic infection of the skin characterised by ulceration with an adherent crust.

Epidemiology

Extremes of age are most commonly affected.

Pathophysiology

Causative organisms include GAS, *Pseudomonas aeruginosa* and *S. aureus*. The infection is much deeper than in impetigo, with loss of the epidermis and dermis, ulceration and scarring. It is more common in immunocompromised patients (HIV, neutropenia), diabetes, high humidity environments and with poor hygiene. Pharyngeal carriers of *S. pyogenes* are more susceptible to recurrent disease.

Clinical features
Small bullae or pustules on an erythematous base are surmounted by a hard crust of dried exudate (Figure 4.5) predominantly on the buttocks, thighs and legs. The crust can only be removed with difficulty to reveal a purulent, irregular ulcer. New lesions may develop by autoinoculation.

Differential diagnosis
Pyoderma gangrenosum, ecthyma gangrenosum, tick bites.

Investigations
Microbiological swabs from affected skin.

Management
Improved hygiene and nutrition, treatment of scabies and any other underlying diseases. Remove crust after soaking with a disinfectant and softening with an oily cream. Topical antibiotics such as fusidic acid and mupirocin can be applied twice daily to localised lesions. Oral antibiotics (flucloxacillin or erythromycin) for 1–2 weeks may be required in the context of multiple lesions or immunocompromised patients.

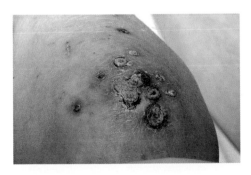

Figure 4.5 Ecthyma. (Source: Courtesy of King's College Hospital Dermatology Department, London, UK.)

Cellulitis and erysipelas

Cellulitis is strictly an acute, subacute or chronic inflammation of loose connective tissue. Erysipelas is a bacterial infection of the dermis and upper subcutaneous tissue involvement. Current usage tends to regard erysipelas as a form of cellulitis rather than a distinct entity.

Epidemiology
Patients most affected are between the fourth and sixth decades. Males are more frequently affected than females.

Pathophysiology
Cellulitis and erysipelas in the immunologically normal patient are predominantly streptococcal diseases, usually involving group A organisms. Group B infections are seen especially under the age of 3 months. *S. aureus* is an occasional cause of cellulitis, but rarely if at all of classical erysipelas. *Haemophilus influenzae* type b is an important cause of facial cellulitis up to the age of 2 years, but this is now rare due to vaccination.

Where there is venous or lymphatic compromise, non-group-A streptococci, especially groups B and G, predominate. Periorbital cellulitis is similar to that in other sites, but orbital cellulitis, usually secondary to sinusitis, involves the major sinus pathogens such as *Streptococcus pneumoniae*, other streptococci, *S. aureus*, *H. influenzae* and penicillin-sensitive anaerobes.

Clinical features
Patients present with redness heat, swelling and pain or tenderness (Figure 4.6). In erysipelas, the edge of the lesion is well demarcated and raised, but in cellulitis it is diffuse, although cases showing both types of edge or an intermediate picture are not uncommon. In erysipelas, blistering is common and there may be superficial haemorrhage into the blisters or in intact skin, especially in the elderly. Severe cellulitis may show bullae (Figure 4.6b) and can progress to dermal necrosis (Figure 4.7), and uncommonly to fasciitis or myositis. Lymphangitis and lymphadenopathy are frequent. Except in mild cases, there is constitutional upset with fever

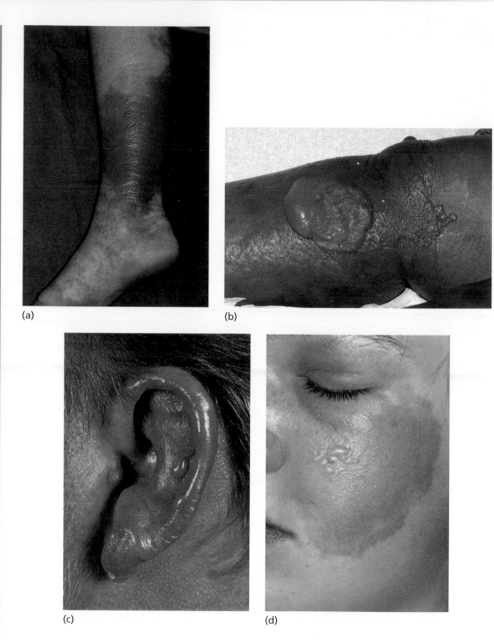

(a) (b) (c) (d)

Figure 4.6 Cellulitis/erysipelas: (a) lower leg; (b) bullous cellulitis of the leg. (Source: Courtesy of King's College Hospital Dermatology Department, London, UK.); (c) pinna; (d) face.

and malaise. Classical erysipelas starts abruptly and systemic symptoms may be acute and severe, but the response to treatment is more rapid.

The leg is the commonest site, normally with a portal of entry such as a wound even if superficial, an ulcer, or an inflammatory lesion including tinea pedis or bacterial infection.

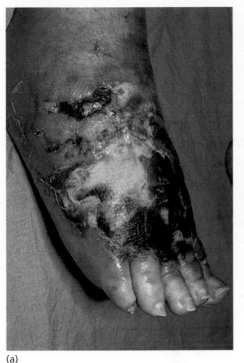
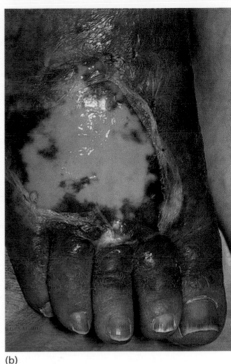

(a)   (b)

Figure 4.7 (a) Cellulitis with early dermal necrosis. (b) The same foot after 11 days; the dermis is forming a black eschar, which eventually sloughed off; the resulting ulcer healed rapidly.

The next most frequent site for classical streptococcal erysipelas is the face, where a traumatic entry site is less common, and where bilateral infection occasionally occurs.

Childhood facial cellulitis is typically unilateral and often associated with ipsilateral otitis media, the presumed source. The patient presents with systemic illness and the affected cheek or periorbital tissue shows induration and discoloration, which is characteristically purplish blue.

Periorbital cellulitis follows trauma to the eyelids or local skin sepsis. If the infection is behind the orbital septum, in the deeper orbital tissues, the term orbital cellulitis applies, and it is commonly a sequel to sinusitis. In addition to cutaneous signs, proptosis, ophthalmoplegia and loss of visual acuity may occur. Periorbital and orbital cellulitis may be complicated by cavernous sinus thrombosis, orbital, subperiosteal or cerebral abscess formation, or meningitis.

Recurrent streptococcal cellulitis (or erysipelas) is attributed to lymphatic damage, which predisposes to further infection and further lymphatic impairment manifesting as lymphoedema.

Inadequately treated cellulitis can lead to fasciitis, myositis, subcutaneous abscesses, septicaemia and, in some streptococcal cases, nephritis.

Differential diagnosis
Necrotising fasciitis, venous insufficiency of the lower leg, acute contact dermatitis.

Investigations
Swabs can be taken from vesicle fluid or eroded or ulcerated surfaces, in addition to blood cultures. In facial infections the pathogen should be sought in nose, throat, conjunctiva and sinuses.

Management
Usually the disease settles over 1–2 weeks with appropriate systemic antibiotics. Initial treatment

should cover streptococci, and for facial infections in young children, *H. influenzae*.

First-line treatment in adults without systemic toxicity or comorbidity is with oral flucloxacillin or clarithromycin in penicillin allergy. In admitted patients a combination of flucloxacillin with benzylpenicillin intravenously is given, or clarithromycin or clindamycin in penicillin allergy. For presumed streptococcal infections, penicillin is the treatment of choice, given as benzylpenicillin intravenously in more severe cases. Anticoagulant therapy should be considered if there is associated thrombophlebitis or reduced mobility.

In recurrent cases of cellulitis, long-term penicillin, 500 mg to 2 g daily, can prevent recurrent attacks; use erythromycin in penicillin allergy. Treatment of any local skin damage is important to prevent recurrent disease.

Folliculitis

Subacute or chronic inflammation of hair follicles in which the inflammatory changes are confined to the ostium or extend only slightly below it, and which heals without scar formation.

Epidemiology
Folliculitis is very common.

Pathophysiology
S. aureus, coagulase-negative staphylococci and physical or chemical irritation are common causes of superficial folliculitis. Other causative organisms include CA-MRSA, *Pseudomonas aeruginosa*, *Pityrosporum* yeast and occasionally dermatophytes. Chemical irritants include mineral oils or tar products. A sterile folliculitis is common beneath adhesive dressings.

Clinical features
Isolated intermittent follicular lesions are frequent on the neck and beard, heal rapidly and are commonly ignored. Also frequent, but more persistent, are papules or pustules on the thighs and buttocks of adolescent and young adult males and occasionally females, especially those with acne. Lesions present as small, follicular papules or pinhead pustules. They are rarely painful. Sometimes small crusts cover a red, pouting, follicular orifice. In *S. aureus* superficial folliculitis, the lesions are domed yellow pustules, sometimes with a narrow red areola. The pustules develop in crops (Figure 4.8) and may heal within 7–10 days, but sometimes become chronic. In older children and adults, the infection may extend more deeply in some follicles as furuncles or as sycosis.

Differential diagnosis
Pustular miliaria, subcorneal pustular dermatosis, pustular psoriasis, tinea infections and pustular drug reaction.

Investigations
When CA-MRSA is suspected, swabs should be taken for sensitivity. In persistent or recurrent cases staphylococcal carriage should be sought in the patient and contacts.

Management
Superficial folliculitis of external chemical or physical origin will settle if the irritant is removed. Mild staphylococcal folliculitis is often self-limiting or responds to daily cleansing with an antiseptic wash; avoid occlusive ointments.

More severe cases require topical antibiotics twice daily to the affected areas, e.g. fuscidic acid, mupirocin or clindamycin 2% cream or oral antibiotics (e.g. flucloxacillin, clindamycin, cephalexin).

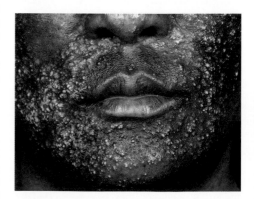

Figure 4.8 Acute folliculitis on the face. (Source: Courtesy of King's College Hospital Dermatology Department, London, UK.)

CA-MRSA can be spread by skin-to-skin contact and appropriate measures should be taken.

Furuncle (boil, abscess)

A furuncle (or boil or abscess) is an acute, usually necrotic, infection of a hair follicle with *S. aureus*. Abscesses are collections of pus in the dermis and adipose tissue that usually result from infection, they are not necessarily centred on the hair follicle.

Epidemiology
Uncommon in early childhood in temperate climates except in atopic subjects. In adolescence, boys are affected more than girls and the peak incidence parallels that of acne vulgaris.

Pathophysiology
Causative organisms include *S. aureus*, which may be meticillin-sensitive *S. aureus* (MSSA) or MRSA, or be PVL positive

Clinical features
A furuncle first presents as a tender, follicular, inflammatory nodule, soon becoming pustular and then necrotic, and healing after discharge of a necrotic core to leave a violaceous macule and, ultimately, a permanent scar. The sites commonly involved are the face and neck, the arms, wrists and fingers, the buttocks and the anogenital region. Attacks may consist of a single crop or of multiple crops, at irregular intervals. There may be fever and mild constitutional symptoms. Pyaemia and septicaemia are favoured by malnutrition. On the upper lip and cheek, cavernous sinus thrombosis is a rare and dangerous complication. Crops may continue to develop for many months or years. In HIV disease, furuncles may coalesce into violaceous plaques.

In patients with multiple and/or recurrent lesions PVL-positive *S. aureus* infections should be suspected (Figure 4.9), or when more than one member of a household is affected either consecutively or simultaneously. PVL lesions tend to be >5 cm in diameter and are more likely to be necrotic and more painful than would normally be expected.

Differential diagnosis
Acne, hidradenitis suppurativa.

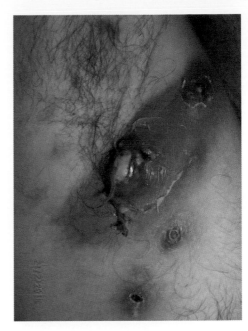

Figure 4.9 Panton–Valentine leukocidin multiple necrotic recurrent abscesses. (Source: Courtesy of King's College Hospital Dermatology Department, London, UK.)

Investigations
Swabs from discharging pus and PVL analysis where appropriate. In recurrent cases nasal and perineal carriage of *S. aureus* in the patient and other household members should be sought.

Management
Simple S. aureus furuncles: Systemic antibiotic, e.g. flucloxacillin or another penicillinase-resistant antibiotic. A topical antibacterial agent reduces contamination of the surrounding skin.

PVL S. aureus furuncles: Optimum management has not been fully determined. Flucloxacillin penetrates poorly into necrotic tissue and results in increased PVL production and is therefore not recommended. Preferred treatment is with a combination of oral clindamycin plus rifampicin or linezolid plus rifampicin. Severe PVL infections may require parenteral antibiotic combinations, including vancomycin, teicoplanin, daptomycin, linezolid, and tigecycline. Large painful abscesses may require incision and drainage in addition to antibiotics. Once the PVL infection has been treated then decolonisation of the index case plus any affected/high-risk close contacts should be undertaken simultaneously. Nasal mupirocin to each nostril three times a day for 5 days plus chlorhexidine 4% or triclosan 1% wash (applied to wet skin, used as a soap, and left on for 1 min) daily for 5 days.

Carbuncle

A deep infection of a group of contiguous follicles with *S. aureus*, larger than abscesses/boils.

Epidemiology
Usually occur in otherwise healthy individuals, predominantly in middle or old age and more common in males. More common in the presence of diabetes, malnutrition, cardiac failure, drug addiction or severe generalised dermatoses, obesity and during prolonged steroid therapy. Nasal *S. aureus* carriers are also at greater risk.

Pathophysiology
The causative organism is *S. aureus*.

Clinical features
Initially smooth, dome-shaped and acutely tender nodule increasing to 3–10 cm diameter. Suppuration begins after 5–7 days and pus is discharged from the multiple follicular orifices. Necrosis of the intervening skin leaves a yellow slough surmounting a crateriform nodule. Most lesions are on the back of the neck, the shoulders or the hips and thighs, and usually solitary. Fever, malaise and prostration may be extreme if the carbuncle is large or the patient's general condition poor. In the frail and ill, death may occur.

Investigations
Skin swabs for microbiology.

Management
Combination of incision/drainage and oral flucloxacillin or another penicillinase-resistant antibiotic. Lesions heal with scarring.

Sycosis

A subacute or chronic pyogenic infection involving the whole depth of the follicle and usually refers to disease in the beard area, sycosis barbae.

Epidemiology
Predominantly post-adolescent males with indoor workers affected more than outdoor.

Pathophysiology
The infecting organism is *S. aureus*.

Clinical features
Many patients are seborrhoeic, with a greasy complexion and chronic blepharitis. An oedematous, erythematous follicular papule or pustule is seen often with some crusting and scaling, but the hairs are retained and there is no scarring. If neighbouring follicles are involved a raised plaque studded with pustules is seen, especially on the upper lip and chin. Attacks of varying duration occur over months or years; more chronic forms may persist for years.

Differential diagnosis
Pseudofolliculitis due to ingrown hairs, and tinea barbae.

Investigations
Bacterial swabs and mycology.

Management
First line: Topical antibiotic or in more chronic forms antibiotic plus steroid combinations. The patient should consider letting beard hair grow. Treat nasal carriage.
Second line: Systemic antibiotics (flucoxacillin, cloxacillin or erythromycin) and oral retinoids.

Staphylococcal scalded skin syndrome

(Syn. Ritter disease)
Staphylococcal scalded skin syndrome (SSSS) SSSS is an exfoliative dermatosis in which most of the body surface becomes tender and

erythematous, and the superficial epidermis strips off (see Chapter 64).

Epidemiology

Children (under the age of 6 years) and neonates are most commonly affected by the generalised form of SSSS; adults are rarely affected.

Renal failure, malignancy, immunosuppression and alcohol abuse predispose adults to the disease.

Pathophysiology

Approximately 5% of *S. aureus* strains produce an exfoliative toxin (ETA or ETB). The initial infection may be very trivial such as a small lesion of impetigo on the face/umbilicus, or a staphylococcal throat/gastrointestinal tract infection. The more extensive and dramatic epidermal changes are then triggered by the ETs, which target the cell adhesion protein desmoglein 1 (DG1) resulting in separation of keratinocytes just beneath the granular layer in the epidermis (intraepidermal). In bullous impetigo, the ETs remain local in the infected skin but in SSSS the ETs are spread haematogenously, resulting in widespread skin involvement.

Histologically, there is splitting of the epidermis between the granular and spinous layers, which do not usually contain inflammatory cells.

Clinical features

Two variants, generalised and localised. The initial event is usually a localised staphylococcal infection (Figure 4.10). After a few days the patient develops fever, irritability and skin tenderness followed by a widespread erythematous eruption accentuated in the flexures and progressing rapidly to superficial blister formation (Nikolsky positive). The condition usually heals within 7–14 days.

Localised SSSS favours the flexures, and healing leaves wrinkled desquamating skin with hyperpigmentation.

Differential diagnosis

Stevens–Johnson/toxic epidermal necrolysis (SJS/TEN) (see Chapter 66). Level of split in a frozen section skin biopsy will aid diagnosis when there is doubt.

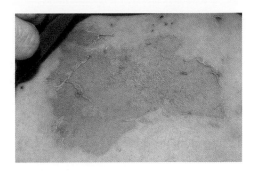

Figure 4.10 Staphylococcal scalded skin syndrome in a child. (Source: Courtesy of King's College Hospital Dermatology Department, London, UK.)

Investigations

Swabs from the original infected site. The blisters are mediated by toxins and swabs will be negative.

Management

Parenteral antibiotics such as flucloxacillin, clindamycin, temocillin, tigecycline or daptomycin. Vancomycin or tobramycin if MRSA is suspected.

If antibiotics are administered early, children usually recover within 7 days and the mortality rate is low at 4%. In adults, the overall mortality rate is higher, around 60%. Patients without underlying disease recover more rapidly.

Toxic shock syndrome

(Syn. Staphylococcal/Streptococcal toxic shock syndrome)

A serious life-threatening illness characterised by fever and acute erythema followed by desquamation, circulatory shock and multisystem disease which is mediated by one or more bacterial toxins produced by *S. aureus* or *S. pyogenes*.

Epidemiology

Toxic shock syndrome (TSS) is rare, affecting 1–17/100 000 tampon users per annum. Early cases were in women using high absorbency tampons in the USA; avoidance of these materials in tampons was followed by a dramatic fall in the incidence.

Recent chickenpox infection, cellulitis and necrotising fasciitis, underlying HIV or internal malignancy, alcohol misuse and diabetes are associated with an increased risk of TSS.

Pathophysiology

TSS toxin 1 is produced by 80–90% of *S. aureus* isolates from affected cases and is believed to be the main bacterial mediator of the disease. Staphylococcal enterotoxin B has also been identified from cases of TSS. A similar disease has been associated with severe infections with *Streptococcus pyogenes.*

Clinical features

Women are usually about 5 days into their menstrual bleeding when they present with fever and a widespread macular erythema which clears within 3 days. Vomiting and diarrhoea are common early features, and involvement of the muscle, liver, kidneys and central nervous system may follow. Circulatory shock (which does not respond to intravenous fluid replacement) is often rapid in onset and severity, frequently with acute renal impairment and multiorgan failure. Oedema of the hands and feet may be marked, with indolent blistering (Figure 4.11). There is generalised mucous membrane erythema, especially intense in the conjunctiva. Oral, oesophageal, vaginal and bladder mucosae may ulcerate. Towards the end of the second week, the majority of patients develop a widespread, itchy, maculopapular, sometimes urticarial, rash. Thrombocytopenia may cause purpura in a retiform pattern at the peripheries. Desquamation is highly characteristic, occurring 10–21 days after onset, and may be confined to the fingertips, affect all the palmar and plantar skin, or be generalised.

Differential diagnosis

Septic shock, Kawasaki disease, staphylococcal scarlatina, Ehrlichosis and *Clostridium sordellii* infection.

Investigations

The diagnosis is clinical, supported by the confirmation of staphylococcal infection in blood cultures and swabs from the wounds and vagina of menstruating or postpartum females. Routine biochemistry may show a raised creatinine, which frequently precedes hypotension.

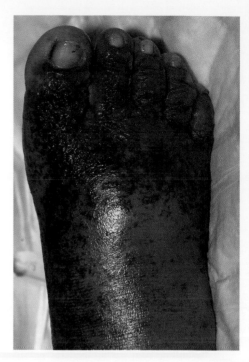

Figure 4.11 Indolent blistering associated with toxic shock syndrome.

Management

Systemic antibiotic therapy (IV clindamycin ± benzylpenicillin sodium (penicillin G) or vancomycin) with haemodynamic resuscitation on a high-dependency unit. Tampons should be removed if present and infected wounds debrided. Patients may require noradrenaline circulatory support and dialysis. For severe cases, consider additional intravenous immunoglobulin (initial dose 2 g/kg, then 4 days of 0.4 g/kg).

Most patients recover over 3 weeks, but the mortality rate remains at about 7%.

Recurrent toxin-mediated perineal erythema

A recurrent perineal erythema mediated by superantigen toxins produced by strains of staphylococci and streptococci, often preceded by a streptococcal throat infection or

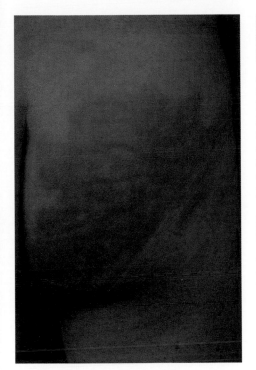

Figure 4.12 Recurrent toxin-mediated perineal erythema.

Perianal streptococcal cellulitis

An uncommon superficial cutaneous infection in the perianal area in young children (6 months to 10 years) due to *Streptococcus pyogenes*. Patients present with perianal soreness or irritation, pain on defecation and sometimes secondary faecal retention. The affected skin is bright red and may be fissured. Responds to 2-week course of oral penicillin.

Blistering distal dactylitis

A distinct entity presenting with localised group A β-haemolytic *Streptococcus* infection of the distal phalanx in children (2–16 years). A large blister or blisters containing thin seropurulent fluid forms on the distal phalanx, usually of a finger, and typically on the palmar pad (Figure 4.13). The organism is cultured from blister fluid and responds to a course of β-lactamase-resistant antibiotics (e.g. flucloxacillin). Differential diagnoses include herpetic whitlow, bullous impetigo and pompholyx eczema.

impetigo. The rash resembles erysipelas (Figure 4.12) with macular erythema but settles quicker with desquamation and few systemic features. Other areas may also be affected, including the hands, feet and axillae. Throat swabs may yield *S. aureus* or *S. pyogenes*. The disease is recurrent but settles rapidly with appropriate antibiotics.

Streptococcal vulvovaginitis

A vaginal infection with GAS mainly affecting prepubescent girls. The patient complains of irritation or soreness in the vaginal area with pain on passing urine. The skin is acutely erythematous and there may be purulent/watery or yellow vaginal discharge. Swabs should be taken for microbiology and to exclude *candida* and sexually transmitted diseases. The infection responds to oral penicillin or erythromycin, but may be recurrent.

Scarlet fever

(Syn. Scarlatina)

A disease manifested by pharyngitis caused by toxin-producing group A β-haemolytic streptococci, with fever and a distinctive scarlatiniform rash.

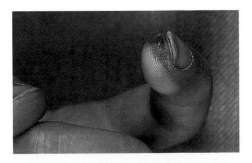

Figure 4.13 Blistering distal dactylitis.

Epidemiology

There has been a dramatic resurgence of cases over the past decade, with most cases occurring between the ages of 5 and 15 years.

Pathophysiology

An acute infection caused by strains of *S. pyogenes* producing pyrogenic exotoxin (erythrogenic toxin, erythrotoxin), of which there are three antigenically unrelated types, A, B and C. Whether an infected individual develops scarlet fever or a septic streptococcal illness, such as tonsillitis or cellulitis, depends on the level of antitoxic immunity, normally acquired by previous exposure. The upper respiratory tract is the usual portal of entry by droplet spread. Overcrowding and poor sanitation are risk factors.

Clinical features

After an incubation period of 2–5 days, fever, anorexia and vomiting occur. If the throat is the portal of entry, there is an acute follicular or membranous tonsillitis, with painful lymphadenopathy. If the infection has entered a wound, there may be increased tenderness and some serous discharge. The rash appears on the second day as a finely punctate erythema on the upper trunk which generalises within a few hours or days. Transverse red streaks in the skin folds due to capillary fragility are known as Pastia lines. The tongue is coated, and by the second or third day swollen red papillae give the 'white strawberry tongue' appearance. As the epithelium is shed, the tongue becomes smooth and dark red ('red strawberry tongue') before returning to normal. The face is flushed and relative pallor around the mouth is characteristic. After 7–10 days, the fever settles and the rash is succeeded by desquamation.

In the severe toxic form, the eruption may be purpuric, fever is high and the patient is delirious or comatose. In the septic forms, the local pharyngeal lesions are severe and there may be extensive oedema. Otitis media and peritonsillar abscesses are frequent.

Complications are either toxic (myocarditis), suppurative (hepatitis, arthritis, meningitis and osteomyelitis) or allergic (rheumatic fever, glomerulonephritis).

Differential diagnosis

Rubella, the early stage of smallpox and some drug reactions.

Investigations

The diagnosis is supported by culture of group A β-haemolytic *Streptococcus* and a rising antistreptolysin-O titre. The peripheral blood usually shows polymorphonuclear leukocytosis.

Management

The prognosis is good and the mortality of treated cases is under 1%. Penicillin should be given in full dosage for 10 days as soon as the diagnosis is suspected.

CORYNEFORM BACTERIA

The term coryneform bacteria is currently used to describe Gram-positive, non-sporing, rod-shaped organisms commonly referred to as diphtheroids. It includes the cutaneous aerobic coryneforms, *Corynebacterium*, and *Brevibacterium* species, as well as the anaerobic *Propionibacterium* species. Diseases caused by Corynebacterium are listed in Box 4.3.

Cutaneous diphtheria

(Syn. Desert sore)

Caused by exotoxin-producing strains of *C. diphtheriae*. While classically a throat and systemic infection, isolated skin infection is seen rarely. Rates of infection are reduced due to immunisation. Although more common in the tropics it does occur in temperate climates, particularly where there is crowding and poor hygiene, and can be travel related.

The typical early lesion is a superficial ulcer with a tough grey adherent membrane. In temperate climates, the lesions occur most commonly at the umbilicus, behind the ears, in the

---

Box 4.3 Diseases caused by *Corynebacterium*

- Diphtheria
- Erythrasma
- Trichomycosis axilliaris
- Pitted keratolysis

genito-crural flexures, in a toe cleft or on a finger or toe. In the tropics they commonly complicate a pre-existing skin lesion described as desert sores. The lesions may simulate impetigo or ecthyma. Diagnosis is made by toxin detection.

Systemic manifestations are characteristically absent or mild in cutaneous diphtheria, but are occasionally severe, especially in infants. In all forms, neurological complications occur in 30% of cases and myocarditis in 5–10%.

Specific intramuscular antitoxin should be administered as soon as the diagnosis is suspected, along with penicillin or erythromycin to treat the carrier status.

Erythrasma

A common disease affecting the axillae, groins and toe webs which may be symptom-free or show mild discomfort and itching.

Epidemiology

Occurs at any age but is more common in adults, within institutions, in warm humid climates and in diabetes.

Pathophysiology

Caused by a group of closely related aerobic coryneform bacteria, usually known as *C. minutissimum*.

Clinical features

Erythrasma occurs most commonly in the groins, axillae (Figure 4.14), toe clefts and intergluteal and submammary flexures. The patches are of irregular shape and sharply marginated, at first red and smooth, but later becoming brown and scaly. In the generalised form, the sharply marginated reddish brown plaques may cover extensive areas of the trunk and limbs.

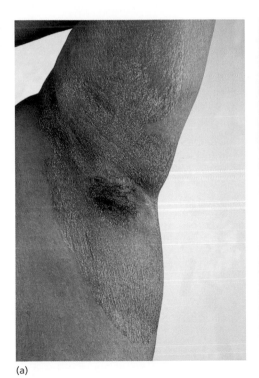

(a)

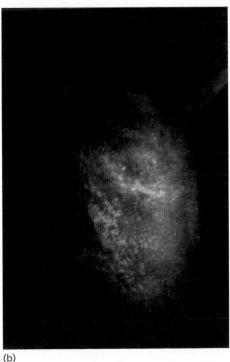

(b)

Figure 4.14 (a) Erythrasma in the axilla. (Source: Courtesy of St John's Institute of Dermatology, London, UK.) (b) Fluorescence with Wood's light. (Source: Courtesy of King's College Hospital Dermatology Department, London, UK.)

Differential diagnosis

Pityriasis versicolor, tinea cruris, tinea pedis or *Candida* infection and flexural psoriasis.

Investigations

Coral-red fluorescence with Wood's light is attributable to coproporphyrin III and strongly suggests erythrasma (Fig 4.14b).

Management

Topical antifungals, such as clotrimazole and miconazole, for 2 weeks. For more extensive lesions, oral erythromycin is effective. Alternatives include topical fucidin and oral tetracycline. In recurrent cases long-term antiseptics, such as povidone–iodine, and drying agents, such as powders, are used.

Trichomycosis axillaris

(Syn. Trichomycosis nodosa)
An asymptomatic superficial infection of axillary and pubic hairs more common in hot and humid environments.

Epidemiology

A common condition.

Pathophysiology

A variety of corynebacteria are involved.

Clinical features

Commonly yellow, or rarely black or red concretions on the hair shaft which may be hard, or soft and nodular, or more diffuse. In the nodular varieties, the hair may be brittle and easily broken. The underlying skin is normal. The axillary sweat may be the colour of the concretions, and the clothing may be stained.

Differential diagnosis

Pediculosis pubis and Piedra.

Investigations

Potassium hydroxide mounts show the bacteria as narrow bacillary organisms in the yellow or red concretions.

Management

Antiperspirant such as aluminium chloride is effective.

Pitted keratolysis

A superficial infection of the soles of the feet caused by a species of *Corynebacterium*.

Epidemiology

A common condition, particularly when there is occlusive footwear and excessive sweating.

Pathophysiology

Caused by several bacteria, including *Streptomyces*, *Corynebacterium*, *Dermatophilus congolensis* and *Kytococcus sedentarius*.

Clinical features (Figure 4.15)

All parts of both soles may be affected, but pressure-bearing or friction areas are most commonly affected. Conspicuous, discrete, shallow, circular lesions with a punched-out appearance coalesce in places to produce irregular erosions. Hyperhidrosis is often associated, sometimes with maceration, stickiness and a foul odour. Irritation is minimal and in most cases patients are unaware of the condition. Changes affecting the palms have been described on rare occasions.

Differential diagnosis

Hyperhidrosis, erythrasma and tinea pedis.

Management

Treatment with topical antibiotics such as fusidic acid. The associated hyperhidrosis should also be treated using potassium permanganate soaks, alu-

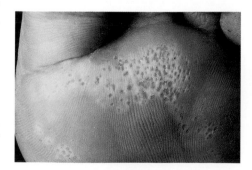

Figure 4.15 Pitted keratolysis. (Source: Courtesy of St John's Institute of Dermatology, King's College London, UK.)

minium chloride, or iontophoresis. Longer term advice on footwear, antiseptics and antiperspirants is important to keep the feet dry and prevent recurrence.

BACILLUS

Bacillus anthracis is a Gram-positive encapsulated organism which can survive as spores for over 20 years in soil and is the cause of anthrax.

Cutaneous anthrax

A zoonotic infection with *B. anthracis*.

Epidemiology
Still a serious problem in Africa, Pakistan, India, Iran, the Middle East and parts of central Asia. Humans are infected from animals or animal products.

Pathophysiology
Cutaneous inoculation by minor trauma or pre-existing skin lesions. Pulmonary and intestinal anthrax are less common and result from the inhalation or ingestion of spores. Systemic anthrax, more common in inhaled and intestinal forms, involves massive bacteraemia and is often fatal.

The major virulence factors are the binary exotoxins: oedema and lethal toxins.

Clinical features
The exposed skin, especially the face, neck, hands or arms are affected most often.

Between 1 and 5 days after infection, an irritable papule develops at the site of inoculation. A bulla follows which ruptures and forms a haemorrhagic crust with surrounding oedema and erythema. In some cases, particularly when the face is involved, malignant oedema, characterised by severe swelling, induration and multiple bullae, may develop.

Constitutional symptoms may begin 3 or 4 days after the onset of the pustule. Anthrax meningitis is a rare complication of cutaneous disease. Overall, the mortality of untreated cutaneous anthrax is between 5 and 20%, but most cases are mild, with resolution after 2–3 weeks.

Differential diagnosis
Staphylococcal infection, ecthyma gangrenosum, cat scratch disease (formerly named paraanthrax), pox infections (e.g. orf), North American blastomycosis and sporotrichosis.

Investigations
Chains of Gram-positive bacilli can be seen in smears of lesions, but skin lesions should be cultured.

Management
Prompt treatment with oral ciprofloxacin or doxycycline prior to bacteriological confirmation. Treatment may be switched to amoxicillin if the infecting strain is susceptible.

Vaccination should be offered to those who are occupationally exposed, alongside control of the disease in animals and disinfection of animal products. Prophylaxis for asymptomatic patients exposed to anthrax spores includes a 6-week course of doxycycline or ciprofloxacin.

ERYSIPELOTHRIX RUSIOPATHIAE

A Gram-positive rod found as a commensal or pathogen in a wide variety of animal species that is the cause of erysipeloid.

Erysipeloid

An acute, rarely chronic, infection with *Erysipelothrix rusiopathiae*. A very rare infection mainly confined to the skin. Human infection is by direct contact, mainly from carcasses, therefore it is more common in slaughtermen, butchers, cooks, fishermen, farmers and veterinary surgeons. Most human infections are localised and self-limiting.

Three days after inoculation, a hot, tender erythema develops around the inoculation site and extends centrifugally with a sharp and sometimes gyrate border, which may be vesicular. Lesions occur on exposed areas, predominantly the hands, fingers or forearms. Approximately 10% of cases have fever and mild constitutional symptoms such as arthralgia. Without treatment, healing normally occurs spontaneously in 2 weeks. Healing is facilitated by antibiotic therapy (penicillins, ciprofloxacin or erythromycin).

For severe or systemic infections, intravenous penicillin is required.

CLOSTRIDIUM

Anaerobic, Gram-positive, spore-forming bacilli, widely distributed in the soil and in the gastrointestinal tracts of humans and other mammals.

Gas gangrene

(Syn. Clostridial myonecrosis)
A potentially fatal infection if unrecognised that occurs when wounds are contaminated with soil or water after trauma.

Pathophysiology
The most important species of *Clostridium* involved are *C. perfringens* (formerly *C. welchii*), *C. oedematicus*, *C. septicum* and *C. histolyticum*. The α-toxin produced by *C. perfringens* is haemolytic and thought to be the main virulence factor in gas gangrene.

Clinical features
The incubation period varies from 12 h to 6 days. Deep, dirty wounds in the muscular regions of the body are most susceptible. The wound becomes painful and swollen with increasing serous discharge. Toxaemia is severe but the patient is often not febrile. The oedema around the wound spreads with brownish staining and mottling, then with bullae and later with the formation of black sloughs. Crepitation from gas in the tissues is classical but inconstant. There is a high mortality where diagnosis is delayed.

Differential diagnosis
Necrotising fasciitis.

Investigations
Clinical diagnosis supported in due course by bacterial examination. Blood cultures should be taken prior to antimicrobial therapy. Radiology confirms gas in the tissues.

Management
Immediate surgical debridement of all damaged tissue along with high-dose intravenous penicillin. Alternatives include clindamycin, metronidazole and imipenem.

GRAM-NEGATIVE BACTERIA

The skin may be infected by Gram-negative bacteria either as a result of systemic spread from another site or through haematogenous dissemination or by direct local invasion.

NEISSERIA MENINGITIDES

Neisseria meningitidis is a Gram-negative coccus. It can be divided into different serotypes on the basis of capsular polysaccharides, types A, B and C being the most important. All types are pathogenic.

Meningococcal septicaemia

(Syn. Meningococcal vasculitis, meningococcal purpura fulminans)
N. meningitidis colonises the human upper respiratory tract and is transmitted by droplets from patients or healthy carriers. It may cause localised infections, such as conjunctivitis and otitis media, or severe and potentially fatal disease with septicaemia and often meningitis.

Epidemiology
An estimated 500 000 cases of meningococcal infection annually worldwide with a case fatality rate of 10%. Infections are more common during the winter and in children aged 0–5 or 15–17 years.

Pathophysiology
N. meningitidis group B is more common in Europe and group A in tropical regions.

Bacteraemia is the primary event in all forms of the infection. The early petechial skin lesions result from the presence of the organisms in capillary endothelium accompanied by disseminated intravascular coagulation, with necrosis of the vessel wall or thrombosis. The later skin lesions show a vasculitis thought to be produced by antigen–antibody complexes.

Clinical features
Acute meningococcal septicaemia with or without meningitis may present as a fulminating illness, and the rash may be a useful clue to early diagnosis. Early skin lesions may be discrete pink macules or papules. Purpura follow, mainly

on the trunk and limbs. In severe cases, there are extensive ecchymoses and necrotic ulceration, particularly in dependent or pressure areas, which are associated with a high mortality.

Vasculitis may occur during the acute illness, beginning 5–9 days after the onset, even with adequate antibiotic treatment.

Differential diagnosis

Causes of acute vasculitis, viral haemorrhagic fevers (e.g. dengue).

Investigations

Isolation of *N. meningitidis* from blood or cerebrospinal fluid or by PCR.

Management

Circulatory support and intravenous fluids with intravenous high-dose benzylpenicillin; ceftriaxone or cefotaxime are suitable alternatives.

Rifampicin for 2 days is recommended as prophylaxis for close family contacts but does not eliminate the need for close clinical surveillance. Vaccines are available for meningococcal infections caused by groups A, C, Y and W-135 organisms but not group B.

Gonococcal infections

Gonococcal infections are discussed under sexually transmitted diseases.

PSEUDOMONAS AERUGINOSA

Pseudomonas infection

(Syn. Gram-negative folliculitis, Ecthyma gangrenosum)

Pathophysiology

Pseudomonas aeruginosa is an aerobic, Gram-negative rod, which occurs only as a transient member of the skin flora, mainly in the anogenital region, axillae and external ear, and is normally kept in check by the dominant Gram-positive cocci.

On the skin surface, the repeated application of bactericidal agents effective against the Gram-positive flora or prolonged maceration favours the establishment of *Pseudomonas* even in previously healthy adults. Typical strains produce two pigments, the blue-green pyocyanin and a greenish yellow pyoverdin.

Clinical features

Pseudomonas species produce a variety of different infections in the skin depending on the site and underlying condition of the patient. Systemic infections are seen frequently, largely in immunosuppressed patients or the acutely sick who have received multiple courses of antibiotics or on neonatal units.

The commonest local infection in infancy is periumbilical, with a foul-smelling bluish green discharge and spreading erythema.

Pseudomonas infection of the toe webs (Figure 4.16), also called tropical immersion foot, is characterised by sharply demarcated areas of maceration and tender erosions, sometimes tinged with green, and showing

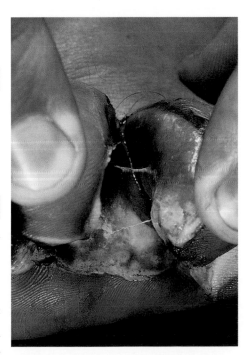

Figure 4.16 *Pseudomonas* infection of the foot. (Source: Courtesy of St John's Institute of Dermatology, King's College London, UK.)

green fluorescence under Wood's light. The presence of *Pseudomonas* spp. beneath nails with onycholysis gives rise to characteristic green discolouration.

Gram-negative folliculitis seen in swimming pool or jacuzzi users can affect any part of the body that has been immersed, but often the worst areas are those in contact with bathing costumes. In most cases, the rash settles spontaneously within 7–10 days in the absence of re-exposure.

Pseudomonas septicaemia most commonly occurs in the severely compromised host. Usually there are no skin lesions, but there may be non-specific erythema, purpura or a cellulitis-like picture. Bullae may form, particularly in moist areas such as the axillae, perineum and the buttocks which rupture to give necrotic ulcers, ecthyma gangrenosum (Figure 4.17).

Investigations
Bacteriological confirmation by cultures from affected skin or blood.

Management
1% acetic acid compresses, potassium permanganate soaks, povidone or silver sulfadiazine cream are used in superficial infections to dry them out.

In septicaemia or where a severely compromised patient has superficial infection, intravenous antibiotics should be started promptly using a combination of ceftazidime, gentamicin, piperacillin, azlocillin, tobramycin and amikacin.

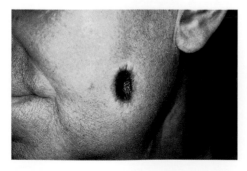

Figure 4.17 Ecthyma gangrenosum. (Source: Courtesy of Dr G. Scott, University College Hospital, London, UK.)

FRANCISELLA TULARENSIS

A pleomorphic non-motile Gram-negative coccobacillus which produces a powerful endotoxin.

Tularaemia

A zoonotic infection caused by *F. tularensis*.

Epidemiology
Wild rodent or other small animal populations are the main reservoir of infection, which is transmitted to humans by the bites of ticks, other arthropods, or by direct contact with infected rodents. The disease is endemic in the USA and many parts of north and east Europe apart from the UK. Sportsmen, sportswomen and campers are most exposed to infection.

Clinical features
The incubation period varies from 1 to 10 days. The clinical manifestations depend on the portal of entry: the skin, eye, respiratory or gastrointestinal tracts. Most sporadic cases are of the ulceroglandular, glandular or oculoglandular type. A red, painful and then ulcerated nodule at the point of inoculation or tick bite is associated with enlargement and tenderness, and later with breakdown of the regional lymph nodes. Systemic symptoms and toxaemia may be severe but are often moderate. During the toxaemic stage cutaneous lesions may develop: a generalised eruption, maculopapular, or resembling erythema multiforme, or profuse crops of nodules, usually on the limbs.

The typhoidal and pulmonary forms, which present with severe generalised or respiratory symptoms, respectively, run a more fulminating course. Untreated, the course may be prolonged; the mortality of the typhoidal and pulmonary forms exceeds 30%, and that of the oculoglandular form is about 5%.

Differential diagnosis
Tick-borne rickettsial infections.

Investigations
The organism may be cultured from the primary lesion, the lymph nodes, or gastric or pharyngeal washings. Specific agglutinins appear in the serum after about 10 days.

Management

All cases require treatment with ciprofloxacin; gentamicin is an alternative. A live attenuated vaccine is available.

PASTEURELLA

Pasteurella multocida and related infections

Pasteurella multocida is a small Gram-negative bacillus found in the normal flora of the respiratory tract or intestines of many domestic and wild animals. Most human infections follow bites by cats, dogs or other animals, or from scratch injuries (usually cats). Lesions are predominantly on the hands, arms or lower legs. Redness and swelling around the wound may spread rapidly over a wide area and break down to discharge greyish yellow, haemorrhagic pus through one or more sinuses. If the bite is deep, there may be osteomyelitis or synovitis. 10–15% of patients are febrile with localised lymphadenopathy. The diagnosis is confirmed by the isolation of the bacillus and the infection responds to penicillin, ampicillin and cephalosporins.

YERSINIA

The main skin pathogens are *Yersinia pestis* and *Y. enterocolitica*.

Plague and *Yersinia* infections

(Syn. Black death, Bubonic/pneumonic plague)
A disease of historical significance, the plague was responsible for several major epidemics in Europe, North Africa and the Middle East in the middle ages and later.

Epidemiology

A zoonotic infection that affects a wide variety of rodents, but particularly the urban and domestic rats, *Rattus rattus* and *R. norvegicus*. It is conveyed from rodent to humans by flea bites or humans may be infected after contact with contaminated material. It is endemic in parts of India and the Far East, and in Madagascar and Southern and Central Africa. Occasional cases occur in travellers from endemic areas.

Pathophysiology

The causative organism is *Y. pestis*.

Clinical (cutaneous) features

The incubation period is 3 or 4 days. A primary cutaneous lesion similar to anthrax may occur in 10% of patients at the site of the flea bite. The regional lymph node becomes swollen (the classic bubo of bubonic plague), and systemic spread, typically with a severe febrile illness, develops, frequently leading to death within days. During the bacteraemic phase, a macular, erythematous or petechial rash may develop; this is sometimes frankly purpuric (the Black Death).

Investigations

Aspiration of a bubo and direct examination of smears and culture confirm the diagnosis. The culture of blood and sputum should also be undertaken.

Management

All cases require antibiotic therapy; streptomycin, gentamicin, doxycycline or chloramphenicol are all effective. Untreated it is fatal.

BRUCELLA

Brucellosis

(Syn. Undulant fever, Mediterranean fever, Malta fever)
A zoonosis and a disease of domestic and farm animals which can be transmitted to humans.

Epidemiology

A widespread infection of cattle and sheep, goats and pigs with *Brucella abortus*, *B. melitensis* and *B. suis*, respectively. Human cases are seen mainly in Mediterranean countries of Europe, the Middle East, North and East Africa, South and Central Asia and Latin America. The incidence is highest in veterinary surgeons and farmers.

Pathophysiology

Humans are infected by the ingestion of contaminated milk or milk products, or by direct contact with infected animals.

Clinical features

After a variable incubation period headache, backache and general malaise accompany the onset of an intermittent fever. The lymph nodes and spleen are enlarged in about 50% of cases and the liver in about 25%. Skin lesions develop in about 5% but are not pathognomonic. Morbilliform, scarlatiniform and roseolar exanthems are described. The illness usually lasts 3 or 4 months, but both acute fulminating and chronic forms occur.

Contact brucellosis. Veterinary surgeons, and others who are in frequent contact with infected animals, may develop a high degree of allergic sensitivity to *Brucella* antigens. Contact with the secretion of an infected animal gives rise to pruritus, erythema and whealing, followed within 48 h by a profuse eruption of fine follicular papules, many of which become vesicular or pustular and heal in 10–14 days to leave small scars. Secondary eruptions of erythema multiforme type may develop remotely from the sites of contact.

Investigations

Specific agglutinins.

Management

The recommended course of treatment for brucellosis includes doxycycline and rifampicin for at least 6 weeks.

BARTONELLA

Bartonella species are regarded as bacteria more closely related to *Brucella* than to other genera. The human diseases associated with these organisms are listed in Table 4.1.

EHRLICHIA

Ehrlichiosis

A tick-borne zoonotic infection caused by *Ehrlichia* spp. (*E. chaffeensis* and *E. sennetsu*) predominantly in the USA. The distribution of the dog tick, *Dermacentor variabilis*, and the lone star tick, *Amblyomma americanum*, coincide with the distribution of human cases. Natural hosts include the white-tailed deer and dogs.

The median incubation period is 7 days and patients generally present with fever, malaise, headache and myalgia. Over 30% of patients have a diffuse maculopapular rash and in some this becomes petechial. Main differential diagnosis is Rocky Mountain spotted fever. Diagnosis confirmed with PCR or a serological assay using immunofluorescence. Treatment with tetracycline or doxycycline.

ANAEROBIC BACTERIA

Tropical ulcers

Tropical ulcers occur in the tropical areas of the Old World and present as acute or chronic ulcers.

Epidemiology

The disease has been described in countries in sub-Saharan Africa, India, South-East Asia and the West Pacific region. Commonest in children.

Pathophysiology

The causative organism is *Fusobacterium ulcerans* plus a variable combination of other bacteria including spiral bacteria.

There is no correlation between nutritional indices and the development of tropical ulcer.

Clinical features (Figure 4.18)

Most tropical ulcers develop at a site of potential trauma, a scratch, cut or insect bite, and are therefore commonest on the lower legs and on the unshod foot.

The floor of the ulcer is covered by a foul-smelling greyish purulent slough. Pain is usual, and there may be fever and constitutional symptoms. There is usually no regional adenitis. If the lesion is treated promptly, the spread is limited and heals slowly.

Differential diagnosis

Yaws, venous ulcers, cutaneous leishmaniasis.

Table 4.1 Diseases caused by *Bartonella* species

	Trench fever	Cat scratch disease	Bacillary angiomatosis	Oroya fever and verruga peruana (Syn. Carrion disease)
Epidemiology	Poor hygiene	Most common in autumn and winter, and in children and teenagers	Uncommon disease in AIDS patients and severe immunosuppression	Rare disease Endemic in Peru
Pathophysiology	*B. quintana*, transmitted to humans by the body louse No animal reservoir	*B. henselae* History of cat contact and a wound	*B. henselae* (transmitted by cat scratch or bite) and *B. quintana* (transmitted by lice) The bacteria enter red blood cells and stimulate angiogenesis in the vascular endothelium	*B. bacilliformis* (transmitted by sandflies of the genus Lutzomyia)
Clinical features	A mild recurrent febrile illness A widespread maculopapular eruption, most prominent on the trunk, fluctuates with the fever	Unilateral lymphadenitis is the usual presenting feature, with a granulomatous nodule distal to the gland at the inoculation site predominantly on the hands and arms and the head and neck Constitutional symptoms are mild; fever is present in 60% of cases	No history of exposure or a primary entry point Friable angiomatous papules and nodules follow a mild septicaemia Local lymphadenopathy is common	Two forms: 1. A febrile illness, Oroya fever, in which the mortality is high; many cases are accompanied by *Salmonella* septicaemia 2. Verruga peruana, multiple small red skin papules, with or without previous Oroya fever
Differential diagnosis		Sporotrichosis, atypical mycobacterial infection	Kaposi sarcoma, pyogenic granuloma, cutaneous lymphomas	Verruga peruana: yaws, acquired haemangiomas and Kaposi sarcoma
Investigation		The clinical picture is diagnostic	Large clusters of bacteria on Warthin–Starry staining	Blood films and blood cultures
Management	Spontaneous recovery	Self-limiting Azithromycin if treatment indicated	Doxycycline or erythromycin for 8 weeks or longer	Chloramphenicol 2 g/day for a week in febrile cases Verruga peruana settle

PART 1: INFECTIONS AND INFESTATIONS

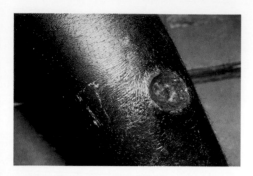

Figure 4.18 Tropical ulcer. (Source: Courtesy of St John's Institute of Dermatology, London, UK.)

Investigations
The mainstays of diagnosis are the rapid onset of lesions, their clinical appearance and the clustering of cases in the locality.

Management
Rest, elevation of the limb and adequate diet.

During the early stages of the disease, penicillin or metronidazole are recommended.

Granuloma inguinale

A sexually transmitted infection (STI), discussed below.

SPIROCHAETES AND SPIRAL BACTERIA

Spirochaetes are long flexible spiral organisms. Three genera exist: *Treponema*, *Borrelia* and *Leptospira*. Syphilis is discussed under STIs.

TREPONEMES

The non-venereal (endemic) treponematoses comprise endemic syphilis or bejel, yaws and pinta.

Endemic syphilis or bejel

A rare disease caused by *Treponema pallidum* subspecies *Endemicum*. Occurs predominantly in the southern border of the Sahara desert and parts of the Middle East. It is spread by non-sexual contact. Histopathological features and serological reactions are identical to those seen in venereal syphilis.

The *primary* lesion, a papule or small ulcer, occurs in the mouth, or on the nipples of breast-feeding women. *Secondary* lesions are similar to those of venereal syphilis. The late (*tertiary*) stage is characterised by gummata of the nasopharynx that may result in destruction of the nose (gangosa), gummatous or plaque-like lesions in the skin, periostitis and bony gummata. Management is similar to venereal syphilis. It responds to parenteral penicillin and azithromycin.

Yaws

(Syn. Framboesia [German and Dutch], Pian [French], Buba [Spanish], Bouba [Portuguese], Parangi [Sinhalese])
An endemic disease caused by *T. pallidum* spp. *pertenue*. A disease of tropical rural populations, occurring in the Caribbean, Central and South America, throughout tropical Africa, South-East Asia and the Pacific islands. Transmission is favoured by overcrowded conditions. Commonest in children.

The initial lesions follow direct entry of bacteria into non-genital skin. In the *primary* stage, the initial lesion ('mother yaw') is a solitary erythematous papule, at the point of entry of the treponemes. This ulcerates and increases in size to resemble a raspberry, and teems with treponemes. The mother yaw lasts for 2–6 months and heals spontaneously to leave an atrophic scar. 'Daughter yaws' are multiple lesions that develop in the *secondary* stage as the initial lesion heals. Early lesions are highly infectious. After several years, the disease enters its late (*tertiary*) stage. The disease can be disabling but is not fatal.

Differential diagnosis includes tropical ulcer and syphilis. Serological tests are as for syphilis. All cases require antibiotic (penicillin or azithromycin) treatment.

Pinta

A disease exclusively of the skin caused by *T. pallidum* subspecies *carateum*. Still thought to be endemic in remote areas of southern Mexico, and central and northern South America.

In the *primary* stage of pinta, a few papules or erythematosquamous plaques develop. After an interval of months or years the *secondary* stage features more extensive lesions known as 'pintids'. Their initial red colour changes to brown, slate blue, black or grey, and eventually there is depigmentation intermixed with hyperpigmentation. Atrophy occurs as the late stage develops. The primary and secondary stages are infectious. In the late (*tertiary*) stage, which takes several years to develop, there is irregular pigmentation, vitiligo-like achromia, areas of hyperkeratosis, and eventually atrophy.

Serological tests are as for syphilis and treatment is with penicillin.

BORRELIA

Relapsing fever

There are two forms of this disease: louse-borne or epidemic relapsing fever due to *Borrelia recurrentis*, for which the human body louse is the vector, and tick-borne endemic relapsing fever caused by various species of *Borrelia*, e.g. *B. duttoni* and *B. hermsi*.

Epidemiology

The louse-borne epidemic form is found in Ethiopia, the Sudan, other parts of Africa and the Far East, while the milder, sporadic tick-borne cases occur worldwide.

Clinical features

High fever, headache, myalgia, vomiting and respiratory symptoms usher in the acute attack. Jaundice and hepatosplenomegaly are common, and a petechial or purpuric rash, predominantly on the trunk, is seen in up to 60% of patients. A remission occurs after a few days to be followed by a relapse, and this pattern may continue for weeks. The cutaneous eruption does not recur after the initial episode.

Investigations

Demonstration of the spirochaete in blood films using stained preparation or dark-ground illumination.

Management

The usual treatment is either tetracycline or erythromycin. Penicillin is an alternative. A severe reaction similar to the Jarisch–Herxheimer reaction is very common at the outset of treatment.

Borrelia burgdorferi and Lyme disease

Lyme disease is a tick-borne zoonotic disease caused by *Borrelia burgdorferi*. Other causes include *B. afzelii* and *B. garinii*.

Epidemiology

The principal vector of *B. burgdorferi* infection is the *Ixodes* tick. Patients usually live close to, or have visited, woodland areas, where small mammals are necessary hosts for immature stages in the life cycle of the tick. Adult ticks may infest in larger mammals, especially deer.

Lyme disease has been reported in most parts of the world but especially in the USA, Central Europe and Scandinavia. Infection may occur at any time of year.

Pathophysiology

The organisms are injected into the skin at the outset and the initial site of proliferation is the dermis. At a varying interval after initial infection, the organism may spread through the bloodstream to other sites such as the central nervous system, joints and heart.

Clinical features

About 50% recall a tick bite.

90% of patients with bite injury develop erythema chronicum migrans (ECM) at the site of inoculation (Figure 4.19). The eruption appears on average 9 days after the bite, and is due to local spread of the spirochaete, usually in a ring formation. The erythema may be intense or barely

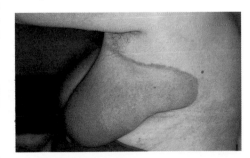

Figure 4.19 Erythema chronicum migrans. (Source: Courtesy of Dr A.S. Highet, York District Hospital, York, UK.)

detectable; it may be entirely flat or show elevation at the centre, the periphery or both. Slight scaling is occasionally seen. There may be a zone of clearing behind the advancing ring producing a target-like morphology. There may be burning or itching. If untreated, the lesion fades, usually within a few weeks. Regional lymphadenopathy and mild constitutional symptoms may occur.

Dissemination of the infection may occur within days or weeks of inoculation. Later manifestations may include arthritis, neurological or cardiac involvement, rarely involving the eyes and liver.

Differential diagnosis

Other forms of insect- or spider-bite reactions, cellulitis and drug eruptions.

Investigations

Confirmation of *B. burgdorferi* by serology, the main tests are an ELISA, an indirect immunofluorescence test and a Western blot. PCR provides a rapid diagnostic test both on serum and tissue. Biopsy of ECM shows a superficial and deep perivascular and interstitial lymphohistiocytic infiltrate containing plasma cells.

Management

Early recognition and treatment prior to serological confirmation are important.

For solitary lesions of ECM, with only regional lymphadenopathy or minor constitutional symptoms, treatment with doxycycline or amoxicillin is recommended for 14–21 days. After dissemination the results of therapy are less impressive. Mild systemic disease is treated as above. More severe cases require intravenous treatment with ceftriaxone 2 g daily IV for 2 weeks but there is still a 15% failure rate.

Careful inspection of the skin after walking in endemic areas and removal of ticks is advised.

MISCELLANEOUS BACTERIAL INFECTIONS

Necrotising fasciitis

A severe infection of the soft tissues of the deep dermis, adipose tissue and subcutaneous fascia, where the hallmark of infection is extensive necrosis accompanying cellulitis.

Epidemiology

Annual incidence of 1/200 000. Rare in children.

Pathophysiology

There are at least two distinct groups of infections.

Type I necrotising fasciitis is the more common type caused by multiple organisms, one of which is an anaerobe (e.g. *Bacteroides*, *Clostridium*) and others include Gram-positive rods (e.g. *S. aureus*, GAS, Enterococci) and Gram-negative rods (e.g. *E. coli*, *P. aeruginosa*). Fournier's gangrene is a term used when the infection is confined to the scrotum or male perineum.

Type II necrotising fasciitis is due to a single organism, usually *S. pyogenes*. *S. aureus*, *Aeromonas hydrophila* and *Vibrio vulnificus* may also be implicated. Zygomycete fungi (mucormycosis) are rarely seen in the immunocompromised patient.

Portal of entry may be a minor break in the skin, trauma or following surgery; it may be difficult to pinpoint in all cases. Infection extends along the fascial planes beyond what is seen on the skin surface delaying a diagnosis. Thrombosis of vessels leads to ischaemia and necrosis. Bacterial toxins produce systemic symptoms.

Predisposing factors include trauma, infection, diabetes, IV drug abuse, chronic systemic diseases, peripheral vascular disease, immunosuppression and previous surgery.

Clinical features

Early recognition is important as the disease progression is fast. The extremities are the most common site along with the perineum, trunk and head and neck. Fever, tachycardia, tachypnoea and hypotension suggest severe disease and require emergency surgical assessment.

Patients present with a hot tender area of swelling, which is erythematous and occasionally dusky with blistering. The skin may look normal and the pain disproportionate. The overlying skin may become anaesthetic. There may be crepitus.

Differential diagnosis

Gas gangrene, mucoromycete infections, cellulitis, pyoderma gangrenosum, ecthyma gangrenosum.

Investigations

Definitive bacteriological diagnosis is best made from tissue specimens obtained from surgical debridement. Plain radiography or CT/MRI may show soft-tissue gas but cannot rule it out and surgical intervention should not be delayed for imaging to be performed.

Management

This is an acute emergency warranting management in an intensive care unit by a multidisciplinary team. The most important step in diagnosis and management is surgical debridement. Broad-spectrum antibiotics should be given until cultures and sensitivities are available.

Mortality from treated necrotising fasciitis is 10–40%, increasing to 70% in severe cases. There may be significant functional and cosmetic sequelae.

RICKETTSIAL INFECTIONS

Rickettsiae are regarded as small bacteria, and most are obligate intracellular parasites. They are spread by the bites of blood-sucking arthropods and cause widespread infection in endothelial cells, which may result in vascular infarcts, extravascular fluid loss and disseminated intravascular coagulation.

Spotted fever group

The infections in this group (Table 4.2) are spread by ticks or mites.

Rocky Mountain Spotted Fever

An acute febrile illness accompanied by an exanthem. The most virulent rickettsial infection.

Epidemiology

Rocky Mountain areas of North America, Maryland, Virginia and North Carolina, and in Mexico, Colombia and Brazil.

Pathophysiology

The organism *R. rickettsii* is transmitted by the bite of the tick, *Dermacentor*.

Widespread inflammatory and destructive changes are produced in the small blood vessels, especially in the skin and central nervous system.

Clinical features

Around 2–14 days after the tick bite, malaise and headache are followed by fever. After 3 or 4 days, a maculopapular eruption appears on the wrists and ankles and spreads centrally to the limbs, trunk and face. The palms and soles are usually involved. Except in the mildest cases, the rash becomes haemorrhagic. The other clinical manifestations depend on the degree of involvement. Gangrene of the fingers, toes, genitalia or nose may result from vascular obstruction.

Differential diagnosis

Viral haemorrhagic fevers, meningococcal septicaemia, other rickettsial infections.

Table 4.2 Classification of the rickettsial spotted fever group

Organism	Main geographical area	Name
Rickettsia rickettsia	Americas (mainly USA)	Rocky Mountain spotted fever
R. conorii	Mediterranean region, South-West Asia, India	Tick typhus
R. sibirica	Russia, Central Asia, China	Tick typhus
R. australis	Australia	Tick typhus
R. felis	Americas, Europe, Australia	Flea-borne spotted fever
R. japonica	Japan	Japanese spotted fever
R. africae	South sub-Saharan Africa	Tick typhus
R. akari	USA, Russia, Central Asia	Rickettsialpox

Investigations

Diagnosis is confirmed serologically or by direct immunfluorescence detection of *R. rickettsii* antigen in the vascular endothelium of a skin biopsy.

Management

Without treatment mortality exceeds 20%. See Box 4.4.

Tick Typhus

(Syn. Mediterranean fever, Fievre boutonneuse, Kenya tick typhus, African and Indian tick typhus, Queensland tick typhus)
An acute febrile illness accompanied by an exanthema often preceded by a primary site of inoculation from a tick bite.

Epidemiology

See Table 4.2. The diagnosis is often not considered in returning travellers.

Pathophysiology

In many countries, tick typhus is caused by *R. conori*, transmitted by the bites ixodid ticks. Other rickettsiae such as *R. africae*, *R. siberica*, *R. felis* and *R. japonica* may also be implicated. The pathological changes follow the usual rickettsial pattern (see Epidemic typhus).

Box 4.4 Management of rickettsial infections

- Doxycycline is the drug of choice given in full dose for 7 days. Epidemic typhus and scrub typhus respond to a single 200 mg dose (100 mg for children).
- Alternative treatments: chloramphenicol is effective and recommended for Rocky Mountain spotted fever in pregnant women and children aged 8 years and under.
- General supportive measures are necessary in severe cases.
- With louse-borne disease (e.g. epidemic typhus, trench fever), isolation and effective delousing are necessary to control the spread of infection.

Clinical features

After an incubation period of 5 to 7 days, fever is accompanied by headache, malaise, joint and stomach pains and, sometimes, mental confusion. In 80% of cases, the onset of fever coincides with the development of a 2–5 mm ulcer (the tache noire) at the site of the tick bite with a black necrotic centre and a red areola. The regional lymph nodes are enlarged and tender. 3–4 days later, a pink maculopapular eruption develops first on the forearms and then generalises, involving the face, palms and soles. In severe cases may be haemorrhagic; rarely more severe reactions such as digital necrosis and pneumonia have been described.

Differential diagnosis

Viral haemorrhagic fevers, meningococcal septicaemia, other rickettsial infections.

Investigations

The diagnosis is confirmed serologically or by tissue-based PCR.

Management

See Box 4.4.

Rickettsialpox
Epidemiology

USA, Central Africa, Europe and Russia.

Pathophysiology

R. akari is a parasite of the house mouse, transmitted to humans by the mite *Allodermanyssus sanguineus.*

Clinical features

After an incubation period of 7–14 days, a papule appears at the site of the mite's bite, enlarges, becomes vesicular and dries to form a crust. The regional lymph nodes are enlarged. The patient often fails to notice the initial lesion. A few days later, influenza-like constitutional symptoms develop and persist for 4 or 5 days accompanied by a generalised eruption of papules surmounted by small vesicles, which crust and heal in a few days. The illness is usually mild and recovery is complete.

Differential diagnosis
Atypical varicella.

Investigations
Laboratory confirmation is by Western blot and PCR.

Management
See Box 4.4.

Scrub Typhus
Epidemiology
Far East and the South-West Pacific.

Pathogenesis
Orientia tsutsugamushi (previously *R. tsutsugamushi*), transmitted to humans from its rodent reservoir by the bites of the mites *Trombicula akamushi* and *T. deliensis*. The pathological changes are a focal vasculitis, involving the skin, lungs, heart, brain and kidneys.

Clinical features
After an incubation period of 6–21 days an acute fever with headache and conjunctivitis accompanies the primary lesion, more frequently seen in white people than in Asian people. The primary lesion, or eschar, is a firm papule up to 1 mm in diameter surmounted by a vesicle, which dries to form a black crust. The regional lymph nodes are enlarged and tender. After a week, a generalised macular or maculopapular eruption develops and may fade rapidly or persist for 7–10 days.

The clinical picture varies with the virulence of the strain. Pneumonitis and myocarditis are frequent; without treatment the mortality reaches 60%.

Investigations
Indirect immunofluorescence.

Management
See Box 4.4.

Epidemic typhus

Caused by *R. prowazeki* and transmitted by the human body louse.

Epidemiology
Occurs worldwide. Epidemics are associated with the displacement of populations by war or natural disasters. Humans are the only reservoir of infection.

Pathophysiology
Multiplication of rickettsiae in the endothelial cells of small blood vessels leads to obstruction, thrombosis, haemorrhage and perivascular inflammatory infiltration.

Clinical features
After an incubation period of 7–14 days the abrupt onset of fever, headache and malaise. Between the fourth and seventh days, a rash develops in over 80% of cases. Pink macules, 5 mm in diameter, appear first on the sides of the trunk and spread centrifugally, sparing the palms and soles. The face is usually flushed with intensely injected conjunctivae. During the second week, the rash becomes deeper red and often purpuric. The other clinical manifestations depend on involvement of the myocardium and the central nervous system. Gangrene of the fingers, toes, genitalia or nose may result from vascular obstruction. Untreated, up to 40% of cases are fatal.

Differential diagnosis
Viral haemorrhagic fevers, meningococcal septicaemia.

Management
See Box 4.4.

Brill–Zinsser disease

(Syn. Sporadic typhus)
This is the recrudescence of epidemic typhus, sometimes after as many as 40 years. Clinical features are milder and less often with a rash.

Murine typhus

(Syn. Endemic typhus)

Caused by *R. mooseri*, spread to humans from the rodent reservoir by the rat flea, *Xenopsylla cheopsis*. The incidence is highest in Central and South America. The clinical features parallel those of epidemic typhus but are much milder.

ACTINOMYCETE INFECTIONS

The actinomycetes are higher bacteria whose members cause two uncommon but important human infections: actinomycosis and nocardiosis.

Actinomycosis

A chronic suppurative and granulomatous disease.

Epidemiology

Higher incidence in rural tropical areas and in agricultural workers.

Pathophysiology

Caused primarily by *Actinomyces israelii*, a normal inhabitant of the human mouth. Trauma provides the portal of entry. Pathologically there is a suppurating fibrotic inflammatory process. Small abscesses and pus-filled sinus tracts are formed. The so-called sulphur granules are lobulated masses of intertwining filaments.

Clinical features

It can affect all organs and tissues of the body. In the skin, draining sinuses are formed through which the characteristic sulphur granules are discharged. Five main clinical types are recognised, depending on the primary site of infection: cervico-facial (lumpy jaw), thoracic, abdominal, primary cutaneous and pelvic.

Differential diagnosis

Tuberculosis, syphilitic gummata, appendicitis, osteomyelitis and liver abscess, and also lung, uterine and intestinal cancer.

Investigations

The diagnosis is established by identifying the granules in the pus and on histological examination and confirmed by culture.

Management

High-dose long-term penicillin and wide surgical excision of the infected tissue.

Nocardiosis

An acute-to-chronic suppurative disease caused by the aerobic actinomycete *Nocardia*.

Epidemiology

A rare sporadic infection. *Nocardia* is an opportunistic pathogen and is often found in immunosuppressed patients, including HIV/AIDS, those receiving anti-TNF antibodies and in solid-organ transplant recipients. Other predisposing factors include Cushing syndrome, diabetes and corticosteroids.

Pathophysiology

Nocardiosis is caused by the bacteria *N. asteroides*, *N. brasiliensis* and *N. otitidis caviarum*.

Clinical features

In systemic nocardiosis, the clinical picture may closely simulate pulmonary or meningeal tuberculosis. Spread to the skin and subcutaneous tissue produces solitary or multiple abscesses, which may involve the muscles and bones.

Direct infection of the skin may result in a solitary cold abscess or a local ulcer with a distal linear arrangement of multiple suppurative nodules, a lymphangitic form.

The prognosis of disseminated nocardiosis without treatment is poor, and even with treatment mortality is over 20%.

Investigations

Pus or sputum smears are examined after staining by Gram, methenamine silver and acid-fast techniques.

Management

All cases require antibiotic treatment with co-trimoxazole; sulphonamides are also active.

SEXUALLY TRANSMITTED BACTERIAL DISEASES

The global health burden of sexually transmitted infections (STIs) and HIV (Chapter 6) is large and increasing. Treatment and prevention of STIs are very cost-effective and the WHO has developed a global strategy for their control.

Syphilis

An infectious disease caused by the spirochaetal bacterium *Treponema pallidum* subsp. *pallidum*. The disease is usually acquired through sexual contact, with the exception of congenital syphilis where the infection occurs through transplacental transmission.

Epidemiology

An annual global incidence of about 10.6 million cases. Most infections occur in developing countries in heterosexual men and women. In developed countries diagnosis of infectious syphilis has increased particularly in men who have sex with men (MSM). This group is characterised by high rates of HIV co-infection and high-risk sexual behaviours.

Pathophysiology

The pathological changes in syphilis are the same in early and late disease. They occur in and around the blood vessels in the form of a perivascular infiltration of lymphocytes and plasma cells, accompanied by intimal proliferation in both the arteries and veins (endarteritis obliterans).

Clinical features

The clinical presentation of syphilis is diverse and may occur decades after the initial infection. Untreated, syphilis may pass through four stages: primary, secondary, latent and late. The first two stages are contagious. They seldom last more than 2 years and do not exceed 4 years. Latency may last from 5 to 50 years.

Incubation period: Most genital primary sores appear 3 weeks after exposure.

Primary syphilis: The primary chancre appears at the site of invasion. Lesions are papular but rapidly ulcerate. They may occur on any skin or mucous membrane surface and are

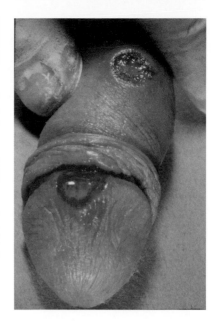

Figure 4.20 Primary syphilis showing chancres on the glans and shaft of the penis.

usually situated on the external genitalia; the anus and rectum in MSM. Unless secondarily infected, primary sores are not painful (Figure 4.20). Without treatment, the chancre heals spontaneously in 3–8 weeks. Regional lymph nodes are enlarged.

Secondary syphilis: The manifestations of generalised treponemal dissemination appear at around 8 weeks. Serological tests are always positive in immunocompetent persons. Rashes are the commonest feature, they are all symmetrical, coppery red and do not itch. The diverse features of secondary syphilis are discussed in Box 4.5. Most patients enter the latency stage within the first year of infection.

Latent syphilis: In latent syphilis there are no clinical stigmata of active disease, although disease remains detectable by positive serological tests. Sexual transmission is less likely in the absence of mucocutaneous lesions.

Tertiary syphilis: Late manifestations arise, often decades later, in about 25% of those who have latent syphilis. Screening for syphilis in blood donors and pregnant women and antibiotic use for unconnected reasons has greatly reduced late syphilis.

Box 4.5 Features of secondary syphilis

- *Constitutional symptoms*: Fever, headache, night-time bone and joint pains
- *Macular syphilide (roseolar rash) (Figure 4.21)*: Symmetrical, coppery red, non-scaly macules; fade to leave depigmented spots, leukoderma syphiliticum (Figure 4.22).
- *Papular syphilide (Figure 4.23)*: Scaly papular eruption. Psoriasiform papules of the palms and soles are especially common in black people (Figure 4.24).
  On the genitals, papules may be eroded or hyperkeratotic and coalesce (condylomata lata) (Figure 4.25). There is predilection for corners of the mouth, angles of the nose, the palms and soles and body folds such as beneath the breasts or in the axillae.
- *Pustular ulcerative syphilide*: Atypical facial plaques or ulcerated nodules; common with coexisting HIV infection.
- *Syphilitic alopecia*: Patchy 'moth-eaten' hair loss.
- *Nails*: Paronychia with secondary onychia.
- *Lesions of the mucous membranes*: Oral mucous patches, 'snail-track' ulcers (Figure 4.26).
- *Other systemic features*: generalised lymphadenopathy, panuveitis, headache, periostitis and joint effusions, glomerulonephritis, hepatitis, gastritis and myocarditis.

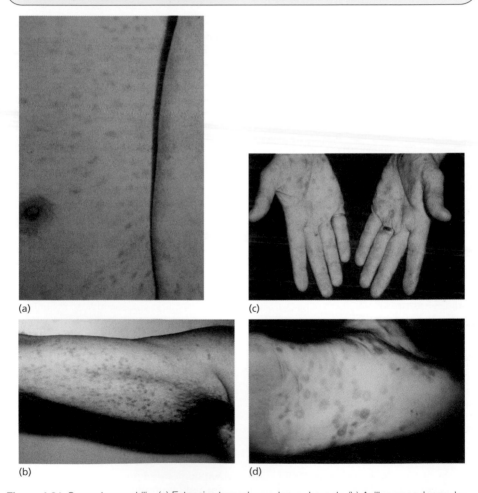

(a)

(b)

(c)

(d)

Figure 4.21 Secondary syphilis. (a) Extensive truncal maculopapular rash. (b) Axillary maculopapular lesions showing a classic coppery colour. (c) and (d) Acral papulosquamous lesions A.

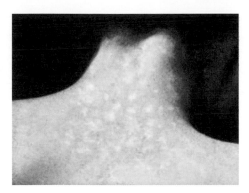

Figure 4.22 Syphilitic leukoderma showing depigmentation at sites of healed secondary lesions on the neck ('necklace of Venus') and upper back.

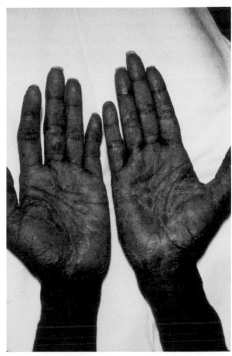

Figure 4.24 Secondary syphilis showing psoriasiform lesions of the palms.

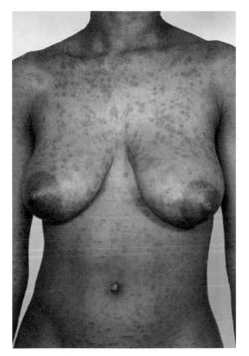

Figure 4.23 Secondary syphilis showing papular syphilides on the trunk.

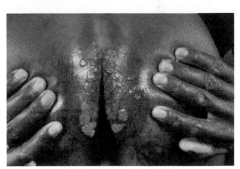

Figure 4.25 Condylomata lata of secondary syphilis: perianal.

Late skin syphilis appears in two types:

- *Nodular or tubercular syphilide*: The lesions are asymptomatic, firm, coppery red nodules (larger than 0.5 cm diameter) which appear in groups with a tendency to a circinate arrange-

ment. Finely wrinkled ('cigarette paper') central scarring is a feature.
- *Gummata*: The characteristic lesions of tertiary syphilis. Painless, cutaneous plaques or nodules with ulceration and peripheral healing with tissue-paper scarring. Lesions may also occur in the mouth (Figure 4.27).

Late syphilis has cardiovascular and neurological complications.

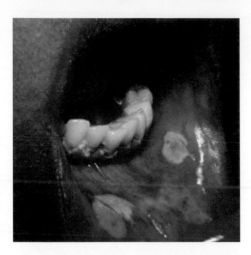

Figure 4.26 Oral lesions of secondary syphilis on the buccal mucosa.

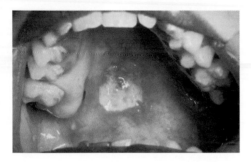

Figure 4.27 Mucosal lesions of tertiary syphilis: early gumma of the hard palate.

Differential diagnosis
Primary syphilis

- *Penile disease*: Genital herpes, chancroid, *Lymphogranuloma venereum* (LGV), granuloma inguinale, scabies, HPV infection, other stages of syphilis, lichen planus, lichen sclerosis, psoriasis, plasma cell balanitis, Behçet disease, fixed drug eruption, squamous carcinoma, Bowen disease.
- *Cervical disease*: Cervical ectopy or metaplasia, cervical cancer or cervical intraepithelial neoplasia.
- *Anal disease*: HPV infection, anal fissure, haemorrhoids, squamous carcinoma.
- *Oral*: Tonsillitis, Behçet syndrome.

Secondary syphilis
Genital herpes, seborrhoeic dermatitis, Behçet syndrome, drug eruptions, squamous carcinoma, scabies, pityriasis rosea, infectious mononucleosis, Stevens–Johnson syndrome, Bowen disease, HPV infection, psoriasis, angular cheilitis, Kaposi sarcoma, circinate balanitis (reactive arthritis), lichen planus, mycoses.

Tertiary syphilis
Lupus vulgaris, psoriasis, chronic venous ulcer, rosacea, mycosis fungoides, Bazin disease, lupus erythematosus, leukaemic infiltrations, neoplasia.

Investigations
Treponema pallidum can be identified from lesions of primary, secondary or early congenital syphilis by dark-field microscopy.

Serological testing remains the bedrock of screening, divided into non-treponemal tests and treponemal tests. There is no test that will differentiate one treponematosis from another. The sensitivity of the different tests varies according to the stage of the syphilis.

Guidelines for serological screening: Screening can be performed by either an enzyme immunoassay (EIA) or the combined Venereal Disease Research Laboratory/ *T. pallidum* haemagglutination assay (VDRL/ TPHA) test. Positive results are confirmed with a treponemal test of a different type.

Non-treponemal tests: Quantitative and useful in assessing treatment response. Reactivity develops 1–4 weeks after the primary chancre. Titres are highest in secondary syphilis. There are four tests available: VDRL, the unheated serum reagin (USR) test, the rapid plasma reagin (RPR) test and the toluidine red unheated serum test (TRUST).

Treponemal antigen tests: Used for confirmatory testing. Remain positive for life. Tests include treponemal EIA, *T. pallidum* particle agglutination assay (TPPA), TPHA and fluorescent antibody absorption (FTA-ABS).

Rapid point-of-care tests for syphilis: Fingerprick blood sample for targeted screening in resource poor areas.. Sensitivity 85–98% and specificity 93–98%.

Biological false positive reactions: All the tests can produce biologically false positive (BFP) results. Common associations with BFP are infections (e.g. malaria, leprosy, infectious mononucleosis), autoimmune disease and dysgammaglobulinaemias.

Management

Treatment is curative and should be given promptly to prevent long-term sequelae. Parenteral penicillin G is the preferred drug at all stages of syphilis; the preparations used, the dosage and the duration of treatment depend on the clinical stage and disease manifestations.

All patients with syphilis should be offered screening for other sexually transmitted infections and HIV.

Jarisch–Herxheimer reaction is an acute febrile reaction that occurs in many patients within 24 h of commencing treatment. Headache, myalgia, bone pains and an exacerbation of skin lesions may accompany the fever. It must be differentiated from penicillin allergy.

Follow-up for clinical and serological assessment should be done at 3, 6 and 12 months after the completion of treatment in early disease. Nontreponemal antibody test titres usually become negative after successful treatment. Attempts should be made to identify, trace and offer further investigation to at-risk sexual contacts.

Congenital syphilis

Transplacental passage of *Treponema pallidum* from an infected pregnant woman to her foetus or during delivery in the presence of maternal genital lesions. If untreated during pregnancy, syphilis can lead to fetal loss or stillbirth or, in a live born infant, neonatal death, prematurity, low birth weight and infant disorders such as deafness, neurological impairment and bone deformities. It is largely preventable by good prenatal care and timely penicillin treatment.

Gonorrhoea

A bacterial infection caused by *Neisseria gonorrhoeae* that causes purulent inflammation of the genital mucous membranes. It is primarily sexually transmitted but vertical transmission during childbirth is important. It is, after *Chlamydia* infection, the second most commonly reported bacterial STI in the UK and other developed countries.

Epidemiology

Estimated 106 million new cases each year worldwide, with a prevalence of 36 million. Rates of the disease and its complications are highest in Africa, Asia and Latin America.

The highest rates of infection occur in young people, especially teenage women and men in their early 20s. Two to three times more frequent in males, with one-third or more homosexually acquired. Those from black ethnic groups are disproportionately affected in the UK and the USA.

Pathophysiology

Caused by the Gram-negative, aerobic, intracellular diplococcus, *Neisseria gonorrhoeae*, which principally infects host columnar epithelium. Humans are the only natural host. Gonorrhoea has a high infectivity and is easily transmitted before symptoms appear.

Predisposing factors for disseminated infection are female, MSM, pregnancy, menstruation, systemic lupus erythematosus, complement deficiency, IV drug use and HIV infection.

Clinical features

Symptoms have their onset 1–5 days after sexual contact with an infectious person. Infection may be asymptomatic and diagnosed as a result of opportunistic testing or contact tracing.

Disseminated infection presents with a dermatitis–arthritis syndrome in a patient with mild fever. The skin lesions are small, tender and initially maculopapular; a central vesicle or pustule (Figure 4.28) appears followed by haemorrhage and necrosis. Lesions occur in crops of 5–40 and seen peripherally near affected joints. Joint or tendon pain is the most common accompanying feature with tenosynovitis of the hands and feet. It may be accompanied by a migratory polyarthralgia. One-third of cases will develop a suppurative arthritis, commonly of the knee. Rarely, pericarditis and

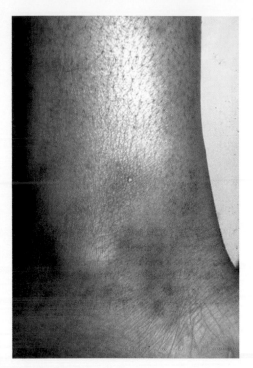

Figure 4.28 Disseminated gonococcal infection showing a pustule surrounded with erythema above the lateral malleolus.

endocarditis may occur at this later stage. Meningitis, similar to that caused by meningococci, but with a less rapid course, is rare but well recognised.

The common presentation in men is with acute urethritis with severe burning dysuria and a purulent discharge. Proctitis may be asymptomatic or present with rectal pain, tenesmus and discharge. Infection of the oropharynx may present with exudative pharyngitis and cervical lymphadenopathy, but is usually asymptomatic. The primary site of infection in women is the cervix, which may be asymptomatic or present with excessive vaginal discharge, dysuria, deep dyspareunia, postcoital bleeding and intermenstrual bleeding.

Complications may occur as a result of local abscess formation, from ascending infections and from haematogenous spread. Figure 4.29 shows the main sites of gonococcal infection. Ophthalmia neonatorum (gonococcal conjunctivitis) occurs in the first week after birth; prompt recognition and treatment are essential to prevent permanent visual damage.

Differential diagnosis
Of skin manifestations: genital herpes, folliculitis.

Investigations
A rapid presumptive diagnosis can be made on Gram stain. Confirmation is by culture of the organism and differentiation from other *Neisseria* species by antigenic or biochemical testing.

Nucleic acid amplification tests (NAATs) are more sensitive than culture but do not produce isolates that allow antimicrobial sensitivity.

Management
In the UK, first-line treatment for uncomplicated infection involves a single dosage regimen with a third-generation cephalosporin (ceftriaxone IM) and oral azithromycin. In complicated infections, more prolonged courses of treatment are employed. These will usually contain an agent effective against *Chlamydia trachomatis*, which often coexists with gonorrhoea.

Patients should be asked to abstain from sexual contact for 7 days after they and their partners have received treatment and their symptoms have resolved. A test of cure using a NAAT should be undertaken 2 weeks after the completion of treatment.

Genital *Chlamydia* infection

Genital *Chlamydia* infection is one of the most commonly reported STIs globally.

Epidemiology
In the UK in 2012 207 000 cases reported. The highest rates of infection are in under 25-year-olds.

Pathophysiology
Caused by *Chlamydia* D–K strain.

Clinical features
Asymptomatic infection occurs in up to 90% of women and more than 50% of men.

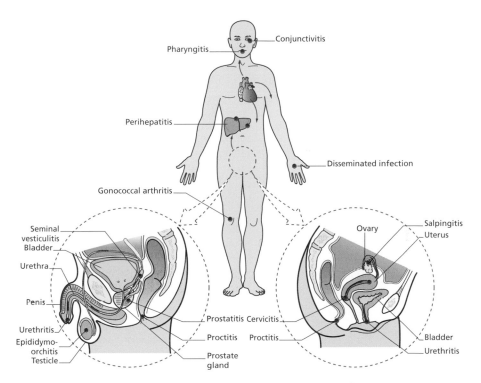

Figure 4.29 The main sites of gonococcal infection.

Chlamydia is strongly associated with reactive arthritis and is termed sexually acquired reactive arthritis (SARA), a seronegative, asymmetrical, spondyloarthropathy with or without:

- Mucocutaneous manifestations including circinate balanitis (Figure 4.30), erosions affecting the buccal and rectal mucosa and keratoderma blenorrhagica (Figure 4.31).
- Iritis and conjunctivitis.

Differential diagnosis
Of skin includes lichen planus, psoriasis, eczema.

Investigations
NAATs are now the only recommended diagnostic test for chlamydia; sensitivity is >90%. NAATs will not differentiate between LGV and non-LGV types, and genotyping should be undertaken. A first-void urine is the sample of choice in men; in females a self-taken vaginal swab or an endocervical swab. In MSM and commercial sex workers, pharyngeal and rectal

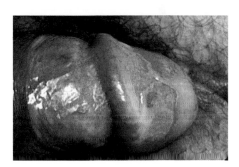

Figure 4.30 Circinate balanitis in Chlamydia infection.

testing may also be indicated. Conjunctival sampling when indicated.

Management
Treatment is indicated if chlamydia is diagnosed or there is a history of contact with an infected person. Patients should be asked to abstain from sexual contact for 7 days after they and their partners have received treatment and their symptoms have resolved.

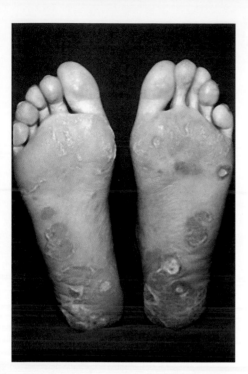

Figure 4.31 Keratodermablenorrhagica sexually acquired reactive arthritis.

In uncomplicated infection, single-dose azithromycin is the treatment of choice, including in pregnancy. In complicated infections, more prolonged courses of treatment are required.

Lymphogranuloma venereum

Lymphogranuloma venereum (LGV) LGV is a sexually transmitted infection caused by the obligate intracellular bacterium *Chlamydia trachomatis*.

Epidemiology
Classic disease is usually acquired heterosexually and prevalent in tropical countries of Africa, Asia, the Caribbean and Central and South America. Prior to 2003 it was rare in industrialised countries, but since then it has re-emerged as a significant disease in MSM. Many are HIV-infected men who also have a high rate of hepatitis C co-infection. Most present with a proctitis syndrome rather than the classic bubonic form.

Pathophysiology
The organism spreads from the site of the initial lesion to the regional lymph nodes. The main pathological process is a thrombolymphangitis and perilymphangitis. Multiple necrotic foci appear within the lymph nodes, which enlarge and coalesce to form stellate abscesses. Fibrosis causes disruption of the lymph node architecture, leading to chronic oedema and induration.

Clinical features
LGV occurs in three stages, as shown in Table 4.3.

Differential diagnosis
Patients presenting with genital ulceration (e.g. genital herpes, primary syphilis or chancroid), inguinal lymphadenopathy or proctitis (e.g. inflammatory bowel disease, enteric infections, other STIs such as gonorrhoea, syphilis, herpes simplex, *C. trachomatis* serovars D–K, human papillomavirus and, in patients who are HIV positive, cytomegalovirus infection).

Investigations
Detection of *C. trachomatis* nucleic acid using NAATs and confirmation by real-time PCR assays for LGV-specific DNA.

Management
There should be detailed investigation to exclude other STIs. Early treatment is important to prevent the chronic phase. Prolonged courses of antibiotics (at least 3 weeks) are required, doxycycline is first line, erythromycin is an alternative. Fluctuant buboes may require aspiration through healthy adjacent skin; surgical incision is usually contraindicated due to risk of complications such as sinus formation. Partner notification should be undertaken.

Chancroid

(Syn. Ducreyi disease)
An acute ulcerative condition affecting the anogenital region often associated with visible lymphadenitis (buboes). The disease has generated renewed interest because of its capacity to facilitate HIV transmission and the organism's resistance to antimicrobial drugs.

Table 4.3 Stages of lymphogranuloma venereum

Stage	Incubation period	Clinical features
Primary	3–30 days	Small papule/pustule/ulcer at the site of inoculation which heals spontaneously with no scarring (Figure 4.32)
		Haemorrhagic proctitis may occur in those engaging in anal intercourse
Secondary	Days to weeks	Lymphatic involvement of nodes that drain the primary lesion
		Classic form: tender unilateral or bilateral inguinal and/or femoral adenopathy ('groove' sign)
		If primary infection is in the rectum the deep iliac lymph nodes are affected but remain unnoticed. This can also occur in women due to drainage of the cervical or upper vaginal area to the perirectal lymph nodes
		The lymph nodes may coalesce to form a 'bubo' or abscesses may rupture spontaneously with the development of fistulae or sinus tracts
		There may be systemic features such as malaise and fever
Tertiary	Years after chronic untreated infection	Chronic granulomatous inflammatory process with lymphatic obstruction, leading to fistula formation, strictures and disfiguring conditions such as genital elephantiasis and esthiomene, which refers to hypertrophic enlargement with ulceration of the external genitalia

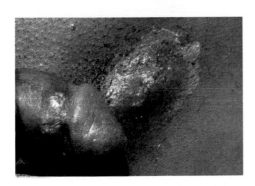

Figure 4.32 Primary stage of lymphogranuloma venereum, showing genital ulceration.

Epidemiology

Found in the developing world where migrant labour is common and in commercial sex workers. Sporadic outbreaks due to infections acquired abroad are occasionally reported in Europe and North America. It is more commonly seen in uncircumcised males.

Pathophysiology

The causative organism is *Haemophilus ducreyi,* a Gram-negative facultative anaerobic coccobacillus. Trauma or microabrasion to the skin or mucosa allows for penetration of the organism into the epidermis.

Clinical features

The incubation period is between 3 and 10 days. There may be a history of recent sexual exposure with someone from an endemic area. Chancroid is characterised by painful anogenital ulceration (Figure 4.33) and lymphadenitis with progression to bubo formation (Figure 4.34). Autoinoculation from the primary ulcer may lead to the development of multiple or kissing ulcers on opposing skin surfaces.

In HIV-infected patients with more advanced immunosuppression, chancroidal lesions may be more persistent, slower to heal, more numerous and fail to respond to single-dose treatment regimens.

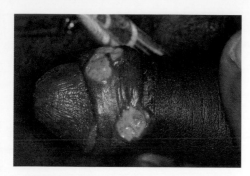

Figure 4.33 Chancroidal penile ulceration. (Source: Courtesy of Dr D. Lewis.)

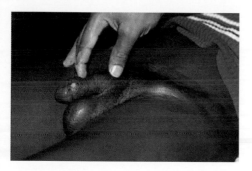

Figure 4.34 Penile chancroid with inguinal bubo.

Differential diagnosis
Syphilis and herpes simplex.

Investigations
PCR should be requested. Genital ulcer disease often has a mixed aetiology so tests for other genital pathogens are essential.

Management
Prompt antibiotic treatment is essential to reduce the risk of complications as well as the risk of acquisition and onward transmission of HIV. Partner notification should be undertaken.

Single-dose treatment with either ciprofloxacin or azithromycin or ceftriaxone. HIV seropositivity is associated with treatment failure and azithromycin should be avoided in co-infected patients. Fluctuant buboes should be aspirated.

Granuloma inguinale

(Syn. Donovanosis)
A genital ulcerative condition found in endemic foci in certain tropical countries.

Epidemiology
The prevalence of granuloma inguinale has decreased markedly in recent times. Usually affects sexually active adults between the ages of 20 and 40 years. It is a risk factor for the acquisition of HIV.

Pathophysiology
The causative organism is *Calymmatobacterium granulomatis*, a Gram-negative coccobacillus. Infection is associated with poor hygienic conditions.

Clinical features
Four types of lesions have been described:

- Ulcerogranulomatous: the most common type with beefy red ulcers that bleed when touched (Figure 4.35).
- Hypertrophic: usually with a raised irregular edge (Figure 4.36).
- Necrotic: offensive smelling ulcer causing tissue destruction.
- Sclerotic or cicatricial: with fibrous or scar tissue.

Lesions commonly occur on the coronal sulcus or inner aspect of the penile prepuce in uncircumcised men, on the anus in MSM and the labia or introitus in females (Figure 4.35). HIV augments continuation of the lesions with persistent ulcers for prolonged periods.

Differential diagnosis
Syphilis, chancroid, chronic herpes simplex, lymphogranuloma venereum (which may co-exist), genital amoebiasis, cutaneous tuberculosis, Crohn disease and genital cancers.

Investigations
The diagnosis is generally made by microscopic identification of Donovan bodies. Specimens may be obtained from pinched-off tissue fragments taken directly from the lesion or from biopsy specimens. HIV test.

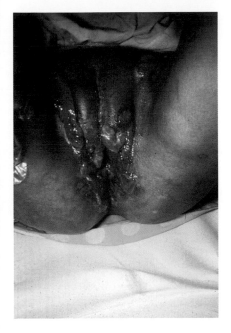

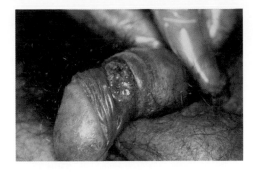

Figure 4.36 Granuloma inguinale with a hypertrophic lesion.

Management

Azithromycin for at least 3 weeks until all lesions have healed; alternative antibiotics include doxycycline, erythromycin, ciprofloxacin and co-trimoxazole. Patients should be thoroughly investigated for accompanying STIs with partner notification.

Figure 4.35 Granuloma inguinale with beefy red granulomata in a female patient.

5

Mycobacterial infections

Mycobacteria are a large group of bacteria producing mould-like pellicles when grown on liquid media. The most important Mycobacteria causing invasion in the skin are infections with *Mycobacterium tuberculosis*, *M. leprae* and atypical (non-tuberculous) mycobacteria. An estimated one-third of the world's population have latent *M. tuberculosis* infection. Immunosuppression caused by HIV infection greatly increases the risk of developing clinical disease. Cutaneous tuberculosis comprises a wide clinical spectrum and presentation is dependent on the route of infection (endogenous or exogenous), the immune status of the patient and whether or not there has been previous sensitisation with tuberculosis.

The diagnosis of skin tuberculosis may be suggested by clinical features and typical histological findings but the only absolute criterium is the demonstration of *M. tuberculosis* in either tissue culture from skin biopsy or cytological smear, or the demonstration of mycobacterial DNA by polymerase chain reaction. Ziehl–Neelsen stain or auramine are used to visualise mycobacteria in specimens. It is not possible to distinguish between different species of mycobacteria using microscopy. The optimal culture temperature for non-tuberculosis mycobacteria is 30°C and for *M. tuberculosis* it is 35°C. Polymerase chain reaction is used for Mycobacterium species identification.

Treatment

General measures

In the UK, all patients with tuberculosis must be notified as this is a statutory requirement and initiates contact tracing if appropriate. It is vital to

Confirm the diagnosis bacteriologically whenever possible and to obtain drug susceptibilities. Tuberculosis, pulmonary or extrapulmonary, is an AIDS-defining illness. HIV testing should be carried out.

Drug therapy

Standard recommended regimen is 6 months of treatment with four first-line drugs: a combination of rifampicin, isoniazid, ethambutol and pyrazinamide. The excision of small lesions of lupus vulgaris or warty tuberculosis, if diagnosed early, may be effective. Surgery may be helpful in scrofuloderma.

CUTANEOUS TUBERCULOSIS

Lupus vulgaris

A chronic, progressive, paucibacillary form of cutaneous tuberculosis, occurring in a previously sensitised individual with a high degree of immunity to tuberculin.

Epidemiology
One of the most prevalent forms of cutaneous tuberculosis; F > M.

Pathophysiology
Originates from an underlying focus of tuberculosis, typically in a bone, joint or lymph node, either by contiguous extension of the disease from underlying affected tissue or haematogenous/lymphatic spread. Can occur at the site of a previous BCG vaccination. Causative organisms are *M. tuberculosis*, *M. bovis* and Bacille Calmette–Guérin (BCG).

Rook's Dermatology Handbook, First Edition. Edited by Christopher E. M. Griffiths, Tanya O. Bleiker, Daniel Creamer, John R. Ingram and Rosalind C. Simpson.
© 2022 John Wiley & Sons Ltd. Published 2022 by John Wiley & Sons Ltd.

Clinical features

The characteristic lesion is a slowly enlarging solitary plaque (Figure 5.1) composed of soft, reddish brown papules, the appearance on diascopy being said to resemble apple jelly. Clinical variants include tumour-like (Figure 5.2), ulcerative, vegetative and papulonodular forms. Sporotrichoid-like spread can occur. The nasal, buccal or conjunctival mucosa may become involved. Nasal lesions can lead to cartilage destruction. Stenosis of the larynx and scarring deformities of the soft palate can also occur. Complications include scarring, contractures, tissue destruction and malignant change (0.5–10% of longstanding lesions).

Differential diagnosis

Leprosy (nodules are firmer) and sarcoidosis (nodules resemble grains of sand rather than 'apple jelly'). Early lesions may be mistaken for lymphocytoma, Spitz naevus, lupus erythematosus (Figure 5.3) or lupoid form of leishmaniasis.

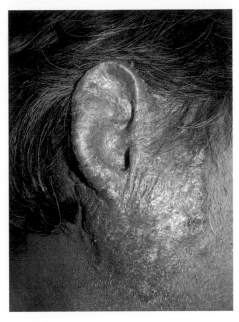

Figure 5.2 Tumour-like form of lupus vulgaris on the ear lobe and face. (Source: Courtesy of Dr V. Ramesh, SJ Hospital and VM Medical College, New Delhi, India, and the Editor of *Paediatric Dermatology*.)

Investigations

Skin biopsy, but paucibacillary so acid-fast bacilli are usually negative. Tissue culture may be helpful. Tuberculin test is usually positive.

Management

Standard multidrug antituberculosis therapy.

Primary inoculation tuberculosis

(Syn. tuberculous chancre)

Inoculation of *M. tuberculosis* into the skin of an individual without natural or artificially acquired immunity leads to a tuberculous chancre.

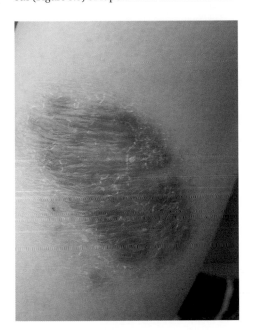

Figure 5.1 Plaque of lupus vulgaris measuring 50 × 30 mm at the site of a previous BCG vaccination. (Source: Courtesy of Dr S.L. Walker, Faculty of Infectious and Tropical Diseases, London School of Hygiene and Tropical Medicine, London, UK, and the Editor of *Clinical and Experimental Dermatology*.)

Epidemiology

An uncommon form of skin tuberculosis that frequently affects children, especially those who have not received BCG vaccination. Also occurs in at-risk occupations, e.g. healthcare workers. Risk factors are overcrowding and low socio-economic status.

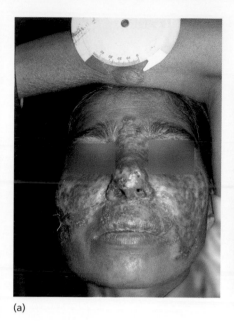
(a)

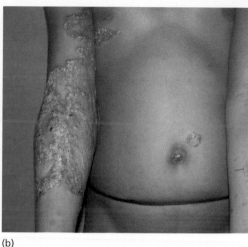
(b)

Figure 5.3 Lupus vulgaris. (a) Lesions of the face resembling discoid lupus erythematosis. Note the strong tuberculin reaction. (b) Lupus vulgaris showing typical central atrophy and a serpiginous edge. (Source: Courtesy of Dr V. Ramesh, SJ Hospital and VM Medical College, New Delhi, India, and the Editor of *Paediatric Dermatology*.)

Lupus vulgaris (Figure 5.1) may develop at the site of inoculation.

Pathophysiology

Causative organisms are *M. tuberculosis, M. bovis* and BCG. The bacillus enters the skin through abrasions and minor injuries, usually on the face or limbs of children.

Histology initially shows acute neutrophilic inflammation with necrosis occurring in both skin and affected lymph nodes. Numerous bacilli are present. After 3–6 weeks the infiltrate becomes granulomatous and caseation appears, coinciding with the disappearance of the bacilli.

Clinical features

A painless, nonhealing ulcer or lesion with localised lymphadenopathy, particularly in children. Lesions are commonest on the face, hands and lower extremities. Initial lesions may be a brownish papule, nodule or ulcer with an undermined edge and a granular haemorrhagic base. 'Apple jelly' nodules may be present on on diascopy. Regional lymphadenopathy develops after 4–8 weeks.

Differential diagnosis

Oother mycobacteria (e.g. *M. marinum*), Buruli ulcers, actinomycosis, cutaneous leishmaniasis and malignancies, sporotrichosis, cat scratch disease, tularaemia.

Investigations

Biopsy of skin and/or lymph nodes. Acid-fast bacilli are seen.

Management

Treatment as per local guidelines. If untreated the chancre will heal slowly over many months. Lupus vulgaris or tuberculosis verrucosa cutis may develop at the site of the original lesion. Occasionally leads to disseminated tuberculosis.

Scrofuloderma

A result of direct invasion of tubercle bacillus into the skin from an underlying contiguous tuberculous focus.

Epidemiology

The commonest form of cutaneous tuberculosis worldwide. Most common in children and young adults.

Pathophysiology

Caused by *M. tuberculosis* usually from a lymph gland, an infected bone or joint, lacrimal gland or duct, breast or testes, which invades overlying skin (Figure 5.4). Histology shows an ulcerated dermal abscess with an ill-defined histiocytic component. Caseating necrosis may be present in deeper structures.

Clinical features

Usually asymptomatic swelling or ulcer or discharging sinus. Bluish red, subcutaneous swellings persist for several months; They break down to form undermined ulceration Fistulae may be present. Extensive ulcerative lesions, particularly on the scalp, may give rise to diagnostic difficulties.

Differential diagnosis

Non-tuberculous mycobacterial infection, *M. avium* complex, lymphadenitis and *M. scrofulaceum* need to be excluded by culture. Other differential diagnoses include sporotrichosis, actinomycosis, syphilitic gummata, hidradenitis suppurativa, melioidosis and bacterial abscess.

Investigations

Skin biopsy from the edge of the sinus or ulcer. Cytology smears from fine-needle aspirations are very useful in a low resource setting and can be used as a first-line investigation.

Management

Spontaneous healing can occur, but the course is very protracted and leaves typical cord-like scars. Antituberculous therapy should be commenced promptly.

Warty tuberculosis

(Syn. Tuberculosis verrucosa cutis)
An indolent, warty, plaque-like form of tuberculosis.

Epidemiology

Incidence variable, commonest in Asia.

Pathophysiology

Exogenous inoculation of *M. tuberculosis* into the skin through open wounds or abrasions in previously sensitised individuals. There are usually few organisms in the lesion (paucibacillary).

Clinical features

Usually a slowly enlarging lesion, may be undiagnosed for many years. Asymptomatic, small, indurated, warty papule which extends to form a verrucose plaque. May have an atrophic centre or may go on to cause a massive, infiltrated, papillomatous plaque (Figure 5.5). Demonstrates sporotrichoid spread (Figure 5.6). There is a destructive form which causes limb deformity. Active disease of other organs may coexist, e.g. bone, tuberculous lymphadenitis or pulmonary tuberculosis.

Differential diagnosis

Viral warts, actinic keratosis (hands), blastomycosis, chromoblastomycosis, actinomycosis, tertiary syphilis, hypertrophic lichen planus.

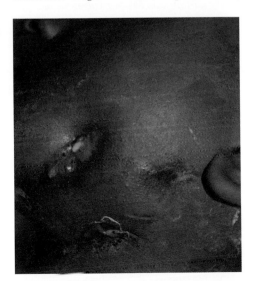

Figure 5.4 Scrofuloderma involving the cervical glands.

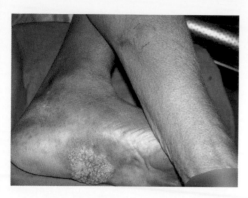

Figure 5.5 Warty tuberculosis with strong tuberculin reactions. (Source: Courtesy of Dr V. Ramesh, SJ Hospital and VM Medical College, New Delhi, India, and the Editor of *Paediatric Dermatology*.)

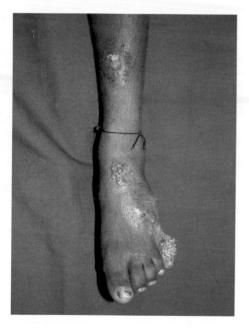

Figure 5.6 Sporotrichoid spread of warty tuberculosis. (Source: Courtesy of Dr V. Ramesh, SJ Hospital and VM Medical College, New Delhi, India, and the Editor of *Dermatologic Clinics*.)

Investigations
Biopsy and/or tissue culture. Assess involvement of other organs.

Management
Follow appropriate guidelines for management of tuberculosis. The condition responds to antituberculosis treatment; without it, extension is usually extremely slow and lesions may remain virtually inactive for months or years. Spontaneous remission may occur and usually results in atrophic scars.

RARER VARIANTS OF CUTANEOUS TUBERCULOSIS

Orificial Tuberculosis

(Syn. Tuberculosis cutis orificialis)
A rare variant of tuberculous infection causing painful ulcerated lesions of the mucosa or the skin adjoining orifices. Caused by autoinoculation of *M. tuberculosis* from internal affected sites; associated with advanced internal tuberculosis. Usually affects middle-aged and elderly males. The most commonly affected area is the oral mucosa, especially the tongue.

Acute Cutaneous Miliary Tuberculosis
Haematogenous spread of tubercle bacilli into the skin seen in advanced pulmonary or meningeal and disseminated tuberculosis. This is a rare variant that usually affects infants/children. Crops of minute bluish papules, vesicles, pustules or haemorrhagic lesions occur in a patient who is obviously ill. Poor prognosis.

Metastatic Tuberculous Abscess

(Syn. Tuberculous gumma)
Disseminated haematogenous spread of mycobacteria causing subcutaneous nodules which may become fluctuant or break down to form ulcers. There is no involvement of underlying tissue. Occurs in malnourished children and immunodeficient adults. Associated with underlying lymphoma and systemic immunosuppressive agents. Presents as either as a firm, subcutaneous nodule(s) or as a nontender, fluctuant abscess (Figure 5.7).

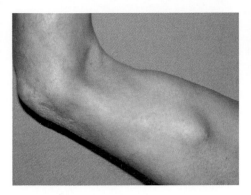

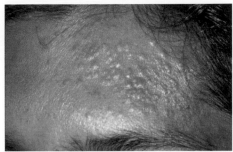

Figure 5.8 Lichen scrofulosorum on the forehead. (Source: Courtesy of Dr Yogesh S. Marfatia, Department of Skin-VD, Medical College and SSG Hospital, Vadodara, Gujarat, India, and the Editor of the *Indian Dermatology Online Journal*.)

Figure 5.7 Tuberculous gumma (metastatic tuberculous abscess) in a patient with a pleural effusion. (Source: Courtesy of Dr V. Ramesh, SJ Hospital and VM Medical College, New Delhi, India, and the Editor of *Paediatric Dermatology*.)

TUBERCULIDS

Cutaneous hypersensitivity reactions to haematogenous dissemination of *M. tuberculosis*. Diagnostic criteria include tuberculoid histology on skin biopsy, a strongly positive Mantoux reaction, the absence of *M. tuberculosis* in the smear and negative culture and resolution of the skin lesions with antituberculous therapy.

Tuberculid classification:

1. *Micropapular*: lichen scrofulosorum.
2. *Papular*: papulonecrotic tuberculid.
3. *Nodular*: erythema induratum of Bazin or nodular tuberculid.

Lichen scrofulosorum

(Syn. Tuberculosis cutis lichenoides)

A rare tuberculid occuring in children and adolescents. It presents as a lichenoid eruption of minute papules occurring predominantly in children and adolescents with active tuberculosis. It is usually associated with a strongly positive tuberculin reaction.

Epidemiology

Rare in Europe, highest incidence is in the Indian subcontinent and sub-Saharan Africa. Commonest in children and adolescents. In one large series from India, 84% of patients were less than 15 years of age.

Pathophysiology

Probably a type III hypersensitivity reaction to a haematogenous spread of mycobacteria from an active internal site of infection. Histology shows superficial periadnexal granulomas without caseation. Epithelioid cells, lymphocytes and occasional giant cells are seen. Mycobacteria are not seen and cannot be cultured from biopsy material.

Clinical features

Lesions are usually subtle and asymptomatic. Skin-coloured 0.5–3.0 mm diameter, closely grouped, lichenoid papules are seen (Figure 5.8). May coalesce into confluent plaques. Lichenoid, psoriasisform and granuloma annulare-like variants have been described.

Differential diagnosis

Lichen nitidus, keratosis spinulosa, keratosis pilaris, papular or lichenoid sarcoidosis, secondary syphilis and drug eruptions.

Investigations

A high index of suspicion is necessary for diagnosis as the lesions may be subtle. Screen for focus of tuberculosis elsewhere. Tuberculin reaction is strongly positive. Mycobacteria are not seen/cultured in a skin biopsy.

Management

Follow the appropriate current guidelines for the treatment of tuberculosis of other organs. Lesions usually clear within 4 weeks and heal without scarring.

Papulonecrotic tuberculid

(Syn. Tuberculosis papulonecrotica)

Epidemiology
Accounts for approximately 4% of patients with cutaneous tuberculosis. Highest incidence in the Indian subcontinent and sub-Saharan Africa. Mainly affects children and young adults.

Pathophysiology
As for the other tuberculids, mainly occurs in patients infected with *M. tuberculosis* but can occur after BCG vaccination. Histology shows sub-acute lymphohistiocytic vasculitis causing thrombosis and destruction of small dermal vessels. These changes lead to a wedge-shaped infarct-like lesion with a large central zone of coagulation necrosis surrounded by inflammation.

Clinical features
Asymptomatic clusters of small, inflammatory, erythematous papules progress to become pustular/necrotic and evolve into discrete crusted ulcers (Figure 5.9). Symmetrical. Heal with varioliform scarring. New crops may continue over months or years. Usually affects ears, acral parts of the limbs and extensor surfaces of the joints. Perniotic areas may be favoured.

Differential diagnosis
Pityriasis lichenoides, leukocytoclastic vasculitis, nodular prurigo.

Investigations
Lesional biopsy and tuberculin testing should be carried out. Screen for an underlying focus of tuberculosis.

Management
Follow the appropriate current guidelines for treatment of tuberculosis of other organs. Lesions clear in 3–4 weeks.

Erythema induratum of Bazin

A tuberculosis-associated panniculitis. See Chapter 51 for full information.

Other nodular tuberculids

Erythema Nodosum
See Chapter 51.

Nodular Vasculitis
Clinically and histologically indistinguishable from erythema induratum, although the lesions do not usually ulcerate.

Tuberculous Mastitis
A cause of granulomatous mastitis. Can be clinically and radiologically indistinguishable from breast cancer. Unilateral ulcerative plaques, nodules, abscesses and sinuses on the breast of young females.

NON-TUBERCULOUS (ATYPICAL) MYCOBACTERIA

Nontuberculous mycobacteria are environmental organisms residing in soil and water. They cause disease much more frequently in the immunocompromised.

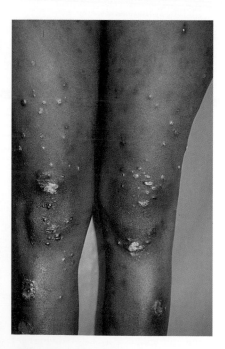

Figure 5.9 Papulonecrotic tuberculid of the legs. (Source: Courtesy of Professor J. Aboobaker, University of Natal, Durban, South Africa.)

M. marinum infection

(Syn. Swimming pool granuloma, fish tank granuloma)
Causes disease in many fish species. Human infection follows contact with fish or contaminated water.

Epidemiology
Occupational or recreational exposure to salt or fresh water has occurred in the majority of cases.

Pathophysiology
M. marinum's natural habitat is fresh or salt water, particularly enclosures of water that are not often replenished, e.g. swimming pools and aquariums or heated water in temperate climates. Vectors include fresh- or saltwater fish, snails, shellfish, dolphins and water fleas. *M. marinum* is probably only pathogenic on abraded skin. Incubation period following inoculation is 2–3 weeks but may be considerably longer.

Early lesions show nonspecific inflammation, while older lesions show well-formed tuberculoid granulomas with fibrinoid masses rather than caseation. Intracellular acid-fast bacilli are only found in approximately 10%.

Clinical features
The commonest presentation is a nodule on the hand or upper limb that may demonstrate sporotrichoid spread (Figure 5.10). Spread of infection to deeper structures occurs in up to a third of patients. Regional lymph glands may be enlarged, but never break down.

Differential diagnosis
Leishmaniasis and sporotrichosis in endemic areas, other atypical mycobacterial infections.

Investigations
A positive culture can be obtained in up to 80% of cases if the organism is grown between 30 and 33°C. Alert the microbiologist to the suspicion of *M. marinum* (or non-tuberculous mycobacterial infection) so that specimens are cultured appropriately as the temperature is lower than that of *M. tuberculosis*.

Management
No randomised trial evidence, therapy should be based upon culture results. Most experts recommend treatment with two active agents for 1–2 months after the resolution of symptoms; clarithromycin and ethambutol are frequently used. Add rifampin if osteomyelitis or other deep structure infection. Public health authorities should be notified when a public source of infection is identified.

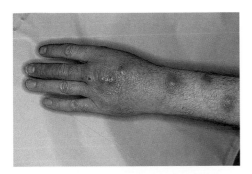

Figure 5.10 *M. marinum* infection showing sporotrichoid spread from the hand to the forearm in an aquarist. (Source: Courtesy of Dr I.H. Coulson, Burnley General Hospital, Burnley, UK.)

Other atypical mycobacterial infections

M. kansasii
A pulmonary pathogen, usually causing a tuberculosis-like illness in patients with underlying pulmonary disease such as chronic obstructive pulmonary disease and cystic fibrosis. Tap water is the major reservoir of infection. Skin lesions include papules, nodules and verrucous plaques, sometimes in a sporotricoid pattern and sometimes also cellulitis and abscesses.

M. ulcerans

(Syn. Buruli ulcer (Uganda), Bairnsdale/ Searls ulcer (Australia), Kasongo (Democratic Republic of Congo))
A slow-growing, environmental *Mycobacterium* that affects the skin and subcutaneous tissues.

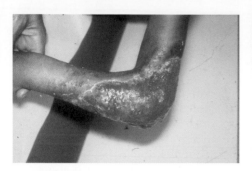

Figure 5.11 Extensive *M. ulcerans* of the elbow in a child. (Source: Courtesy of Dr P.L.A. Niemel, Surinam.)

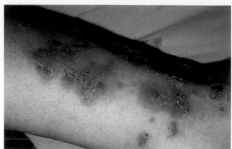

Figure 5.12 *M. abscessus* infection causing abscesses. (Source: Courtesy of Dr A.G. Smith, North Staffordshire Hospital, Stoke-on-Trent, UK, and the Editor of the *British Journal of Dermatology*.)

Most common in rural tropical wetlands, especially areas with stagnant water. Children (5–15 years old) have the highest incidence. Transmission is through minor skin trauma that permits inoculation of *M. ulcerans*. There is a latent period of around 4 months. *M. ulcerans* proliferates and produces a toxin which causes local apoptosis and necrosis, and suppresseses host immune responses. Skin lesions begin as nodules and then develop into large, indolent ulcers with undermined edges usually on the arm or leg. Satellite lesions may develop and surrounding induration can occur (Figure 5.11). Treatment is with rifampicin plus streptomycin for 8 weeks (WHO recommendation).

M. avium complex (M. avium and M. intracellulare)

The commonest cause of cervical lymphadenitis in children. *M. avium* and *M. intracellulare* found in tap water, soil, dairy products, animals and house dust. Infection occurs in immmnocompromised individuals or immunocompetent hosts with predisposing lung conditions, such as pneumoconiosis, silicosis and cystic fibrosis. Skin involvement occurs following traumatic skin inoculation in cervical lymphadenitis or dissemination from primary visceral lesions. Clinical features are variable and include multiple ulcers, nodules abscesses and plaques resembling lepromatous leprosy or lupus vulgaris. Treatment is with surgical excision of the affected nodes and/or excision of localised skin lesions in conjunction with a macrolide + ethambutol.

M. haemophilum

An increasingly recognised pathogen in immunocompromised patients. Erythematous or violaceous papules and nodules that enlarge to become painful abscesses or ulcers; occasionally presents as annular plaques or panniculitis. Lesions usually situated over joints. Systemic features are common. No standardised guidelines. Usually treat with multiple antibiotics for 12–24 months.

M. szulgai

Fast-growing mycobacteria that are very common in the environment. Includes the *M. abscessus* group, *M. chelonae*, *M. fortuitum* group and *M. smegmatis* infection. These organismas are widely distrubuted in the environment, they are found in soil and water and may be commensal organisms of human skin. In the immunocompetent host, a traumatic injury (including tattooing and surgical procedures) is followed by the development of localised abscess formation (Figure 5.12). In the immunocompromised individual disseminated disease, with multiple subcutaneous nodular lesions, can occur without history of trauma. Skin biopsy and culture are required to guide therapy.

Leprosy

(Syn. Hansen's disease)

A chronic granulomatous disease with a long incubation period caused by *M. leprae*, mainly affecting peripheral nerves and skin.

Epidemiology

About 4 million people have, or are disabled by, leprosy. 86% of cases are in India, Brazil, Indonesia, Nigeria, Ethiopia and Bangladesh. Peak incidence is in the teens and early 20s.

Pathophysiology

Living in an endemic area, age, sex and household contact predispose to acquiring leprosy. Haematogenous spread of bacilli occurs to cool, superficial sites, including eyes, upper respiratory mucosa, testes, small muscles and bones of hands, feet, face, peripheral nerves and skin.

Clinical expression of leprosy is due to the type of host immune response elicited by the organism. *Lepromatous* and *tuberculoid* leprosy represent the extreme ends ('poles', also known as 'polar leprosy') of immune response. Between these 'poles' are a spectrum of borderline patients. Types of leprosy are:

- *Lepromatous leprosy* (LL) represents a failure of cell mediated immunity specifically towards *M. leprae* with resultant bacillary multiplication, spread and accumulation of antigen in infected tissues.
- *Tuberculoid leprosy* (TT) is a result of strongly expressed cell-mediated immunity. The infection is therefore restricted to one or a few skin sites and peripheral nerves.
- *Borderline patients* (borderline tuberculoid, BT; borderline borderline, BB; borderline lepromatous, BL) are immunologically unstable and may upgrade towards the tuberculoid end or downgrade towards the lepromatous end of the spectrum.

Lepra reactions are immune-mediated reactions that occur in patients with leprosy:

- Type 1 (reversal) reactions are delayed hypersensitivity reactions caused by increased recognition of *M. leprae* antigens in skin and nerve sites. These occur in patients with borderline disease and are common following commencement of therapy.
- Type 2 reactions occur in BL and LL patients. These reactions are due in part to immune complex deposition. The most common manifestation is erythema nodosum leprosum (ENL).

Nerve damage occurs in skin lesions and in peripheral nerve trunks causing anaesthesia, muscular weakness/contracture and autonomic dysfunction. These permit trauma, bruising, burns, cuts and, especially, tissue necrosis from prolonged, inappropriate or repetitive trauma, which in turn lead to ulceration, secondary cellulitis and osteomyelitis and loss of tissue, so that deformity is added to disability. Histology shows small nerve fibre loss, with segmental demyelination and remyelination. Different forms of leprosy show different types of histological features with compact epithelioid granulomas in tuberculoid leprosy and diffuse foamy macrophages in the lepromatous spectrum.

Nasal discharges from untreated LL patients (often undiagnosed for several years) are the main source of infection in the community.

Clinical features

Early lesions and presenting symptoms

The commonest early lesion is an area of numbness on the skin, or a visible skin lesion. The classic early skin lesion is 'indeterminate' leprosy, which is usually found on the face, extensor surface of the limbs, buttocks or trunk (Figure 5.13).

Established leprosy (see Table 5.1)

Patients frequently present with signs of nerve damage; weakness or anaesthesia due to a peripheral nerve lesion.

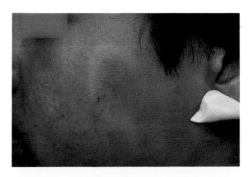

Figure 5.13 Indeterminate leprosy: early skin lesions. Face of a Nepali child showing vague hypopigmented patch with some central healing. Note the mark of a recent slit-skin smear.

Table 5.1 Characteristics of lesions of polar leprosy

	Tuberculoid leprosy	Lepromatous leprosy
Number of lesions	1–10	Hundreds, confluent
Distribution	Asymmetrical, anywhere	Symmetrical, avoiding 'spared' areas
Definition and clarity	Erythematous, copper coloured or purple, well defined edges, flattened and hypopigmented centre (Figure 5.14)	Vague edge, slight hypopigmentation (Figure 5.15)
Anaesthesia	Early, marked, defined, localised to skin lesions or major peripheral nerve	Late, initially slight, ill-defined, but extensive, over 'cool' areas of body
Autonomic loss	Early in skin and nerve lesions	Late, extensive as for anaesthesia
Nerve enlargement	Marked, in a few nerves	Slight but widespread
Mucosal and systemic	Absent	Common, severe during type 2 reactions
Number of *M. leprae*	Not detectable	Numerous in all affected tissues

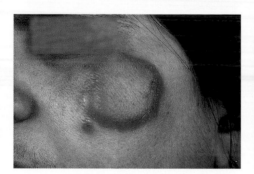

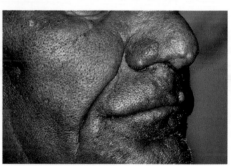

Figure 5.14 Tuberculoid leprosy. Face of Pakistani woman showing erythematous plaque with a well-defined active edge and a small satellite lesion. On the face, such lesions may not be anaesthetic.

Figure 5.16 Lepromatous leprosy. Face of a man showing diffuse infiltration of the skin and appearance of nodules on the nose and lip.

Late changes of LL

Leonine facies (Figure 5.16), eyebrows/eyelash thinning, misshapen nose, hoarse voice, ichthyotic legs, 'glove and stocking' anaesthesia.

Borderline leprosy

Skin lesions represent stages on a clinical spectrum between the two polar types. Towards the tuberculoid end of the spectrum, lesions are fewer and drier, and have fewer bacilli in smears and biopsies, and vice versa towards the lepromatous pole.

Lucio leprosy presents with thickened smooth skin like scleroderma while histoid leprosy presents with well-defined widespread cutaneous nodules.

Figure 5.15 Lepromatous leprosy (borderline lepromatous/lepromatous). Back of a Bangladeshi boy showing numerous, often confluent hypopigmented macules, with relative sparing of the midline.

Type 1 reactions

Clinical features are acute neuritis and/or acutely inflamed skin lesions (Figure 5.17).

Type 2 reactions

ENL presents as painful red nodules develop on the face and extensor surfaces (Figure 5.18). Fever and malaise are common and may be associated with systemic involvement including uveitis, dactylitis, arthritis, neuritis, lymphadenitis, myositis and orchitis. Peripheral nerve neuritis and uveitis are the most serious complication of type 2 reactions.

The Lucio reaction is a potentially fatal deep cutaneous vasculitis causing infarction with painful ulcers.

Differential diagnosis

Macular lesions

Vitiligo, hypopigmented eczema, pityriasis alba in children, pityriasis versicolor is not always scaly, tinea corporis.

Plaques/annular lesions

Ringworm, granuloma multiforme, sarcoidosis and cutaneous tuberculosis.

Nodules

Cutaneous leishmaniasis.

Investigations

Diagnosis requires two out of three of:

- Anaesthesia of a skin lesion, or in the distribution of a peripheral nerve, or over dorsal surfaces of hands and feet.
- Thickened nerves.
- Typical skin lesions.

Alternatively, the demonstration of acid-fast bacilli in slit-skin smears, or the typical histology on skin and nerve biopsies can make the diagnosis.

Management

See World Health Organization guidance on multidrug therapy for leprosy.

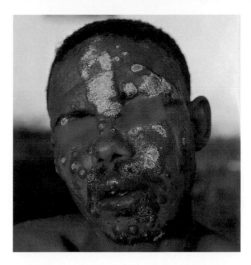

Figure 5.17 Type 1 reaction: borderline leprosy in an Ethiopian man. Existing lesions become acutely inflamed, scale and threaten ulceration. Many small new lesions have appeared.

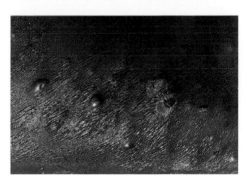

Figure 5.18 Type 2 reaction in lepromatous leprosy in a Nigerian man: erythema nodosum leprosum. Several of the reaction nodules have broken down, releasing pus.

The principles of treating reactions are controlling acute inflammation, easing pain and reversing nerve and eye damage. Multidrug therapy must be continued. For neuritis and inflamed lesions a tapering course of oral prednisolone is given. Erythema nodosum leprosum requires high-dose steroids.

6

HIV and the skin

Human immunodeficiency virus (HIV) infection is acquired sexually, from blood or blood products, or vertically from an infected mother during pregnancy, birth or breastfeeding. The virus infects immunocompetent cells, including CD4+ T cells and macrophages. It creates variable patterns of disease, but all are characterised by evolving, sometimes fulminant, immunodysfunction affecting many systems of the body. AIDS (acquired immune deficiency syndrome) is a term used for the most advanced stages of HIV infection.

Epidemiology

AIDS was first described as a distinct clinical entity in 1981. HIV-1 infection now represents a global pandemic. Of AIDS cases, 95% occur in non-industrialised countries and 75% in sub-Saharan Africa. HIV infection in children is increasing.

Pathophysiology

HIV is a single-stranded RNA virus. Two main types of HIV infect humans: HIV-1 and HIV-2. Worldwide, HIV-1 is the commonest cause of AIDS. HIV-2, found predominantly in West Africa, causes immune deficiency and AIDS more slowly than HIV-1 and is less infectious. The immunosuppressive nature of HIV infection is due to infection and destruction of CD4+ T cells with loss of cell-mediated immunity. This results in increased susceptibility to opportunistic infections and certain cancers.

Clinical features

HIV disease should be viewed as a continuum including primary infection, symptomatic infection, early symptomatic state (previously known as AIDS-related complex), late symptomatic disease and advanced disease.

Acute primary HIV infection may be clinically silent but up to 90% of patients develop a non-specific, symptomatic illness 1–6 weeks after exposure that usually lasts less than 2 weeks. Symptoms and signs are those of a non-specific viral infection with lassitude, fever, arthralgia, myalgia and lymphadenopathy. Weight loss, nausea, vomiting and diarrhoea are common. 75% have a rash which may be exanthematous, urticarial, erythema multiforme or a toxic erythema. Other dermatological manifestations include orogenital ulceration, acute genito-crural intertrigo and oro-pharyngeal candidosis.

Differential diagnosis

Toxic erythema, urticaria, erythema multiforme, orogenital ulceration, pityriasis rosea, guttate psoriasis, Still disease, infections (e.g. Epstein–Barr virus).

Investigations

HIV diagnosis can be established through a variety of tests detecting the presence of HIV in the serum, saliva or urine. These tests detect antibodies, viral antigens or viral RNA. CD4+ T-cell counts is often associated with viral load testing to measure the progression of HIV.

Management

The care of patients with HIV should be by a clinician with appropriate expertise and training and follow local/national guidance. Treatment includes HIV prevention and antiretroviral treatment (ART).

Rook's Dermatology Handbook, First Edition. Edited by Christopher E. M. Griffiths, Tanya O. Bleiker, Daniel Creamer, John R. Ingram and Rosalind C. Simpson.
© 2022 John Wiley & Sons Ltd. Published 2022 by John Wiley & Sons Ltd.

ART and subsequent immune restoration may reactivate the host response to latent infections or unmask autoimmune diseases in genetically susceptible individuals, the immune reconstitution inflammatory syndrome (IRIS). Other terms include immune restoration disease (IRD) and immune reconstitution associated disease (IRAD). Half of all IRIS events are dermatological, including infections (e.g. herpes simplex virus [Figure 6.5], varicella zoster virus, candidosis, atypical mycobacterium), inflammatory reactions (e.g. lupus erythematosus, sarcoidosis, oral ulceration, seborrheic dermatitis, eosinophilic folliculitis) and tumours (e.g. Kaposi sarcoma).

DERMATOLOGICAL MANIFESTATIONS OF HIV INFECTION

Skin disease may provide the first suspicion of the diagnosis of HIV infection, cause significant morbidity as the disease progresses or point to a diagnosis with important systemic implications. The number of mucocutaneous diseases, like the CD4+ T-cell count, is a prognostic indicator of the development of AIDS and overall survival.

The commonest dermatological conditions associated with HIV infection are listed in Box 6.1.

Seborrhoeic dermatitis

Patients with HIV commonly develop seborrheic dermatitis, severity is increased when CD4+ T cell $<100 \times 10^6$/L. Itchy, scaly patches are found at the classic sites for seborrhoeic dermatitis (Figure 6.1) and elsewhere.

Eosinophilic folliculitis

An HIV-specific disorder related to Ofuji disease. It occurs at CD4+ T-cell counts of 250–300 $\times 10^6$/L, identifying patients at immediate risk of developing opportunistic infections, and can present during the immune reconstitution syndrome.

> **Box 6.1 Common dermatological conditions in HIV infection**
>
> - Pruritus/xerosis/ichthyosis
> - Nodular prurigo
> - Folliculitis
> - Eosinophilic folliculitis
> - Pruritic papular eruption
> - Seborrhoeic dermatitis
> - Psoriasis (often florid or atypical)
> - Granuloma annulare
> - Drug eruptions
> - Herpes simplex
> - Herpes zoster
> - Viral warts
> - Mollusca
> - Oral and vaginal candidosis
> - Tinea (including onychomycosis)
> - Scabies
> - Basal cell carcinoma
> - Squamous cell carcinoma
> - Kaposi sarcoma
>
> Source: Data from Bunker CB, Male Genital Skin Disease. London: Saunders, 2004.

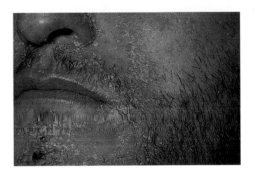

Figure 6.1 Seborrhoeic dermatitis on the face. (Source: Courtesy of Medical Illustration UK Ltd, Chelsea and Westminster Hospital, London, UK.)

There is clinical and histological overlap with the pruritic papular eruption (PPE) of HIV and bacterial, seborrhoeic or acneiform folliculitis. Eosinophilic folliculitis presents as a centripetal (face and trunk) eruption of pruritic, erythematous, perifollicular papules and pustules (Figure 6.2). Histology can be characteristic, with degranulating eosinophils and mast cells in a perifollicular distribution. There may be a

Figure 6.2 Eosinophilic folliculitis: excoriated papules on the trunk. (Source: Courtesy of Medical Illustration UK Ltd, Chelsea and Westminster Hospital, London, UK.)

peripheral eosinophilia and elevated levels of IgE. Swabs are negative as the lesions are sterile. The disease has virtually disappeared in the developed world with the introduction of ART, although immune reconstitution exacerbations can occur. Treatment can be difficult; phototherapy can be successful.

Pruritic papular eruption

A common cutaneous manifestation of HIV, the prevalence varying between 10% and 60% depending on geographical area. It is common in Africa and Asia. Insect bite hypersensitivity, as in papular urticaria, is the likely pathomechanism. PPE is a sign of an advanced degree of immunosuppression and may be the first sign of HIV, occurring at CD4+ T-cell counts $<100–200 \times 10^6$/L.

It presents as excoriated, erythematous, urticarial papules associated with eosinophilia and elevated IgE. Phototherapy may be helpful.

Drug reactions

Drug reactions are a common challenge in HIV dermatology. A morbilliform toxic erythema is the usual reaction seen (with fever, arthralgia, abnormal liver function tests and eosinophilia), but all forms of drug reactions are encountered.

All protease inhibitors and some nucleoside reverse transcriptase inhibitors (NRTIs) cause lipodystrophy. Protease inhibitors develop retinoid-like side effects of paronychia, periungual

pyogenic granuloma-like lesions, xerosis and cheilitis and curly hair.

Infections

There should be a high index of suspicion and a low threshold for performing microbiological investigations and skin biopsies.

Bacterial infections (see Chapter 4)
Staphylococcus aureus (including MRSA), *Pseudomonas* species, *Escherichia coli* and *Streptococcus pyogenes* are the commonest isolates. Clinical differentiation of folliculitis between staphylococcal folliculitis, *Malassezia* folliculitis, dermatophyte folliculitis, eosinophilic folliculitis, demodex folliculitis and acne vulgaris or rosacea may be challenging, and these entities may coexist.

Bacillary angiomatosis is caused by *Bartonella* infection and presents with purple, popular and nodular vascular lesions resembling Kaposi sarcoma (KS) (Figure 6.3).

Syphilis may present atypically in HIV infection, and serological tests may be false negative. Dermatologists should regard all genital, perianal and oral ulceration and any papulosquamous eruption with suspicion and investigate appropriately.

Reinfection with, or reactivation of, *Mycobacterium tuberculosis* occurs early in HIV infection, and extrapulmonary, including cutaneous, tuberculosis is common.

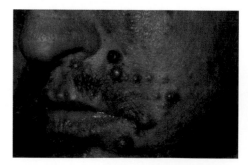

Figure 6.3 Bacillary angiomatosis: purple nodules on the face. (Source: Courtesy of Medical Illustration UK Ltd, Chelsea and Westminster Hospital, London, UK.)

Viral infections (see Chapter 3)

Herpes simplex: HSV-2 causes severe, chronic, ulcerative, perianal disease (Figure 6.4). Although anogenital involvement is frequent, any site can be affected with acute lesions that are vesicobullous which become chronic, eroded and crusted, vegetative or ulcerating. HSV infection may not be self-limiting, as it is in normal individuals. HSV as a manifestation of IRIS can present with chronic erosive disease, which may be difficult to diagnose (Figure 6.5).

Varicella-zoster virus (VZV) reactivation frequently occurs and can be severe. Intractable post-herpetic neuralgia may require specialised pain control. Disseminated VZV infection can be severe with a poor prognosis.

Cytomegalovirus: Reactivation of CMV occurs with a CD4+ count below $50\times 10^6/L$. Skin involvement with CMV is relatively uncommon in HIV, but when it occurs the mortality is 85% at 6 months. Purpura, papules, nodules, verrucous plaques, painful ulcers (Figure 6.6) and nodular prurigo (Figure 6.7) have been described.

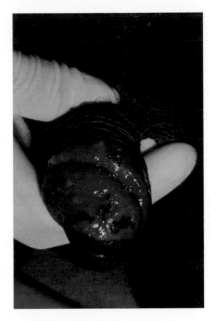

Figure 6.5 Herpes simplex immune restoration disease: chronic erosions on the penis. (Source: Courtesy of Medical Illustration UK Ltd, Chelsea and Westminster Hospital, London, UK.)

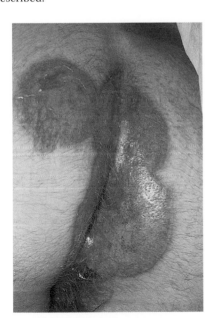

Figure 6.4 Chronic perianal ulceration in herpes simplex infection before the era of highly active antiretroviral therapy.

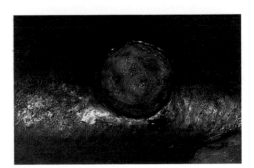

Figure 6.6 Cytomegalovirus vasculitis: leg ulcers. (Source: Courtesy of Medical Illustration UK Ltd, Chelsea and Westminster Hospital, London, UK.)

Human papillomavirus: Around 40% of men who have sex with men (MSM) diagnosed with HIV may have genital warts at presentation, they may be extensive, numerous and exuberant. Human papillomavirus 6 (HPV-6) and HPV-11 are most frequently found. Anal cancer is 50 times and penis cancer 5–6 times commoner in HIV. A pattern resembling the rare, inherited condition,

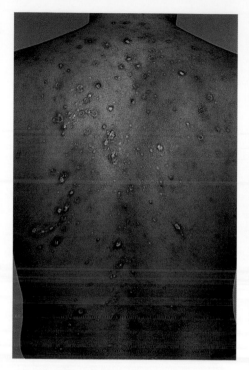

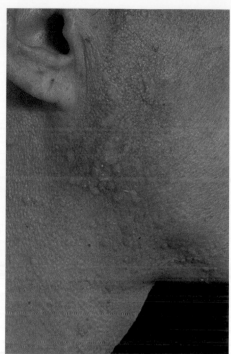

Figure 6.7 Cytomegalovirus infection: nodular prurigo-like eruption on the back. (Source: Courtesy of Medical Illustration UK Ltd, Chelsea and Westminster Hospital, London, UK.)

Figure 6.8 Epidermodysplasia verruciformis in human papillomavirus infection: discrete and confluent warty papules on the right cheek and neck. (Source: Courtesy of Imperial College School of Medicine, London, UK.)

epidermodysplasia verruciformis, can occur (Figure 6.8), presenting in some patients as a pityriasis versicolor-like eruption.

Mollusca frequently affect the skin of patients with HIV, particularly homosexual seropositive patients. Lesions may lack the characteristic central umbilication.

Fungal infections (see Chapter 7)
Candidosis: Oral candidosis has classically been associated with immunosuppressive states and is commoner in homosexual seropositive patients than intravenous drug users.

Histoplasmosis: In endemic areas, such as North, Central and Latin America, Africa, India or the Far East, 20–50% of patients with AIDS will develop histoplasmosis at CD4+

counts below 200×10^6/L. The systemic presentation can mimic tuberculosis. A spectrum of lesions is seen: macules, papules, plaques, crusted/eroded/ulcerated papules and plaques mainly located on the face and chest, as well as oral involvement with erosions and ulcers.

Cryptococcosis: Cryptococcus neoformans infection affects 5–10% of patients with AIDS in the UK and USA and 30–40% in Africa. The brain, lung and skin are sites of predilection. Up to 20% of patients with disseminated disease may have skin involvement. In HIV/AIDS, cryptococcal skin involvement should be suspected when papulonodular necrotising skin lesions with central umbilication are encountered in the context of neurological or pulmonary disease (Figure 6.9).

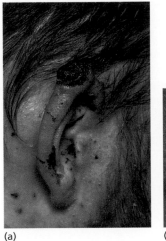
(a)

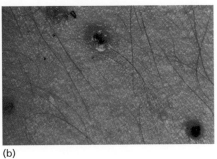
(b)

Figure 6.9 Cryptococcosis. (a) Necrotising papules and nodules on the right ear and neck. (b) Close up of necrotising papules. (Source: Courtesy of Medical Illustration UK Ltd, Chelsea and Westminster Hospital, London, UK.)

Other fungal infections: Penicilliosis causes fever, lymphadenopathy, hepatosplenomegaly, skin lesions (Figure 6.10) and anaemia. *Malassaezia* species may cause a folliculitis and pityriasis versicolor may be more extensive in HIV.

Miscellaneous infections

Scabies (Chapter 9) occurs frequently in HIV-infected patients and may have unusual clinical features (Figure 6.11), often involving the head and neck. Norwegian/crusted scabies should arouse suspicion of underlying HIV infection.

Demodex can cause a pruritic, papulonodular follicular eruption of the face, neck and torso.

AIDS-related Kaposi sarcoma (Chapter 77)

Kaposi sarcoma (KS) KS is caused by infection with HHV-8 (KS herpesvirus). It is probably transmitted sexually more by the faecal–oral route or ejaculate than by blood, in HIV-positive MSM. It occurs mainly in patients with low CD4+ counts and high viral loads. Cutaneous

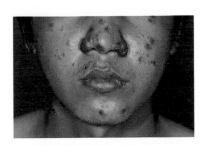
Figure 6.10 Penicilliosis (Source: Courtesy of Professor Vesarat Wessagowit, Bangkok, Thailand.)

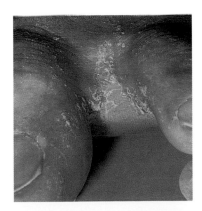
Figure 6.11 Norwegian scabies: interdigital scale.

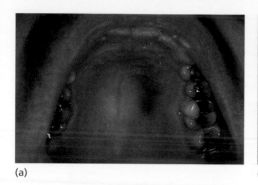
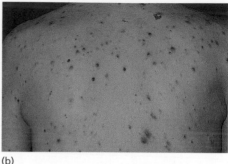

(a)   (b)

Figure 6.12 Kaposi sarcoma. (a) Purple nodules on the palate. (b) Multiple purple nodules and plaques on the back. (Source: Courtesy of Medical Illustration UK Ltd, Chelsea and Westminster Hospital, London, UK.)

KS is multicentric and often involves the face, oral mucosa, palate (Figure 6.12a) and genitalia. Lesions may be multiple (Figure 6.12b), follow skin creases and may be grouped or linear and koebnerize. The classic lesion in HIV is a purple patch, plaque or nodule, which may ulcerate. A high index of suspicion and skin biopsy is important. ART is very effective for early stage KS.

Other cutaneous malignancies

HIV/AIDS patients have a 2–5-fold increased risk of developing keratinocyte cancer. Melanoma is probably more common. Sun exposure is possibly more important in the causation than immunosuppression. HPV has a role in anogenital and oral cancer, epidermoplasia verruciformis and nail unit squamous cell carcinoma (SCC).

SCC may present atypically, at a younger age, at unusual sites (e.g. the digit and nail fold), be multifocal and be aggressive with a high risk of recurrence, metastasis and a high mortality. Basal cell carcinoma (BCC) presents at a younger age, may be multiple and eruptive and is commonly of the superficial type. Melanoma may present atypically and behave more aggressively with decreased disease-free and overall survival rates. Low CD4+ counts indicate a poorer prognosis.

Castleman disease is a rare HIV-associated atypical cutaneous lymphoproliferative disorder (ACLD) presenting as an itchy, generalised eruption (patches, plaques, erythroderma). It is a rare condition clinically suggestive of mycosis fungoides or Sézary syndrome. A polyclonal CD8+ T-cell infiltrate on biopsy is seen: the condition usually responds to ART.

Hair abnormalities

Abnormalities of the hair associated with HIV include patchy and diffuse alopecia/telogen effluvium, fine hair, eyelash trichomegaly (marker of advanced HIV infection), alopecia areata and universalis.

Nail abnormalities

Up to 70% of HIV-infected individuals can have nail changes. Grey nails and distal banded nails are associated with low CD4+ counts of <200 × 10^6/L. Paronychia and ingrown toenails are particular complications of indinavir.

Other findings include clubbing, half and half nails, transverse (Beau) lines, longitudinal ridging, loss of the lunula, leukonychia, blue nails, longitudinal melanonychia, yellow nail syndrome, periungual erythema, onycholysis, onychoschizia and onychomycosis (*Trichophyton rubrum*).

Oral abnormalities

HIV patients should have their oral cavity examined regularly. Smoking and alcohol ingestion contribute to the morbidity. Oral hyperpigmentation is a sign of low CD4+ counts ($<200 \times 10^6$/L). Distressing mouth ulceration occurs frequently.

Hairy leukoplakia is a clinical entity that has emerged during the HIV epidemic and is probably associated with Epstein–Barr virus infection. It is particularly important because it is an early specific sign of HIV infection and is usually asymptomatic (Figure 6.13).

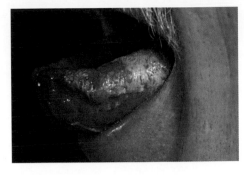

Figure 6.13 Hairy leukoplakia. (Source: Courtesy of Media Resources UCL Trust, London, UK.)

7

Fungal infections

Fungi are broadly divided into two basic forms: moulds and yeasts (Table 7.1). Drug doses are standard unless detailed in the text.

Table 7.1 Morphology and diseases caused by the two main forms of fungi: yeasts and moulds

Features	Yeasts	Moulds	Dimorphic fungi
Physical forms	Single-celled organisms that usually reproduce by budding	Multicellular fungi that often have complex life cycles and forms and produce different types of conidia (spores)	Fungi that can exist as either moulds or yeast or yeast-like forms The mould form seen at environmental temperature and the yeast or yeast-like form associated with human body temperature
Examples of diseases associated with these forms	*Candida*: candidosis, including superficial oral or cutaneous disease and systemic candidosis *Malassezia*: pityriasis versicolor, seborrhoeic dermatitis, *Malassezia* folliculitis *Cryptococcus*: cryptococcosis; including cryptococcal meningitis	*Aspergillus*: aspergillosis; dermatophytes (including *Trichophyton, Microsporum, Epidermophyton*); dermatophytosis of skin, hair and nail Mucoraceous moulds (including *Mucor, Rhizopus, Lichtheimia*); causes of mucormycosis	*Histoplasma*: histoplasmosis *Coccidioides*: coccidioidomycosis *Blastomyces*: blastomycosis

Rook's Dermatology Handbook, First Edition. Edited by Christopher E. M. Griffiths, Tanya O. Bleiker, Daniel Creamer, John R. Ingram and Rosalind C. Simpson.
© 2022 John Wiley & Sons Ltd. Published 2022 by John Wiley & Sons Ltd.

SUPERFICIAL MYCOSES

Fungal infections of the skin and mucosal surface.

SKIN DISEASE CAUSED BY *MALASSEZIA* SPECIES

Pityriasis versicolor

A mild, chronic infection of the skin caused by *Malassezia* yeasts.

Epidemiology
Rare in childhood; more common in the late teens, with a peak in the early 20s. More common in tropical climates. A positive family history among relations and conjugal cases also occur.

Pathophysiology
The normal flora of the skin includes a number of yeasts in the genus *Malassezia*. colonisation is especially dense in the scalp, the upper trunk and flexures; areas rich in sebaceous glands. Pityriasis versicolor in most cases represents a shift in the relationship between the host and the resident yeast flora. The causative organism is usually *M. globosa* and possibly *M. sympodialis* and *M. furfur*. Factors contributing to the change are probably multiple.

Clinical features
Patchy change of skin colour sometimes with mild irritation. Lesions are sharply demarcated macules, sometimes erythematous with fine scaling (Figure 7.1), often becoming confluent.

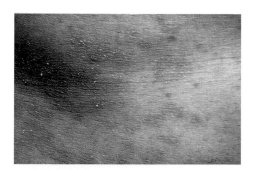

Figure 7.1 Pityriasis versicolor showing typical fine scaling.

Predominantly over the upper trunk with spread to the upper arms, neck and abdomen. Scaling may be emphasised by firm scraping or stretching of the skin.

In untanned white skin, the affected areas are darker than normal and fail to respond to light exposure; in the suntanned subject, the abnormal skin is commonly paler, as in black people. After resolution, depigmentation may remain for many months without any scaling.

Differential diagnosis
Vitiligo, pityriasis rosea and secondary syphilis.

Investigations
Under Wood's light the scaly lesions may show pale yellow fluorescence. Light microscopy shows coarse mycelium, together with spherical, thick-walled yeasts has been likened to 'spaghetti and meatballs' or 'bananas and grapes'.

Management
Relapse is common, whatever the primary treatment. Patients should be warned that repigmentation may take several months.
First line: Topical azoles, terbinafine 1% cream, ketoconazole shampoo, 2.5% selenium shampoo.
Second line: Oral itraconazole.

Malassezia folliculitis

(Syn. Pityrosporum folliculitis)
A clinically distinct form of folliculitis on the back and upper trunk associated with *Malassezia* yeasts.

Epidemiology
Teenagers or young adult males. Often reported following a sunny holiday or in patients who are acutely ill such as in an intensive care unit.

Pathophysiology
Biopsies show clusters of yeasts within follicles surrounded by inflammatory cells.

Clinical features
Itchy papules and pustules scattered on the shoulders and back. The itching and distribution distinguish them from acne vulgaris.

Management

Responds well to oral itraconazole and less well to ketoconazole shampoo.

DERMATOPHYTOSIS

Dermatophytes are related fungi causing skin changes of the type known as ringworm or dermatophytosis. The traditional division of ringworm is according to the site of the body (Box 7.1). The ringworm species are all moulds belonging to three asexual genera: *Microsporum*, *Trichophyton* and *Epidermophyton*.

Box 7.1 Ringworm syndromes

- Tinea corporis
- Tinea capitis
- Tinea barbae
- Tinea faciei
- Tinea pedis
- Tinea manuum
- Tinea cruris
- Onychomycosis caused by dermatophytes
- Steroid-related tinea
- Dermatophytide reactions

Investigation relies on the collection of adequate material (Chapter 1) which is then examined by direct microscopy, culture and molecular techniques such as polymerase chain reaction (PCR) analysis.

Tinea corporis

(Syn. Tinea circinate)
Ringworm of the body skin.

Epidemiology

Commoner in the tropics.

Pathophysiology

The most common are *Trichophyton. rubrum* and *Microsporum canis*. The source of infection is an active lesion on an animal or human; fomite transmission can occur.

Clinical features

Lesions occur on the trunk and limbs, excluding specialised sites such as the scalp, feet and groin. Lesions are single or multiple annular plaques, usually sharply marginated with a raised edge and often with central clearing (Figure 7.2); they may coalesce. The degree of inflammation is variable depending on the species of the fungus, the host immune status and extent of follicular invasion. Pustules or vesicles may dominate in inflammatory lesions. In less inflammatory infections, scaling is common.

T. verrucosum from cattle, *T. erinacei* from hedgehogs, *T. mentagrophytes* from small rodents and *M. persicolor* from voles are all likely to cause inflammatory lesions of exposed skin.

T. rubrum can be extensive and the inflammatory margin difficult to distinguish. Typical lesions on the legs extend from the feet with raised margins and perifollicular granulomatous papules. Tinea cruris may extend onto the buttocks and lower back, as well as more distant sites of the trunk.

Differential diagnosis

Psoriasis, discoid eczema, lichen simplex, seborrheic dermatitis, pityriasis rosea (herald patch), candidosis and pityriasis versicolor.

Management

Localised disease: topical terbinafine *or* azole.
Widespread disease:
First line: Oral terbinafine *or* itraconazole.
Second line: Griseofulvin 1 g/day for 4 weeks.

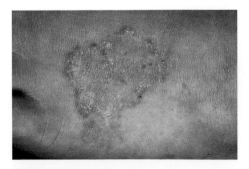

Figure 7.2 Tinea corporis: characteristic ringworm lesions.

Tinea capitis

Ringworm of the scalp.

Epidemiology
Predominantly an infection of children, although adult cases are seen, particularly with *T. tonsurans* infections. *T. tonsurans* show a predilection for African/Caribbean hair type.

Pathophysiology
Most species of dermatophyte are capable of invading hair but some species (e.g. *T. tonsurans, T. schoenleinii* and *T. violaceum*) have a distinct predilection for the hair shaft. *E. floccosum, T. concentricum* and *T. interdigitale* are exceptional in never causing tinea capitis. There are several distinct types of hair invasion:

- *Ectothrix type*: Hyphae inside the hair and a sheath of spores outside the hair. *M. audouinii, M. canis, M. equinum* or *M. ferrugineum*. Fluorescence under the Wood's light is characteristically present.
- *Endothrix type*: Fungus confined to the inside of a hair. *T tonsurans, T. soudanense, T. violaceum, T. yaoundei, T. gourvilii* or *T. rubrum* (rare). Hair is especially fragile and breaks off close to the scalp surface. This type is non-fluorescent.
- *Favus*: Caused by *T. schoenleinii*. It is now seen rarely and sporadically in countries such as South Africa and Ethiopia, where it is still endemic.

Clinical features
The clinical appearance is variable, depending on the type of hair invasion, the level of host resistance and the degree of inflammatory host response. In all types, the cardinal features are partial hair loss with inflammation of some degree, itching is variable. There are several basic clinical pictures.

Ectothrix type: In *M. audouinii* and *M. ferrugineum* infections, there are patches of partial alopecia with numerous dull grey broken-off hairs, fine scale, a well-defined margin and minimal inflammation. There may

be several random patches. In *M. canis* the picture is similar but there is typically more inflammatory change (Figure 7.3). Green fluorescence under the Wood's light is usual.

Kerion: A painful inflammatory mass; any hairs remaining are loose (Figure 7.4). There may be pus and sinus formation, crusting and matting of adjacent hairs. Lymphadenopathy is frequent. Usually caused by one of the zoophilic species, typically *T. verrucosum* or *T. mentagrophytes*. Secondary bacterial infection may be present.

Endothrix type: In *T. tonsurans* and *T. violaceum* infections, a relatively non-inflammatory type of patchy baldness occurs. The common clinical types are gray patch (scaling with patchy hair loss), black dot

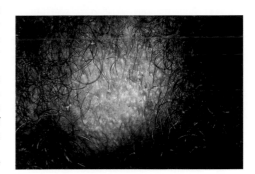

Figure 7.3 Tinea capitis caused by *Microsporum canis*.

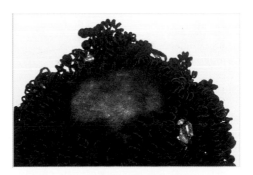

Figure 7.4 Kerion in a patient with *Trichophyton tonsurans* infection of the scalp.

and diffuse alopecia. Black dots (swollen hair shafts) occur when the affected hair breaks at the surface of the scalp. The patches are usually multiple, sometimes mimicking discoid lupus erythematosus or seborrhoeic dermatitis. A low-grade folliculitis may also be seen.

Management
Oral terbinafine, itraconazole or griseofulvin.

Ketoconazole shampoo or selenium sulphide can be used to prevent spread in the early phases of therapy when used in combination with oral treatment. For outbreaks in schoolchildren careful investigation and treatment is recommended; exclusion of children from school is not needed. Identification and treatment of potential source of the infection is also required, e.g. domestic pets.

With kerions, remove crusts using wet compresses and consider coexisting bacterial infection. Permanent hair loss from scarring is usually less than would be expected. Severe inflammatory forms should be reviewed early after starting antifungal therapy and consider oral steroids when there is a widespread Id reaction.

Tinea barbae

Ringworm of the beard and moustache areas of the face with the invasion of coarse hairs.

Epidemiology
Adult males. Commonly farm workers due to cattle ringworm *T. verrucosum*.

Pathophysiology
Ectothrix infections with *T. verrucosum* and *T. mentagrophyte*.

Clinical features
An inflammatory, pustular folliculitis of the beard area, similar to a kerion. Hairs are loose and easily removed without causing pain. Lesions often persist for some months, but tend to settle spontaneously. Some infections are less severe with dry, circular, reddish, scaly lesions enclosing hair stumps which are either broken off close to the surface of the skin or plug the follicles.

Differential diagnosis
The classic, highly inflammatory lesions are distinguished from boils by their relative lack of pain.

Management
Oral itraconazole or terbinafine, sometimes in combination with topical therapy. A vaccine against *T. verrucosum* in cattle is available.

Tinea faciei

Infection of the face with a dermatophyte fungus (excluding moustache and beard areas of the adult male).

Pathophysiology
T. mentagrophytes and *T. rubrum* predominate, but *T. tonsurans*, *M. audouinii* and *M. canis* are also common causes worldwide. Facial skin may be infected either by direct inoculation from an external source (e.g. *T. mentagrophytes* from an infected pet mouse) or by secondary spread from pre-existing tinea of another body site.

Clinical features
The clinical features vary considerably, but complaints of itching, burning and exacerbation after sun exposure are common. There will often be a history of exposure to animals.

Erythema is usual, but scaling is present in less than two-thirds of cases. Lesions are commonly annular or circinate with induration and a raised margin (Figure 7.5). Papular lesions and flat patches of erythema also occur. The use of topical steroids frequently alters the appearance.

Differential diagnosis
Discoid lupus erythematosus (DLE), psoriasis, impetigo, rosacea and seborrhoeic dermatitis.

Management
In localised cases, topical antifungals. therapy with tolnaftate or one of the imidazoles. Consider oral terbinafine or itraconazole when diagnosis delayed and when steroid therapy has modified the condition.

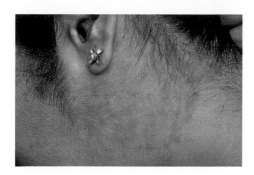

Figure 7.5 Tinea faciei caused by *Trichophyton rubrum*.

Tinea pedis

(Syn. Athlete's foot, foot ringworm)
Infection of the feet or toes with a dermatophyte fungus.

Epidemiology
Tinea pedis is the most common form of dermatophyte infection in the UK and North America. Living in an institution where washing facilities are shared increases the chances of infection.

More common in adults than children; mean age of onset 15 years. Adult males have ~20% chance of developing tinea pedis compared to 5% of women.

Pathophysiology
T. rubrum, *T. interdigitale* and *Epidermophyton floccosum* are responsible for the majority of cases of foot ringworm throughout the world. Occlusion of toe clefts through wearing shoes predisposes to this condition, which is in most cases initially a lateral web space infection, where moist conditions favour growth of the fungus directly and damage the stratum corneum at the same time.

Clinical features
Itching is a common complaint in warm weather. The condition is highly persistent and the history is long. The most common form of tinea pedis is an intertriginous dermatitis charaterised by peeling, maceration and fissuring affecting the lateral toe clefts and sometimes spreading to involve the undersurface of the toes.

In *T. rubrum* infections an often chronic and resisitant scaling, hyperkeratotic type, affects the soles, heels and sides of the feet. If the foot is extensively involved, the term 'moccasin foot' or dry-type infection is used (Figure 7.6). The patient may also complain of the smell and secondary bacterial infection, with fissuring in the toe clefts, may aggravate symptoms.

T. interdigitale features vary from mild, insignificant scaling in the toe clefts to severe, acute, inflammatory reactions affecting all parts of the feet (Figure 7.7). Vesicles may become pustules, and when they rupture leave collarettes of scaling. This frequently goes on to apparent spontaneous cure, but tends to recur in warm weather. There may be associated hyperhidrosis.

Apart from mild toe cleft intertrigo, *E. floccosum* may produce a similar picture to *T. interdigitale* and *T. rubrum*, but with less toenail involvement.

The presence of interdigital tinea pedis is a risk factor for cellulitis in patients with lymphoedema. Other complications include a vesicular allergic reaction (ide) on the uninfected hands in patients with acute vesicular tines pedis.

Differential diagnosis
Erythrasma is usually asymptomatic and rarely causes fissures. Candidosis causes a build-up of white, macerated skin. Bacterial infections with staphylococci or streptococci or Gram-negative organisms, including *Acinetobacter* species, can produce inflammation and often odour. Other differentials include soft corns or callonition, eczema, psoriasis and contact dermatitis.

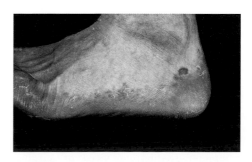

Figure 7.6 Dry-type *Trichophyton rubrum* infection.

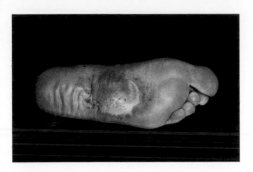

Figure 7.7 *Trichophyton interdigitale* infection: bullous lesion on the sole.

Management

Mild and moderate interdigital disease: topical imidazole twice daily for 4 weeks *or* topical terbinafine twice daily for 7 days.

Dry type tinea pedis: oral terbinafine *or* itraconazole 400 mg/day for 1–2 weeks.

Permanganate or aluminium chloride solution 20–30% twice daily can ease secondary infection. Confirmed bacterial infection or cellulitis should be treated with oral antibiotics.

Tinea manuum

Ringworm of the palmar skin and infections beginning under rings.

Pathophysiology

T. rubrum is the most common causative organism. In most cases, apart from animal infections, there is pre-existing foot infection with or without toenail involvement. Infections beginning under rings and wrist watches, and where there is maceration between the fingers, are particular susceptibility to *T. interdigitale* infections, and may occur without obvious foot involvement. Poor peripheral circulation and palmar keratoderma are also predisposing factors.

Clinical features

Palmar involvement is often subtle and chronic, commonly passing unnoticed or misdiagnosed. Diffuse hyperkeratosis of the palms and fingers is the commonest pattern and is unilat-

eral in half of cases. The accentuation of the flexural creases is a characteristic feature. Modification by inappropriate use of topical steroids leads to further diagnostic difficulties.

Differential diagnosis

Contact dermatitis, especially primary irritant, psoriasis, constitutional eczemas and keratoderma. In ring infections, candidosis and bacterial intertrigo.

Investigation

Unilateral palmar scaling should always alert the clinician to taking scrapings. Subungual hyperkeratosis if present should be scraped.

Management

Chronic ringworm infections of the palm are not easily cleared, and oral itraconazole or terbinafine is always needed.

Tinea cruris

(Syn. Dhobi itch)
Ringworm of the groins.

Epidemiology

Commoner in male adults and in hot and humid climates.

Pathophysiology

T. rubrum is the main cause. Apart from numerous cases of autoinfection from the foot to the groin, the sharing of towels and sports clothing is important.

Clinical features

Itching is a predominant feature. The lesions in the early stages are erythematous plaques, with curved sharp margins extending from the groin down the thighs. Scaling is variable and occasionally may mask the inflammatory changes. Vesiculation is rare, but dermal nodules forming beading along the edge are commonly found in older lesions. Central clearance is usually present.

Spread to the scrotum is common, but scaling is minimal and inflammation is inconspicuous against a background erythema. An extension of infection from the groin to other sites is common, in *T. rubrum* classically to the buttocks, the lower back and the abdomen. The penis is occasionally affected.

Differential diagnosis
Candidosis, erythrasma, flexural seborrhoeic dermatitis, psoriasis, mycosis fungoides, atopic eczema, clothing or deodorant contact dermatitis.

Management
Recent-onset disease: Topical terbinafine or imidazoles twice daily for 2 weeks.
Chronic or extensive disease: Oral terbinafine or itraconazole.

Steroid-modified tinea

(Syn. Tinea incognito)
Ringworm infections modified by corticosteroids (systemic or topical).

Clinical features
The usual sites are the groin, lower legs, face and hands. The patient is often satisfied initially with the treatment. Itching is controlled and the inflammatory signs settle, but they relapse on stopping treatment, with varying rapidity.

The raised margin is diminished, scaling is lost and the inflammation is reduced to a few nondescript nodules and pustules (Figure 7.8). Often, a bruise-like brownish discoloration is seen, especially in the groin. On the face, the picture may be modified by a superimposed perioral dermatitis with papules and pustules. Steroid-modified eyelid infection may resemble a sty. With chronic use there may be atrophy, telangiectasia and, in the groin and axillae, striae.

Management
Oral terbinafine or itraconazole.

Dermatophytide reactions

(Syn. Id reaction)
A non-infective cutaneous eruption representing an allergic response to a distant focus of dermatophyte infection.

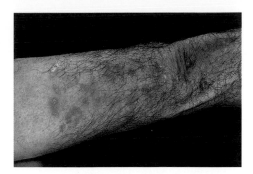

Figure 7.8 Tinea corporis in a patient on systemic corticosteroids.

Pathophysiology
The criteria required for the diagnosis of an Id reaction to a dermatophyte infection are:

- Proven dermatophyte infection.
- A distant eruption, which is demonstrably free of ringworm fungus.
- Spontaneous disappearance of the rash when the ringworm infection settles, with or without treatment.

Clinical features
The main Id reactions include:

1. A widespread symmetrical eruption of follicular papules grouped or diffusely scattered usually on the trunk, but may spread to limbs and occasionally face. Scalp ringworm kerion, caused by *T. verrucosum*, is the commonest cause. Treatment of the original ringworm lesion may trigger the process.
2. A pompholyx-like Id affecting the web spaces and palmar surfaces of the fingers, the palms and sometimes the dorsal surfaces of the hands is associated with acutely inflammatory tinea pedis, which is indistinguishable from pompholyx.

OTHER HYPHAL FUNGI

Superficial mycoses caused by *Neoscytalidium dimidiatum*

A common infection mainly seen in those born in a tropical envionment but has also been seen in Europeans who have visited an endemic area. Examination reveals ringworm-like infections of the palms, soles, toe webs and nails. There is no effective therapy; some patients may respond to treatment with topical azoles.

ONYCHOMYCOSIS

Fungal nail disease or onychomycosis is divided into those caused by dermatophytes, *Neoscytalidium*, other non-dermatophyte moulds and *Candida* (Table 7.2).

A wide variety of other non-dermatophyte moulds have been reported from abnormal nails (mostly toenails). As these are common in the environment and may be isolated as contaminants, their significance needs very careful reassessment before they can be considered significant. A primary dermatophyte infection may also be secondarily invaded by moulds.

CANDIDOSIS

(Syn. Candidiasis, moniliasis, thrush)
An infection caused by the yeasts of the genus *Candida*, predominantly the species *Candida albicans*. *C. albicans* is a frequent normal commensal of the gastrointestinal and vaginal tracts; a number of factors increase the risk of carriage and infection (Box 7.2).

A wide variety of different skin conditions are seen, including disease of the oral mucous membranes (Chapter 59), the anogenital area (Chapter 61), the nails (see above) and paronychium (Chapter 48), congenital/neonatal candidosis (Chapter 63) and chronic mucocutaneous candidiasis.

Candidosis of the skin and genital mucous membranes

Most cases of cutaneous candidosis occur in the skin folds or where occlusion from clothing or medical dressings produces abnormally moist conditions. Areas close to the body orifices and the fingers, which are frequently contaminated with saliva, are also at risk. For vulvo-vaginal candidosis, Candida balanitis and perianal and scrotal candidosis see Chapter 61.

Candida Intertrigo
(Syn. Flexural candidosis)

Clinical features
Any skin fold may be affected, especially in obese subjects. Patients present with soreness and itching. Clinically there is early erythema deep in the fold (Figure 7.12) which spreads beyond the area of contact, with an irregular edge and subcorneal pustules which rupture to give tiny erosions and then peeling. Satellite lesions, pustular or papular, are classic. Topical steroids may modify the inflammatory signs and cause diagnostic confusion. Where the web spaces of the toes or fingers are affected, marked maceration with a thick, white, horny layer is usually prominent. In the case of the hands, some abnormality, including wide, fat fingers, appears to predispose to infection. Interdigital infections of the feet may occur in very hot climates, particularly in those with heavy footwear. Apart from skin folds, macerated skin under rings and dressings may become infected with *Candida*.

Box 7.2 Factors that increase risk of *Candida* infection

Host factors

Age (elderly and very young)
Inadequate oral hygiene: severely ill patients/dentures/orthodontic devices
Maceration of skin/occlusion, e.g nappy area, occlusive footwear (worse in hot climates)
Oral antibiotics
Pregnancy, oral contraceptives, intrauterine devices

Endocrine factors

e.g. diabetes, Cushing syndrome

Immunological factors

Systemic steroids
Immunosuppressive treatment
Neutropenia
Severely ill patients with leukemia/lymphoma/cancer
HIV patients

	Dermatophyte	Candidal	Neoscytalidium	Other non-dermatophyte moulds
Epidemiology	Rare in children			
Pathophysiology				
Causative organism	(i) *T. rubrum, T. interdigitale* are rarely *E. floccosum* associated with foot and hand infections (ii) *T. tonsurans, T. violaceum* and *T. soudanense* associated with scalp infections	*Candida albicans*	*Neoscytalidium dimidiatum*	*Scopulariopsis brevicaulis, S. acremonium, Fusarium,* and *Aspergillus, Onychocola cana*
Predisposing factors	Poor peripheral circulation, Raynaud phenomenon, trauma and the elderly (where linear growth is slow)			
Clinical features	Asymmetrical Commonly with evidence of tinea pedis/ manuum (Figure 7.9)	Commonly with paronychia (Figure 7.10)	Commonly with paronychia and infection of palms, soles and toe webs, but not groin, or dorsum of hand/foot	Indistinguishable from *T. interdigitale* but no concurrent skin infection *S. brevicaulis* (Figure 7.11) may give a cinnamon colour Great toenails most often affected
Differential	Psoriasis, eczema, lichen planus, other causes of onycholysis, onychogryphosis, bacterial infection (pseudomonas causes black or green discolouration)			
Management	**First line** *Mild infections of distal nail plate or non-linear superficial onychomycosis* Topical amorolfine or ciclopirox olamine *All other* Oral terbinafine 6 weeks fingernails, 3 months toenails *or* itraconazole 1 week in 4; 2–3 months fingernails, 3–4 months toenails **Second line** Griseofulvin dose for 4–8 months (longer for toenails) 15% treatment failures more in elderly, traumatic dystrophy and poor peripheral circulation Early treatment of tinea pedis and tinea manuum reduces the prevalence	Oral fluconazole or itraconazole	No effective treatment	*S. brevicaulis:* Difficult; search and treat co-dermatophyte infection Consider: 40% urea paste chemical nail avulsion followed by topical azole antifungal daily to nail bed until new nail formed. Itraconazole for 1 week in 4 for 3–4 months may help Other non-dermatophytes: Difficult; amorolfine 5%, tioconazole 28% or removal of the nail with 40% urea may be tried

PART 1: INFECTIONS AND INFESTATIONS

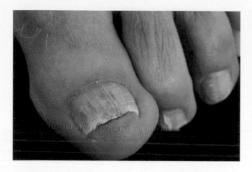

Figure 7.9 Onychomycosis caused by *Trichophyton rubrum*.

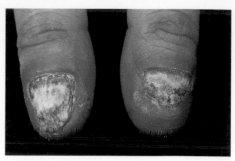

Figure 7.10 Candida onychomycosis in a patient with chronic mucocutaneous candidosis.

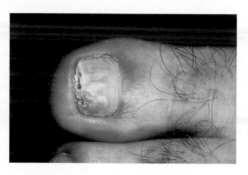

Figure 7.11 Onychomycosis caused by *Scopulariopsis brevicaulis*.

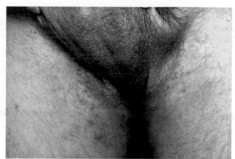

Figure 7.12 *Candida* infection of the groins.

Differential diagnosis

Tinea, seborrhoeic dermatitis, bacterial intertrigo, flexural psoriasis, Hailey–Hailey disease and flexural Darier disease.

Investigations

Skin scraping and swab.

Management

Topical azole or polyene for 2 weeks, along with careful drying of the area and, for toe web infections, open footwear. In some patients with moist *Candida* intertrigo, potassium permanganate soaks are more effective.

Perineal Candidosis of Infancy
(Syn. Diaper candidiasis, nappy candidiasis)

C. albicans infection predominantly of the napkin area with erythema and, in some, the classic subcorneal pustules, a fringed irregular border and satellite lesions. Steroid creams modify the clinical features and topical antibiotic use favours yeast growth.

Rashes in the napkin area should be investigated for *Candida* and, if present, this can be treated with topical antifungals combined with with frequent nappy changes.

Nodular or Granulomatous Candidosis of the Napkin Area
(Syn. Granuloma gluteale infantum)
A rare condition. The primary napkin dermatitis may clear leaving only the nodules.

Management involves the removal of microorganisms, avoidance of topical steroids and general measures to keep the area dry.

Chronic mucocutaneous candidosis

Persistent *Candida* infection of the mouth, the skin and the nails, refractory to conventional topical therapy, is a distinct clinical pattern of infection. Most chronic mucocutaneous candidosis (CMC) patients develop signs in early childhood, and usually *Candida* infection is the presenting feature. Those patients with an underlying immune defect, such as severe combined immunodeficiency or agammaglobulinaemia, are not included in this group. The syndrome comprises a heterogeneous group classified into several distinct categories using genetic and clinical criteria (autosomal recessive, autosomal dominant, idiopathic, CMC associated with endocrinopathy, and late-onset), although there is overlap between the groups.

Treatment with systemic anti-*Candida* therapy (fluconazole, itraconazole or voriconazole) may have to be prolonged and repeated. Endocrine screening tests should be repeated, even if initially negative, as patients with endocrinopathy may develop endocrine disease years after the first appearance of candidosis. Where appropriate, parents should be given genetic counselling.

SUBCUTANEOUS MYCOSES

Subcutaneous mycoses, or mycoses of implantation, are caused by fungi present in the natural environment that are directly inoculated through a penetrating injury. They are mainly seen in the tropics.

The most common of these infections are sporotrichosis, mycetoma and chromoblastomycosis. Rarer infections are phaeohyphomy-cosis, lobomycosis, rhinosporidiosis and subcutaneous mycosis caused by *Conidiobolus* or *Basidobolus*.

Sporotrichosis

Infection caused by *Sporothrix schenckii* and closely related species. There are both cutaneous and systemic forms of sporotrichosis.

Epidemiology
Sporotrichosis is mainly seen in the tropics and subtropics. The fungus grows on decaying vegetable matter.

Pathophysiology
Causative organisms include *S. schenckii*, *S. braziliensis*, *S. mexicana*, *S. globose* and *S. lurei* introduced into the skin or mucous membrane by trauma: a thorn, a splinter or an insect bite. Sporotrichosis is not contagious. The incubation period is around 8–30 days.

Infection may remain localised in the subcutaneous tissue, spread locally in the subcutaneous lymphatics or, rarely, be widely disseminated in the bloodstream after pulmonary infection. The underlying host immunity probably determines the form that the infection assumes.

The fungus provokes a mixed granulomatous reaction with neutrophil foci. The fungus is present in the tissue, usually in the form of small cigar-shaped or oval yeasts, surrounded by a thick, radiate, eosinophilic substance that forms the distinctive asteroid bodies.

Clinical features
Cutaneous sporotrichosis is normally divided into two main types, the lymphangitic and fixed forms.

The most common type of sporotrichosis is the localised lymphatic variety, which follows the implantation of spores in a wound. Predominantly on exposed skin, often on the upper extremity and known as lymphangitic sporotrichosis (Figure 7.13). A nodule or pustule forms, which may break down into a small ulcer. Untreated, the disease usually follows a chronic course, which is characterised by involvement of the lymphatics from the draining area; a chain of lymphatic nodules

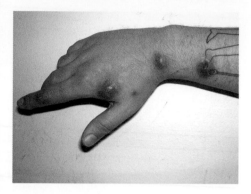

Figure 7.13 Lymphangitic sporotrichosis

develops connected by tender lymphatic cords. New nodules appear at intervals of a few days. As the disease becomes chronic, the regional lymph nodes become swollen and may break down.

The fixed variety, where the pathogen remains localised at the point of inoculation, is less common. The lesions may be acneform, nodular, ulcerated or verrucous.

Differential diagnosis

Mycobacterial infections, leishmaniasis.

Investigations

Samples from exudates and skin biopsy both from the edge and from the centre of the lesion for culture and histology. Biopsy specimens intended for culture must be placed in sterile saline or wrapped in moistened sterile gauze if they cannot be processed immediately. Delays in processing samples will increase the likelihood of bacteria or saprophytic fungi contaminating the samples.

Management

Itraconazole *or* terbinafine until clinical recovery (at least 3 months).

Mycetoma

(Syn. Maduromycosis, Madura foot, eumycetoma, actinomycetoma)

A localised chronic infection caused by various species of fungi (eumycetoma) and aerobic actinomycetes (actinomycetoma), which occur as saprophytes in soil or on plants. They are implanted subcutaneously, usually after a penetrating injury, resulting in the formation of aggregates of the causative organisms (grains) within abscesses. This results in severe damage to the skin, subcutaneous tissues and bones of the feet, hands and other parts of the body.

Epidemiology

Actinomycetomas caused by *Nocardia* species are most common in Central America and Mexico. In other parts of the world, the most common organism is a eumycetoma agent, *Madurella mycetomatis*. The actinomycete, *Streptomyces somaliensis*, is most often isolated from patients originating from Sudan and the Middle East.

Pathophysiology

The main aetiological agents are listed in Box 7.3 and characterised by the presence of different coloured grains, which represent microcolonies of the organisms. It is not contagious.

Clinical features

The clinical features are the same no matter which fungus or actinomycete is concerned. Because trauma favours infection, most lesions are on the foot and lower leg. The earliest stage

---

Box 7.3 Main aetiological agents of mycetoma

Fungi: dark grain

- *Madurella* spp.
- *Leptosphaeria* spp.
- *Cochliobolus* (formerly *Curvularia*) *lunata*

Fungi: pale grain

- *Scedosporium apiospermum*
- *Neotestudina rosatii*
- *Sarocladium* (formerly *Acremonium*) spp.

Actinomycetes

- *Actinomadura madurae*
- *Actinomadura pelletieri* (red grain)
- *Streptomyces somaliensis*
- *Nocardia* spp.

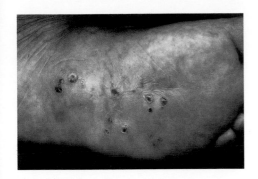

Figure 7.14 Mycetoma caused by *Madurella grisea*.

is a firm, painless nodule but with time papules and pustules, which break down to form draining sinuses, appear on the skin surface (Figure 7.14). The colour of the grain squeezed from the sinus relates to the different causative organism. The whole area becomes hard and swollen, often without significant pain. Extension to underlying bones and joints gives rise to periostitis, osteomyelitis and arthritis. In advanced cases, there may be destruction of bone within an infected area and gross deformity may result.

Differential diagnosis
Chronic osteomyelitis of bacterial or tuberculous aetiology.

Investigations
Histopathology is very important in diagnosis. Pus should be examined under the microscope for the presence of grains, which may then be processed for histology or examined directly in potassium hydroxide. A tentative diagnosis sufficient to initiate treatment may be made on the basis of grain colour, texture and direct microscopic appearance; black grains are always caused by fungi and red grains by an actinomycete.

Management
First line: Dapsone plus streptomycin or rifampicin *or* co-trimoxazole plus streptomycin or rifampicin.
Second line: Surgical excision.

Chromoblastomycosis

(Syn. Chromomycosis, verrucous dermatitis)
A chronic fungal infection of the skin and subcutaneous tissues caused by pigmented fungi. It is characterised by the production of slow-growing exophytic lesions, usually on the feet and legs.

Epidemiology
Usually found in the tropics, but occasionally seen as an imported infection in Europe and the USA. Adult male agricultural workers are most often affected.

Pathophysiology
Chromoblastomycosis is caused by several fungi, the most common of which are *Phialophora verrucosa*, *Fonsecaea pedrosoi*, *F. compacta* and *Cladophialophora carrionii*. The causal fungi have been isolated from wood and soil, and the infection usually results from trauma, such as a puncture from a splinter of wood.

Histology is that of a foreign-body granuloma, with isolated areas of microabscess formation. In the organised granuloma, mainly within giant cells, groups of fungal cells may be seen which are chestnut or golden brown in colour.

Clinical features
The lesions are usually found on exposed sites, particularly the feet, legs, arms, face and neck (Figure 7.15). The disease develops over years. A warty papule slowly enlarges to form a hypertrophic plaque, which gradually expands with central scarring. After months or many years, large hyperkeratotic masses are formed, and these may be as large as 3 cm thick (Figure 7.16). Secondary ulceration may occur. The lesion is usually painless unless the presence of secondary infection causes itching and pain. Satellite lesions are produced by scratching, and there may be lymphatic spread to adjacent areas.

The course is chronic but non-fatal. Squamous cell carcinomas may develop in chronic lesions.

Differential diagnosis
Blastomycosis, cutaneous tuberculosis, leishmaniasis, syphilis and yaws.

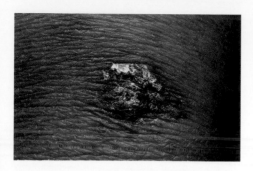

Figure 7.15 Early lesion of chromoblastomycosis.

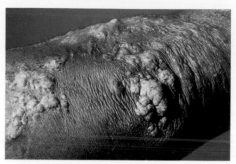

Figure 7.16 Plaque-type chromoblastomycosis.

Investigations
Biopsy and culture of material.

Management
First line: Itraconazole or terbinafine daily until clinical recovery.
Second line: Heat application.

SYSTEMIC MYCOSES

The systemic mycoses are fungal infections that involve deep structures and have the propensity to disseminate, usually via the bloodstream, from the original focus of infection. They include two main groups of disease: the endemic mycoses and the opportunistic systemic mycoses.

Endemic mycoses are usually acquired via inhalation of the causative organisms. The main endemic mycoses are histoplasmosis (classic and African types), blastomycosis, coccidioidomycosis, paracoccidioidomycosis and infection caused by *Talaromyces marneffei*. The clinical manifestations of these infections are affected by the underlying state of the patient, and many of them develop in the presence of particular immunodeficiency states, notably AIDS.

Cryptococcosis shares features of both endemic mycoses and the opportunistic infections. The opportunistic systemic mycoses are those systemic infections that only occur in patients with some underlying predisposition. In contrast to the endemic mycoses, they may occur in any geographical area and their clinical manifestations are very variable, depending on the predisposition and mode of entry of the fungus.

Histoplasmosis

A highly infectious mycosis caused by *Histoplasma capsulatum* affecting primarily the lungs.

Epidemiology
Small-form histoplasmosis is caused by *H. capsulatum* var. *capsulatum*, occurring in the Americas, Africa and Australasia. *H. duboisii* causes African or large-form histoplasmosis and is uncommon.

Infants and children are frequently infected. The rate is highest in male agricultural workers. Patients with lymphoma and AIDS are more at risk.

Pathophysiology
H. capsulatum is a saprophyte, often isolated from soil, particularly when contaminated with chicken feathers or bird or bat droppings. Histoplasmosis is normally a pulmonary infection which spreads through the bloodstream to affect other sites.

Clinical features
The four main clinical varieties of histoplasmosis are acute pulmonary, acute disseminated, chronic pulmonary and chronic disseminated forms. The skin is rarely affected except in AIDS patients and in African histoplasmosis; papules, ulcers, nodules, granulomas, abscesses, fistulae, scars and pigmentary changes may be seen.

Differential diagnosis

Tuberculosis, *Talaromyces* infections and cryptococcosis. Skin lesions may resemble molluscum contagiosum.

Investigations

Identification of the small intracellular yeast cells of *Histoplasma* in sputum, peripheral blood, bone marrow or biopsy specimens.

Management

First line: Itraconazole until clinical remission. For patients who are severely ill, amphotericin B and/or itraconazole for a further period depending on clinical response.
Second line: Fluconazole until clinical remission.

Blastomycosis

A *Blastomyces dermatitidis* infection that can affect otherwise healthy individuals as well as the immunosuppressed. It affects primarily the lungs but disseminating forms also affect the skin, bones, central nervous system and other sites.

Epidemiology

Commonest in North America and Africa. The incidence of infections highest in rural areas and in agricultural workers. Human–human transmission unusual. Adult males, 30–50 years, are most commonly affected.

Pathophysiology

The tissue reaction, and ultimately the course and prognosis, are determined by the immunological response of the patient.

Clinical features

There are three forms of blastomycosis: primary cutaneous, pulmonary and disseminated.

Primary cutaneous blastomycosis: Very rare and follows trauma to the skin. After inoculation, an erythematous, indurated area with a chancre appears in 1–2 weeks with associated lymphangitis and lymphadenopathy. Tends to recover spontaneously.

Pulmonary blastomycosis: Similar to pulmonary tuberculosis.

Disseminated blastomycosis: The infection spreads from the chest, commonly to the skin, bones and central nervous system. One or many skin lesions may be present, often symmetrical, usually on the trunk. Each consists of a papule or nodule that may ulcerate and discharge pus. The lesions enlarge at the periphery with central scarring, resulting in a serpiginous outline with raised, warty borders (Figure 7.17) and a violaceous margin studded with miliary abscesses containing the organisms.

Differential diagnosis

Tuberculosis, syphilis, leprosy, pyoderma gangrenosum and drug reactions resulting from bromides and iodides.

Investigations

Direct microscopy of pus in 10% potassium hydroxide and confirmed by culture or biopsy.

Management

Itraconazole until clinical remission. For patients who are severely ill, amphoterocin B for 2 weeks followed by itraconazole for a further period depending on clinical response.

Coccidioidomycosis

A (primary) respiratory fungal infection caused by *Coccidioides immitis* and *C. posadasii*, which may become progressive and disseminated, with severe or fatal forms.

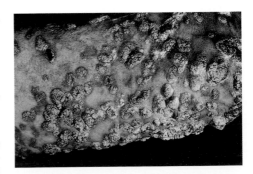

Figure 7.17 Cutaneous blastomycosis (Source: Courtesy of Dr M. James, Royal Berkshire Hospital, Reading, UK.)

Epidemiology

Endemic in desert areas of the southwestern states of the USA, and in parts of Central and South America. There are two species of *Coccidioides*: *C. immitis* which occurs only in California and *C. posadasii* which occurs elsewhere. With increasing travel, cases of coccidioidomycosis are found in many parts of the world.

Pathophysiology

The fungus is a soil inhabitant; infection of humans and a wide variety of domestic and wild animals is acquired by inhalation of fungus-laden dust particles. Between 2 and 6 weeks after exposure, the patient becomes sensitive to an intradermal skin test using the fungal antigen, coccidioidin.

Clinical features

Severity varies from a very mild upper respiratory tract infection to an acute, disseminated fatal disease. Erythema multiforme or erythema nodosum occurs from the third to the seventh week in up to 25% of patients, particularly in females. There may be accompanying uveitis, arthralgia, generalised aches, malaise and severe headaches. An early, generalised, macular erythematous rash is seen in 10% of patients. Regional lymphadenopathy develops but resolves after a few weeks.

Disseminated coccidioidomycosis is very uncommon and develops in fewer than 0.5% of infected individuals, usually in black, Filipino or immunosuppressed patients including patients with AIDS. The death rate in acute disseminated disease, or with meningitis, is very high. Lesions may occur in the skin, subcutaneous tissues, bones, joints and all organs. The skin lesions may appear as abscesses, granulomas, ulcers or discharging sinuses, particularly if there is underlying bone or joint disease.

The prognosis for the primary form is excellent; untreated, acute disseminated forms are fatal.

Differential diagnosis

Chronic infectious conditions.

Investigations

The large globular spherules may be seen in potassium hydroxide mounts of sputum, cerebrospinal fluid or pus. Confirmation depends on the isolation of the fungus in culture.

Management

In the primary pulmonary infection, no specific therapy apart from rest is necessary.

Oral itraconazole or fluconazole are effective in some forms of localised infection such as solitary disseminated skin lesions. For disseminated disease, the approach depends on the form of disease.

Infections caused by *Talaromyces marneffei*

(Syn. Penicilliosis, talaromycosis)

Talaromyces marneffei is a recently recognised fungal pathogen that causes a disseminated mycosis in both healthy and immunocompromised patients, particularly those with AIDS. Normally confined to South-East Asia, particularly Thailand, southern China and Vietnam, but also seen in travellers to the endemic area.

Patients present with respiratory symptoms or with signs of dissemination such as anaemia, multiple skin papules and hepatosplenomegaly. Skin lesions occur in over 50% of cases with small papules, ulcers or molluscum-like lesions on the face and trunk. Left untreated it is fatal.

The diagnosis can be made from appropriately stained biopsies, smears and blood films.

Treatment with itraconazole is given until clinical remission. In severe cases, amphotericin B is necessary.

Cryptococcosis

An acute, subacute or chronic infection caused by the encapsulated yeast *Cryptococcus neoformans*.

Epidemiology

Occurs throughout the world. Usually between 30 and 60 years old; uncommon in childhood. The incidence in patients with AIDS varies from 3–5% in the USA and UK to over 12% in parts of Africa (e.g. Zaire) and Thailand. Susceptibility is also increased by lymphomas, sarcoidosis, collagen disease, carcinoma, immunosuppressive treatments and systemic corticosteroid therapy.

Pathophysiology
Caused by *C. neoformans* and *C. gattii*. The respiratory tract is the usual portal of entry, but primary cutaneous lesions may occur. Histologically, the characteristic lesion consists of encapsulated budding cells mixed with a network of connective tissue, which enlarges and compresses the surrounding tissues.

Clinical features
The central nervous system manifestations predominate, presenting as a chronic meningitis or as focal brain lesions simulating a tumour. In disseminated disease, the most frequent types of skin lesions are firm or cystic, slow-growing, subcutaneous, erythema nodosum-like swellings; acneiform papules or pustules around the nose and mouth are characteristic of widespread systemic infection.

Differential diagnosis
Histoplasmosis and infections caused by *Talaromyces marneffei*.

Investigations
Cryptococci may be recognised in smears of pus and of cerebrospinal fluid. Biopsy and culture of skin lesions.

Management
Non-AIDS patients: Intravenous amphotericin B combined with flucytosine.
AIDS patients: Amphotericin B with or without flucytosine or fluconazole to induce remission, followed by long-term oral maintenance with fluconazole.

Systemic candidosis

Systemic candidosis is an infection of deep organs, including the bloodstream, caused by *Candida* species.

Pathophysiology
In most cases of systemic candidosis, the causal organism originates in the gastrointestinal tract, and in patients with leukaemia or other serious illness a history of mucocutaneous candidiasis in the past is the indication for vigilance. Invasion by *Candida* along intravenous infusion lines is also important; signs suggestive of cutaneous candidosis on adjacent skin should not be ignored. Drug addicts are particularly at risk.

Clinical features
Typical lesions start as macules, become papular or nodular, and may show a pale centre. Some are haemorrhagic and break down to form ecthyma gangrenosum-like lesions. Subcorneal pustules are not a feature, but follicular invasion by *Candida* leading to pustules and nodules in the coarse hair-bearing areas of the scalp, beard, axilla and pubis may be characteristic of *Candida* septicaemia in heroin abusers. Fever, diffuse muscle tenderness and an erythematous macular rash are regarded as an indication for prompt skin biopsy in any compromised patient.

Investigations
The histology of a skin lesion showing *Candida* cells in the dermis provides a rapid diagnosis, often before a blood culture is positive.

Management
Intravenous amphotericin B, caspofungin or azole drugs is necessary.

8

Parasitic diseases

This chapter considers infections with the following types of parasites:

- *Nematodes*: worms; the human is an obligatory host at some stage of the life cycle of the parasite.
- *Trematodes*: non-segmented single-sex worms, also known as flukes or flatworms.
- *Protozoa*: single-celled microscopic organisms.

NEMATODE INFECTIONS

Onchocerciasis

(Syn. River blindness)
Caused by the filarial nematode, *Onchocerca volvulus*. Second commonest infectious cause of blindness worldwide.

Epidemiology
Most cases (>99%) are in rural communities in sub-Saharan Africa. Approximately 500 000 are blind due to onchocerciasis.

Pathophysiology
See Figure 8.1 for lifecycle. Blackfly bites deposit infective *O. volvulus* larvae into human skin, which mature over 6–12 months into mature adult parasites (macrofilariae).

Microfilariae also invade the eye, which can lead to blindness. Free microfilariae also penetrate superficial lymphatic vessels and may be found in the urine, tears, sputum, cerebrospinal fluid and, occasionally, in vaginal smears or irrigation sediment.

Clinical features
Typical signs and symptoms are pruritus, dermatitis, nodules and blindness.

Acute papular onchodermatitis (APOD): early changes confined to one skin area, often accompanied by small itching papules or pustules (Figure 8.2).

Chronic papular onchodermatitis (CPOD): later disease, localised areas of scarring, excoriated papules and flat-topped scars with hyperpigmentation and lichenification. Common on buttocks and shoulders (Figure 8.3).

Lichenified onchodermatitis (LOD): late stage disease, associated with gross enlargement of regional lymph nodes (Figure 8.4).

Atrophy ('lizard skin', Figure 8.5) and depigmentation ('leopard skin', Figure 8.6) are also a consequence of long-standing disease.

Differential diagnosis
Leprosy, *Loa loa* infection, lymphatic filariasis, scabies, syphilis and yaws.

Investigations
Excision of nodules for histological examination for worms and microfilariae. Skin 'snips' can be shaved off with a very sharp blade without bleeding, placed in normal saline and examined microscopically 1–4 h later. Filarial immunofluorescence or enzyme-linked immunosorbent assay (ELISA) is positive in 60–90% of cases.

Rook's Dermatology Handbook, First Edition. Edited by Christopher E. M. Griffiths, Tanya O. Bleiker, Daniel Creamer, John R. Ingram and Rosalind C. Simpson.
© 2022 John Wiley & Sons Ltd. Published 2022 by John Wiley & Sons Ltd.

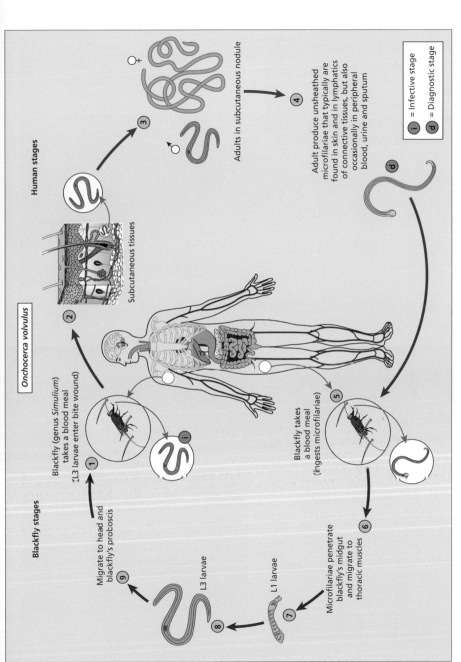

Figure 8.1 Life cycle of *O. volvulus*. (Source: Courtesy of the Centers for Disease Control and Prevention. http://www.cdc.gov/dpdx/onchocerciasis/, last accessed December 2014, Public Domain.)

Figure 8.2 Acute papular onchodermatitis. Early in the disease the papules are usually urticarial.

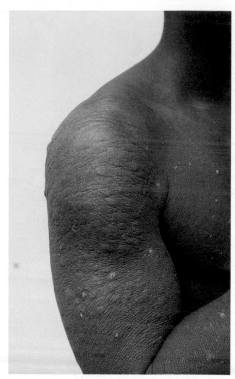

Figure 8.4 Late lichenified onchodermatitis (pachyderma).

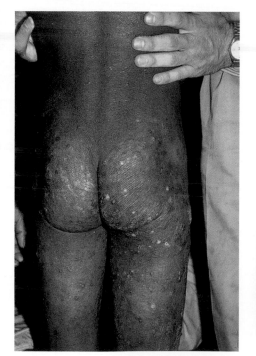

Figure 8.3 Chronic papular onchodermatitis with early lichenification.

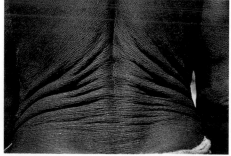

Figure 8.5 Late onchocerciasis. Atrophy of skin and damage to supporting tissue cause the skin to sag in folds (lizard skin).

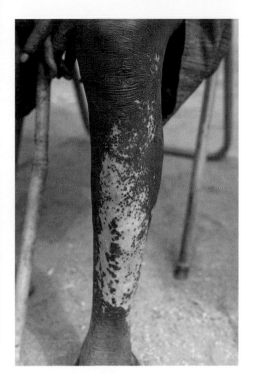

Figure 8.6 Depigmentation over the shin in late onchocerciasis (leopard skin).

Management
First line: Doxycycline, PO × 6 weeks, followed by ivermectin, retried every 6–12 months until asymptomatic.

Second line: Ivermectin, retried every 6–12 months until asymptomatic.

Third line: Suramin, nodulectomy.

Lymphatic filariasis

(Syn. Tropical elephantiasis)
Nematode infection whereby organisms occupy the lymphatic system in humans and can lead to the disease elephantiasis.

Epidemiology
The highest incidence is in South-East Asia and sub-Saharan Africa. An estimated 250 million people are infected.

Pathophysiology
Causative organisms are *Wuchereria bancrofti* (most common), *Brugia malayi* and *Brugia timori*, transmitted by mosquitos. The presence of adult worms in the lymphatics with the resulting inflammatory response causes lymphatic obstruction. Leakage of lymph may contribute to tissue damage. Microfilariae in lungs may cause tropical pulmonary eosinophilia. See Figure 8.7 for lifecycle of *W. bancrofti*.

Clinical features
Initial signs are often swelling, tenderness and erythema on the arms, legs or scrotum. Cellulitis is common and may be recurrent. In the severest form, it presents with fever, sweats and the painful enlargement of inguinal lymph nodes and/or lymphangitis. Other complications include orchitis, recurrent epididymitis, deep limb muscle abscesses or lymphatic abscesses.

Lymphatic obstruction occurs over many years following repeated cellulitis. In males, these commonly present as hydroceles, but lower leg oedema and elephantiasis may also develop. Limb oedema of a varying extent and nature is also common and passes through several grades of severity before becoming gross elephantiasis.

Investigations
Clinical diagnosis can be made in endemic areas. Biopsy of an enlarged lymph node may be diagnostic. Clinical diagnosis and microfilariae are found on blood film. ELISA is often positive.

Differential diagnosis
Bacterial lymphadenitis, lymphogranuloma venereum (genital lesions).

Management
First line: Diethylcarbamazine for 12 days, repeat 10 days later. Contraindicated in patients co-infected with onchocerciasis as a severe inflammatory response can occur.

Second line: Ivermectin (treatment of choice for patients with concurrent onchocerciasis).

Cutaneous larva migrans

Nematode infection. Distinctive creeping/ migrating cutaneous eruption due to the presence of moving parasites in the skin.

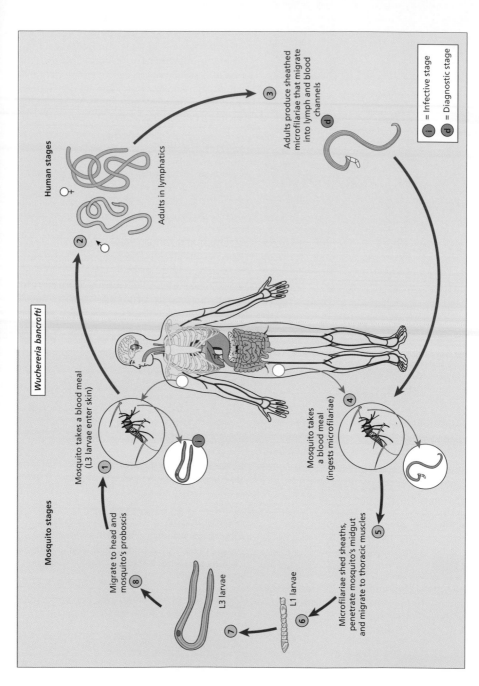

Figure 8.7 Life cycle of *W. bancrofti*. (Source: Courtesy of DPDx, Centers for Disease Control and Prevention. http://www.cdc. gov/dpdx/onchocerciasis/, last accessed October 2019, Public Domain.)

Epidemiology

Infection is found most commonly in tropical and subtropical climates of Africa, South America, South-East Asia, the Caribbean and the south-eastern USA.

Pathophysiology

Causes include the hookworms *Ancylostoma brasiliense*, *A. caninum*, *A. ceylonicum*, *Uncinaria stenocephala* and *Bubostomum phlebotomum*. *Strongyloides stercoralis* causes a distinctive form of cutaneous larva migrans. *Dirofilaria repens* and *Spirometra* spp. cause a subcutaneous granuloma that may migrate very slowly. *Gnathostoma* spp. and *Loa loa* cause migratory evanescent subcutaneous swellings. Cutaneous myiasis due to larvae of flies of the genera *Gasterophilus* and *Hypoderma* may cause a creeping eruption similar to that caused by the animal hookworms (Figure 8.8).

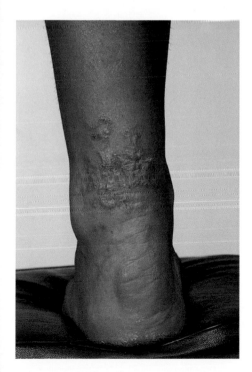

Figure 8.8 Cutaneous larva migrans (creeping eruption). There are several tortuous indurated inflamed worm tracks, in some of which is seen a blister that marks the head of the track.

Clinical features

A pruritic erythematous papule may occur at the site of penetration where the skin has been in contact with infected soil or sand from beach holiday (commonly feet, hands and buttocks). They can lie quiet for weeks or months, or immediately begin creeping activity with the production of a wandering thread-like line about 3 mm wide. This is exceedingly itchy, slightly raised, flesh-coloured or pink and forms bizarre, serpentine patterns.

Differential diagnosis

Larva currens (strongyloidiasis).

Investigations

Clinical diagnosis, biopsy is of little value as the larva is usually ahead of the clinical rash.

Management

First line: Ivermectin.
Second line: Albendazole.

TREMATODE INFECTIONS

Schistosomiasis

(Syn. Bilharziasis, swimmer's itch)
Trematode infection. A serious systemic disease due to different species of human schistosomes or blood flukes. A second group of non-human schistosomes cause cutaneous symptoms only.

Epidemiology

The commonest agent, *S. mansoni*, is endemic in Africa and South America. *S. japonicum* occurs in the Far East, and *S. haematobium* in Africa, Arabia, Madagascar and south-west India. Common and rare forms of cutaneous schistosomiasis are increasingly being described in non-endemic regions of the world.

Pathophysiology

See Figure 8.9 for the lifecycle of Schistosoma.

Clinical features

Skin manifestations vary:

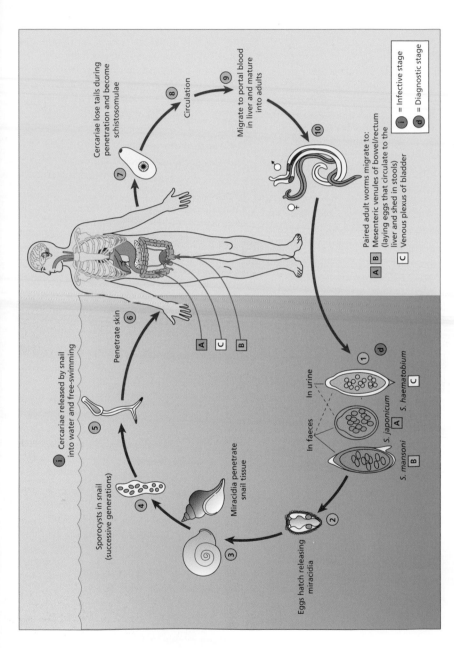

Figure 8.9 Life cycle of the *Schistosoma*. (Source: Courtesy of DPDx, Centers for Disease Control and Prevention http://www.cdc.gov/parasites/schistosomiasis/biology.html, last accessed October 2019, Public Domain.)

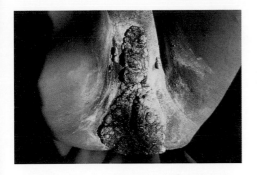

Figure 8.10 Schistosomiasis of the vulva and anus. Condylomatous lesions containing granulomas around schistosome ova. (Source: Courtesy of Professor G. Nelson, Liverpool School of Tropical Medicine, Liverpool, UK.)

1. *Schistosomal dermatitis*: itchy papular eruption in parts of the skin in contact with infected water. May only last a few hours.
2. *Urticarial reactions in the early weeks of the disease*: occurs 4–8 weeks after infection. May be associated with eosinophilia, fever, purpura, malaise, arthralgia, abdominal cramps, diarrhoea and enlargement of the liver and spleen. Lasts 4–6 weeks.
3. *Paragenital granulomas and fistulous tracts* (Figure 8.10).
4. *Ectopic cutaneous schistosomiasis*: 2–3 mm firm papules on trunk, often paraumbilical.

Complications occur due to infections affecting the liver (fibrosis), intestinal involvement and bladder infection, which may lead to carcinoma.

Investigations
Ova are found in stools or urine. Ectopic cutaneous schistosomiasis is diagnosed by biopsy.

Management
Praziquantel.

PROTOZOAL INFECTIONS

Cutaneous leishmaniasis

A protozoal disease transmitted by sandfly vectors. Usually classified as cutaneous or visceral, but the species that cause visceral disease may also cause skin lesions. Clinical manifestations of disease range from aggressive cutaneous ulcers to systemic multiorgan disease. 'Old World' leishmaniasis is responsible for all the cutaneous disease on the northern Mediterranean littoral west of Greece and for some of the disease in North Africa. 'New World' leishmaniasis occurs in South and Central America.

Epidemiology
1.5 million new cases of cutaneous leishmaniasis occur annually.

Pathophysiology

Old World disease **is due to** *L. major, L. tropica, L. aethiopica* **and** *L. donovani infantum.*
Sandflies inoculate when taking a blood meal. Inoculated promastigotes are taken up by histiocytes and monocytes, in which they multiply. After a period of time, a clinical lesion appears comprising parasitised macrophages, lymphocytes and plasma cells. Focal necrosis of parasitised cells then occurs. The overlying epidermis becomes hyperkeratotic and breaks down, causing an ulcer.

New World disease - American cutaneous leishmaniasis and mucocutaneous leishmaniasia
The pathology of the skin lesions is similar to Old World disease. However, *L. brasiliensis* demonstrates blood borne spread to the mucosa of the nose, mouth, palate or larynx. Here, they may later start to multiply and cause severe destructive lesions. Histology of the mucosal lesion shows lymphocytes and plasma cells around small arterioles in the nasal submucosa.

Clinical features
Clinical features of leishmaniasis, both Old World and New World type, are summarised in Table 8.1.

Diffuse cutaneous leishmaniasis
In the Old World this form of the disease is due to *L. aethiopica* and has characteristic features:

- There is an initial lesion, which spreads locally, and from which the disease disseminates to other parts of the skin, often involving large areas (Figure 8.16).
- The lesions are nodules that do not ulcerate.

Table 8.1 Clinical features of cutaneous leishmaniasis (Adapted from Weatherall *et al.*)

Parasite and lesion	Natural outcome	Treatment
Old World Leishmaniasis		
Leishmania major (Figures 8.11–8.13)		
Self-healing sores	3–5 months	Physical/topical/IL/nil
	Disabling scars	Sb
		(?Some unresponsive)
L. tropica		
Self-healing sores	10–14 months	Physical/topical/IL/nil
		Sb
Leishmaniasis recidivans	>10 years destructive	Sb
L. aethiopica (Figures 8.14–8.16)		
Self-healing, nodular	2–5 years	Physical/topical/nil
Mucocutaneous	>10 years destructive	Pentamidine
DCL	Persists, disfiguring	Pentamidine
New World Leishmaniasis		
L. m. Mexicana		
Self-healing	6–8 months	Physical/topical/IL/nil
Chiclero ear	>10 years, destructive	Sb
L. m. amazonensis		
Self-healing	?Duration	?Sb
DCL	Persists, relapses, disfiguring	Sb
L. b. brasiliensis		
Self-healing	?Duration, later mucocutaneous	Sb
Mucocutaneous	Persists, destructive	Sb
L. b. guyanensis		
Self-healing	?6–8 months	Sb
Lymphatic nodules 'pian bois'	?Late espundia	If poorly responsive to Sb, use pentamidine
L. b. panamensis		
Self-healing	?Duration	Sb
	?Late espundia	
L. b. peruviana		
Self-healing	?Duration	Physical/topical/nil
		Sb

m., Mexicana; b., brasiliensis; DCL, diffuse cutaneous leishmaniasis; IL, intralesional injection; Sb, antimony as pentavalent antimonial. Source: Adapted from Weatherall DJ, Ledingham JGG, Warrell DA, eds. Oxford Textbook of Medicine, 2nd edn. Oxford: Oxford University Press, 1987.

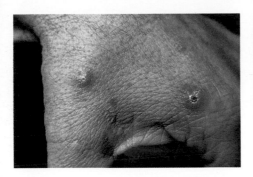

Figure 8.11 Cutaneous leishmaniasis due to *Leishmania major*: early papules, one of which is starting to show central crusting.

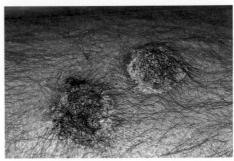

Figure 8.12 Cutaneous leishmaniasis due to *Leishmania major* from Saudi Arabia, showing marked and persistent crusting.

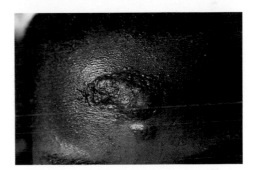

Figure 8.14 Cutaneous leishmaniasis due to *Leishmania aethiopica* from Kenya. A large nodule with many satellite papules and abundant parasites.

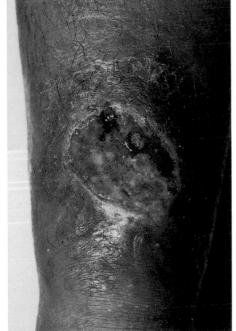

Figure 8.13 Cutaneous leishmaniasis due to *Leishmania major* from Sudan. An ulcer with a raised edge.

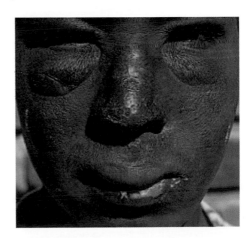

Figure 8.15 Nasal involvement and marked inflammatory oedema in leishmaniasis due to *Leishmania aethiopica* in Ethiopia.

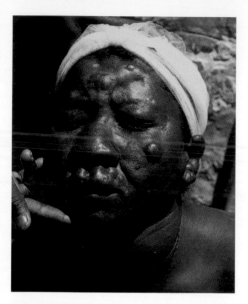

Figure 8.16 Diffuse cutaneous leishmaniasis due to *Leishmania aethiopica* in Ethiopia. The face is covered with infiltration and nodulation but there is no ulceration.

- There is a superabundance of parasites in the lesions.
- The histology is characteristic in that macrophages full of amastigotes predominate.
- Internal organs are not invaded and there is no history of kala-azar.
- The leishmanin test and other tests of specific cellular immunity are negative.
- The disease progresses slowly and becomes chronic.
- Treatment produces only gradual improvement and relapse is the rule.

Investigations

A positive diagnosis of cutaneous leishmaniasis (Old World and New World types) can be suggested by one or more of the following diagnostic criteria:

- History of exposure to an endemic area in the previous weeks or months.
- History of sandfly bites in the previous weeks or months.
- History of high-risk activities such as sleeping outdoors, jungle or desert trekking.
- Non-healing chronic nodular violaceous ulcer for 4–6 weeks or longer.

- Demonstration of amastigotes in Giemsa-stained smears from infected skin by direct microscopy.
- Demonstration of intracellular amastigotes in the dermis of H&E sections of skin.
- Presence of leishmanial granulomas in the dermis in H&E specimens.
- Growth of promastigotes in Nicolle–Novy–MacNeal (NNN) culture medium from lesional specimens.
- Demonstration of leishmanial DNA by PCR.

Management
Old World
See Table 8.1. Most sores heal spontaneously, but their duration cannot be predicted. Systemic treatment should be reserved for problematic sores: these include sores where scarring would be disabling or severely disfiguring; sores that will not heal easily, for example on the lower leg or over a joint, sores involving mucosa or cartilage, or sores that might be due to parasites of the *L. brasiliensis* group.

American cutaneous leishmaniasis and mucocutaneous leishmaniasis
See Table 8.1. In particular, lesions due to *L. b. brasiliensis* should be treated systemically for a week beyond parasitological cure to prevent mucocutaneous leishmaniasis from developing.

Visceral leishmaniasis

(Syn. Kala-azar)
A systemic form of leishmaniasis causing a severe systemic infection, which may be accompanied by cutaneous manifestations.

Pathophysiology
Caused by *Leishmania donovani donovani and Leishmania donovani infantum*. See Figure 8.17.

Clinical features
Characterised by fever fatigue, abdominal discomfort, cough, diarrhoea and epistaxis. Gross splenomegaly occurs. A primary skin sore has been described in some African cases. Rarely, there may be an accompanying mucosal lesion. In Indian people especially, the skin of the face,

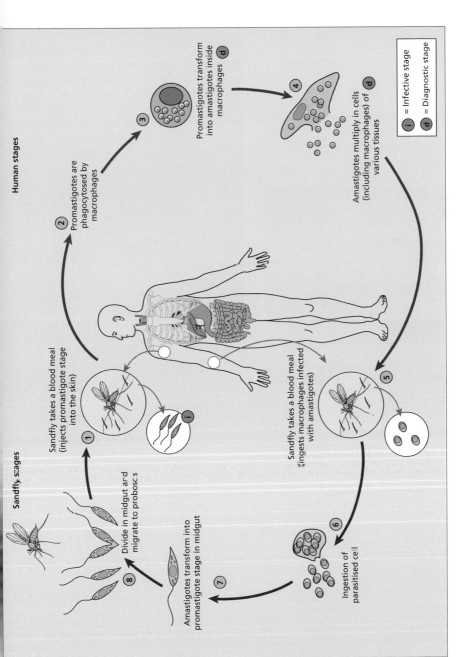

Figure 8.17 Life cycle of leishmaniasis parasite. (Source: Courtesy of DPDx, Centers for Disease Control and Prevention http://www. cdc.gov/parasites/leishmaniasis/biology.html, last accessed October 2019, Public Domain.)

Human stages

2 Promastigotes are phagocytosed by macrophages

3 Promastigotes transform into amastigotes inside macrophages d

4 Amastigotes multiply in cells (including macrophages) of various tissues d

i = Infective stage
d = Diagnostic stage

Sandfly stages

1 Sandfly takes a blood meal (injects promastigote stage into the skin)

5 Sandfly takes a blood meal (ingests macrophages infected with amastigotes)

6 Ingestion of parasitised cell

7 Amastigotes transform into promastigote stage in midgut

8 Divide in midgut and migrate to proboscis

PART 1: INFECTIONS AND INFESTATIONS

hands, feet and abdomen becomes hyperpigmented. Post-kala-azar dermal leishmaniasis (PKDL, Figure 8.18) is a rash that develops after the visceral disease has healed. A few patients develop widespread hypopigmentation (especially in India) during the recovery phase (Figure 8.19).

Treatment

Liposomal amphotericin B, sodium stibogluconate and meglumine antimoniate remain the most widely used agents. Case fatality without treatment is over 90%.

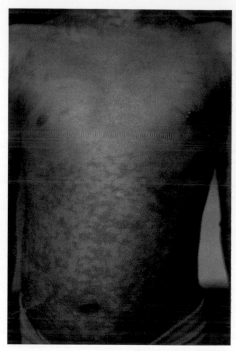

Figure 8.19 Post-kala-azar dermal leishmaniasis in an Indian person showing the extensive hypopigmented macular rash.

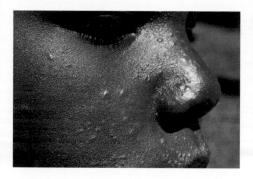

Figure 8.18 Post-kala-azar dermal leishmaniasis. Typical facial papules in a Kenyan arising 6 weeks after treatment and healing spontaneously. (Source: Courtesy of Dr J.D. Chulay.)

Arthropods, stings and bites

9

Arthropods can be divided into two groups: mandibulates with antennae and chelicerates without antennae. The mandibulates include insects, Chilopoda and Diplopoda. The chelicerates include scorpions, spiders and mites. Arthropods are characterised by segmented bodies, paired, jointed appendages, an exoskeleton and a bilateral symmetry. They go through the following life stages: egg, larva or nymph and finally mature adult (male or female).

Pathophysiology

Cutaneous effects occur by a variety of mechanisms, including mechanical trauma, injection of irritant, cytotoxic or pharmacologically active substances and injection of potential allergens. The reaction type depends on previous exposure to the same or related species with the development of host-specific antibodies to antigenic substances in the arthropod saliva or venom.

'Exaggerated reaction of insect bite', also called 'insect-bite-like reaction' or 'eosinophilic eruption of haematoproliferative disease', is a relatively common and disturbing skin reaction in chronic lymphocytic leukaemia patients. Other reactions to arthropod bites are secondary infection, invasion of the host's tissues (myiasis), contact reactions, reactions to retained mouthparts and transmission of disease.

Histopathological changes include a superficial and deep, wedge-shaped inflammatory infiltrate of lymphocytes and eosinophils.

Clinical features

Table 9.1 shows the clinical and epidemiological features of the main arthropod bites.

Papular urticaria is the most commonly seen clinical feature (Figure 9.1). An extremely itchy urticarial weal develops at the site of the bite, followed by a firm pruritic papule, which usually persists for several days. The weal and papule may show a central haemorrhagic punctum and the papule may be surmounted by a tiny vesicle. Lesions are often grouped in clusters and develop in crops at irregular intervals.

Bullous reactions are common on the lower legs (Figure 9.2).

Secondary infection is a common complication. Bite reactions may persist for months. Tick attachment sites, in which the mouthparts may be retained, are the most likely to persist.

Investigations

Usually a clinical diagnosis based on history.

Management

Prevention: Insect repellents.

General management

- Local wound care by cleansing, removing of remaining arthropod parts.
- Management of pain and patient discomfort by using ice packs, application of topical corticosteroid, systemic antihistamine, injection of local anaesthetics or sometimes the use of systemic analgesic.

Rook's Dermatology Handbook, First Edition. Edited by Christopher E. M. Griffiths, Tanya O. Bleiker, Daniel Creamer, John R. Ingram and Rosalind C. Simpson.
© 2022 John Wiley & Sons Ltd. Published 2022 by John Wiley & Sons Ltd.

Table 9.1 Arthropod bites: main clinical and epidemiological features

Arthropod	Clinical feature on examination	Location	Timing of pruritus	Context
Bedbugs	Three or four bites in a line or curve	Uncovered areas	Morning	Travelling
Fleas	Three or four bites in a line or curve	Potentially anywhere	Daytime	Pet owners or rural living
Mosquitoes	Non-specific papules	Potentially anywhere	*Anopheles* spp. night, *Culex* spp. night, *Aedes* spp. day	Worldwide distribution
Head lice	Eggs attached to hairs Live lice on the head associated with itchy, excoriated lesions	Scalp, ears and neck	Any	Children, parents, or contact with children
Body lice	Excoriated papules and hyperpigmentation; live lice inside clothes	Back	Any	Homeless people, developing countries
Scabies	Vesicles, burrows, nodules and non-specific secondary lesions	Interdigital spaces, forearms, breasts, genitalia	Night	Sexually transmitted, households or institutions
Ticks	Erythema migrans or ulcer	Potentially anywhere	Asymptomatic	Pet owners or hikers
Pyemotes ventricosus	Comet sign, a linear erythematous macular tract	Under clothes	Any time when inside habitat	People exposed to woodworm contaminated furniture (*P. ventricosus* is a woodworm parasite)
Spiders	Necrosis (uncommon)	Face and arms	Immediate pain, no itching	Rural living

Source: Bernardeschi, C., Le Cleach, L., Delaunay, P., & Chosidow, O. (2013). Bed bug infestation. BMJ, 346(jan22 1), f138-f138. © 2013 BMJ Publishing Group Ltd.

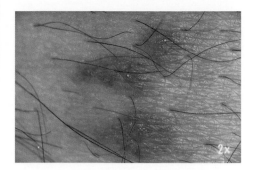

Figure 9.1 Typical papular urticaria. In this case, in response to flea bites.

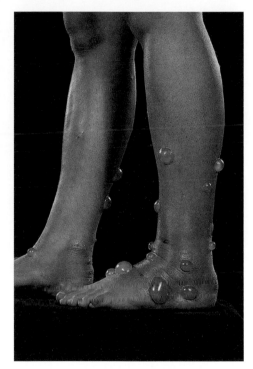

Figure 9.2 Bullous lesions in response to arthropod bites. (Source: Courtesy of Dr F.A. Ive, Durham, UK.)

- Institution of supportive measures in case of allergic (anaphylaxis) or toxic reaction.
- Antibiotic therapy in case of secondary infection.
- Tetanus prophylaxis if necessary.

MYIASIS

Infestation of body tissues of animals by the larvae of Diptera (mosquitoes, gnats, midges and flies). The Diptera are important as biting insects and as the cause of myiasis, in addition to their capacity to transmit disease.

Pathophysiology

Classified according to the part of the body affected. Cutaneous myiasis: *Cochliomyia hominivorax*, *Chrysomya bezziana* and *W. magnifica* cause a serious complication of war wounds in tropical areas, and they are sometimes seen in neglected ulcers or wounds in most parts of the world. Obligatory cutaneous myiasis is classified as furuncular and migratory. Furuncular myiasis is caused by *Dermatobia hominis*, *Cuterebra*, *Cordylobia anthropophaga*, *Cordylobia* (*Stasisia*) *rodhaini*, *Wohlfahrtia* species and *Hypoderma* species. Migratory myiasis is produced by *Gasterophilus* or *Hypoderma* species larvae.

Other types are cavitary myiasis (rare) and intestinal and urogenital myiasis.

Clinical features

Cutaneous myiasis occurs on exposed skin, often the face, scalp, arms or legs. In the furuncular form, boil-like lesions develop gradually over a few days. Each lesion has a central punctum, which discharges sero-sanguinous fluid. The posterior end of the larva, equipped with a group of spiracles, is usually visible in the punctum (Figure 9.3). The lesions are often extremely painful. Lymphangitis, regional lymphadenopathy, systemic symptoms or secondary bacterial infection may occur. Lesions rapidly resolve once the larva emerges/is removed.

Migratory myiasis resembles cutaneous larva migrans (Chapter 8), in which a tortuous thread-like red line with a terminal vesicle marks the passage of the larva through the skin. The larva lies ahead of the vesicle in apparently normal skin. Infestation may present with pustules, nodules or recurrent swelling.

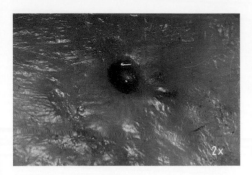
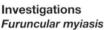

Figure 9.3 Furuncle-like lesion produced by *Dermatobia hominis*. The tail of the larva is visible in the centre of the lesion.

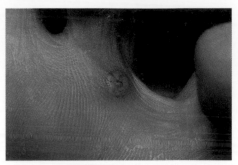

Figure 9.4 Tungiasis, showing a characteristic lesion on the sole of the foot. (Source: Courtesy of Dr N.H. Cox, Cumberland Infirmary, Carlisle, UK.)

Investigations

Furuncular myiasis

Clinical features are often sufficient. Dermoscopy may be helpful in difficult cases, showing a yellowish structure with black barb-like spines. Ultrasound or colour Doppler sonography may be helpful.

Migratory myiasis

Clinical identification of the larva, magnification is used to visualise the parasite.

Wound myiasis

Diagnosis is easily made by the clinical inspection of the wound.

Management

Some larvae can be expressed by firm pressure around the edges of the lesion. Others require surgical management. Ivermectin is used if surgery is unsuccessful. Infected wounds require surgical debridement and irrigation to remove larvae, plus treatment of secondary infection.

TUNGIASIS

Caused by the sand flea *Tunga penetrans*, also known as the jigger or chigoe.

Epidemiology

Occurs in South America, Africa, the Caribbean, India and Mexico.

Pathophysiology

The impregnated female *Tunga penetrans* flea is picked up from dry, sandy soil and burrows into the feet of mammals. In humans, the fleas predominantly stay between the toes, under the nails and on the soles (Figure 9.4). Once established in the skin, large numbers of eggs are produced and extruded over 2 weeks, following which the female flea dies and is sloughed from the skin.

Clinical features

Lesions initially show a black dot surrounded by a halo of erythema, followed by enlargement to form a mother of pearl-coloured papule with a central dark punctum. Intense irritation occurs. Secondary infection or tetanus can occur.

Differential diagnosis

Myiasis, verruca vulgaris, ingrowing toenail, acute paronychia, mycotic granuloma, malignant melanoma and arthropod bites.

Management

Blunt dissection of the intact parasite.

LICE

(Syn. Pediculosis)

Wingless insects which are obligate ectoparasites of birds and mammals. Humans are parasitised by two species of Anopleura (lice): *Pediculus humanus*, divided into *Pediculus humanus capitis* (the head louse) and *Pediculus humanus humanus* (the clothing or body louse), and *Pthirus pubis*, the pubic or crab louse.

Head lice

(Syn. Pediculus capitis)

Epidemiology
Occurs most commonly in children 3–11 years, girls > boys.

Pathophysiology
The empty egg case or 'nit' appears white and is easier to see than the intact eggs close to the scalp surface. The louse reaches maturity in approximately 10 days.

The majority of infestations are acquired by direct head to head contact. In developing countries, spread of lice is encouraged by poverty, poor hygiene and overcrowding. Lack of hygiene alone does not encourage infection.

Clinical features
Scalp pruritus is characteristic, some may be asymptomatic. Secondary bacterial infection may occur from scratching, concomitant head louse infection must always be considered in cases of scalp impetigo. Pruritic papular lesions may occur on the nape of the neck.

The empty egg cases occur in greatest density on the parietal and occipital regions (Figure 9.5).

Investigations
The most reliable method of diagnosing current active infestation is by detection combing.

Management
Live head lice can be treated by wet combing with fine-toothed comb; chemical treatment if ineffective, e.g malathion. Important to consult local policies as resistance to treatments exist. Treat all affected contacts and repeat after 7–10 days.

Causes of therapeutic failure for head lice include misunderstanding of instructions, non-adherence, resistance, failure to retreat after 7–10 days and reinfestation.

Clothing/body lice

(Syn. Pediculus corporis)

Epidemiology
Associated with poor socioeconomic conditions. Body lice may transmit epidemic typhus (*Rickettsia prowazekii*), spirochete infection (*Borrelia recurrentis*) and 'trench fever' (*Bartonella quintana*).

Pathophysiology
The natural habitat is the clothing of its host, and lice only visit the skin to feed. Eggs are cemented to clothing fibres.

Clinical features
Itching is the main complaint. The body is often covered in excoriations and/or secondary bacterial infection. Post-inflammatory pigmentation occurs in longstanding disease.

Investigations
Lice and eggs should be sought in the clothing.

Management
Bed linens and clothes should be decontaminated by hot washing. Infested materials sealed

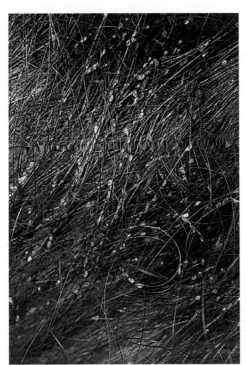

Figure 9.5 Numerous head louse eggs and empty egg cases.

in plastic bags may be used safely after 3 days. Infested furniture, mattresses and box springs should be discarded or fumigated to destroy lice and nits.

Crab lice

(Syn. Phthiriasis pubis)

Epidemiology

Most common in sexually active young adults. Prevalence has decreased, possibly due to pubic hair removal practices. Other sexually transmitted infections often coexist.

Pathophysiology

Transmitted by close physical contact, usually sexual. May affect areas of hair with reduced density in addition to pubic hair (axillary, eyebrows, eyelashes, beard hair and hair on the trunk and limbs). Infection in children is usually acquired by close physical contact with infected parents and is not necessarily indicative of sexual abuse.

Clinical features

Itching, mainly in the evening and at night, is the main symptom. Inspection of affected areas will reveal lice on hairs close to the skin surface, and louse eggs attached to the hair shafts (Figure 9.6). When pubic crab lice are identified other hairy areas of the body should be examined.

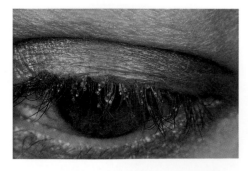

Figure 9.6 Crab louse eggs on the eyelashes.

Management

All hairy areas of the body should be treated at the same time. Pubic lice are treated with the same insecticidal creams or lotions as pediculosis capitis, with a second application after 7–10 days. Eyelash infestations should be treated with permethrin 5% cream (washed off after 10 min) or only with petrolatum (applied twice a day for 8–10 days), followed by mechanical removal of the nits. Screen for associated sexually transmitted disease.

CLASS ARACHNIDA

Arachnida are readily distinguished from insects, as the adults have no wings or antennae and possess four pairs of legs. The body of arachnids is divided into two, the cephalothorax, from which the legs arise, and the abdomen.

The Arachnida are classified into seven orders, only three of which have medical importance: Araneae (spiders), Scorpiones (scorpions) and Acari (ticks and mites).

Spiders

(Syn. Araneae)

Very few of the many thousands of species are dangerous to humans. The clinical syndrome following the bite of a spider is known as arachnidism. The diagnosis of spider bite is based on a clear history of a spider biting.

Pathophysiology

Latrodectus (widow spiders) are widely distributed throughout the world. *Latrodectus* venom is considered to be one of the most potent toxins, *Latrodectus hasselti*, the red-back spider, is common in Australia.

Genera *Atrax/Hadronyche* (Australia and south Pacific) and *Macrothele* (Taiwan and parts of eastern Asia) are known as funnel web spiders.

Genus *Loxosceles* ('fiddleback' spider, 'violin' spider, 'brown recluse' spider). The majority are in North and South America. Several species induce human skin necrosis: *L. reclusa, L. laeta, L. deserta, L. arizonica* and *L. rufescens*. There are two distinct clinical forms of loxoscelism:

necrotic cutaneous loxoscelism and the much less frequent viscerocutaneous loxoscelism.

Clinical features

Latrodectus bite is fairly painless but within a few minutes increasingly severe pain develops. Cramp-like or colicky abdominal pain is common. Puncta may be visible at the site of the bite, and there is local erythema and oedema. There is frequently profuse sweating, and neuromuscular involvement causes paraesthesiae, incoordination and paralysis. Myocardial damage, occasionally fatal, has been reported.

The bite of funnel web spiders is painful. From the majority of bites, especially those of female spiders, no general symptoms follow, but the large amount of venom from male spiders may cause severe systemic symptoms.

In necrotic cutaneous loxoscelism, there is local damage to the skin and subcutaneous tissues, but systemic symptoms are mild. In severe envenomation, a 'target' lesion is seen: central blue/purple discoloration surrounded by an ischaemic halo and an outer ring of erythema After 3 or 4 days, the central area becomes necrotic and an eschar develops.

Management

Symptomatic management, antivenom if available.

Scorpions

(Syn. Scorpiones)

Scorpions are widely distributed in the tropics and subtropics. Approximately 1500 species of scorpions are described. Venom is carried in the curved sting at the tip of the tail.

Pathophysiology

The principal components of the venom are neurotoxins.

Clinical features

Local effects are usually immediate severe burning pain and hyperaesthesia, and there may be marked swelling. Systemic effects include restlessness, profuse sweating, muscle spasms, difficulty with speech, marked increase in salivary and lacrimal secretion, nausea, vomiting, convulsions, hypertension, cardiac arrhythmias, myocarditis and pulmonary oedema. Death is usually due to respiratory or cardiac failure.

Management

Early treatment includes neutralising the circulating toxin, treating symptoms of envenomation and general supportive measures. Specific antivenoms are available and indicated in all severe cases.

Ticks

(**Syn. Acari**)

Ticks are important vectors of diseases such as tick-borne relapsing fever, and in a number of viral, rickettsial and *Borrelia* infections (Lyme disease). There are two major types: the Ixodidae (hard ticks) and the Argasidae (soft ticks). Humans usually become accidental hosts when walking through, or sitting in, an area that contains ticks. At the point of penetration of the tick mouthparts there is coagulation necrosis of the epidermis and papillary dermis. Hard ticks are visible attached to the skin. Bites from soft ticks are usually painful. Acute lesions include erythematous macules, papules or nodules, tissue necrosis and ulcers. The reaction at the site of the bite is mild oedema, vesiculation or bullae formation. Chronic lesions due to tick bite granuloma include plaques, papules and nodules. Auto-eczematisation may occur. Temporary alopecia may occur in the scalp. Secondary infection is common. Non-dermatological disease such as anaphylaxis, paralysis and other systemic symptoms may be seen. The tick should be removed intact using tweezers or another special device. The risk of vector-borne disease transmission is minor if the tick is removed within 24 h. Tetracycline is the antibiotic of choice for most tick-borne diseases.

Mites

(**Syn. Acari**)

Classical Scabies

Scabies in humans and other animals is caused by mites of the family Sarcoptidae, which includes *Sarcoptes scabiei*, the scabies mite, and *Notoedres cati*, a mange mite of cats.

Epidemiology

Affects around 100–300 million people worldwide, including all age and ethnic groups. Most frequent in the elderly in residential and nursing homes.

Pathophysiology

Usually transmitted by close physical contact. Away from the host, scabies mites survive for 24–36 h. Allergic sensitivity plays an important role.

Clinical features

Itch (onset occurs 3–4 weeks after infection occurs) is the classical symptom. Typical locations of lesions are the finger webs (Figure 9.7a), the flexor surfaces of the wrists, the elbows, the axillae, the buttocks and genitalia (Figure 9.7b) and the breasts of women (Figure 9.7c). The face is often spared. The typical lesions of scabies are burrows (Figure 9.7d). Inflammatory pruritic papules or nodules, sometimes surmounted by burrows, on the male genitalia are characteristic.

Scabies in infants and young children show more extensive distribution of burrows, vesicular and vesiculopustular lesions, extensive eczematisation is often present, and multiple crusted nodules on the trunk and limbs (Figure 9.8). In the elderly, burrows commonly

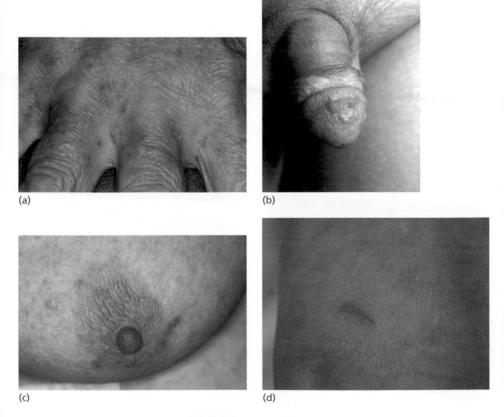

(a)   (b)

(c)   (d)

Figure 9.7 (a) Typical scabies in the finger webs. (b) Pruritic papules and nodules on the penis in scabies infestation. (c) Papular lesions on the nipples and areolae are a common location for scabies in women. (d) A typical linear burrow. (Source: Monsel, G., Delaunay, P. and Chosidow, O. (2016). Arthropods. In Rook's Textbook of Dermatology, Ninth Edition (eds C.E.M. Griffiths, J. Barker, T. Bleiker, R. Chalmers and D. Creamer). doi:10.1002/9781118441213.rtd0035.)

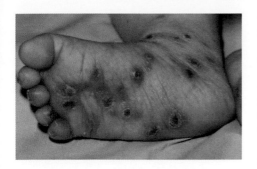

Figure 9.8 The foot of an infant with scabies superinfection presenting as impetigo. (Source: Monsel, G., Delaunay, P. and Chosidow, O. (2016). Arthropods. In Rook's Textbook of Dermatology, Ninth Edition (eds C.E.M. Griffiths, J. Barker, T. Bleiker, R. Chalmers and D. Creamer). doi:10.1002/9781118441213.rtd0035.)

occur on the palms and soles, and may be very numerous. Secondary eczematisation is often troublesome. Crusted scabies is discussed separately (see below).

The inappropriate use of topical steroids may modify the clinical picture. Secondary infection, manifest as folliculitis or impetigo, may also be severe and extensive. There is a risk of poststreptococcal glomerulonephritis and systemic sepsis in supetinfected scabies.

Investigations

Diagnosis is usually clinical. Genital lesions in men or breast nodules in women are strongly suggestive. Absolute confirmation can only be made by the discovery of burrows and/or microscopic examination or on dermoscopy. A skin biopsy may confirm the diagnosis of scabies if a mite or parts can be identified.

Management

Treatment should be prescribed to the patient and close physical contacts, even those without pruritus or cutaneous lesions. Patients should be advised to avoid close physical contact until they, their household members and sexual partners have been treated. All clothes and bedding must be washed at high temperature (>50°C) or kept in a plastic bag for up to 72 h. See Table 9.2 for specific treatments. Itching may persist several weeks after scabies. The persistence of itching after 4 weeks should be reinvestigated. Consider cutaneous irritation (over treatment,

eczematisation, contact dermatitis), treatment failure and psychogenic pruritus.

Human Crusted Scabies
(Syn. Norwegian scabies)

Crusted scabies is a rare and severely debilitating form of the disease characterised by the infestation of up to millions of mites and the development of hyperkeratotic skin crust.

Epidemiology

Occurs in patients with learning disability, dementia, immunosuppression or HIV. Down syndrome is a frequent association.

Pathophysiology

An inadequate immune response to the mite, allows the mites to multiply. It is a severe disease with a significantly higher morbidity than ordinary scabies.

Clinical features

Large warty crusts form on the hands (Figure 9.9a) and feet (Figure 9.9b). The palms and soles may be irregularly thickened and fissured. The nail apparatus is frequently affected (Figure 9.9c). Erythema and scaling occur on the face, neck, scalp and trunk, and may generalise. Itching is often absent or slight but may be severe. Generalised lymphadenopathy is present in some cases, and blood eosinophilia and elevated IgE levels are common.

Differential diagnosis

Hyperkeratotic eczema, psoriasis.

Investigations

Skin scrapings show mites and eggs on microscopy.

Management

Isolation of the patient is required to manage crusted scabies because of the risk of transmission to people in physical contact. Simultaneously treat all cases and all exposed people. A keratolytic agent (e.g. salicylic acid preparation) should be used to treat hyperkeratosis. Nails should be cut short and brushed with a scabicidal agent Expert consensus recommends combining topical and oral therapy (Table 9.2).

PART 1: INFECTIONS AND INFESTATIONS

Table 9.2 Drugs commonly used to treat scabies

Treatment	Dosage and treatment regimen	Recommended group	Contraindication	Advantages	Disadvantages
Permethrin	5% cream rinsed off after 8–12 h	Classical scabies Children<2 years old Pregnancy Crusted scabies (± ivermectin)	–	Effective, well tolerated, safe	Itching and stinging on application
Lindane	1% lotion or cream rinsed off after 6 h		Pregnant women, infants, seizure disorders	Effective, inexpensive	Cramps, dizziness, seizures in children
Benzyl benzoate	25% ointment rinsed off after 24 h (one or several times)	Classical scabies	Pregnant women and infants (only 12-h application)	Effective, inexpensive	Can cause severe skin irritation
Esdepalletrin (bioallethrin)	0,6% aerosol rinsed off after 12 h		People with asthma	–	–
Crotamiton	10% ointment rinsed off after 24 h then reapplied for an additional 24 h	Scabies nodules in children	–	Well tolerated, safe for infants	Questionable efficacy
Precipitated sulphur	2–10% precipitate in petroleum base; rinsed off after 24 h and then reapplied every 24 h for the next 2 days (with a bath taken between each application)		–	Safe for infants, pregnant and breastfeeding women	Questionable efficacy, skin irritation
Ivermectin	Tablets, 200 μg/kg repeated on day 7–14	Superinfected scabies Crusted scabies (± permethrin)	Children <15 kg; pregnant or breastfeeding women	Good patient compliance	Expensive

Source: Adapted from Chosidow, O. (2006). Scabies. New England Journal of Medicine, 354(16), 1718–1727. doi:10.1056/nejmcp052784

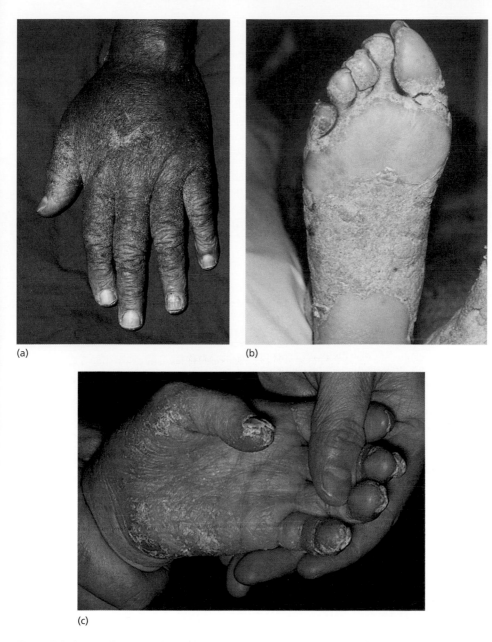

(a)

(b)

(c)

Figure 9.9 Crusted (Norwegian) scabies of (a) the hand and (b) the foot. (c) Grossly dystrophic nails in crusted scabies.

Other Mites That Cause Infection

Storage mite allergy

Well-recognised in certain occupations, including farmers, grain elevator workers and bakers. Respiratory allergy and skin lesions can occur, secondary to bites or contact with allergens.

House-dust mite

Dermatophagoides pteronyssinus (the house-dust mite) is widely distributed in the human environment in house dust and beds. The largest numbers of mites are found in houses that are damp and inadequately heated. Numbers vary seasonally, increasing in early summer to reach a maximum by early autumn. House dust mite allergens are thought to play a role in the sensitisation and induction of clinical symptoms of atopic eczema.

Cheyletiella mites

Obligatory parasites of certain mammals, predominantly dogs, cats and rabbits. Causes intensely itchy papules distributed in areas of contact with an infested animal; the abdomen and thighs are frequently involved.

Harvest mites

Humans are infested while working in or walking through grass or low vegetation; larvae (most commonly from rabbits) may cause troublesome dermatitis (trombidiosis; scrub itch), and some are important vectors of rickettsial disease. Lesions commonly occur around the feet and ankles, the groins and genitalia, the axillae, the wrists and antecubital fossae and areas constricted by clothing, such as the waistline.

Follicle mites

Demodex folliculorum (see Chapter 45).

STINGS AND BITES

Stings: marine injuries

The main types of marine stings and bites are shown in Table 9.3.

Bites

The main types of bites are shown in Table 9.4.

Table 9.3 Main types of marine stings and bites

	Jellyfish, sea anemones and corals	Sponges	Sea urchins	Sea mats	Venomous fish
Description	Marine organisms with 'jellyfish' lifecycle. Classes of causative organisms are Hydroza (includes fire corals), Cubozoa (box jellyfish), Scyphozoa (jellyfish distributed worldwide), Anthozoa (including sea anemones, soft corals and true corals);	Contact with certain sponges typically occurs in divers in Australia and New Zealand	Spherical organisms whose shell has numerous moveable spines, some of which are venomous	Form mat-like encrustations on rocks, seaweeds or other surfaces	Numerous fish species are capable of inflicting painful or dangerous stings from dorsal or caudal spines which have venom glands
Pathophysiology	Tentacles bearing batteries of stinging cells (nematocysts) which inject venom. The venom effects vary with species. Classes of causative organisms are Hydroza (includes fire corals), Cubozoa (box jellyfish), Scyphozoa, Anthozoa (including sea anemones, soft corals and the stony or true corals)	Spicules becoming lodged in the skin	Envenomation by sea urchin spines causes symptoms and clinical effects	Causes an allergic contact dermatitis (rather than a physical dermatosis or sting) occurring during summer months	Most injuries by venomous fish are from stingrays, catfish and scorpionfish. Usually results from stepping on the fish; the fish tail drives its spines into the skin

(Continued)

PART 1: INFECTIONS AND INFESTATIONS

PART 1: INFECTIONS AND INFESTATIONS

Table 9.3 (Continued)

	Jellyfish, sea anemones and corals	Sponges	Sea urchins	Sea mats	Venomous fish
Clinical features	Contact with tentacles causes a painful linear erythematous eruption Corals cause urticarial lesions which may turn vesicobullous 'Seabather's eruption' (Figure 9.10) describes itchy, red papules and weals occurring under swimwear Fatalities have been reported	Initial pruritus and burning may progress to erythema with papules, vesicles or bullae Nausea and vomiting may be present Erythema multiforme has been described	Immediate burning pain, local swelling Puncture wound heals within 1–2 weeks May become infected Delayed granulomatous reactions can occur	Acute, papular, occasionally bullous, contact dermatitis on the hands, arms and face May have a photoallergic component	Painful lacerations or puncture wounds with surrounding swelling and erythema Severe stingray wounds may become dusky or cyanotic with subsequent necrosis Fatalities have been reported
Management	Vinegar stops discharge of nematocysts of box jellyfish Cold packs improve pain Antivenom is available for some stings	Wound irrigation with normal saline or sea water Adhesive tape to remove spicules NSAIDs for pain relief	Removal of spines (surgical exploration may be needed) Hot water inactivates toxins Intralesional steroid to granulomatous lesions	Emollients and potent topical steroids	Hot water inactivates toxins and diminishes pain Antivenom is available for some stings

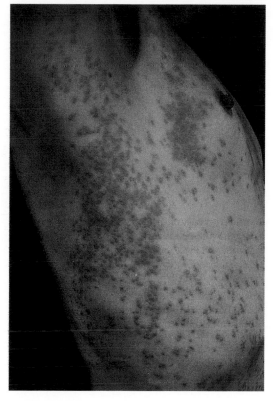

Figure 9.10 Seabather's eruption. (Source: Courtesy of Dr R. MacSween, Kingston, Ontario, Canada.)

Table 9.4 Main types of bites

	Rodent (Syn. Haverhill fever)	Snake	Dog or cat	Human bites
Description	Rat-bite fever febrile illness from scratch/bite from infected rat	The majority of snake bites do not result in envenomation; effects depend upon the type of venom	Most infections that develop from dog and cat bites are polymicrobial	Human bites are quite common, clenched fist injuries ('fight bites') being the most prevalent
Epidemiology	Risk factors for rat-bite fever are handling an infected rat, or contact with infected rat faeces	Highest incidence in South America, West Africa, the Indian subcontinent and South-East Asia	Highest incidence of dog bites occurs in school-aged children, usually on the extremities	Common
Pathophysiology	Caused by *Streptobacillus moniliformis* or *Spirillum minus*	Envenomation may cause neurotoxicity, systemic toxicity, coagulopathy, rhabdomyolysis and renal failure	Most infections are polymicrobial, including aerobic and anaerobic bacteria. Approximately 80% of dog bites lead to infection with *Capnocytophaga canimorsus*. *Pasteurella multocida* is frequently isolated from infected dog or cat bites	Infection with aerobic Gram-positive cocci may complicate. *Eikenella corrodens* is recovered from 7–29%
Clinical features	2–10 days after exposure: fever, myalgia and arthralgia, nausea, vomiting, headache, maculopapular, petechial or pustular rash on extremeties (sometimes palms and soles). Polyarthritis (50%)	Local tissue necrosis is varied, fang marks may be present. Initially non-specific malaise, nausea, vomiting. Specific signs and symptoms of envenomation may occur	Dog bites: skin lesions include a localised eschar at the bite site, cellulitis, non-specific maculopapular lesions, erythema multiforme petechiae, purpura fulminans and symmetrical peripheral gangrene. Cat bites: deep puncture wounds; hand bites are prone to osteomyelitis or septic arthritis	Semicircular or oval area of erythema or bruising and/or broken skin. Necrotising fasciitis, transmission of herpes virus and hepatitis B/C viruses have been reported
Management	Wound care. *First line:* intravenous penicillin for 5–7 days. *Second line:* tetracycline orally or doxcycline intravenously for 7 days. 25% fatality if untreated	Antivenom is the specific treatment if signs of systemic envenomation or local tissue destruction	Wound care; primary closure for simple dog wounds. Most cat wounds should be left to heal by secondary intention. Prophylactic antibiotics with co-amoxiclav. May need tetanus vaccine or rabies post-exposure prophylaxis	Wound care, leave to heal by secondary intention. Prophylactic antibiotics with co-amoxiclav if bite extends through dermis

Part 2
Inflammatory Dermatoses

Psoriasis

10

Epidemiology

Psoriasis affects 2–3% of the population in Europe and the USA. There are wide variations in the reported prevalence of psoriasis. It is more common in countries that are further from the equator and in white people, and is very rare in Native Americans and in Latin American Indians. It has two peak ages of incidence: 16–22 years and 57–62 years. This has led to the concept of type I and type II or early and late-onset psoriasis. In 35% of patients, disease onset is before the age of 20 years. M = F; earlier age of onset in women.

Based on population data, lifetime risks of psoriasis are 4%, 28% and 65% if neither, one or both parents are affected. Type I is hereditary, strongly HLA associated (particularly HLA-C:06:02), early onset and more likely to be severe and linked with guttate psoriasis. Type II is sporadic, HLA unrelated, of late onset and often mild.

There is concordance for psoriasis in 20% of monozygotic twins compared to 9% for dizygotic twins, corresponding to an estimated heritability of 68%.

Triggers include streptococcal infection, HIV infection, excessive alcohol, stress, withdrawal of systemic or potent topical corticosteroids, and drugs including lithium salts, synthetic antimalarials, interferon α and tumour necrosis factor-α (TNF-α) inhibitors, β-blockers, non-steroidal anti-inflammatory drugs and angiotensin-converting enzyme inhibitors. Psoriasis can occur in sites of cutaneous trauma and old scars (Koebner phenomenon). Cigarette smoking can exacerbate; sunlight is generally beneficial but in 5–20% of patients (predominantly young women) it may provoke psoriasis (Figure 10.1).

Psoriatic arthritis is the most frequent inflammatory disease associated with psoriasis. Inflammatory bowel disease, both Crohn disease and ulcerative colitis, is frequent, 1 in 10 people with psoriasis. Other associated immune-mediated diseases include autoimmune thyroid disease, type 1 diabetes, alopecia areata and vitiligo.

Severe psoriasis is associated with the metabolic syndrome (truncal obesity, hyperlipidaemia, hypertension and insulin resistance). The strongest of these associations is with obesity, which can be seen in childhood psoriasis and tends to predate the onset of psoriasis. There is also an increased association with chronic obstructive pulmonary disease and chronic kidney disease.

Patients with severe psoriasis die at a younger age than unaffected people and cardiovascular disease accounts for the majority of this excess mortality. There is also an increased risk of peripheral vascular disease and atrial fibrillation.

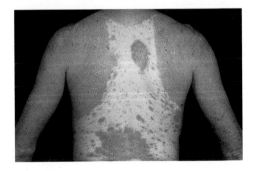

Figure 10.1 Although sunlight is generally beneficial, psoriasis may be provoked by sunlight in a minority. (Source: Courtesy of St John's Institute of Dermatology, London, UK.)

Rook's Dermatology Handbook, First Edition. Edited by Christopher E. M. Griffiths, Tanya O. Bleiker, Daniel Creamer, John R. Ingram and Rosalind C. Simpson.
© 2022 John Wiley & Sons Ltd. Published 2022 by John Wiley & Sons Ltd.

Non-alcoholic fatty liver disease is the most frequently identified liver pathology, present in up to 50%. Alcoholic liver disease is common.

Pathophysiology

Activation of T cells of the adaptive immune system, specifically Th17 cells, which in turn activate keratinocytes to proliferate and produce multiple chemokines and antimicrobial peptides. Activated T cells are of the Th1, Th17 and Th22 phenotype. In psoriasis plaques there are increased levels of IL-2, IL-8, interferon-γ, TNF-α, IL-15, IL-17, IL-22 and IL-23. There is a distinct absence of Th2 cytokines such as IL-4 and IL-10.

The three key pathological features are epidermal hyperproliferation, marked dermal and epidermal inflammatory infiltrate and increased dermal angiogenesis. In psoriasis, progression of basal cell keratinocytes through the epidermis takes only 4–5 days as opposed to 30 days in normal skin. Histology shows parakeratosis, focal orthokeratosis, and the accumulation of neutrophils in the stratum corneum (Munro microabscesses), near absence of the granular layer, spongiform pustules in the Malpighian layer, hyperplasia with elongation of rete ridges and suprapapillary epidermal thinning. There are dilated, tortuous papillary blood vessels which are surrounded by a mixed mononuclear and neutrophil infiltrate. Tissue destruction and scarring do not occur in psoriasis.

Clinical features

Pruritus is present although not as severe as in atopic eczema. Skin tightness and burning are frequent in unstable, erythrodermic or pustular psoriasis and pain may be experienced in areas of fissure formation, particularly in palmoplantar or flexural disease. Shedding of scale can be a significant symptom. It is a relapsing and remitting disorder the course of which varies between individuals.

Plaque psoriasis is the most common type, accounting for about 80–90% of all cases. Typical lesions are red scaly plaques which are well demarcated with sharply delineated edges (Figure 10.2). Plaques may be encircled by a clear peripheral zone, the halo or ring of Woronoff (Figure 10.3). When multiple, lesions are usually monomorphic and

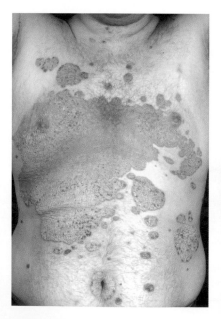

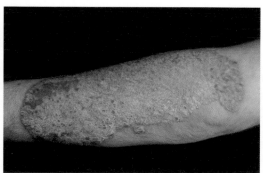

Figure 10.2 Psoriasis is characterised by well-demarcated red scaly plaques.

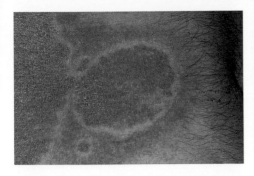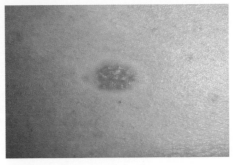

Figure 10.3 Plaques may be encircled by a clear peripheral zone, the halo or ring of Woronoff.

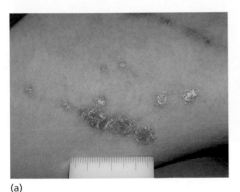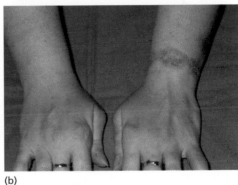

(a)   (b)

Figure 10.4 (a) Koebner phenomenon. Psoriasis appearing in the line of a scratch. (b) Psoriasis provoked by the friction of wearing a watch.

distributed symmetrically over the scalp, trunk and extensor surfaces of the limbs. They vary in diameter from one to several centimetres and are oval or irregular in shape. Large plaques may form by coalescence of smaller plaques and are commonly seen on the legs and sacral region. Involuting lesions often clear from the centre initially, producing annular or arcuate shapes. Linear and geometric configurations may arise at sites of trauma as an isomorphic (Koebner) phenomenon (Figure 10.4).

The colour of the plaques is a full rich red (sometimes referred to as 'salmon pink') (Figure 10.5). This quality of colour is of particular diagnostic value in lesions on the palms, soles and scalp. In darker skin the quality of the colour is lost (Figure 10.6). Erythema may

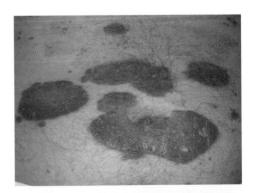

Figure 10.5 The colour of the plaques, a full rich red. (Source: Courtesy of St John's Institute of Dermatology, London, UK.)

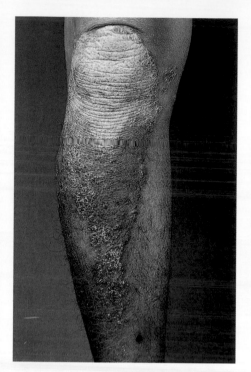

Figure 10.6 In black skin the quality of the colour is lost. (Source: Courtesy of St John's Institute of Dermatology, London, UK.)

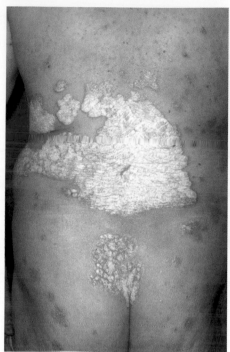

Figure 10.8 Most plaques of psoriasis are surmounted by silvery white scaling, which varies considerably in thickness.

persist at the site of a previously treated plaque for many months. Post-inflammatory hypopigmentation or hyperpigmentation are frequent and occasionally lentigines may persist following clearance of a plaque (Figure 10.7).

Plaques are covered in silvery white scales, which vary considerably in thickness (Figure 10.8). The amount of scaling may be

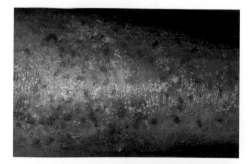

Figure 10.7 Lentigines in a plaque of psoriasis.

minimal in partially treated disease and in the flexures. The successive removal of scales usually reveals an underlying smooth, glossy red membrane with small bleeding points where the thin supra-papillary epidermis has been torn off (Auspitz sign; Figure 10.9).

The scalp is one of the first and commonest areas to be affected. The scalp may be diffusely involved, or multiple discrete plaques of varying size may be seen. Plaques tend to be restricted to hair-bearing areas, extending a short distance beyond the hairline and around the ears. May be associated with reversible hair loss. Pityriasis amiantacea (Figure 10.10) may occur (see Chapter 31).

Follicular psoriasis affecting the hair follicles on the trunk and limbs may occur as an isolated phenomenon or in association with plaque psoriasis (Figure 10.11).

Sebopsoriasis presents as plaques of thin. sharply demarcated erythema with variable scale in the typical distribution of seborrhoeic

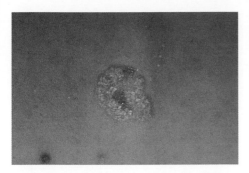

Figure 10.9 Auspitz sign: removal of the thinned suprapapillary epidermis by entle scraping reveals vascular bleeding points. (Source: Courtesy of St John's Institute of Dermatology, London, UK.)

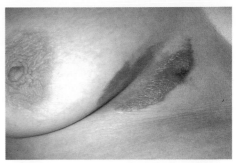

Figure 10.12 Submammary flexural psoriasis.

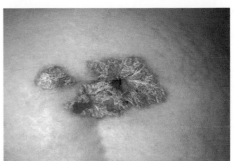

Figure 10.13 Flexural psoriasis affecting the umbilicus.

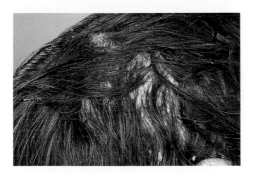

Figure 10.10 The disease often first appears in the scalp, where it may present as pityriasis amiantacea. (Source: Courtesy of St John's Institute of Dermatology, London, UK.)

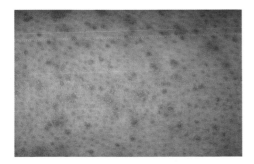

Figure 10.11 Psoriasis around hair follicle openings (follicular psoriasis).

Flexural psoriasis (Syn. Inverse psoriasis) involves the inguinal creases, axillae, submammary folds (Figure 10.12), gluteal cleft and umbilicus (Figure 10.13). It is commoner in older adults and associated with obesity. Flexural plaques are thin, scaling is greatly reduced or absent with glazed appearance. Involvement of the napkin area may be the first presentation of psoriasis in infancy.

Genital psoriasis

Genital skin is considered a flexural site. Skin of the scrotum and penile shaft may be affected, the glans penis is the most frequently affected part. In circumcised men, lesions on the glans are similar in appearance to plaques at other sites. In the uncircumcised, the plaques lack scale but the colour and well-defined edge are usually distinctive (Figure 10.14). Women with vulval involvement often complain of marked pruritus. The most common vulval presentation is a symmetrical, erythematous, non-scaly, well-demarcated thin plaque affecting the labia majora (Figure 10.15).

dermatitis, involving paranasal areas, external ears, medial eyebrows, hairline, presternal and interscapular chest wall.

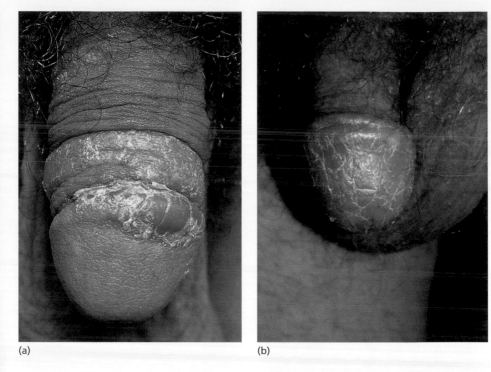

(a)   (b)

Figure 10.14 (a) Penile psoriasis in a circumcised man. (Source: Courtesy of St John's Institute of Dermatology, London, UK.) (b) Penile psoriasis in a circumcised man retaining its typical psoriatic morphology.

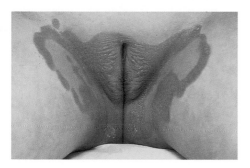

Figure 10.15 Well-demarcated thin plaques of psoriasis affecting the labia majora. (Source: Courtesy of St John's Institute of Dermatology, London, UK.)

Non-pustular palmoplantar psoriasis

On the palms and soles (Figure 10.16), psoriasis may present as typical scaly patches; less well-defined plaques resemble lichen simplex or hyperkeratotic eczema. A sharply defined edge at the wrist, forearm or palm (Figure 10.17) and absence of vesiculation are helpful to distinguish from eczema. On the dorsal surface, the knuckles frequently show a dull-red thickening of the skin. There may be a relationship to trauma or occupational irritants.

Nail psoriasis

Nail changes are present in about 40% of cases and may be seen in association with all types of psoriasis or occasionally as an isolated feature. They are associated with more extensive psoriasis, longer disease duration, family history of psoriasis and the presence of psoriatic arthritis (twice as common in the presence of nail disease).

Psoriasis may affect any part of the nail unit, including the nail matrix, nail bed and hyponychium. Nail matrix disease presents with pits, ridges and grooves of the nail plate. Pitting (Figure 10.18) is the most frequent change seen in fingernails, individual pits being uniform in

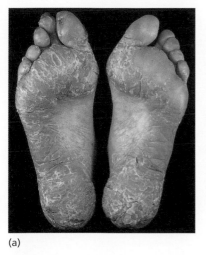

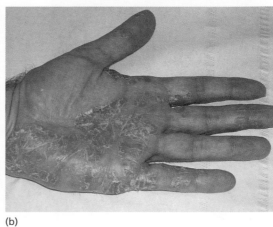

(a)   (b)

Figure 10.16 (a) On the palms and soles, psoriasis may present as typical scaly plaques. (Source: Courtesy of St John's Institute of Dermatology, London, UK.) (b) Typical psoriatic plaques on the palm.

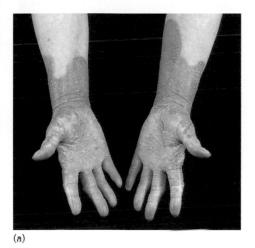

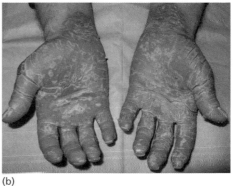

(a)   (b)

Figure 10.17 (a) A sharply defined edge at the wrist or forearm and absence of vesiculation are helpful diagnostic features. (Source: Courtesy of St John's Institute of Dermatology, London, UK.) (b) Severe confluent palmar psoriasis.

size at about 1 mm diameter and sometimes arranged longitudinally. Nail bed disease can be seen as subungual 'oil drops' which are highly specific for psoriasis (Figure 10.19). Nail bed disease also causes subungual hyperkeratosis, splinter haemorrhages and distal onycholysis (Figure 10.20). It can be difficult to distinguish clinically between toenail bed psoriasis and onychomycosis.

Mucosal lesions
True mucosal involvement is very rare. There may be an association with benign migratory glossitis (geographic tongue).

Ocular lesions
Direct involvement of the eyelids or eyelid margins may cause blepharitis. Uveitis is an important complication and is associated with more extensive psoriasis and psoriatic arthritis.

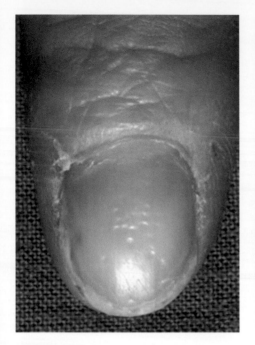

Figure 10.18 Psoriatic nail pitting. (Source: Courtesy of St John's Institute of Dermatology, London, UK.)

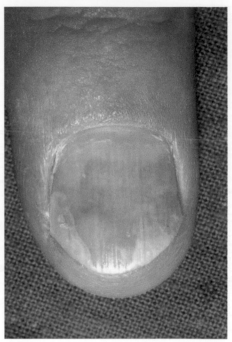

Figure 10.19 Salmon patches ('oil drops'), with distal onycholysis.

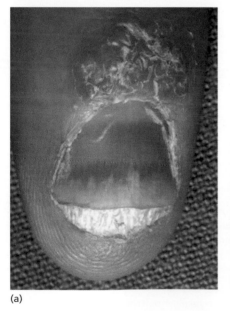

(a)

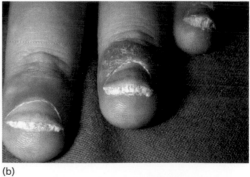

(b)

Figure 10.20 (a) Psoriatic subungual hyperkeratosis with distal onycholysis. (b) Marked psoriatic subungual hyperkeratosis.

Acute guttate psoriasis

Sudden onset of a shower of small lesions, appearing diffusely over the body (Figure 10.21). It should be distinguished from small plaque psoriasis and follicular psoriasis, which follow a more chronic course. It is more common in children and young adults, in whom it may be the first presentation of psoriasis. It frequently follows several weeks after pharyngitis caused by group A streptococci, serological evidence for which can be found in about 60% of individuals.

The lesions are from 2 or 3 mm to 1 cm in diameter, round or slightly oval often with minimal scaling. They are scattered evenly over the body with a predominant centripetal distribution. Lesions on the face are often sparse and disappear quickly. Lesions usually resolve over 3 months. Approximately one-third of patients with acute guttate psoriasis subsequently develop plaque psoriasis.

Unstable psoriasis

In some individuals and in some phases of the disease there is marked activity in the form of increasing numbers of plaques which become more inflamed (Figure 10.22). Patients complain of more pain or pruritus. The Koebner phenomenon is more frequent. The immediate outcome is unpredictable. Lesions may return to the inactive state or progress to erythrodermic psoriasis. Patients may develop such unstable phases repeatedly.

Erythrodermic psoriasis

Greater than 90% of body surface area is affected (Figure 10.23). It occurs in 1–2% of patients.

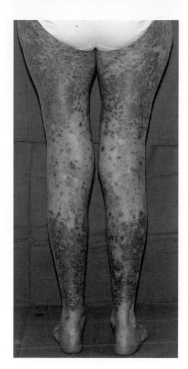

Figure 10.22 Extensive tender fiery red plaques of unstable psoriasis.

Psoriasis is the underlying cause of about 25% of cases of erythroderma. Erythroderma in psoriasis may be chronic due to the gradual extension of plaque psoriasis or acute as part of the spectrum of 'unstable' psoriasis. In the chronic form, the individual may be systemically well, the clinical characteristics of psoriasis are retained, and there are usually some areas of uninvolved skin.

The patient may be febrile and systemically ill. Dependent oedema is common. Itching is often severe. There may be clinical overlap with generalised pustular psoriasis. Untreated, the course is prolonged, relapses are frequent and there is an appreciable mortality. Complications are those of skin failure, including sepsis, hypothermia or hyperthermia, hypoalbuminaemia, anaemia, dehydration, acute kidney injury and high output cardiac failure

Atypical forms of psoriasis

Verrucous lesions particularly affect the legs. Rupioid, elephantine. and ostraceous psoriasis are terms sometimes used to describe plaques

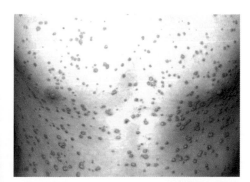

Figure 10.21 Extensive lesions of guttate psoriasis in a young man.

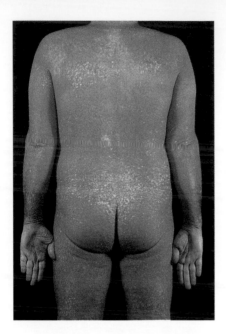

Figure 10.23 Acute erythrodermic psoriasis. (Source: Courtesy of St John's Institute of Dermatology, London, UK.)

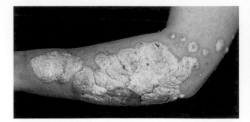

Figure 10.24 Elephantine psoriasis: large plaques with gross hyperkeratosis. (Source: Courtesy of St John's Institute of Dermatology, London, UK.)

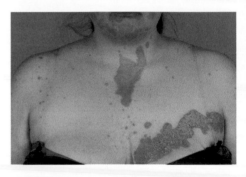

Figure 10.25 Segmental psoriasis.

associated with gross hyperkeratosis. Rupioid psoriasis refers to limpet-like cone-shaped lesions. The term elephantine psoriasis describes unusual but very persistent, thickly scaled, large plaques that sometimes occur on the back, limbs or hips (Figure 10.24). Ostraceous psoriasis refers to a ring-like hyperkeratotic lesion with a concave surface, resembling an oyster shell. True linear or segmental psoriasis, with unilateral or Blaschko linear lesions, is unusual (Figure 10.25). It is called isolated linear psoriasis when alone, or superimposed linear psoriasis when, as occurs more frequently, associated with non-segmental plaque psoriasis (Figure 10.26). Segmental manifestations are thought to represent genetic mosaicism.

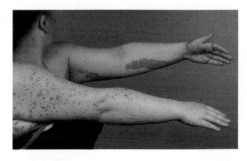

Figure 10.26 Linear psoriasis on the left arm associated with small plaque psoriasis on the right arm.

Psoriasis in childhood and old age

Psoriasis is common in children (F > M) with a cumulative prevalence up to 18 years of 0.71%. Congenital psoriasis is very rare. Psoriasis in children is significantly associated with several co-morbidities, including obesity and diabetes. There is no evidence that onset of psoriasis in childhood predicts severe disease in adult life.

All of the clinical variants of psoriasis described in adults are recognised in childhood. Establishing the diagnosis in infancy can be challenging because of limited involvement or an atypical appearance. The napkin area, frequently the first site affected under the age of 2 years, with or without disseminated lesions, presents with well-defined erythema devoid of scale. At this site, psoriasis must be differentiated from irritant contact dermatitis and seborrhoeic dermatitis.

In older children, plaque psoriasis is the most frequent presentation, and the face and ano-genital sites are affected more frequently than in adults. The disease often first appears in the scalp, where it may present as pityriasis amian-tacea. Interdigital tinea is uncommon in children and a toe cleft intertrigo may be psori-atic. Other flexural forms also occur. Although localised pustular psoriasis is extremely rare in children, parakeratosis pustulosa (an indolent and recurrent scaling pustular acrodermatitis, sometimes around the nail of only one digit) usually proves to be psoriasis. Psoriatic arthritis is uncommon in childhood.

In older age groups, psoriasis that starts for the first time after the age of 65 years tends to be less extensive than early-onset disease. Plaque psoriasis with prominent scalp involvement is the commonest phenotype. Inverse psoriasis and erythrodermic psoriasis may be more com-mon than in early-onset disease whereas gut-tate and generalised pustular psoriasis are rare.

HIV-induced or exacerbated psoriasis

Plaque psoriasis may be the first presentation of HIV infection, as may the deterioration in previously stable disease. Sebopsoriasis, rupi-oid psoriasis and erythrodermic psoriasis are also common. Psoriasis tends to be more preva-lent in the later stages of HIV-related immunod-ysfunction. Psoriasis tends to improve with a reduced viral load, especially on treatment with highly active antiretroviral therapy.

Psoriasis and mental health

Psoriasis is associated with significant psycho-logical distress, including dysfunctional thought, pathological worrying, fear of stigmati-sation and effects on self-image, personality and temperament. Excessive alcohol consump-tion has been found significantly more com-monly in men with severe psoriasis than in other groups with the disease.

Psoriasis is also associated with a significant psychiatric morbidity, with higher risk of anxiety, depression and suicide. The risk of depression in those with severe psoriasis is more frequent in younger people.

Complications

High-dose psoralen and ultraviolet A (PUVA) is known to increase the risk of cutaneous squa-mous cell carcinoma and basal cell carcinoma, and this may be compounded by immunosup-pressive treatments.

In severe disease pregnancy is associated with increased risk of spontaneous abortion, pre-eclampsia and low birth weight.

Differential diagnosis

The diseases that need to be distinguished from psoriasis vary depending on the clinical variant of psoriasis and the site affected:

- *Chronic plaque psoriasis*: lichen simplex, discoid eczema, lichen planus, pityriasis rubra pilaris, Bowen disease, tinea corporis, cutaneous lupus erythematosus and mycosis fungoides.
- *Guttate psoriasis*: pityriasis rosea, lichen planus, pityriasis lichenoides chronica and secondary syphilis.
- *Flexural psoriasis:* seborrheic dermatitis, can-didiasis, tinea cruris, bacterial intertrigo, allergic contact dermatitis and Hailey-Hailey disease.
- *Erythrodermic psoriasis*: drug-induced, eczema, cutaneous T-cell lymphoma/Sezary syn-drome and pityriasis rubra pilaris.

Investigations

The diagnosis of psoriasis is usually clinical and there is no reliable diagnostic test. A skin biopsy of lesional skin may occasionally be helpful in atypical cases. There is no constantly present laboratory abnormality in uncomplicated psoriasis. Screening for known comorbidities should also be undertaken, which will include assessments for psoriatic arthritis, metabolic syndrome and depression.

The Psoriasis Area Severity Index (PASI; Table 10.1) is the most widely used clinical measure of psoriasis severity. PASI is not appro-priate in forms of psoriasis other than plaque disease. The static Physician Global Assessment (sPGA) may be more appropriate in a non-specialist environment. There remains a need for further assessment tools for use in site-specific psoriasis, pustular psoriasis and psoria-sis in children and in pigmented skin types.

Table 10.1 Erythema, scaling and induration are graded in each region and a combined score ranging from 0 to 72 calculated as the PASI

	Thickness 0–4	Scaling 0–4	Erythema 0–4	× Area 0–6	Total
Head	a	b	c	$d(a + b + c)$	$\times 0.1 = A$
Upper limbs	e	f	g	$h(e + f + g)$	$\times 0.2 = B$
Trunk	i	j	k	$l(i + j + k)$	$\times 0.3 = C$
Lower limbs	m	n	o	$p(m + n + o)$	$\times 0.4 = D$
					$PASI = A + B + C + D$

Severity: 0, none; 1, mild; 2, moderate; 3, severe; 4, very severe.
Area: 0, no involvement; 1, 0 < 10%; 2, 10 < 30%; 3, 30 < 50%; 4, 50 < 70%; 5, 70 < 90%; 6, 90 < 100%.
Axillae, upper limb; neck/buttocks, trunk; genito-femoral, lower limb.

The most frequently used measure of health-related quality of life is the skin-specific tool the Dermatology Life Quality Index (DLQI).

Severe psoriasis has been variously defined as PASI > 12, PASI ≥ 10 with DLQI > 10 or a score of 10 or more in either PASI or DLQI.

Staphylococci are often grown from a skin swab but are rarely locally pathogenic, but this may be a concern if orthopaedic surgery is being considered.

Management

Plaque psoriasis is chronic and persistent, changing little over years. In between a third and a half of patients spontaneous remission may occur. Guttate attacks carry a better prognosis than those of a slower and more diffuse onset, and have longer remissions after treatment. Conversely, erythrodermic and pustular forms carry an appreciable mortality and arthropathic forms a considerable morbidity.

The importance of talking to patients, trying to allay their concerns, coupled with advice on how to handle negative beliefs about their disease cannot be overestimated. Cognitive behavioural therapy is a useful adjunct to pharmaceutical therapies.

Attention to the patient's general, physical and psychological health is always worthwhile. Known comorbidities, for instance psoriatic arthritis and cardiovascular disease, should be actively looked for and treated. Lifestyle and behaviours that contribute to general health and treatment responsiveness such as weight management and smoking cessation should be addressed.

The disease remains incurable and there is no current evidence that treatment alters its natural history.

Mild plaque psoriasis without psoriatic arthritis. *First line*: Coal tar, dithranol, potent topical corticosteroid or vitamin D analogue often combined with corticosteroid.
Second line: Local narrow band UVB or PUVA, excimer laser.

Moderate to severe plaque psoriasis without psoriatic arthritis. *First line*: Narrow band UVB or PUVA.
Second line: Acitretin, apremilast, ciclosporin, fumaric acid esters (where available), methotrexate.
Third line: Anti-TNF; anti-IL23/12, anti-IL17, anti-IL23 biologics.

Moderate to severe plaque psoriasis with psoriatic arthritis. *First line*: Apremilast, methotrexate.
Second line: anti-TNF, anti-IL23/12, anti-IL17 and anti-IL23 biologics.
Third line: Combination therapy.

PUSTULAR PSORIASIS

Pustules may be provoked within plaques of psoriasis as part of an unstable phase of the disease: this is better considered 'plaque psoriasis with pustules' rather than a form of pustular psoriasis per se (Figure 10.27). Under these circumstances, pustules can often more readily be seen by dermoscopy (Figure 10.28).

Pustular psoriasis consists of a clinically heterogeneous group of diseases and their place within the spectrum of psoriatic disease is being refined as their molecular genetic basis is further resolved. It is useful to separate these

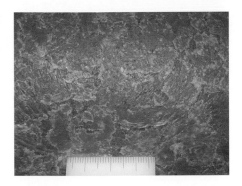

Figure 10.27 Pustulation in unstable psoriasis – 'psoriasis with pustules' – rather than pustular psoriasis.

conditions into localised and generalised pustular psoriasis, but there is clinical overlap and recent molecular genetic studies have revealed mutations in *IL36RN* at varying frequencies in both localised and generalised pustular psoriasis. In the localised forms, the disease is usually confined largely to the hands and feet, and tends to be chronic. In the generalised forms, the whole body may be involved and the course is subacute, acute or even fulminating and life threatening.

The conventional classification is shown in Box 10.1.

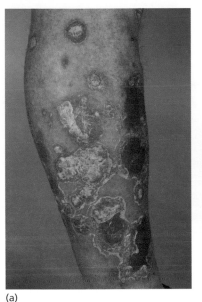

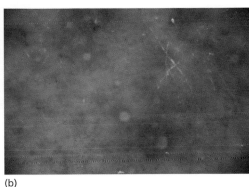

(a)   (b)

Figure 10.28 (a) Inflammatory unstable psoriasis. (b) Close-up of pustules on dermoscopy.

Box 10.1 Classification of pustular psoriasis

Generalised pustular psoriasis

Clinical variants (based on morphology and natural history):
  i) Acute generalised pustular psoriasis (von Zumbusch)
  ii) Subacute annular and circinate pustular psoriasis (Lapière)

Other specified forms (based on age or precipitants):

  i) Acute generalised pustular psoriasis of pregnancy (impetigo herpetiformis)
  ii) Infantile and juvenile generalised pustular psoriasis

Localised pustular psoriasis

  i) Palmoplantar pustulosis
  ii) Acrodermatitis continua of Hallopeau

Generalised pustular psoriasis

An acute, subacute or occasionally chronic eruption with generalised sterile pustulosis as its central feature.

Epidemiology

Generalised pustular psoriasis (GPP) is rare. The incidence peaks between 40 and 59 years of age, but infantile and juvenile cases are also reported. The age at onset tends to be earlier in those with pure GPP without plaque psoriasis. F:M = 2:1.

Inflammatory polyarthritis is common. The metabolic syndrome is also frequently associated.

Pathophysiology

Triggers are the same as for chronic plaque psoriasis, see above.

In acute GPP there is intense inflammation with a mixed inflammatory infiltrate and spongiform pustule formation (Kogoj pustules). Microabscesses are present along with acanthosis with elongation of rete ridges. The stratum corneum soon becomes parakeratotic and the subcorneal pustule is shed as epidermal turnover is accelerated.

Deleterious germline mutations in *IL36RN* have been reported in familial and sporadic GPP in certain populations. *IL36RN* encodes the IL-36 receptor antagonist (IL36-Ra), which is expressed primarily in the skin and is an antagonist of three pro-inflammatory cytokines of the IL-1 family (IL-36α, -β and -γ). There is some evidence for genotype–phenotype correlation as *IL36RN* mutations are present in a lower proportion of GPP patients with concomitant or prior plaque psoriasis than in those with 'pure' GPP.

Clinical features

Some patients may have phases of plaque psoriasis before or after the GPP, but in others it occurs as the sole phenotype without plaque psoriasis at any time. In the acute stage, there is a burning painful sensation in the skin, usually without a prodrome. Fever and malaise accompany the development of waves of pustules. About a third of patients complain of arthralgia.

Acute GPP (von Zumbusch)

This is the most acute and severe form and is clinically and genetically heterogeneous. It may occur as the sole phenotype or arise following plaque psoriasis, acrodermatitis continua of Hallopeau or palmoplantar pustulosis. It may manifest only in pregnancy, when it has been referred to as impetigo herpetiformis, and may be the phenotype in infantile and juvenile generalised pustular psoriasis. Diagnostic criteria have been proposed consisting of recurrent episodes of fever with general malaise, multiple isolated sterile pustules and laboratory abnormalities (leukocytosis, elevated erythrocyte sedimentation rate or C-reactive protein), supported by Kogoj's spongiform pustules on histopathology.

It may be atypical initially, restricted to acral or flexural sites but rapidly and spontaneously progresses to the generalised pustular form. Pre-existing lesions become fiery and develop pinpoint pustules (Figure 10.29) or sheets of

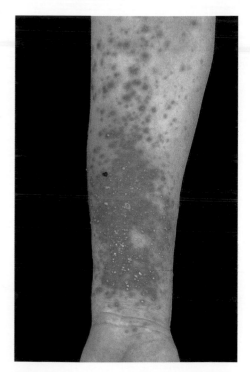

Figure 10.29 Acute generalised pustular psoriasis: pre-existing psoriasis plaques become fiery and develop pinpoint pustules. (Source: Courtesy of St John's Institute of Dermatology, London, UK.)

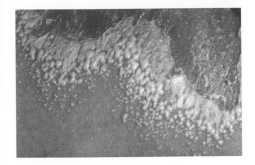

Figure 10.30 Acute generalised pustular psoriasis of von Zumbusch.

erythema and pustulation spread to involve previously unaffected skin, the flexures and genital regions being particularly involved (Figure 10.30). Any configuration or variety of pustular exanthem may occur, for instance isolated pustules, lakes of pus, circinate lesions, plaques of erythema with pustular collarettes or a generalised erythroderma. Waves of pustulation may succeed each other, subsiding into exfoliation of the dried pustules. The nails become thickened or separated by subungual lakes of pus. The buccal mucosa and tongue may be involved. Remission may occur within days or weeks, the psoriasis returning to its normal state, or erythroderma develops. Relapses are common.

Subacute annular GPP

Annular and other patterned lesions are more characteristic of the rarer subacute or chronic forms of widespread pustular psoriasis. This is a common presentation of GPP in infancy and early childhood. Lesions begin as discrete areas of erythema, which become raised and oedematous. Slow centrifugal spread may mimic erythema annulare centrifugum (Lapiere). Pustules appear peripherally on the crest of the advancing edge, become desiccated and leave a trailing fringe of scale as the lesion slowly advances (Figure 10.31). There are no systemic symptoms.

Acute GPP of pregnancy
(Syn. Impetigo herpetiformis)

This is a rare entity that presents in pregnancy (usually last trimester). The disease tends to persist until delivery. The features are of GPP, usually of flexural onset and with a marked tendency to symmetry, and sometimes grouping of areas of pustulation. Usually starts in the inguinogenital region and other flexures, with minute pustules arising on an acutely inflamed area of skin. These extend centrifugally, drying in the centre, or form plaques, which may become widespread. As individual areas heal, they leave a reddish brown pigmentation. The tongue, buccal mucosa and even the oesophagus may be involved, with circinate or erosive lesions following short-lived pustules.

PART 2: INFLAMMATORY DERMATOSES

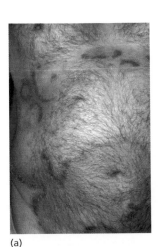

(a)

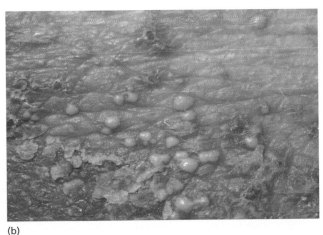

(b)

Figure 10.31 (a) Subacute annular generalised pustular psoriasis. (b) Monomorphic non-follicular pustules of generalised pustular psoriasis (von Zumbusch).

Constitutional disturbance is characteristically severe with fever, and death may occur due to cardiac or renal failure. The more severe and longstanding the disease, the greater the risks of placental insufficiency leading to stillbirth, neonatal death or fetal abnormalities. Characteristically, the disease recurs in subsequent pregnancies.

Infantile and juvenile GPP. All forms of pustular psoriasis are rare in childhood, accounting for about 1% of severe psoriasis in this age group; in over 25% of cases onset has been in the first year of life.

When the onset is in infancy, systemic symptoms are often absent and spontaneous remissions may occur. In at least one-third of infantile cases a history of an eruption diagnosed as seborrhoeic dermatitis, napkin dermatitis or sudden-onset napkin psoriasis is obtained. Often localised to flexural areas, for instance the neck.

The majority of children are aged 2–10 years at onset. Annular and circinate forms are commonest in this age group. Attacks often settle within a few days, but repeated waves of inflammation may follow.

Complications of GPP

In the acute phase, the affected individual is systemically unwell. Hypovolaemia and oligaemia can cause acute kidney injury. Hypoalbuminaemia in the acute episode may be profound, perhaps because of a sudden loss of plasma protein into the tissues and intestinal malabsorption. Hypocalcaemia may arise as a consequence of the hypoalbuminaemia and malabsorption. Abnormalities of liver enzymes are common. Staphylococcal infection may complicate GPP.

Differential diagnosis

Systemic infection, acute generalised exanthematous pustulosis, pemphigus foliaceus, bowel bypass syndrome, Sweet syndrome and Behçet syndrome.

Investigations

Skin biopsy may be needed when diagnosis is uncertain. ESR rate and CRP are usually raised. Check FBC (neutrophilia), plasma albumin, zinc and calcium.

Management

There is a paucity of data on the long-term prognosis of GPP. The prognosis is good for subacute annular and circinate GPP and, as a consequence, for GPP in infants and children.

The treatment of acute GPP often requires in-patient dermatological management with topical and usually systemic drug therapy, general supportive measures and removal of possible provocative factors. Excessive heat loss must be prevented by maintaining an adequate ambient temperature. Fluid balance should be monitored so that the daily urine volume remains adequate. Infection, where present, should be treated rigorously with the appropriate antibiotics.

First line: Bed rest in hospital, mild sedation, greasy emollients with fluid and protein replacement, acitretin (avoid in pregnancy), ciclosporin, methotrexate (avoid in pregnancy).

Second line: Infliximab, adalimumab, etanercept, prednisolone (special circumstances only), anti-IL-36.

Palmoplantar pustulosis

Palmoplantar pustulosis (PPP) is a common condition in which erythematous and scaly plaques studded with sterile pustules persist on the palms or soles. It is chronic and very resistant to treatment. It is a distinct entity, but one-fifth of patients may develop chronic plaque psoriasis.

Epidemiology

Prevalence is up to 0.05%. Onset may be in early adult life, but peaks between the ages of 30 and 50 years. F:M = 5:1.

There is an association with autoimmune thyroid disease and thyroid antibodies have been found in association. Some patients also have antigliadin antibodies.

Pathophysiology

Usually starts without obvious provocation. Cigarette smoking has been reported to be strongly associated: more than 90% of patients are current or previous smokers and in some instances the disease improves in those who manage to stop smoking. PPP is one of the commonest morphologies seen in patients who develop psoriasiform rashes on exposure to TNF inhibitors for the treatment of rheumatoid arthritis or Crohn disease.

Histology is similar to GPP, but early lesions are vesicles that develop into pustules containing mononuclear cells and neutrophils as they become more superficial. Keratinocytes from the interductal epidermis of PPP show an altered staining pattern for nicotinic acetylcholine receptors. The pustules in palmoplantar pustulosis are sterile.

Molecular genetic studies have demonstrated that it is genetically distinct from plaque psoriasis. There is no association with the major psoriasis susceptibility locus *PSORS1* or *HLA-C:06:02*.

Clinical features

Itching is variable; the patient complains of 'burning' discomfort in the lesions. The disease presents with one or more well-defined plaques. On the hands, the thenar eminence is the most common site involved. Less commonly, the hypothenar eminence or the central palm or the distal palm are involved. On the feet, the instep, the medial or lateral border are affected. Striking symmetry of the lesions on the hands or feet is common, but sometimes a solitary lesion persists for months before others appear.

The affected area is dusky red and scaly, and fissures may develop. Within this plaque, numerous pustules are present, usually 2–5 mm in diameter. In early disease, dermoscopy can help to identify vesicles, or vesicopustules within plaques, the lesions arising at the top of dermatoglyphic ridges. Fresh pustules are yellow; older ones are yellow-brown or dark brown as the pustule dries. Normally, pustules in all stages of evolution are seen (Figures 10.32 and 10.33). Eventually, the desiccated pustule is exfoliated. Plaques of psoriasis may be present elsewhere on the body in a minority of patients and may be mild and atypical.

PPP is the commonest cutaneous manifestation of a group of rare diseases characterised by sterile osteitis or synovitis known as SAPHO syndrome (synovitis, acne, pustulosis, hyperostosis and osteitis; Syn. Pustulotic arthroosteitis). This most frequently involves the anterior chest wall but may also involve the axial skeleton.

Differential diagnosis

Tinea, vesicular dermatitis and allergic contact dermatitis. Tinea is usually unilateral and the toe clefts may be involved.

Investigations
Clinical diagnosis

Skin scrapings for mycological examination may be needed, and occasionally bacterial swabs or patch testing may be indicated.

Management

The course is usually prolonged. Remission is rare. Effective therapy is elusive and treatment often disappointing.

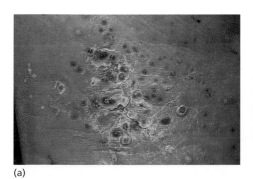

(a)

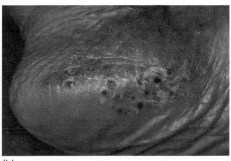

(b)

Figure 10.32 (a) Palmoplantar pustulosis. Normally, pustules in all stages of evolution are seen. (Source: Courtesy of St John's Institute of Dermatology, London, UK.) (b) Palmoplantar pustulosis of the heel.

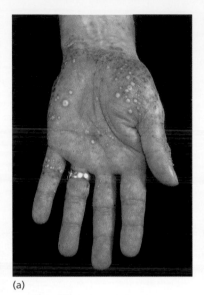

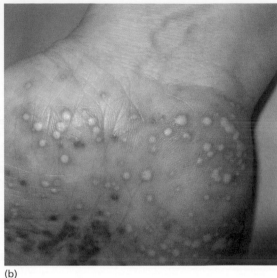

(a) (b)

Figure 10.33 (a) Acute palmoplantar pustulosis. (Source: Courtesy of St John's Institute of Dermatology, London, UK.) (b) Acute palmoplantar pustulosis.

First line: Super-potent topical corticosteroid, ± occlusion.

Second line: Acitretin; ciclosporin; oral or topical PUVA ± acitretin.

Third line: Methotrexate, fumaric acid esters, alitretinoin, adalimumab, infliximab, ustekinumab.

Acrodermatitis continua of Hallopeau

A rare chronic sterile pustular eruption affecting initially the tips of the fingers or toes that tends slowly to extend locally but which may evolve into GPP.

Epidemiology

Commoner in older adults, may be seen in children. F > M.

Pathophysiology

The features are similar to those of GPP. In the epidermis, there are numerous subcorneal neutrophilic pustules and spongiform pustules with hypergranulosis and parakeratotic hyperkeratosis.

There is a lymphocytic infiltrate in the dermis, which in chronic disease may become atrophic.

Clinical features

The distribution of lesions is distinctive, as is the local destruction of soft tissue, nail apparatus and sometimes the terminal digit. The first lesion starts on a finger or thumb more often than on a toe. The skin over the distal phalanx becomes red and scaly, and pustules develop. The nail folds and nail bed may be involved, leading to nail dystrophy. The proximal edge of the lesion is bordered by a fringe of undermined epidermis, irregular, often sodden and sometimes preceded by a line of vesiculopustules. Removal of scale or desiccation of pustules may leave a brighter red, glazed, very sore and painful digit. Slow proximal extension is the rule, but this may take several years. Eventually, other digits may be involved. The nail plate may be completely destroyed (Figure 10.34). Bone changes can occur with osteolysis of the tuft of the distal phalanx. The free end of the digit may become wasted and tapered, mimicking scleroderma.

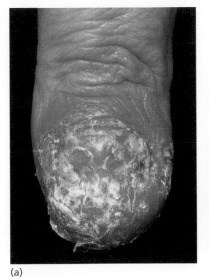

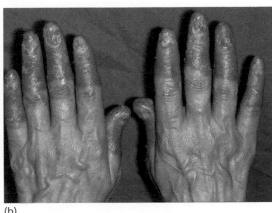

(a)   (b)

Figure 10.34 (a) Acrodermatitis continua with destruction of the nail plate. (Source: Courtesy of St John's Institute of Dermatology, London, UK.) (b) Acrodermatitis continua in the acute phase.

In such digits, the circulation may be secondarily affected so that discomfort is greatest in cold weather. Acrodermatitis continua of Hallopeau may evolve into GPP, especially in the elderly.

Differential diagnosis
In the earliest stage, staphylococcal infection, pulp infection, herpetic whitlow, tinea or contact dermatitis may be suspected.

Investigations
The diagnosis can usually be made clinically. Swabs should be taken for bacterial culture.

Management
The usual course is prolonged. Slow spread or extension may be refractory to all treatment. Spontaneous remission can occur but is more often temporary than permanent.

First line: Super-potent topical corticosteroid ± occlusion.
Second line: Acitretin; ciclosporin.
Third line: Adalimumab.

PSORIATIC ARTHRITIS

A seronegative inflammatory arthritis, which occurs in up to 40% of patients with moderate to severe psoriasis. It can be destructive to joints and adds considerably to the impairment of quality of life and symptoms such as fatigue suffered by patients with psoriasis. In 70% of patients the skin features of psoriasis develop prior to joint disease, in 20% of patients the joint disease presents first, and in 10% the skin and joints are affected concurrently. In rheumatology practice, psoriatic arthritis can be differentiated from other forms of arthritis according to the Classification Criteria for Psoriatic Arthritis (CASPAR), with 99% sensitivity and 91% specificity (Table 10.2).

Table 10.2 CASPAR criteria for psoriatic arthritis. To be characterised as having psoriatic arthritis, a patient with inflammatory articular disease (joint, spine or entheseal) must have three or more points from five categories. Each category scores a maximum of 1 point, except category 1, which scores 2 points for current psoriasis.

Psoriasis	Current psoriasis	2
	Personal history of psoriasis	1
	Psoriasis in a first- or second-degree relative	1
Typical psoriatic nail involvement		1
A negative test for rheumatoid factor		1
Dactylitis (Figure 10.35), interphalangeal joint involvement (Figure 10.36), arthritis mutilans (Figure 10.37)	Current dactylitis	1
	History of dactylitis	1
Radiological evidence of juxta-articular new bone formation		1

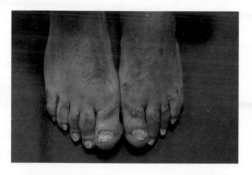

Figure 10.35 Dactylitis.

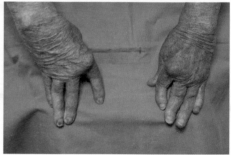

Figure 10.37 Arthritis mutilans.

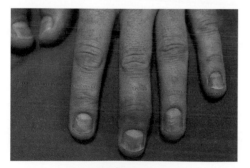

Figure 10.36 Distal interphalangeal involvement.

Pityriasis rubra pilaris

11

Pityriasis rubra pilaris (PRP) is a papulosquamous dermatosis of unknown cause. It is divided into five clinical types and a sixth type related to HIV infection.

Epidemiology

Uncommon, occurring in less than 1 in 5000.

A rare familial form starts in early childhood. The acquired forms have a bimodal age distribution with peaks in the first and fifth decades. M = F.

Pathophysiology

Pathogenesis is unknown. The rare genetic form has been linked to gain-of-function mutations in the *CARD14* gene. It has been associated with HIV infection.

The histological features are not pathognomonic but allow discrimination from psoriasis and other causes of erythroderma.

Hyperkeratosis occurs with follicular plugging. Ortho- and parakeratosis may alternate and the follicles can show foci of parakeratosis in the perifollicular shoulder. Patchy or confluent hypergranulosis may occur. Dermal capillaries are dilated but are not tortuous as seen in psoriasis. Acantholysis may be present, often restricted to adnexal epithelium.

Associated with various autoimmune diseases, including systemic sclerosis and autoimmune thyroiditis.

Clinical features

The more common generalised sporadic forms (types I and III) tend to have an acute onset. The rare familial form of PRP (type V) generally has a slow and gradual onset.

Patients typically present with well-defined salmon-red or orange-red dry scaly plaques, which may coalesce and become widespread. Patches of normal skin are present, 'islands of sparing'. Pruritus may be present in the early stages.

The disease often starts on the scalp before spreading down the rest of the body. Some patients may become erythrodermic. There is dependent oedema and risk of high-output cardiac failure in erythrodermic patients.

On the elbows, wrists and the backs of the fingers characteristic follicular hyperkeratosis may be present, 'nutmeg grater' papules. Palms and soles may become thickened and fissured with an orange discolouration. In type IV, the disease is largely limited to the extremities.

Clinical variants

Six clinical variants have been described.

Classical adult-onset PRP (type I)

This is the most common and recognisable form, representing some 50% of cases. It usually starts as an erythematous slightly scaly macule on the head, neck or upper trunk. Further macules appear within a few weeks and at this stage it may be mistaken for seborrhoeic dermatitis. The true diagnosis becomes apparent with the appearance of a profusion of erythematous perifollicular papules, each with a central acuminate keratotic plug. Follicular lesions are initially discrete but then coalesce to form groups of two, three or more. Irritation may be pronounced as the disease spreads (Figure 11.1a).

Interfollicular erythema appears and the follicular lesions are gradually submerged in sheets of erythema of a slight orange hue, which typically spreads from the head to the feet. The face becomes uniformly erythematous and mild ectropion may follow (Figure 11.2a). There is diffuse bran-like scaling on the scalp. Erythroderma frequently develops within 2–3 months

Rook's Dermatology Handbook, First Edition. Edited by Christopher E. M. Griffiths, Tanya O. Bleiker, Daniel Creamer, John R. Ingram and Rosalind C. Simpson.
© 2022 John Wiley & Sons Ltd. Published 2022 by John Wiley & Sons Ltd.

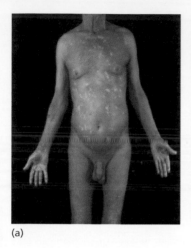 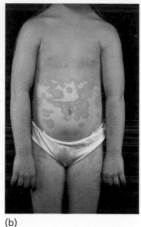 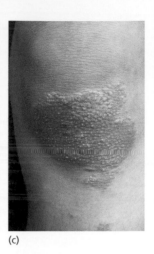

(a) (b) (c)

Figure 11.1 PRP: (a) classical adult-onset, type I; (b) classical juvenile-onset, type III; and (c) circumscribed juvenile-onset, type IV. Note: 'islands of sparing' in erythrodermic type I PRP (a), orange-red erythema with cephalocaudal downward extension in type III PRP (b) and prominent 'nutmeg-grater' keratotic follicular spines in type IV PRP (c).

(Figure 11.1a). Island sparing is usually present (Figure 11.1a). The palms and soles become hyperkeratotic and yellow (Figure 11.2b–d). The nails are thickened and discoloured distally, showing splinter haemorrhages, but unlike psoriasis there is no dystrophy of the nail plate and pitting is minimal (Figure 11.2e).

Untreated, type I PRP eventually resolves in an average of 3 years.

Atypical adult-onset PRP (type II)
A more chronic form, which may last many years. The scaling is more variable and many patients show eczematous features and the keratoderma is coarser than in other types. The rapid progression of inflammation from the head down towards the feet as occurs in type I PRP does not occur and erythroderma is less common.

Classical juvenile-onset PRP (type III)
The most common childhood form of PRP, considered to be the counterpart of type I PRP but

with an onset between the ages of 5 and 10 years (Figure 11.1b). Usually undergoes spontaneous resolution in 1–2 years.

Circumscribed juvenile PRP (type IV)
This type occurs in prepubertal children under 12 years of age. Commonest features are well-circumscribed plaques of erythema and follicular hyperkeratosis occurring on the elbows and knees (Figures 11.1c and 11.3a,b). Scattered erythematous scaly macules may be present on the trunk and scalp. Palmoplantar keratoderma may be observed (Figure 11.3c–d). The prognosis is uncertain but may remit in teenage years.

Atypical juvenile PRP (type V)
Familial PRP is most often of this type, which may be genetically heterogeneous and difficult to distinguish from ichthyoses and erthyrokeratoderma. It may be present at birth or start in early childhood with erythema and hyperkeratosis.

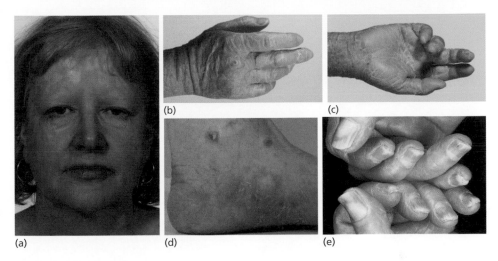

Figure 11.2 Classical adult-onset PRP: (a) confluent orange-red erythema on the face and neck with prominent 'islands of sparing'; (b)–(d) prominent erythema and scale on the dorsa of the hands and wrists with marked orange-yellow palmoplantar keratoderma; (e) thickening of the nails, subungual hyperkeratosis and splinter haemorrhages.

Follicular hyperkeratosis is a prominent feature and keratoderma is common.

HIV-related PRP (type VI)

This form tends to resemble type I PRP and to be resistant to treatment. It may, however, respond to antiretroviral therapy.

Differential diagnosis

Dermatoses with erythema and follicular hyperkeratosis should be considered. These include psoriasis, erythrokeratoderma variabilis, Sézary syndrome and other T-cell lymphomas, and other forms of erythroderma.

Type IV PRP shares many clinical features with keratosis circumscripta.

Investigations

Diagnosis is made on clinical features and supported by histology. No other tests are indicated.

Management

In a disease in which spontaneous resolution is the norm (Figure 11.4), claims of treatment success must be balanced against this. Patients who are erythrodermic may need intense supportive care to prevent hypothermia, electrolyte imbalance, protein loss and sepsis.

First line: Emollients, topical corticosteroids, acitretin.

Second line: Methotrexate, ustekinumab.

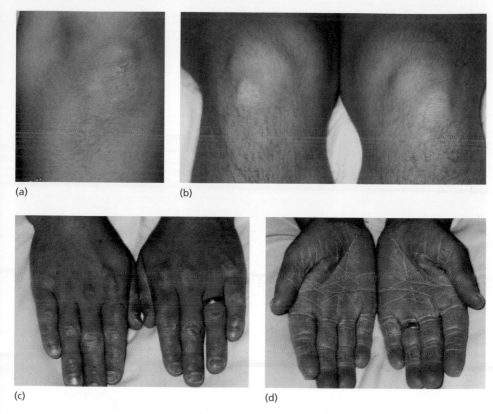

(a)   (b)

(c)   (d)

Figure 11.3 Juvenile-onset circumscribed PRP may persist into adulthood, as here: (a), (b) circumscribed areas of hyperkeratosis over the elbows and knees may not show prominent follicular hyperkeratosis; (c), (d) there may be prominent involvement both of the dorsa of the hands and feet and of the palms and soles.

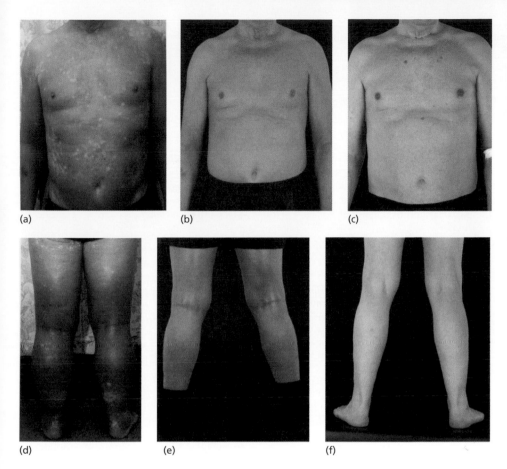

(a) (b) (c)

(d) (e) (f)

Figure 11.4 Resolution of type I PRP: (a), (d) erythrodermic PRP at presentation 6 months after initial onset in a 60-year-old male: note 'islands of sparing' and dramatic oedema of lower extremities; (b), (e) significant improvement over ensuing 12 weeks with acitretrin therapy; (c), (f) complete resolution and off therapy 18 months after presentation.

12

Lichen planus and lichenoid disorders

Lichenoid disorders are inflammatory dermatoses characterised clinically by flat-topped, papular lesions and histologically by a lymphocytic infiltrate with a band-like distribution in the papillary dermis. Lichen planus (LP) is the prototype.

Lichen planus

The most typical and best characterised lichenoid dermatosis is an idiopathic inflammatory disease affecting the skin and mucosal membranes.

Epidemiology

Incidence varies between 0.22% and 1% of the adult population worldwide. Oral LP has a reported incidence between 1% and 4% of the population. Rare in children; commonly affects adults during the fourth to sixth decade. F = M.

Pathophysiology

A T-cell-mediated autoimmune disease, targeting the basal keratinocytes, which has a variety of triggers, including viruses, drugs and contact allergens.

The lymphocytic infiltrate of LP is composed of CD8+ T cells with a significant proportion of γ-δ T cells. CD1a+ Langerhans cells and factor XIIIa+ cells are increased and may be involved in antigen presentation to T cells.

Environmental factors associated with LP:

- Drugs include antimicrobials, antihypertensives, antimalarials, antidepressants, anticonvulsants, diuretics, metals, non-steroidal anti-inflammatory drugs imatinib,

intravenous immunoglobulin, TNF-inhibitor biologics.
- Dental amalgam and Betel nut.
- Radiotherapy confined to the radiation field.
- Hepatitis B vaccines.

Histology demonstrates an increase in epidermal Langerhans cells associated with a superficial perivascular infiltrate of lymphocytes and histiocytes, impinging on the dermal–epidermal junction (DEJ). A focal increase in the thickness of the granular layer and infiltrate corresponds to the presence of Wickham's striae. Degenerating basal epidermal cells are transformed into *colloid bodies* (15–20 μm diameter), which appear singly or in clumps. The rete ridges may appear flattened or effaced (*'saw-tooth' appearance*), and focal separation from the dermis may lead to Max Joseph spaces. In older or hypertrophic lesions, the number of colloid bodies is considerably reduced. In 'active' LP, a *band-like infiltrate* of lymphocytes and histiocytes, rarely admixed with plasma cells, obliterates the DEJ. Epidermal melanocytes are absent or considerably decreased in number, while *pigmentary incontinence* with dermal melanophages is characteristic. Benign lichenoid keratoses are usually solitary but may be multiple and show characteristic lichenoid infiltrates of lymphocytes, occasional parakeratosis and apoptotic bodies in the epidermis without nuclear atypia of keratinocytes.

Clinical features

The classic clinical presentation of LP includes primary lesions consisting of firm, flat-topped, shiny, polygonal, 1–3 mm diameter papules with a red to violet colour. More closely, a

Rook's Dermatology Handbook, First Edition. Edited by Christopher E. M. Griffiths, Tanya O. Bleiker, Daniel Creamer, John R. Ingram and Rosalind C. Simpson.
© 2022 John Wiley & Sons Ltd. Published 2022 by John Wiley & Sons Ltd.

tracery of thin white lines can be seen on the surface of the lesions, known as Wickham's striae (Figure 12.1). Papules can be isolated or grouped, in a linear or annular distribution. Typically, a greyish brown pigmentation can be observed in lesions that have resolved due to deposition of melanin in the superficial dermis. Annular lesions are common on the penis (Figure 12.2) and rarely may be the predominant type of lesion present, later leading to atrophy. It can affect any part of the body surface, but is most often seen on the volar aspect of the wrists (Figure 12.3), the lumbar region and around the ankles. The ankles and shins are the commonest sites for hypertrophic lesions. When the palms and soles are affected, the lesions tend to be firm and rough with a yellowish hue (Figure 12.4). Linear LP occurring on Blashko's lines can also be observed.

Mucous membrane lesions are very common, occurring in 30–70% of cases, and may be present without evidence of skin lesions. They are, however, much less common in black people. The buccal mucosa and tongue are most often involved, but lesions may be found around the anus, on the genitalia, in the larynx and, very rarely, on the tympanic membranes or in the oesophagus. White streaks, often forming a lacework, on the buccal mucosa are highly characteristic (Figure 12.5). They may be seen on the inner surface of the cheeks, on the gum margins or on the lips. On the tongue, the lesions are usually in the form of fixed, white plaques, often slightly depressed below the surrounding normal mucous membrane, especially on the upper surface and edges (Figure 12.6). Ulcerative lesions can occur in the mouth (Figure 12.7).

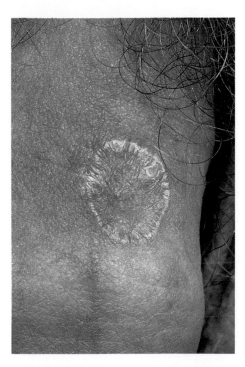

Figure 12.2 Lichen planus showing annular lesion on the shaft of the penis. (Source: Courtesy of St John's Institute of Dermatology, King's College London, UK.)

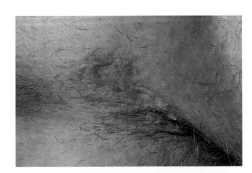

Figure 12.1 Lichen planus. Close up to show Wickham's striae. (Source: Courtesy of the Welsh Institute of Dermatology, University Hospital of Wales, Cardiff, Wales, UK.)

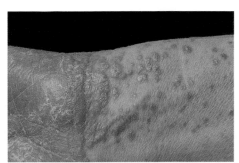

Figure 12.3 Lichen planus. Classic eruption on the volar aspect of the wrist. (Source: Courtesy of the Welsh Institute of Dermatology, University Hospital of Wales, Cardiff, Wales, UK.)

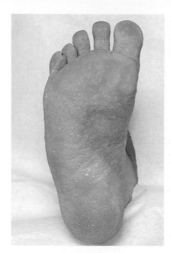
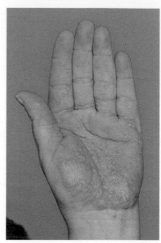

Figure 12.4 Lichen planus of the palms and feet showing hyperkeratosis and a yellow colour. (Source: Courtesy of the Welsh Institute of Dermatology, University Hospital of Wales, Cardiff, Wales, UK.)

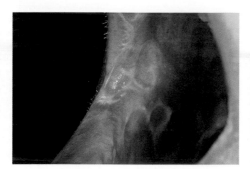

Figure 12.5 Lichen planus on the buccal mucosa showing a lacework of white streaks. (Source: Courtesy of the Welsh Institute of Dermatology, University Hospital of Wales, Cardiff, Wales, UK.)

Pruritus ranges from occasional mild irritation to more or less continuous, severe itching. Hypertrophic lesions usually itch severely. Paradoxically, there is seldom evidence of scratching, as the patient tends to rub to gain relief. Oral lesions may produce discomfort, stinging or pain; ulcerated lesions are especially painful.

LP principally involving mucous membranes

Lesions confined to the mouth, or with minimal accompanying skin involvement, account for

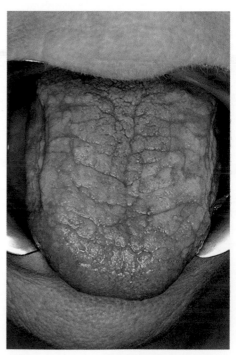

Figure 12.6 Lichen planus of the tongue showing irregular, fixed, white plaques. (Source: Courtesy of the Welsh Institute of Dermatology, University Hospital of Wales, Cardiff, Wales, UK.)

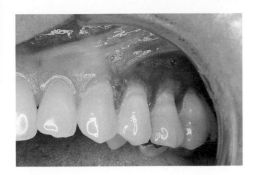

Figure 12.7 Erosive lichen planus of the buccal mucosa. (Source: Courtesy of the Welsh Institute of Dermatology, University Hospital of Wales, Cardiff, Wales, UK.)

15% of cases. Lesions do not differ from those found in connection with skin lesions. Distinct clinical subtypes such as reticular, atrophic, hypertrophic and erosive forms occur either together or in isolation. Differential diagnosis includes lichenoid drug eruption, leukoplakia on the tongue and buccal mucosa, gingivitis or chronic candidiasis on the gum margin, 'smoker's patches' on the palate and white-sponge naevi, which occur mainly on the floor of the mouth. Oesophageal LP may result in dysphagia and benign strictures.

In young men, the lesions are sometimes restricted to the genitalia and/or mouth. Genital lesions, which are usually characteristic, may be present on the penile shaft (Figure 12.2), glans penis, prepuce or scrotum. The presence of buccal mucosal lesions will usually confirm the diagnosis. Lesions on the female genitalia are common, occurring alone or combined with lesions in the mouth or more extensive disease. Involvement of the vulva spans a spectrum from subtle, fine, reticulate papules to severe erosive disease accompanied by dyspareunia, scarring and loss of the normal vulvar architecture. Diagnostic criteria include well-demarcated erosions/erythematous areas at the vaginal introitus, the presence of a hyperkeratotic border to lesions and/or Wickham's striae in the surrounding skin, symptoms of pain/burning, scarring/loss of normal architecture, the presence of vaginal inflammation and involvement of other mucosal surfaces. The association of erosive LP of the vulva and vagina with desquamative gingivitis has been termed the vulvovaginal–gingival syndrome (Figure 12.8).

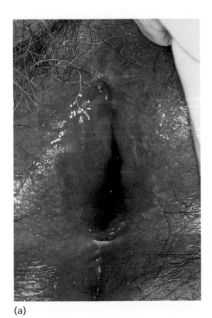

(a)

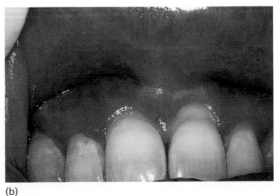

(b)

Figure 12.8 Vulvo-vaginal–gingival syndrome showing (a) vulvitis and (b) gingivitis in the same patient. (Source: Courtesy of Dr S. Neill, St John's Institute of Dermatology, King's College London, UK.)

Nail involvement occurs in up to 10% of cases, but is usually a minor feature of the disease. The majority of cases present during the fifth or sixth decades. Long-term permanent damage to the nails is rare. Fingernails are more frequently affected than toenails. The most common changes are exaggeration of the longitudinal lines and linear depressions due to slight thinning of the nail plate (Figure 12.9). These changes usually occur in the context of severe generalised LP, although skin lesions may not be seen in the vicinity of the affected nail. Elevated nail ridges may occur. Adhesion between the epidermis of the dorsal nail fold and the nail bed may cause partial destruction of the nail (pterygium unguis; Figure 12.10a). Rarely, the nail is completely shed; there is usually clinical evidence of LP at the base of the nail before shedding. Nails may partially regrow or be lost permanently (Figure 12.10b); the nails of the great toes are most often affected. LP is a cause of childhood idiopathic atrophy of the

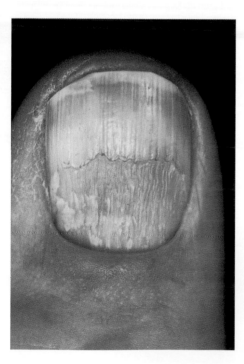

Figure 12.9 Lichen planus of the thumbnail showing thinning of the nail plate and longitudinal lines. (Source: Courtesy of St John's Institute of Dermatology, King's College London, UK.)

nails. LP of the nail bed may give rise to longitudinal melanonychia, hyperpigmentation, subungual hyperkeratosis or onycholysis, or changes mimicking yellow nail syndrome.

Lichen planopilaris
(Syn. Follicular lichen planus)

Follicular lesions usually appear during the course of typical LP, but occasionally they predominate. A variant in which groups of 'spiny' lesions resembling keratosis pilaris develop around hair follicles (lichen planopilaris) is common (Figure 12.11). Follicular lesions occurring in the scalp are accompanied by scaling and are likely to lead to a scarring alopecia (Figure 12.12). Very rarely, the scalp alone is involved. The characteristic histopathological features are an absence of arrector pili muscles and sebaceous glands, a perivascular and perifollicular lymphocytic infiltrate in the reticular dermis and mucinous perifollicular fibroplasia within the upper dermis with an absence of interfollicular mucin, and superficial perifollicular wedge-shaped scarring.

Graham Little–Piccardi–Lassueur syndrome

Comprises the triad of multifocal scalp cicatricial alopecia, non-scarring alopecia of the axillae and/or groin and keratotic lichenoid follicular papules.

Frontal fibrosing alopecia

Is a scalp condition that affects elderly women in particular and frequently involves the eyebrows. It is regarded as a clinically distinct variant of lichen planopilaris and is associated with mucocutaneous LP. A genome-wide scan has shown strong association with HLA-B*07:02.

Hypertrophic LP

Hypertrophic or warty lesions most often occur on the lower limbs, especially around the ankles; venous stasis has been put forward as an explanation (Figure 12.13). The lesions may persist for many years.

Differential diagnosis: Lichen simplex chronicus and lichen amyloidosus (papular).

LP of the palms and soles

Lesions on the palms and soles are uncommon, lack the characteristic shape and colour of lesions elsewhere and are firm to the touch and

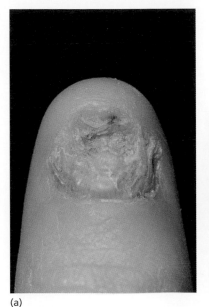

(a)

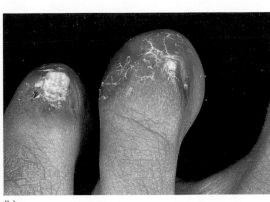

(b)

Figure 12.10 (a) Severe lichen planus of the fingernails showing involvement of the nail fold areas and early pterygium formation. (Source: Courtesy of the Welsh Institute of Dermatology, University Hospital of Wales, Cardiff, Wales, UK.) (b) Severe, destructive lichen planus of the toenails. (Source: Courtesy of St John's Institute of Dermatology, King's College London, UK.)

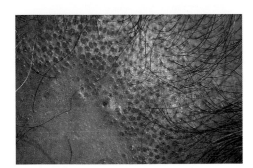

Figure 12.11 Lichen planopilaris showing hyperpigmented, follicular, 'plugged' lesions in the frontal scalp hairline. (Source: Courtesy of St John's Institute of Dermatology, King's College London, UK.)

yellow (Figure 12.5). They may be broad sheets or punctate keratoses.

Actinic LP

Usually occurs in children or young adults; virtually all cases originate from the Middle East, East Africa or India. Lesions occur on exposed skin (usually the face) as well-defined annular or discoid patches, which have a deeply hyperpigmented centre surrounded by a striking hypopigmented zone (Figure 12.14). Sunlight exposure appears to be central to the pathogenesis. It may mimic melasma.

LP pigmentosus

A pigmentary disorder seen in India and the Middle East that may be associated with typical LP papules. Macular hyperpigmentation involves chiefly the face, neck and upper limbs, although it can be more widespread, and varies from slate grey to brownish black. It is mostly diffuse, but reticular, blotchy and perifollicular forms occur. Occasionally, lesions may predominate at intertriginous sites, especially the axillae. The mucous membranes, palms and soles are usually not involved.

Annular LP

Although small annular lesions are common in LP, cases showing a few large annular lesions only are unusual. They may be widely scattered, and have a very narrow rim of activity and a

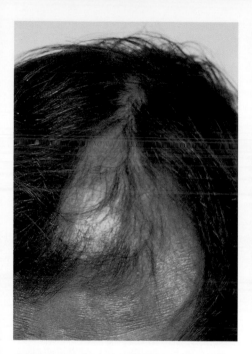

Figure 12.12 Lichen planus of the scalp leading to large areas of cicatricial alopecia. (Source: Courtesy of St John's Institute of Dermatology, King's College London, UK.)

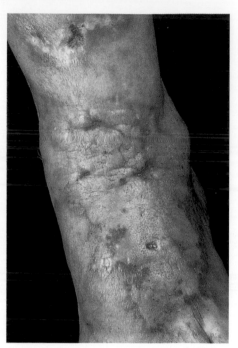

Figure 12.13 Hypertrophic lichen planus of great chronicity occurring on the lower leg and ankle. (Source: Courtesy of St John's Institute of Dermatology, King's College London, UK.)

depressed, slightly atrophic centre (Figure 12.15). Annular lesions are characteristically found on the penis (see Figure 12.2), sometimes associated with lesions on the buccal mucosa. The differential diagnosis includes granuloma annulare.

Guttate LP

Lesions are widely scattered and discrete, may be small (1–2 mm) or larger (up to 1 cm); individual lesions seldom become chronic (Figure 12.16).

Differential diagnosis: Guttate psoriasis.

Bullous LP and LP pemphigoides

In bullous LP blisters arise only on or near the lesions of LP as a result of severe liquefaction degeneration of the basal cell layer. Histologically, there is subepidermal bulla formation with typical changes of LP, and direct and indirect immunofluorescence (IMF) are negative. The eruption is usually only of short duration. In LP pemphigoides

the LP tends to be acute and generalised and is followed by the sudden appearance of large bullae on both involved and uninvolved skin (Figure 12.17). In LP pemphigoides, the histology shows a subepidermal bulla with no evidence of associated LP. Direct IMF shows linear basement membrane zone deposition of IgG and C3 in perilesional skin. Immunoelectron microscopy reveals deposition of IgG and C3 in the base of the bulla and not in the roof as is found in bullous pemphigoid.

Immunoblotting data have revealed that circulating autoantibodies in LP pemphigoides react with an epitope within the C-terminal NC16A domain of bullous pemphigoid 180 kDa antigen, and also with a 200 kDa antigen detected in bullous pemphigoid. The mean age of patients with LP pemphigoides is lower than that of those with classic bullous pemphigoid, and the disease tends to be less severe.

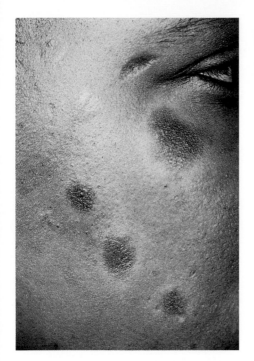

Figure 12.14 Lichen planus actinicus showing well-defined, pigmented, nummular patches on the face. (Source: Courtesy of St John's Institute of Dermatology, King's College London, UK.)

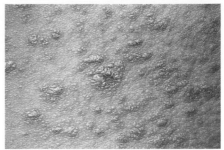

Figure 12.16 Guttate lichen planus. (Source: Courtesy of St John's Institute of Dermatology, King's College London, UK.)

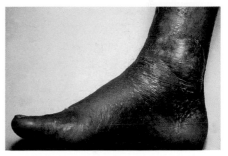

Figure 12.17 Lichen planus pemphigoides showing large bulla arising on and around the vicinity of lichen planus around the ankle. (Source: Courtesy of St John's Institute of Dermatology, King's College London, UK.)

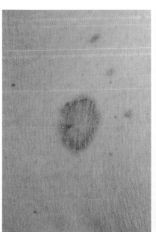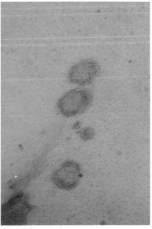

Figure 12.15 Annular lichen planus. (Source: Courtesy of the Welsh Institute of Dermatology, University Hospital of Wales, Cardiff, Wales, UK.)

PART 2: INFLAMMATORY DERMATOSES

Lichen nitidus

A rare variant of LP characterised by the presence of pinpoint to pinhead-sized papules, which are usually asymptomatic and flesh-coloured, with a flat, shiny surface. Most cases occur in children or young adults. They usually remain discrete, although they may be closely grouped (Figure 12.18). They are found on any part of the body but the sites of predilection are the forearms, penis (Figure 12.19), abdomen, chest and buttocks. The eruption is sometimes generalised. When the palms or soles are involved the changes can be those of a confluent hyperkeratosis resembling chronic fissured eczema, or there may be multiple, distinctive, minute papules. On the palms, the minute papules can become purpuric and may occasionally resemble pompholyx. Such cases may lack lesions of lichen nitidus elsewhere.

Nail pitting may coexist with lichen nitidus, or the affected nails may appear rough due to increased linear striations and longitudinal ridging. Mucous membrane lesions are much rarer than in LP.

Differential diagnosis: lichen scrofulosorum and keratosis pilaris.

In most cases, the papules eventually flatten after a few months, often to be replaced by an area of pigmentation that retains the shape of the papule and persists for months or years. There may be a gradual change in colour from pink to blue to black. The residual pigmentation may be intense, especially in black skin, or almost imperceptible in fair-skinned individuals.

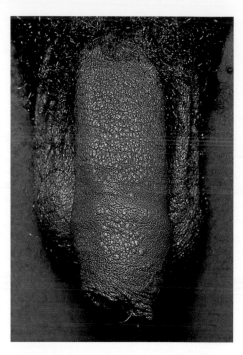

Figure 12.19 Lichen nitidus showing aggregates of pinhead-sized papules on the shaft of the penis. (Source: Courtesy of St John's Institute of Dermatology, King's College London, UK.)

Squamous cell carcinoma developing on oral lesions is uncommon but is particularly associated with ulcerated lesions. Lesions may occur on the lip, the buccal mucosa or the gum margin.

Idiopathic LP has been reported in association with diseases of altered or disturbed immunity, including ulcerative colitis, alopecia areata, vitiligo, dermatomyositis, morphoea and lichen sclerosus, systemic lupus erythematosus, pemphigus and paraneoplastic pemphigus.

Investigations

Skin biopsy for histology and if bullous direct IMF may be helpful.

Management

Treatment of LP can represent a challenge and depends on the localisation, clinical form and severity. For cutaneous LP, which can clear spontaneously within 1–2 years, the aim of

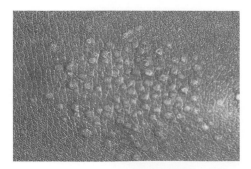

Figure 12.18 Lichen nitidus showing a close-up of aggregated, pinhead-sized papules. (Source: Courtesy of St John's Institute of Dermatology, King's College London, UK.)

treatment is to reduce pruritus and time to resolution. However, painful, erosive LP may need aggressive and long-term treatments. Nail or scalp involvement, which may induce scars, genital LP and oesophageal and conjunctival involvement, which may induce strictures and fibrosis, may require rapid treatment to avoid scarring.

Cutaneous LP
The goals of therapy are to improve itching and reduce time to resolution of the lesions.
First line:

- *Limited cutaneous LP:* very potent corticosteroids (clobetasol propionate ointment 0.05%); potent topical corticosteroids in less severe forms or during maintenance therapy.
- *Widespread cutaneous LP*: prednisolone.

Second line: Prednisolone, ciclosporin, azathioprine, psoralen and UVA (PUVA) or UVB ± systemic retinoids.
Third line: Methotrexate, hydroxychloquine.

Oral LP
The aims of treatment are to heal erosive lesions to reduce pain and permit normal food intake. Education of the patient should emphasise that oral LP frequently has a chronic course marked by treatment-induced remission followed by relapse. Alcohol and tobacco should be avoided as well as spicy or acidic foods and drinks. Good oral hygiene and professional dental care are recommended.
First line:

- *Symptomatic oral LP:* very potent corticosteroids (clobetasol propionate ointment 0.05%); potent topical corticosteroids in less severe forms or during maintenance therapy; soluble prednisolone tablets; an alternative to prednisolone tablets is betamethasone soluble tablets (Betnesol).
- *Severe erosive LP:* prednisolone.

Second line: Azathioprine, mycophenolate mofetil, methotrexate, ciclosporin, topical ciclosporin.

Anogenital LP
Very potent corticosteroid treatment (0.05% clobetasol propionate ointment). Hydrocortisone suppositories, foam or cream every other day are used for vaginal lesions. Potent corticosteroids used daily during the initial phase until symptom resolution. Foreskin retraction or removal surgery in uncircumcised men and vaginal dilators in women are used to prevent synechiae formation. Surgery is required after complete resolution of the active lesions if adhesion occurs.

Lichen planopilaris
First line: Very potent corticosteroids (e.g. 0.05% clobetasol propionate ointment).
Second line: Monthly intralesional triamcinolone acetonide injections or systemic oral corticosteroids.

Frontal fibrosing alopecia
Treatments can be of limited efficacy but include topical and intralesionaltramcinolone, doxycycline, hydroxychloroquine, topical and oral immunomodulators, tacrolimus and 5α-reductase inhibitors.

Nail LP
If fewer than four nails involved, topical very potent corticosteroids (e.g. 0.05% clobetasol propionate ointment); if lesions are more severe, monthly intralesional injection of triamcinolone acetonide in the periungual sites. If more than two or three nails involved, prednisolone.

Lichen nitidus
As the disease is often asymptomatic and eventually self-limiting, no treatment is required in most cases. Potent topical corticosteroids for lesions on the penis. PUVA, narrow-band UVB phototherapy. Acitretin for palmoplantar lichen nitidus.

Actinic LP
Acitretin and topical corticosteroids, ciclosporin.

Bullous LP planus and LP pemphigoides
Combination of prednisolone and acitretin.

Lichen striatus

A distinctive, usually self-limiting and asymptomatic inflammatory dermatosis characterised by pink or red papules in a linear distribution that develop in the lines of Blaschko.

PART 2: INFLAMMATORY DERMATOSES

Epidemiology

The incidence and prevalence are unknown.

Over 50% of cases occur in children, usually between ages 5 and 15 years. F > M = 2:1.

It occurs more often in individuals with atopy.

Pathophysiology

It is proposed that lichen striatus arises due to cutaneous antigenic mosaicism and a localised inflammatory T-cell response potentially related to viral infection or injury.

The histological appearances are variable and depend on the stage of disease. Usually, a band-like infiltrate composed of lymphocytes and histiocytes is observed with associated overlying epidermal change, including parakeratosis and hyperkeratosis, resembling LP. Like the spongiosis, acanthosis is variable in degree. Dyskeratotic keratinocytes, like the 'corps ronds' of Darier disease, are seen in about 50%. There is focal liquefactive degeneration of the basal layer. The dermis is oedematous, and the vessels and appendages are surrounded by an infiltrate of lymphocytes and histiocytes, which may be dense and extend deeply.

Clinical features

The initial presentation is characterised by the sudden appearance of small, discrete, pink, flat-topped, lichenoid papules in a typical linear distribution. The lesions extend over the course of a week or more and rapidly coalesce to form a dull-red to brown, slightly scaly, linear band, usually 2 mm to 2 cm in width, and often irregular. Occasionally, the bands broaden into plaques, especially on the buttocks. The lesion may be only a few centimetres in length or may extend the entire length of the limb and may be continuous or interrupted (Figure 12.20).

The lesions occur most commonly on one arm or leg, or the neck, occasionally the trunk. Nails may have longitudinal ridging, splitting or onycholysis, or be lost altogether.

Parallel linear bands or zosteriform patterns can occur (Figure 12.21). The majority of episodes are solitary, but occasionally repeated episodes can occur in different locations.

Differential diagnosis

Linear inflammatory eruptions that are distributed along Blaschko's lines or show a zosteriform

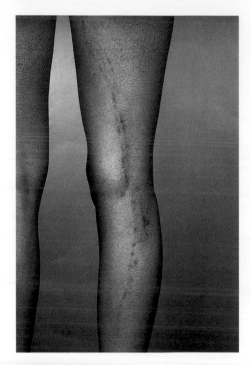

Figure 12.20 Lichen striatus of the inner thigh in a girl aged 16 years. (Source: Courtesy of Dr R.A. Marsden, St George's Hospital, London, UK.)

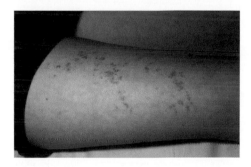

Figure 12.21 Lichen striatus showing parallel linear bands in a zigzag distribution on the thigh of a 15-year-old girl.

distribution, including linear psoriasis, linear Darier disease, linear LP, linear porokeratosis and inflammatory linear verrucous epidermal naevus, should be considered in the differential diagnosis.

Investigations
Skin biopsy.

Management
The disease course is variable. The majority of lesions last for at least 6 months and resolve within 1 year. It may follow a prolonged and/or relapsing course, particularly in adults. Post-inflammatory hypopigmentation may last for years, particularly in black skin.

Usually no treatment is necessary in childhood cases.

First line: Observation and reassurance, topical corticosteroids.

Second line: Topical calcineurin inhibitors.

Third line: Photodynamic therapy.

Nékam disease

(Syn. Keratosis lichenoides chronica)
A rare disease, possibly an unusual variant of LP. The great majority of cases are adults between the ages of 20 and 40 years, although children are occasionally affected.

It is characterised by violaceous, papular and nodular lesions typically arranged in a linear and reticulate pattern (Figure 12.22), most marked on the extremities and buttocks, and accompanied by a seborrhoeic dermatitis-like eruption on the face. The individual lesions are erythematous, verrucous papules covered by a hyperkeratotic plug that can only be removed with difficulty, revealing irregular indentations and prominent capillary loops. In extensive disease, the lesions tend to be symmetrical, mainly involving the antecubital fossae, extensor forearms, lumbosacral area and buttocks, posterior thighs, popliteal fossae and less commonly the oral cavity and genitalia. Oral involvement occurs in 50%, recurrent aphthous ulcers, larger chronic ulcers or erythrokeratotic papules being the commonest oral features. The nails can be thickened, longitudinally ridged and prone to paronychia. Cases have followed trauma and erythroderma. Histologically, changes are often non-specific and consistent with a chronic dermatitis, but lichenoid features can occur.

Management
The course is chronic, progressive and very resistant to therapy.

PUVA ± acitretin has been successful.

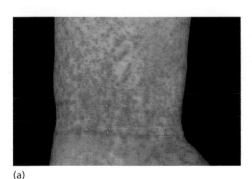
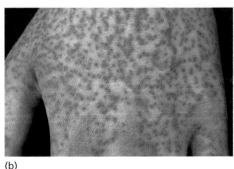

(a)

(b)

Figure 12.22 Nékam disease. Reticulate keratotic erythematous papules on (a) the volar aspect of the wrist and (b) the dorsum of the hand. (Source: Courtesy of St John's Institute of Dermatology, King's College London, UK.)

13 Graft-versus-host disease

Graft-versus-host disease (GvHD) is a multiorgan disease process that results from the action of donor-derived immunocompetent T lymphocytes against antigens expressed on the cells of the immunocompromised recipient host. The main organs affected are the skin, liver and gastrointestinal (GI) tract.

GvHD is a major complication of allogeneic haematopoietic stem cell transplantation (HSCT).

Synonyms and inclusions

- Acute graft-versus-host disease, acute GvHD (aGvHD).
- Chronic graft-versus-host disease, chronic GvHD (cGvHD).
- GvHD overlap syndrome, sometimes called acute on chronic GvHD.

GvHD is the major cause of morbidity and non-relapse-related mortality following allogeneic HSCT. The first and commonest site affected is the skin.

GvHD has classically been divided into acute and chronic based on time of onset but clinicians now prefer to define acute (aGVHD) and chronic (cGvHD) based on the distinctive clinical features. An overlap syndrome for GvHD is also included in the National Institutes of Health consensus diagnostic criteria in which clinical features of aGVHD and cGvHD appear together.

Epidemiology
Incidence and prevalence
Approximately 10–80% of HSCT recipients will develop aGVHD, depending on the risk factors present. Recipient HLA mismatching, the use of unrelated donors, gender mismatch, total body irradiation and older recipient age confer a greater risk of aGvHD.

Pathophysiology
Acute graft-versus-host disease
It is likely that aGvHD arises from a three-stage process:

- Toxicity from conditioning chemotherapy or radiotherapy causes tissue damage in the host and release of inflammatory cytokines.
- Mature donor lymphocytes from the graft are recruited, leading to their activation and proliferation when contact is made with host and donor antigen-presenting cells expressing disparate host antigens.
- Alloreactive T cells expand to form cytotoxic effector T cells that, in turn, induce further tissue injury and release more inflammatory cytokines.

Pathology
aGVHD, skin histopathology shows a lichenoid inflammatory process with a linear arrangement of lymphocytes along the basement membrane zone. The hallmark change is satellite cell necrosis consisting of apoptotic keratinocytes with tightly associated lymphocytes seen in the epidermis and associated interface vacuolar change. Histology can be indistinguishable from a lichenoid drug eruption

In cGVHD, histological changes depend on the type of skin involvement, i.e. lichenoid or sclerodermatous.

Rook's Dermatology Handbook, First Edition. Edited by Christopher E. M. Griffiths, Tanya O. Bleiker, Daniel Creamer, John R. Ingram and Rosalind C. Simpson.
© 2022 John Wiley & Sons Ltd. Published 2022 by John Wiley & Sons Ltd.

Acute graft-versus-host disease

Clinical features (Figures 13.1 and 13.2)
Acute GvHD usually occurs 2–4 weeks after HSCT. Pruritus or a burning sensation can precede the skin eruption with or without oral or genital ulceration.

Typically, erythematous blanching macules develop on the palms, soles or ears. The eruption may appear photoaggravated in distribution affecting the neck, upper back and face, or it may be folliculocentric.

In severe cases, there may be generalised erythroderma, bullae and extensive Nikolsky sign-positive epidermal skin loss with a toxic epidermal necrolysis-like picture.

Xerostomia, erythema and ulcers occur but may be difficult to distinguish from chemotherapy-induced mucositis.

Differential diagnosis
Adverse drug reaction, viral exanthema and engraftment syndrome.

Complications and comorbidities
Oral ulceration and diarrhoea can lead to weight loss and dehydration. Skin erosions can lead to secondary infection.

Disease course and prognosis
The severity grade of aGvHD correlates with overall survival. The transplant-related mortality rates for grades 0–IV aGvHD are 28%, 27%, 43%, 68% and 92%, respectively (see Box 13.1).

Investigations
Diagnosis of acute cutaneous aGvHD can be challenging and is based on clinical findings.

Management (Figure 13.3)

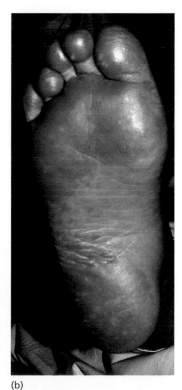

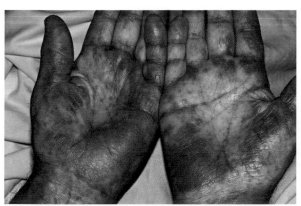

(a)   (b)

Figure 13.1 Clinical features of aGvHD. (a) Acute palmar erythema. (b) Plantar erythema.

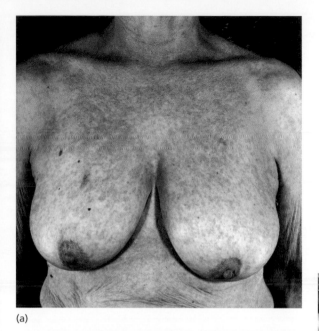

(a)

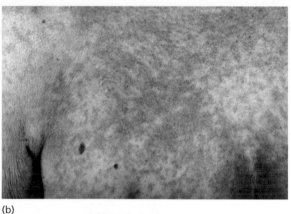

(b)

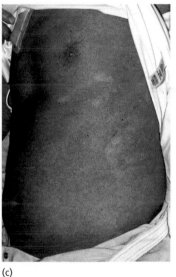

(c)

Figure 13.2 Clinical features of aGvHD. (a) Morbilliform exanthem with photoexposed accentuation. (b) Morbilliform exanthem with telangiectasia in close up. (c) Confluent erythroderma.

Box 13.1 International Bone Marrow Transplant Registry (IBMTR) severity index for acute graft-versus-host disease

The severity is the highest level which the patient reaches based on separate skin, liver and gastrointestinal staging.

A – Stage 1 skin involvement; no liver or gut involvement

B – Stage 2 skin involvement; stage 1–2 gut or liver involvement

C – Stage 3 skin, liver or gut involvement

D – Stage 4 skin, liver or gut involvement

Source: Adapted from Rowlings PA, Przepiorka D, Klein JP, et al. IBMTR Severity Index for grading acute graft-versus-host disease: retrospective comparison with Glucksberg grade. Br J Haematol 1997, 97, 855–864.

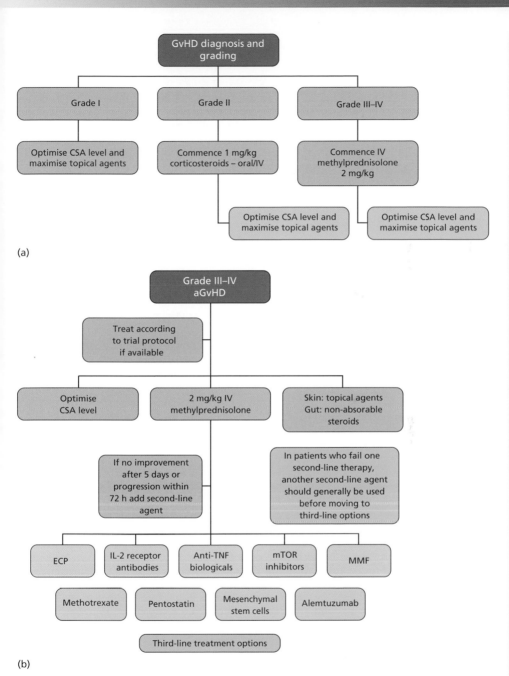

(a)

(b)

Figure 13.3 (a) Treatment algorithm summarising initial treatment of aGvHD. CSA, ciclosporin. (b) Treatment algorithm for grade III–IV aGvHD (third-line agents). ECP, extracorporeal photopheresis; IL-2, interleukin 2; TNF, tumour necrosis factor; mTOR, mammalian target of rapamycin; MMF, mycophenolate mofetil. (Source: Adapted from Dignan FL, Amrolia P, Clark A, et al. Diagnosis and management of chronic graft-versus-host disease. Br J Haematol 2012, 158(1), 46–61.)

Chronic graft-versus-host disease

Clinical features
The skin is the most common site involved, followed by mucosa, but virtually any organ can be affected. Patients can report the insidious onset of dry, tight or itchy skin. Ocular discomfort and dryness as well as oral discomfort may occur as can genital symptoms such as vulvovaginal dryness, itch and discomfort. Nausea, diarrhoea and vomiting, shortness of breath and muscle weakness are important in this multisystem disease.

Presentation
Clinical variants of chronic graft-versus-host disease (Figures 13.4–13.7)
Cutaneous features

1. Sclerotic:
   - Sclerodermoid, deep sclerosis/eosinophilic fasciitis-like.
   - Lichen sclerosus-like.
   - Morpheaform.
2. Lichenoid.
3. Epidermal – eczematoid, papulosquamous.
4. Associated features:
   - Oral lesions – lichenoid, microstomia, mucoceles, sicca symptoms, oral verruciform xanthoma (rare).
   - Hair – scarring or non-scarring alopecia.
   - Nails – dystrophy, anonychia, pterygium.

- Ocular and genital mucosa – erosions, pain, lichen planus-like or lichen sclerosus-like lesions.
5. Extracutaneous manifestations:
   - Liver.
   - GI.
   - Lung.
   - Musculoskeletal (fasciitis, myositis).
   - Other, e.g. demyelination.

Differential diagnosis
Drug-induced lichenoid eruptions, radiation-induced fibrosis and skin sclerosis and morphoea.

Complications and co-morbidities
Sclerotic disease and fascial contractures can cause severe limitation of movement and disability along with other issues such as difficult venous access. Dyspigmentation and poikiloderma can cause profound changes of appearance.

Disease course and prognosis
cGvHD is the major cause of mortality and morbidity in long-term survivors of HSCT. Severity grading predicts prognosis. Chronic GVHD is associated with a higher treatment-related mortality post-allogeneic transplant despite a slightly lower rate of disease relapse. Overall survival at 2 years is 97%, 86% and 62% for patients with mild, moderate and severe cGVHD, respectively.

Management (Figure 13.8)

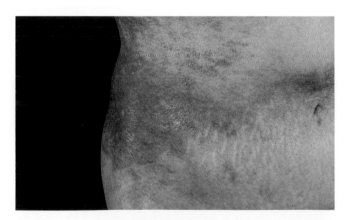

Figure 13.4 Clinical features of lichenoid cGvHD. Lichenoid skin change accentuated on the flanks, along the waistband site.

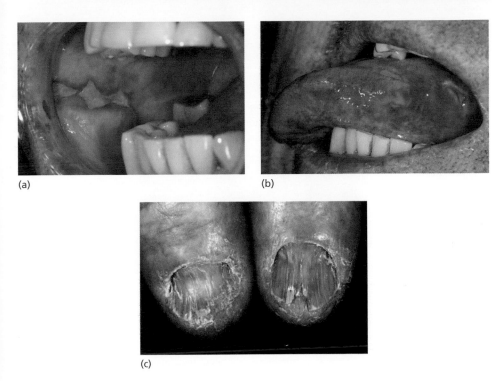

(a)

(b)

(c)

Figure 13.5 Clinical features of lichenoid cGvHD. (a) Oral cGVHD with lichenoid buccal change and hyperkeratosis along the bite line. (b) Lichenoid change and ulceration of the tongue. (c) Lichenoid nail changes of cGvHD.

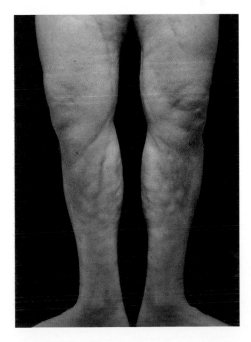

Figure 13.6 Clinical features of chronic sclerodermoid GvHD. cGvHD showing extensive sclerodermoid changes of the legs with orange peel-like change, woody induration of the skin and venous guttering. (Source: Courtesy of Dr F. Child, St John's Institute of Dermatology, London, UK.)

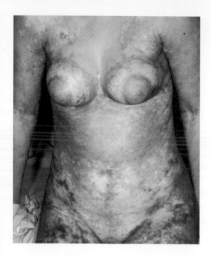

Figure 13.7 Clinical features of chronic sclerodermoid GvHD. (Source: Courtesy of Dr C. Kennedy, Bristol Royal Infirmary, UK.)

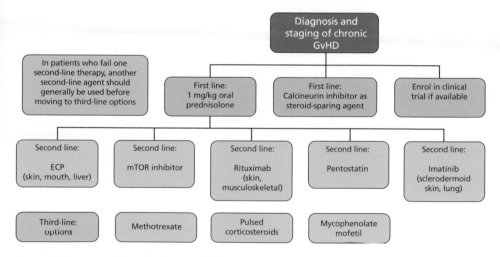

Figure 13.8 An algorithm to show treatment options in cGvHD to show first-, second- and third-line treatment options. ECP, extracorporeal photopheresis; mTOR, mammalian target of rapamycin. (Source: Dignan FL, Amrolia P, Clark A, et al. Diagnosis and management of chronic graft-versus-host disease. Br J Haematol 2012, 158(1), 46–61. © 2012 John Wiley & Sons.)

Eczematous disorders

14

ECZEMA

(Syn. Dermatitis)

Eczema, a term derived from the Greek word $\varepsilon'\kappa\zeta\varepsilon\mu\alpha$ meaning 'to boil'. Box 14.1 provides a list of the eczematous dermatoses split into those with a known exogenous trigger and those that are thought to be more endogenous.

Epidemiology

Incidence and prevalence

Eczematous dermatoses account for a large proportion of all skin disease. The point prevalence of all forms of eczema is 18 per 1000 (seven accounted for by atopic eczema, whereas hand eczema, dyshidrotic eczema and nummular eczema are two each).

Consultations for eczema are a major part of the workload in primary care, accounting for 19–25% of dermatological consultations, the majority of which (60%) are exogenous in nature.

Eczematous dermatoses are reported in all ethnic groups, but data are limited regarding ethnic differences for non-atopic eczema.

Filaggrin mutations are linked to hand eczema, irritant contact dermatitis and allergic contact dermatitis due to nickel and possibly other allergens.

Irritants and allergens may act as triggers for irritant contact dermatitis and allergic contact dermatitis, respectively.

Clinical features

The hallmark of eczema is pruritus, which may disturb sleep and other elements of quality of life and can affect other family members profoundly as well. When taking the history, it is important to note occupation and recreational activities because these may be relevant in terms of irritant and allergen exposures.

Acute eczema presents as an eruption that is typically oedematous, vesicular and may be exudative. In chronic eczema, these features give way to a more stable picture of erythema, scaling, excoriation and lichenification.

A characteristic feature of eczematous inflammation is its tendency to spread far from its point of origin and to become generalised. This phenomenon is often termed autosensitisation or, more specifically,

---

Box 14.1 Classification of the principal forms of eczema

Exogenous eczemas

- Allergic contact eczema
- Dermatophytide
- Eczematous polymorphic light eruption Infective dermatitis
- Irritant eczema
- Photoallergic contact eczema
- Post-traumatic eczema

Endogenous eczemas

- Asteatotic eczema
- Atopic eczema

- Chronic superficial scaly dermatitis
- Eyelid eczema
- Hand eczema
- Juvenile plantar dermatosis
- Nummular dermatitis
- Pityriasis alba
- Metabolic eczema or eczema associated with systemic disease
- Seborrhoeic eczema
- Venous eczema

Rook's Dermatology Handbook, First Edition. Edited by Christopher E. M. Griffiths, Tanya O. Bleiker, Daniel Creamer, John R. Ingram and Rosalind C. Simpson.
© 2022 John Wiley & Sons Ltd. Published 2022 by John Wiley & Sons Ltd.

autoeczematisation. Generalised spread is especially likely when the primary site of the eczema is on the legs or the feet. Conditioned hyper-irritability is the phenomenon whereby an area of inflamed skin on one part of the body results in a generalised hyperirritability of the skin at distant sites.

Differential diagnosis

This will be discussed in relation to each non-atopic eczema subtype.

Disease course and prognosis

Eczema tends to follow a chronic, relapsing remitting course.

Investigations

Most cases of eczema can be diagnosed clinically. It can sometimes be helpful to measure the total IgE level in order to determine whether an individual is atopic. Biopsy can occasionally be helpful in confirming the eczematous nature of the eruption, and immunofluorescence can help identify less common conditions such as dermatitis herpetiformis or, in older patients, a non-bullous presentation of bullous pemphigoid.

Management

Some frequently used treatments are listed in Table 14.1. When an extrinsic cause is identified or suspected this should be removed. In all cases, exposure to irritants should be carefully avoided and the skin should be protected using emollients and appropriate dressings. Psychological support is an important aspect of management at all stages.

Table 14.1 Management of eczema

Therapeutic agent	Acute	Subacute	Chronic
Rest, sedation	++	+	±
Wet dressings and soaks	++	±	−
Wet wrap bandaging	++	+	±
Paste bandages	±	+	++
Sedative antihistamines	++	++	+
Emollients	++	++	++
Corticosteroids, local	+	++	+
Pimecrolimus (topical)	+	++	++
Tacrolimus (topical)	+	++	++
Tar, ichthammol, etc.	±	+	++
Polythene occlusion	±	+	+
Intralesional steroids	−	±	+
Habit reversal therapy	−	±	+
X-ray therapy	−	−	±
UVB phototherapy	−	+	+
PUVA phototherapy	−	+	+
UVA1 phototherapy	−	+	+
Systemic corticosteroids	+	+	±
Ciclosporin	+	+	±
Azathioprine	−	+	+
Methotrexate	−	+	+
Alitretinoin (hand eczema)	−	+	+

PUVA, psoralen and UVA; UV, ultraviolet.

Subacute eczema

If an acute eczema has failed to clear almost completely in 3–4 weeks, perpetuating factors such as exposure to a sensitising agent and concordance with treatment should be considered.

Management

First line: Avoidance of irritants and allergens, emollients and soap substitutes
Second line: Topical corticosteroids and topical calcineurin inhibitors
Third line: Phototherapy, oral immunosuppressants and alitretinoin (hand eczema)

Nummular dermatitis

(Syn. Discoid eczema, nummular eczema)

Definition and nomenclature

Nummular dermatitis is characterised by a single, non-specific morphological feature, namely circular or oval plaques of eczema with a clearly demarcated edge. It should be distinguished from an irregular, patchy form of eczema in which lesions are not clearly demarcated. It tends to be a chronic problem, undergoing relapses and remissions.

Epidemiology

The prevalence of nummular dermatitis is two per 1000. In women, onset is usually in early adulthood, whereas in men onset is commonest in the older age groups.

Genetics

There may be an indirect link via atopy.

Environmental factors

There may be a clinically relevant underlying allergic contact dermatitis in about one-third of patients.

Dry skin due to low environmental humidity is sometimes associated with nummular dermatitis, particularly in the elderly. An association between excessive alcohol intake and nummular dermatitis has been reported.

Pathophysiology

Histology usually shows a subacute dermatitis indistinguishable from other forms of eczema, with spongiotic vesicles and a predominantly lymphohistiocytic infiltrate. Eosinophils may also be present in the upper dermis.

Clinical features

The diagnostic lesion of nummular dermatitis is a coin-shaped plaque of closely set, thin-walled vesicles on an erythematous base. This arises, quite rapidly, from the confluence of tiny papules and papulovesicles. In the acute phase the lesions are dull red, very exudative or crusted and highly pruritic (Figure 14.1). They progress towards a less vesicular and more scaly stage, often with central clearing, and peripheral extension, causing ring-shaped or annular lesions.

After any period of between 10 days and several months, secondary lesions occur, often in a

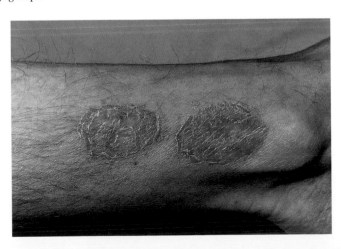

Figure 14.1 Nummular dermatitis of the lower leg. (Source: Courtesy of Dr W. A. D. Griffiths, Epsom Hospital, Surrey, UK.)

mirror-image configuration on the opposite side of the body. It is characteristic that patches which have apparently become dormant may become active again, particularly if treatment is discontinued prematurely.

There are a number of variants of nummular dermatitis:

- Exudative type.
- Dry type.
- Nummular dermatitis of the hands.
- Exudative discoid and lichenoid chronic dermatosis.

In 'exudative' nummular dermatitis the skin lesions resemble the acute phase of the more typical form of the condition, with leakage of serous fluid and crust formation. This variant may require oral antibiotic treatment.

'Dry' nummular dermatitis is uncommon, consisting of multiple, dry, scaly, round or oval discs on the arms or legs, but also with scattered microvesicles on an erythematous base on the palms and soles. Pruritus is minimal, in contrast with other forms of nummular dermatitis, and the condition persists for several years, with fluctuation or remission.

Nummular dermatitis of the hands affects the dorsa of the hands or the backs or sides of individual fingers. It often develops as a single plaque, which may occur at the site of a burn or a local chemical or irritant reaction. An atopic history appears to be more frequent in young women with discoid hand eczema than in other forms of the disease.

Exudative discoid and lichenoid chronic dermatosis is a widespread, extremely pruritic eruption, characterised by discoid lesions with 'lichenoid' and exudative phases (Figure 14.2).

Differential diagnosis

Tinea corporis, psoriasis and pityriasis rosea. (Table 14.2).

Management

General considerations apply, such as avoidance of irritants, as with other forms of eczema. Bed rest and removal from a stressful environment can be helpful. Ambient conditions of low humidity should be corrected.

First line: Emollient, topical corticosteroid ± topical or oral antibiotic.

Second line: Topical calcineurin inhibitor.

Third line: Phototherapy (narrow-band UVB/PUVA), oral immunosuppressants including methotrexate or oral steroids.

Asteatotic eczema

(Syn. Eczéma craquelé, winter eczema)

Asteatotic eczema usually affects the legs, arms and hands in the context of dry skin. A characteristic 'crazy-paving' pattern is observed on the legs in particular (eczéma craquelé).

Epidemiology

Elderly people are predominantly affected and prevalence increases with increasing age.

All ethnicities can be affected.

Asteatotic eczema may be a presenting sign of myxoedema and can also be due to zinc deficiency.

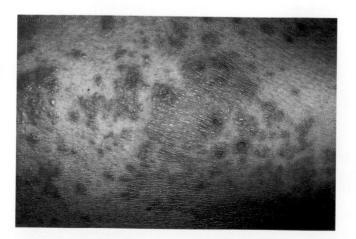

Figure 14.2 Exudative discoid and lichenoid chronic dermatitis. (Source: Courtesy of Dr A. Warin, Royal Devon and Exeter Hospital, Exeter, UK.)

Table 14.2 Diagnosis of some discoid skin lesions

Disease	Distribution	Features	Histology	Course and evolution
Tinea corporis	Limbs or trunk	Oval or round, itchy Scraping produces scale for mycology	PAS stain shows fungus	Progresses and spreads steadily until treated
Nummular dermatitis	Limbs more than trunk	Oval or round, very itchy	Eczema, often intense changes	Variable, fluctuant or intermittent
Pityriasis alba	Face, proximal limbs	Depigmentation	Very mild eczema	Spontaneous remission after 1 or more years
Chronic superficial dermatitis	Limbs more than trunk	Oval or round, no infiltration	Epidermal eczematous	Very chronic, benign, no fluctuations
Prelymphomatous eruption	Flank, trunk, proximal limbs	Angular, bizarre, infiltrated, itchy	Dermal infiltrate	Persistent, may change to lymphoma

PAS, Periodic acid-Schiff.

Environmental factors

A patient will often ascribe the onset to an event or change in life, e.g. the installation of central heating or a particularly cold, dry winter. In industry, years of contact with degreasing agents may be tolerated until, usually in the 50–60-year age group, some small additional hazard precipitates a disabling dermatitis.

Diuretics may be a contributory factor in elderly people. Cimetidine has also been reported to cause the condition.

Pathophysiology

The histopathological features are those of a mild, subacute eczema, with a varying amount of dermal infiltrate. When vesicular or nummular dermatitis supervenes, the changes are more marked and are as seen in the latter disease.

Clinical features
History

Irritation in this form of eczema is often intense and worse with changes of temperature, particularly at night.

Presentation

The condition occurs particularly on the legs, arms and hands. The asteatotic skin is dry and slightly scaly (Figure 14.3). The surface of the backs of the hands is marked in a criss-cross

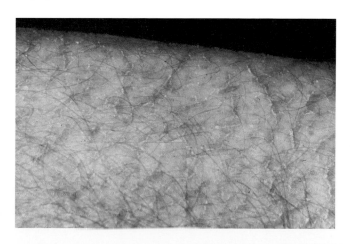

Figure 14.3 Asteatotic eczema.

fashion. The finger pulps are dry and cracked, producing distorted prints and retaining a prolonged depression after pressure ('parchment pulps'). On the legs the pattern of superficial markings is more marked and deeper ('crazy-paving' pattern or eczéma craquelé). Fissures may become haemorrhagic.

Clinical variants

Extensive or generalised forms involving the trunk as well as the legs are rare but should raise the suspicion of malignancy. Cases have been reported in association with malignant lymphoma, angioimmunoblastic lymphadenopathy, anaplastic gastric adenocarcinoma and spheroidal cell carcinoma of the breast.

Differential diagnosis

The differential diagnosis is limited to other forms of eczema.

Complications and co-morbidities

As with all forms of eczema, secondary infection is possible due to a reduction in skin barrier function.

Disease course and prognosis

Without treatment, the condition is usually chronic, relapsing each winter and clearing in the summer, but eventually becoming permanent.

Management

First line: Humidify environment and avoid sudden temperature changes.

Second line: Emollients, with or without urea, bath oil and soap substitute.

Third line: Mild topical corticosteroids; a randomised, vehicle-controlled trial of 40 patients with asteatotic eczema found pimecrolimus 1% cream to be effective after 4 weeks of treatment.

Dermatitis and eczema of the hands

(Syn. Hyperkeratotic palmar eczema is also known as 'tylotic eczema', Pompholyx hand eczema is also known as 'vesicular eczema of palms and soles'. When pompholyx occurs on the palms, it may be called 'cheiropompholyx', and when on the soles, 'podopompholyx')

The term hand eczema implies that the dermatitis is largely confined to the hands (Box 14.2). Up to 30% of occupational medical practice relates to hand eczema, with important issues regarding medical litigation, worker's compensation and disability.

Epidemiology
Incidence and prevalence

Minor degrees of hand eczema are very common (Box 14.3).

Hand eczema point prevalence is about 4%, 1-year prevalence 10%. and lifetime prevalence 15%.

In high-risk groups the figures are even higher.

Box 14.2 Hand eczema: aetiology

Exogenous

- Contact irritants:
  - Chemical (e.g. soap, detergents, solvents)
  - Physical (e.g. friction, minor trauma, cold dry air)
- Contact allergens:
  - Delayed hypersensitivity (type IV) (e.g. chromium, rubber)
  - Immediate hypersensitivity (type I) (e.g. seafood)
- Ingested allergens (e.g. drugs, possibly nickel, chromium)
- Infection (e.g. following bacterial infection of hand wounds)
- Secondary dissemination (e.g. dermatophytide reaction to tinea pedis)

Endogenous

- Idiopathic (e.g. discoid, hyperkeratotic palmar eczema)
- Immunological or metabolic defect (e.g. atopic)
- Psychosomatic: stress aggravates, but may not be causative
- Dyshidrosis: increased sweating aggravates, but may not be causative

> ### Box 14.3 Morphological patterns of hand eczema
>
> - Apron eczema
> - Chronic acral dermatitis
> - Nummular dermatitis (discoid eczema)
> - Fingertip eczema
> - 'Gut' eczema
> - Hyperkeratotic palmar eczema
> - Pompholyx
> - Recurrent focal palmar peeling
> - Ring eczema
> - 'Wear and tear' dermatitis (dry palmar eczema)
> - Other patterns (e.g. patchy vesiculosquamous)

F:M 2:1. Common in all ethnic groups. It is more common if previous history of atopic eczema.

Pathophysiology

In general, the differences between the various forms of hand eczema are clinical rather than histological, but the considerably thickened horny layer and the presence of numerous sweat glands modify the histological features of eczema on the hands. Atopy, a naturally dry skin, or a superadded contact allergic or irritant dermatitis are all predisposing factors. The common link is now known to be filaggrin gene mutations. Many patients give a convincing account of exacerbations at times of acute anxiety, frustration or grief. The role of hormonal factors is also difficult to assess. Occasionally, there is a history of premenstrual exacerbation or deterioration during pregnancy.

Twin studies suggest hereditary factors play a role in the development of hand eczema, with the atopic diathesis as the commonest endogenous cause. Filaggrin gene mutations are linked with an increased susceptibility to chronic irritant contact dermatitis and chronic hand eczema.

Contact irritants are the commonest exogenous cause of hand eczema, but contact allergens including chromate, epoxy glues and rubber are also important (Figure 14.4).

Type 1 allergic reactions to certain proteins may also give rise to hand eczema.

Clinical features

Particular attention should be given to the patient's occupational and recreational activities. Occupational involvement is suggested by improvement associated with leave from work.

Clinical variants

Hyperkeratotic palmar eczema

This common condition is a distinct form of hand eczema characterised by highly irritable, scaly, fissured, hyperkeratotic patches on the palms and palmar surfaces of the fingers (Figure 14.5).

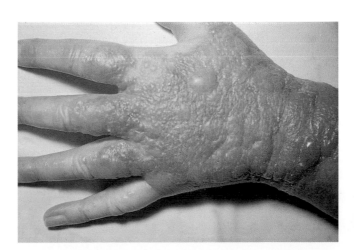

Figure 14.4 Bullous eczema due to contact allergy to rubber gloves.

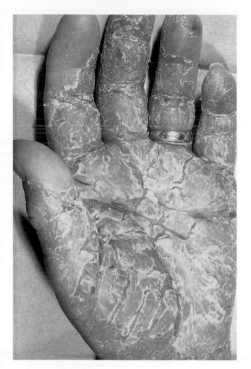

Figure 14.5 Hyperkeratotic palmar eczema.

Pompholyx

A form of eczema of the palms and soles in which oedema fluid accumulates to form visible vesicles or bullae (Figure 14.6). As a result of the thick epidermis in these sites, the blisters become relatively large before they burst. Pompholyx probably accounts for about 5–20% of all cases of hand eczema.

Apron eczema

Involves the proximal palmar aspect of two or more adjacent fingers and the contiguous palmar skin over the metacarpophalangeal joints, thus resembling an apron (Figure 14.7).

Chronic acral dermatitis

This distinctive syndrome affects patients in middle age. A chronic, intensely pruritic, hyperkeratotic, papulovesicular eczema of the hands and feet, is associated with grossly elevated IgE levels in subjects with no personal or family history of atopy.

Nummular dermatitis

This is also known as discoid eczema (see previous section).

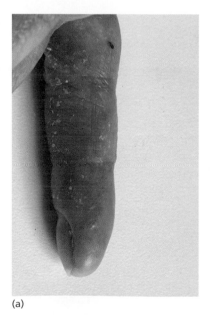

(a)

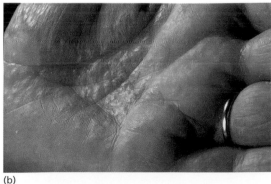

(b)

Figure 14.6 Pompholyx eczema. (a) Small vesicles coalescing into blisters on the lateral aspect of a finger. (b) Confluent vesicles of the palm.

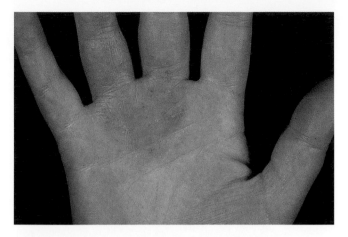

Figure 14.7 Apron eczema, showing the characteristic distribution.

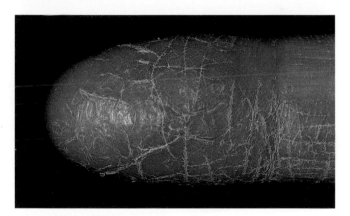

Figure 14.8 Fingertip eczema in a patient with wear and tear eczema. (Source: Courtesy of Dr D. A. Burns, Leicester Royal Infirmary, Leicester, UK.)

Fingertip eczema

This condition presents a characteristic pattern, involving the palmar surface of the tips of some or all of the fingers. The skin is dry, cracked and sometimes breaks down into painful fissures (Figure 14.8). Two patterns may be distinguished. The first and most common involves most or all of the fingers, mainly those of the dominant hand, and particularly the thumb and forefinger. The second pattern involves preferentially the thumb, forefinger and third finger of one hand. This is usually occupational. The condition usually involves the dominant hand, but there may be allergy to onions, garlic and other kitchen products held in the non-dominant hand when being cut.

'Gut'/slaughterhouse eczema

Workers who eviscerate and clean pig carcasses are at risk of developing vesicular eczema which starts in the finger webs and spreads to the sides of the fingers. This is a mild, self-limiting condition.

Patchy vesiculosquamous eczema

A mixture of irregular, patchy, vesiculosquamous lesions occur on both hands, usually asymmetrically. Nail changes are common if the nail folds are affected.

Recurrent focal palmar peeling

Also known as desquamation en aires, keratolysis exfoliativa or ringed keratolysis of the palms. During the summer months, small areas of superficial, white desquamation develop on the sides of the fingers and on the palms or on the feet (Figure 14.9). They appear abruptly and expand before peeling off.

Ring eczema

This characteristic pattern particularly affects young women, rarely men. The condition usually starts soon after marriage or childbirth. An irritable patch of eczema begins under a ring – usually a broad wedding ring – and typically spreads to involve the adjacent side of the middle finger and the adjacent area of the palm.

Differential diagnosis

Psoriasis, Tinea manuum

Lichen planus and pityriasis rubra pilaris may resemble eczema on the hands.

Pompholyx eczema can resemble palmoplantar pustulosis. Pemphigoid, linear IgA disease and pemphigoid gestationis occasionally present with blisters on the palms that mimic pompholyx.

Following an acute attack of pompholyx, about one-third of patients experience no further episodes, one-third suffer from recurrent episodes, and in the remainder the condition develops into a chronic, possibly hyperkeratotic phase.

Management

First line: Hand care advice, irritant and allergen avoidance, emollients, soap substitute.

Second line: Potent or very potent topical corticosteroids.

Third line: Alitretinoin/PUVA/azathioprine/ciclosporin/methotrexate.

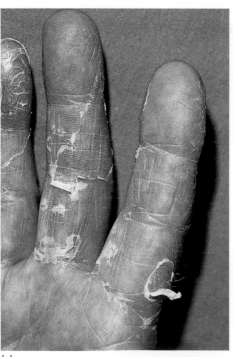

(a)

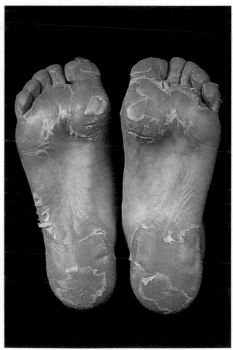

(b)

Figure 14.9 Recurrent focal palmar peeling. (a) Well-established lesions on the hands. (Source: Courtesy of Dr A. Marsden, St George's Hospital, London, UK.) (b) Lesions on the feet.

Dermatitis and eczema of the lower legs

(Syn. Venous eczema is also known as varicose eczema, eczema and dermatitis are used interchangeably)

Definition and nomenclature

Dermatitis and eczema of the lower legs is subclassified as venous eczema, stasis dermatitis and allergic contact dermatitis. Venous eczema and stasis dermatitis both result from dysfunctional venous drainage of the lower legs.

Epidemiology

The combined prevalence of venous eczema and venous stasis is estimated to be between 3% and 11% of the population.

Venous eczema patients are usually middle-aged or elderly. F > M.

There is an association between venous eczema and allergic contact dermatitis.

Pathophysiology

Venous eczema is more likely after a previous deep vein thrombosis and in the presence of venous stasis, which is itself linked to obesity, immobility and previous cellulitis.

Clinical features

Venous eczema may develop suddenly or insidiously. Venous eczema and stasis dermatitis are erythematous, scaly and often exudative eruptions usually seen around the ankle and lower leg (Figure 14.10). The eczema is often accompanied by other manifestations of venous hypertension, including dilatation or varicosity of the superficial veins, oedema, purpura, haemosiderosis and ulceration (Figure 14.11), or small patches of white, atrophic, telangiectatic scarring ('atrophie blanche'). Leashes of dilated venules around the dorsum of the foot or ankle are particularly common. There may be a subepidermal vascular proliferation producing purple papules around the ankle, which may resemble Kaposi sarcoma.

Secondary patches of eczema may develop on the other leg, even when it is not affected by obvious venous insufficiency. Generalised secondary dissemination may occur and occasionally this can progress to erythroderma.

Differential diagnosis

Most cases of eczema of the lower leg are secondary to venous hypertension or stasis dermatitis but many other types of eczema may affect this region and often there are multiple causative factors. Psoriasis, hypertrophic lichen planus, dermatophyte infection and profuse actinic keratoses.

Secondary infection occasionally leading to cellulitis.

Lipodermatosclerosis

Chronic venous insufficiency may result in lipodermatosclerosis.

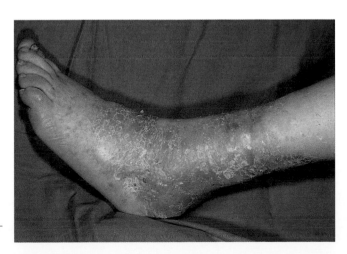

Figure 14.10 Venous (gravitational) eczema.

Venous ulceration

There is an association between venous eczema and venous ulceration because these are both the result of venous hypertension.

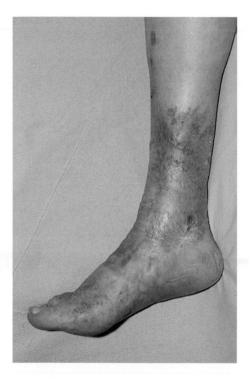

Figure 14.11 Venous eczema of the ankle with ulceration at the medial malleolus.

Investigations

Ankle brachial pressure index (ABPI) measurement is required prior to consideration of compression therapy.

Management

First line: Skin care, including leg elevation, emollients and topical corticosteroids.

Second line: Compression hosiery.

Third line: Referral to vascular surgeon to consider surgical intervention.

Dermatitis and eczema of the eyelids

Eczema affecting predominantly the eyelids.

Eyelid involvement is a very common feature of atopic eczema (Figure 14.12) and it is likely that many cases represent mild atopic eczema without other manifestations. Seborrhoeic dermatitis may also underlie the presentation. Contact allergy to various components of eye makeup, nail varnish, fragrance, rubber or ophthalmic medicaments are responsible for some cases. Allergy to nickel in spectacle frames may cause eczema near the lower eyelids.

Management

First line: Avoid allergens/irritants (if relevant), emollient.

Second line: Hydrocortisone 1% cream.

Third line: Tacrolimus ointment or pimecrolimus 1% cream.

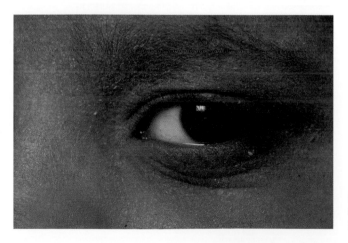

Figure 14.12 Eyelid atopic eczema (note the infra-orbital Dennie–Morgan fold).

Juvenile plantar dermatosis

(Syn. Forefoot eczema, peridigital dermatosis, dermatitis plantaris sicca, atopic winter feet)

Definition and nomenclature
This condition is characterised by shiny, dry, fissured dermatitis of the plantar surface of the forefoot.

Epidemiology
Occurs mainly in children (commoner in boys) aged 3–14 years.

Pathophysiology
Histology shows a mild, non-specific eczema.

Environmental factors
The use of synthetic materials such as nylon and plastics, compared with more porous natural materials such as cotton, wool and leather in footwear, may be responsible. Many of the affected children are keen on dancing or sports, suggesting friction and enhanced sweating may be important.

Clinical features
The presenting features are symmetrical redness and soreness on the plantar surface of the forefeet, which assumes a shiny, 'glazed' and cracked appearance (Figure 14.13). The condition is most severe on the ball of the foot and toe pads, and tends to spare the non-weight-bearing instep. The toe clefts are normal. Occasionally, the disease can affect the hands.

Most cases will clear spontaneously during childhood or adolescence.

Management
First line: Change to leather footwear and cotton socks/open sandals.

Second line: Emollients, including urea-containing preparations.

Third line: Lassar's paste/tar/tacrolimus ointment.

MISCELLANEOUS SPECIFIED ECZEMATOUS DERMATOSES

Infective dermatitis

(Syn. Microbial eczema)
Infective dermatitis is a controversial entity and some dermatologists never make the diagnosis. It is caused by microorganisms or their products, and that by definition clears when the organisms are eradicated (Figure 14.14). This should be distinguished from infected eczema

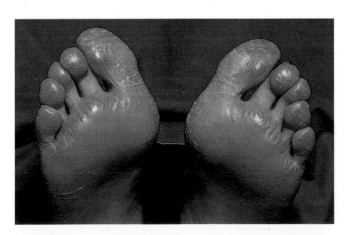

Figure 14.13 Juvenile plantar dermatosis, showing the characteristic glazed appearance of the forefoot skin.

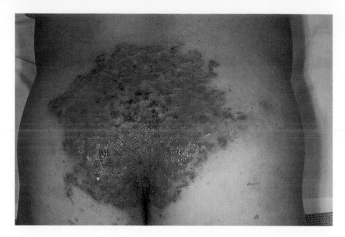

Figure 14.14 Infective dermatitis in a non-atopic man. Histology of this localised rash showed eczema, and *Staphylococcus aureus* was repeatedly isolated.

in which eczema due to some other cause is complicated by secondary bacterial or viral invasion of the skin (Figure 14.15)

Pathophysiology

The histological picture of infective eczema is in general that of subacute or chronic dermatitis. The dermis shows inflammatory changes, with polymorphonuclear and lymphocytic infiltration that invades the epidermis to a variable extent. In some stages, subcorneal pustulation may be conspicuous.

Clinical features

Infected eczema

Infected eczema shows erythema, exudation and crusting. The margin is characteristically sharply defined, and the horny layer is often split to form an encircling collarette. There may be small pustules in the advancing edge.

Infective eczema

Infective dermatitis usually presents as an area of advancing erythema, sometimes with microvesicles. It is seen predominantly around discharging wounds or ulcers, or moist skin lesions of other types. Infective dermatitis is relatively common in patients with venous leg ulcers.

Tinea pedis may also become eczematous due to the overgrowth of Gram-negative

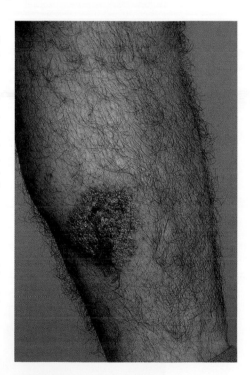

Figure 14.15 Infected eczema. This man had a patch of nummular dermatitis that became secondarily infected with *Staphylococcus aureus*.

organisms. Infective dermatitis may also complicate chronic threadworm infestation, pediculosis or scabies.

Infective dermatitis of the forefeet is a distinctive pattern of eczema that mainly affects the interdigital spaces on the dorsum of the medial toes.

Management

First line: Treat primary cause (e.g. ulcer) or modify footwear if relevant.

Second line: Topical antibiotics (for mild presentations).

Third line: Systemic antibiotics (also potassium permanganate soaks for forefeet variant).

Infective dermatitis of children associated with human T-cell leukaemia virus 1 infection

(Syn. **Infective dermatitis of Jamaican children**)
Severe, exudative eczema with crusting involving the scalp, eyelid margins, perinasal skin, retroauricular areas, axillae and groins in Jamaican children.

Human T-cell leukaemia virus 1 (HTLV-1) infection has been associated with this pattern of dermatitis.

Post-traumatic eczema

Eczema may develop at sites of trauma (Koebner) in individuals who have no past history of eczematous dermatosis. Eczema can also occur in burn scars.

Pityriasis alba

A pattern of dermatitis in which hypopigmentation is the most conspicuous feature.

Epidemiology

Pityriasis alba occurs predominantly in children between the ages of 3 and 16 years. It is often a manifestation of atopic eczema but it is not confined to atopic individuals.

Pathophysiology

The histological changes are unimpressive: acanthosis and mild spongiosis, with moderate hyperkeratosis and patchy parakeratosis. Although pigment is reduced, melanocyte numbers are not and may even be increased relative to healthy skin.

Clinical features

The individual lesion is a rounded, poorly marginated, oval or irregular hypopigmented patch. Lesions are often slightly erythematous and have fine scaling. Initially, the erythema may be conspicuous and there may even be minimal serous crusting. Later, the erythema subsides completely leaving only persistent fine scaling and hypopigmentation. Hypopigmentation is most conspicuous in pigmented skin, and in lighter skins may become more evident after sun tanning (Figure 14.16).

There are usually several patches ranging from 0.5 to 2 cm in diameter, but they may be larger, especially on the trunk. In children the lesions are often confined to the face and are most common on the cheeks and around the mouth and chin. Less commonly the face is spared and there are scattered lesions on the trunk and limbs.

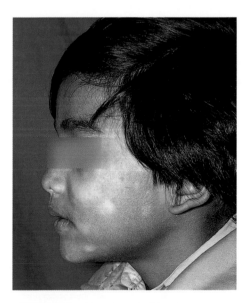

Figure 14.16 In pityriasis alba the failure of the affected patches to tan may first bring them to the patient's notice. (Source: Courtesy of Dr A. Marsden, St George's Hospital, London, UK.)

PART 2: INFLAMMATORY DERMATOSES

Differential diagnosis

Vitiligo, naevus depigmentosus, psoriasis (if on the trunk) and mycosis fungoides.

Recurrent crops of new lesions may develop at intervals. The average duration of the common facial form in childhood is a year or more.

Management

First line: Emollient.
Second line: Mild topical corticosteroids.
Third line: Topical tacrolimus or pimecrolimus.

Chronic superficial scaly dermatitis

(Syn. Benign form of parapsoriasis-en-plaques, chronic superficial dermatitis, digitate dermatosis, persistent superficial dermatitis, small plaque parapsoriasis, xanthoerythroderma perstans of Radcliffe–Crocker)

A chronic condition characterised by the presence of round or oval erythematous, slightly scaly patches on the limbs and trunk, which histologically show mild eczematous changes with little or no dermal infiltrate (Table 14.3). The condition is clinically benign by definition, but in some cases clonality of the lymphocytic infiltrate can be demonstrated.

Epidemiology

In most cases the onset is in middle-age. M > F.

Pathophysiology

The histology is not characteristic. It usually shows the changes of a very mild eczematous eruption, consisting of patchy parakeratosis, mild spongiosis and a slight, mainly perivascular, infiltrate in the dermis, chiefly composed of lymphocytes.

Clinical features

The disease begins insidiously with one or more erythematous, slightly scaly patches. The legs, trunk and arms are most often affected (Figure 14.17). It seldom involves the face, palms or soles. The patches are generally round or oval, but finger-like processes are also common, especially on the trunk, giving rise to the alternative name 'digitate dermatosis'. The patches are usually about 2.5 cm across, although much larger areas occur at times, especially on the legs. Individual patches are often slightly wrinkled and appear like cigarette paper. Itching may occur.

Differential diagnosis

Nummular dermatitis, eczematides, poikiloderma in its early phase and the early stages of the classic (Alibert) form of mycosis fungoides.

The patches are more prominent in winter than in summer, and may clear temporarily with natural or artificial sunlight. In a few patients the condition clears permanently.

Management

Only symptomatic treatment is required to allay irritation.

First line: Emollient.

Second line: Mild topical corticosteroids.

Third line: Phototherapy (narrow-band UVB/PUVA).

Table 14.3 Features that distinguish between a pre-lymphomatous (pre-reticulotic) eruption and chronic superficial scaly dermatitis

pre-lymphomatous eruption	Chronic superficial scaly dermatitis
Bizarre or angulated shape	Regular, round or oval shape
Fine scale	Coarser scale
May be irritable	Little or no irritation
Progresses to cutaneous lymphoma	Does not become malignant
Histology	
Absence of epidermal eczema	May be eczematous changes
Dermal infiltrate	Little or no dermal infiltrate

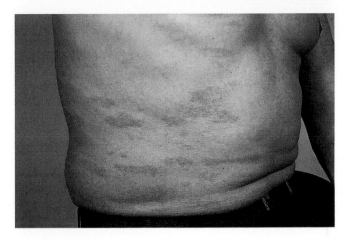

Figure 14.17 Chronic superficial scaly dermatitis.

DERMATOPHYTIDE

This is a reaction, at a remote site, to a dermatophyte infection.

This diagnosis should be suspected when the presence of a dermatophyte infection has been established and no fungus can be demonstrated in the dermatophytide lesions. A dermatophytide is thus a secondary, distant, aseptic skin lesion.

Epidemiology
Probably a rare condition.

Clinical features
Various clinical patterns of dermatophytide can occur. On the hands, eczematous vesicles may occur symmetrically on the sides of the fingers, usually as a reaction to tinea pedis. An eczematous dermatophytide can also mimic pityriasis rosea. Treatment of the dermatophyte leads to resolution of the secondary rash.

Halo dermatitis

Definition and nomenclature
(Syn. **Meyerson** **naevus,** **Meyerson** **phenomenon**)
Halo dermatitis is the occurrence of an eczematous ring surrounding a melanocytic naevus.

Histology shows a benign naevus surrounded by a dermal lymphocytic and eosinophilic infiltrate, with overlying acanthosis, spongiosis and parakeratosis (Figure 14.18). It differs from

Sutton halo depigmentation. Similar changes may be seen around seborrhoeic keratoses and other elevated skin lesions and are termed the Meyerson phenomenon.

Murray Williams warts

Multiple seborrhoeic keratoses occurring in areas of resolved eczema. They arise in the few months following resolution of the eczema and tend to gradually resolve by 6 months.

OTHER RELATED DERMATOSES

Lichen simplex and lichenification

(Syn. **Circumscribed neurodermatitis**)
An eczematous dermatosis characterised by a small number of heavily lichenified plaques or, very often, a single lesion.

Mild or early lichenification presents as a rather subtle coarsening of the skin surface markings on a background of dry and usually erythematous skin. As the condition progresses, the skin becomes markedly thickened and hyperkeratotic (Figure 14.19). Lichenification may occur spontaneously, when it is known as lichen simplex, or may occur as a secondary consequence of eczema and other inflammatory dermatoses.

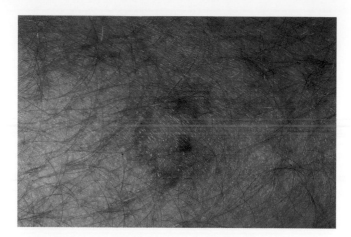

Figure 14.18 Halo dermatitis showing eczema around a nevus.

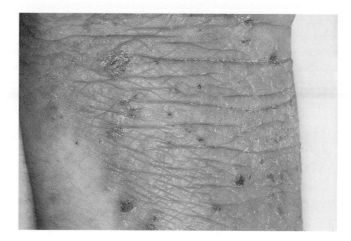

Figure 14.19 Lichenification of the arm in a patient with atopic eczema.

Epidemiology

The peak incidence is between 30 and 50 years of age, but it is seen at any age from adolescence onwards. F > M.

Patients with lichen simplex are more readily conditioned to scratch following an itch stimulus than are control subjects.

Pathophysiology

The histological changes of lichen simplex vary with site and duration. Acanthosis and variable degrees of hyperkeratosis are usually observed. The rete ridges are lengthened. Spongiosis is sometimes present and small areas of parakeratosis are occasionally seen. There is hyperplasia of all components of the epidermis.

The dermis contains a chronic inflammatory infiltrate and in very chronic lesions there may be some fibrosis.

In very chronic lesions, especially in giant lichenification, the acanthosis and hyperkeratosis are gross, and the rete ridges are irregularly but strikingly elongated and widened.

Lichenification can arise as a result of allergic contact dermatitis.

Clinical features

In all forms of lichenification, pruritus is a prominent symptom, and is often out of proportion to the extent of the objective changes.

In lichen simplex, single and multiple sites are involved with about equal frequency. Almost any area may be affected, but the commonest sites are those that are conveniently reached. The usual sites are the nape of the neck, lower legs (Figure 14.20a) and ankles (Figure 14.20b), sides of the neck, scalp, upper thighs, vulva, pubis or scrotum and extensor forearms.

Follicular eczematous papules may be seen, particularly on the forearms and elbow regions of children (Figure 14.21).

Lichen simplex of the nape of the neck (lichen nuchae) is usually confined to women. Scaling is often profuse and psoriasiform, and episodes of secondary infection are frequent. Post-auricular involvement may occur.

If lichenification occurs at sites where the subcutaneous tissues are lax and excoriation continues for many years, solid tumour-like plaques may be formed, with a warty, cribriform surface. This variant is known as giant lichenification of Pautrier and occurs mainly in the genito-crural region.

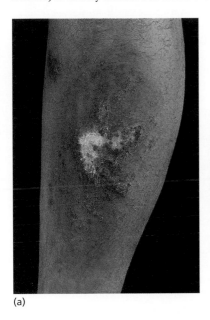
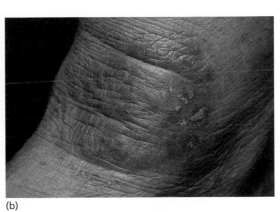

(a) (b)

Figure 14.20 Lichen simplex. (a) On the lower leg. (Source: Courtesy of Dr D. A. Burns, Leicester Royal Infirmary, Leicester, UK.) (b) On the ankles.

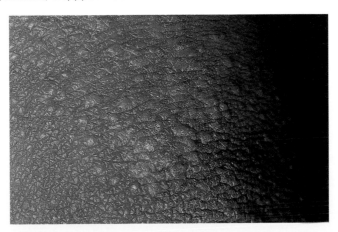

Figure 14.21 Follicular papules of lichenification adjacent to the elbow.

Pebbly lichenification is a distinctive clinical variant, consisting of discrete, smooth nodules, seen occasionally in atopic and seborrhoeic subjects, and in photodermatitis.

Differential diagnosis

Lichen planus, lichen amyloidosis and psoriasis should be excluded.

Management

A careful psychological history should be taken to elucidate any underlying problems.

First line: Patient education.

Second line: Topical corticosteroids, including impregnated adhesive tape.

Third line: Zinc paste bandages for limbs or intralesional triamcinolone for solitary lesions.

Erythroderma

(Syn. Exfoliative dermatitis, although the degree of exfoliation is sometimes quite mild) Erythroderma is the term applied to any inflammatory skin disease that affects more than 90% of the body surface. It may be the initial presentation of eczema in an individual or, more commonly, arises in the context of longstanding eczema.

Epidemiology

Incidence and prevalence
Annual incidence at 0.9 per 100 000 population.

Associated diseases
This will vary depending on the underlying cause of the erythroderma.

Pathophysiology

The main causes of erythroderma in adults are listed in Table 14.4.

Histopathology can help identify the cause of erythroderma in up to 50% of cases.

Clinical features

Erythroderma developing in primary eczema or associated with a lymphoma is often of sudden onset. Patchy erythema, which rapidly generalises, may be accompanied by fever, shivering and malaise. Hypothermia may develop.

The erythema extends rapidly and may be universal in 12–48 h. Scaling appears after 2–6 days, often first in the flexures, but it varies greatly in degree and character from case to case. The scales may be large or fine and bran-like. At this stage the skin is bright red, hot and dry, and palpably thickened. Many patients complain of feeling cold, especially when the erythema is increasing.

When the erythroderma has been present for some weeks, the scalp and body hair may be shed, the nails become ridged and thickened, and may also be shed. The periorbital skin is inflamed and oedematous, resulting in ectropion, with consequent epiphora. In very chronic cases there may be pigmentary disturbances, especially in black skin where patchy or widespread loss of pigment is often seen.

Table 14.4 Causes of erythroderma and relative prevalence in adults

Condition causing erythroderma	Relative prevalence (%)
Eczema of various subtypes	40.0
Psoriasis	25.0
Lymphoma and leukaemias	15.0
Drugs (including phenylbutazone, phenytoin, carbamazepine, gold salts, lithium, cimetidine)	10.0
Unknown	8.0
Hereditary disorders (ichthyosiform erythroderma, pityriasis rubra pilaris)	1.0
Pemphigus foliaceus	0.5
Other skin diseases (lichen planus, dermatophytosis, crusted scabies, dermatomyositis)	0.5

It is important that dermatopathic lymphadenopathy is not mistaken for lymphoma. In difficult cases, lymph node biopsy may be advisable.

Clinical variants are considered in terms of the underlying cause of the erythroderma.

Eczematous dermatoses

Generalisation of an eczema occurs most frequently in the sixth and seventh decades when venous eczema is a common precedent. However, atopic erythroderma may occur at any age. Pruritus is often intense. Some elderly patients have increased serum IgE and lactic dehydrogenase levels, with eosinophilia.

Psoriasis

In erythrodermic psoriasis (Figure 14.22) the clinical picture may be highly desquamative but when the erythroderma is fully developed the specific features of psoriasis are often lost. In some cases, crops of miliary pustules may develop at intervals and transition to generalised pustular psoriasis may occur.

Lymphoma, leukaemia and other malignancy

Cutaneous T-cell lymphoma is the commonest malignancy to cause erythroderma (Figure 14.23), followed by Hodgkin disease. Non-Hodgkin lymphoma, leukaemias and myelodysplasia have also been reported as causes.

Drugs

A wide range of drugs can cause erythroderma. Among the more commonly implicated are phenylbutazone, phenytoin, carbamazepine, cimetidine, gold salts and lithium. Erythema may first appear in the flexures or over the whole skin (Figure 14.24). This group has the best prognosis of all the causes of erythroderma, often resolving in 2–6 weeks.

Erythroderma of unknown origin

The percentage of cases in which no underlying disease is demonstrable diminishes with the thoroughness of investigation and the duration of observation, but in any series of cases it is rarely below 10%.

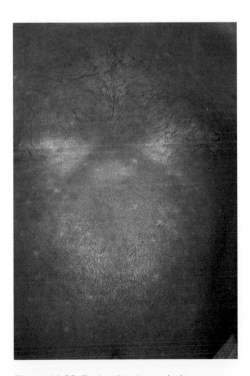

Figure 14.22 Erythrodermic psoriasis.

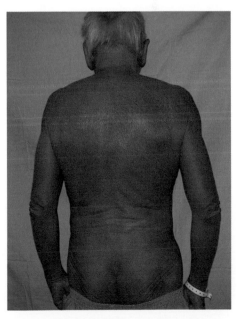

Figure 14.23 Erythroderma in Sézary syndrome. (Source: Courtesy of Dr B. Dharma, University Hospitals Coventry and Warwickshire, UK.)

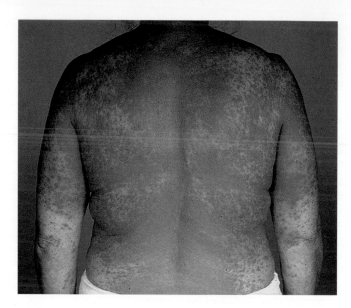

Figure 14.24 Widespread drug rash. This will progress rapidly to erythroderma if the drug is continued.

The three commonest causes of idiopathic protracted erythroderma are atopic eczema of the elderly, intake of drugs overlooked by the patient and prelymphomatous eruptions.

Histological features are usually non-specific. Immunofluorescence is negative.

It begins with an eruption of brownish red, flat-topped papules that become confluent (Figure 14.25a). The limbs and trunk are affected, and the face and flexures tend to be spared. A characteristic and distinctive pattern of sparing of the abdominal flexures has been termed the 'deck chair sign' (Figure 14.25b). The lesions sometimes develop along scratch marks. Pruritus is a consistent feature. Additional features include hyperkeratosis and fissuring of the palms and soles, and benign lymphadenopathy. There is usually circulating eosinophilia and a raised IgE. In terms of prognosis, papuloerythroderma typically persists for many years, although some cases have remitted.

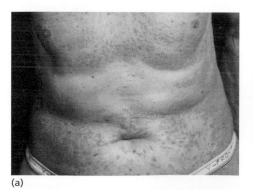

(a)

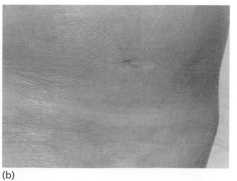

(b)

Figure 14.25 Papuloerythroderma of Ofuji. (a) The papules. (b) The 'deck-chair sign' (sparing of the body folds). (Source: Courtesy of Dr M.J. Tidman, Edinburgh Royal Infirmary, Edinburgh, UK.)

Reports of papuloerythroderma occurring in association with malignancies, which have included T-cell and B-cell lymphomas and gastric, lung, colon, prostate and hepatocellular carcinomas, would suggest that this eruption may sometimes occur as a paraneoplastic phenomenon. There are also several reports that papuloerythroderma may progress into mycosis fungoides. In terms of management, emollients, topical corticosteroids and antihistamines have produced a slow response in some cases. The condition can respond well to oral prednisolone, although high doses are sometimes required. PUVA, including bath PUVA, has proved effective, but papuloerythroderma is sometimes very refractory to treatment.

Papuloerythroderma of Ofuji

This distinctive pattern of erythroderma was described by Ofuji in 1984. It differs from ordinary erythroderma in that papulation is prominent, it spares the face and flexures, and is often intensely pruritic. Papuloerythroderma occurs in later life many cases occur in the eighth or ninth decades. M:F 4.7:1.

Differential diagnosis

See Table 14.4 for possible underlying causes.

The main complications of erythroderma are haemodynamic (high-output cardiac failure, especially in elderly patients) and metabolic disturbances. Cutaneous, subcutaneous and respiratory infections are common and pneumonia remains the commonest cause of death.

Management

First line: Consider hospital or day unit admission, withdraw or switch medications that may be implicated as a cause, monitor and correct loss of homeostasis, including temperature and fluid balance, treat any secondary infection, frequent application of greasy emollients.

Second line: Systemic therapy dependent on underlying cause.

PART 2: INFLAMMATORY DERMATOSES

Seborrhoeic dermatitis (SD) is a common, relapsing dermatitis; dandruff is a mild form affecting the scalp only.

(Syn. Seborrhoeic eczema, dandruff)

Epidemiology

Affects 1–3% of the adult population. Dandruff affects up to half of the world's population post puberty. M > F; presents around the age of 30 years in men, with a later peak in women.

The prevalence of SD is higher in patients with HIV infection. Iatrogenic immunosuppression also increases the rate of SD, e.g. in renal transplant recipients the overall prevalence is 9.5%. It is commoner in patients with chronic neurological disease, including Parkinson disease.

Pathophysiology

Malassezia globosa and *M. restricta* are most commonly associated with SD and dandruff.

Reported to occur more commonly in winter and improves with sun exposure; it is associated with stress, anxiety and depression and alcoholism.

Histology is not diagnostic and usually shows overlapping features of psoriasis and chronic dermatitis.

Clinical features

Onset is usually in early adult life with localised inflammation and superficial flaking of the skin. Affected areas may be asymptomatic or intensely itchy, and symptoms may be disproportionate to the clinical signs, especially on the scalp.

Facial SD typically affects the cutaneous folds – naso-labial, post-auricular, eyelids and glabellar area – and medial eyebrows (Figures 15.1 and 15.2). Hypopigmentation may be a prominent feature in dark-skinned individuals. Fine flaking of the skin with localised erythema is often present around the alar creases and nasal side walls, with scaling in the external ear canals or a more inflammatory otitis externa. Secondary bacterial or *Candida*

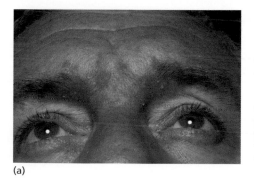
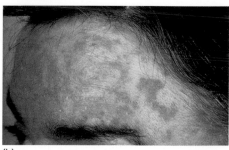

(a) (b)

Figure 15.1 Facial seborrhoeic dermatitis. (a) Characteristic redness and scaling of the medial eyebrows and glabellar folds. (b) Diffuse involvement of the forehead, eyebrows, and scalp margin.

Rook's Dermatology Handbook, First Edition. Edited by Christopher E. M. Griffiths, Tanya O. Bleiker, Daniel Creamer, John R. Ingram and Rosalind C. Simpson.
© 2022 John Wiley & Sons Ltd. Published 2022 by John Wiley & Sons Ltd.

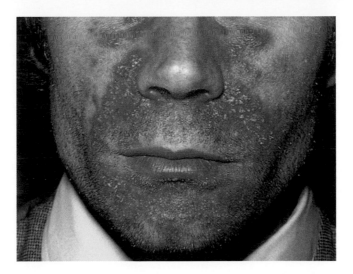

Figure 15.2 Severe facial seborrhoeic dermatitis with prominent involvement of the naso-labial grooves.

infection may occur (Figure 15.3). Scalp involvement ranges from mild flaking without underlying erythema to a more inflammatory eruption with thicker, yellow, greasy scales and crusts; similar changes can occur in the beard. Inflammation of the anterior eyelid margin (anterior blepharitis) can result in conjunctival irritation and red eye.

In men, involvement of the presternal area is typical with petaloid (petal-shaped) lesions that may be localised (Figure 15.4). More widespread involvement may extend to the upper back, umbilicus, axillae, groins and submammary area. In the large flexures, the affected areas may appear glazed and pink (Figure 15.5). The 'pityriasiform' variant of SD comprises a generalised erythematosquamous eruption, similar to but more extensive than pityriasis versicolor, with involvement of the neck up to the hair margin. Anogenital involvement may occur in both sexes.

Widespread SD may rarely evolve into an exfoliative dermatitis with erythroderma.

Infantile SD presents primarily with cradle cap and/or napkin dermatitis. It usually appears by 3 months and disappears spontaneously by 8 months of age. Additional involvement of the eyebrows, paranasal areas and large flexures is often present; this distribution is helpful in distinguishing infantile SD from atopic eczema.

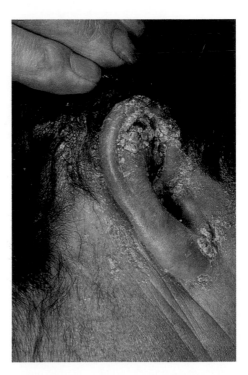

Figure 15.3 Seborrhoeic dermatitis of the ears with secondary bacterial infection.

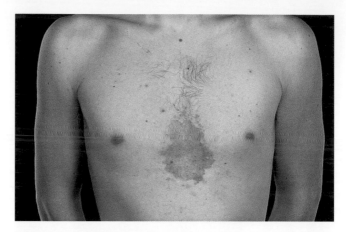

Figure 15.4 Seborrhoeic dermatitis of the presternal area. (Source: Courtesy of Dr D.A. Burns, Leicester Royal Infirmary, UK.)

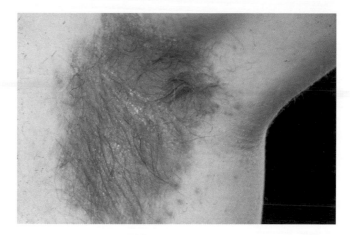

Figure 15.5 Seborrhoeic dermatitis of the axilla. The large flexures may become secondarily infected.

Differential diagnosis

In atypical cases the differential diagnosis is wide, including psoriasis, contact dermatitis, mild cases of Darier disease and Hailey-Hailey disease, perioral dermatitis, pemphigus foliaceus, pemphigus erythematosus, pityriasis rosea, early cutaneous T-cell lymphoma and erythrasma. Drugs may produce SD-like eruptions.

Differential diagnoses in infants include histiocytosis, zinc deficiency, acrodermatitis enteropathica and Leiner disease. In prepubertal children exclude tinea capitis and pediculosis.

Management

The diagnosis is usually made on clinical grounds without the need for diagnostic tests. HIV testing should be considered.

SD is generally considered to be chronic, punctuated by flares and requiring long-term treatment (Table 15.1).

Table 15.1 Summary of NICE recommendations for the treatment of seborrhoeic dermatitis

Type of seborrhoeic dermatitis	First-line therapy	Second-line therapy	Additional therapy
Scalp and beard	2% ketoconazole shampoo or selenium sulphide shampoo twice a week for a month, then once or twice a week for symptom control 0.1% tacrolimus cream b.d.	Medicated shampoos with zinc pyrithione, coal tar or salicylic acid	Topical keratolytic or mineral/olive oil for the removal of scale and crust Potent topical corticosteroid scalp application for 4 weeks if there is severe scalp itch
Face and body in adults	2% ketoconazole cream o.d./b.d., clotrimazole 1% cream b.d./t.d.s., econazole 1% cream b.d., miconazole 2% cream b.d. 0.1% tacrolimus cream b.d.	Mild topical corticosteroids for 1–2 weeks	Antifungal shampoo, e.g. 2% ketoconazole, as a body wash Hygiene measures for eyelid involvement using cotton buds moistened with baby shampoo
	Use as above for at least 4 weeks, then less frequently		
Severe	Review diagnosis, consider specialist referral, HIV testing		
In infants	Removal of scalp crusts with baby shampoo and gentle brushing Overnight soak of petroleum jelly or warmed vegetable oil if needed Daily bathing with soap substitute	Topical imidazole cream: clotrimazole 1% cream b.d./t.d.s., econazole 1% cream b.d., miconazole 2% cream b.d.	Topical corticosteroids not routinely advised but may be used for certain infants with nappy rash

Source: Adapted from the National Institute for Health and Care Excellence (NICE).

PART 2: INFLAMMATORY DERMATOSES

Atopic eczema

(Syn. atopic dermatitis)

Atopic eczema (AE) is an itchy, chronic or chronically relapsing inflammatory skin condition that often starts in early childhood (usually before 2 years of age; Box 16.1).

Box 16.1 The UK refinement of Hanifin and Rajka's diagnostic criteria of atopic dermatitis (eczema)

In order to qualify as a case of AE with the UK diagnostic criteria, the child must have:
- An itchy skin condition (or parental report of scratching or rubbing in a child)
  Plus three or more of the following:

1. Onset below age of 2 years (not used if child is under 4 years)
2. History of skin crease involvement (including cheeks in children under 10 years)
3. History of a generally dry skin
4. Personal history of other atopic disease (or history of any atopic disease in a first-degree relative in children under 4 years)
5. Visible flexural dermatitis (or dermatitis of cheeks/forehead and outer limbs in children under 4 years)

From Williams HC, Burney PG, Pembroke AC, Hay RJ. The U.K. Working Party's Diagnostic Criteria for Atopic Dermatitis. III. Independent hospital validation. Br J Dermatol. 1994 Sep;131:406-16

Atopic and nonatopic eczema

Epidemiology

AE has a lifetime prevalence over 20% in many affluent countries. There is good evidence for an increase in prevalence in low-income countries, in particular in Africa and East Asia. The prevalence of AE in adults declines gradually from 10% at age 20–29 to less than 5% after 50 years of age. In the majority of cases, AE starts during infancy usually before the age of 2, typically between 2 and 6 months.

Pathophysiology

Recently, there has been a growing realisation that, as with asthma and bronchial epithelial dysfunction, AE involves abnormalities not only of immune regulation but also a range of primary functions of the epidermis. Filaggrin insufficiency predisposes to barrier dysfunction but additionally T helper 2 (Th2) cytokines [interleukin (IL)-4 and IL-13] can also downregulate filaggrin expression, indicating a complex interplay in which the epithelia and the immune system regulate each other.

Monozygotic twins have a concordance rate of 0.72, whereas in dizygotic twins it is 0.23. Therefore, although an undoubted central genetic effect is clear, almost one-third of cases have strong environmental factors important in causality.

Rook's Dermatology Handbook, First Edition. Edited by Christopher E. M. Griffiths, Tanya O. Bleiker, Daniel Creamer, John R. Ingram and Rosalind C. Simpson.
© 2022 John Wiley & Sons Ltd. Published 2022 by John Wiley & Sons Ltd.

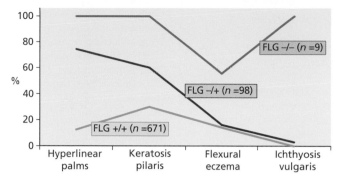

Figure 16.1 Filaggrin (FLG). A representation of the clinical features identified in *FLG* homozygote or compound hetrerozygote mutations (FLG –/–) versus heterozygotes (FLG –/+) versus wild-type status (FLG +/+). (Source: Adapted from Brown SJ, Relton CL, Liao H, et al. Filaggrin haploinsufficiency is highly penetrant and is associated with increased severity of eczema: further delineation of the skin phenotype in a prospective epidemiological study of 792 school children. Br J Dermatol 2009; 161: 884-9.)

Environmental influences on skin barrier integrity, such as frequent use of detergents and water hardness, are associated with an increase in AE risk, probably through induction of skin barrier impairment by a reduction in natural moisturising factor, increase in skin pH and a subsequent upregulation in protease activity.

Data demonstrate that skin barrier function is defective in lesional more than nonlesional AE, and that impaired barrier function parallels disease severity. This supports the view that the skin barrier is critical in AE pathogenesis. The clinical phenotype of *FLG* loss-of-function variants is described in Figure 16.1.

AE symptoms correlate positively with latitude and negatively with annual outdoor temperature. There is good evidence of higher eczema burden in cities compared to the countryside, particularly in less affluent settings.

There is an inverse association between AE prevalence and per capita consumption of vegetables, protein from cereal and nuts as well as all fresh and frozen fish, even after adjustment for Gross National Product. There is a positive association between outdoor pollution and AE.

Large sibships, daycare attendance, living on a farm, pets and helminth infection might be protective of developing AE but the effects are not clearcut. Early gut microflora of children who later develop AE has more *Staphylococcus aureus* and coliforms, and less lactobacilli and bifidobacteria.

A variety of primary immune deficiencies, including Wiskott-Aldrich syndrome, hyper-IgE (Job) syndrome and Omenn syndrome, give rise to eczematous lesions, which suggests that immunological dysfunction alone can result in cutaneous inflammation typical of AE. However, individuals with AE are not systemically immuno-compromised and show balanced profiles of immunological subsets in blood as compared to controls.

The term 'atopic march' describes the progression within an individual from AE to other atopic diseases, including allergic rhinitis, food allergy and asthma. Whether this progression from AE to other atopic conditions is causal or reflects co-manifestation is unknown.

The prevalence of associated food allergy is approximately 30–40% of unselected infants with AE, but the prevalence of food allergy *induced* AE is far less.

Patients with AE are particularly susceptible to certain cutaneous infections. The most common skin infection is with *S. aureus*. However, human papillomavirus-induced warts, fungal infections and viruses (such as HSV-1 and -2, vaccinia, coxsackie A and the poxvirus of molluscum contagiosum) are also frequent pathogens.

Innate immunity is compromised in AE, as demonstrated by reductions in keratinocyte-derived antimicrobial peptides (cathelicidin LL-37, β-defensin 2 and β-defensin 3).

Many patients are aware that sweating induces itching and aggravates their condition.

Patients with AE commonly complain that their condition is exacerbated by episodes of psychological stress.

> **Box 16.2 Clinical features of AE**
>
> - Itching
> - Macular erythema
> - Papules or papulovesicles
> - Eczematous areas with crusting
> - Lichenification and excoriation
> - Hyper- or hypopigmentation
> - Dryness of the skin
> - Secondary infection
>
> Source: Adapted from Brown SJ, Relton CL, Liao H, et al. Filaggrin haploinsufficiency is highly penetrant and is associated with increased severity of eczema: further delineation of the skin phenotype in a prospective epidemiological study of 792 school children. Br J Dermatol 2009; 161: 884-9.

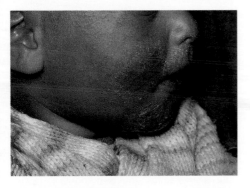

Figure 16.2 Atopic eczema: infantile phase.

Clinical features

The cardinal symptom is itch associated with a chronic fluctuating rash with a range of features (see Box 16.2). Itch may cause sleep disturbance, irritability and distress, and can be aggravated by warmth, sweating, bathing, exercise, emotional upset and woollen clothes worn against the skin. The skin is inflamed and painful.

The pattern of the rash varies with age (Figure 16.2).

Infantile phase

The lesions most frequently start on the face (Figure 16.2), but may occur anywhere on the skin surface. Often, the napkin area is relatively spared. When the child begins to crawl, the exposed surfaces (Figure 16.3a), especially the extensor aspect of the knees and elbows (Figure 16.3b), are most involved. The lesions consist of erythema and discrete or confluent oedematous, intensely itchy papules. Secondary infection and lymphadenopathy are common. The disease runs a chronic fluctuating course, varying with such factors as teething, respiratory infections, emotional upsets and changes in humidity.

Childhood phase

From 18 to 24 months onwards, the sites most characteristically involved are the elbow and knee flexures (Figure 16.4a); a mixture of erythema, crusting, excoriation, hyper- and hypopigmentation and warty lichenification

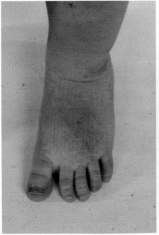

(a)

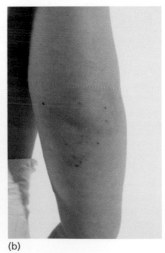

(b)

Figure 16.3 (a) Dermatitis causing hypopigmentation. (b) Extensor dermatitis in an infant.

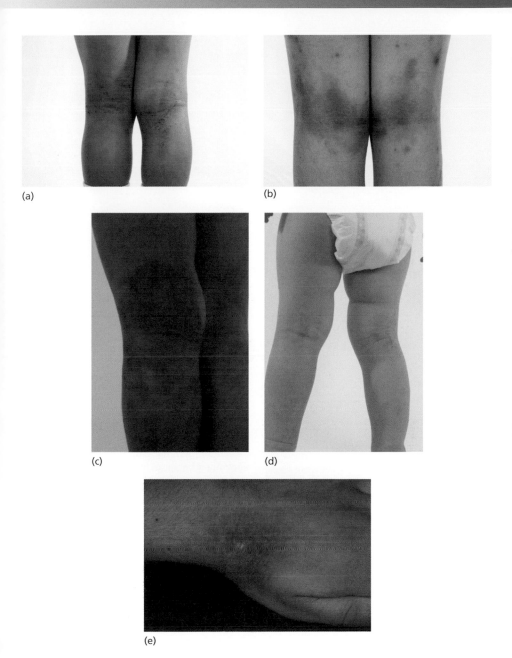

(a)

(b)

(c)

(d)

(e)

Figure 16.4 (a) Lichenification, crusting and excoriation in the popliteal fossae. (b) Postinflammatory pigmentation. (c) Flexural dermatitis causing hypopigmentation. (d) Flexural dermatitis. (e) Warty lichenification.

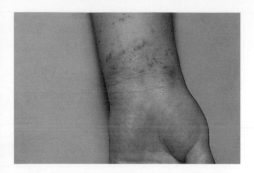

Figure 16.5 Flexural AE of the wrist in a child.

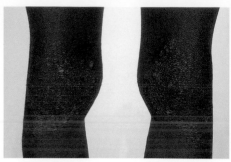

Figure 16.8 Marked lichenification on the knees of an African child.

Figure 16.6 Atopic 'dirty neck'; reticulate pigmentation on the neck of a patient with longstanding AE.

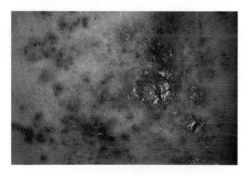

Figure 16.7 Atopic eczema: erythema, papules, excoriations, crusting and secondary infection but, in this case, little lichenification.

may be seen depending on the skin type (Figure 16.4b–d) on the sides of the neck, wrists and ankles (Figure 16.4e and Figure 16.5). The sides of the neck may show a striking reticulate pigmentation, sometimes referred to as 'atopic dirty neck' (Figure 16.6). Some patients with AE may not lichenify, even after prolonged rubbing (Figure 16.7). Patients with an extensor distribution of eczema in later childhood are uncommon and may take longer to remit. This distribution is commoner in black or Asian children (Figure 16.8). As well as the typical mixture of papules and lichenification, true eczematous lesions with vesiculation may occur, often in discoid patches (Figure 16.9). Involvement of the hands, often with exudative lesions, and sometimes with nail changes, is common (Figures 16.10 and 16.11). Acute generalised or localised vesiculation should suggest the possibility of secondary bacterial or viral infection.

Adult phase

Presentation similar to that in later childhood, with lichenification, especially of the flexures and hands (Figure 16.12). Localised patches of AE can occur on the nipples, especially in adolescent and young women. Involvement of the vermilion of the lips and the adjacent skin is commonly an atopic manifestation. Follicular lichenified papules (Figure 16.13a) are a frequent feature in black people and the Japanese. Photosensitivity may occur in adults with AE.

The hands may be affected in more than 50% of patients with active AE and the prevalence increases with age. A more diffuse, chronic lichenified eczema of the hands is frequently found in cases of extensive AE which persist into adult life (Figure 16.13b). Involvement of the feet is also common.

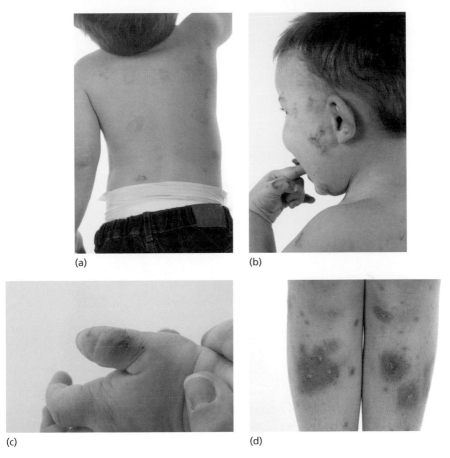

(a)

(b)

(c)

(d)

Figure 16.9 (a) Discoid eczema lesions in an atopic child. (b) Discoid lesions on the face. Saliva is a common irritant in young children. (c) Discoid lesion aggravated by thumb sucking. (d) Severe postinflammatory hyperpigmentation and lichenification in a discoid pattern.

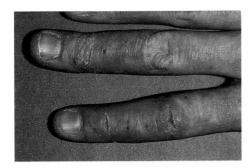

Figure 16.10 AE of the fingers of a child.

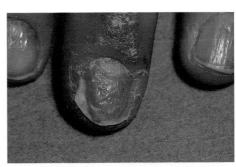

Figure 16.11 Nail involvement in AE in childhood.

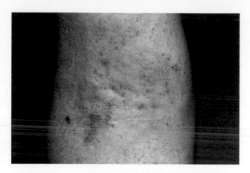

Figure 16.12 Adult flexural dermatitis.

> ### Box 16.3 Rare disorders that may have an AE-like rash
>
> - Hyper-IgE syndrome
> - Hypereosinophilic syndrome
> - Agammaglobulinaemia
> - Anhidrotic ectodermal dysplasia
> - Ataxia telangiectasia
> - Netherton syndrome (ichthyosis, bamboo hairs)
> - Phenylketonuria
> - Wiskott–Aldrich syndrome (infections and thrombocytopenia)

A previous history of AE, and more particularly hand involvement, is a highly significant risk factor for the development of occupational dermatitis, particularly if associated with loss-of-function filaggrin mutations and occupational food-related hand dermatoses.

The diagnosis of AE is based on history and clinical examination. The UK diagnostic criteria (see Box 16.1) have been rigorously validated for both adults and children of white and non-white groups.

Differential diagnosis

Infants: scabies, infantile seborrhoeic dermatitis, immunodeficiency states if the disease is severe in infants with recurrent systemic or ear infections and failure to thrive. Recurrent infected eczema in Jamaican children may be associated with human T-lymphotropic virus 1 (HTLV-1) infection. An eruption resembling AE, with or without other atopic disorders, and sometimes with raised IgE levels may be found in several rare disorders (Box 16.3).

Adults: nickel allergy and occupational contact dermatitis.

There are numerous proposed scoring systems for assessing the severity of AE. The three that have been most appropriately tested and validated [SCORing Atopic Dermatitis (SCORAD), Eczema Area and Severity Index (EASI) and Patient Orientated Eczema Measure (POEM)] are predominantly used in research and clinical trials.

AE has a profound effect, equal to or greater than that of asthma and diabetes, on many aspects of patients' lives and the lives of their

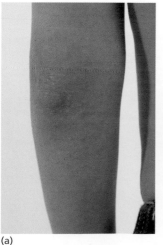

(a)

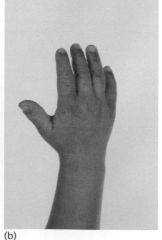

(b)

Figure 16.13 (a) Follicular lichenification on the surface. (b) Atopic hand eczema.

families. The psychological disturbance caused by eczema is increasingly recognised and may be amenable to specific interventions.

Growth delay may be associated with AE but usually only in severely affected children.

Secondary bacterial infection with staphylococci or streptococci is virtually an integral part of the clinical picture.

Patients with AE, both active and quiescent, are liable to develop acute generalised infections with herpes simplex virus (eczema herpeticum) to produce the clinical picture of Kaposi varicelliform eruption (Figure 16.14). Such episodes may present as a severe systemic illness with high fever and a widespread eruption.

Similarly, the frequency of warts and molluscum contagiosum is increased in children with AE.

A number of ocular changes can occur in AE. The Dennie–Morgan fold (Figure 16.15) is often present as a fold of skin under the lower eyelids. This change is not specific to AE, and is

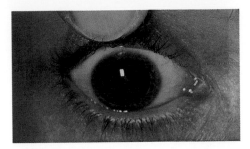

Figure 16.16 Atopic cataract.

commonly seen in nonatopic black children. Conjunctival irritation is common.

Keratoconus, or conical cornea, is rare and may occur in the absence of any other disease or in association with AE.

Cataract associated with AE (Figure 16.16) is thought to arise due to a combination of rubbing and the use of topical coticosteroids. Posterior cataract occurs more commonly than anterior in AE although the prevalence of anterior cataract is significantly more common in AE than in the population as a whole.

There is an increased risk of a variety of cancers, including both systemic and cutaneous lymphomas in AE, which is greater in more severe cases.

Allergic rhinitis (hay fever) and asthma occur in 30–50% of cases of AE.

Dry skin **is** a common feature of AE and figures prominently in its management. Ichthyosis vulgaris and keratosis pilaris may also be present.

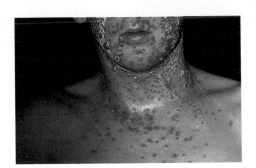

Figure 16.14 Kaposi varicelliform eruption: eczema herpeticum.

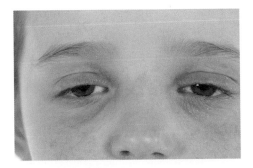

Figure 16.15 Periorbital dermatitis with Dennie–Morgan fold.

Infantile seborrhoeic dermatitis
Starts earlier than AE. There are a number of children who present with what appears to be seborrhoeic dermatitis and then progress to typical AE.

Lip-lick cheilitis
(Syn. Perioral eczema)
Moist or fissured eczema around the mouth is common in children with AE. It can also occur as a result of food allergy, and in children with no known atopy or allergy. Frequently spreading some distance around the mouth, it may become secondarily infected and crusted, and causes hyperpigmentation in darker skin (Figure 16.17). Its

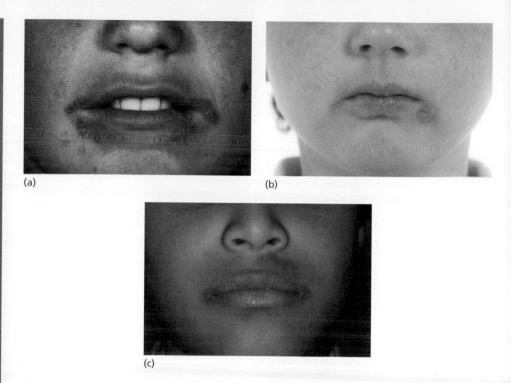

Figure 16.17 (a) Lip-lick cheilitis. (b) Lip-lick dermatitis with mild impetiginisation. (c) Lip-lick dermatitis with hyperpigmentation.

persistence, and perhaps its origin, is attributable to habits of lip licking, thumb sucking, dribbling or chapping. It is easily transformed into true perioral dermatitis by the application of potent corticosteroids.

Abdominal symptoms due to food allergy are more frequent in patients with atopic disorders, but are not restricted to them.

Those cases of urticaria in which an allergic basis is found occur more often in atopic individuals.

Spring and summer flare, often in association with hay fever, can be related to exposure to grass and tree pollens. This pattern is often associated with a facial distribution in the older child.

Investigations
The initial diagnosis of AE is rarely aided by investigations.

Management
Factors that indicate a worse prognosis include severe childhood disease, early onset and a concomitant or family history of asthma or hay fever. Children with raised IgE antibodies to foods and inhalant antigens at 2 years of age may also have a poorer prognosis. Poor prognostic factors may be underpinned by abnormalities of filaggrin structure and function. Teenage patients with dermatitis have a high risk of persistent disease in adult life.

Probiotics before and after pregnancy shows some benefit. Use of once-daily emollients from 3 weeks for 6 months in high-risk infants showed a 67% reduction in the development of active eczema.

AE is a chronic condition that is variable in severity and age of onset. Treatment should be tailored to an individual's needs, bearing in mind age, sex, social conditions, sites of involvement and severity.

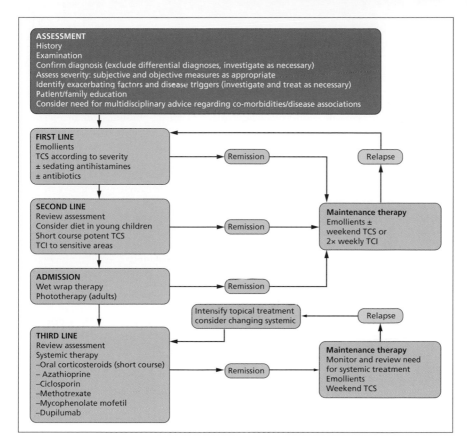

Figure 16.18 AE treatment algorithm. TCI, topical calcineurin inhibitors; TCS, topical corticosteroids.

In all settings, the initial assessment is very important. Although over 80% of sufferers have mild disease it is important to take a comprehensive history of the patient's disease, family history and recognised trigger factors.

Examination should include an assessment of the whole skin to assess severity, complications, and co-morbidities, including eyes and lymph nodes, and if required general medical examination of the respiratory and gastrointestinal systems.

For treatment see Figure 16.18.

A disease that may present with short-lived itchy weals, angio-oedema or both. It may be spontaneous or inducible.

(Syn. Angio-oedema (angioneurotic oedema, Quincke's oedema), Spontaneous (ordinary or idiopathic) urticaria, Inducible (physical, cholinergic and contact) urticarias)

Classification of urticaria

The main types of urticaria are shown in Box 17.1.

Box 17.1 Main subtypes of urticaria

- Spontaneous urticaria (previously 'ordinary urticaria')
  - Acute (the disease resolves in less than 6 weeks)
  - Intermittent (episodic)
  - Chronic (previously known as 'idiopathic'; continuous disease lasting for 6 weeks or more)
- Inducible urticarias (previously 'physical' and 'contact' urticarias)

Epidemiology

One in five of the general population may develop some form of urticaria over their lifetime. The point prevalence for acute and chronic urticariais is 0.11–0.14%.

May occur at any age. Acute spontaneous urticaria often presents in childhood but the peak incidence of chronic spontaneous urticaria is in the fourth to fifth decades.

F > M 2:1 for chronic spontaneous urticaria but F = M for acute spontaneous urticaria and inducible urticarias.

Autoimmune urticaria has an association with autoimmunity, especially autoimmune thyroid disease. Higher frequency of autoimmune disease in patients with autoimmune urticaria. *Helicobacter pylori* infection is linked to chronic urticaria. Bowel helminth infection should always be considered in countries where it is endemic. There is an increased risk of haematological malignancies including lymphoma.

Pathophysiology

A mast cell driven disease. A range of immunological and nonimmunological stimuli can degranulate cutaneous mast cells *in vivo* and *in vitro*. Cross-linking of mast cell bound specific immunoglobulin E (IgE) by exogenous allergens may be relevant to acute spontaneous urticaria but type I allergy is not the cause of chronic spontaneous disease; functional IgG autoantibodies against IgE or the high-affinity IgE receptor occur in 25–30% of patients with chronic spontaneous urticaria.

Weals and angio-oedema result from transient vasopermeability and vasodilatation of the dermal and subcutaneous vasculature following the release of preformed and newly synthesised mast cell mediators. Histamine is the major preformed mediator in most patients. Activation of H_1 receptors in the skin induces itch, flare, erythema and wealing whereas activation of H_2 receptors contributes to erythema and wealing. The histology of weals is usually nonspecific, with vascular and lymphatic dilatation, oedema and a variable perivascular

Rook's Dermatology Handbook, First Edition. Edited by Christopher E. M. Griffiths, Tanya O. Bleiker, Daniel Creamer, John R. Ingram and Rosalind C. Simpson.
© 2022 John Wiley & Sons Ltd. Published 2022 by John Wiley & Sons Ltd.

cellular dermal infiltrate consisting of lymphocytes, neutrophils and eosinophils. In the majority of weals, there is a sparse perivascular infiltrate, predominantly of helper T lymphocytes with a TH_0 cytokine profile expressing mRNA for interleukin (IL)-4, IL-5 and interferon-γ (IFN-γ).

Acute spontaneous urticaria

Although some cases of acute urticaria can be ascribed to immediate hypersensitivity, infection, or food or drug intolerance, the cause in at least 60% of patients remains unknown and may be multifactorial.

Potential causes are listed in Box 17.2.

Box 17.2 Potential allergic causes of acute urticaria

- Idiopathic
- Infections
  - Viral, e.g. upper respiratory tract infections, hepatitis B and C
  - Bacterial, e.g. *Streptococcus pyogenes*
  - Parasitic, e.g. *Anisakis simplex*
- Foods, e.g. cow's milk, hen's egg, nuts, seeds
- Drugs, e.g. β-lactam antibiotics
- Stings, e.g. bee, wasp venoms
- Blood products, e.g. transfusions
- Vaccines
- Contactants, e.g. latex

Acute urticarial reactions to food are common and many go unreported. The reaction may not be to the main food itself but to other ingredients, such as seeds or spices. Rarely, allergic reactions to food occur only if intake is followed by exercise, with neither food nor exercise alone inducing weals (food-dependent exercise-induced anaphylaxis), e.g. wheat, hazelnuts and shellfish. Wheat-dependent exercise-induced anaphylaxis is associated with IgE against omega-5-gliadin.

Not all acute urticaria is allergic. Food may contain vasoactive amines, including histamine (such as in cheese, fish, processed meat, tomatoes, pineapple, avocados and red wine) or histamine-releasing substances (such as in strawberries). Histamine generated in scombroid fish (underprocessed tuna, mackerel, swordfish) by histidine decarboxylase from bacteria can cause acute flushing, urticaria, vomiting and diarrhoea. High levels of histamine can usually be found in affected fish. Alcohol-induced urticaria is rare, but appears not to be allergic. Sulphites in white wine have been reported to cause urticaria and anaphylaxis.

Chronic spontaneous urticaria

Approximately 50% of patients with chronic spontaneous urticaria will react with a red weal response to intradermal injection of their own serum, known as the autologous serum skin test (ASST) response. These patients are said to show autoreactivity. Around half of these will have functional autoantibodies on the basophil histamine release assay. A much smaller number will show evidence of dietary pseudoallergens or chronic infection as aggravating factors that may be driving their illness. Chronic urticaria is often a multifactorial disease and its day-to-day activity is determined by exogenous aggravating factors.

Food additives, natural salicylates, amines, spices, green teas and alcohol may aggravate existing chronic spontaneous urticaria in up to 30% of patients, but are rarely the cause.

There is a highly significant linkage of human leukocyte antigen (HLA) DRB1*04 (DR4) and its associated allele DQB1*0302 (DR8) with histamine-releasing autoantibody-positive chronic spontaneous urticaria.

Clinical features

A *weal* is a descriptive term for transient, well-demarcated, superficial pink or pale swellings of the dermis due to reversible exudation of plasma in the skin that fade, usually within hours, without leaving a mark (Figure 17.1). Weals are usually very itchy and associated with a surrounding red flare when they arise.

Angio-oedema is a descriptive term for deep swellings of the dermis, subcutaneous or submucosal tissues (Figure 17.2). They are usually painful, rather than itchy, poorly defined and normal in colour. They can occur anywhere on the skin or in the mouth and usually last longer than weals.

PART 2: INFLAMMATORY DERMATOSES

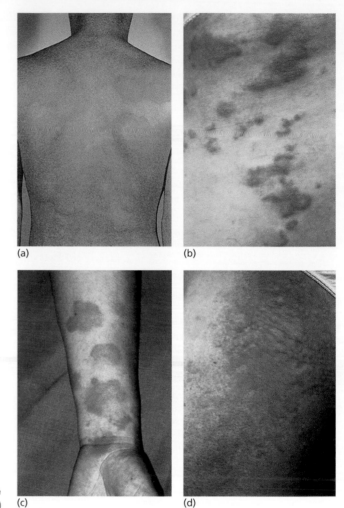

(a)

(b)

(c)

(d)

Figure 17.1 (a)–(d) Different morphology of urticarial weals. (Source: (a) Courtesy of Addenbrooke's Hospital, Cambridge, UK; (b)–(d) courtesy of St John's Institute of Dermatology, London, UK.)

Anaphylaxis is a sudden, severe, life-threatening, systemic reaction often involving the skin due to mast cell mediator release that may be allergic or nonallergic.

Itchy red macules develop into weals consisting of pale to pink, oedematous, raised areas of the skin often with an initial surrounding red flare. They may occur anywhere on the body, including the scalp, palms and soles, in variable numbers and sizes, ranging from a few millimetres to lesions covering large areas, and of varying shapes including rounded, annular, serpiginous and bizarre patterns due to confluence of adjacent lesions (Figure 17.1). Very rarely, bullae may form. Patients tend to rub rather than scratch, so excoriation marks are unusual, but occasionally bruising may result which may be seen particularly on the thighs. Weals may be more pronounced in the evenings or premenstrually.

50% of patients with spontaneous urticaria describe angio-oedema associated with wealing at some point in the illness (Figure 17.2); about 10% describe angio-oedema without weals. These deep swellings, which may be the same colour as normal skin, occur most frequently on the face, affecting the eyelids and lips, but ears, neck, hands, feet and genitalia may be affected. Mucosal swellings may also occur inside the oral cavity on the buccal

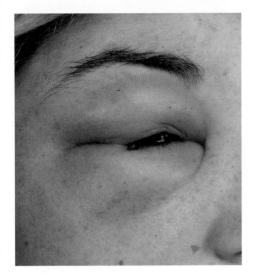

Figure 17.2 Angio-oedema of the eyelid. (Source: Courtesy of St John's Institute of Dermatology, London, UK.)

mucosa, tongue and pharynx but laryngeal involvement is rare. Angio-oedema may be preceded by an itching or tingling sensation, but it is not always itchy and may be painful. It may last from hours to days and the swellings resolve without skin dryness, unlike acute contact dermatitis.

It is often possible to identify nonspecific aggravating factors in chronic urticaria (Box 17.3).

Box 17.3 Aggravating factors for spontaneous urticaria

- Physical
  - Pressure
  - Overheating (passive or active)
- Infections, e.g. upper respiratory tract
- Drugs
  - Nonsteroidal anti-inflammatory drugs (common)
  - Opiates (rarely)
- Dietary pseudoallergens
  - Natural salicylates
  - Histamine
  - Food additives (tartrazine, azo dyes, e.g. E110)
  - Spices
  - Alcohol
- Menses (premenstrual especially)
- Stress

Inducible urticarias

The inducible urticarias are a distinct subgroup in which a specific stimulus induces reproducible wealing; this accounts for 19% of cases of uricaria. This feature is the basis of diagnosis and classification (Box 17.4).

Box 17.4 Classification of inducible urticarias by eliciting stimulus

Mechanical

- Skin stroking
  - Immediate
    - Symptomatic dermographism (itchy)
    - Simple dermographism (physiological, no itch)
    - Cholinergic dermographism
    - Red dermographism
  - Delayed
- Vibration
  - Acquired vibratory angio-oedema
  - Familial vibratory angio-oedema

Thermal

- Cold contact
  - Immediate
    - Primary cold contact urticaria (idiopathic)
    - Secondary cold contact urticaria (to cryoproteins)
  - Delayed (rare)
  - Localised
- Heat contact (rare)
- Generalised chilling
  - Reflex cold urticaria (drop in body core temperature)
  - Cold-dependent cholinergic urticaria (exercise in the cold)
- Generalised overheating
- Exercise-induced anaphylaxis (active overheating only)
- Food- and exercise-induced anaphylaxis (e.g. after gluten or shrimp)

Cholinergic urticaria (sweating induced)

- Overheating (passive or active)
- Stress
- Spicy foods

Others

- Solar
- Aquagenic
- Contact urticaria
  - Allergic (immunological)
  - Non-allergic (non-immunological)

Wealing caused by inducible stimuli usually occurs within minutes at the site of contact with the skin and persists for less than 30–60 min (immediate contact type, e.g. dermographism and most cold urticarias). Sometimes a generalised stimulus affecting the whole body is necessary (reflex type, e.g. cooling body core temperature to induce reflex cold urticaria and a rise in core temperature to induce cholinergic urticaria). In a few forms of physical urticaria, there is a delay of several hours from when the physical stimulus occurs before weals appear, for example delayed dermographism, delayed pressure urticaria and the rare delayed cold urticaria.

Angio-oedema and systemic reactions may occur from mediator release in many forms of inducible urticaria, but this is not seen in symptomatic dermographism.

Symptomatic dermographism (factitious urticaria)

The triple response of local erythema followed by oedema and a surrounding flare after stroking the skin is commonly elicited in chronic urticaria patients. This is known as simple dermographism. In <5% it is accompanied by severe itching (symptomatic dermographism).

Commonest in young adults. Wealing and itching at sites of trauma, friction with clothing or scratching the skin. Itching is disproportionately severe compared with wealing and is often most severe at night. The eliciting stimulus determines the shape of the weals (Figure 17.3), usually linear. It is usually idiopathic, but may sometimes follow a drug reaction (e.g. penicillin) or an infestation, including scabies. Dermographism may last for months or years, or be present intermittently.

Delayed pressure urticaria

Accounts for 2% of cases; patients nearly always have a component of chronic spontaneous urticaria. Wealing occurs at sites of sustained pressure applied to the skin after a delay of 4–8 h and lasts 12–72 h. Causes include tight clothing, manual work, sitting and walking (Figure 17.4). Lesions may be itchy, but are often tender or painful. May be accompanied by systemic symptoms of malaise, flu-like symptoms, arthralgia, myalgia and leukocytosis.

The diagnosis can usually be made by careful questioning; objective testing is performed by using a dermographometer.

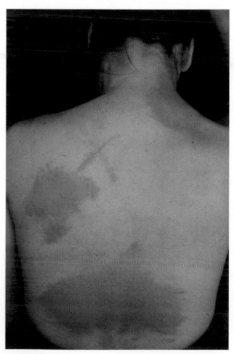

Figure 17.4 Extensive delayed pressure urticaria over the back after sitting against a hard surface. Induced delayed dermographism is also seen on the upper back. (Source: Courtesy of St John's Institute of Dermatology, London, UK.)

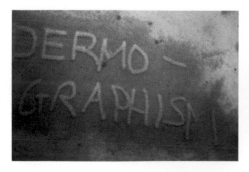

Figure 17.3 Dermographism, meaning 'skin writing'. (Source: Courtesy of St John's Institute of Dermatology, London, UK.)

Symptoms fluctuate in severity; they may show spontaneous improvement or last for many years.

Vibratory angio-oedema

Very rare. Any vibratory stimulus such as jogging, vigorous towelling or using lawnmowers induces a localised red itchy swelling within minutes and that lasts less than a few hours, but if the stimulus is severe, generalised erythema and headache may occur.

Heat contact urticaria

One of the rarest forms. Localised warming of skin at temperatures from 38 to 44°C for 2–5 min induces wealing at the test site lasting 1 h.

Cold contact urticaria

Encompasses a variety of syndromes in which cold induces urticaria. Idiopathic cold contact urticaria is the most common. It is important to warn against cold water bathing due to the risk of anaphylaxis and drowning. Treatment with low-sedation antihistamine is helpful. Induction of tolerance by repeated graduated exposures to cold can be helpful for selected patients, but it is time-consuming and not always effective.

Primary cold contact urticaria

Includes immediate and delayed urticaria.

Immediate urticaria

By far the commonest form, occurring at any age but most frequently in young adults. Itching and wealing of the skin occur on cold exposure within minutes and last up to 1 h. Cold winds and cold rain are particularly effective stimuli. Sometimes the mouth and pharynx may swell after drinking cold liquids. Systemic symptoms include flushing, palpitations, headache, wheezing and loss of consciousness, and drowning has occurred after cold water bathing.

Dermographism and cholinergic urticaria are frequently associated with cold urticaria. Diagnosis is made by application of a melting ice cube, in a thin plastic bag, onto the skin for 5–20 min and wealing occurs within 10 min, usually during rewarming (Figure 17.5).

Delayed urticaria. This form, where wealing occurs after a delay of hours after cold contact, is very rare

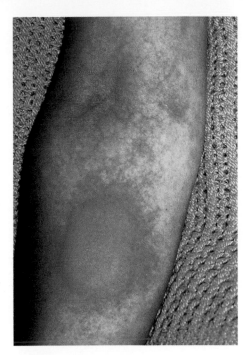

Figure 17.5 Wealing following application of a melting ice-pack for 20 min. (Source: Courtesy of St John's Institute of Dermatology, London, UK.)

Secondary cold urticaria

Secondary to cryoproteins is rare. It was found in only 1% of one series. It is usually associated with other manifestations such as Raynaud phenomenon, purpura or skin necrosis. Widespread wealing occurs in response to cooling of the core body temperature.

Familial cold autoinflammatory syndrome

Rare. Inherited as an autosomal dominant trait and is now known to be caused by the same gene mutation as Muckle–Wells syndrome.

Cholinergic urticaria

Very distinctive type in which characteristic small weals appear in association with sweating. It accounts for about 5% of chronic urticaria. Typically occurs in adolescents of either sex and may be worse in the winter months. The patient complains of itching weals that appear within minutes of exertion, when overheated or after emotional disturbances or even after eating spicy food. The weals characteristically are small,

1–3 mm across, with or without a well-marked flare. Cholinergic pruritus without weals can occur.

The diagnosis of cholinergic urticaria is best confirmed by provocation, with the appearance of typical itchy weals on an eythematous background after warming.

Exercise-induced anaphylaxis

Does not appear to be associated with cholinergic urticaria and cannot be reproduced by hot bathing. It occurs in patients sporadically and unpredictably, and appears to be a distinct entity. It is possible that some are examples of unrecognised food-dependent exercise-induced anaphylaxis.

Solar urticaria. Weals develop within minutes of exposure to visible, long- or short-wave UV radiation and fade within 2 h (Figure 17.6).

Aquagenic urticaria

Contact with water at any temperature induces an eruption resembling cholinergic urticaria, although the weals are few in number and are surrounded by a wide flare This is a different entity from aquagenic pruritus, in which there is water-induced itching but no wealing.

Contact urticaria

Common, but is not usually a cause of hospital referral unless there is an occupational problem, for instance latex allergy due to glove use. The term simply means urticaria resulting from skin or mucosal contact with the provoking substance. It may be *allergic* or *nonallergic*. The range of chemical, plant, animal and food exposures causing contact urticaria is very wide (Box 17.5).

> **Box 17.5 Some causes of contact urticaria**
>
> - Allergic contact urticaria (immunological)
>   - Foods
>   - Cow's milk
>   - Cod
>   - Kiwi fruit
>   - Peanuts
>   - Spices
>   - Celery
>   - Animals
>   - Saliva
>   - Moths/caterpillars
>   - Urine
>   - Human
>   - Semen
>   - Other
>   - Fragrance
>   - Latex
> - Nonallergic contact urticaria (nonimmunological)
>   - Histamine liberators
>   - Cobalt
>   - Dimethyl sulphoxide
>   - Vasoactive
>   - Nettle stings
>   - Jellyfish stings
> - Undetermined action
>   - Bleaching agent
>   - Ammonium persulphate
>   - Fragrance
>   - Balsam of Peru
>   - Flavouring agents
>   - Cinnamic acid
>   - Cinnamic aldehyde
>   - Preservatives
>   - Benzoic acid
>   - Sorbic acid

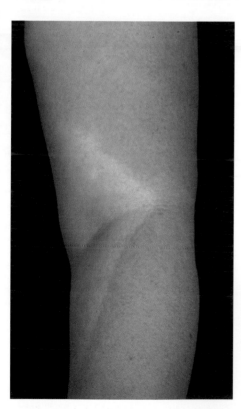

Figure 17.6 Solar urticaria.

Allergic percutaneous or mucosal penetration of an allergen to which the individual has already developed specific IgE will provoke a type I hypersensitivity response involving mast cell degranulation with histamine release resulting in an immediate, localised weal and flare resolving within 2 h.

Oral allergy syndrome

A form of allergic contact urticaria involving the mouth, characterised by immediate itching, swelling and burning after eating a wide range of fresh fruits, including apples, pears, cherries, plums, celery, spices and hazelnuts.

Nonallergic contact urticaria

May be caused by direct injection of vasoactive chemicals by plants (e.g. nettles) or animals (e.g. caterpillars, jellyfish). A more common form is from exposure to cosmetics (e.g. cinnamic aldehyde, balsam of Peru) or food additives (e.g. sorbic acid or benzoic acid) in foods such as tomato ketchup.

Occupational exposures include ammonium persulphate in hairdressing.

Differential diagnosis

Papular urticaria, erythema multiforme and prebullous eruptions. Acute contact dermatitis, lymphoedema and connective tissue disease (such as dermatomyositis) may mimic angio-oedema, but these conditions last longer than 24–48 h.

Investigations

See Box 17.6.

A full blood count and erythrocyte sedimentation rate (ESR) should be performed routinely. Thyroid function tests and thyroid autoantibodies, as around 14% of patients with chronic spontaneous urticaria have thyroid autoimmunity. There is currently no simple clinical test for serum histamine-releasing autoantibodies, although the ASST appears to be a reasonably sensitive and specific marker for them. If angio-oedema is the major component of the disease, measuring plasma C4 complement should be performed as a screening test for hereditary or acquired C1-esterase inhibitor deficiency. It is reduced and rarely, if ever, reaches normal values even between

---

Box 17.6 Investigation of spontaneous urticaria

Acute

- Infection
  - Throat swab if pharyngeal symptoms
  - Other appropriate samples for suspected viral or bacterial infection
- Foods
  - Investigate for IgE sensitisation (skin prick tests or ImmunoCAP where appropriate)

Chronic

- H_1 antihistamine responsive
  - Full blood count, erythrocyte sedimentation rate
  - Others as indicated by the presentation
- H_1 antihistamine unresponsive
  - Thyroid autoantibodies (all patients)
  - Thyroid function tests (all patients)
  - Additional tests dependent on clinical presentation
    - C4 complement (angio-oedema without weals)
    - Nonorgan-specific autoantibodies (if associated autoimmune disease possible)
    - Basophil histamine release assay or basophil activation tests (if functional autoantibodies suspected)
    - *Helicobacter pylori* (stool antigen or urea breath test)
    - Stool for ova, cysts and parasites (foreign travel)
    - Chest X-ray (if lymphoma considered)

---

attacks of C1-esterase deficiency angio-oedema. Functional C1-esterase inhibitor is reduced in hereditary and acquired disease. A skin biopsy may be helpful if urticarial vasculitis or delayed pressure urticaria are suspected.

Management

Acute attacks may last a few hours or days and be of great severity (Figure 17.7). There is no way of predicting the duration of an initial attack. Chronic cases where no diagnosis is established may last for weeks, months or even years, or be intermittent with repeated episodes occurring over decades. The severity is often

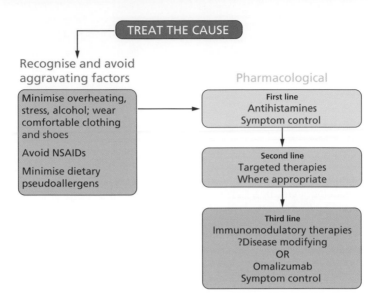

Figure 17.7 Management algorithm of chronic urticaria.

greatest at the onset, with subsequent waning. In general, spontaneous improvement occurs even in the absence of diagnosis or treatment. 50% of those with weals alone attending a specialist clinic can be expected to be clear within 6 months of onset, but 50% of those with associated angio-oedema can still be expected to have their condition 10 years later.

Explanation and nonspecific measures, including the wearing of loose-fitting clothing and application of soothing creams with menthol may be helpful. Patients should minimise aggravating factors, including overheating, stress and alcohol. Aspirin, aspirin-containing compounds and other NSAIDs should be avoided if possible. Selective COX-2 inhibitors may be tolerated by aspirin-sensitive patients if an anti-inflammatory drug is essential. If food additives, colourings or preservatives have been proven to be a problem, diets excluding these substances may be of value. Drug therapies can be first, second or third line, the choice of treatment depending on response to previous measures and degree of impairment in quality of life.

First line (antihistamines): H_1 antihistamines, hydroxyzine is the most potent of the classical antihistamines. The second generation of potent specific low-sedation H_1 antihistamines such as cetirizine; fexofenadine or loratadine is now the treatment of choice. Low-sedation antihistamines are used to control the symptoms of urticaria but do not influence the disease course. A combination of an H_1 antihistamine with an H_2 antagonist may be more effective than H_1 antihistamines alone. Ranitidine is preferable to cimetidine, which has more antian-drogenic side effects and potential drug interactions. Increasing the dose of second-generation H_1 antihistamines up to fourfold above licence in adults has become common practice.

Antihistamines in childhood

The principles of prescribing of antihistamines in childhood are the same as for adults. Doses should follow the relevant manufacturer's recommendations.

Second line (targeted therapy): Oral corticosteroids are effective in severe urticaria at high doses and may be used as rescue treatment over 1–3 days. The choice of other second-line therapies will be influenced by the clinical situation. Leukotriene receptor antagonists benefit aspirin-sensitive urticaria and may be of value in delayed pressure urticaria and autoimmune urticaria when added to antihistamines. Doxepin may be used for pruritus at night. Danazol may be beneficial for refractory cholinergic urticaria, but it is more likely to be tolerated by men than women because of unwanted virilising effects. Sulphasalazine and dapsone may be useful for delayed pressure urticaria, especially when oral corticosteroids are otherwise required for disease control. Tranexamic acid may suppress nonhistaminergic idiopathic angio-oedema. Narrow-band UVB can also be useful, especially in symptomatic dermographism. The emergency treatment for histaminergic nonhereditary angio-edema with oropharyngeal-laryngeal obstruction is intramuscular epinephrine.

Third line (immunomodulatory): For severe unremitting spontaneous urticaria not responding to conventional therapy, ciclosporin or omalizumab (anti-IgE).

Recurrent angio-oedema without weals

Angio-oedema is a deep, localised and self-limiting swelling of the skin and submucosal tissues due to a temporary increase in vascular permeability resulting from vasoactive mediators.

Angio-oedema *without* weals should be considered separately from angio-oedema *with* weals which falls within the spectrum of spontaneous or inducible urticarias (Table 17.1).

C1INH: C1-esterase inhibitor

Angio-oedema without weals involves the subcutaneous and submucosal tissues, rather than the dermis. Almost any part of the body may be involved, but the most common sites are the lips (Figure 17.8), eyelids and genitalia. The tongue and pharynx may also be affected, but this is much less common in mast cell mediator-induced angio-oedema than bradykinin-induced angio-oedema. Individual lesions may be either single or multiple and may appear suddenly. Itching is often absent. The lesions last from a few hours to several days.

Mast cell mediator-induced angio-oedema

Less than 10% of patients with chronic spontaneous urticaria develop angio-oedema alone. Delayed pressure urticaria weals are often deep and may resemble angio-oedema.

Hereditary angio-oedema (HAE)

A rare disorder, accounting for less than 2% of all cases of angio-oedema without weals. A family history is usual and up to 25% of cases result from a *de novo* mutation of the gene controlling

Table 17.1 The different types of angio-oedema presenting without weals

Mast cell mediator induced	Bradykinin induced
Chronic spontaneous urticaria • *Known causes* (autoreactivity, infection, food intolerance) • *Unknown cause* (idiopathic)	Hereditary angio-oedema • Type I (C1INH *concentration* low • Type II (C1INH *activity* low • Type III normal C1INH
Chronic inducible urticarias (only rarely present with pure angio-oedema) • Vibratory angio-oedema • Cholinergic urticaria	Acquired angio-oedema • Acquired C1INH deficiency • Drug induced (e.g. ACE inhibitor) • Idiopathic non-mast cell mediator-induced angio-oedema

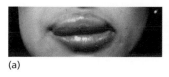
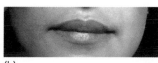

(a) (b)

Figure 17.8 Angio-oedema of the lips (a) during and (b) 3 days after an attack. (Source: Courtesy of St John's Institute of Dermatology, London, UK.)

C1INH (*SERPING1*). HAE is divided into three types (see Table 17.1).

Mast cell mediator-induced angio-oedema can present at any age but more often in the fourth or fifth decades of life. Over 75% of patients with HAE will have had their first attack by the age of 15 years. ACE inhibitor-induced angio-oedema is predominantly a problem of older people requiring antihypertensive treatment.

Mast cell mediator-induced angio-oedema and ACE inhibitor-induced angio-oedema F > M.

ACE inhibitor-induced angio-oedema has highest incidence in Afro-Caribbeans

Mast cell mediator-induced angio-oedema is associated with thyroid autoimmunity in common with spontaneous urticaria.

Pathophysiology
Mast cell mediator-induced angio-oedema
Most cases are due to mast cell degranulation.

ACE inhibitor-induced angio-oedema
Although ACE inhibitors mainly inhibit kininase II, resulting in an increase in bradykinin, several enzymatic pathways are involved and the pathophysiology is more complicated than is often assumed).

HAE. Patients with HAE types I and II are deficient in a natural inhibitor of C1INH. It has an autosomal dominant pattern of inheritance.

Angio-oedema due to acquired C1INH deficiency
Two types are recognised. Type 1 is due to continuous activation of complement by lymphoproliferative disease, including paraproteinaemia due to increased catabolism of C1INH. Type 2 is due to autoantibodies that recognise C1INH and inactivate it without triggering its target proteases. Both forms will have reduced antigenic and functional C1INH levels. All types of HAE are aggravated by oestrogen in contraceptive and hormone replacement therapies, but not NSAIDs.

Clinical features
Mast cell mediator-induced angio-oedema
Presentation is the same as angio-oedema in patients with spontaneous urticaria who also exhibit weals. Oro-pharyngeal involvement is unusual and laryngeal oedema is exceptional.

ACE inhibitor-induced angio-oedema
Swellings are confined to the face and oropharynx. Larnygeal angio-oedema may occur and may be fatal without prompt recognition and treatment. Recurrent swellings of the skin and mucous membranes throughout life, often associated with nausea, vomiting, colic and urinary symptoms. These attacks may occur regularly every few days or weeks. Abdominal symptoms may occur in the absence of skin changes and cause great diagnostic difficulty. The skin and mucosal lesions are often solitary and may be painful. They seldom itch and they may occur spontaneously or after trauma, dental trauma and intubation being especially hazardous. Weals do not occur, but many patients exhibit a distinctive reticulate erythema which occurs prodromally (Figure 17.9).

Systemic capillary leak syndrome (Syn. Clarkson syndrome)
A rare syndrome with dramatic recurrent episodes of exudation of fluid into various organs and may involve the skin. Angio-oedema can occur. A severe shock-like state may ensue and the eventual mortality is high. There is an immunoglobulin G (IgG) paraproteinaemia.

Episodic angio-oedema with eosinophilia (Syn. Gleich syndrome)
Recurrent episodes of angio-oedema associated with pyrexia, blood eosinophilia and infiltration of the dermis with eosinophils. No systemic involvement. Each episode resolves with prednisolone treatment.

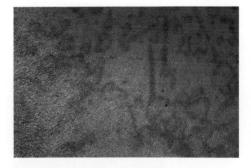

Figure 17.9 Reticulate prodromal erythema seen in some families with hereditary angio-oedema. (Source: Courtesy of Dr A. P. Warin, Royal Devon and Exeter Hospital, UK.)

Differential diagnosis

Oro-facial granulomatosis, dermatitis (especially of the eyelids), cellulitis and idiopathic scrotal oedema.

Investigations

Severe inflammatory disorders should be ruled out by checking C-reactive protein and a white blood cell differential. Patients with frequent attacks and/or longstanding disease should be checked for underlying causes.

C_4 complement screening for HAE types I and II, especially during attacks. The laboratory profile of the different types of angio-oedema without weals is shown in Figure 17.10.

Management

Chronic mast cell mediator-induced angio-oedema usually lasts for several months to years. Spontaneous resolution is the rule. HAE is lifelong with variations in activity corresponding to environmental factors, lifestyle, drugs (especially exogenous oestrogens and ACE inhibitors) and endogenous factors (e.g. puberty and pregnancy). The main risk of HAE is suffocation and death.

Management of mast cell mediator-induced angio-oedema as for chronic spontaneous urticaria.

Management of bradykinin-induced angio-oedema requires the input of clinical immunologists.

Urticarial vasculitis

A rare disease characterised clinically by persistent urticarial lesions with histological evidence of leucocytoclastic vasculitis.

Epidemiology

Rare. The lifetime prevalence of urticarial vasculitis is approximately 0.025% (estimated as 5% of the prevalence of chronic urticaria).

It occurs with peak incidence in the fourth decade. The incidence of hypocomplementaemic urticarial vasculitis syndrome (HUVS) peaks in the fifth decade. F > M. Both forms are rare in children.

Common associations are connective tissue diseases, including systemic lupus erythematosus and Sjögren disease, chronic hepatitis B and C, haematological disorders (essential

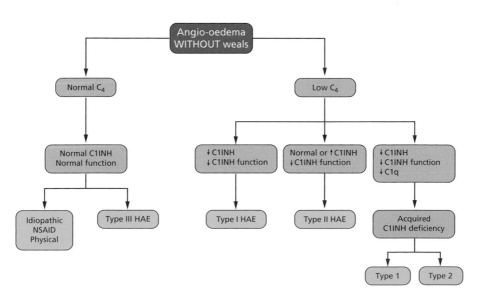

Figure 17.10 Laboratory profiles of different types of angio-oedema without weals. HAE, hereditary angio-oedema; NSAID, non-steroidal anti-inflammatory drugs.

cryoglobulinaemia and idiopathic thrombocyto-penia) and malignancies (Hodgkin lymphoma, acute myeloid leukemia, immunoglobulin A myeloma). Serum sickness represents an acute form of urticarial vasculitis.

Pathophysiology

Vascular endothelial damage is thought to be mediated by circulating immune complexes: deposition of IgG, IgM and C3 within and around the vessel wall and at the dermal-epidermal junction is a common feature.

Histopathology is consistent with a small vessel leucocytoclastic vasculitis. Potential causes include drugs, infections and physical factors. Drugs implicated in the development of urticarial vasculitis include cimetidine, diltiazem, procarbazine, potassium iodine, fluoxetine, procainamide, cimetidine and etanercept. Infections include hepatitis B and C, infectious mononucleosis and Lyme disease. Rarely, the disease is caused by physical factors such as exercise and exposure to sun or cold.

Clinical features

In some cases, infection or drug intake may precede onset. Patients complain of recurrent weals which are typically painful rather than itchy, lasting longer than 24 h and leaving residual hyperpigmentation (Figure 17.11). Fatigue, malaise or fever may be associated with weals.

In some patients, weals in urticarial vasculitis are indistinguishable from those in chronic urticaria. In addition to weals, other cutaneous signs may include livedo reticularis and Raynaud

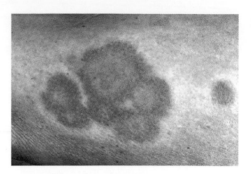

Figure 17.11 Urticarial vasculitis lesions resembling weals of chronic spontaneous urticaria. These sometimes fade leaving bruising.

phenomenon and very occasionally bullous lesions. Angio-oedema frequently occurs.

Joint involvement is common, usually arthralgia. Transient or persistent microscopic haematuria and proteinuria may occur. Pulmonary symptoms may include cough, dyspnoea or haemoptysis.

Hypocomplementaemic urticarial vasculitis

See Chapter 54 for differential diagnosis.

Investigations

See Table 17.2.

Management

In most patients, urticarial vasculitis is a self-limiting disease. Patients with normocomplementaemic urticarial vasculitis limited to the

Table 17.2 Diagnostic work-up in urticarial vasculitis

Initial work-up	Extended work-up (dependent on clinical presentation)
Lesional skin biopsy (diagnostic)	Direct immunofluorescence studies of skin biopsy
Full blood count	CH50, anti-C1q antibodies
Erythrocyte sedimentation rate	Cryoglobulins
Biochemical profile	24-h urine protein and creatinine clearance
C3, C4 complement components (serial testing)	Serum protein electrophoresis
Antinuclear antibodies	Chest X-ray, lung function tests
Antiextractable nuclear antigens	Assessment of visual acuity and slit lamp examination
Hepatitis B and C serology	
Circulating immune complexes	
Urinalysis	

skin tend to have a benign disease with a good prognosis. Conversely, hypocomplementaemic urticarial vasculitis is associated with a more severe course and more frequent systemic involvement (see Chapter 54).

First line: Non-sedating H1 antihistamines, NSAIDS.

Second line: Dapsone, colchicine, hydroxy-chloroquine, short trials of corticosteroids.

Third line: Azathioprine, ciclosporin, mycophenolate mofetil, methotrexate, omalizumab, intravenous immunoglobulins, cyclophosphamide, IL-1RA.

PART 2: INFLAMMATORY DERMATOSES

18

Mastocytosis

Mastocytosis is a rare acquired condition characterised by too many mast cells in the skin and other tissues.

Epidemiology

Mastocytosis is uncommon; lifetime prevalence is in the region of 1:10 000 to 1:30 000. The incidence of new cases of mastocytosis is bimodal, with about one-third presenting in childhood, usually in the first 2 years of life. Adults generally present between their third to sixth decades. There is no gender difference.

About 20% of adults with indolent systemic mastocytosis (ISM) have osteoporosis. The lifetime risk of adults developing an associated nonmast cell haematological disorder is estimated to be 20% of adults with ISM.

Pathophysiology

Mast cells accumulate in tissues as a direct consequence of acquiring a gain of-function mutation of *KIT,* which encodes the transmembrane receptor for stem cell factor (KIT).

Mast cell numbers are increased in the dermis of all types of mastocytosis. The epidermis is normal apart from an increase in melanin. They are also well demonstrated by Giemsa, tryptase or chloroacetate esterase stains in formalin-fixed biopsies. Mast cell infiltrates are predominantly found around blood vessels and skin appendages in the papillary dermis. In urticaria pigmentosa, they are increased up to 15-fold above normal. Full-thickness infiltration of the skin or a band-like involvement of the upper dermis are seen in mastocytomas and diffuse cutaneous mastocytosis. There are a number of degranulating stimuli for mast cells (Box 18.1).

Clinical features

Most cases presenting to dermatology clinics will be cutaneous in children or systemic indolent in adults. Distinguishing between cutaneous and systemic mastocytosis in patients presenting with skin lesions depends on further investigation, including bone marrow biopsy and blood tryptase measurements. Most adult cases will have systemic disease when investigated by bone marrow biopsy but other tissues, including the gut and liver, may be involved.

Box 18.1 Potential mast cell degranulating stimuli

- Physical triggers (especially rubbing, heat or exertion)
- Nonsteroidal anti-inflammatory drugs, e.g. aspirin, ibuprofen, diclofenac
- Some general anaesthetic drugs
  - Some nondepolarising muscle relaxants, e.g. atracurium, mivacurium
  - Opiates, e.g. morphine, codeine
  - Plasma volume expanders, e.g. dextrans
  - Anticholinergics, e.g. hyoscine
- Radiocontrast media (especially iodine-based ionic agents)
- Insect and snake venoms (allergic and nonallergic effects)
- Other allergens, e.g. latex
- Alcohol

Rook's Dermatology Handbook, First Edition. Edited by Christopher E. M. Griffiths, Tanya O. Bleiker, Daniel Creamer, John R. Ingram and Rosalind C. Simpson.
© 2022 John Wiley & Sons Ltd. Published 2022 by John Wiley & Sons Ltd.

Urticaria pigmentosa

The commonest pattern of cutaneous mastocytosis in adults and children (Figure 18.1). Numerous reddish-brown or pale monomorphic maculopapules, plaques or nodules appear in a symmetrical distribution anywhere on the body except the palms and soles, with the highest concentration usually being on the trunk (Figure 18.2) and thighs (Figure 18.3). Lesions may be seen in the hairline of children and on the neck of adults, but it is unusual for the face to be affected. They characteristically urticate within minutes of gentle rubbing (Darier sign) in children (Figure 18.4). Lesions may blister in infancy or childhood and this may be the presenting feature. Bullous mastocytosis is most often seen in infants with mastocytomas and diffuse cutaneous mastocytosis due to intense subepidermal oedema resulting from mast cell degranulation.

Flushing occurs in about 50% of patients, alcohol intolerance and pruritus in slightly less. Other symptoms may include heat or cold intolerance, recurrent diarrhoea, acid dyspepsia and urinary frequency.

Telangiectasia macularis eruptiva perstans

Patients are usually adults presenting with persistent red macules that may or may not show obvious telangiectasia, especially on the trunk,

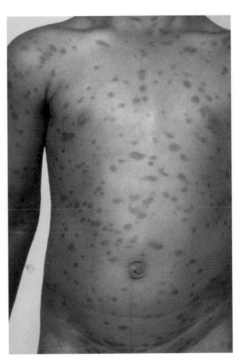

Figure 18.2 Urticaria pigmentosa lesions on the trunk of a child. (Source: Courtesy of St John's Institute of Dermatology, London, UK.)

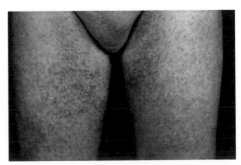

Figure 18.3 Urticaria pigmentosa on the thighs of an adult. (Source: Courtesy of St John's Institute of Dermatology, London, UK.)

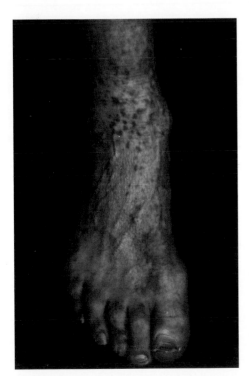

Figure 18.1 Patient with urticaria pigmentosa, extensive erythema and telangiectasia resembling telangiectasia macularis eruptive perstans.

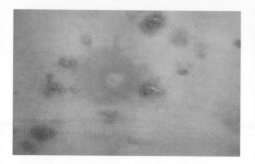

Figure 18.4 Positive Darier's sign in a nodule of urticaria pigmentosa in a young child. (Source: Courtesy of Norfolk and Norwich University Hospital, UK.)

Figure 18.5 Telangiectasia macularis eruptive perstans. (Source: Courtesy of St John's Institute of Dermatology, London, UK.)

which flush but usually do not urticate on rubbing (Figure 18.5).

Mastocytoma

Cutaneous mastocytosis may present with red, pink or yellowish nodules or plaques in infancy or early childhood, measuring up to 3–4 cm in diameter (Figure 18.6). They are usually solitary. If multiple, the lesions can be difficult to distinguish from nodular urticaria pigmentosa. They tend to blister if rubbed, especially in the napkin area of infants and, occasionally, attacks of flushing can be induced by rubbing a solitary mastocytoma. Nearly all mastocytomas involute over the first few years of childhood.

Diffuse cutaneous mastocytosis

A very rare form of mastocytosis in which mast cells infiltrate the entire skin diffusely (Figure 18.7). Blistering after minor trauma or scratching is common and pruritus for the child may be intense. The epidermis may be lost over a large area and can resemble impetigo. Patients are at risk of systemic disease and severe complications, including anaphylaxis and diarrhea.

Management

Most patients presenting to dermatology clinics with cutaneous mastocytosis or ISM will have an excellent prognosis, particularly children.

Most mastocytomas resolve in childhood. Around 50% of children with urticaria pigmentosa clear by adolescence. Prognosis of advanced mastocytosis with an associated

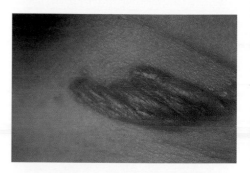

Figure 18.6 Pink mastocytoma in an infant. (Source: Courtesy of St John's Institute of Dermatology, London, UK.)

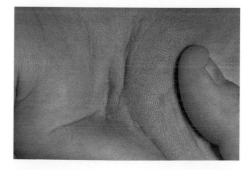

Figure 18.7 Diffuse cutaneous mastocytosis on the back.

blood disorder will relate to the associated haematological disorder, and management will be directed primarily towards this (Figure 18.8).

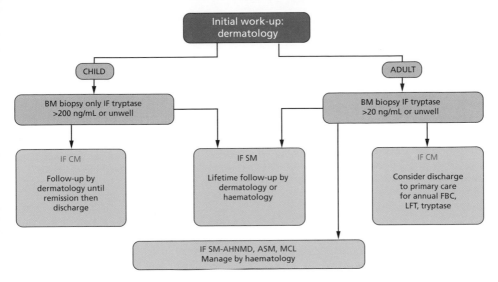

Figure 18.8 Algorithm for reviewing adults and children with mastocytosis. ASM, aggressive systemic mastocytosis; BM, bone marrow; CM, cutaneous mastocytosis; FBC, full blood count; LFT, liver function test; MCL, mast cell leukaemia; SM, systemic mastocytosis; SM-AHNMD, systemic mastocytosis associated haematological non-mast cell disease.

Box 18.2 Summary of management options for mastocytosis

- Avoid triggers of mast cell degranulatioan (see Box 18.1)
- Treat systemic and skin symptoms due to mast cell mediator release
  - H1 antihistamines (up-dosing allowed in line with urticaria)
  - H2 antihistamines (hyperacidity)
  - Proton pump inhibitors
  - Sodium cromoglycate (orally for bowel symptoms)
- Consider skin-directed treatments for symptoms and for improving the appearance of lesion
  - Topical corticosteroids (e.g. 0.05% clobetasol propionate twice daily for up to 6 weeks for urticaria pigmentosa on the body in adults but not the face)
  - Topical 4% sodium cromoglycate cream for children (if available)
  - Narrow-band ultraviolet B phototherapy or photochemotherapy (PUVA)
- Cytoreductive treatments for systemic mastocytosis with organ dysfunction or failure

- Oral corticosteroids
- Interferon-α
- Cladribine
- KIT tyrosine kinase inhibitors
  - Imatinib (not effective for D816V-positive systemic mastocytosis)
  - Midostaurin
  - Masitinib (ongoing phase III study for cutaneous mastocytosis, ISM and smouldering systemic mastocytosis [SSM with handicap])
- Manage complications
  - Osteopenia and osteoporosis
    - Vitamin D and calcium supplements
    - Bisphosphonates
  - Haematological (chemotherapy protocols for associated haematological non-mast cell disease, AHNMD)
  - Anaphylaxis (epinephrine autoinjectors should be offered to adults with systemic mastocytosis and children with extensive cutaneous mastocytosis)

19 Reactive inflammatory erythemas

A group of skin conditions that present with ring-like or annular lesions that do not necessarily lead to a specific underlying diagnosis and may pose diagnostic and therapeutic problems.

Erythema multiforme

Erythema multiforme (EM) is a self-limiting cytotoxic dermatitis resulting from cell-mediated hypersensitivity most commonly to drugs or infection.

Pathophysiology

The clinical reaction pattern of EM is associated with many different triggering factors and probably has an immunological basis. Human leukocyte antigen (HLA) studies have shown an association with HLA-B62 (B15), HLA-B35 and HLA-DR53 in recurrent cases. There are a variety of triggers of EM (see Box 19.1).

Pathophysiology

The most important histological changes are necrotic keratinocytes in the epidermis, which can be zonal and in the upper dermis, that is, a spectrum belonging to the lichenoid, band-like or cytotoxic reaction patterns. Some cases have prominent dermal inflammatory changes, with an interstitial and perivascular lymphohistiocytic infiltrate, sometimes with eosinophils if drug-related, papillary oedema and vasodilatation. If chronic, individually necrotic apoptotic cells and pigmentary incontinence with papillary melanophages. Such changes occur especially in classic EM with 'target' lesions. In more severe bullous cases, there are subepidermal bullae and necrosis of the whole epidermis.

Clinical features

EM can occur at any age, including in neonates or young children. In general, the course is that of an eruption developing over a few days and

---

Box 19.1 Triggers of erythema multiforme

Viral infections
Bacterial infections
Fungal infections
Contact hypersensitivity reactions
- *Primula obconica*,
- Poison ivy
- Laurel oil,
- *Alpinia galanga* (spicy edible Thai ginger)
- Diphenylcyclopropenone
- Bromofluorene
- Latex glove
- Blister beetle

Miscellaneous
- Carcinoma, lymphoma, leukaemia
- Granulomatosis with polyangiitis
- Lupus erythematosus (Rowell syndrome)
- Polyarteritis nodosa
- Polymorphic light eruption
- Pregnancy, premenstrual, 'autoimmune progesterone dermatitis'
- Sarcoidosis
- X-ray therapy

Drug reactions
Metals and other elements

Rook's Dermatology Handbook, First Edition. Edited by Christopher E. M. Griffiths, Tanya O. Bleiker, Daniel Creamer, John R. Ingram and Rosalind C. Simpson.
© 2022 John Wiley & Sons Ltd. Published 2022 by John Wiley & Sons Ltd.

resolving in 2–3 weeks. Repeated attacks associated with recurrent herpes simplex are frequent.

EM minor, papular or simplex form

This accounts for approximately 80% of cases. Clinically, macular, papular or urticarial lesions, as well as the classic iris or 'target lesions' (Figures 19.1 and 19.2), are distributed preferentially on the distal extremities., The lesions are dull red, flat or slightly raised maculopapules. Target lesions are less than 3 cm in diameter, rounded and have three zones: a central area of dusky erythema or purpura, a middle paler zone of oedema and an outer ring of erythema with a well-defined edge. Lesions appear in successive crops for a few days and fade in 1–2 weeks. Lesions may be few or profuse. Characteristically, the dorsa of the hands, palms, wrists, feet and extensor aspects of the elbows and knees are affected; less commonly the face as well as the oral and genital mucous membranes (Figures 19.3–19.5). The Koebner phenomenon is not uncommon. Photoaggravation of EM is well recognised.

Localised vesiculobullous form

This is intermediate in severity. Lesions present as erythematous macules or plaques, often with a central bulla and a marginal ring of vesicles (herpes iris of Bateman). Lesions tend to occur in the classic acral distribution, but may be few in number.

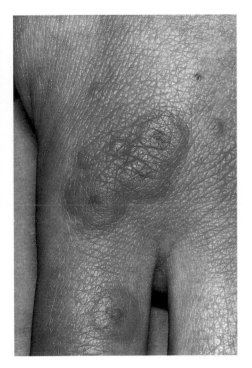

Figure 19.1 Classic target lesion in EM.

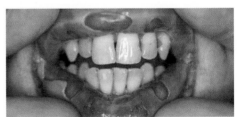

Figure 19.3 Mucosal lesions in EM.

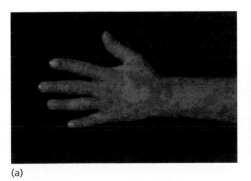

(a)

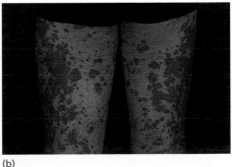

(b)

Figure 19.2 (a) Widespread acutely inflamed target lesions, including blisters, in EM on the hands and arm in a 33-year-old Asian man. (b) Classic target lesions in EM on the thighs in an adult white man.

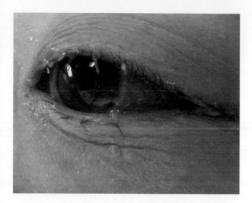

Figure 19.4 Eye involvement in EM.

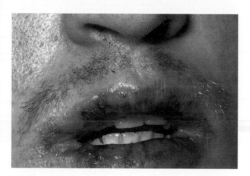

Figure 19.5 EM minor. Mucosal lesions.

EM major

A severe illness associated with more extensive target lesions and mucous membrane involvement. Onset is usually sudden, a prodromal systemic illness of 1–13 days may be present.

Atypical cases

EM-like lesions have been reported in the setting of acute generalised exanthematous pustulosis. EM along Blaschko's lines has been reported.

Rowell syndrome

This syndrome comprises lupus erythematosus associated with EM-like skin lesions and immunological findings of speckled antinuclear antibodies, anti-La or anti-Ro antibodies and a positive test for rheumatoid factor.

Differential diagnosis

Vancomyin-induced linear IgA disease and lupus erythematosus, pemphigoid and other autoimmune bullous conditions, toxic erythemas of unknown cause, stem cell transplantation erythematous eruptions, urticarial vasculitis and Kawasaki disease.

Management

Investigation of underlying cause and symptomatic treatment only is more often necessary in the limited papular and localised bullous forms. Ocular involvement requires early referral to an ophthalmologist. For more severe cases, prednisolone at an initial dosage of 30–60 mg/day, decreasing over a period of 1–4 weeks, may be used.

Erythema annulare centrifugum

(Syn. Erythema perstans, erythema gyratum perstans, annular erythema of infancy, erythema figuratum perstans, erythema simplex gyratum)

Erythema annulare centrifugum (EAC) is a gyrate erythema that is typically characterised by annular, polycyclic, erythematous plaques with scaling behind the advancing edge (Figure 19.6a).

EAC is considered to include all the gyrate erythemas except for erythema marginatum, erythema chronicum migrans and erythema gyratum repens.

Epidemiology

There is approximately one case per 100 000 population per year. It can occur at any age with no gender bias.

Associated diseases

EAC is a reactive process which may be precipitated by drugs or malignancy but a concurrent infection is the most common underlying association, including viral (Epstein–Barr virus), bacterial (streptococcal infections, *Escherichia coli*), mycobacterial, fungal (dermatophytes, 48% of cases) or parasitic.

Pathophysiology

A spectrum of nonspecific histological findings is seen in EAC and it is critical to have clinicopathological correlation. The characteristic

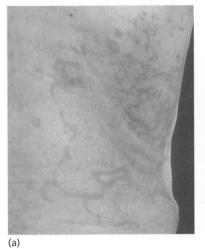
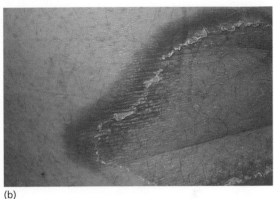

(a)   (b)

Figure 19.6 Erythema annulare centrifugum. (a) Multiple polyclic annular lesions, some of which have a urticated edge. (b) Close up view of a lesion.

histological feature in EAC is a perivascular 'sleeve-like' lymphohistiocytic infiltrate which may be mainly superficial, mainly deep or mixed.

Clinical features
Presentation is with expanding polycyclic, annular, erythematous plaques that may expand by up to 2–3 mm per day with central clearing.

EAC may be of variable duration, lasting from days to decades, with a mean of 2.8 years.

Differential diagnosis
Tinea corporis, subacute cutaneous lupus erythematosus, annular sarcoidosis, necrotic migratory erythema, granuloma annulare, cutaneous T-cell lymphoma, granuloma faciale, drug eruptions, EM, erythema gyratum repens, erythema marginatum and Wells syndrome (eosinophilic cellulitis).

Management
Investigations are aimed at excluding alternative diagnoses and identifying an underlying cause. As fungal infections are the commonest cause, a culture of affected skin and nails should be undertaken if a dermatophyte infection is suspected.

First line: The first goal should be to identify and treat any underlying condition but if this is not possible treatment with moderately potent or potent topical corticosteroids or topical calcipotriol would be appropriate.

Second line: Topical tacrolimus, phototherapy.

Third line: Chloroquine or hydroxychloroquine, systemic corticosteroids.

Annular erythema of infancy

Annular erythema of infancy was first described as a distinct dermatosis in 1981.

Pathophysiology
The appearances are typically the same as in cases of EAC with a dermal perivascular and interstitial lymphocytic infiltrate.

Clinical features
The lesions are identical to those of EAC with polycyclic annular, erythematous, maculopapular lesions enlarging and evolving into variably sized, single or grouped annular plaques predominantly localised to the face, trunk and proximal limbs (Figure 19.7). Individual lesions last from two to several days and there may be a cyclical pattern of new lesions appearing every

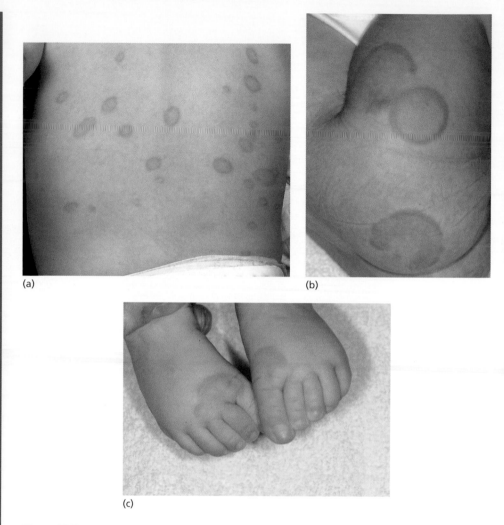

Figure 19.7 Scattered lesions of annular erythema of infancy on (a) the back, (b) the upper leg and (c) the feet. (Source: (b) and (c) Courtesy of Dr Jane Ravenscroft, Consultant Dermatologist, Queen's Medical Centre, Nottingham, UK.)

5–6 weeks. The eruption may start in infancy or in teenage years, is self-limiting and has no associated systemic symptoms.

Differential diagnosis

Familial annular erythema, urticaria, erythema gyratum atrophicans, neonatal lupus erythematosus, erythema chronicum migrans, tinea corporis, mycosis fungoides and annular lichenoid dermatitis of youth.

Management

Investigations include microscopy and culture of skin scrapings, antinuclear antibodies, including antibodies to dsDNA, and extractable nuclear antigen (ENA) (Ro, La, Sm, and RNP), and skin biopsy if indicated.

First line: Any associated infection should be treated.

Second line: Topical corticosteroids.

Third line: Topical tacrolimus.

Erythema gyratum repens

Erythema gyratum repens is a rare, distinctive, figurate eruption.

Epidemiology

It usually occurs in patients older than 40 years, usually in the seventh decade.

M:F = 2:1.

Pathophysiolology

The histological features are not diagnostic.

Clinical features

Regular waves of erythema spread over the body to produce a series of concentric, figurate bands in a pattern resembling the grain of wood. The characteristic feature is the way the rings, swirls or waves appear within existing lesions to form a concentric pattern of sequential eruptions, with day-to-day migration of the leading edge by about 1 cm. Scaling, usually at the trailing edge, and itch are usually prominent. Hyperkeratosis of palms occurs in about 10% and has been reported in both paraneoplastic and idiopathic cases.

Erythema gyratum repens is considered in the majority of patients (80%) to be a paraneoplastic dermatosis and may precede the diagnosis of malignancy or may post-date such a diagnosis. The most frequent underlying malignancy in descending order is carcinoma of the lung (47%) followed by oesophagus, breast, stomach, kidney, cervix, pharynx, urinary bladder, uterus and/or cervix, pancreas, prostate and haematological neoplasia.

Prognosis is dependent on the underlying disease.

Differential diagnosis

EAC, EM, necrolytic migratory erythema, subacute cutaneous lupus erythematosus, lupus erythematosus gyratum repens, erythema chronicum migrans, tinea corporis, erythrokeratoderma variabilis, subacute annular (Lapière) variant of psoriasis and pityriasis rubra pilaris.

Management

Useful investigations include a full blood count, biochemistry, antinuclear antibody profile, chest X-ray, mammogram, cervical smear, prostate-specific antigen, CT scan of the thorax, abdomen and pelvis, and, if indicated, endoscopy or colonoscopy.

First line: Identify the underlying disease.

Second line: Treat the underlying disease.

Erythema marginatum

Erythema marginatum is an annular and sometimes polycyclic, serpiginous, erythematous eruption.

Epidemiology

Erythema marginatum as a manifestation of rheumatic fever is predominantly a disease of developing countries.

It is most common in children between the ages of 5 and 15 years.

Together with carditis, migratory polyarthritis, chorea and subcutaneous nodules, it is one of the Duckett Jones major criteria for the diagnosis of rheumatic fever in which it occurs in about 10% of cases.

A firm diagnosis of rheumatic fever requires that two major or one major and two minor criteria are satisfied (Box 19.2), in addition to evidence of recent streptococcal infection.

Pathophysiology

The histological features are nonspecific and include a perivascular polymorphous infiltrate of neutrophils and mononuclear cells in the papillary dermis and upper portion of the reticular dermis.

It is predominantly associated with a β-haemolytic streptococcal infection.

Clinical features

The annular rash commonly occurs over the trunk and inner aspects of the upper arms and thighs, but rarely if ever on the face. The rash is nonpainful and rarely pruritic, and typically appears in crops as erythematous macules or papules (which may be urticated) that rapidly spread peripherally and may merge to produce the typical serpiginous, polycyclic annular eruption lasting hours to several days. The rash blanches on pressure, is transient and tends to migrate from one part of the body to another.

PART 2: INFLAMMATORY DERMATOSES

Box 19.2 Duckett Jones criteria for the diagnosis of rheumatic fever

Major criteria

- Carditis
- Polyarthritis
- Chorea: also known as Sydenham's chorea or St Vitus' dance
- Erythema marginatum
- Subcutaneous nodules: usually located over bones or tendons, these nodules are painless and firm

Minor criteria

- Fever
- Arthralgia
- Previous rheumatic fever or rheumatic heart disease
- Raised acute phase reactants, e.g. leukocytosis, elevated erythrocyte sedimentation rate and C-reactive protein
- Prolonged P-R interval on electrocardiogram

It is associated with rheumatic fever but only occurs in 1–18% of patients.

Differential diagnosis

Annular erythema, urticaria, toxic erythema, and EM.

Management

Erythema marginatum is part of a clinical syndrome for which no specific tests exist.

First line: Aspirin or nonsteroidal anti-inflammatory drugs; penicillin or erythromycin,

Necrolytic migratory erythema

(**Syn. Glucagonoma syndrome, pancreatic islet cell tumour, pseudoglucagonoma syndrome, pancreatic neuroendocrine tumours**) Necrolytic migratory erythema (NME) is, in most cases, considered to be a paraneoplastic cutaneous eruption.

Epidemiology

The key features of the 'glucagonoma syndrome' are NME and diabetes.

The estimated incidence has been reported to be 2.4/100 000 000 population per year.

Median age at diagnosis has been reported at 53.5 years and the median time from onset of symptoms to diagnosis is 39 months.

Pathophysiology

A skin biopsy should be taken from the edge of early lesions and, in view of the evolving nature of the eruption, serial biopsies may be required.

Histology shows parakeratosis with loss of the granular cell layer, necrosis and separation of the papillary epidermis with vacuolar degeneration of the keratinocytes, dyskeratotic keratinocytes and the presence of neutrophils.

Clinical features

Most cases of NME have an underlying glucagonoma. In those patients with NME in the absence of a glucagon-secreting tumour (pseudoglucagonoma syndrome) underlying diseases include chronic pancreatitis, alcoholic liver disease, gastrointestinal malabsorption, hepatic cirrhosis and aberrant glucagon-secreting tumours such as bronchial or naso-pharyngeal carcinomas.

NME may present initially with a nonspecific itchy or tender macular erythema with a predilection for the groin, genitalia or buttocks (Figure 19.8). It then evolves to form a centrifugally extending, annular, erythematous eruption having a crusted edge which may be itchy, burning, painful, blistered or eroded. It often displays a fluctuating or cyclical pattern and predominantly affects the flexural sites on the lower abdomen, groins, buttocks and thighs.

NME may present with well-demarcated, acral (mainly hands and feet but can affect forearms, knees and lower legs), dusky discoloration with peripheral blister formation progressing to form keratotic erythrokeratoderma-like chronic inflammation.

Differential diagnosis

Eczema, impetiginised eczema, psoriasis, pemphigus foliaceus, annular lesions of pustular psoriasis and subcorneal pustular dermatosis.

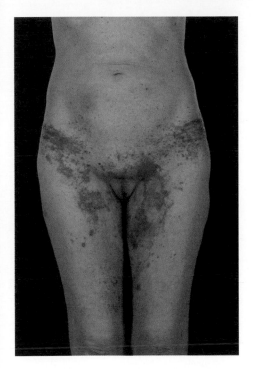

Figure 19.8 Necrolytic migratory erythema in the groin area.

51% of patients with NME secondary to glucagonoma will have metastastic disease (to liver, regional or cervical lymph nodes, bone and lung) at the time of diagnosis, in part because of the invariable delay in reaching a diagnosis.

Management

Investigations include a full blood count, biochemistry and glucose, serum glucagon level, skin biopsy, abdominal ultrasound, CT scan of the chest, abdomen and pelvis, PET CT scan, coeliac axis angiography and single photon emission CT (SPECT). Somatostatin receptor imaging using ^{111}In-octreotide (octreotide is a somatostatin analogue and is taken up by neutrophil extracellular traps as they overexpress somatostatin receptors) can also be useful. Management of the tumour by surgery and/or chemotherapy is the cornerstone of management. There are no specific treatments for the skin lesions other than emollients.

PART 2: INFLAMMATORY DERMATOSES

20

Behçet disease

Behçet disease (BD) is a multisystem inflammatory disease of unknown aetiology, classified as a systemic vasculitis and as a neutrophilic dermatosis.

(Syn. **Adamantiades–Behçet disease, Behçet syndrome, Malignant aphthosis**)

Epidemiology

BD has a worldwide occurrence, being endemic in eastern and central Asian and the eastern Mediterranean countries and rare in northern European countries, central and southern Africa, the Americas and Australia. It most often affects patients in their 20s and 30s. Both genders are equally affected; a male predominance is still observed in Arab populations, whereas female predominance is evident in Korea, China, some northern European countries and the USA.

Pathophysiology

The aetiology of the disease remains unknown. Characteristic histopathological features of BD are vasculitis and thrombosis. Biopsies from early mucocutaneous lesions show a neutrophilic vascular reaction with endothelial swelling, extravasation of erythrocytes and leukocytoclasia or a fully developed leukocytoclastic vasculitis with fibrinoid necrosis of the blood vessel walls.

The major microscopic finding at most sites of active disease is an immune-mediated occlusive vasculitis. Disease activity has been known to correlate with bacterial infection, particularly streptococcal.

Immunological mechanisms are considered to play a major role in the pathogenesis of BD; the disease is classified as an autoinflammatory disorder.

Clinical features

Recurrent oral aphthous and genital ulcers, skin manifestations, ocular lesions and arthritis/arthropathy are the most frequent clinical features. Vascular, neurological, gastrointestinal, psychiatric, pulmonary, renal and cardiac manifestations, epididymitis and other findings can also occur.

Diagnosis of BD is based on clinical signs as neither a pathognomonic laboratory test nor histological characteristics are available. The Revised International Criteria for BD provide the most accurate criteria for diagnosis (Table 20.1).

Mucocutaneous lesions

Recurrent oral aphthous and genital ulcers are the most frequently observed mucosal manifestations. Oral aphthous ulcers are the presenting sign in more than 80% of patients (Figure 20.1). Typically, lesions are multiple, painful, 1–3 cm in diameter and sharply margined with a fibrin-coated base and surrounding erythema (Figure 20.2). Oral aphthous ulcers usually heal without scarring (92%). Genital ulcers may not recur as often and usually heal with a characteristic scar (64–88%) (Figure 20.3). Spontaneous healing of aphthae occurs within 4 days to 1 month; genital ulcers may persist longer. Genital ulcers can occur on the penis, scrotum, vagina, labia and urethra, and also in the anal, perineal and inguinal regions.

Skin lesions accepted as diagnostically relevant in BD are pustular vasculitic lesions (including pathergy lesions), erythema nodosum-like lesions, Sweet disease-like lesions, pyoderma gangrenosum-like lesions and palpable purpuric lesions of necrotising venulitis.

Rook's Dermatology Handbook, First Edition. Edited by Christopher E. M. Griffiths, Tanya O. Bleiker, Daniel Creamer, John R. Ingram and Rosalind C. Simpson.
© 2022 John Wiley & Sons Ltd. Published 2022 by John Wiley & Sons Ltd.

PART 2: INFLAMMATORY DERMATOSES

Table 20.1 Revised International Criteria for Behçet disease

Clinical feature	Points[a]
Ocular lesions (recurrent)	2
Oral aphthosis (recurrent)	2
Genital aphthosis (recurrent)	2
Skin lesions (recurrent)	1
Central nervous system lesions	1
Vascular manifestations	1
Positive pathergy test[b]	1

[a] Score ≥4 indicates Behçet disease.
[b] Though the main scoring system does not include a pathergy test, where pathergy testing is conducted a positive result may be included for one extra point.
Source: The International Criteria for Behçet's Disease (ICBD): a collaborative study of 27 countries on the sensitivity and specificity of the new criteria. J Eur Acad Dermatol Venereol 2013, 28, 338–347. © 2013 John Wiley & Sons.

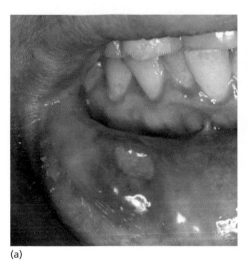
(a)

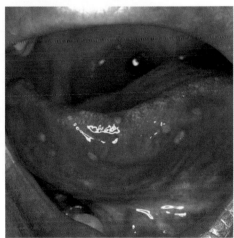
(b)

Figure 20.1 (a) Single and (b) multiple oral aphthous ulcers in BD. (Source: (a) from Altenburg A, Papoutsis N, Orawa H, et al. Epidemiology and clinical manifestations of Adamantiades–Behçet disease in Germany – current pathogenetic concepts and therapeutic possibilities. J Dtsch Dermatol Ges 2006, 4, 49–66.)

Systemic lesions

Ocular involvement is the major cause of morbidity in patients with BD. The most diagnostically relevant lesion is posterior uveitis (also called retinal vasculitis). Other ocular lesions include anterior uveitis, hypopyon and secondary complications such as cataract, glaucoma and neovascular lesions. Recurrent vasculitic changes can ultimately lead to ischaemic optic nerve atrophy.

The characteristic arthritis is a nonerosive, asymmetrical, sterile, seronegative oligoarthritis, but symmetrical polyarticular involvement is common. An HLA-B27-positive erosive sacroiliitis has to be excluded.

Systemic vascular involvement can be significant and includes venous occlusions and varices, arterial occlusions and aneurysms, often migratory. Pulmonary artery aneurysms are the principal feature of pulmonary

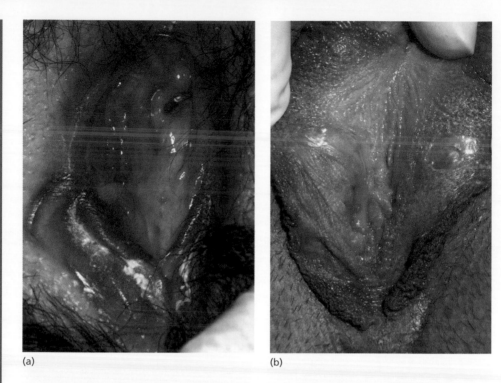

(a)   (b)

Figure 20.2 (a) Genital ulcer of BD healing with (b) a demarcated flat scar.

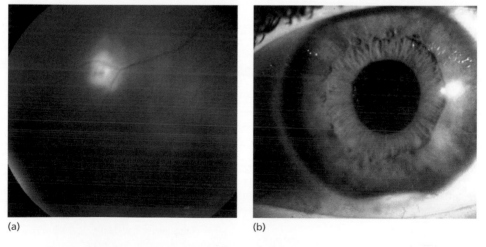

(a)   (b)

Figure 20.3 (a) Posterior uveitis. (b) Hypopyoniritis. (Source: From Altenburg A, Papoutsis N, Orawa H, et al. Epidemiology and clinical manifestations of Adamantiades–Behçet disease in Germany – current pathogenetic concepts and therapeutic possibilities. J Dtsch Dermatol Ges 2006, 4, 49–66.)

involvement in BD. Cardiac involvement can include myocarditis, coronary arteritis, endocarditis and valvular disease. A wide spectrum of renal manifestations can occur, varying from minimal change disease to proliferative glomerulonephritis and rapidly progressive crescentic glomerulonephritis. Gastrointestinal complaints can be a symptom for aphthae throughout the gastrointestinal tract. Sterile prostatitis and epididymitis can be present in male patients without genital ulcers.

Significant neurological manifestations such as meningoencephalitis occur in approximately 10% of patients and may be delayed in onset. Psychiatric symptoms, such as depression, insomnia or memory impairment, are also signs of neurological involvement.

Ophthalmic and neurological sequelae are leading causes of morbidity, followed by severe vascular and gastrointestinal manifestations. The clinical course is variable: there can be a delay of up to several years before the diagnosis is made and this may influence the prognosis. Mucocutaneous and joint manifestations usually occur first. Blindness can often be prevented with early aggressive therapy of posterior uveitis. Markers of severe prognosis include HLA-B51 positivity, male gender and early development of systemic signs. Onset in childhood does not necessarily predict a poor prognosis. Spontaneous remissions of certain or all manifestations of the disease can occur.

Differential diagnosis

- Oculocutaneous/mucocutaneous syndromes
- Erythema multiforme exudativum and variants, including Stevens–Johnson syndrome
- Vogt–Koyanagi–Harada syndrome
- Reactive arthritis
- Bullous autoimmune diseases: pemphigus vulgaris, cicatricial mucous membrane pemphigoid, epidermolysis bullosa acquisita
- Viral infections (herpes, coxsackie, echo)
- Syphilis
- Articulomucocutaneous syndromes
- Systemic lupus erythematosus
- MAGIC syndrome (*m*outh *a*nd *g*enital ulcers with *i*nflamed *c*artilage)
- Yersiniosis
- Arthropathic psoriasis
- Gastrointestinal/mucocutaneous syndromes
- Ulcerative colitis, Crohn disease
- Tuberculosis
- Bowel-associated dermatitis–arthritis syndrome
- Aphthae
- Recurrent aphthous stomatitis
- Cyclic neutropenia

- Herpes oralis/labialis/genitalis recidivans
- Genital ulcers
- Ulcus vulvae acutum (Lipschütz ulcer)
- Sexually transmitted infections
- Uveitis
- Other forms of uveitis
- Arthritis
- Ankylosing spondylitis
- Juvenile rheumatoid arthritis
- Central nervous system manifestation
- Multiple sclerosis
- Neuro-Sweet disease
- Lung manifestation
- Sarcoidosis

Pathergy test

A positive pathergy test (hyper-reactivity reaction) manifests within 48 h as an erythematous papule (>2 mm) or pustule at the site of a skin needle prick. A positive pathergy reaction is a sign of BD, but is not pathognomonic, as it can also occur in patients with pyoderma gangrenosum, rheumatoid arthritis, Crohn disease and genital herpes infection.

Management

The choice of treatment for patients with BD depends on the site and severity of the clinical manifestations of the disease. Recurrent aphthae are most often treated with palliative agents, such as mild diet, avoidance of irritating agents and potent topical glucocorticoids and local anaesthetics. Topical hyaluronic acid 0.2% gel applied twice a day over 30 days has been found to be effective. For the topical treatment of genital ulcers and skin lesions, corticosteroid and antiseptic creams can be applied for up to 7 days. Painful genital ulcerations can be managed by topical anaesthetics in cream. Corticosteroid injections (triamcinolone acetonide 0.1–0.5 mL/lesion) can be helpful in recalcitrant ulcerations.

Patients with mucocutaneous lesions resistant to topical treatment, those with systemic involvement and patients with markers of poor prognosis are candidates for systemic treatment. Oral and intravenous prednisolone can be combined with other immunosuppressants, colchicine, dapsone, sulfasalazine or interferon-α (IFN-α). A synergistic effect with ciclosporin has been described in patients with ocular involvement. Colchicine can be combined with immunosuppressants and IFN-α. A rapid relapse often occurs after discontinuing dapsone, ciclosporin, IFN-α or infliximab.

Male patients with systemic involvement as a presenting sign should be treated systemically because of the poor prognosis.

Patients with severe or progressive recurrent aphthous stomatitis should be followed up for years as potential candidates for BD, particularly those with familial occurrence of the disease.

A collection of skin conditions characterised by a dense, inflammatory infiltrate comprised mainly of neutrophils.

Pyoderma gangrenosum

Pyoderma gangrenosum (PG) is a rare noninfectious neutrophilic dermatosis commonly associated with underlying systemic disease.

Epidemiology

Incidence is 0.63 per 100 000 person-years.

The incidence of PG increases with age, with a median age of 59. F > M.

As with other neutrophilic dermatoses there are classical accepted diseases that occur in association with PG in 33–50% of cases. The *pustular form* of PG is mainly associated with inflammatory bowel disease (IBD) and the *bullous form* with haematological malignancies; the *vegetative form* is usually not associated with underlying disease.

Estimates vary but the most frequent disease associations include IBD, with a similar incidence of Crohn disease and ulcerative colitis, present in 20–30% of cases. Rheumatoid arthritis and other seronegative arthritides occur in about 10% of cases, haematological malignancy or monoclonal gammopathy in approximately 5% and other visceral malignancies in 5%.

Recently, the association of PG, cystic acne and hidradenitis has been suggested as a distinct entity (PASH) that lacks the genetic abnormalities and arthritis which are a feature of the pyogenic arthritis pyoderma and acne (PAPA) syndrome.

Pathergy, in common with other vasculitides, is the phenomenon whereby skin trauma provokes lesions or the first onset of the disease at a site of injury. In patients with ulcerative colitis, the incidence of extra-intestinal manifestations, including PG, is independently promoted by smoking and appendicectomy.

Pathophysiology

Pathergy, in common with other vasculitides, is the phenomenon whereby skin trauma provokes lesions or the first onset of the disease at a site of injury. In patients with ulcerative colitis, the incidence of extra-intestinal manifestations, including PG, is independently promoted by smoking and appendicectomy.

Skin biopsies should be taken to exclude other causes of ulceration. There is no typical histopathology of PG. In the *ulcerative* variant of PG, there is a massive dermal–epidermal neutrophilic infiltrate with suppuration/ abscess formation. In *pustular* PG, there is a perifollicular neutrophilic infiltrate with subcorneal pustule formation; the *bullous* variant shows a neutrophilic infiltrate with intraepidermal vesicle formation. In *vegetative* PG, there is a granulomatous reaction with peripheral palisading histiocytes and giant cells.

Once the skin becomes ulcerated, the appearance of acute and chronic perivascular inflammatory cell infiltrates may be secondary to the ulceration rather than a primary event. PG is not usually associated with vasculitis, but patients with positive tests for either C-antineutrophil cytoplasmic antibody (ANCA) or P-ANCA are occasionally reported in drug-induced PG, typically with thio-uracils.

Rook's Dermatology Handbook, First Edition. Edited by Christopher E. M. Griffiths, Tanya O. Bleiker, Daniel Creamer, John R. Ingram and Rosalind C. Simpson.
© 2022 John Wiley & Sons Ltd. Published 2022 by John Wiley & Sons Ltd.

Clinical features

PG is a chronic condition often taking many months or years to completely resolve and has a significant mortality of 16% over 8 years. Once healed, it may be recurrent in up to 60% of cases.

It has a variety of clinical presentations.

Classical ulcerative PG

This is the commonest and best recognised variant, presenting with small, tender, red-blue papules, plaques or pustules that evolve into painful ulcers with characteristic violaceous undermined edges (Figure 21.1). There may be granulation tissue, necrosis or purulent exudate at the ulcer base. Lesions may be solitary or multiple, and occur most commonly on the legs (in 70%), but may affect any body site, including the genitals and mucosae. Healing usually occurs with an atrophic cribriform scar. Associated symptoms include fever, malaise, myalgia and arthralgia.

Parastomal or peristomal PG

May arise as a pathergy response to the trauma of appliances and faecal irritation. It is most common with ileostomy for active IBD and the risk is greater with high body mass index, female sex and autoimmune disorders (Figure 21.2).

Pustular PG

A variant that often occurs during acute exacerbations of IBD. Discrete painful pustules, with a surrounding halo of erythema, develop on normal skin. Pustules commonly arise with a scattered distribution on the extensor aspects of the limbs. Other painful pustular eruptions in this spectrum of IBD need to be distinguished, including bowel-associated dermatitis–arthritis syndrome (BADAS), subcorneal pustular dermatosis and pyostomatitis vegetans where the pustules are predominantly mucosal.

Bullous PG

Presents with rapidly arising, superficial, haemorrhagic bullae, often located on the arms. It typically ulcerates and heals with scarring. Areas of concentric bullae that rapidly become confluent and ulcerate may occur. This form is particularly associated with myeloproliferative disorders.

Granulomatous superficial PG

A variant with superficial lesions with a granulomatous histology. Most cases begin as a single superficial ulcer with granulations and an elevated edge. This form has a lower incidence of associated conditions and is more responsive to therapy.

Differential diagnosis

PG is a diagnosis of exclusion. In nonclassical PG, skin biopsy and culture are important as are targeted enquiry, examination and investigation for differential diagnoses. These include vascular occlusive or venous disease, vasculitis, cancer, primary infection, exogenous tissue injury and other inflammatory disorders, fungi, atypical mycobacteria and opportunistic infections, sporotrichosis, fusariosis, mycosis fungoides, mucormycosis, histoplamosis, blastomycosis and drug-induced ulceration, including nicorandil.

Management

Often complex and will depend on comorbidities, associated diseases and the site and extent of the lesions.

Due to the range of underlying conditions and potential for involvement of other systems, a thorough work-up is important.

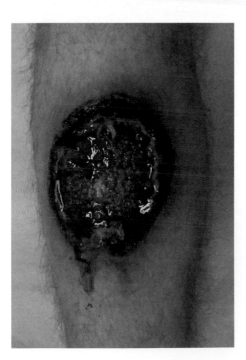

Figure 21.1 Classical pyoderma gangrenosum.

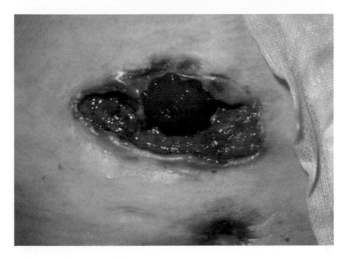

Figure 21.2 Parastomal pyoderma gangrenosum.

Limited ulceration

Supportive therapy will include attention to dressings, pain relief and topical agents for cleansing, debriding and keeping the wound moist. Potent topical corticosteroids, intralesional corticosteroids and topical tacrolimus can be used.

Extensive ulceration

Potent topical corticosteroid combined with prednisolone (0.5–1 mg/kg daily or ciclosporin up to 5 mg/kg daily. Other systemic agents may be tried, including dapsone or teyracyclines in the setting of malignancy-associated PG. For recalcitrant cases the tumour necrosis factor-α inhibitors infliximab and adalimumab are effective.

Sweet syndrome

(Syn. Acute febrile neutrophilic dermatosis)
An inflammatory dermatosis characterised by fever and tender, erythematous plaques and papules. Three main types of Sweet syndrome are recognised: classical, malignancy associated and drug-induced.

Epidemiology

Occurs worldwide. 16% of cases have an associated malignancy. May occur at any age but most commonly between 30 and 60 years. F:M of 4:1.

Numerous diseases have been associated with both classical and malignancy-associated Sweet syndrome (Table 21.1)

Pathophysiology

The classical and diagnostic histopathological features are a dense dermal infiltrate of neutrophils and prominent dermal papillary oedema. Subepidermal vesicles may be seen. Other cells involved in the infiltrate can include lymphocytes, eosinophils and histiocytes. The cell infiltrate is usually diffuse but perivascular and dermal band patterns are seen. Genuine vasculitis is not seen, although leukocytoclasis is a common finding and endothelial swelling without fibrinoid necrosis is also seen.

Most patients presenting with classical Sweet syndrome have a fever and a history of infection. Upper respiratory tract infections commonly precede the appearance of the skin lesions by 1–3 weeks.

Drug-induced Sweet syndrome is an established phenomenon.

Clinical features

The classical appearance is of tender red papules, nodules and eventually plaques distributed over the head, neck, upper trunk and upper arms. Cases of malignancy-associated Sweet syndrome may have a more widespread

Table 21.1 Diseases associated with Sweet syndrome

Category	Examples
Infections	Streptococcal and upper respiratory tract Gastrointestinal (especially *Salmonella, Yersinia*) Mycobacterial infections (including vaccinations)
Inflammatory bowel disease	Ulcerative colitis Crohn disease
Endocrine	Pregnancy Autoimmune thyroid disease
Immunological disorders	Collagen vascular disorders: lupus erythematosus, Sjögren's syndrome, autoimmune thrombocytopenic purpura, pemphigus
Haematological malignancy and related conditions, immunodeficiencies	Acute myelogenous leukaemias Myelodysplastic conditions, polycythaemia Aplastic anaemia Fanconi anaemia Monoclonal gammopathy Lymphomas (various, less common) Chronic granulomatous disease
Other malignancies Other medical conditions	Genitourinary, breast, gastrointestinal, prostate, larynx Sarcoidosis Rheumatoid arthritis Still disease SAPHO
Medications	Numerous; the most consistently associated agents are: • Colony-stimulating factors • All-*trans* retinoic acid imatinib mesylate, bortezomib, contraceptives and propylthiouracil
Unusual consequences of Sweet syndrome	Acquired cutis laxa, mid-dermal elastolysis, elastophagocytosis

SAPHO, synovitis, acne, pustulosis, hyperostosis, osteomyelitis.

distribution. The plaques are often oedematous and as the process develops they may become studded with pseudovesicles (Figures 21.3 and 21.4) or pseudopustules. Definite vesicles and pustules with subsequent ulceration may occur. An associated arthralgia occurs in approximately one-third of patients. Ocular involvement is also relatively common, with conjunctivitis and episcleritis occurring. Oral and genital involvement are uncommon.

Spontaneous resolution may occur, often within 3 months, or a pattern of fluctuating exacerbations may be seen in untreated cases.

Diagnostic criteria for Sweet syndrome indicate that patients must meet the two major and two of the four minor criteria (Box 21.1).

Neutrophilic dermatosis of the dorsal hands

Generally accepted as a variant of Sweet syndrome with identical clinical lesions, histology,

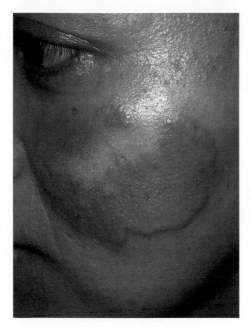

Figure 21.3 Sweet syndrome. The face is often affected.

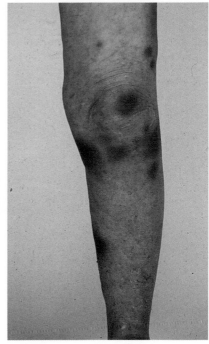

Figure 21.4 Sweet syndrome. Multiple large erythematous lesions on the leg.

Box 21.1 Diagnostic criteria for Sweet syndrome: both major and at least two minor criteria should be present

Major

1. Acute onset of typical lesions
2. Histopathological findings consistent with Sweet syndrome

Minor

1. Fever >38°C
2. Association with malignancy, inflammatory disorder or pregnancy, or antecedent respiratory or gastrointestinal infection
3. Excellent response to systemic corticosteroids or potassium iodide (KI)
4. Abnormal laboratory values at presentation (three of four required: ESR > 20 mm, leukocytes > 8000, neutrophils > 70%, elevated C-reactive protein)

---

demographic features and disease associations. It is characterised by bluish or haemorrhagic papules, bullae and nodules on the dorsal hands (Figures 21.5 and 21.6). In 50% of cases, typical Sweet syndrome lesions are seen at other sites and the condition responds promptly to prednisolone or dapsone. Clinical distinction from PG, especially the bullous variant, and pustular vasculitis may be difficult. Cases have been associated with myeloproliferative disorders, occult malignancy, IBD and rheumatoid arthritis.

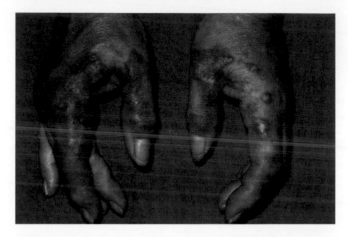

Figure 21.5 Neutrophilic dermatosis of the dorsal hands.

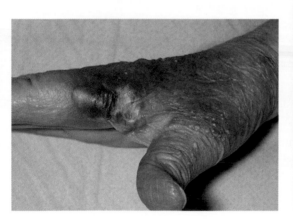

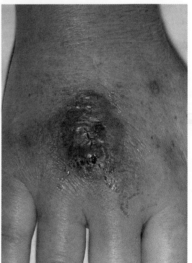

Figure 21.6 Bullous variants of neutrophilic dermatosis of the dorsal hands.

Subcutaneous Sweet syndrome

Presents with erythema nodosum-like, tender subepidermal nodules on the extremities, usually the legs.

Histiocytoid Sweet syndrome

Characterised by a dermal infiltrate composed of large histiocytoid mononuclear cells. Haematological malignancy-associated, idiopathic and drug-induced cases have been reported. Clinically, they may resemble classi-cal Sweet syndrome or may present with subcutaneous erythema nodosum type lesions.

Differential diagnosis

The following conditions should be considered:

- Infectious disorders: erysipelas, cellulitis, herpes simplex.
- Inflammatory: panniculitides, pyoderma gangrenosum, syphilis, tuberculosis.
- Neoplastic: metastases.

- Reactive erythemas: erythema nodosum, erythema multi-forme, urticarial.
- Systemic disease: Behçet disease, lupus, bowel bypass syndrome.
- Vasculitis: erythema elevatum diutinum, polyarteritis nodosa, granuloma faciale.

Management

Investigations include ESR, full blood count, C-reactive protein, chest X-ray and a screen for malignancy if indicated. Without treatment, the disease will often resolve within 3 months. Approximately one-third of cases will recur. The response to corticosteroids is usually rapid.

First line: Systemic corticosteroids (0.5–1 mg/kg for 4–6 weeks); potent topical or intralesional corticosteroids may be tried for mild localised disease.

Second line: Dapsone; potassium iodide or colchicine

Third line: Ciclosporin; clofazimine or intravenous immunoglobulin.

BADAS is defined by the presence of pustular vasculitic lesions associated with blind loops of bowel or other causes of stasis of bowel content.

Subcorneal pustular dermatosis

(Syn. Sneddon–Wilkinson disease)
Subcorneal pustular dermatosis is a rare neutrophilic dermatosis, with sterile subcorneal pustules typically affecting the flexural areas of the trunk and proximal extremities.

Epidemiology

Subcorneal pustular dermatosis occurs most frequently in adults aged 40–60 years. F:M 4:1. It is associated with benign monoclonal gammopathy, more commonly IgA, IBD, multiple myeloma, lymphomas, PG, rheumatoid arthritis and connective tissue disease, including systemic lupus erythematosus.

Pathophysiology

Biopsies from early lesions show a perivascular inflammatory infiltrate with occasional eosinophils. The pustules, subcorneal accumulation of neutrophils, sit on the surface of the epidermis, rather than within it, spongiosis and spongiotic

pustules are absent, and acantholysis is only seen in old lesions. Culture of the pustules is sterile.

Clinical features

The eruption occurs with acute flares lasting for several days or weeks. The distribution is mainly in the flexures of the trunk and proximal limbs, including axillae, groins, submammary area, neck and inframammary and apron area, sparing the face and mucous membranes. Lesions are oval, pea-sized flaccid pustules on a normal or erythematous base (Figure 21.7). A characteristic fluid level with pus in the lower half and clear fluid in the upper half may be seen. Pustules may be isolated or grouped and coalescent to form annular or serpiginous patterns. Successive waves may pass over the same area. In the flexures, these pustules may rupture thereby becoming indistinct (Figure 21.8).

Differential diagnosis

The differential diagnosis includes impetigo, pustular psoriasis, pemphigus foliaceus, dermatitis herpetiformis, intercellular IgA pemphigus and acute generalised exanthematous pustulosis (AGEP).

The condition is benign but chronic with an average duration of 6 years.

Management

Investigations should include skin biopsy. It is important to biopsy early pustules and to avoid sampling later lesions where blisters have burst and also perform immunofluorescence. Bacterial culture of skin swabs should be taken to exclude impetigo.

As with other neutrophilic dermatoses, therapy for the condition needs to be considered along with therapy directed at any associated disease.

First line: Dapsone 50–150 mg daily is the treatment of choice, leading to either a partial or a complete response.

Pyodermatitis: pyostomatitis vegetans

(Syn. Pyoderma vegetans)
Pyostomatitis vegetans is a disorder distinct from PG in which there is oral mucosal thickening with multiple pustules and 'snail track' superfi-

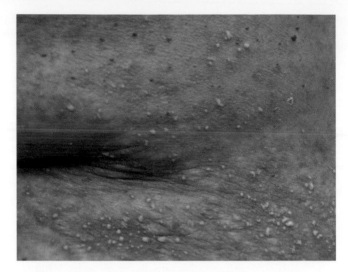

Figure 21.7 Typical appearance of pustules in subcorneal pustular dermatosis.

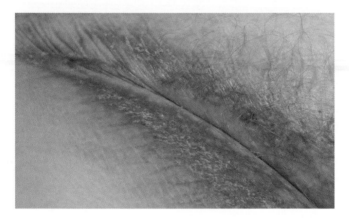

Figure 21.8 Subcorneal pustular dermatosis. Pustules may rupture and be inconspicuous in the skin folds.

cial ulceration on an erythematous base (at any site, although the tongue is less affected).

The strongest association, particularly for oral lesions, is with IBD, particularly ulcerative colitis. Leukaemias, lymphoma, diabetes, acne conglobata, hidradenitis suppurativa and dissecting cellulitis, immunosuppression and malnourishment are also associated.

Pathophysiology

Histology shows intraepithelial and/or subepithelial abscesses containing large numbers of eosinophils. Although deeper tissues have a mixed infiltrate, including neutrophils, eosinophils are prominent and there is often an associated peripheral blood eosinophilia.

Eosinophilia is present in 50–90% of cases.

Clinical features

The skin lesions are often flexural and clinically suggestive of pemphigus vegetans with verrucous plaques studded with pustules. There may be associated dorsal hand lesions that are morphologically very similar to neutrophilic dermatosis, and a rash resembling Sweet syndrome. Lesions may display pathergy.

Management

First line: Antimicrobials, rather than corticosteroids or antineutrophil therapies, are indicated if the cause is uncertain; oral disease may respond to topical corticosteroids or tacrolimus; systemic prednisolone is often effective where topical therapies fail.

Amicrobial pustulosis of the skin folds

A condition of rapidly evolving small semi-confluent pustules that predominantly affects the flexures, with one major or minor skin fold usually affected, i.e. the face or scalp.

22 Immunobullous diseases

The immunobullous disorders represent a group of blistering conditions characterised by antibody-mediated autoimmune responses against structural elements of the skin.

INTRAEPIDERMAL IMMUNOBULLOUS DISEASES

Pemphigus

This is characterised by the presence of antibodies against desmosomal adhesion proteins. Clinical and immunopathological features of the various pemphigus disorders are summarised in Table 22.1.

Epidemiology
The incidence of pemphigus is low but variable worldwide, ranging from 0.05 to 2.7/100 000/year. Pemphigus vulgaris (PV) is the commoner form. PV is commoner in Europe, the US and India whereas pemphigus foliaceus (PF) is commoner in Brazil and Africa. M = F.

PV can occur at any age but usually between the fourth and sixth decades of life. Children usually develop PV rather than PF. PV is more common in Ashkenazi Jews, and Mediterranean, Iranian and Indian populations. It is associated with other autoimmune diseases, particularly thyroid disease and rheumatoid arthritis. Paraneoplastic pemphigus occurs in association with haematological malignancy.

An endemic form of the disease (fogo selvagem) occurs in several parts of the world, most notably rural Brazil and Tunisia. The disease is clinically and immunological similar to PF, though it tends to affect children and young adults rather than the older population affected by sporadic PF.

Drug-induced pemphigus is rare, mostly in association with drugs containing a thiol group such as penicillamine (pemphigus which may occur in 3–10% of patients on the drug typically after 1 year of exposure).

Black flies (*Simulium* spp.) maybe involved in the pathogenesis of fogo selvagem.

Pathophysiology
The principal target antigens in pemphigus are desmogleins (Dsg) 1 and 3, which are expressed in the skin and mucosal tissue (see Table 22.1).

The predominant class of tissue-bound pemphigus antibody is immunoglobulin G (IgG), which can be demonstrated on direct and indirect immunofluorescence (IF) testing (Figure 22.1).

In paraneoplastic pemphigus, antibodies develop against multiple epidermal antigens in addition to Dsg 1 and 3.

The key pathological process in all types of pemphigus, is acantholysis: separation of keratinocytes from one another.

Clinical features
PV
Nearly all patients have mucosal lesions, predominantly oral but genital and ocular mucosae are involved in some patients. These may precede cutaneous lesions by months or be the only manifestation of the disease. Intact bullae are rare in the mouth; there are ill-defined irregularly shaped buccal or palatal erosions which are slow to heal (Figure 22.2).

Rook's Dermatology Handbook, First Edition. Edited by Christopher E. M. Griffiths, Tanya O. Bleiker, Daniel Creamer, John R. Ingram and Rosalind C. Simpson.
© 2022 John Wiley & Sons Ltd. Published 2022 by John Wiley & Sons Ltd.

Table 22.1 The intraepidermal immunobullous diseases: immunopathology

Disease	Direct IMF	Isotype	Target antigens	Antigens (kDa)	Location	Immunogenetics
Pemphigus vulgaris/ pemphigus vegetans	Intercellular	IgG (occasionally IgM, IgA), C3	Dsg 3, sometimes Dsg 1, desmocollins	130	Desmosome	DRB1*0402 DRB1*1401
Pemphigus fciliaceus	Intercellular	IgG, C3	Dsg 1, sometimes desmocollins	160	Desmosome	HLA-DRB1*14
Endemic pemphigus foliaceus	Intercellular	IgG, IgM	Dsg 1, sometimes desmocollins	160	Desmosome	Several susceptibility alleles, all with the same amino acid sequence in DRB-1 gene DRB1*0102 DRB1*0404, *1402 or *1406
Paraneoplastic pemphigus	Intercellular and subepidermal	IgG	Multiple (desmogleins, desmoplakin, envoplakin, periplakin, BP230)	Various	Desmosomes, BMZ; stratified, simple and transitional epithelia	Unknown

BMZ, basement zone; C3, complement 3; Dsg, desmogleins; IgA, immunoglobulin A; IgG, immunoglobulin G; IgM, immunoglobulin M; IMF, immunofluorescence.

PART 2: INFLAMMATORY DERMATOSES

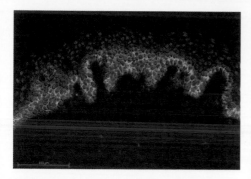

Figure 22.1 Direct immunofluorescence of pemphigus vulgaris. Antibody is deposited around the cell membrane of epidermal keratinocytes.

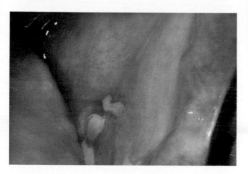

Figure 22.2 Pemphigus vulgaris. Mucosal erosions are an early sign in pemphigus vulgaris, often preceding the cutaneous changes. (Source: Courtesy of Dr R.J. Pye, Addenbrooke's Hospital, Cambridge, UK.)

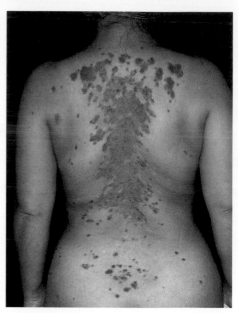

Figure 22.3 Pemphigus vulgaris. Cutaneous lesions typically affect the chest and back in addition to the scalp. (Source: Courtesy of Dr R.J. Pye, Addenbrooke's Hospital, Cambridge, UK.)

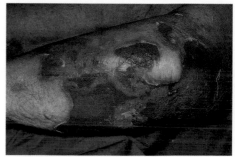

Figure 22.4 Pemphigus vulgaris. Because bullae occur within the epidermis, they are fragile and frequently break down to leave widespread erosions. (Source: Courtesy of Dr R.J. Pye, Addenbrooke's Hospital, Cambridge, UK.)

Cutaneous lesions may be localised to one site but more commonly become widespread. The disease has a predilection for the scalp, face, neck, upper chest and back (Figure 22.3). Flaccid blisters filled with clear fluid arise on either normal skin or an erythematous base. The contents may become turbid or the blisters rupture, producing painful erosions which extend at the edges as more epidermis is lost (Figure 22.4). Nikolsky sign is positive. Healing occurs without scarring but with hyperpigmentary change.

Lesions in skin folds may form vegetating granulations (Figure 22.5); flexural PV merges with its variant pemphigus vegetans. Nail dystrophies, acute paronychia and subungual haematomas occur. Pemphigus may deteriorate in pregnancy and the puerperium.

Pemphigus foliaceous

Less severe than PV. Onset is insidious with scattered, scaly lesions involving 'seborrhoeic' areas of the scalp, face, chest and upper back (Figures 22.6 and 22.7). Individual lesions typically have a fine collarette of scale. Blistering

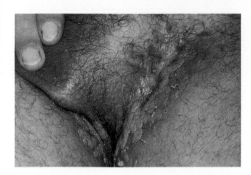

Figure 22.5 Pemphigus vegetans. Vegetating lesions typically occur in the flexures, often without evident blistering. (Source: Courtesy of Dr R.J. Pye, Addenbrooke's Hospital, Cambridge, UK.)

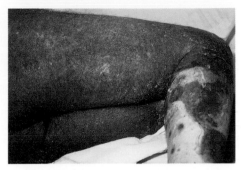

Figure 22.8 Pemphigus foliaceus. Occasionally, pemphigus foliaceus becomes widespread and can result in erythroderma.

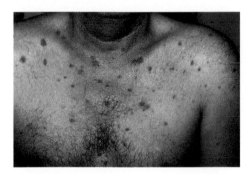

Figure 22.6 Pemphigus foliaceus. There are superficial erosions, frequently without obvious bullae.

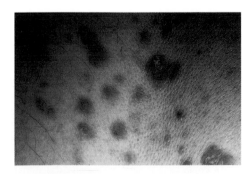

Figure 22.7 Pemphigus foliaceus. Lesions frequently have a fine superficial scale, sometimes as a collarette.

may not be obvious because cleavage is superficial and the small flaccid blisters rupture easily. Scales separate leaving well demarcated crusted erosions surrounded by erythema. In severe cases the patient may become erythrodermic (Figure 22.8).

Pemphigus vegetans

A rare variant of PV characterised by vegetating erosions, primarily in the flexures (Figure 22.5). Two subtypes are recognised: the severe Neumann type and the milder Hallopeau type.

The disease chiefly affects middle-aged adults. Involvement of oral mucosa is almost invariable, often with cerebriform changes on the tongue. Lesions are primarily flexural, although vegetations may occur at any site. In the Neumann type, vesicles and bullae rupture to form hypertrophic granulating erosions, which bleed easily. Lesions evolve into vegetating masses exuding serum and pus. The edges are studded with small pustules. In the Hallopeau type, pustules rather than vesicles characterise early lesions but progress to vegetating plaques.

Pemphigus erythematosus

A localised variant of PF, originally described by Senear and Usher. Erythematous scaly lesions over the nose and cheeks in a butterfly distribution simulate cutaneous lupus erythematosus or seborrhoeic dermatitis. Sunlight may exacerbate the disease. Lesions on the trunk, either localised or generalised, are similar to those in PF.

PART 2: INFLAMMATORY DERMATOSES

Paraneoplastic pemphigus

Has been reported in association with neoplasms, almost exclusively of haematological origin. The commonest is non-Hodgkin lymphoma but chronic lymphocytic leukaemia, Castleman disease, thymoma and Waldenström macroglobulinaemia have been associated.

Clinical features include severe stomatitis, conjunctivitis which may be scarring and oesophageal, genital mucosal and flexural involvement together with bullous and erosive lesions elsewhere. The respiratory tract may be severely affected. Cutaneous lesions may be erosive or blistering as in PV, though tense pemphigoid-like blisters may occur as well as erythema multiforme or lichenoid changes.

IgA pemphigus

Mainly affects adults. Two histological forms occur: an intraepidermal neutrophilic type and a subcorneal pustular dermatosis type, both of which may be clinically indistinguishable from subcorneal pustular dermatosis (Sneddon–Wilkinson disease). Patients have flaccid vesicles or pustules arising on either erythematous or normal skin. Lesions may be intensely pruritic and show a circinate or annular configuration with central clearing, evolving to crusted or scaly erythematous macules. Sites of predilection are axillae and groin though the trunk, face, scalp and proximal limbs may be affected. Whilst some patients are indistinguishable from Sneddon–Wilkinson disease, others may resemble PF. Mucosal involvement is unusual. Most run a chronic indolent course.

The most frequently reported association is with monoclonal IgA gammopathy in the subcorneal type, a feature in common with classical subcorneal pustular dermatosis.

Differential diagnosis

PV

Erosions may simulate acute herpetic stomatitis, erythema multiforme, aphthous ulcers, lichen planus or mucous membrane pemphigoid. Vegetating, pustular lesions in flexures must be differentiated from chronic infections or Hailey–Hailey disease (benign familial pemphigus).

Vegetating plaques mimicking pemphigus vegetans may occur in IgA pemphigus and paraneoplastic pemphigus. The hyperkeratotic lesions of chronic pemphigus vegetans may simulate cutaneous tumours.

PF

May resemble seborrhoeic dermatitis, impetigo and dermatitis herpetiformis. Pemphigus erythematosus should be distinguished from both seborrhoeic dermatitis and chronic cutaneous lupus erythematosus.

Paraneoplastic pemphigus differential diagnosis includes PV, erythema multiforme, graft-versus-host disease, lichen planus and viral infections, including herpes simplex.

Investigations

Skin biopsy from the edge of an active lesion for histology and from uninvolved skin for direct IF. Blister cavities contain rounded-up acantholytic cells found in smears taken from the base of a blister or an oral erosion (Tzank preparation).

Direct IF is the most accurate way to diagnose mucosal pemphigus. Specimens may be posted to a suitable laboratory in Michel's medium if facilities for snap freezing and storage of the tissues are not available.

The diagnosis of pemphigus is confirmed by direct IF (Figure 22.1) Circulating pemphigus autoantibodies are detected by indirect IF in over 80% of patients.

Using ELISA, over 95% of PV patients have detectable Dsg 3 antibodies and around 50% have Dsg 1 antibodies.

Management

Pemphigus typically has a chronic course. Early age of onset and Asian ethnicity are associated with more prolonged disease activity.

Potent topical or intralesional steroids may reduce the requirement for oral steroids. Good oral hygiene, including treatment of periodontal disease, is important. An ophthalmology opinion should be sought at the outset of treatment.

In patients with widespread blistering, intensive nursing care is mandatory. Opportunist infection is the major cause of death; potassium permanganate and topical antiseptics may help reduce the risk of cutaneous infection. Liberal use of emollients reduces frictional stress on affected skin.

First line: Prednisolone together with a steroid-sparing agent, e.g. azathioprine or mycophenolate mofetil, and topical therapy is the initial treatment for most patients. IV pulses methylprednisolone or IV dexamethasone are safer alternatives, often used together with intravenous immunoglobulin (IVIG), immunoabsorption or plasmapheresis.

Second line: Rituximab, two infusions of 1 g, 2 weeks apart. IVIG at a dose of 2 g/kg split over 3–5 days may need to be continued monthly for prolonged periods.

Cyclophosphamide is generally reserved for patients who have failed to respond to conventional immunosuppression with azathioprine or mycophenolate mofetil.

SUBEPIDERMAL IMMUNOBULLOUS DISEASES

These bullous disorders include pemphigoid diseases and dermatitis herpetiformis.

Bullous pemphigoid

Bullous pemphigoid (BP) is the most common disorder within the group of subepidermal immunobullous disorders and the most frequent autoimmune blistering disease in general.

Epidemiology
Predominantly a disease of the elderly with mean age at onset 69–83 years. F > M.

Triggers include trauma, burns, skin grafting, radiotherapy and UV radiation including sunlight, UVA1, psoralen and UVA (PUVA), and photodynamic therapy.

It may be triggered by drugs, most frequently furosemide.

Pathophysiology
For target antigens see Table 22.2. Autoantibodies bind to BP180 (also termed type XVII collagen) and BPAG2.

Light microscopy of *lesional* skin shows a subepidermal blister with a dense eosinophil-rich infiltrate, including neutrophils, macrophages and T lymphocytes within the papillary dermis and along the dermal–epidermal junction (DEJ).

Tissue-bound autoantibodies can be visualised by direct IF microscopy of a *perilesional*

Table 22.2 Pemphigoid diseases

Disease	Target antigen	Clinical signs of diagnostic relevance
Bullous pemphigoid (BP)	*BP180 NC16A, BP230*	Tense blisters, erosions, intense pruritus, old age (>75 years); no predominant mucosal involvement
MMP	BP180, laminin 332, *BP230*, α6β4 integrin, laminin 311	Predominant mucosal involvement
Linear IgA disease	LAD–1, BP230 (IgA reactivity)	Tense blisters, erosions; no predominant mucosal involvement
Pemphigoid gestationis	*BP180 NC16A, BP230*	Erythema, papules, rarely vesicles, intense pruritus; pregnancy or postpartum period
Anti-p200/laminin γ1 pemphigoid	p200 antigen laminin γ1	Tense blisters, erosions; <75 years of age; no predominant mucosal involvement
Epidermolysis bullosa acquisita	*Type VII collagen*	Mechanobullous (like epidermolysis bullosa) and inflammatory variant (like BP or MMP)
Bullous SLE	Type I: *type VII collagen* Type II: BP180, BP230, laminin 332	SLE present; tense blisters, erosions; no predominant mucosal involvement; excellent response to dapsone
Lichen planus pemphigoides	*BP180 NC16A, BP230*	Tense blisters independent of lichen planus lesions
Cicatricial pemphigoid	BP180, *BP230*, laminin 332	Blisters and erosions that heal with scarring and/or milia formation; no predominant mucosal involvement

BP, bullous pemphigoid; IgA, immunoglubulin A; MMP, mucous membrane pemphigoid; SLE, systemic lupus erythematosus. Source: Adapted from Schmidt E and Zillikens D. Pemphigoid diseases. Lancet 2013, 381, 320–332.

biopsy in almost all patients. Linear deposits of IgG and/or C3, and to a lesser extent IgA and IgE, along the DEJ.

Circulating autoantibodies can be detected by indirect IF and/or ELISA.

Splitting of the DEJ can be induced by incubation in 1 M NaCl solution. In this technique, BP autoantibodies bind to the roof of the artificial split and can therefore be differentiated from autoantibodies in antilaminin 332 pemphigoid, anti-p200 pemphigoid and epidermolysis bullosa acquisita (EBA).

Clinical features

A prodromal nonbullous phase usually precedes development of tense generalised blisters. Pruritus is typical and may occur without skin lesions. Excoriated papules, eczematous or urticarial lesions, haemorrhagic crusts and excoriations prevail.

The bullous stage is characterised by intense pruritus accompanied by widespread tense blisters and vesicles on apparently normal or erythematous skin (Figure 22.9). Partly haemorrhagic crusts and urticated and infiltrated erythematous plaques with an occasionally annular or figurate pattern are present (Figure 22.10). Blisters may be many centimetres in diameter and contain a clear sometimes haemorrhagic exudate. Nikolsky sign is negative. Pruritus is constant. Blisters are typically symmetrically distributed and may persist for several days. After mechanical irritation erosions and yellowish or haemorrhagic crusts develop. Predilection sites involve the flexural aspects of the limbs and abdomen. In the intertriginal areas, vegetating plaques may occur and oral lesions develop in 10–20% of cases. Mucosae of the eyes, nose, pharynx, oesophagus and anogenital areas are rarely affected. Without severe superinfection all lesions heal without scarring. Erythema may persist at the sites of previous blisters for many weeks or months. Milia formation is rare.

Patients with BP are at high risk for pulmonary infection and embolism.

Several clinical variants of BP are described (see Figures 22.11 and 22.12).

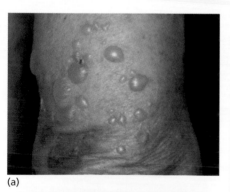

(a)

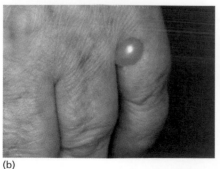

(b)

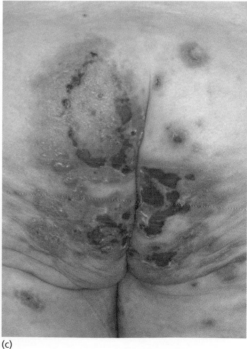

(c)

Figure 22.9 Classical bullous pemphigoid. Tense blisters and erosions on (a) the arm, (b) the hand and (c) the gluteal region. Blisters may arise on erythematous (a, c) or otherwise normal skin (b).

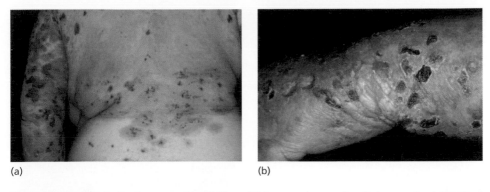

(a)   (b)

Figure 22.10 Classical bullous pemphigoid. Tense blisters, erosions and partly haemorrhagic crusts on (a) the back and left arm, and (b) the left hand.

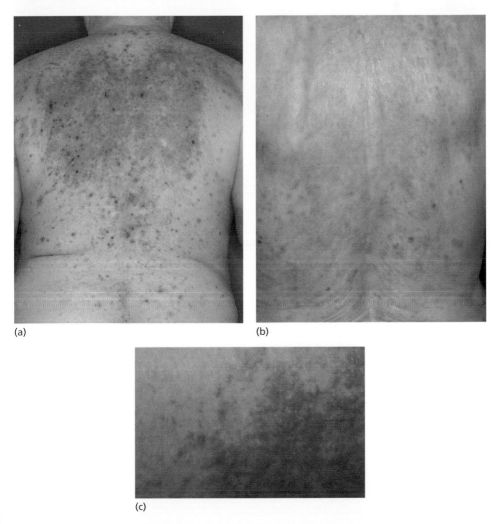

(a)   (b)

(c)

Figure 22.11 Clinical variants of bullous pemphigoid. (a), (b) Eczematous lesions with some erosions and crusts, and (c) papular variant.

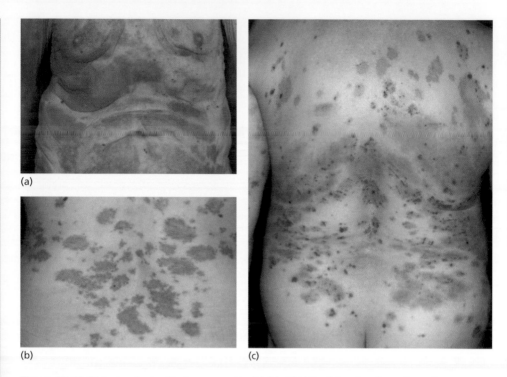

(a)

(b)

(c)

Figure 22.12 Clinical variants of bullous pemphigoid. (a), (b) Urticarial and erythematous plaques accompanied by (c) erosions and excoriations.

Localised BP

The disease can be limited to certain body parts, mostly the pretibial area. Flexures, palms, soles, genital area and umbilicus have been described as well as around stomata and haemodialysis fistulae (Figure 22.13). Localised lesions may persist or develop into classical BP.

Childhood BP

There are two peaks of incidence: in the first year of life (infantile BP) and around the age of 8 years. There are no immunopathological differences between BP in childhood and adults. Close association with preceding vaccinations has been reported, most of them in infants. In infants, the distribution of the lesions is often acral, in particular palmar and plantar. In older children, involvement of the genital region occurs in almost half of the cases (Figure 22.14). Generally, infants and children with BP have a good prognosis with remissions within weeks to a few months under therapy.

Differential diagnosis

Diseases of the *pemphigus group* have distinctive clinical (positive Nikolsky sign) and immunopathological features. *Mucous membrane pemphigoid* is differentiated from BP by its predominant involvement of mucosal surfaces. Distinction of BP from *linear IgA disease*, *EBA* and *anti-p200/laminin γ1 pemphigoid* based on clinical and histopathological features. In dermatitis herpetiformis, direct IF microscopy findings, particularly the presence of antitransglutaminase 1 and 2 as well as antigliadin IgA antibodies, are often required for diagnosis.

In the nonbullous prodromal stage or in atypical presentations, BP can closely resemble localised or generalised drug reactions, contact and allergic dermatitis, prurigo, urticaria, urticarial vasculitis, arthropod reactions, scabies, ecthyma and pityriasis lichenoides.

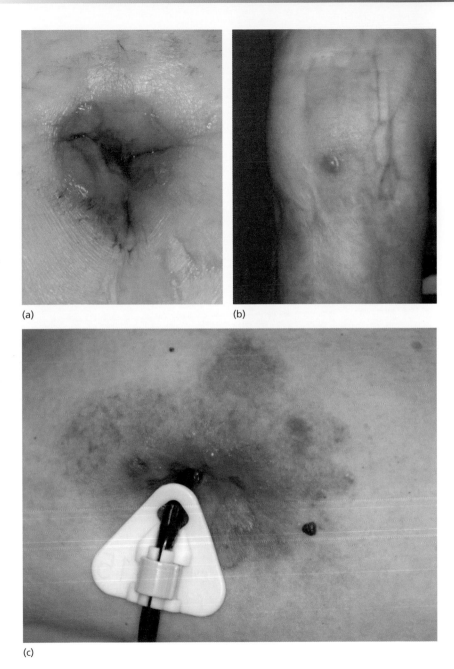

(a)

(b)

(c)

Figure 22.13 Localised bullous pemphigoid. (a) Tense blisters and erosions limited to the umbilical area. (b) Single tense blister at the site of major surgery. (c) Eczema, erosions and tense blisters restricted to the site of percutaneous endoscopic gastrostomy.

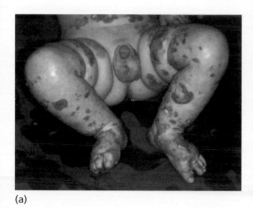

(a)

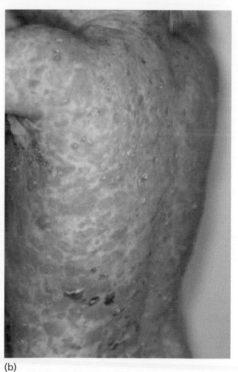

(b)

Figure 22.14 Childhood bullous pemphigoid. (a) Disseminated tense blisters, erosions and crusts on the lower abdomen, genitalia and lower extremities in an infant. (b) Generalised erythema, numerous tense vesicles and some erosions on the back of a 3-year-old boy.

Investigations

The diagnosis is based on the combination of the clinical picture, direct IF microscopy and serology (Figure 22.15).

Management

Untreated BP runs a chronic, self-limiting course over a number of months or years. Remission may occur within a few months or eruptions may continue for many years. Relapses are frequent and appear in about half. Disease duration is usually 3–6 years, with most patients achieving complete remission off treatment.

Localised and mild disease. Lesional very potent topical corticosteroids.

Moderate disease. *First line:* Very potent topical corticosteroids on whole body surface.
Second line: Very potent topical corticosteroids on the whole-body surface plus doxycycline ± nicotinamide; azathioprine *or* dapsone *or* methotrexate *or* mycophenolate mofetil, *or* prednisolone tapering, *with or without* azathioprine, dapsone, doxycycline, methotrexate, mycophenolate.

Extensive disease. *First line:* Very potent topical corticosteroids on the whole-body surface twice daily, plus azathioprine, dapsone, doxycycline, methotrexate, mycophenolate mofetil (see earlier), or very potent topical corticosteroids on the whole-body surface twice daily plus prednisolone tapering, with or without azathioprine, dapsone, doxycycline, methotrexate, mycophenolate.
Second line: In case of insufficient response treat with oral prednisolone, increase dose to 0.75 mg/kg/day and, if still insufficient, to 1.0 mg/kg/day.
Third line: IVIG, immunoadsorption or rituximab.

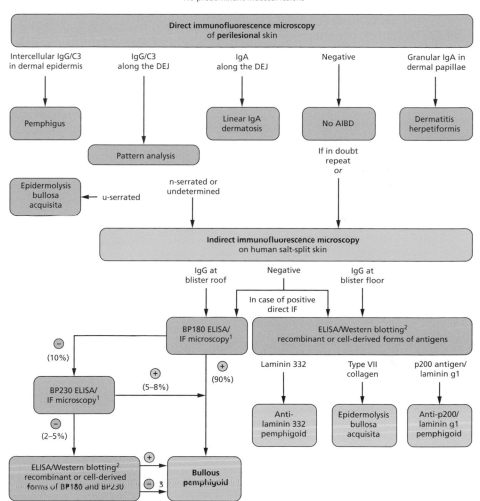

Figure 22.15 Diagnostic pathway for bullous pemphigoid. The diagnostic gold standard is still direct IF microscopy of a perilesional biopsy. About 90% of patients can be diagnosed based on the clinical picture and serological tests. [1]Commercially available assay; [2]only available in specialised diagnostic centres; [3]with positive direct IF microscopy and epidermal binding of IgG by indirect IF microscopy on salt-split skin *or* n-serrated/undetermined IgG binding by direct IF microscopy and no reactivity against laminin 332, p200 antigen, laminin γ1 and type VII collagen. AIBD, autoimmune bullous dermatoses; DEJ, dermal–epidermal junction; ELISA, enzyme-linked immunosorbent assay.

PART 2: INFLAMMATORY DERMATOSES

Mucous membrane pemphigoid

(Syn. Cicatricial pemphigoid)

Mucous membrane pemphigoid (MMP) is an immunobullous disease with predominant mucosal involvement and autoantibodies against components of the DEJ

Epidemiology

A disease of late middle to old age with a mean age of onset of 60–65 years. F > M.

Pathophysiology

Six different target antigens in patients with MMP have been identified (see Table 22.2).

Autoantibodies in MMP may be IgG, IgA or both isotypes.

Blisters in the mouth and on the skin show subepithelial or subepidermal blister formation, but often lack diagnostic features. There are usually fewer eosinophils present in the cutaneous lymphohistiocytic infiltrate than in BP. At a later stage, fibrosis, the distinctive feature of MMP, may develop. The conjunctiva shows epithelial metaplasia, reduced numbers of goblet cells, a lymphocytic infiltrate with plasma cells and mast cells in the substantia propria, fibrosis of the lamina propria accompanied by inflammatory cells and an appearance of granulation tissue in the submucosa.

Tissue-bound autoantibodies can be visualised by direct IF microscopy of a perilesional biopsy. Linear deposits of IgG, C3 and/or IgA at the DEJ are diagnostic together with a compatible clinical phenotype.

Clinical features

Affected sites include oral cavity (in 85% of patients) followed by conjunctivae (65%), skin (25–30%), nasal cavity (20–40%), anogenital area (20%), pharynx (20%), larynx (5–10%) and oesophagus (5–15%). At all affected body sites except the oral cavity, lesions tend to heal with scarring.

The extent of oral lesions may vary considerably from mild almost asymptomatic erosions and chronic gingivitis to extensive extremely painful ulcers (Figure 22.16). Nasal lesions may present as haemorrhagic crusts and epistaxis, and can lead to disfiguring fibrosis and septum perforation. Pharyngeal lesions manifest with odynophagia, with initial involvement of the larynx as hoarseness. Oesophageal disease becomes symptomatic with dysphagia, odynophagia (painful swallowing) and heartburn. Genital lesions usually present with erosions (Figure 22.17). Scarring may lead to labial fusion and introital shrinkage with end-stage scarring indistinguishable from lichen sclerosus. Skin lesions may either resemble BP or heal with scarring and milia formation.

Ocular lesions, usually unilateral initially, with subtle symptoms such as burning, dryness and foreign-body sensation and may proceed to scar formation causing shortening of the inferior fornix, symblepharon, trichiasis, neovascularisation and finally blindness (Figure 22.18). Within 2 years, the disease is usually bilateral. All patients with MMP should be examined by an ophthalmologist to detect subtle changes by slit-lamp examination and measurement of the fornix depth. Of note, a solid cancer is present in about 30% of patients with antilaminin 332

Differential diagnosis
Oral lesions

PV, paraneoplastic pemphigus, oral lichen planus, Behçet disease, Stevens–Johnson syndrome/toxic epidermal necrolysis and bacterial gingivitis.

Ocular lesions

Rosacea, chronic anti-glaucoma therapy, conjunctival lichen planus, Stevens–Johnson syndrome/toxic epidermal necrolysis, Sjögren syndrome, graft-versus-host disease, chronic allergic conjunctivitis, severe atopic eczema, trauma and viral and bacterial infections.

Investigations

Diagnosis is based on the combination of the clinical picture, direct IF microscopy and indirect IF serology.

Management

MMP is typically a chronic, progressive disease. Spontaneous remission is rare except in localised

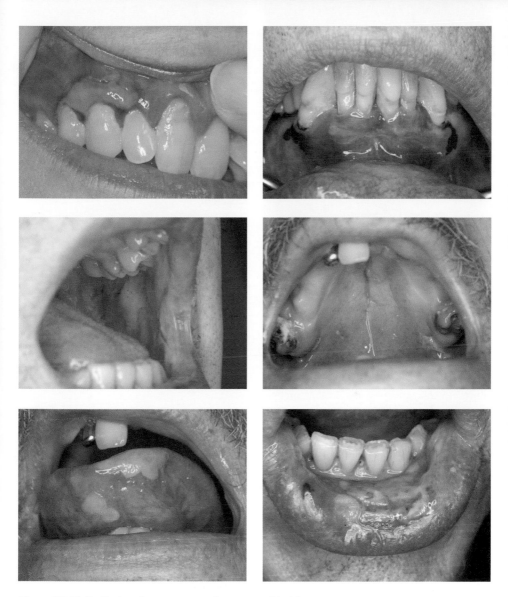

Figure 22.16 Oral lesions in mucous membrane pemphigoid.

oral disease. Patients with dual IgG and IgA anti-DEJ autoantibodies have more severe and persistent disease. Conjunctival scarring may continue for some time after inflammation has been successfully treated. MMP, a solid cancer is present, a thorough search for malignancy is required in patients with this subtype.

Oral MMP. *First line:* Professional oral hygiene; topical moderate or potent topical corticosteroids.
Second line: Plus dapsone *and/or* sulfapyridine/sulfamethoxypyridazine *or* anti-inflammatory antibiotics, e.g. doxycycline or minocycline.
Third line: Plus prednisolone tapering.

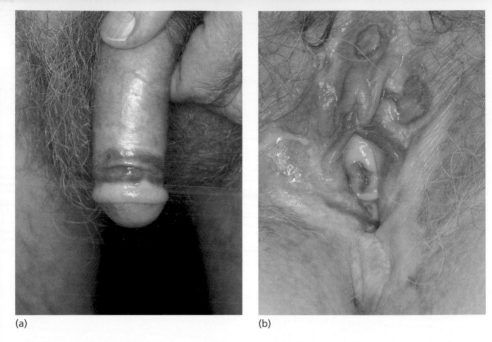

(a)

(b)

Figure 22.17 Genital involvement in mucous membrane pemphigoid: (a) male and (b) female.

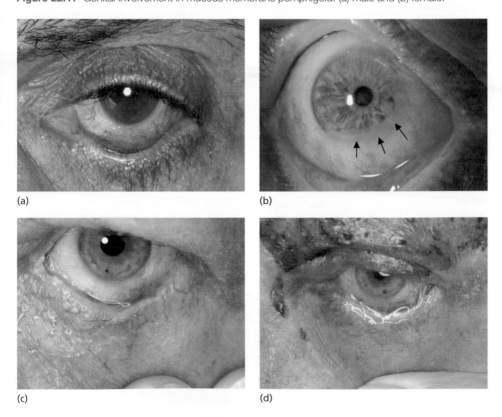

(a)

(b)

(c)

(d)

Figure 22.18 Ocular disease in mucous membrane pemphigoid. (a) Conjunctival hyperaemia, inferior fornix shortening and loss of the plica in early disease. (b) Conjunctival inflammation and limbal scarring (black arrows) in early disease. (Source: Courtesy of Dr J.K.D. Dart, Moorfields Eye Hospital, London, UK.) (c) Loss of the temporal fornix and symblepharon with loss of lashes. (d) Complete loss of inferior fornix with some symblephara and loss of lashes.

Generalised MMP without rapid progression in conjunctivae, larynx or oesophagus. *First line:* Dapsone plus prednisolone tapering.
Second line: Mycophenolate mofetil *plus* prednisolone 0.5 mg/kg/day tapering.
Third line: As for rapid progression.

Generalised MMP with rapid progression in conjunctivae, larynx or oesophagus. *First line:* Cyclophosphamide plus prednisolone tapering.
Second line: Mycophenolate mofetil *plus* prednisolone tapering.
Third line: Plus immunoadsorption; rituximab *or* IVIG.

Linear iga disease

(Inc. Chronic bullous disease of childhood)
A subepidermal blistering disease defined by its main immunopathological feature, the exclusive or predominant binding of IgA along the DEJ.

The clinical features and immunopathology are summarised in Table 22.2.

Epidemiology
Most patients are adults. The incidence is higher in developing countries.

It is the most frequent immunobullous disorder in children. Two peaks of onset, below the age of 5 and between the ages of 60 and 65 years. F ≥ M

Pathophysiology
Histopathology of a lesional biopsy typically shows subepidermal splitting and an infiltrate with neutrophils in the papillary dermis sometimes forming microabscesses, as typically seen in dermatitis herpetiformis.

Tissue-bound autoantibodies can be visualised by direct IF microscopy of a perilesional biopsy. Linear deposits of IgA, frequently accompanied by weaker staining of IgG and/or C3, at the DEJ are diagnostic.

The major target antigen is the ectodomain of BP180.

The majority of linear IgA disease (LAD) sera, in addition to IgA anti-BP180 antibodies, also contain IgG antibodies against BP180.

It can be triggered by various drugs, most frequently vancomycin, followed by nonsteroidal anti-inflammatory drugs and penicillins. Patients with LAD have a higher frequency of lymphoproliferative disorders and nonlymphoid malignancies as well as ulcerative colitis compared to the general population.

Clinical features
In both children and adults, the individual lesions are similar, including tense blisters and vesicles, urticated plaques, erosions and erythema (Figures 22.19 and 22.20). Blisters and vesicles frequently arise in an annular pattern with blistering along the edge of lesions forming the so-called 'string-of-pearls', 'crown of jewels' or 'cluster of jewels' sign (Figure 22.21a). This sign is not pathognomonic for LAD and may also be seen in BP (Figure 22.21b). In children, lesions arise more abruptly and tend to involve the perioral area and perineum in addition to the other predilection sites, trunk and limbs. Latter localisations are mainly involved in adult patients. Mucosal, mostly oral, involvement is common (in about 70%); nasal crusting and genital lesions may also occur. When mucous membrane lesions are predominant there is a diagnostic overlap with MMP. As in BP, lesions tend to heal without scarring. Milia are uncommon.

Differential diagnosis
Children: Bullous impetigo, epidermolysis bullosa.

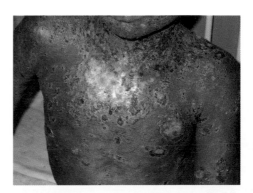

Figure 22.19 Linear IgA disease. Erosions and tense blisters on the trunk in a child. Lesions were also present on the face.

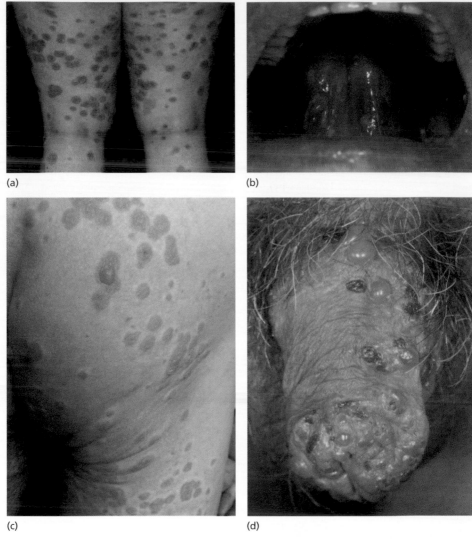

(a)

(b)

(c)

(d)

Figure 22.20 Linear IgA disease. (a) Tense blisters in an annular pattern on the thighs, (b) erosions on the tongue, (c) erythema and blisters on the right gluteal region and (d) tense blisters and crusted erosions on the penis in adult patients.

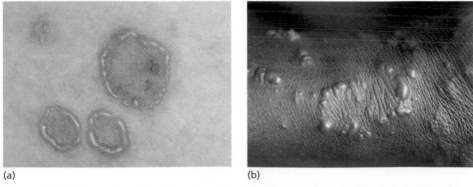

(a)

(b)

Figure 22.21 'Cluster of jewels' or 'ring of pearls' sign. (a) The peculiar appearance of vesicles in an annular pattern or along the edge of a lesion is frequently seen in linear IgA disease, but it is not pathognomonic and may also be observed in bullous pemphigoid (b).

Adults: BP, MMP, dermatitis herpetiformis, atypical erythema multiforme, pemphigus vulgaris and prurigo.

Investigations

Diagnosis is based on the combination of the clinical picture and direct IF microscopy When scarring ocular disease or laryngeal and oesophageal lesions are present most clinicians would diagnose MMP (with predominant IgA reactivity).

Management

Patients with LAD almost always respond well to treatment. Relapses may occur over the next 2–4 years but are usually less severe than the initial disease episode. Most children go into complete remission within 2 years of disease onset and only very rarely does the disease persist after puberty. Drug-induced LAD usually heals within 4–8 weeks after discontinuation of the drug. Involve ophthalmologists in management.

First line: Dapsone + very potent topical corticosteroids ± prednisolone.

Second line: Other sulfa drugs (sulfapyridine, sulfamethoxypyridazine); anti-inflammatory antibiotics (e.g. oxytetracycline, doxycycline) ± nicotinamide.

Third line: Mycophenolate mofetil; IVIG; immunoadsorption.

Epidermolysis bullosa acquisita

A clinically heterogeneous subepidermal blistering disease defined by autoantibodies against type VII collagen.

Epidemiology

An estimated incidence of between 0.2 and 0.5 new cases per million per year.

The disease occurs at any age, with reported mean ages of disease onset of 44 and 54 years.

It occurs more frequently in black patients of African descent.

Pathophysiology

The autoantigen of EBA is homotrimeric type VII collagen, a constituent of anchoring fibrils.

Penicillin, vancomycin in conjunction with gentamycin, UV radiation and contact allergy to metals have been implicated as precipitating factors. There is an association with Crohn disease and haematological malignancies, i.e. lymphoma.

The histopathological hallmark is subepidermal blistering. Depending on the clinical subtype, the inflammatory infiltrate in the dermis is variable, scarce in the mechanobullous variant and dense with predominant neutrophils, eosinophils, monocytes and lymphocytes reminiscent of BP in the inflammatory subtype. Serum autoantibodies label the dermal side of human salt-split skin by indirect IF microscopy.

Tissue-bound autoantibodies can be detected by direct IF microscopy of a perilesional biopsy as linear deposits of IgG and/or C3 at the DEJ.

EBA is associated with HLA-DRB1*15

Clinical features

Two main clinical forms can be differentiated: the classical mechanobullous variant, in about a third of patients, and the inflammatory subtype. The classical mechanobullous phenotype mimics dystrophic hereditary EB when severe and porphyria cutanea tarda when mild. Clinical characteristics are skin fragility, erosions, blisters, crusts and scars on trauma-prone areas such as the hands, knuckles, elbows, knees and toes (Figures 22.22 and 22.23). Scarring alopecia and nail loss may occur. The inflammatory variant resembles other pemphigoid diseases such as BP, MMP or LAD (Figures 22.24 and 22.25). However, both the classic and the inflammatory forms may coexist in the same patient and the clinical presentation of a given EBA patient may change during the disease course. Both subtypes may occur in adults (Figures 22.22 and 22.24) and children (Figures 22.23). Mucous membranes are affected in about half.

Differential diagnosis

Mechanobullous subtype: Dystrophic EB (family history, direct IF microscopy) and porphyria cutanea tarda (porphyrins in urine, direct IF microscopy).

Inflammatory subtype: BP, MMP and LAD.

PART 2: INFLAMMATORY DERMATOSES

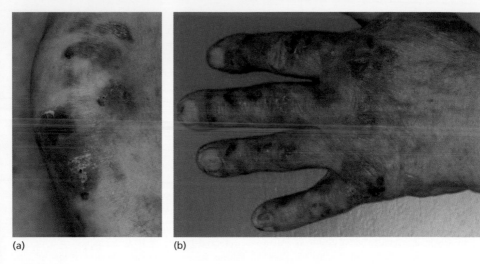

(a) (b)

Figure 22.22 Epidermolysis bullosa acquisita, mechanobullous variant. (a) Erythema, erosions and crusts on the left knee and (b) erythematous plaques, atrophic scars, milia, crusts and a tense blister on trauma-prone extensor surface of the left hand of a 75-year-old man.

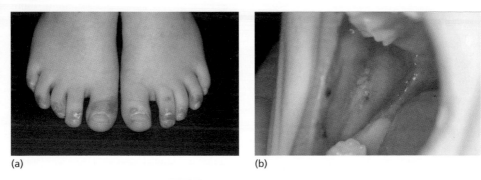

(a) (b)

Figure 22.23 Childhood epidermolysis bullosa acquisita, mechanobullous variant. (a) Erythema, erosions and tense blisters on the trauma-prone dorsal aspects of the toes and (b) erosions of the buccal mucosa in a 5-year-old boy.

Investigations

Diagnosis is based on the combination of the clinical picture, direct IF microscopy and serology.

Management

Chronic relapsing disease is difficult to treat compared to other pemphigoid disorders. There is a better overall prognosis in children compared to adults. No difference with respect to response to treatment occurs between the mechanobullous and the inflammatory variants.

First line: Prednisolone + colchicine ± dapsone.

Second line: + Mycophenolate mofetil *or* + ciclosporin.

Third line: Rituximab *or* IVIG.

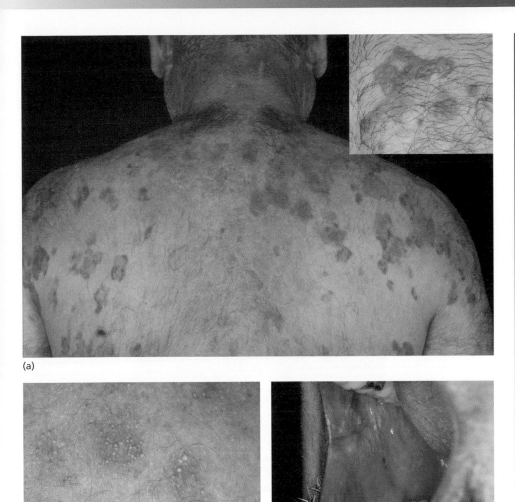

(a)

(b)

(c)

Figure 22.24 Epidermolysis bullosa acquisita, inflammatory variant. (a) Erosions and tense blisters (insert) on the upper back, (b) milia and (c) erosions of the buccal mucosa.

Most children are treated with a combination of systemic corticosteroids and dapsone.

Bullous systemic lupus erythematosus

An autoimmune subepidermal blistering disease that occurs in patients with SLE. For a detailed description see Chapter 23.

VERY RARE PEMPHIGOID DISORDERS

Lichen planus pemphigoides

Always arises in conjunction with lichen planus and can affect both adults and children, in contrast to BP.

Diagnosis is made by the presence of tense blisters close to lichen planus lesions (Figure 22.25). There are linear deposits of IgG

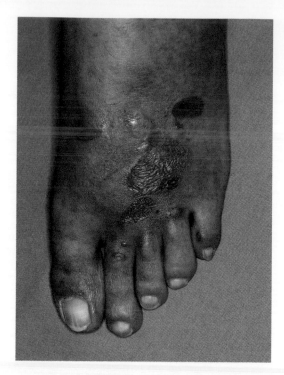

Figure 22.25 Lichen planus pemphigoides. Erosions, erythema, partly ruptured and subsequently desiccated blisters and a tense vesicle on the left foot. In addition, a lichen planus lesion is seen. Of note, erosions and blisters are separate from the lichen planus lesion.

and/or C3 at the DEJ by direct IF microscopy of a perilesional biopsy and circulating IgG antibodies against BP180 NC16A.

Brunsting–Perry pemphigoid

A clinical subtype of cicatricial pemphigoid. This rare disease occurs in middle-aged and elderly populations. Skin lesions are characteristically confined to the head, neck and upper trunk (Figures 22.26 and 22.27). Mucous membranes can also be involved. Direct IF microscopy shows linear deposits of IgG and/or C3 at the DEJ. Differential diagnosis includes squamous cell carcinoma, basal cell carcinoma, erosive pustular dermatosis of the scalp and dermatitis artefacta. Treatment usually comprises topical corticosteroids.

Anti-p200 pemphigoid

A distinct subepidermal bullous skin disease characterised by autoantibodies against a 200 kDa protein, p200, of the DEJ. The mean age is 69 years. M > F.

The C terminus of laminin γ1 is the immunodominant region in anti-p200 pemphigoid.

Histopathology does not differentiate anti-p200 pemphigoid from other pemphigoid diseases. Most patients present with tense blisters on erythematosus or normal skin resembling BP. Management is as for BP.

Dermatitis herpetiformis

Dermatitis herpetiformis (DH) is a chronic, intensely pruritic, skin condition associated with gluten-sensitive enteropathy (GSE).

Epidemiology

Most common in people of northern European descent.

Onset is most commonly in adult life, typically in the fourth decade, though cases have been reported from childhood to old age. M > F.

The commonest association is with GSE, the severity of which is variable and may be

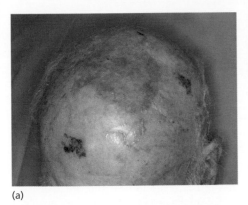

(a)

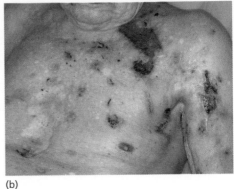

(b)

Figure 22.26 Brunsting–Perry pemphigoid. Erosions on the scalp (a), chest and upper left arm as well as atrophic scars (b) in a 95-year-old man. Linear staining of IgG and C3 was seen at the DEJ by direct IF microscopy. Serum autoantibodies exclusively labelled the epidermal side by indirect IF microscopy on salt-split skin and reacted with BP180 NC16A.

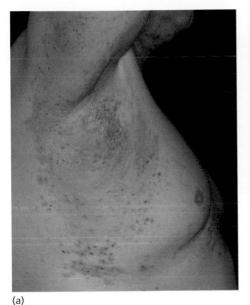

(a)

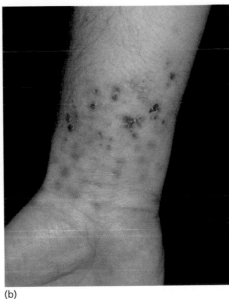

(b)

Figure 22.27 Anti-p200 pemphigoid. Erythematous partly excoriated papules and erythema on (a) the right axilla and (b) vesicles and erythematosus papules on the right wrist in a 52-year-old patient.

clinically silent or mild. First-degree relatives of patients with GSE or DH are significantly more likely to be affected by one or other disorder and thus family screening may be indicated. Monozygotic twins have a disease concordance rate >0.9.

Pathophysiology

The pathology in DH and GSE results from an IgA dominant autoimmune response to transglutaminase molecules. In GSE, the principal target is tissue transglutaminase (tTG); in DH it is epidermal transglutaminase 3 (TG3). Asian

PART 2: INFLAMMATORY DERMATOSES

patients have a distinct fibrillar pattern of IgA deposition in the skin, only very rarely associated with GSE.

The histopathology of an intact vesicle demonstrates subepidermal blister formation with neutrophils located at the tips of the dermal papillae. There is frequently perivascular inflammatory cell infiltrate. Because vesicles may not survive the pruritus, clefting may not be seen.

Complement 3 may also be found in association with the IgA deposits.

There is an association with HLA-DQ2.

Dietary gluten and its constituent gliadin are the principal environmental factors involved in DH and GSE. Iodine exposure can precipitate flares of DH. Increased risk of small bowel lymphoma. Particularly associated with autoimmune thyroid disease but also type 1 diabetes, Addison disease and vitiligo.

Clinical features

The principal symptom is itch with grouped erythematous papules and vesicles located over extensor sites: elbows, knees, buttocks and scalp (Figure 22.28). Because the condition is so pruritic, intact vesicles are rarely seen and the patient may simply present with excoriations. Lesions tend to be symmetrical and heal without scarring. Punctate purpura may develop on palms and soles. Mucosal change may occur.

The principal complications and comorbidities of DH relate to GSE and the associated risk of small bowel lymphoma. GSE may lead to malabsorption resulting in anaemia, weight loss and osteoporosis. In children, short stature is a consequence. Rarely, GSE (and consequently DH) may be associated with neurological changes including ataxia and neuropathy.

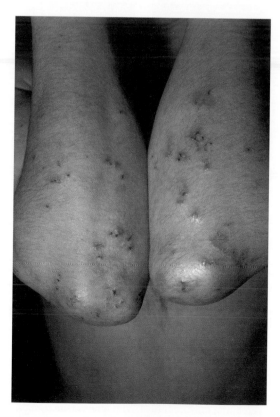

Figure 22.28 Dermatitis herpetiformis. Intact tense bullae and erosions on the elbows. (Source: ISM/CID/Medical Images.)

Differential diagnosis

Includes many pruritic and vesiculobullous disorders, including LAD, pemphigoid, eczema and scabies.

Investigations

Direct IF samples are best taken from nonlesional skin as characteristic changes may be lost in lesional tissue. The diagnostic finding is that of deposition of IgA in the papillary dermis in a granular or fibrillar pattern (Figure 22.29).

Management

Strict adherence to a gluten-free diet is crucial. Not only does this improve skin changes over time but it is essential in the management of associated GSE. Because of the slow response to gluten-free diet, most patients with DH require pharmacological intervention to control their disease in the short to medium term. Dapsone is highly effective, often suppressing pruritus within days of initiation of treatment. If patient is dapsone intolerant sulphamethoxypyridazone can be used. Dapsone does not impact on the gastrointestinal aspects of associated GSE. All patients with DH should be reviewed by a gastroenterologist and investigated accordingly.

Dapsone should always be used in combination with a gluten-free diet. With time, it may be possible to decrease and potentially withdraw dapsone without relapse, as long as the patient is able to adhere to the diet. Remission is recognised and seems to be more common in adult patients over the age of 40 years.

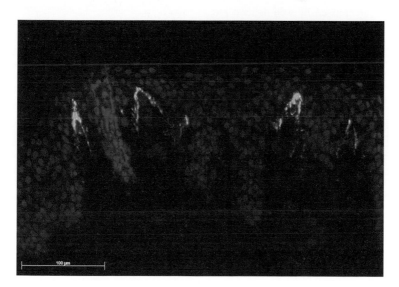

Figure 22.29 Dermatitis herpetiformis. Direct immunofluorescence demonstrating granular IgA deposition in the dermal papillae.

Lupus erythematosus (LE) is divided into two main types, discoid LE (DLE) and systemic LE (SLE), and a third group, subacute cutaneous LE (SCLE).

Discoid lupus erythematosus

(Syn. Chronic cutaneous lupus erythematosus) DLE is a benign inflammatory disorder of the skin, most frequently involving the face and scalp, and characterised by well-defined red, scaly patches of variable size, which heal with atrophy, scarring and pigmentary changes.

Epidemiology
Incidence 4/100 000. There is a peak age of onset in the fourth decade in females and slightly later in males, although it can occur at any age. F > M = 2:1 The disease is more common and more severe in Asians, African Americans, Afro-Caribbeans and Hispanic Americans.

Pathophysiology
Cutaneous inflammation in DLE is a process in which interferons (IFNs), type I and type 3, induce Th1-biased inflammation, with a predominantly lymphocytic infiltration. Predisposing factors are shown in Box 23.1.

The various clinical types of LE show an essentially similar histological picture. The salient features are shown in Box 23.2.

Clinical features
Most patients have disease limited to the head and neck (localised DLE), but a few have much more extensive disease, potentially affecting any area of the skin (disseminated DLE). Some patients have a history of Raynaud phenomenon, chilblains or poor peripheral circulation. Joint pains may occur. Most patients have no symptoms of systemic upset, even with widespread cutaneous disease, although fatigue is common.

Localised DLE
Face and scalp are most commonly affected. The circumscribed or discoid form is the most frequent type (Figure 23.1), and occurs particularly

---

Box 23.1 Predisposing factors to discoid lupus erythematosus

- Trauma, including X-rays and diathermy
- Stress
- Ultraviolet light exposure, including psoralen with UVA and laser light
- Infection, including herpes zoster and old smallpox vaccination
- Drugs: many drugs are associated with the precipitation or exacerbation of DLE,

including isoniazid, penicillamine, griseofulvin and dapsone
- Seasonal exacerbation in both winter (10%) and summer (50%)
- Cold exposure

Unpublished Chapel Allerton Hospital at Leeds data.

Rook's Dermatology Handbook, First Edition. Edited by Christopher E. M. Griffiths, Tanya O. Bleiker, Daniel Creamer, John R. Ingram and Rosalind C. Simpson.
© 2022 John Wiley & Sons Ltd. Published 2022 by John Wiley & Sons Ltd.

> **Box 23.2 Histological features of cutaneous lupus erythematosus**
>
> - Lymphocytic interface dermatitis with basal layer degeneration
> - Apoptotic keratinocytes
> - Basement membrane thickening (greatest in DLE)
> - Perivascular and periadnexal lymphohistiocytic infiltrate
> - Follicular plugging
> - Dermal mucinosis
> - Epidermal atrophy

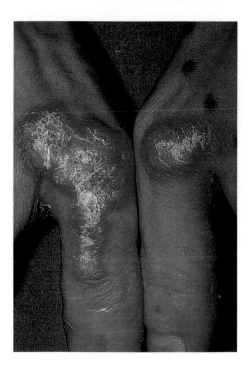

Figure 23.1 Localised DLE showing typical scaling on the fingers.

on the cheeks, bridge of the nose, ears, side of the neck and scalp. Alopecia occurs in the scalp lesions in approximately one-third, and is usually permanent (Figure 23.2). The eyebrows may be sparse, with erythema of the eyebrow skin. Lesions occur as well-defined erythematous patches, varying in size from a few millimetres to

10–15 cm. There is adherent scale in many cases, and when this is removed its undersurface shows horny plugs that have occupied dilated pilosebaceous canals. The 'tin-tack' sign. The surface may present a dirty, brownish yellow appearance that is rough to the touch because of follicular plugging. Warty lesions of LE may occur on the face and scalp, but also on the palms and soles (Figure 23.3). Lesions flatten and may clear completely, without much scarring, with treatment. More frequently, a thin, white scarred area remains (Figure 23.4a). Localised cribriform scarring occurs, particularly on the face (Figure 23.4b). Wide follicular pits occur mainly in the concha or triangular fossa of the ear (Figure 23.5) in up to one-third of cases of DLE but they also occur in SLE. The lesions on the face can resemble rosacea (Figure 23.6).

Tumid lesions in which the tissues are swollen, brawny, warm and tense (Figure 23.7) may be many centimetres in diameter and involve the whole of one cheek, or even the whole of a limb. Another clinical type of DLE results in annular atrophic plaques on the face, neck and behind the ears. The centre of the plaques is depressed and sclerotic, and lesions resemble morphoea, lichen sclerosus or annular atrophic plaques.

Scarring is common and may be atrophic, hypertrophic, cribriform or acneiform. Pigmentary disturbances are common, especially in dark-skinned people (Figure 23.8). Patches of leukoderma may be interspersed with hyperpigmented areas. Once scarring has occurred, no further inflammation is seen. Calcification may occur in plaques. Lesions on the ear lead to considerable atrophy and scarring (Figure 23.9).

Disseminated DLE

Characteristic lesions of DLE may occur in a widespread pattern on the trunk and limbs. This occurs most often in women, usually cigarette smokers. This may be indistinguishable from the papulosquamous type of SCLE, but scarring occurs in most patients. Lesions on the dorsa of the hands (Figure 23.10a), palms or toes (Figure 23.10b) occur in a minority. Nonitching, hyperkeratotic, papulonodular lesions on the arms and hands, resembling keratoacanthoma, hypertrophic lichen planus or nodular prurigo, also occur. It may resemble psoriasis. Another disseminated variety results in a reticulate telangiectasia, usually on the arms, legs and back of the calves. This type of telangiectasia is

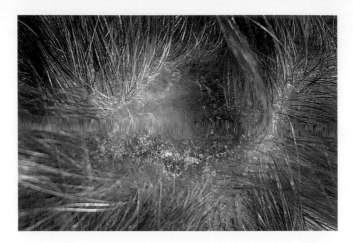

Figure 23.2 Localised DLE of the scalp showing follicular plugging.

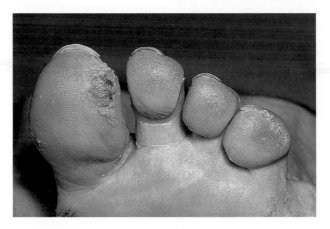

Figure 23.3 Warty lesions of the feet in chronic lupus erythematosus.

probably similar to lupus erythematosus telangiectoides (Figure 23.11). A further, more annular variant, lupus erythematosus gyratus repens, consists of a migratory gyrate annular erythema with the histological features of LE (Figure 23.12); there may be an underlying carcinoma. Rarely, bullous lesions may occur.

Chilblain lupus

May occur in patients with either DLE or SLE. Approximately 6% of patients with cutaneous lupus, predominantly female, develop chilblain-like lesions chiefly on toes and fingers (Figure 23.13). It can be precipitated by pregnancy. Some patients may have cryofibrinogenaemia or cold agglutinins and are often Ro antibody positive. They are also either smokers or have markedly abnormal peripheral circulation. Occasionally, one or more fingers may show a curious atrophic spindling, sometimes with hyperextension of the terminal phalanges and dystrophy of the nails (Figure 23.14). The fingers and toes may become markedly atrophic, with patchy erythema and tuft resorption on X-ray. 15% develop SLE.

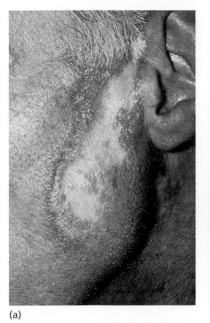

(a)

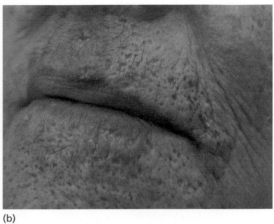

(b)

Figure 23.4 Scarring in DLE. (a) Preauricular DLE with pigmentation around the scarred area. (b) Cribriform scarring in DLE.

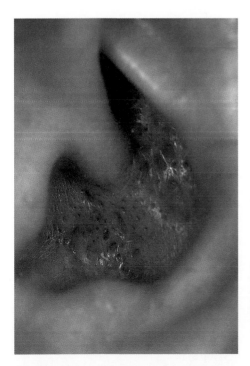

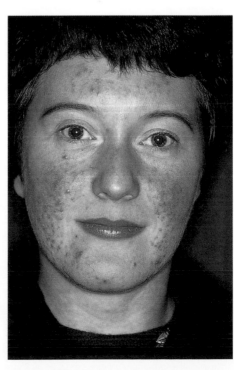

Figure 23.5 Typical lesions in the ear in DLE.

Figure 23.6 Rosaceous pattern of DLE.

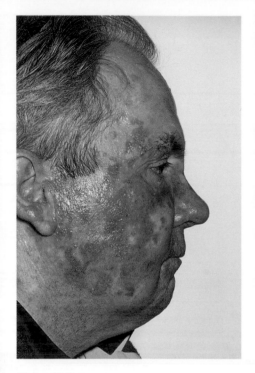

Figure 23.7 Tumid lesions of the face in DLE.

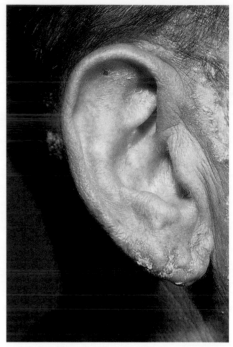

Figure 23.9 DLE of the ear with scarring and atrophy.

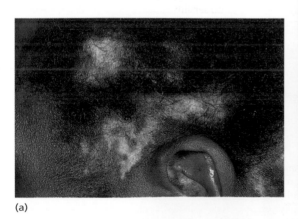

(a)

(b)

Figure 23.8 Pigmentary changes in DLE. (a) Patches on the scalp of a black patient. (b) DLE in an Asian patient showing marked hyperpigmentation at the border of the affected area.

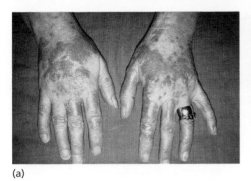

(a)

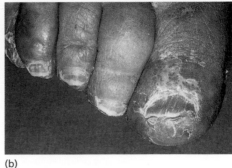

(b)

Figure 23.10 Disseminated DLE. (a) Plaques on the back of the hands. (b) Characteristic redness and scaling of the toes.

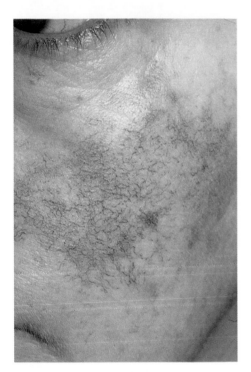

Figure 23.11 Telangiectatic LE of the cheek.

Lupus erythematosus profundus (panniculitis)

The cutaneous infiltrate occurs primarily in deeper portions of the skin, giving rise to firm, sharply defined nodules from 1 to several centimetres in diameter, lying beneath clinically normal skin with atrophy of fat (Figure 23.15).

Differential diagnosis

Morphoea, lichen sclerosus, Jessner's lymphocytic infiltration, contact eczema, seborrhoeic dermatitis, psoriasis and lupus vulgaris.

Reticular erythematous mucinosis, which can show clinical and histological features similar to DLE, may also be induced by UV radiation but is a discrete clinical entity.

Necrobiosis lipoidica can give facial lesions similar to those in DLE. The rosaceous type of LE can usually be differentiated from true rosacea by the absence of pustules.

Lesions on the lips, tongue, scalp and buccal mucosa may be confused with lichen planus. Overlap cases, in addition to LE-like lesions, have lichenoid papules, verrucous lesions, anonychia and oral and vulval lesions resembling lichen planus.

Sun sensitivity can cause diagnostic difficulty with polymorphic light eruption and Bloom syndrome.

Investigations

Diagnostic skin biopsy to confirm the diagnosis. Baseline investigations should include ANA and ENA, haematology and biochemistry and urine testing for proteinuria. Baseline ophthalmology assessment if systemic antimalarials to be considered.

Management

A complete medical assessment of the patient is necessary to establish a diagnosis of the subtype

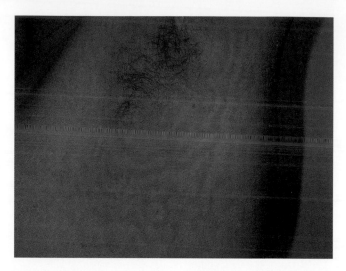

Figure 23.12 Gyrate erythema in LE.

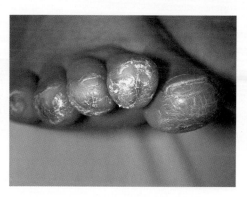

Figure 23.13 'Chilblain' lesions in a patient with Ro-positive SLE.

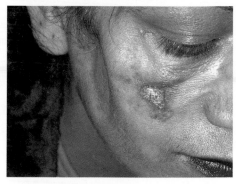

Figure 23.15 LE profundus.

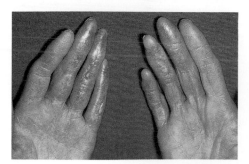

Figure 23.14 Unusual spindling of the fingers and hyperextension of the distal phalanges in DLE.

of DLE, a likely prognosis, and a baseline by which later progress may be judged. Appropriate sun protection against UVA and UVB should be advised. Vasodilator drugs, particularly calcium-channel blockers such as nifedipine, are helpful in those with Raynaud phenomenon and chilblain lesions. Scarred lesions may be camouflaged.

First line: Topical potent corticosteroids. Intralesional corticosteroid injections in resistant cases. Topical calcineurin inhibitors, such as tacrolimus, provide a useful alternative to corticosteroids.

Second line: Hydroxychloroquine is the first-line systemic treatment of choice. Chloroquine phosphate is an alternative. Mepacrine is also useful, and is safe from an ophthalmological point of view, but limited because of yellow discolouration of the skin.

For patients with severe, extensive or scarring disease, particularly affecting the scalp, a tapering course of oral prednisolone is often the most helpful initial treatment and allows the slower acting agents such as antimalarials to work. Pulsed intravenous methylprednisolone may help resistant cases.

Third line: Thalidomide, methotrexate and mycophenolate mofetil. IV immunoglobulin and IV pulses of cyclophosphamide may also be used in resistant cases.

Subacute cutaneous lupus erythematosus

SCLE is a specific subset of lupus, often drug-induced. Patients exhibit mainly cutaneous disease and usually have a good prognosis. Antibodies to the Ro/Sjögren's-syndrome-related antigen A (SS-A) are often found.

Epidemiology

Prevalence is estimated to be 6.2–14 per 100 000. It affects adults of all ages; F > M = 4:1. Drug-induced SCLE occurs in older patients (mean age 59 years) and is generally milder.

Pathophysiology

UVR increases Ro/SS-A antigen expression on the surface of keratinocytes, which is enhanced by oestrogen.

Drug-induced SCLE is common, the onset is often delayed after the introduction of the drug. Resolution is slow after discontinuation of the drug. Antihypertensive agents, such as thiazides and calcium channel blockers, and terbinafine are the commonest causes. It may occur during PUVA treatment of psoriasis, radiation therapy and IFN-1α therapy Homogeneous antinuclear antibodies (ANAs) are found in 60% and anti-Ro/SS-A antibodies in 80%; higher levels in females. Anticardiolipin antibodies occur in approximately 16%.

Histologically SCLE can be differentiated from DLE by the presence of more epidermal atrophy and less hyperkeratosis, basement-membrane thickening, follicular plugging and inflammatory infiltration. Colloid bodies and epidermal necrosis are present in more than 50% of cases, especially in those with Ro/SS-A antibodies. Lesional subepidermal immunoglobulin is found in approximately 60%.

Clinical features

Patients may have a history of previous sun-induced skin problems, and often classical polymorphic light eruption. Raynaud phenomenon may occur before the characteristic skin rash, and patients may have mild arthralgia, although arthritis is unusual before the onset of rash.

Two-thirds of patients present with a nonscarring papulosquamous eruption (Figure 23.16a); one-third present with annular polycyclic lesions. Lesions usually occur above the waist and particularly around the neck, on the trunk, on the outer aspects of the arms (Figure 23.16b), and sometimes along the lines of Blaschko. The borders may show vesiculation, crusting and occasionally bullae, which may be associated with coexistent porphyria cutanea tarda. Lesions resolve to leave grey-white hypopigmentation and telangiectases. Diffuse nonscarring alopecia and photosensitivity occur in approximately half of patients; other features include mouth ulceration (palate), reticular livedo and periungual telangiectasia.

Differential diagnosis

Dermatomyositis, LE or DLE, erythema annulare centrifugum, erythema gyratum repens, erythema multiforme, granuloma annulare, lichen planus, psoriasis and tinea corporis.

Investigation

As for DLE.

Management

Avoidance of UV exposure.

First line: Sunscreens, topical or intralesional corticosteroids or the topical macrolides pimicrolimus and tacrolimus.

Second line: Antimalarials, usually hydroxychloroquine (less effective in smokers).

PART 2: INFLAMMATORY DERMATOSES

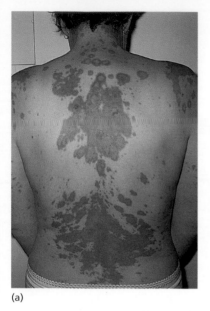

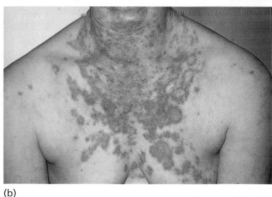

(a)   (b)

Figure 23.16 Subacute cutaneous LE. (a) Papulosquamous eruption on the back. (b) Annular polycyclic lesions on the chest.

Third line: Oral corticosteroids or pulsed intravenous methylprednisolone, acitretin, isotretinoin, dapsone, oral, intravenous and subcutaneous methotrexate, thalidomide, UVA, mycophenolate mofetil, intravenous immunoglobulin and etanercept.

Systemic lupus erythematosus

A systemic disease characterised by multisystem organ inflammation, most commonly the skin, joints, and vasculature and associated immunological abnormalities.

Epidemiology

Uncommon. Prevalence of 30 per 100 000 in white people and 200 per 100 000 in Afro-Caribbeans. Incidence estimated at 3.8 per 100 000 per year. Black Americans have an earlier age of diagnosis and renal disease is more common.

Occurs in early adult life: peak age of onset in females is approximately 38 years, earlier in black women, later in white women and in men. Serositis and Sjögren syndrome are more common in the elderly. F > M = 10:1. Onset in

childhood occurs in 15%. Children usually have more severe disease.

Pathophysiology

There is no single diagnostic pathological feature for SLE in the skin, but a combination of features aids diagnosis. The histopathology of the skin is similar in each of the different forms of LE-specific skin disease (Box 23.1) The primary histology comprises fibrinoid necrosis, collagen sclerosis, necrosis and basophilic body formation and vascular endothelial thickening. The LE cell is a neutrophil that has engulfed nuclear material from dying cells

Immunoglobulins, predominantly IgG, but less frequently IgM and IgA, together with complement (C1q, C3) can be demonstrated at the dermal–epidermal junction by immunofluorescence techniques. Such deposits are also present in clinically normal skin.

Many autoimmune diseases, including rheumatoid arthritis, systemic sclerosis, type 1 diabetes, inflammatory bowel disease and Behçet disease, share risk loci. A range of autoantibodies may be present in SLE, although some are more disease-specific (anti-dsDNA and anti-Smith (Sm) antibodies)

and some are much more common (antinuclear and anti-Ro antibodies).

Environmental factors include exposure to sunlight and UV radiation, smoking, infections and medications such as TNF inhibitor biologics, which are linked more to arthritis than cutaneous changes. Other factors include bacterial infection, virus infection and mental or physical stress. Oestrogen-containing contraceptive compounds, early menarche and post-menopausal oestrogen use all increase the risk of SLE.

The precipitation of SLE by drugs, especially the antihypertensive hydralazine, is well known. Drug-induced SLE is uncommon in black people. It occurs in an older age group, renal and central nervous system involvement are infrequent, antihistone antibodies are frequent, anti-DNA antibodies are absent and serum complement is normal.

Clinical features

See Table 23.1.

The most commonly observed presenting symptoms are arthralgias followed by cutaneous involvement. The evolution can be gradual, starting with localised skin lesions and systemic involvement developing later. As most patients are female, sex is an important diagnostic point. Fatigue is reported in up to 80% of patients. Approximately 57–85% of patients have cutaneous findings at some stage (Figure 23.17). The typical cutaneous findings are shown in Table 23.2.

Patients with any of the LE-specific features described under the cutaneous subtypes may have skin disease alone or SLE if they fulfil the new Systemic Lupus International Collaborating Clinics (SLICC) criteria (Table 23.3). The risk of SLE with localised versus generalised DLE is 5% versus 20% over time. Patients with lupus panniculitis may have up to 35% chance of a preceding, concurrent or subsequent diagnosis of SLE, thus these patients should be followed closely for the development of systemic disease. Similarly, although the incidence of SLE in patients with SCLE is approximately 50%, only 10–15% have serious organ involvement.

Acute cutaneous lupus erythematosus (ACLE) is often associated with active SLE; some patients can experience recurrent ACLE in an isolated fashion over years. Cutaneous erythema is the most common feature, particularly on light-exposed areas (Figure 23.18a). In localised ACLE, a blush or discrete maculopapular eruption with fine scaling or oedema on the butterfly area of the cheeks, typically sparing the nasolabial folds, is common (Figure 23.18b). In generalised LE, a diffuse or papular erythema of the face, upper trunk and extremities can resemble a viral exanthem or a drug eruption. Photosensitivity is very common. UV radiation from fluorescent lighting and UVA from photocopiers may cause exacerbations, as well as chronic exposure to indoor light sources. A negative history of photosensitivity does not exclude sensitivity to light as there is a latency period of several weeks. Systemic disease activity

Table 23.1 Clinical features of SLE

Clinical feature	Occurrence in SLE (%)
Fever	90
Arthritis and arthralgia	90
Skin lesions	80
Renal involvement	67
Lymphadenopathy	50
Pleurisy	40
Raynaud phenomenon	35
Pericarditis	25
Hepatomegaly	25
Central nervous system involvement	25
Abdominal symptoms	20
Splenomegaly	15

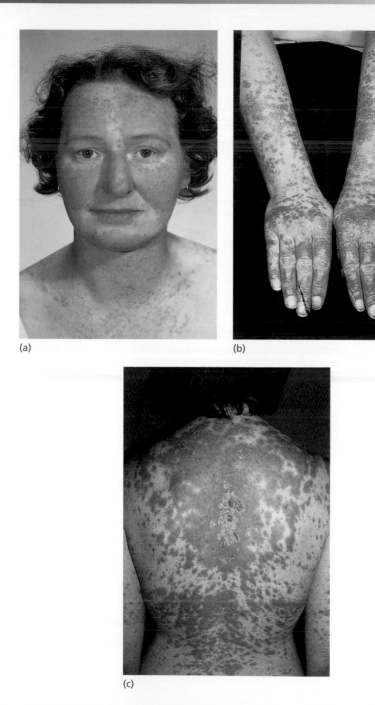

(a)

(b)

(c)

Figure 23.17 SLE. (a) Typical symmetrical, slightly scaling erythema of the face and neck. (b) Erythema of the dorsa of the hands and forearms. Identical changes may occur in DLE. Note the chloroquine pigmentation of the distal part of the nails. (c) Gross involvement of the back.

Table 23.2 Cutaneous features of SLE in 73 patients

Cutaneous feature	Occurrence in SLE (%)
Butterfly rash as part of ACLE	51
Subacute cutaneous LE	7
Chronic DLE	25
Scarring DLE alopecia	14
Facial oedema	4
Non-scarring alopecia	40
Chilblain lupus	20
Mouth ulceration	31
Bullous eruptions	8
Photosensitivity	63
Raynaud phenomenon	60
Chronic urticaria (>36 h)	44
Cutaneous vasculitis	11
Livedo reticularis	4
Episcleritis	4
Cheilitis	4

The cutaneous features in italic are considered LE-specific skin changes, with the characteristic histology of cutaneous lupus. The other cutaneous features are considered lupus nonspecific cutaneous features. ACLE, acute cutaneous lupus erythematosus; DLE, discoid lupus erythematosus; LE, lupus erythematosus; SLE, lupus erythematosus systemic. Source: Adapted from Yell JA, Mbuagbaw J, Burge SM. Cutaneous manifestations of of systemic lupus erythematosus. Br J Dermatol 1996; 135: 355–62.

is increased in the 3–6 months following maximal sun exposure. Occasionally, more acute lesions with bullae may follow sun exposure. The rash in generalised LE and the generalised form of chronic cutaneous lupus erythematosus usually spares the distal interphalangeal, proximal interphalangeal and metacarpophalangeal joints, an important distinguishing feature from dermatomyositis (Figure 23.19).

Erythema can occur over the hyperthenar and hypothenar eminences of the palms and may be confused with palmar erythema of liver disease. Reticulated palmar erythema may also be associated with vasculopathy of the antiphospholipid syndrome.

Nail changes include nail fold erythema, splinter haemorrhages, red lunulae and nail fold hyperkeratosis (Figure 23.20a). Other findings include nail ridging, onycholysis, onychomadesis and punctate or striate leukonychia caused by altered keratinisation of the nail matrix (Figure 23.20b). Blue-black nail pigmentation due to increased melanin deposition may also be observed, most commonly in African-American patients with SLE. This may also be caused by medications, most frequently antimalarials (Figure 23.21).

Telogen effluvium occurs in more than 60% of cases. Alopecia can be chronic and associated with disease activity, leading to coarse, dry and fragile hair along the peripheral hairline during a systemic flare 2–3 months later, so-called 'lupus hair' (Figure 23.22). Permanent scarring alopecia is similar to that found in DLE.

Vascular reactions can be divided into vasculitis or vasculopathy.

Vasculitis in the context of SLE most commonly affects the skin, usually as a small-vessel leukocytoclastic vasculitis with palpable petechiae or purpura in dependent areas. The involvement of medium and/or large vessels may manifest as retiform or stellate purpura with or without necrosis and ulceration or as subcutaneous nodules (Figure 23.23). Other manifestations include gangrene, periungual infacts, splinter haemorrhages and urticarial and bullous changes. Raynaud phenomenon occurs in up to 60%.

Livedo reticularis occurs in approximately 35% with and without the antiphospholipid syndrome. It is most common on buttocks, legs and outer aspects of the arms (Figure 23.24). Livedo racemosa has a 'broken net' type of pattern and is a sign of more severe disease due to the presence of cholesterol and fibrin thrombi in the vessels. Livedo reticularis in patients with SLE and antiphospholipid syndrome may associate with central nervous system involvement. Patients with both antiphospholipid antibodies (APA) and SLE may present with retiform purpuric plaques. Atrophie blanche-type lesions (painful, ivory, stellate scars on the lower extremities) may occur. Lesions similar to those in Degos disease (malignant atrophic papulosis) may also occur in patients with APA (Figure 23.25).

PART 2: INFLAMMATORY DERMATOSES

Table 23.3 Systemic Lupus International Collaborating Clinics classification criteria for SLE, 2012[a]

Clinical criteria	Definition
1. Acute cutaneous lupus	Including lupus malar rash (do not include if malar discoid), bullous lupus, toxic epidermal necrolysis variant of SLE, maculopapular rash, photosensitive lupus rash in the absence of dermatomyositis; *or* subacutue cutaneous lupus
2. Chronic cutaneous lupus	Including classic discoid rash, hypertrophic (verrucous) lupus, lupus panniculitis (profundus), mucosal lupus, lupus erythematosus tumidus, chilblain lupus, discoid lupus/lichen planus overlap
3. Oral ulcers	Palate, buccal, tongue or nasal ulcers in the absence of other causes
4. Nonscarring alopecia	Diffuse thinning or hair fragility with broken hairs in the absence of other causes
5. Synovitis	Involving two or more joints characterised by effusion or swelling *or* tenderness in two or more joints and at least 30 min of morning stiffness
6. Serositis: pleurisy or pericarditis	More than 1 day duration of pleural/pericaridal effusions or pleural/pericardial rub
7. Renal disorder: persistent proteinuria (>0.5 μg/day) or cellular casts	
8. Neurological disorder	Seizures, psychosis, mononeuritis multiplex, myelitis or acute confusional state in the absence of other causes
9. Haemolytic anaemia	
10. Leukopenia (<4000/mm³ at least once) *or* lymphopenia (<1000/mm³)	
11. Thrombocytopenia (<100 000/mm³ at least once)	

Immunological criteria
1. ANA above reference laboratory range
2. Anti-dsDNA antibody above reference laboratory range (or more than twofold the reference range if tested by ELISA)
3. Anti-Sm: presence of antibody to Sm nuclear antigen
4. Antiphospholipid antibody positivity
5. Low complement (low C3, C4 or CH50)
6. Direct Coombs test in the absence of haemolytic anaemia

[a] Criteria are cumulative and need not be present concurrently. Classify a patient as having SLE if he or she satisfies four of the clinical and immunological criteria, including at least one clinical criterion, *or* if he or she has biopsy-proven nephritis compatible with SLE in the presence of ANAs or anti-dsDNA antibodies.
ANA, antinuclear antibody; anti-dsDNA, anti-double-stranded DNA; ELISA, enzyme-linked immunosorbent assay.
Source: Adapted from Petri, M., Orbai, A.-M., Alarcón, G. S., Gordon, C., Merrill, J.T., Fortin, P.R., . . . Nived, O. Derivation and validation of the Systemic Lupus International Collaborating Clinics classification criteria for systemic lupus erythematosus. Arthritis Rheum 2012; 64:2677–87.

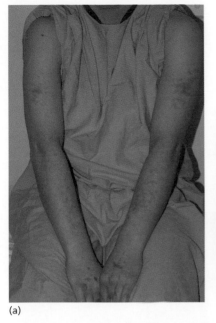

(a)

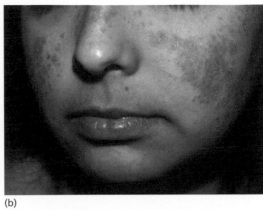

(b)

Figure 23.18 SLE showing acute cutaneous lupus of (a) the arms and (b) the face.

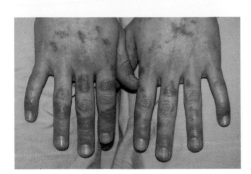

Figure 23.19 SLE showing discoid lesions on the hands characteristically sparring the interphalangeal joints.

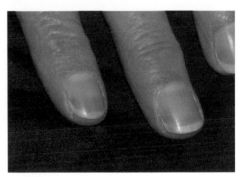

Figure 23.21 Blue nail discolouration as a result of antimalarial therapy.

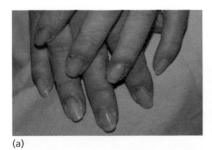

(a)

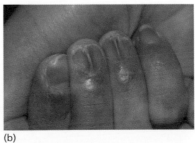

(b)

Figure 23.20 (a) Extensive nail fold necrosis and (b) nail ridging in SLE.

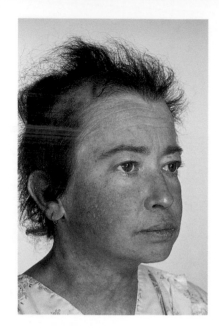

Figure 23.22 Unruly 'lupus hair' with diffuse alopecia.

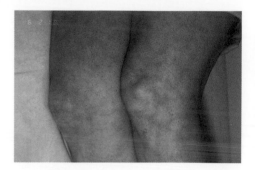

Figure 23.24 Extensive livedo reticularis in the setting of SLE.

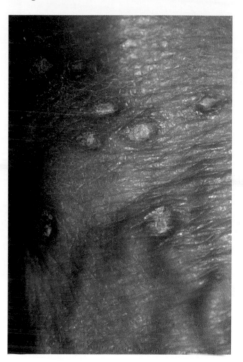

Figure 23.25 Degos like lesions in a patient with SLE.

Cryoglobulins occur in 25% of patients with SLE, type II or III cryoglobulinaemia, associated with palpable purpura of a small-vessel vasculitis, with ulceration and necrosis in severe cases. Calciphylaxis may also occur.

Papulonodular mucinosis, multiple, asymptomatic, flesh-coloured papules, usually on the trunk, arms or head and neck, from mucinous deposits in the dermis may be a presenting feature of LE (Figure 23.26).

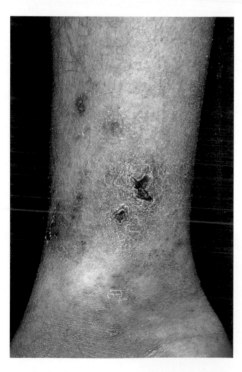

Figure 23.23 Necrotic crusted leg ulcers in SLE.

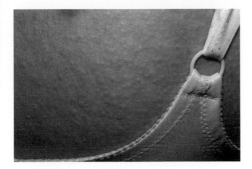

Figure 23.26 Multiple papules on the back due to mucinosis in SLE.

Pigmentary disturbances and hypopigmentation may result from both SCLE and DLE.

Bullous lesions

Blistering SLE can be divided into three categories:

1. Subepidermal bullae in SCLE and ACLE lesions.
2. SLE-associated autoimmune bullous disease.
3. Bullous SLE (BSLE), a distinct type of non-specific, autoantibody-mediated, cutaneous SLE that results in a subepidermal blister.

The diagnosis of BSLE requires the presence of (i) SLE, (ii) a vesiculobullous eruption arising but not limited to sun-exposed skin, (iii) histopathological subepidermal blisters and neutrophilic upper dermal infiltrates and (iv) immunoglobulin and complement deposition at the basement-membrane zone. The bullous lesions arise predominantly on normal or erythematous sun-exposed or flexural skin and can heal with milia (Figure 23.27). Blistering often parallels systemic flares of SLE, particularly affecting the kidneys.

Pemphigus erythematosus

Combines the immunological features of pemphigus and LE and presents with erythematous, scaly, hyperkeratotic or crusted lesions, sometimes adversely affected by the sun. See Chapter 22 for further details.

Oral and naso-pharyngeal ulcers are associated with increased disease activity (Figure 23.28), are usually nonpainful and commonly affect the hard palate.

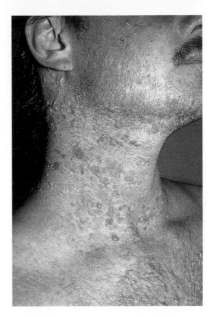

Figure 23.27 Bullous LE of the face and neck.

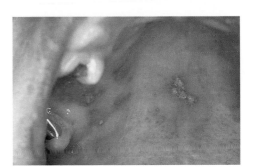

Figure 23.28 SLE involving the palate.

Differential diagnosis

Other connective tissue diseases such as rheumatoid arthritis, mixed connective tissue disease, undifferentiated connective tissue disease, Kikuchi–Fujimoto disease, acute viral syndromes (parvovirus, Epstein–Barr virus, infectious mononucleosis, HIV), Behçet disease, familial Mediterranean fever, amyopathic dermatomyositis and drug-induced lupus.

Involvement of the joints occurs at some time in approximately 90% of patients, arthralgia being more common than arthritis. It is usually rheumatoid-like and a severe form, Jacoud arthropathy, may occur.

Table 23.4 Circulating antibodies in SLE

Antibody	Frequency in SLE	Other features
Anti-DNA	Approx. 100%	Levels correlate with clinical activity
Anti-Smith	30%	Specific for SLE
Anti-RNP	23–40%	Black patients > white; missed connective tissue disease
Anti-Ro	30–40%	SCLE 60–90%; neonatal lupus
Anti-La	10–15%	Sjogren syndrome; neonatal lupus

Cardiovascular disease is one of the main prognostic predictors in SLE. Transient pleurisy is the most common pulmonary feature; acute pneumonitis may be a presenting manifestation of SLE. Renal changes are important in assessing prognosis and may result in end-stage renal failure.

The prevalence of neuropsychiatric disease varies from 37% to 95%. It includes cognitive dysfunction headache, mood disorders, cerebrovascular disease, seizures, polyneuropathy and psychosis. Peripheral sensorimotor and autonomic neuropathy occurs.

The most common ocular manifestation is dry eyes caused by secondary Sjögren syndrome. Retinal vasculopathy is the next most common manifestation and suggests active SLE and lupus cerebritis.

There is a higher risk of complicated pregnancies in SLE, regardless of whether or not SLE is active. Oestrogen-containing contraceptives should be avoided in lupus patients with positive anticardiolipin ± lupus anticoagulant.

Kikuchi–Fujimoto disease

A benign and usually self-limiting histiocytic necrotising lymphadenitis of unknown aetiology that has been found with autoimmune diseases including SLE. There is an increased risk of haematopoetic malignancy, particularly non-Hodgkin lymphoma, as well as an elevated risk of lung and hepatobiliary cancers.

Investigations

Skin biopsy is often necessary to confirm the diagnosis. Biopsy for DIF is unnecessary if the case is characteristic and may be false-positive if taken from photo-exposed skin.

Diagnosis is made using the SLICC (see Figure 23.3).

Testing for circulating antibodies is recommended (see Table 23.4).

Management

General measures include sun avoidance and smoking cessation. Because patients with SLE are advised to avoid UV radiation, it is important to monitor serum 25-hydroxy vitamin D.

Skin disease is managed as described for cutaneous forms of LE.

Antiphospholipid syndrome

(Syn. Hughes syndrome)

Antiphospholipid syndrome (APLS) is diagnosed in a patient with thrombosis and/or defined pregnancy morbidity in the presence of persistent antiphospholipid antibodies (APA). Primary APLS occurs in the absence of any other related disease. Secondary APLS is when the condition occurs in the context of other autoimmune diseases, such as SLE.

Epidemiology

One in four patients with a venous thromboembolism exhibit APA and one in 10 women with recurrent miscarriage are diagnosed with APLS. F > M; commonest in young to middle-aged adults.

APA can be detected in about one in five patients who have had a stroke at less than 50 years of age. About 40% of patients with SLE have APA but of them less than 40% will have thrombotic events.

Pathophysiology

Histologically, noninflammatory thrombosis of small dermal blood vessels can be demonstrated, but necrotising vasculitis is not a feature. Many mechanisms for thrombosis in APLS have been suggested. β2-glycoprotein-1 (apolipoprotein H) is a cofactor required for APA to bind to cardiolipin.

Clinical features

Patients have one or more clinical episodes of arterial, venous or small vessel thrombosis. Venous thrombosis in APLS is most commonly lower limb deep-vein thrombosis or pulmonary embolism. The most frequent site of arterial thrombosis in APLS is in the cerebral vasculature, resulting in transient cerebral ischaemia/stroke. Myocardial infarction is less common.

Pregnancy morbidities include unexplained death of a normal foetus after the 10th week of gestation and preterm birth of a normal foetus before the 34th week of gestation because of eclampsia or recognised features of placental insufficiency and unexplained consecutive spontaneous miscarriages.

Cutaneous lesions include thrombophlebitis, purpura and ecchymoses, livedo reticularis, leg ulcers, cutaneous necrosis, gangrene and subungual splinter haemorrhages.

In addition to thrombosis and pregnancy morbidity, thrombocytopenia, occult heart valve disease, chorea, cognitive impairment, haemolytic anaemia and nephropathy are potential complications of APLS. Transverse myelopathy occurs in SLE and may be more frequent in those with APLS.

The long-term prognosis is dictated by the risk and effects of recurrent thrombosis and any underlying autoimmune condition in those with secondary APLS. Those with primary APLS have a poor prognosis, with one-third having organ damage.

Differential diagnosis

Conditions presenting with thrombocytopenia and thrombosis include heparin-induced thrombocytopenia, thrombotic thrombocytopenic purpura and disseminated intravascular coagulation.

Investigations

A diagnosis of APS depends on patients having one or more clinical criteria (vascular thrombosis or pregnancy morbidity) together with laboratory evidence for the presence of antiphospholipid antibodies. The three tests used to identify antiphospholipid antibodies are (i) enzyme immunoassays for antibodies to cardiolipin, (ii) enzyme immunoassays for antibodies to β2-glycoprotein I and (iii) tests for lupus anticoagulant activity (usually dilute Russell viper venom time). All three blood investigations should be assayed in patients with suspected APS. The diagnosis relies on two abnormal tests spaced at least 12 weeks apart.

Management

Treatment and prevention of thrombosis is a major goal of therapy; this includes modifying lifestyle factors such as smoking, obesity and diabetes.
First line: Anticoagulation with heparin or warfarin in the nonpregnant patient. Heparin ± low-dose aspirin should be considered in the pregnant patient.

Neonatal lupus erythematosus

A well-recognised subtype of lupus erythematosus caused by the transplacental passage of maternal antibodies (see Chapter 63).

Dermatomyositis (DM) is an autoimmune disorder predominantly affecting skin and skeletal muscle. It is classified alongside polymyositis in the idiopathic inflammatory myopathies (IIMs).

Epidemiology

The IIMs are rare, annual incidence varying from 0.1 to 6.7 per 100 000 person-years. Higher incidence in African Americans than in white Americans.

Prevalence is 5.1–22 per 100 000. The relative proportion of DM within IIM appears to increase with increasing southerly latitude in Europe; UV radiation may influence the presentation and phenotype of DM. Peak incidence occurs around 50–60 years of age; much rarer in children. F > M - 2:1 in adults, 5:1 in children.

Pathophysiology

The histology of DM is often subtle. A lichenoid tissue reaction with vacuolar changes in the basal layer and occasional Civatte bodies is typical. Often only a sparse superficial perivascular infiltrate of lymphocytes with upper dermal oedema and mucinous change. The basement membrane may be thickened. In acute DM the changes resemble those of subacute lupus erythematosus, although the dermal oedema may be more extensive and involve all layers of the dermis. In poikilodermatous DM there is epidermal atrophy, dilatation of superficial vessels and melanin incontinence. Hyperkeratosis, acanthosis and mild papillomatosis are seen in Gottron papules.

Muscle contains cellular infiltrates of B cells and CD4+ cells predominantly in the perivascular and perifascicular areas. There is perifascicular atrophy; an early change is C5b-9 deposition on the capillary walls.

The majority of patients have disease-associated autoantibodies. These may be myositis-specific antibodies (MSAs), such as anti-Mi-2, anti-transcription intermediary factor 1γ (TIF-1γ), antimelanoma differentiation-associated gene (MDA)-5 and antismall ubiquitin-like modifier (SUMO)-activating enzyme, which are only found in myositis patients, or myositis-associated antibodies (MAAs), such as anti-52kD Ro, U1 ribonucleoprotein (RNP), PM-Scl and Ku, which also occur in myositis-overlap syndromes and in other diseases.

For two of the MSAs, MDA-5 and anti-Jo-1, antibody titres show some correlation with disease activity.

Clinical features

DM has a broad spectrum of cutaneous manifestations commonly involving the face, hands and extensor surfaces of the limbs. In the early phase most patients develop a facial dermatosis. One pattern is characterised by confluent erythema of the whole face, extending onto the neck and upper chest. Alternatively, a lupus erythematosus-like malar rash can occur with fixed erythema over the nose and cheeks (Figure 24.1). Some patients have a seborrhoeic dermatitis-like eruption, with involvement of the hairline, facial margins and naso-labial folds. Scalp involvement in DM is common and is characterised by erythema (sometimes poikiloderma) and a diffuse nonscarring hair loss. The facial eruption may be accompanied by slight scaling; scalp involvement may also be scaly.

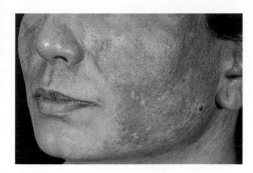

Figure 24.1 Facial erythema in DM is often widespread and can mimic many dermatoses, including lupus erythematosus.

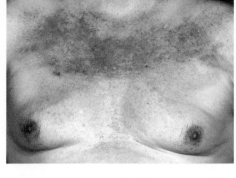

Figure 24.3 The upper chest is a common site of skin involvement in DM.

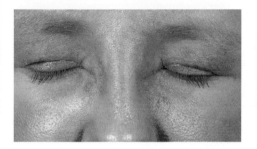

Figure 24.2 Eyelid involvement in DM. There is lilac erythema of the upper eyelids, which are also oedematous. In this patient with DM the facial skin is generally red.

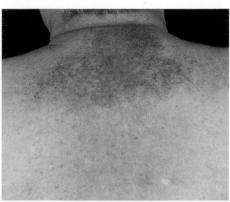

Figure 24.4 Erythema of the upper central back is known as the shawl sign.

Involvement of the upper eyelids is characteristic with an erythema that is lilac (or heliotrope) in colour often with oedema and involvement of perioribital skin (Figure 24.2). The presence of the eyelid dermatosis with oedema often reflects activity of the myositis. Fixed macular erythema commonly appears on the upper torso, both the V of the chest (Figure 24.3), and across the shoulders, where it is termed the 'shawl sign' (Figure 24.4). If untreated the rash of DM often becomes poikilodermatous, with a prominent telangiectatic component.

Nail fold changes consist of periungual erythema with visible dilated capillary loops in the proximal nail fold (Figure 24.5a). The periungual vessels are best appreciated when viewed with a dermatoscope. Small haemorrhagic infarcts are also sometimes seen within the hyperaemic nail folds. Hypertrophic cuticles,

which are dystrophic (ragged), are typical (Figure 24.5b). The nail fold changes in DM are indistinguishable from those seen in other connective tissue diseases.

Gottron papules are inflammatory, flat-topped, lichenoid, red or lilac lesions that occur on the skin overlying the distal and proximal interphalangeal and metacarpophalangeal joints (Figure 24.6). Similar larger lesions may develop over the elbows and knees. Linear red streaks may occur on the skin overlying the extensor tendons (Figure 24.7). Hand oedema may complicate acute disease. The rash of DM preferentially affects the extensor surfaces and is characterised by zones of livid erythema with mild scaling. The buttocks are often involved; erythema over the

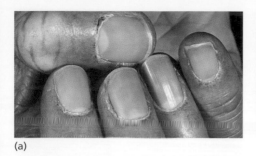
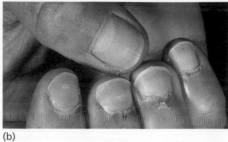

(a)   (b)

Figure 24.5 The nail folds and cuticles are usually affected in DM. (a) Dilated nail fold capillary loops are visible. (b) The cuticles are hypertrophic and ragged. There are infarcts within the cuticles.

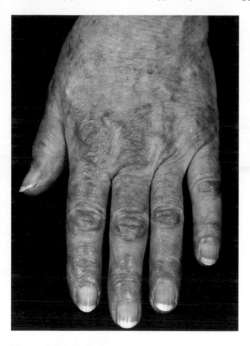

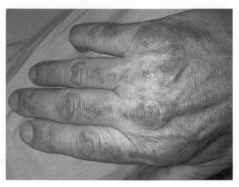

Figure 24.7 There are streaks of erythema on the dorsal aspects of the fingers, extending onto the backs of the hands.

Figure 24.6 Gottron papules: violaceous, flat topped, shiny papules on the skin overlying the interphalangeal joints and metacarpophalangeal joints.

hips and lateral thighs has been termed the 'holster sign' (Figure 24.8). In extremely active disease, lesional skin may become eroded. Distinctive vasculopathic ulcers, which tend to be punched-out and surrounded by a zone of dusky erythema, may occur on the fingers, dorsal aspect of the hands and extensor surfaces of the elbows and knees (Figure 24.9). Vasculopathic ulcers are particularly associated with the presence of anti-MDA-5 antibody.

Flagellate erythema is a striking cutaneous sign that is strongly associated with a diagnosis of DM although it is also seen as a side effect of bleomycin and as a toxicity manifestation of the ingestion of Shitake mushrooms. It is characterised by multiple, red, macular streaks occurring on the trunk and proximal limbs. The eruption may be sore or pruritic. Erythema on the torso can become confluent and extensive (Figure 24.10).

Calcinosis cutis (cutaneous calcinosis) is a complication in which insoluble calcified material is deposited in the skin and subcutaneous tissue. Calcinosis occurs in around 10% of adult DM patients and is more common in patients with longer periods of sustained disease activity, digital ulceration and antinuclear matrix protein 2 (anti-NXP2) antibodies.

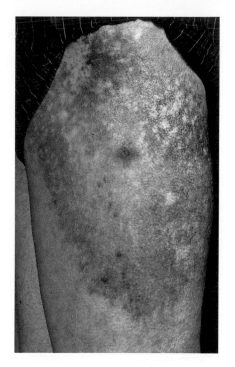

Figure 24.8 The dermatosis of DM can affect the gluteal skin and proximal thighs. Involvement of the skin overlying the hips is known as the holster sign.

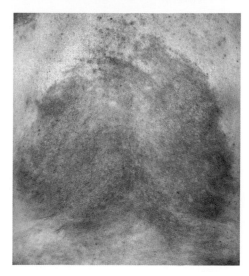

Figure 24.10 Flagellate and confluent erythema on the torso in severe DM.

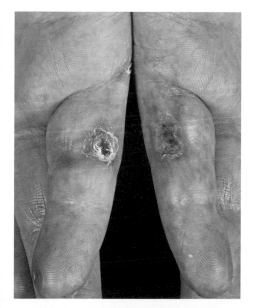

Figure 24.9 Vasculopathic ulcers on the fingers.

Muscle disease usually becomes clinically apparent after the onset of skin signs. The initial symptoms of myositis are proximal muscle weakness and fatigue. Patients have difficulty in climbing stairs, raising their arms and standing from a sitting position. There may be myalgia but muscle tenderness is relatively rare.

Respiratory compromise in DM may be caused by interstitial lung disease (ILD), respiratory muscle weakness or aspiration in patients with dysphagia or immunosuppression. ILD is found in 20–40% of IIM. The majority of ILD is nonspecific interstitial pneumonitis. The oropharynx and the upper oesophageal sphincter are frequently affected, causing dysphagia, which is associated with a poor prognosis. Cardiac abnormalities such as minor rhythm disturbances can frequently be found.

Reynaud phenomenon is particularly associated with the antisynthetase syndrome and mixed connective tissue disease, but is rare in children. A symmetrical, nondeforming arthritis may develop, usually affecting the small joints of the hands, wrists and ankles.

Internal malignancy and adult DM
There is a strong association between internal malignancy and adult DM. Approximately a third of adult DM patients have an associated

malignancy, with a standard incident ratio of 3 compared to the general population. Unlike adult DM, juvenile DM is not associated with an increased risk of malignancy.

The risk of malignancy rises with increasing age, severe skin disease with necrosis, dysphagia, diaphragmatic weakness, lack of extramuscular systemic features and antibodies to anti-transcription intermediary factor 1γ (anti-TIF1γ) or NXP-2. Malignancies may be identified in patients before, at, or after the onset of DM. The risk of cancer is greatest in the first few years after the diagnosis of DM, but there remains an increased, albeit lower, risk more than 5 years after diagnosis.

Tumours of many types have been associated with DM, although the majority are adenocarcinomas of the breast and ovary in women; lung cancer is the leading malignancy both overall and in men. In the Far East naso-pharyngeal carcinoma is commonest.

Antisynthetase syndrome

Occurs in the presence of antisynthetase antibodies, most commonly anti-histidyl tRNA synthetase (anti-Jo-1) antibody, which is found in 10–20% of DM cases. It is characterised by myositis, arthritis, Raynaud phenomenon, ILD, fever and 'mechanic's hands' (Figure 24.11).

Juvenile dermatomyositis (JDM)

May be superficially considered as DM presenting in childhood. There are a few subtle but important distinctions. Unlike adult DM there is not an increased risk of malignancy. Calcinosis, which is relatively rare in adults, is found in 6–50% of JDM; this is associated with increased disease activity. Acquired lipodystrophy is a relatively common finding, occurring in 10%. It is associated with insulin-resistant type 2 diabetes and acanthosis nigricans. It may be general, partial or focal. In focal disease there may be an associated panniculitis. Antibody frequency and phenotype association differ somewhat between adult DM and JDM. Anti-Jo-1 occurs in around 20% of adult myositis cases but occurs in very few JDM patients.

Clinically amyopathic DM (CADM; DM sine myositis)

Characterised by the presence of cutaneous manifestations of DM in the absence of clinical signs of muscle involvement. Despite the lack of myositis, patients with CADM appear to be at risk for developing cancer and ILD. Consequently, it is important to make a thorough assessment for ILD in patients with amyopathic disease.

Drug-induced DM

Hydroxycarbamide is the commonest cause and is not associated with myositis, whereas myositis occurs in 80% of nonhydroxycarbamide cases. Most reports occur in patients who have received hydroxycarbamide for many years, the commonest indication being

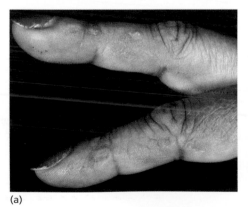

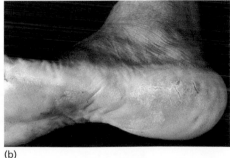

(a) (b)

Figure 24.11 Noninflammatory hyperkeratosis occurring on (a) the fingers and (b) the feet may be seen in Jo-1-positive DM. Involvement of the radial surfaces of the fingers resembles the callosities seen in manual workers, so-called mechanic's hands.

myeloproliferative disorders such as polycythemia vera. Hydroxycarbamide-induced DM usually improves within 12 months of drug discontinuation.

Differential diagnosis

The skin signs in DM can mimic a number of other dermatoses. When myositis is prominent the diagnosis of DM is usually straightforward. However, in CADM a number of differential diagnoses should be considered: lupus erythematosus, seborrheic dermatitis, rosacea, allergic contact dermatitis, psoriasis, lichen planus, lichenoid drug eruption and cutaneous T-cell lymphoma.

Investigations

For baseline investigations see Box 24.1.

MAAs can support the diagnosis, not confirm it. Anti-52kD Ro antibodies are the commonest MAA, found in 20% of IIM cases, and may be found in conjunction with other myositis antibodies, particularly anti-Jo-1. Anti-Ku, anti-U1-RNP, U3-RNP and PM-Scl antibodies may occur in myositis, usually in the context of overlap syndromes with sclerodermatous features.

MSAs are specific for myositis and help define phenotype. The antisynthetase antibodies are the commonest, occurring in approximately 20% of IIM patients, with anti-Jo-1 being by far the commonest and the other seven antisynthetase antibodies accounting for only a small percentage of cases. Antisynthetase antibodies are extremely rare in JDM.

In the anti-MDA-5-positive patients (commoner in the Far East) there is a high incidence of clinically amyopathic disease (50%) and ILD (67%). Anti-TIF-1γ antibodies are specific to DM and are found in around 15–20% of cases.

> ### Box 24.1 Baseline investigations in suspected DM
>
> - Full biochemical profile
> - Full blood count
> - Muscle enzymes (may be normal in amyopathic DM)
> - ANA, ENA, dsDNA, lupus anticoagulant, complement levels, anticardiolipin antibodies and β_2-glycoprotein 1 antibodies to exclude lupus which may include an inflammatory myosistis

They are associated with severe skin disease and a high incidence of cancer. As such, these patients should have a thorough screen for malignancy.

Anti-NXP2 antibodies are frequent in JDM (11–23%), where they are associated with calcinosis. In JDM, patients with anti-NXP2 appear to have a more severe disease course and worse functional status. Anti-NXP2 antibodies are rare in adults.

Anti-Mi-2 antibodies are specific to DM and are found in around 10–20% of cases. Patients with this antibody generally have classic cutaneous features of DM. Muscle disease tends to be mild and ILD rare in patients with anti-Mi-2 antibodies.

Anti-SUMO-activating enzyme antibodies occur in approximately 8% of adult DM patients.

Investigation of myositis includes electromyography. Magnetic resonance imaging of the proximal muscles may show oedema suggestive of muscle inflammation, muscle biopsy only required if the rash isn't typical of DM. Muscle biopsies should be assessed in an experienced specialist laboratory where immunohistochemistry can be performed on frozen muscle tissue.

Plain radiography is an effective method of detecting and monitoring calcinosis.

ILD is a major cause of mortality in DM and should be actively screened for. Lung function tests should be performed at presentation.

In view of the increased risk of an underlying tumour in DM, screening for malignancy is necessary. There is no agreed protocol on the set of investigations needed. CT scans of the neck, thorax, abdomen and pelvis should be performed on all adult patients. Further investigations should be organised as indicated following a full clinical assessment.

Higher rates of malignancy are found in the elderly and those with severe skin disease, dysphagia, diaphragmatic weakness and anti-TIF1γ and NXP-2 antibodies. If there is a high index of suspicion for an underlying malignancy a positron emission tomography scan should be performed.

Management

Multidisciplinary care is required including dermatology, rheumatology and respiratory.

IIM has a 10-year survival of up to 90%, with slightly higher mortality in DM than polymyositis. The main causes of death are cardiac disease, respiratory disease and malignancy.

For skin-limited disease: Potent topical corticosteroid ointment or topical tacrolimus 0.1% ointment *plus* hydroxychloroquine (± mepacrine)

First line: Pulsed IV methylprednisolone followed by oral prednisolone or a disease-modifying antirheumatic drug such as methotrexate, azathioprine, ciclopsorin and cyclophosphamide.

Second line: Mycophenolate mofetil *or* oral tacrolimus.

Third line: Rituximab.

Sclerosis and morphoea 25

Systemic sclerosis

(Syn. Scleroderma)
A multisystem autoimmune disease that causes fibrosis in the skin and internal organs with associated vascular and inflammatory manifestations, including Raynaud phenomenon. Systemic sclerosis (SSc) is rare but important because it has the highest case-specific mortality of any autoimmune rheumatic disease. It is divided into limited and diffuse disease.

Epidemiology
Prevalence in Europe approximately 1 in 10 000. Mean age of onset 50–55 years, rare in children. F:M = 4:1. The highest risk factor for developing SSc is having a sibling or first-degree relative with the disease (13–15-fold increased risk).

Those presenting >60 years of age more frequently develop the limited subtype, pulmonary hypertension and cardiovascular disease. Males are more likely to have diffuse disease and interstitial lung disease and have a higher mortality. Childhood onset is most likely to have limited or overlap forms of the disease and a better overall survival.

Associated with other autoimmune diseases in one-fifth of patients, particularly Sjögren syndrome, autoimmune thyroiditis and primary biliary cholangitis. Systemic sclerosis can occur as a component of an overlap connective tissue disorder such as mixed connective tissue disease.

Associated with malignancy in up to 10% of patients (M > F); increased risk of lung cancer, non-Hodgkin lymphoma and haematopoietic cancers.

Pathophysiology
Genetic factors that have been identified comprise a strong human leukocyte antigen (HLA) association, particularly with DRB1 and DQB1 haplotypes, and also altered immune inflammatory genes, especially within the innate immune system.

The pathology of SSc includes three major facets: vasculopathy, inflammation and fibrosis or scarring. Histological appearances depend upon the stage and subset of disease and on the affected organ. In the early stages of the disease both inflammation and fibrosis predominate; at later stages tissue atrophy, failed healing of ulcers and other pathologies may occur. The earliest pathological change in skin is microvascular injury with a reduction in capillary density and evidence of endothelial cell activation (Figure 25.1).

Clinical features
SSc is a clinical diagnosis and can be reliably defined using classification criteria (Table 25.1).

Typical presenting features are Raynaud phenomenon, symptoms of gastro-oesophageal reflux and swelling or discomfort in the extremities. This is followed by specific skin manifestations such as puffiness, tightness, hardening or itching. Cutaneous manifestations of SSc are demonstrated in Figure 25.2. Thickening or fibrosis occur mostly over the extremities and face in limited forms of SSc and much more extensively in diffuse cases. Telangiectasia and calcinosis tend to occur later in the disease, as do features of internal organ manifestations, including cardiorespiratory and more severe gastrointestinal tract involvement. Skin sclerosis leads to

Rook's Dermatology Handbook, First Edition. Edited by Christopher E. M. Griffiths, Tanya O. Bleiker, Daniel Creamer, John R. Ingram and Rosalind C. Simpson.
© 2022 John Wiley & Sons Ltd. Published 2022 by John Wiley & Sons Ltd.

PART 2: INFLAMMATORY DERMATOSES

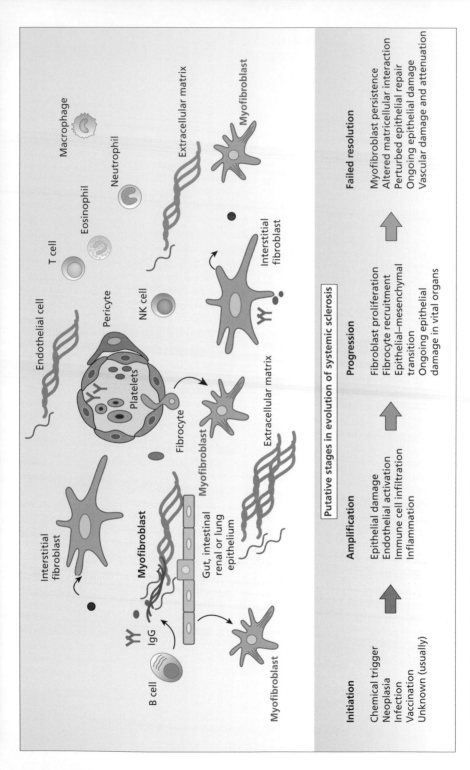

Figure 25.1 The cellular and molecular pathogenesis of SSc: the complex and pathogenesis of SSc that involves cells and mediators of the innate and adaptive immune system, vasculature and mesenchymal compartments as well as epithelial structures and more specialist organotypic cell types.

Table 25.1 Classification criteria for SSc

Item	Subitem	Score
Skin thickening of the fingers of both hands extending proximal to the MCP joints (sufficient criterion)		9
Skin thickening of the fingers (only count the highest score)	Puffy fingers	2
	Whole finger, distal to MCP	4
Fingertip lesions (only count the highest score)	Digital tip ulcers	2
	Pitting scars	3
Telangiectasia		2
Abnormal nail fold capillaries		2
Pulmonary arterial hypertension and/or interstitial lung disease		2
Raynaud phenomenon		3
Scleroderma-related antibodies (any of anticentromere, antitopoisomerase 1 (anti-Scl-70) or anti-RNA polymerase III)		3
Total score		
Add the maximum score in each category to calculate total score		
Patients having a total score of 9 or more are classified as having definite systemic sclerosis		

MCP, metacarpophalangeal.
Source: Adapted from Van den Hoogen F, Khanna D, Fransen J, et al. 2013 Classification criteria for systemic sclerosis: an American College of Rheumatology/European League Against Rheumatism collaborative initiative. Arthritis Rheum 2013; 65: 2737–47.

progressive loss of skin appendages, reduced hair growth, reduced sweating and joint contractures. Mask-like facies develop. Nasal 'beaking' and radial furrowing of perioral skin, reduced oral aperture and sclerosis of the frenulum may be present. The extent of skin sclerosis can be measured in a standardised and reproducible manner using the modified Rodnan skin score (MRSS).

Mat-like telangiectases on the face, upper trunk and limbs, and cutaneous calcinosis, most often on the fingers over joints and at pressure points, develop in the later stages, particularly in limited SSc.

Internal organ involvement is common and may be present at the time of presentation. Manifestations include the following:

- Gastrointestinal tract manifestations are almost universal, especially gastro-oesophageal reflux.
- Pulmonary manifestations: pulmonary fibrosis, pulmonary artery hypertension.
- Cardiac disease.

- Scleroderma renal crisis (SRC) is an important complication of SSc occurring in 5 10% of patients, usually within the first 5 years.
- Digital vascular disease is almost universal and, in addition to Raynaud phenomenon, structural vascular damage is associated with ischaemia and digital ulceration.
- Musculoskeletal manifestations:
  - Inflammatory muscle involvement plus contractual changes in the skin and tendons causes major functional limitations.
  - Myositis and arthritis occur in SSc overlap with systemic lupus or dermatomyositis.
  - Tendon friction rubs over the finger flexors and extensors, wrists, elbows, knees and ankle joints occur in approximately 10% of patients at presentation.
  - Muscle weakness is common (90% cases).

SSc can be classified into limited or diffuse subsets, based on the extent of skin involvement (Table 25.2).

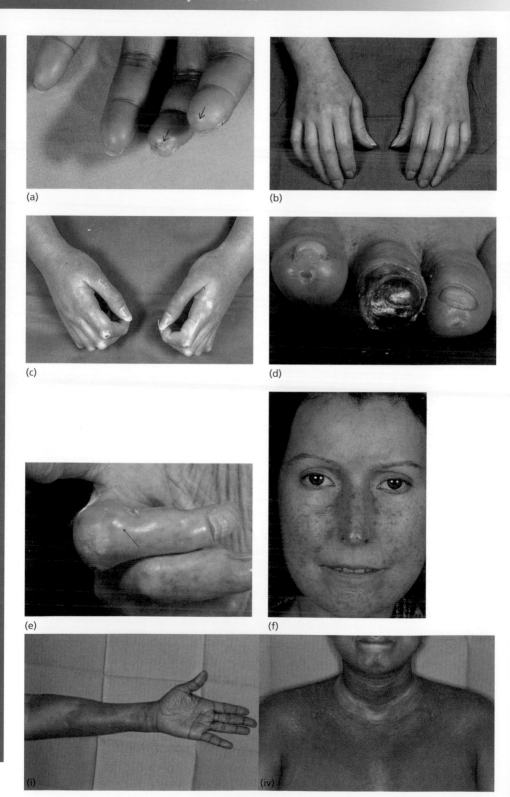

(a)

(b)

(c)

(d)

(e)

(f)

(i)

(iv)

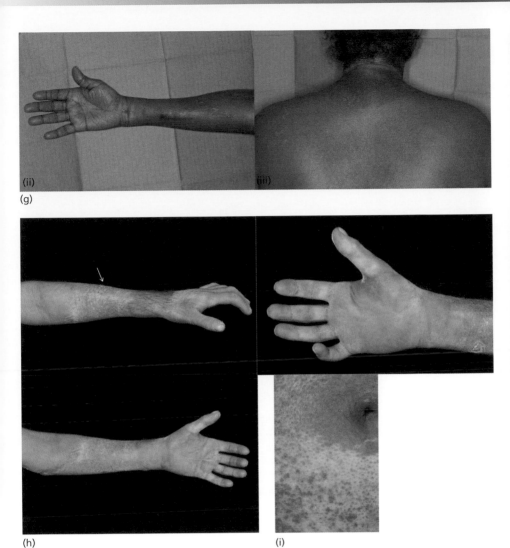

Figure 25.2 Cutaneous features of systemic sclerosis. (a) Raynaud phenomenon showing bluish discoloration of the fingertips (ring and middle fingers) with digital pitted scars (arrows). (b) Sclerodactyly and sclerosis extending proximal to the metacarpophalangeal joints. (c) Advanced-stage sclerodactyly with contractures and vasculopathic ulcers over the bony prominences. (d) Digital ulceration and necrosis. (e) Advanced disease showing severe flexion contractures and calcinosis (arrow). (f) Typical facial features: note the expressionless facies, mat-like telangiectases, microstomia, perioral furrowing and beak-like nose. (g) Sclerosis of the forearms (i), (ii), back (iii) and chest (iv) in early progressive antitopoisomerase (Scl-70) positive diffuse disease. (h) Severe sclerosis with contractures and cobblestone appearance (arrow). (i) The abdomen in a white patient with dSSc (diffuse disease) showing mixed hyper- and hypopigmentation.

Table 25.2 Typical features of limited and diffuse forms of SSc

Limited SSc	Diffuse SSc
ACA+ in 50% of cases	RNAP+ in 25% or ATA+ in 30% of cases
Skin sclerosis: extremities and face	Skin sclerosis: extends to proximal limbs, trunk and face
Long history of pre-existing Raynaud phenomenon	Short history or concomitant-onset Raynaud phenomenon
Slower onset and progression	Rapid onset and progression skin signs in first 6–18 months; skin disease may plateau and improve in years 2 and 3
Peak skin sclerosis score (MRSS) <14	Peak skin sclerosis score (MRSS) >14
Gastrointestinal disease (especially GORD) is universal	High-risk of organ-based complications
Isolated/primary PAH Lung fibrosis half as common as in dSSc	Lung fibrosis, secondary PH (especially in the ATA+ group)
Low-risk scleroderma renal crisis and cardiac disease	Scleroderma renal crisis (especially in the RNAP+ group)
Digital ulcers, calcinosis	Digital ulcers

ACA, anticentromere antibody; ATA, antitopoisomerase; dSSc, diffuse systemic sclerosis; GORD, gastro-oesophageal reflux disease; MRSS, modified Rodnan skin score; PAH, pulmonary arterial hypertension; PH, pulmonary hypertension due to left heart disease or lung disease/hypoxia; RNAP, anti-RNA polymerase.

Diffuse systemic sclerosis (dSSc)
Proximal extension above the knees or elbows or involvement of the anterior chest or abdominal skin then cases. These cases have a higher frequency generally of major internal organ disease, a greater overall mortality and a tendency to maximal activity of the disease within the first 3 years and then often greater stability and even improvement of the skin sclerosis.

Limited systemic sclerosis (LSSc)
Skin changes occur distally on the limbs, and on the head and neck.

Overlap features of another autoimmune rheumatic disease
These cases represent up to one-fifth of SSc patients and are important because the overlap manifestations need to be treated in the context of SSc.

Differential diagnosis
See Table 25.3 for the main differentials.

Investigations
The most important generic tests are ANA reactivity, nail fold capillaroscopy and investigations to exclude or confirm other autoimmune rheumatic diseases including arthritis or other forms of connective tissue disease (see Table 25.4 for autoantibody tests).

All patients should have these standard tests to identify internal involvement within the first 12 months of diagnosis and every 1–2 years in follow-up independently of subset.

- Routine assessment of biochemical and haematological laboratory tests.
- Electrocardiogram and echocardiography.
- Chest X-ray.
- Lung function tests (if abnormalities detected progress to high-resolution CT scanning).
- Annual echocardiography and lung function testing together with systematic symptom assessment is recommended.

Other tests may be indicated by clinical developments such as muscle weakness, arthritis or nutritional problems.

Management
Multidisciplinary management is essential (see Figure 25.3 and Boxes 25.1 and 25.2).

Table 25.3 Comparative features of generalised morphoea, eosinophilic fasciitis, scleredema, scleromyxoedema and nephrogenic systemic fibrosis

Feature	Generalised morphoea	Eosinophilic fasciitis	Scleredema	Scleromyxoedema	Nephrogenic systemic fibrosis
Hypercellular dermis (CD34+ fibrocytes)	No	No	No	Yes	Yes
Mucin	+	No	++	++++	++/+++
Depth of skin involvement	Into subcutis fascia and muscle	Fat and deep fascia	Into subcutis (fat replaced by collagen)	To mid-reticular dermis	Into panniculus (thickened septae)
Inflammation	Perivascular lymphocytic prominent early	Yes ± eosinophils	No	Perivascular upper dermis	No/less obvious
Typical site and clinical features	Can be generalised; spares hands, feet and nipples	Extremities (lower limbs especially); spares fingers and toes; typical 'groove sign'	Back, sides of neck, face; can be generalised; spares hands and feet	Face, neck, hands and forearms (waxy papules, leonine facies); normal hair growth	Extremities, trunk (brawny induration, burning sensation)
ANA	ANA±	ANA ± eosinophilia	No	ANA±	No
	SSc specific AA rare				
Other associations	Absent Raynaud phenomenon, normal nail fold capillaries	Polyclonal hypergammaglobulinaemia, immune morphoea, haematological cytopenias, malignancy	Diabetes, infection (especially streptococcal), paraprotein, IgG-κ, IgA, myeloma	Paraprotein IgG-λ	Renal failure, gadolinium exposure

AA, autoantibody; ANA, antinuclear antibody; Ig, immunoglobulin; SSc, systemic sclerosis.

Table 25.4 Autoantibodies in systemic sclerosis and their common clinical associations

Autoantibody	Target antigen	Frequency	Clinical features
Anti-topoisomerase (ATA, Scl-70)	Topoisomerase 1	30% dSSc 10% lSSc	Diffuse skin sclerosis > limited (60%/40%) Severe digital vasculopathy ILD and pulmonary fibrosis ±Severe cardiac disease Secondary PAH Highest overall mortality
Antiribonucleoprotein ARA, RNAP)	RNA polymerase III	25% dSSc 2% lSSc	Rapidly progressive diffuse skin sclerosis Hypertensive renal crisis Risk of isolated PAH Lower overall mortality
Anti-centromere (ACA)	CENP-B protein (centromere protein B)	50% lSSc 5–7% dSSc	Limited skin sclerosis Severe gastrointestinal disease
Anti-polymyositis-scleroderma (anti-PM-Scl)	PM-Scl-75 and -100	5% SSc 33% of patients with SSc/ myositis overlap	Limited or diffuse skin sclerosis Myositis Pulmonary fibrosis Arthritis
Anti-fibrillarin (U3-RNP)	Fibrillarin	5% SSc	Diffuse skin sclerosis > limited Isolated PAH, myositis and vasculopathy ±Cardiac disease
Anti-U1RNP	nRNP	15% SSc 44% SSc/SLE overlap	Limited skin sclerosis >> diffuse Overlap syndromes, arthritis
Th/To	Ribonucleoprotein	5% SSc	Limited skin sclerosis PAH and pulmonary fibrosis Poor prognosis

CTD, connective tissue disease; dSSc, diffuse SSc; DM, dermatomyositis; HLA, human leucocyte antigen; ILD, interstitial lung disease; lSSc, limited SSc; PAH, pulmonary arterial hypertension; PF, pulmonary fibrosis; PM, polymyositis; RNP, ribonucleoprotein; SSc, systemic sclerosis; SLE, systemic lupus erythematosus; SRC, scleroderma renal crisis.

In all cases of diffuse skin disease systemic immunosuppression should be considered and this should include either methotrexate or mycophenolate mofetil. For refractory or severe skin disease, cyclophosphamide may be considered.

It is important to minimise glucocorticoid exposure as it may be associated with risk of SRC. *Avoid systemic steroids in diffuse SSc as these can precipitate renal crisis.*

There is a large variation in disease course and prognosis. Reduced life expectancy by 16–34 years. The case-specific mortality is high. Pulmonary fibrosis, pulmonary hypertension and cardiac disease are the most common causes of disease-related death in SSc. Patients

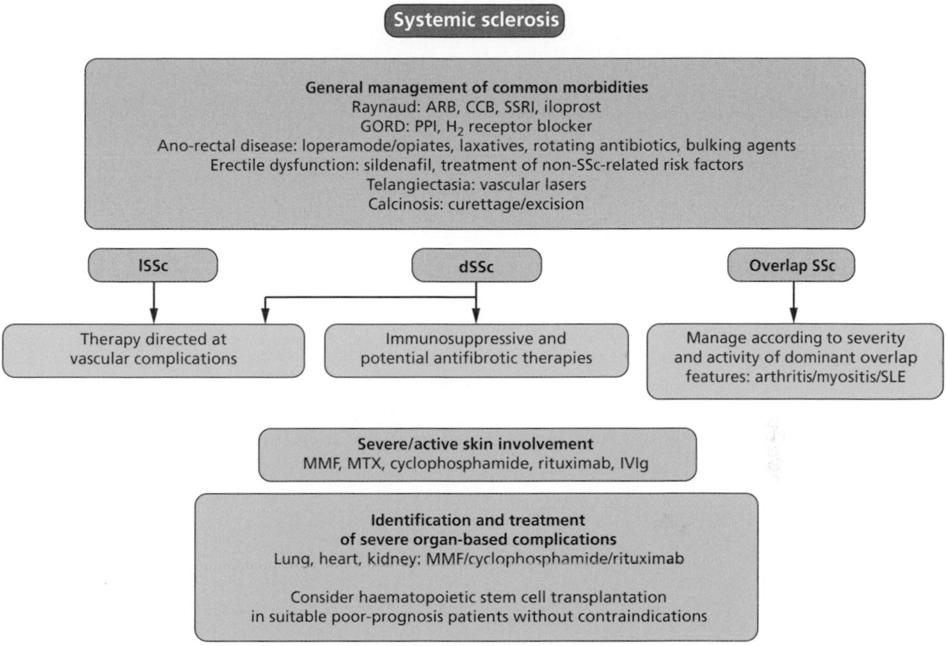

Figure 25.3 Management of systemic sclerosis. ARB, angiotensin receptor blocker; CCB, calcium channel blocker; dSSc, diffuse SSc; GORD, gastro-oesophageal reflux disease; IVIg, intravenous immunoglobulin; lSSc, limited SSc; MMF, mycophenolate; MTX, methotrexate; PPI, proton pump inhibitor; SLE, systemic lupus erythematosus; SSRI, selective serotonin reuptake inhibitor.

Box 25.1 Management of skin manifestations in systemic sclerosis

General
- Manual lymphatic drainage
- Physiotherapy

Topical
- Emollients
- Topical corticosteroids
- Calcineurin inhibitors (evidence in morphoea)
- Vitamin D analogues (evidence in morphoea)
- Phototherapy PUVA, UVA1 (in SSc)

Diffuse or progressive skin sclerosis
- Methotrexate
- Mycophebolate mofetil
- Azathioprine

Diffuse or progressive skin sclerosis *with* lung involvement
- IV cyclophosphamide

Systemic sclerosis with associated myositis
- Consider intravenous immunoglobulin

Management of digital vasculopathy in systemic sclerosis

Raynaud phenomenon
- Supportive measures: warm clothing, avoid cold, stop smoking and caffeine
- Topical GTN microemulsion
- Angiotensin receptor blockers
- Calcium channel blockers
- Iloprost

Critical digital ischaemia/digital ulceration
- Hydrocolloid occlusion, wound care, pain control, antibiotics
- PDE5 inhibitors (sildenafil)
- Endothelin receptor blocker (bosentan)

> **Box 25.2 Management of organ-based complications of SSc**
> - PAH: prostacyclin and prostacyclin analogues, endothelin receptor blockers and phosphodiesterase type 5 inhibitors
> - SRC requires early diagnosis; ACE inhibitors supplemented by other antihypertensives remain the cornerstone of management. May require dialysis.
> - Lung fibrosis needs to be carefully assessed because mild or stable disease may not require intensive treatment. Severe or progressive cases are usually treated with pulsed IV cyclophosphamide for at least 6 months
> - Inflammatory arthritis can be managed with TNF inhibition with infliximab or etanercept may improve

with the highest MRSS at baseline have a worse overall outcome.

Morphoea

(Syn. Localised scleroderma)

Localised form of systemic sclerosis comprising a group of conditions characterised by varying degrees of sclerosis, fibrosis and atrophy in the skin and subcutaneous tissues. Extracutaneous manifestations occur in up to 25% of cases but in contrast to SSc, no internal organ fibrosis or vascular changes occur.

Epidemiology

Rare, overall incidence of 4–27 per million per year. Prevalence of 0.05% at age 18 years and 0.22% at age 80 years. More common in white people.

Peak age of onset differs for the different clinical subtypes of disease. 75% of plaque disease occurs between 40 and 50 years, whereas 75% of linear disease occurs between 2 and 14 years. F:M = 7:1 in adults, 3:1 in children. Exception is adult pansclerotic morphoea, which appears to be more common in males. An association with HLA-DRB1*04:04 and HLA-B*37 has been demonstrated, particularly for the linear and generalised subtypes.

Plaque morphea is the commonest subtype (56% of cases), followed by linear (20%), generalised (13%) and deep (11%) subtypes.

Linear morphoea is the most frequent childhood subtype (65%).

Associated with increased prevalence of autoimmune disease, particularly in adults, and most commonly associated with generalised morphoea. Associated with both extragenital and genital lichen sclerosus, occurring in conjunction with plaque morphoea.

Also associated with breast cancer; occurs in 1/500 breast cancer patients, suggesting radiotherapy as a causative factor. Most cases develop within a year of completing radiotherapy and in most cases morphoea develops within the radiotherapy field.

A variety of drugs have been implicated in the development of morphoea-like lesions. The delay in onset ranges from 1 to 30 months and resolution on withdrawal, although reported, is not invariable.

Although the classic description of morphoea suggests no internal organ or systemic manifestations, small series in adults and children have found extracutaneous features in 21–27% of patients.

Pathophysiology

Aetiology is uncertain, but it is probably autoimmune disease due to reported autoantibody and autoimmune disease associations. ANA positivity is common.

It has been proposed that Th1 and Th17 cytokines are activated during the early inflammatory stages of morphoea, whereas Th2 cytokines correlate with later stages of damage and fibrosis. Endothelial cell swelling and apoptosis have been identified in early morphoea lesions. Direct immunofluorescence studies have shown immunoglobulin M (IgM) and C3 staining in the small blood vessels of the papillary dermis. Fibrosis is thought to result from a combination of increased collagen deposition by fibroblasts and reduced extracellular matrix turnover in morphoea.

All subtypes of morphoea share similar histopathological findings of an early active inflammatory phase, in which newer lesions demonstrate a lymphocytic infiltrate, with a variable number of plasma cells and eosinophils. As lesions evolve, the numbers of inflammatory cells are reduced as collagen bundles thicken and skin sclerosis increases in the later fibrotic phase. Histopathological changes are similar in all subtypes of morphoea, but vary in relation to the depth of involvement. In the sclerotic stage there are few recognisable fibroblasts and little inflammation. Collagen bundles are closely packed, highly eosinophilic and orientated horizontally. The dermal appendages and subcutaneous fat are progressively lost. Reduced numbers of eccrine glands are entrapped by collagen, and thus appear higher in the dermis. Fewer blood vessels are seen within the thickened hyalinised collagen.

Clinical features

Individual lesions generally begin with an erythematous, oedematous, inflammatory phase, which may be subtle and 'bruise-like' in appearance. The onset is often slow and insidious. This is followed by the development of central sclerosis associated with a change in skin colour and texture to thickened, waxy, yellowish white. There may be loss of hair and absent sweating. This central sclerotic area may be surrounded by an erythematous to violaceous so-called 'lilac

ring', widely thought to reflect ongoing active disease. Over months or years, lesions become atrophic and hyper- or hypopigmented. Depending on the depth and type of lesion, changes in the subcutis, muscle, fascia, bone and underlying brain may be present. Cutaneous features can be scored using the localised scleroderma cutaneous assessment tool.

Morphoea has a number of clinical variants which can be categorised into limited, generalised and linear.

Limited type
Limited plaque morphoea
This commonest form of morphoea presents with round to oval lesions >1 cm in diameter, in up to two of seven anatomical regions (head–neck, each limb, anterior trunk, posterior trunk) (Figures 25.4 and 25.5). Plaques are most frequently located on the trunk. The breasts are often involved, but the nipples and areolae are uniformly spared.

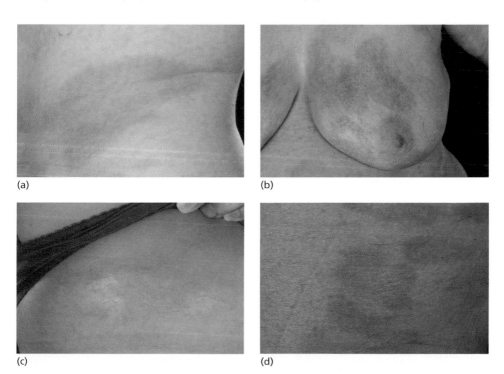

(a)   (b)

(c)   (d)

Figure 25.4 (a) and (b) Early, inflammatory, superficial plaque of morphoea with erythema and bruise-like appearance. (c) Sclerotic centre with inflammatory, peripheral lilac ring. (d) Hyperpigmented, atrophic late-stage disease.

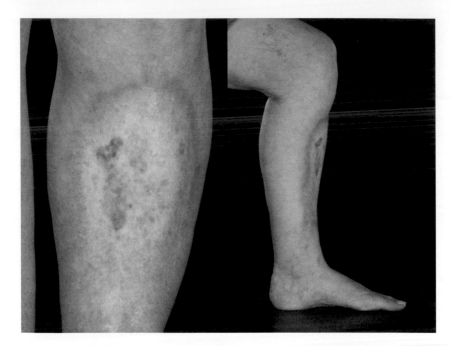

Figure 25.5 Plaque morphoea with deep involvement.

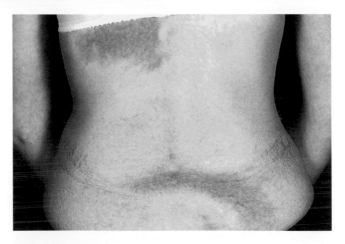

Figure 25.6 Atrophoderma of Pasini and Pierini. (Source: Courtesy of Dr D. A. Burns, Leicester Royal Infirmary, Leicester, UK.)

Guttate morphoea

A rare variant in which multiple, small (<1 cm), erythematous or yellowish white, mildly indurated lesions develop, most frequently on the trunk. Lesions are superficial and may have a shiny, crinkled surface, clinically resembling extragenital lichen sclerosus.

Atrophoderma of Pasini–Pierini (Figure 25.6)

Probably a primarily superficial and atrophic variant of morphoea. A rare condition representing 0.1% of childhood morphoea cases that usually occurs in adolescence and young adult life. Symmetrically distributed truncal lesions are the most common but single lesions and zosteriform distributions are described. Lesions are nonindurated, blue-grey to brown, hyperpigmented and sharply demarcated depressed patches, with a 'cliff-drop' border.

Keloidal/nodular morphoea

. A rare subtype is characterised by the presence of keloid-like nodules in patients with previous or coexistent morphoea or, in a majority of cases, SSc (Figure 25.7).

Limited deep morphoea (Syn. Morphoea profunda)

Inflammation and sclerosis are found in the deep dermis, panniculus, fascia or muscle.

Generalised type
Disseminated plaque morphoea

Gradual development of multiple plaques of morphoea at several anatomical sites, some of which may coalesce. Most frequently located on the trunk, thighs and lumbosacral area in adults.

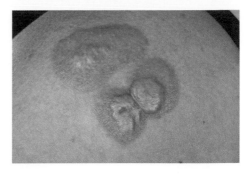

Figure 25.7 (a) Keloidal morphoea in a patient with limited cutaneous systemic sclerosis. (Source: Courtesy of Dr F. Deroide, Department of Histopathology, Royal Free London NHS Foundation Trust, UK.)

Pansclerotic morphoea

Very rare, characterised by extensive, often circumferential involvement of the majority of body surface areas with sparing of the fingers and toes (Figure 25.8). A widespread and severe progressive

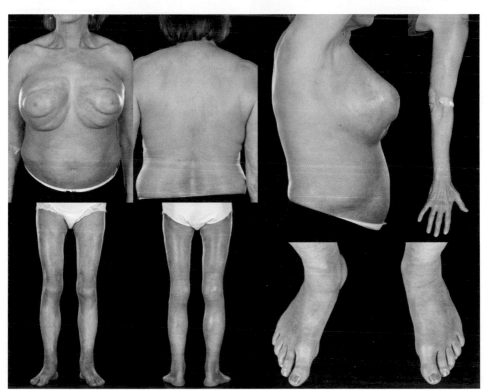

Figure 25.8 Pansclerotic morphoea in one patient showing circumferential involvement of the lower limbs and trunk with sparing of the areolae and hands.

PART 2: INFLAMMATORY DERMATOSES

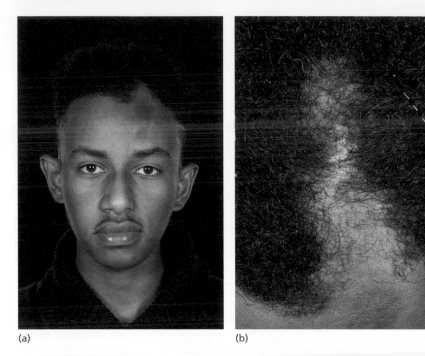

(a)   (b)

Figure 25.9 Linear morphoea en coup de sabre. (a) Hyperpigmention on the forehead with subcutaneous atrophy and a subtle indentation of bone. (b) Alopecia with sclerotic changes on the scalp.

disease occurring predominantly in children in which deep fibrosis progresses rapidly to involve muscle, fascia and underlying bone.

Eosinophilic fasciitis

Usually extensive and involves deep tissues. It symmetrically involves the extremities, particularly the lower limbs, sparing the fingers and face. In the early stages there is painful, burning erythema and pitting oedema of the limbs. This is replaced by induration and fibrosis resulting in a 'peau d'orange' appearance. It can result in severe joint contractures and associated morbidity.

Linear type
Morphoea en coup de sabre

Morphoea usually begins in childhood but occasional adult-onset cases are described. It most frequently involves the frontoparietal area of the face and scalp in a paramedian distribution and follows Blaschko's lines (Figure 25.9). Scarring alopecia of the eyelashes, eyebrows and scalp occur if they are involved in the band. Linear depressions in the skull bones are a common consequence. Neurological, ocular and auditory complications are well recognised.

Progressive hemifacial atrophy

A unilateral, progressive, primary atrophic disorder of the skin, subcutaneous tissue, muscle and underlying cartilage and bone (Figure 25.10). Altered pigmentation, usually a brownish or bruise-like change, but occasionally hypopigmentation, occurs at the affected sites. A progressive facial asymmetry develops as a result of a gradual loss of fat and muscle, and atrophy of the frontal, maxillary and/or mandibular bones. The mouth and nose become deviated towards the affected side. Enophthalmos is caused by a combination of progressive fat atrophy, shrinkage of the eyeball and thinning of the extraocular muscles.

Trunk/limb variants

Linear bands follow Blaschko's lines and may exhibit varying degrees of erythema, sclerosis, atrophy and hyperpigmentation. Coexistent or preceding plaque morphoea, most often on the trunk, is commonest in this form of linear disease.

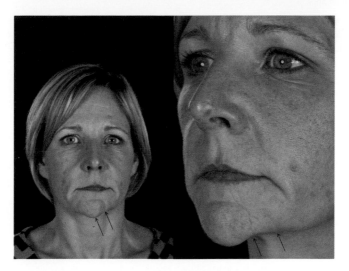

Figure 25.10 Progressive hemifacial atrophy involving the left side of the mandible and chin. Normal skin overlies atrophic deeper structures (arrows). Note the facial asymmetry. The patient had noticed progressive changes in facial contours for over 5 years before a diagnosis was reached.

Mainly unilateral. May result in flexion contractures. Myopathic changes, atrophy and weakness of involved and adjacent muscles may occur. Joint contractures, muscle atrophy and limb shortening cause pain and significant functional limitations.

Linear atrophoderma of Moulin
Unilateral, depressed, hyperpigmented Blaschkoid plaques on the trunk and limbs, with onset between 6 and 20 years of age.

Linear deep atrophic morphoea
Linear primary atrophic morphoea with no preceding clinical inflammation or sclerosis, involving the subcutis and deep dermis and resembling progressive hemifacial atrophy on a limb.

Mixed type
4% of adults and up to 23% of children have coexistence of more than one subtype of morphoea. The commonest combination is linear limb/trunk and plaque morphoea, but any combination can occur.

Extracutaneous manifestations
Overall, one-fifth to one-quarter of patients experience extracutaneous manifestations:

- *Oral and dental problems*: malocclusion (94%), an overgrowth tendency of the anterior lower third of the face (82%), abnormal mastication (69%), dental anomalies (63%), skeletal asymmetry (56%), bone involvement (50%) and temporomandibular joint involvement (19%).
- *Vascular complaints* (mainly Raynaud phenomenon, 31%).
- *Musculoskeletal*: arthralgia/arthritis (24%), myositis.
- *Respiratory*: dyspnoea (20%), mild gas transfer defects and restrictive changes in lung function.
- *Gastrointestinal complications*: asymptomatic oesophageal dysmotility, dysphagia (14%).
- *Cardiovascular*: electrocardiogram abnormalities, particularly incomplete right bundle branch block.
- *Neurological*: seizures and headache particularly in children with linear disease involving the head.
- *Ocular*: episcleritis, anterior uveitis and keratitis.
- *Psychological morbidity*.

Differential diagnosis
Limited morphoea:

- *Early inflammatory phase*: granuloma annulare, early extragenital lichen sclerosus,

erythema migrans, mycosis fungoides, cutaneous mastocytosis, radiation dermatitis, fixed drug eruption.
- *Sclerotic phase*: necrobiosis lipoidica, pretibial myxedema.
- *Hyperpigmented phase*: post-inflammatory hyperpigmentation, actinic lichen planus, café au lait macule.
- *Atrophic phase*: lipodystrophy, steroid-induced atrophy, lupus profundus, acrodermatitis chronica atrophicans, panniculitis (late stage).

Pansclerotic morphoea and eosinophilic fasciitis: systemic sclerosis, sclerodermoid graft-versus-host disease, scleredema, scleromyxoedema, porphyria cutanea tarda, primary systemic amyloidosis, nephrogenic systemic fibrosis, carcinoid syndrome, drug-induced morphoea and chemical and occupational causes of skin sclerosis.

Investigations

The diagnosis of morphoea is largely clinical, but a number of investigations can be helpful in guiding management.

- Clinical photography is important for monitoring purposes.
- Skin biopsy: deep incisional ellipse (to include fascia and muscle if deep involvement suspected).
- MRI (images brain and depth of extent on limbs), CT (images bony contours) for linear lesions.
- Routine blood investigations are usually normal in limited subtypes. In patients with generalised, deep or linear disease, it may be helpful to measure eosinophils, serum immunoglobulins, creatine kinase (if muscle involvement suspected), inflammatory markers (ESR/CRP), ANA and rheumatoid factor.

- If there is concern about the possibility of SSc (e.g. in cases of pansclerotic morphoea or eosinophilic fasciitis) evidence of Raynaud phenomenon, puffy fingers, sclerodactyly, nail fold capillaroscopic abnormalities, and SSc-specific antibodies (anticentromere, anti-topoisomerase and anti-RNA polymerase) should be requested.

Management

Multidisciplinary management as appropriate. See Figure 25.11 for management of morphoea.

Limited/superficial morphoea. *First line:* Tacrolimus ointment 0.1% (± occlusion); topical/intralesional corticosteroids.
Second line: Calcipotriol-betamethasone.
Third line: Phototherapy (UVA-1, broad-band UVA, narrow-band UVB).

Disseminated plaque disease. *First line:* UVA-1 phototherapy.
Second line: PUVA, Narrow-band UVB.

Pansclerotic, linear or deep disease or disease unresponsive to other treatments and with significant impact on quality of life. First line: Methotrexate (MTX) + IV corticosteroids or MTX + oral corticosteroids.
Second line: Mycophenolate mofetil.
Third line: Combination oral medication, e.g. MTX + mycophenolate mofetil, ciclosporin, abatacept, combination oral medication with phototherapy, extracorporeal photopheresis.

Mixed forms of disease are more likely to run a more protracted and complicated course; relapse following treatment is more frequent in generalised, deep and mixed forms. Transition from morphoea to SSc has been reported in 0.13–1.3%. Patients with SSc-specific antibodies should be kept under review, but in the absence of nail fold capillary abnormalities and sclerodactyly a transition to SSc is extremely unlikely.

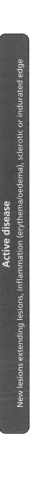

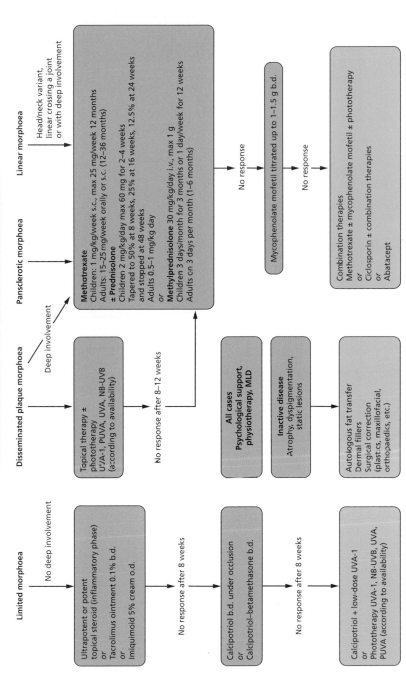

Figure 25.11 Therapeutic algorithm for morphoea based on existing evidence. b.d., twice a day; IV, intravenous; MLD, manual lymphatic drainage; NB, narrow band; o.d., once a day; PUVA, psoralen and UVA; s.c., subcutaneous; UV, ultraviolet.

Part 3
Metabolic and Nutritional Disorders Affecting the Skin

Cutaneous amyloidoses

26

The key feature of amyloidoses is the extracellular deposition of autologous proteins as morphologically characteristic amyloid fibrils. The amyloidoses may be localised to the skin or systemic and either primary in origin or secondary to systemic disease.

Epidemiology

Amyloidoses are rare in Europe and usually affect those of South-East Asian, Chinese and South American ethnic origin. The commonest cutaneous amyloidosis is primary localised cutaneous amyloidosis (PLCA), accounting for 85% of total cases. F > M = 2–3:1 for PLCA. Most PLCA is acquired rather than hereditary.

Pathophysiology

The principle pathogenesis is extracellular fibrillar protein aggregation. Once amyloid has aggregated, serum amyloid P component stabilises the aggregates together with other molecules like glycosaminoglycans and collagen fibres. See Table 26.1 for amyloid precursor details.

Clinical features

The clinical features of localiaed cutaneous amyloidoses and cutaneous amyloidoses due to systemic disease are summarised in Tables 26.1 and 26.2, respectively. Skin lesions include papules, nodules and plaques.

Typical features of systemic amyloidosis are petechiae or haemorrhages, often in the periorbital region (Figure 26.2a), mucocutancous infiltrates, especially macroglossia (Figure 26.2b), and sometimes nail dystrophy (Figure 26.2c).

Investigations

The most important diagnostic step is a lesional skin biopsy. Using Congo red stain, amyloid exhibits characteristic apple-green birefringence when viewed under polarised light.

Management

See Figure 26.3.

Rook's Dermatology Handbook, First Edition. Edited by Christopher E. M. Griffiths, Tanya O. Bleiker, Daniel Creamer,
John R. Ingram and Rosalind C. Simpson.

PART 3: METABOLIC AND NUTRITIONAL DISORDERS AFFECTING THE SKIN

Table 26.1 Localised cutaneous amyloidoses

Type of amyloidosis	Amyloid fibril precursor	Clinical features	Differential diagnosis
Acquired localised cutaneous amyloidosis			
Papular (lichenoid) PLCA = lichen amyloidosus (Figure 26.1a)	Predominantly cytokeratin 5	Soft or hyperkeratotic, partially confluent papules On lower leg, forearm, trunk	Lichen simplex chronicus, hypertrophic lichen planus
Macular PLCA (Figure 26.1b)	Predominantly cytokeratin 5	Vaguely demarcated, pigmented plaques; lesions often associated with areas of friction or excoriations	Atopic eczema, postinflammatory hyperpigmentation Lichen simplex chronicus, fixed drug eruption, atrophoderma of Pasini and Pierini, morphoea
Nodular (tumefactive) PLCA (Figure 26.1c)	Immunoglobulin light chains	Solitary or multiple, waxy nodules with atrophic epidermis and/or telangiectasia On feet, nose, genitals	Naevus lipomatosus, cutaneous lymphomas
SLCA	Predominantly cytokeratin 5	Associated with skin tumours[a], discoid lupus erythematosus	Depends on clinical presentation (see associations)
Hereditary localised cutaneous amyloidosis			
Familial PLCA	apolipoprotein E4, cytokeratin	Papules (often tiny and dome-shaped), macules Distribution similar to that in papular or macular PLCA	See differentials under PLCA/macular amyloidosis

[a] Skin tumours: naevi, sweat gland tumours, pilomatrixomas, actinic keratoses and seborrhoeic keratoses, porokeratosis of Mibelli, Bowen disease, basal cell carcinoma and trichoepithelioma. PLCA, primary localised cutaneous amyloidosis; SLCA, secondary localised cutaneous amyloidosis.

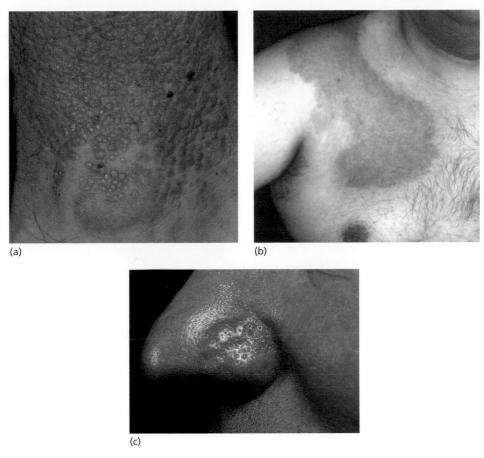

(a)

(b)

(c)

Figure 26.1 Acquired localised cutaneous amyloidosis. (a) Lichenoid primary localised cutaneous amyloidosis on the ankle of a male patient. (b) Macular cutaneous amyloidosis on the chest. (Source: (a) and (b) Schreml, S. Cutaneous amyloidoses. In Griffiths CEM, Barker J, Bleiker T, Chalmers R, Creamer D, eds. Rook's Textbook of Dermatology, 9th edn. Oxford: Wiley, 2016. Reproduced with permission from John Wiley & Sons. (c) Nodular (tumefactive) primary localised cutaneous amyloidosis on the side of the nose. (Source: Courtesy of St John's Institute of Dermatology, London, UK.)

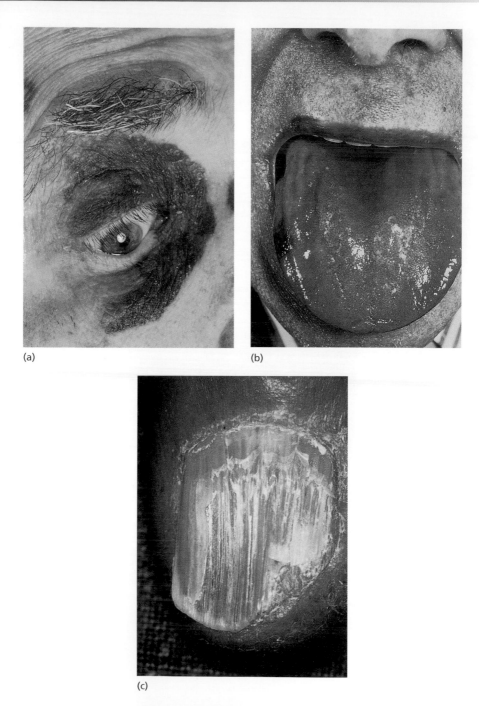

(a)

(b)

(c)

Figure 26.2 Cutaneous amyloidosis due to systemic disease. (a) Primary systemic amyloidosis with cutaneous involvement showing prominent periorbital bleeding following coughing. (b) Macroglossia in a patient with primary systemic amyloidosis. (c) Nail dystrophy in a patient with primary systemic amyloidosis. (Source: Courtesy of St John's Institute of Dermatology, London, UK.)

Table 26.2 Cutaneous amyloidoses due to systemic disease

Type of amyloidosis	Amyloid fibril precursor	Clinical features	Extracutaneous findings
Non-hereditary systemic amyloidoses with cutaneous involvement			
Primary systemic and myeloma- or plasmocytoma-associated amyloidosis	Immunoglobulin light chains (AL)	Petechiae, haemorrhages, nail dystrophy, waxy papules/nodules/plaques, tumid lesions, scleroderma-like infiltration, purpura, papules, nodules, bullous lesions, alopecia, cutis laxa	Macroglossia (Figure 26.2b), nephropathy, cardiomyopathy, neuropathy, intestinal involvement, CTS
Secondary systemic amyloidosis associated with inflammation/tumour	Serum amyloid A	Minor cutaneous involvement, sometimes petechiae, purpura and alopecia	Nephropathy, hepatosplenomegaly, gastrointestinal disorders (bleeding, motility disorders)
Secondary haemodialysis-associated systemic amyloidosis	β₂-microglobulin	Soft plaques	CTS, bone cysts, destructive arthropathy
Hereditary systemic amyloidoses with cutaneous involvement			
Hereditary transthyretin amyloidosis/familial amyloid polyneuropathy	Transthyretin	Atrophic scars, nonhealing ulcers, petechiae	Peripheral and autonomic neuropathy, CTS, cardiomyopathy, nephropathy
Hereditary ApoA1 amyloidosis	Apolipoprotein A1	Maculopapular lesions, petechiae	Cardiomyopathy
Hereditary cystatin C amyloidosis	Cystatin C	Clinically asymptomatic, but positive histology	Multiple cerebral haemorrhages
Hereditary gelsolin amyloidosis (Meretoja syndrome)	Gelsolin	Cutis laxa, pruritus, petechiae, ecchymoses, hypotrichosis, alopecia	Corneal dystrophy, neuropathy often with cranial nerve involvement, CTS, minor nephropathies
Hereditary systemic diseases with secondary cutaneous amyloidosis			
Muckle–Wells syndrome	Serum amyloid A	Cold sensitivity, pruritus, cold urticaria-like lesions	Fever, chills, arthralgia, leukocytosis, limb pain
TNF receptor 1 associated periodic fever syndrome	Serum amyloid A	Periorbital oedema, migrating cutaneous erythemas, conjunctivitis	Prolonged episodic fever periods, abdominal pain, myalgia

CTS, carpal tunnel syndrome; TNF, tumour necrosis factor.

PART 3: METABOLIC AND NUTRITIONAL DISORDERS AFFECTING THE SKIN

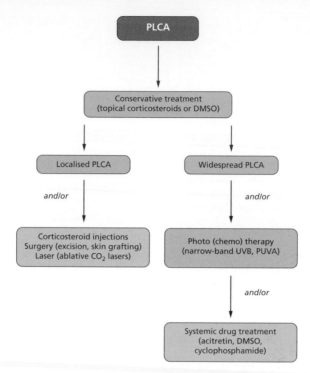

Figure 26.3 Treatment options for primary localised cutaneous amyloidosis (PLCA). DMSO, dimethyl sulfoxide; PUVA, psoralen and long-wave UVA radiation; UV, ultraviolet.

Cutaneous mucinoses 27

Cutaneous mucinoses are a heterogeneous group of disorders defined by increased mucin deposition in skin. Mucin is a jelly-like amorphous mixture of acid glycosaminoglycans that holds large quantities of water, hence excess mucin is characterised by cutaneous oedema.

Localised (pretibial) myxoedema

An infiltrative dermopathy due to mucin deposition, usually arising on the shins and typically associated with hyperthyroidism due to Graves disease.

Epidemiology
Present in 1–5% of patients with Graves disease and in up to 25% of patients who have associated exophthalmus. F > M, 3:1, with a peak incidence in the sixth decade of life.

Pathophysiology
Histopathology reveals hyperkeratosis with follicular plugging, acanthosis and sometimes papillomatosis. The reticular dermis, particularly the mid to lower part, shows separation of collagen bundles by large quantities of mucin.

Clinical features
Pretibial myxoedema is one of the signs of Graves disease and, uncommonly, may occur with no thyroid dysfunction. It is characterised by bilateral thickening and induration of the skin on the shins and dorsa of the feet. The four main clinical variants are shown in Figure 27.1. Other features of Graves disease include goitre, exophthalmos, thyroid acropathy and elevated thyroid-stimulating hormone levels.

Differential diagnosis
Lichen simplex chronicus, hypertrophic lichen planus, obesity-associated lymphoedematous mucinosis.

Investigations
Skin biopsy, thyroid-stimulating hormone level, thyroid stimulator antibody levels.

Management
Refer to endocrinology to treat any thyroid gland dysfunction. Compression stockings are beneficial, as well as the following options

Rook's Dermatology Handbook, First Edition. Edited by Christopher E. M. Griffiths, Tanya O. Bleiker, Daniel Creamer, John R. Ingram and Rosalind C. Simpson.
© 2022 John Wiley & Sons Ltd. Published 2022 by John Wiley & Sons Ltd.

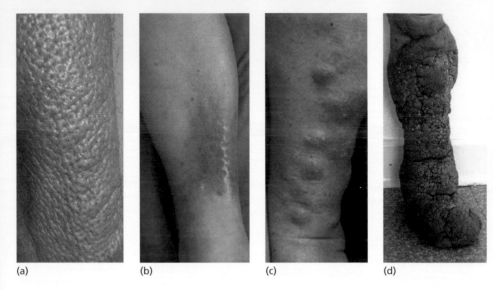

(a) (b) (c) (d)

Figure 27.1 Clinical variants of pretibial myxoedema. (a) Diffuse non-pitting oedema, with orange peel appearance (most common). (Source: Courtesy of S. Verma, MD, Vadodara, Gujarat, India.) (b) Plaque type. (c) Nodular. (d) Elephantiasis (least common). (Source: Courtesy of B. Cribier, MD, Strasbourg, France.)

(third-line therapies are usually reserved for the elephantiasic sub-type).

First line: Potent/super potent topical corticosteroid under occlusive dressing.

Second line: Intralesional corticosteroid.

Third line: Rituximab/plasmapheresis/intravenous immunoglobulin/octreotide.

Rare dermal mucinoses not associated with thyroid disease

See Table 27.1.

Table 27.1 Subtypes of rare dermal mucinoses

Condition ...	Lichen myxoedematosus		Reticular erythematous mucinosis	Scleredema	Papular and nodular mucinosis in connective tissue diseases
	Scleromyxoedema	Localised LM			
Pathophysiology	Histopathological triad of mucin deposition, fibroblast proliferation, fibrosis	Dermal mucin, variable fibroblast proliferation, minimal fibrosis	Interstitial deposits of mucin in the upper dermis, perivascular (and perifollicular) T-cell infiltrate	The dermis is three to four times thicker than normal Collagen fibres appear swollen and are separated by wide spaces	Mucin deposition through-out dermis and sometimes the subcutaneous fat
Epidemiology	Associated with monoclonal gammopathy	F > M for discrete papular LM subtype	F > M	Associated with diabetes, infection (streptococcal), haematological malignancy	Associated with or predates connective tissue disease, usually lupus erythematosus, rarely dermatomyositis/scleroderma
Clinical features	Widespread eruption of 2–3 mm, firm, waxy, closely spaced, dome-shaped papules of upper body and thighs (Figure 27.2a) May progress to affect other organs, including central nervous system	Small firm waxy papules confined to a few sites: (i) acral persistent papular mucinosis (Figure 27.2b), (ii) discrete papular lichen myxoedematosus, (iii) cutaneous mucinosis of infancy, (iv) nodular	Erythematous macules, indurated papules or plaques with a reticular configuration and lack of surface scale in the midline of the chest or back (Figure 27.2c)	Firm, non-pitting oedema and induration of upper body (Figure 27.2d) May cause restriction of movement	Skin-coloured papules, nodules and plaques on trunk and upper extremities (Figure 27.2e)
Differential diagnosis	Scleroderma (systemic sclerosis), scleredema	Granuloma annulare, lichen amyloidosus, lichen planus/lichenoid eruptions, eruptive collagenoma	Lupus erythematosus tumidus, seborrhoeic dermatitis, pityriasis versicolor	Myxoedema, amyloidosis, lymphoedema, cellulitis, dermatomyositis, trichinosis, oedema of cardiac or renal origin	Lupus erythematosus tumidus
Management	Intravenous immunoglobulin/thalidomide	Benign condition often managed conservatively	Antimalarials, topical/systemic corticosteroids	No effective treatment known Phototherapy generally first option	Therapy is the same as for the connective tissue disease

LM, lichen myxoedematosus.

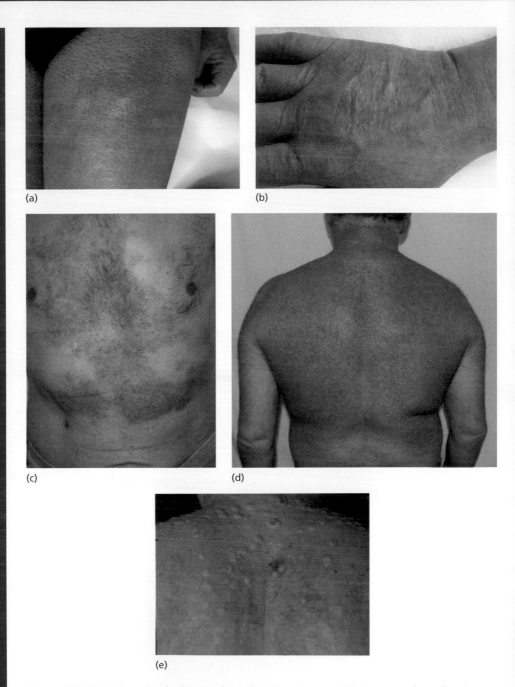

Figure 27.2 Clinical images of subtypes of rare dermal mucinoses. (a) Scleromyxoedema. Papules on the thigh. (b) Acral persistent papular mucinosis. Multiple skin-coloured papules on the dorsal aspect of the hand. (c) Reticular erythematous mucinosis in the midline of the chest and abdomen. (d) Scleredema in a diabetic patient with firm non-pitting oedema and induration on the upper back, neck and shoulders on erythematous background, with a peau d'orange appearance. (e) Papular and nodular mucinosis in connective tissue disease.

Porphyrias

28

The porphyrias are a group of disorders caused by defects in the biosynthesis of haem. Porphyrins have phototoxic properties and cause photosensitivity when they accumulate. In any porphyria, a partial enzyme deficiency causes the accumulation of porphyrins (Figure 28.1). The majority are inherited.

Porphyrias can be classified into those that cause acute attacks only, skin disease only, or both.

Cutaneous disease only:

- *Porphyria cutanea tarda (PCT)*: commonest porphyria.
- *Congenital erythropoietic porphyria (CEP)*: also known as Günther disease. Autosomal recessive severe and rare childhood porphyria causing lifelong mutilating photosensitivity and haematological disease.
- *Erythropoietic protoporphyria (EPP)*: an autosomal dominant hereditary porphyria characterised by painful, lifelong photosensitivity and occasionally liver disease.

Cutaneous disease and acute attacks:

- *Hereditary coproporphyria (HC)*: a rare inherited disease characterised by acute attacks that only involves the skin in a minority of patients.
- *Variegate porphyria (VP)*: a rare inherited disease usually characterised by photo-induced skin fragility.

Acute attacks only:
- *Acute intermittent porphyria (AIP)*: the commonest acute porphyria.

This chapter will only focus on the porphyrias that cause skin disease.

Pathophysiology: general
All cutaneous porphyrias are caused by violet light (Soret wavelength, 408 nm), which leads to a local porphyrin phototoxicity reaction.

Investigations: general
Biochemical analysis is the only way of reliably diagnosing the individual porphyrias. All specimens should be kept at room temperature or at 4°C in the dark and analysed within 48 h of collection to prevent spontaneous oxidation of porphyrinogens. For urine and faecal analysis, fresh random specimens are required. Table 28.1 summarises the main biochemical findings in the cutaneous porphyrias.

Histology from affected skin in all the cutaneous porphyrias shows homogeneous material within the vessel walls of the upper dermal and papillary vascular plexus. In bullous porphyrias and pseudoporphyria subepidermal bullae are seen. Direct immunofluorescence shows IgG in a vascular distribution and at the dermal–epidermal basement membrane zone.

Management
Apart from PCT, where effective specific treatments exist, skin management is based on preventing Soret wavelength light penetrating the epidermis (Table 28.2). Basic measures include sun avoidance behaviour, and sun-protective clothing and hats. Sunscreens containing reflectant particles, e.g. Dundee sunscreen, effectively protect against Soret wavelength light. Window films to absorb violet light are useful on car and home windows, and may be needed on theatre lights if the patient requires a surgical procedure.

Rook's Dermatology Handbook, First Edition. Edited by Christopher E. M. Griffiths, Tanya O. Bleiker, Daniel Creamer, John R. Ingram and Rosalind C. Simpson.
© 2022 John Wiley & Sons Ltd. Published 2022 by John Wiley & Sons Ltd.

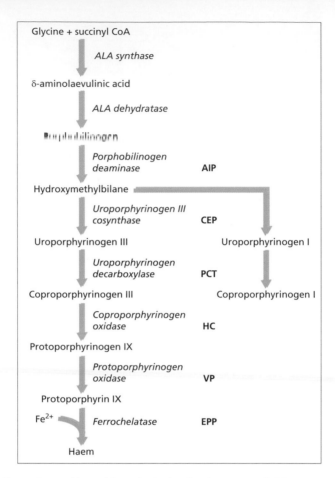

Figure 28.1 The pathway of haem biosynthesis showing the enzyme deficiency associated with each porphyria. Abbreviations of the disease names are defined in the text.

Table 28.1 Investigations for cutaneous porphyrias

	Urine	Faeces	Red cell	Plasma fluorimetry
Porphyria cutanea tarda	Uroporphyrin III, heptacarboxyporphyrin	Isocoproporphyrin, heptacarboxy-porphyrin	Normal	Peak at 615–620 nm
Variegate porphyria	Coproporphyrin III	Protoporphyrin, coproporphyrin III, X-porphyrin	Normal	Peak at 624–627 nm
Erythropoietic protoporphyria	Normal	Protoporphyrin (not diagnostically helpful)	Free protoporphyrin	Peak at 626–634 nm
Pseudoporphyria	Normal	Normal	Normal	Not applicable

Table 28.2 Management of cutaneous porphyrias

	Photoprotection	Medical treatment	Follow up	Genetic testing
PCT	Sun-protective clothing, including hats, reflectant sunscreen (e.g. Dundee formulation), window films, monitor for vitamin D deficiency	Chloroquine 125 or 250 mg twice weekly until biochemical remission (approx. 6–15 months) Venesection if ferritin high (stop when biochemical remission) Erythropoietin if renal failure	Long-term to monitor for relapse (by measuring urinary porphyrin excretion) and for the management of coexisting liver disease	No, detection of latent PCT does not alter outcomes
VP	As above	No specific medical therapy Avoid drugs that can induce attacks or cholestasis, avoid alcohol and cannabis	Long-term to monitor for development of hepatocellular carcinoma	Yes, to identify relatives with latent disease due to risk of acute attacks
EPP	As above, plus films on theatre lights if liver transplant required	Oral β-carotene (180 mg o.d. in adults, 90 mg o.d. in children) May require admission for opioid analgesia during acute attack	Annual liver function tests and red cell protoporphyrin Protoporphyric liver failure is rare but requires liver transplant	No, EPP is rarely life-threatening therefore antenatal diagnosis not required
Pseudoporphyria	Broad-spectrum UV protection required until sunbed-related disease resolves	Removal of cause is curative in drug and sunbed-induced pseudoporphyria Dialysis-related pseudoporphyria persists until renal transplantation	Nil	No

Porphyria cutanea tarda

PCT is the commonest porphyria. It is characterised by fragility and blistering of exposed skin.

Epidemiology

The prevalence is around 1 in 10 000.

Pathophysiology

Deficiency of uroporphyrinogen decarboxylase (UROD) causes accumulation of uroporphyrin and other highly carboxylated porphyrins. These cause a phototoxic reaction in the upper dermis in sun-exposed skin. There are two types: type I (acquired, 75%) and type II (autosomal dominant inherited, 25%). The latter has a low penetration genetic mutation and family history is positive in less than 7% of cases. Major risk factors are subclinical genetic haemochromatosis, hepatitis C infection, alcohol and oestrogens. They all predispose to the inhibition of UROD in the liver.

Clinical features

Acquired PCT usually presents in middle age; inherited PCT occurs at a younger age. Increased fragility of light-exposed skin with minor trauma, particularly the backs of the hands and forearms, is common (Figure 28.2). Bullae leave atrophic scars, milia and pigmentary changes. Other common features are scarring alopecia, hypertrichosis (Figure 28.3), usually on the upper face and forehead, melasma-like hyperpigmentation, or diffuse hyperpigmentation on light-exposed skin (Figure 28.4). Photo-induced onycholysis, accelerated solar elastosis and morphoea-like plaques may also be seen.

The homozygous form of familial PCT, hepato-erythropoietic porphyria causes a severe disease, with photosensitivity during infancy causing immediate pain on sun exposure, blisters on sun-exposed skin and mutilating scarring of the face and fingers. Life expectancy is normal.

Differential diagnosis

PCT can be clinically indistinguishable from other porphyrias that cause skin disease, pseudoporphyria and other blistering disorders (see Chapter 87).

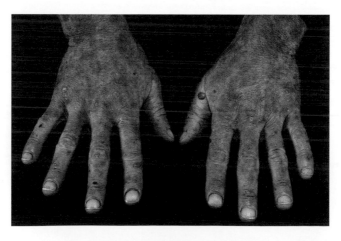

Figure 28.2 PCT: erosions, blisters, pigmentary changes and scarring.

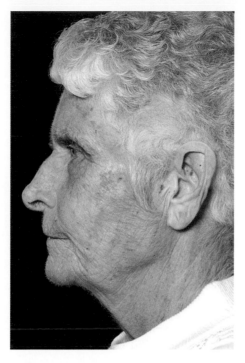

Figure 28.3 Hypertrichosis. (Source: Courtesy of Cardiff archives.)

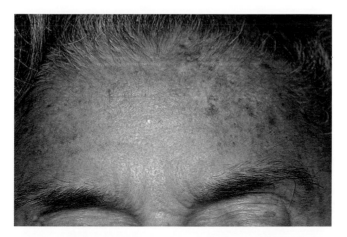

Figure 28.4 Pigmentation in light exposed skin. (Source: Courtesy of Cardiff archives.)

Investigations

See Table 28.1. It is essential to investigate for risk factors in all patients diagnosed with PCT.

Management

See Table 28.2. Definitive treatment with venesection or low-dose antimalarials is required in almost all cases. Venesection is first-line therapy if there is pathologically high serum ferritin, homozygous Cys282Tyr mutation or significant hepatitis C liver disease. Around 500 mL of blood is removed every 1–2 weeks, aiming to decrease transferrin saturation to 15%, haemoglobin to 11–12 g/dL and plasma ferritin to below 25 μg/L. Erythropoeitin is first-line for PCT in renal failure where patients are too anaemic for venesection and cannot excrete chloroquine.

Erythropoietic protoporphyria

EPP is characterised by painful, lifelong photosensitivity and occasionally liver disease.

Epidemiology

The incidence of EPP in Europe varies between countries (from 0.03 new cases/million per year in Spain to 0.36 in the UK).

Pathophysiology

EPP results from deficient activity of ferrochelatase, the final enzyme of haem biosynthesis. This causes accumulation of protoporphyrin in erythroid cells, which causes a phototoxic reaction as they pass through the small upper dermal blood vessels and are exposed to sunlight.

It is an autosomal dominant hereditary porphyria with incomplete penetrance.

Clinical features

EPP causes immediate pain on exposure to bright sunlight. It usually presents in the first year and affected babies cry when exposed to sunny weather. Onset in adulthood is rare. In spring and summer, after varying duration of sun exposure, patients describe discomfort, tingling or itching in exposed skin. If exposure continues, severe burning pain follows. Lack of physical signs often leads to delay in diagnosis. Psychosocial issues and social isolation occur as children cannot go outside in spring/summer months.

Usually the only physical sign during an attack is subtle oedema. Physical signs that may develop during childhood include slight thickening over the metacarpophalangeal and interphalangeal joints, superficial waxy scarring on the nose and shallow scars on the cheeks, forehead and lips (Figure 28.5). 15% have no physical signs.

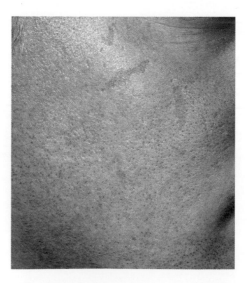

Figure 28.5 Typical scars on the cheeks in EPP.

Investigations

See Table 28.1. Additionally, gallstones occur in around 12% due to protoporphyrin excretion into bile. Protoporphyrin causes severe liver damage in 1% of patients. Vitamin D deficiency is common.

Management

See Table 28.2. For an acute reaction, complete sun avoidance leads to earlier resolution. For severe attacks, hospital admission may be necessary for light avoidance and opiate analgesia. Oral β-carotene is the most widely used specific treatment, although the evidence for its use is poor.

Variegate porphyria

VP causes photo-induced skin fragility and blistering, it may also cause acute attacks.

Epidemiology

VP is common in South Africa, with prevalence in whites and Afrikaner-descended non-whites of 1/200. At least 80% of South African carriers of a pathogenic VP mutation are completely asymptomatic.

The incidence in Europe is reported between 0.01 and 0.26 new cases/million/year. Elsewhere the prevalence is around 0.5–1/100 000.

Acute attacks are three times more common in women than men and occur between 20 and 40 years of age.

Pathophysiology

An autosomal dominant inherited deficiency of protoporphyrinogen oxidase leads to accumulation of copro- and protoporphyrinogen. These predominate in the skin to cause PCT-like upper dermal blistering. Skin disease may be exacerbated in pregnancy or females taking the oral contraceptive pill.

Clinical features

Approximately 70% have cutaneous involvement. Symptoms begin in adolescence or early adulthood with fragility of sun-exposed skin, particularly on the backs of the hands. However, a significant number of patients have their worst problems in late summer and autumn

rather than high summer. Acute photosensitivity can occur in patients with disturbed liver function. Skin signs show painful tense bullae, scarring, pigmentary abnormalities, pseudosclerodermatous changes of the hands and fingers and occasionally photo-onycholysis.

Only around 17% of patients with cutaneous VP will ever suffer an acute attack. These range from mild abdominal pain, sometimes accompanied by vomiting and constipation, through to very severe attacks with bulbar palsy and respiratory paralysis.

Differential diagnosis

VP is similar to PCT, late-onset CEP, HC and pseudoporphyria. Biochemical analysis is required to diagnose VP.

Investigations

See Table 28.1.

Management

See Table 28.2. Liver transplantation may be curative in cases where acute attacks are frequent, severe and uncontrollable by medical means. VP sometimes goes into remission in old age.

Pseudoporphyria

A non-porphyric dermatosis clinically and histologically indistinguishable from PCT.

Pathophysiology

The causes of pseudoporphyria are photosensitising drugs, haemodialysis for chonic renal failure and UVA sunbeds. The most common causes of pseudoporphyria are non-steroidal anti-inflammatory drugs.

Clinical features

Cutaneous features are indistinguishable from PCT. However, hypertrichosis, hyperpigmentation, sclerodermoid changes and dystrophic calcification are much less commonly seen than in PCT. In children, facial scarring can resemble that seen in EPP, although pseudoporphyria is painless. There are no internal manifestations of pseudoporphyria.

PART 3: METABOLIC AND NUTRITIONAL DISORDERS AFFECTING THE SKIN

Differential diagnosis

The main differential diagnoses are PCT and EPP where there is EPP-type scarring.

Other relevant blistering diseases such as epidermolysis bullosa acquisita and bullous pemphigoid may be considered (see Chapter 87).

Investigations

The diagnosis requires the presence of clinical features of PCT in the skin, with normal urine, faecal and plasma porphyrin concentrations (Table 28.1).

Diagnosis is more complex in patients in renal failure as haemodialysis is associated with increased plasma porphyrin concentrations. Conclusive differentiation of PCT from pseudoporphyria in the context of renal failure and dialysis is not always possible, but can sometimes be achieved on the basis of the degree of increase in porphyrin concentrations in plasma, faeces and (where available) urine.

Management

See Table 28.2.

Nutritional disorders affecting the skin

29

Malnutrition

Malnutrition is an imbalance between the intake of necessary nutrients and physiological needs that leads to derangements of normal physiological processes. Two phenotypic forms are recognised: *kwashiorkor* and *marasmus*. They typically affect infants and younger children who present with failure to thrive. The elderly, people with chronic illness, hospitalised individuals and people with AIDS can also be affected.

Kwashiorkor

Prolonged disproportionate intake of carbohydrate in excess of other macronutrients, specifically protein. Skin findings characteristically include a dermatosis (Figure 29.1) with scale and irregular fissuring (Figure 29.2). Hair and nails grow slowly and are brittle. Hair develops a lustreless, red-brown colour. Skin biopsies show psoriasiform hyperplasia, hyperkeratosis and epidermal pigmentation. Other clinical features are loss of subcutaneous fat, peripheral oedema and abdominal distention.

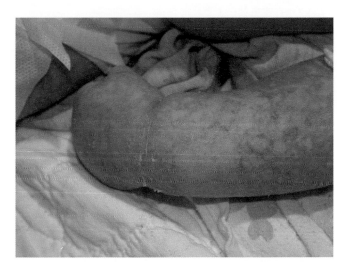

Figure 29.1 Kwashiorkor manifesting as peripheral oedema and a 'flaky paint' dermatitis.

Rook's Dermatology Handbook, First Edition. Edited by Christopher E. M. Griffiths, Tanya O. Bleiker, Daniel Creamer, John R. Ingram and Rosalind C. Simpson.

Marasmus

Globally decreased intake of all macronutrients, including carbohydrate, protein and fat. Loss of subcutaneous fat results in a prematurely aged appearance with dyspigmentation and desquamative changes. The abdomen may become distended, skin is typically wrinkled, loose and dry (Figure 29.3).

Differential diagnoses include atopic eczema, seborrhoeic dermatitis and acrodermatitis enteropathica/acquired zinc deficiency. Refeeding syndrome is a potentially fatal complication that can arise when a malnourished patient is given nutrients enterally or parenterally after a period of prolonged deprivation. During this phenomenon, acute electrolyte disturbances can occur, leading to hypophosphataemia, hypomagnesaemia and hypokalaemia. A multidisciplinary approach to management is required.

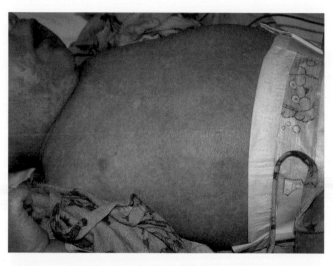

Figure 29.2 Erythrodermic findings in kwashiorkor. This patient was fed rice 'milk' as a primary food source due to parental concerns over presumed food allergies.

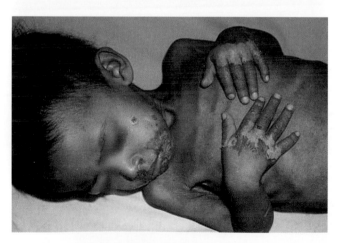

Figure 29.3 Marasmus. Note the loss of subcutaneous tissue, dyspigmentation and desquamative changes. (Source: From Irvine AD, Hoeger PH, Yan AC (eds) Harper's Textbook of Dermatology, 3rd edn, 2011. Oxford: Wiley Blackwell.)

Vitamin abnormalities

Table 29.1 summarises findings seen with specific vitamin deficiency or excess. Those without skin manifestations are not listed. See Box 29.1 for a summary of key cutaneous features associated with vitamin and mineral abnormalities.

B-complex vitamin abnormalities

B-complex vitamins are water soluble and deficiency of these is summarised in Table 29.2. See also Box 29.1.

Minerals

Diseases of mineral deficiency and excess are summarised in Table 29.3. For zinc deficiency (acrodermatitis enteropathica) see Chapter 64, for copper deficiency (Menkes disease) see Chapters 31 and 39. Management of all mineral abnormalities is by correcting the underlying cause, removing the source of excess or supplementing with the deficient mineral. See also Box 29.1.

Box 29.1 Key cutaneous features of vitamin and mineral abnormalities

Vitamin A deficiency:	Phrynoderma
Vitamin A excess:	Carotenaemia
Vitamin D deficiency:	Alopecia (acquired type), atrychia, facial/scalp papules (type II vitamin D-dependent rickets)
Vitamin E excess:	Easy bleeding/bruising
Vitamin K deficiency:	Easy bleeding/bruising
Vitamin C deficiency:	Hyperkeratotic hair follicles, corkscrew hairs, perifollicular haemorrhage and purpura, phyrnoderma
Vitamin B1 deficiency:	Red burning tongue
Vitamin B2 deficiency:	Acute: erythema, epidermal necrolysis and mucositis; chronic: angular stomatitis, cheilitis, glossitis
Vitamin B3 deficiency:	Photodistributed dermatitis, especially on hands
Vitamin B6 deficiency:	Seborrhoeic dermatitis-like eruption involving the face, scalp, neck, shoulders, buttocks and perineum
Vitamin B9 deficiency:	Glossitis, angular cheilitis, oral ulceration, perineal seborrhoeic dermatitis, hair depigmentation, mucocutaneous hyperpigmentation
Vitamin B12 deficiency:	Similar to vitamin B9 deficiency
Iron deficiency:	Koilonychia, glossodynia, aphthous stomatitis, angular stomatitis, brittle hair
Zinc deficiency:	Psoriasiform dermatitis hands/feet/knees
Selenium deficiency:	White nail beds, hypopigmentation of skin and hair, non-specific cutaneous findings
Selenium excess:	Brittle nails with white horizontal streaks, brittle hair, scalp exfoliative dermatitis, reddish hue to teeth, hair and nails

PART 3: METABOLIC AND NUTRITIONAL DISORDERS AFFECTING THE SKIN

Table 29.1 Findings seen with specific vitamin deficiency or excess

	Vitamin A (retinol) deficiency	Vitamin A excess (Syn. Hypervitaminosis A, vitamin A toxicity, carotenaemia, carotenoderma)	Vitamin D (calcitriol) deficiency (Syn. Hereditary vitamin D-dependent rickets type I and II)	Vitamin E (tocopherol or tocotrienol) excess	Vitamin K (phytonadione) deficiency (Syn. Vitamin K deficiency bleeding)	Vitamin C (ascorbic acid) deficiency (Syn. Scurvy)
Introduction	Fat-soluble; needed for keratinisation, epithelial proliferation, vision and development	Fat-soluble; needed for keratinisation, epithelial proliferation, vision and development	Fat-soluble; essential in the regulation of calcium and phosphorus metabolism	Fat-soluble; potent antioxidant	Fat-soluble; cofactor in the synthesis of coagulation factors II, VII, IX and X, proteins C and S	Water-soluble; antioxidant and cofactor for collagen biosynthesis, carnitine and catecholamine metabolism and dietary iron absorption
Epidemiology	Estimated 5.2 million preschool-aged children have night blindness	Potential association with increased risk of gastric and lung cancer	1 billion people worldwide; higher risk in newborns and institutionalised elderly	Rare	Neonatal VKDB incidence 6–12% within 24 h after birth and 0.25–1.5% within 7 days after birth	Prevalence 7.1% in the USA
Pathophysiology	Predisposed by poor dietary intake, malnutrition, fat malabsorption, chronic intestinal inflammation and liver disease	Increased dietary intake can cause toxicity, increased absorption in certain medical conditions, e.g. hypothyroidism, can lead to carotenaemia (a benign disorder)	Vitamin D deficiency leads to hypocalcaemia and consequently stimulation of parathyroid hormone secretion and release of calcium from bone	Usually arises due to oversupplementation; vitamin E has inherent antiplatelet effects	Neonates: poor transplacental transfer, lack of gastrointestinal flora to generate vitamin K, inadequate maternal dietary intake Adults: decreased dietary intake, malabsorption; liver disease and various medications cause vitamin K deficiency	Decreased intake (elderly, alcoholics, presumed food allergies) or increased requirements (smoking, certain medications) or losses (dialysis patients)

Clinical features	Night blindness, corneal xerosis, generalised xerosis, phrynoderma (keratotic papules with intrafollicular plugging on extensor surfaces) (Figure 29.4)	Carotenaemia: yellow discoloration of the skin (mucous membranes spared) (Figure 29.5) Toxicity: headaches, vision changes, fatigue, anorexia, nausea, vomiting, myalgia/arthralgia	Acquired vitamin D deficiency: alopecia Type II vitamin D-dependent rickets: generalised atrychia; papules on face and scalp Both types have various skeletal defects	Easy bruising or bleeding	Easy bruising or bleeding, particularly gingival bleeding, epistaxis and genitourinary or gastrointestinal bleeding	Phrynoderma (Figure 29.4), corkscrew hairs, perifollicular haemorrhage (Figure 29.6), purpura, peripheral oedema, splinter haemorrhages, oral disease, musculoskeletal disease, lethargy
Differential diagnosis	Phrynoderma occurs with vitamin B, C, E and essential fatty acid deficiency	Jaundice; medication-induced pigmentation	Osteomalacia, osteopenia and/or osteoporosis	Other causes of haemorrhage	Anticoagulation, liver disease, haematological malignancies, inherited coagulapathies	Trauma, medications, haematological abnormalities, collagen vascular diseases
Investigations	Serum retinol level	Serum vitamin A levels if suspect toxicity Carotenaemia: elevated serum carotene level greater than 250 µg/dL	Low serum 25-hydroxyvitamin D, hypocalcaemia, hypophosphataemia, increased alkaline phosphatase and increased parathyroid hormone	Plasma α-tocopherol concentration	Prolonged prothrombin and activated partial thromboplastin times; low serum vitamin K level	Clinical diagnosis Serum ascorbic acid levels can be measured
Management	Vitamin A supplementation	Discontinuation of excess vitamin A and β-carotene intake	Vitamin D replacement	Discontinue excess intake	Intramuscular or parenteral vitamin K	Ascorbic acid replacement

VKDB, vitamin K deficiency bleeding.

Table 29.2 B-complex vitamin abnormalities

Vitamin abnormality	Vitamin B1 (thiamine) deficiency (Syn. Beriberi)	Vitamin B2 (riboflavin) deficiency (Syn. Oculo-orogenital syndrome)	Vitamin B3 (niacin/nicotinic acid) deficiency (Syn. Pellagra, Hartnup disease)	Vitamin B6 deficiency	Vitamin B9 (folate) deficiency	Vitamin B12 (cobalamin) deficiency (Syn. Pernicious anaemia)
Introduction	Co-enzyme for the metabolism of carbohydrates, lipids and branched chain amino acids	Essential for cellular oxidation-reduction reactions and vitamin B6 metabolism	Important component of NAD and NADP	Essential co-enzyme for various metabolic processes Three forms: pyridoxine, pyridoxamine and pyridoxal	Co-enzyme for amino acid, purine and pyrimidine metabolism	Critical co-enzyme involved in DNA, protein, lipid and carbohydrate metabolism
Epidemiology	Rare in developed countries	Endemic in populations where diets rely on unenriched cereals or lack dairy products and meats	Pellagra is rare in developed countries; endemic in areas with a high grain (unfortified), low meat diet Can be associated with carcinoid syndrome	The elderly are at higher risk	Prevalence 0.2%; pregnant women are at increased risk	Estimated 3.2% of US adults older than 50 years have a low serum vitamin B12 level Pernicious anaemia prevalence ranges from 50 to 4000 cases/100 000 persons
Pathophysiology	Seen with poor dietary intake, inadequately supplemented parenteral nutrition, gastrointestinal malabsorption and increased metabolic requirements	May develop as a result of decreased dietary intake, malabsorption and phototherapy (e.g. in neonatal hyperbilirubinaemia)	Alcoholism, eating disorders and presumed food allergies put people at risk for inadequate intake Hartnup disease is a rare autosomal recessive disorder (see Chapter 39)	Contributory factors are decreased dietary intake, malabsorption, and medications particularly alcoholics and inflammatory bowel disease	Alcoholics, malabsorption, antifolate medications, e.g. methotrexate	Deficiency results from inadequate intake, malabsorption and inborn errors of transport and metabolism

Clinical features	'Wet beriberi' has prominent cardiovascular involvement and red burning tongue has been described 'Dry beriberi' has prominent neurological manifestations	Acute: presents with deep red erythema, epidermal necrolysis and mucositis Chronic: findings include angular stomatitis, chelitis, glossitis, dyssebacia of the nose and a seborrhoeic dermatitis-like eruption	Photodistributed dermatitis (painful, erythema and oedema, especially on hands, Figure 29.7), diarrhoea and dementia	Seborrhoeic cermatitis-like eruption involving the face, scalp, neck, shoulders, buttocks and perineum; neuropsychiatric symptoms	Mucocutaneous: glossitis with atrophic filiform papillae, angular chelitis, oral ulceration, perineal seborrhoeic dermatitis, hair depigmentation, mucocutaneous hyperpigmentation Haematological: megaloblastic anaemia	Similar mucocutaneous and haematological findings to folate deficiency, distinguished by development of neurological symptoms
Differential diagnosis	Glossitis due to other B vitamin deficiencies	Other B-complex vitamin deficiencies have similar clinical features	Porphyrias, polymorphous light eruption, chronic actinic dermatitis, photosensitive drug eruptions, cutaneous lupus	Significant overlap with niacin deficiency	Vitamin B12 deficiency	Folate deficiency
Investigations	Low blood thiamine levels; erythrocyte thiamine transketolase level before and after thiamine pyrophosphate stimulation	Measure erythrocyte glutathione reductase activity	Mainly clinical diagnosis; reduced niacin urinary metabolites	Low plasma pyridoxal-5-phosphate is indicative of vitamin B6 deficiency	Serum and red blood cell folate levels (megaloblastic anaemia with hypersegmented neutrophils)	Serum cobalamin level less than 200 pg/mL
Management	Intravenous or intramuscular thiamine	Riboflavin supplementation	Nicotinamide or nicotinic acid; untreated pellagra can be fatal	Pyridoxine supplementation	Folate supplementation	Vitamin B12 either parenterally or orally

NAD, nicotinamide-adenine dinucleotide; NADP, nicotinamide-adenine dinucleotide phosphate.

PART 3: METABOLIC AND NUTRITIONAL DISORDERS AFFECTING THE SKIN

Table 29.3 Diseases of mineral deficiency and excess

Vitamin abnormality…	Iron deficiency	Zinc deficiency	Selenium deficiency (Syn. Keshan disease, Kashin–Beck disease)	Selenium excess
Introduction	Essential for multiple metabolic pathways, including collagen synthesis, haem synthesis and oxidation-reduction reactions	Plays an important role in many of the body's biochemical processes	Necessary component of several proteins, known as selenoproteins	Necessary component of several proteins, known as selenoproteins
Epidemiology	14% of 1–4-year-olds; 9% of menstruating females	17% of the world's population has inadequate dietary zinc intake	Uncommon; the highest incidence is in parts of China with selenium-deficient soil	Uncommon
Pathophysiology	Infants, menstruating or pregnant females, people with conditions resulting in chronic bleeding are all at risk	Decreased dietary intake, decreased absorption, or increased elimination can lead to zinc deficiency; biopsy shows psoriasiform hyperplasia	Caused by inadequate intake, defective absorption or increased losses	Excess ingestion of selenium from supplements or exposure during some occupations
Clinical features	Koilonychia, glossodynia, aphthous stomatitis; angular stomatitis; brittle hair	Psoriasiform dermatitis (Figure 29.8) on the hands, feet and knees, growth retardation, hypogonadism	Non-specific cutaneous findings: white nail beds, hypopigmentation of skin and hair Characterised by multifocal myocarditis	Brittle nails with white horizontal streaks, brittle hair, scalp exfoliative dermatitis, reddish hue to teeth, hair and nails Neurological signs, acute toxicity can be fatal
Differential diagnosis	Folate, riboflavin, niacin and vitamin B12 deficiency	Seborrhoeic dermatitis, biotin deficiency, kwashiorkor and irritant dermatitis	Hepatic cirrhosis, kwashiorkor	
Investigations	Microcytic anaemia; low serum iron, low ferritin and high total iron binding capacity	Low serum zinc levels	Plasma selenium levels and glutathione peroxidase activity	Plasma selenium levels

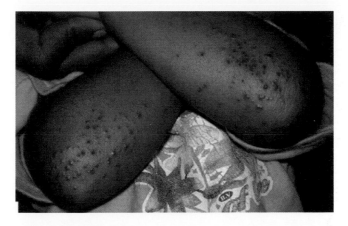

Figure 29.4 Phrynoderma: keratotic papules with intrafollicular plugging on extensor surfaces of the forearms of a 3-year-old Indian girl presenting with night blindness. Both conditions responded within 1 month to vitamin A supplementation. (Source: Murthy SR, Prabhakaran VC. Phrynoderma and night blindness. Indian J Ophthalmol 2010;58:175-6) http://www.ncbi.nlm.nih.gov/pmc/articles/ PMC2854467/ last accessed October 2019 copyright of the *Indian Journal of Ophthalmology*.)

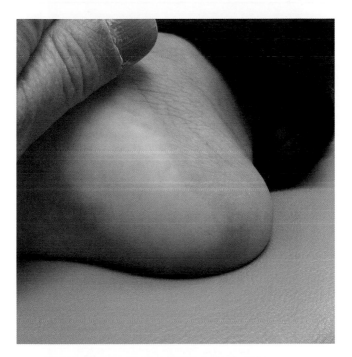

Figure 29.5 Carotenoderma. Note the yellow colour of the plantar foot.

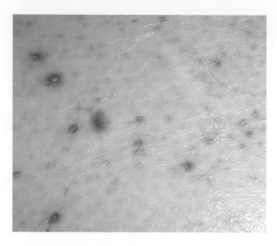

Figure 29.6 Scurvy. Note the corkscrew-like hairs and the perifollicular purpura.

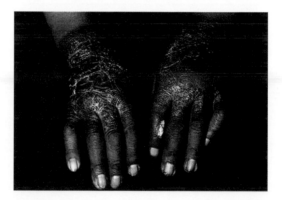

Figure 29.7 Pellagra. (Source: From Irvine AD, Hoeger PH, Yan AC (eds) Harpers Textbook of Dermatology, 3rd edn, 2011. Oxford: Wiley Blackwell.)

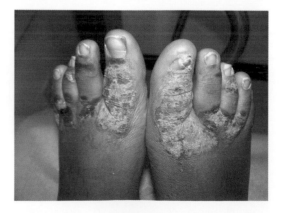

Figure 29.8 Psoriasiform plaques on the extremities of this patient with acquired zinc deficiency associated with nephrotic syndrome.

Part 4
Genetic Disorders Involving the Skin

Inherited disorders of epidermal keratinisation

30

Ichthyosis vulgaris

The word 'ichthyosis' is derived from the Greek word *ichthys*, which means fish and refers to excessive skin scale. Ichthyosis vulgaris (IV) is a relatively mild scaling disorder inherited as an autosomal semidominant trait.

Epidemiology
The prevalence of IV in Europe is 1%. There is an association with typically mild atopic eczema.

Pathophysiology
Although inherited as an autosomal dominant trait, two filaggrin (*FLG*) gene mutations are required for the full clinical IV phenotype. In the one third of patients who have only one *FLG* mutation, the phenotype is limited to accentuated palmar and plantar creases, and somewhat dry skin. Filaggrin mutations result in impaired epidermal barrier formation and a marked reduction of natural moisturizing factors, which play an important role in hydration of the stratum corneum and also predispose to atopic eczema (see Chapter 16).

Clinical features
IV usually develops during the first months of life. Scaling may resolve or be reduced markedly in the summer due to seasonal variation and increased humidity. Individuals with IV present with light grey scales covering mainly the extensor surfaces of the extremities and the trunk (Figure 30.1a). The scales tend to be smaller than in recessive X-linked ichthyosis, and the groin and larger flexures are spared. Almost all IV patients exhibit hyperlinear palms (Figure 30.1b), and this clinical feature is not influenced by factors such as season or humidity. Patients may report hypohidrosis and lack of tolerance to high temperatures.

Differential diagnosis
The differential diagnosis of IV includes other forms of ichthyosis, distinguished by clinical phenotype, family history, histology and, if necessary, genetic testing.

Investigations
The diagnosis can usually be made from clinical phenotype and family history. If there is diagnostic doubt, the following investigations may be considered:

- Histology reveals orthohyperkeratosis with a diminished or absent granular layer.
- Immunohistochemical studies demonstrate an absent or markedly reduced filaggrin.
- Ultrastructure from electron microscopy shows scarce and crumbly keratohyalin granules.
- *FLG* mutation analysis.

Management
Treatment is focused on emollients, particularly ointments that hydrate the stratum corneum or creams containing glycerol. In those patients without concomitant atopic eczema, urea containing creams (up to 10%) or creams containing lactic acid (up to 12%) also work well. In contrast to autosomal recessive congenital ichthyosis, daily bathing is not necessary, but showering and subsequent application of emollients is advisable.

Rook's Dermatology Handbook, First Edition. Edited by Christopher E. M. Griffiths, Tanya O. Bleiker, Daniel Creamer, John R. Ingram and Rosalind C. Simpson.
© 2022 John Wiley & Sons Ltd. Published 2022 by John Wiley & Sons Ltd.

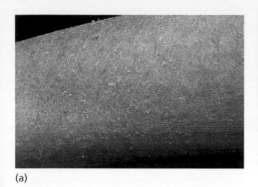
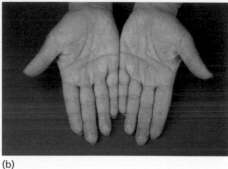

(a)   (b)

Figure 30.1 Ichthyosis vulgaris. (a) Fine scaling and (b) hyperlinear palms. (Source: Courtesy of the Department of Dermatology, University Hospital Münster, Münster, Germany.)

Recessive X-linked ichthyosis

Recessive X-linked ichthyosis (RXLI) is a relatively mild scaling disorder caused by mutations in the *STS* gene encoding steroid sulphatase.

Epidemiology

The disease affects boys almost exclusively. Based on systematic screening of pregnancies for steroid sulphatase deficiency, the prevalence in males is 1: 1500. RXLI may be associated with cryptorchidism in up to 20%, with attention-deficit hyperactivity syndrome in up to 40% and autism in around 25%.

Pathophysiology

In 90% of cases the *STS* gene mutation is a deletion, which often spans the entire gene. High concentrations of cholesterol sulphate accumulate, inhibiting proteases such as kallikrein 5 and kallikrein 7 that are important for normal degradation of corneodesmosomes. This in turn leads to decreased desquamation, and as a consequence hyperkeratosis. Histology from a skin biopsy is expected to show orthohyperkeratosis and a well-maintained, often thickened, stratum granulosum. Ultrastructurally, a marked increase of persistent corneodesmosomes can be seen.

Clinical features

Mothers of affected children may have birth complications such as prolonged delivery necessitating caesarean section, relating to the presence of the enzyme defect in the placenta. Directly after birth, most affected infants exhibit very fine scaling or peeling of the skin that often goes unnoticed and soon resolves. At the age of 2–6 months, large thick dark brown to yellow-brown hyperkeratoses develop covering the trunk, the extremities and the neck (Figure 30.2). The antecubital and popliteal fossae are usually spared. The palms of the hands and the soles remain unaffected. In around 30% of patients the colour of the scale is light grey (Figure 30.2d). These patients may be misdiagnosed as having IV. Dark hyperkeratosis of the lateral aspects of the trunk and the back of the neck is a feature which is typical of RXLI and is usually not present in IV.

Differential diagnosis

Other forms of ichthyosis are distinguished by clinical phenotype, family history, histology and, if necessary, genetic testing.

Investigations

Usually, the diagnosis can be made from clinical phenotype and family history. The existence of an affected male relative on the maternal side is suggestive of the diagnosis of RXLI. If there is diagnostic doubt, a skin biopsy may be necessary. Steroid sulphatase activity measured from plasma and mutation analysis of *STS* gene is possible.

Management

Emollient therapy is the mainstay of treatment. Systemic retinoids such as acitretin may be given at low dosage during periods of disease exacerbations, e.g. during winter.

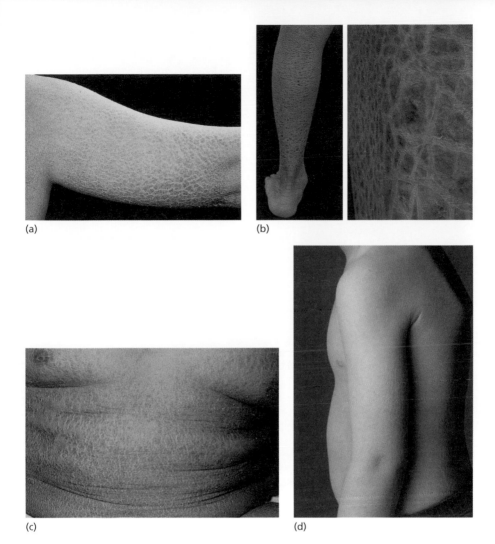

(a)

(b)

(c)

(d)

Figure 30.2 Recessive X-linked ichthyosis. Scaling on (a) the arm, (b) the legs and (c) the trunk and (d) a patient with light grey scaling. (Source: parts (a)–(c) Courtesy of Dr M. Judge, Salford Royal NHS Trust, UK; part (d) Courtesy of the Department of Dermatology, University Hospital Münster, Münster, Germany.)

Lamellar ichthyosis and congenital ichthyosiform erythroderma

(Lamellar ichthyosis, Syn. Non-bullous ichthyosiform erythroderma)
Lamellar ichthyosis (LI) and congenital ichthyosiform erythroderma (CIE) are examples of autosomal recessive congenital ichthyosis (ARCI), representing the mild and severe ends of the phenotypic spectrum, respectively.

Epidemiology
Prevalence of ARCI in Europe is approximately 1.6:100 000.

Pathophysiology
Deficiency of the enzyme transglutaminase-1 (TG1) is the most frequent cause of ARCI. TG-1 contributes to assembly of the cornified envelope by catalysing calcium-dependent crosslinking of proteins, such as involucrin and loricrin.

Clinical features

LI is characterised by large plate-like dark-brown hyperkeratoses covering the entire body, with mild palmoplantar involvement (Figure 30.3a). At the other end of the clinical spectrum, ARCI patients may exhibit severe erythroderma, mostly fine white or grey scales and often pronounced palmoplantar keratosis, with the phenotype known as CIE (Figure 30.3b).

At birth most ARCI patients present as 'collodion babies', encased in a shiny parchment-like membrane. The membrane is transient, cracking a few days after birth (Figure 30.4) and peeling off within 4 weeks. Initially, the clinical presentation may include ectropion and everted lips. Subsequently, several different clinical phenotypes may develop, including LI, CIE, bathing suit ichthyosis, or self-improving congenital ichthyosis. The most severe subtype

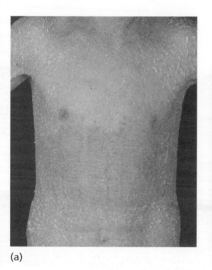
(a)

(b)

Figure 30.3 Autosomal recessive congenital ichthyosis. (a) Lamellar ichthyosis. (b) Congenital ichthyosiform erythroderma. (Source: Courtesy of the Department of Dermatology, University Hospital Münster, Münster, Germany.)

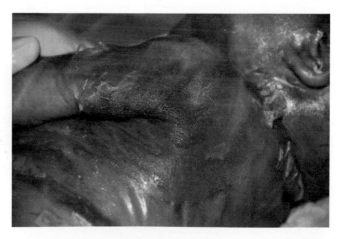

Figure 30.4 Autosomal recessive congenital ichthyosis. Shedding of collodion membranes after 1 week.

of ARCI, harlequin ichthyosis, is the exception that does not present as a collodion baby.

Differential diagnosis

Other subtypes of ARCI, including LI, CIE, bathing suit ichthyosis, harlequin ichthyosis and self-improving congenital ichthyosis, as well as other types of ichythosis.

Investigations

See Figure 30.5.

Management

ARCI requires lifelong management based on the establishment of the correct molecular diagnosis, as summarised in Figure 30.5.

Collodion baby management is best regarded as a dermatological emergency, requiring a multidisciplinary approach. Neonates should be nursed in a high humidity incubator in a neonatal intensive care unit, with close monitoring of body temperature. Emollients should be applied at least twice daily. Topical salicylic acid is contraindicated to avoid metabolic acidosis. Complications include infection, ectropion, poor feeding and restricted pulmonary ventilation.

The subsequent general management approaches for ARCI are:

- *Emollient therapy:* high water content ointment/petrolatum-like ointments, bandage wraps, urea or lactic acid additives; salicylic acid contraindicated.
- *Bathing:* daily, with sodium bicarbonate additive.
- *Systemic therapy:* retinoids, including acitretin or isotretinoin.

There are also some specific management issues:

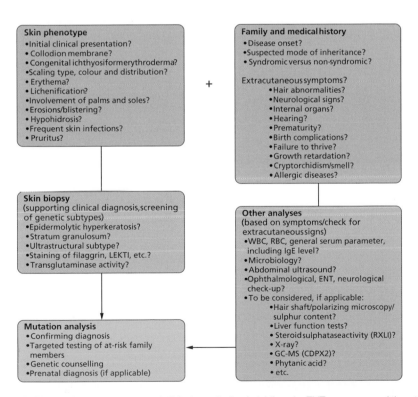

Figure 30.5 Diagnostic management and clinical monitoring in ichthyosis. ENT, ear, nose and throat; GC-MS, gas chromatography–mass spectrometry; IgE, immunoglobulin E; LEKTI, lymphoepithelial Kazal-type related inhibitor; RBC, red blood cell; RXLI, recessive X linked ichthyosis; WBC, white blood cell.

- *Eye:* severe ectropion may lead to corneal perforation, surgical correction may be needed.
- *Ear:* input from ear, nose and throat (ENT) specialist, frequent clearance of keratin material may be needed.
- *Hypohydrosis:* reduced tolerance of warm environments, may improve with oral retinoid therapy.
- *Musculoskeletal:* consider physiotherapy for infants and children, check for vitamin D deficiency.

Epidermolytic ichthyosis

(Syn. Bullous congenital ichthyosiform erythroderma)
Epidermolytic ichthyosis (EI) is one of the keratinopathic ichthyoses, which are rare cornification disorders due to mutations in keratin genes.

Epidemiology
Keratinopathic ichthyoses are rare, with a prevalence of 1:350 000.

Pathophysiology
EI is usually inherited as an autosomal dominant trait (occasionally autosomal recessive). It is due to mutations in *KRT1 or KRT10* genes encoding epidermal keratins that are intermediate filaments which contribute to the formation of the keratinocyte cell cytoskeleton. Histology shows epidermolytic hyperkeratosis and electron microscopy demonstrates cytoplasmic keratin aggregates (keratin clumps) or perinuclear shell formation.

Clinical features
Patients usually present at birth with erythroderma, multiple blisters and erosions. Resolution of erosions occurs, which are replaced by hyperkeratosis in the first few months of life. Subsequent white-brown scaling is generalised and may be particularly prominent on frictional areas and over joints (Figure 30.6a,b). Skin fragility remains and when patients experience pyrexia, skin infections, warmer temperatures or mechanical friction, bouts of blistering can occur. The older child and adult patients usually present with marked keratotic lichenification seen as rippled keratotic ridges in the axilla, elbows and popliteal fossae. Patients with *KRT1* mutations usually have severe involvement of the palms and soles (Figure 30.6c), in some cases impairing walking, while in those with *KRT10* mutations the palms and soles are usually spared (Figure 30.6d).

Differential diagnosis
Other keratinopathic ichthyoses
Superficial epidermolytic ichthyosis, ichthyosis Curth–Macklin, congenital reticular ichthyosiform erythroderma.

Other ichthyoses, including the autosomal recessive congenital ichthyoses.

Investigations
See Figure 30.5 for an outline of relevant investigations.

Management
Patients with *KRT10* mutations exhibiting sparing of the palms and soles tend to respond well to moderate dosages of systemic retinoids. In contrast, systemic retinoids in patients with *KRT1* mutations may worsen the skin problems.

Epidermolytic palmoplantar keratoderma

Palmoplantar keratodermas form a heterogeneous group of disorders defined by excessive epidermal thickening of the palms and soles. One of the inherited conditions in the group, epidermolytic palmoplantar keratoderma (EPPK), is probably the most common form of diffuse keratoderma.

Epidemiology
Prevalence of 4.4/100 000.

Pathophysiology
EPPK is usually due to mutations in *KRT9*, which is a keratin gene preferentially expressed in palmoplantar skin. Disruption of intermediate filament integrity due to these mutations is predicted to reduce the resilience of the

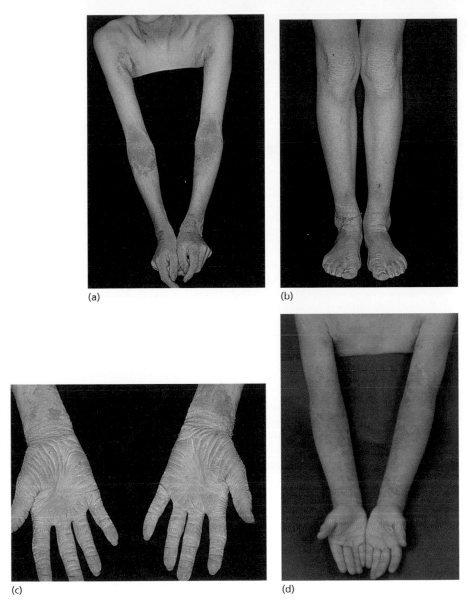

(a)

(b)

(c)

(d)

Figure 30.6 Epidermolytic ichthyosis. (a) Arms, (b) legs, (c) severe palm involvement indicative of *KRT1* mutation and (d) sparing of the palms indicative of *KRT10* mutations. (Source: parts (a)–(c) Courtesy of Dr M. Judge, Salford Royal NHS Trust, UK.)

cytoskeleton to minor external trauma, leading to blistering and hyperkeratosis as well as epidermolysis with tonofilament clumping.

Histologically, EPPK shows epidermolytic change in suprabasal keratinocytes. Round or ovoid eosinophilic inclusions may be detected. Electron microscopy may show the characteristic finding of whorls of keratins containing tubular structures observed in transverse and longitudinal sections ('tonotubules').

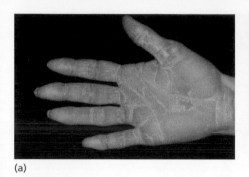
(a)

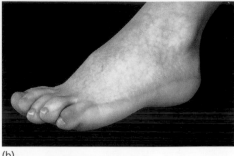
(b)

Figure 30.7 Epidermolytic palmoplantar keratoderma. (a) Confluent keratoderma of palm. (b) Hyperkeratosis of the sole spares the dorsa surface, with a sharp demarcation.

Clinical features

Diffuse keratoderma develops in infancy. In adults, there is confluent keratoderma (Figure 30.7a), sparing dorsal surfaces, with a sharp demarcation and erythematous edge (Figure 30.7b). Blistering is not a major feature, but some patients may give a history of blisters or fissuring of the palms. Hair, teeth and nails are normal.

Differential diagnosis

Pachyonychia congenital, non-epidermolytic palmoplantar keratoderma, other non-syndromic forms of palmoplantar keratoderma (PPK), syndromic forms of PPK.

Investigations

Skin biopsy.

Management

First line: Mechanical debridement of scale.

Second line: Topical keratolytics.

Third line: Low-dose oral retinoids.

Pachyonychia congenita

Pachyonychia congenita (PC) is a rare palmoplantar keratoderma, inherited as an autosomal dominant trait, due to mutation in one of five keratin genes.

Pathophysiology

The keratin gene mutations disrupt cytoskeletal function via dominant-negative interference, leading to cell fragility. The variable distribution of lesions in PC corresponds to different expression patterns of the mutant keratins: PC-K6a (most common and most severe form), PC-K6b, PC-K6c (the mildest form), PC-K16 and PC-K17 (severe form).

On histology, palmoplantar epidermis shows marked hyperkeratosis with alternating ortho- and parakeratosis. Acanthosis is present with patchy hypergranulosis, in which large and malformed keratohyalin granules are present, without epidermolysis. Tonofilament aggregates are seen on electron microscopy.

Epidemiology

Prevalence is unknown due to rarity.

Clinical features

Three clinical features are reported in more than 90% of patients across all mutation subtypes: toenail dystrophy, plantar keratoderma and plantar pain, which in patients older than 3 years are highly diagnostic for PC (Figure 30.8). Hyperkeratosis of the toenail bed first appears from less than a year old, up to 9 years old. Plantar keratoderma manifests as calluses, fissures and thickened skin. Thick yellow keratoses are found on sites of pressure. Frictional blisters may occur, especially in hot weather in childhood. Plantar pain is a very common symptom of PC and has an important impact on quality of life. Additional diagnostic findings include follicular hyperkeratoses on the knees and elbows, oral leukokeratosis, palmoplantar hyperhidrosis, epidermoid and other cysts and natal teeth.

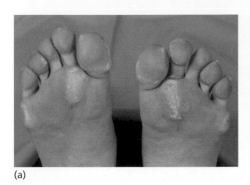
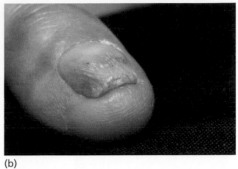

(a)   (b)

Figure 30.8 Pachyonychia congenita. (a) Focal keratoderma on mechanically stressed areas.
(b) Typical curvature of nail ('covered wagon').

Differential diagnosis
See EPPK section.

Investigations
Skin biopsy. Mutational analysis of keratin genes can be considered.

Management
Nails
Nail care, orthotic input for footwear.

Skin
Emollients and keratolytics may help milder cases, systemic retinoids can thin callouses but may increase plantar skin pain.

Hyperhidrosis
Standard treatments to reduce secondary blistering.

Cysts
Surgical excision.

Darier disease

Darier disease (DD) is an autosomal dominant genodermatosis characterised by a chronic eruption of keratotic papules, the histology of which shows acantholysis and dyskeratosis.

Epidemiology
DD has a worldwide distribution; reported prevalence in northern European populations is between 1:100 000 and 1:30 000, M = F. The rash usually first appears in early teenage years, but patients may not present until their sixth or seventh decade. Penetrance is complete in adults although phenotypic expression may be variable, with some patients featuring nail changes only. In some families plane wart-like keratoses known as acrokeratosis verruciformis predominate.

Pathophysiology
Histologically, DD shows epidermal acantholysis. Lacunae appear suprabasally in the earliest lesions and extend irregularly throughout the Malpighian layer. In the overlying epidermis, rounded dyskeratotic cells with eosinophilic cytoplasm, 'corps ronds', give rise to small cells with shrunken cytoplasm ('grains') and the stratum corneum is hyperkeratotic.

DD is caused by mutations in *ATP2A2*, which encodes an intracellular calcium pump. Altered intracellular Ca^{2+} concentrations interfere with epidermal keratinocyte differentiation and adhesion.

Clinical features
Discrete or confluent rough, greasy, skin-coloured or yellowish-brown papules are commonest on the seborrhoeic areas of the trunk, face, ears, scalp, neck and flexural sites, including the perineum, axillae and groin (Figure 30.9a,b). Hair growth is unaffected. The disease often begins with small groups of keratotic papules on sun-exposed sites such as the neck. Isolated hyperkeratosis of the nipples may precede other signs of disease. Coalescing papules, particularly in the axillae, perineum, groin,

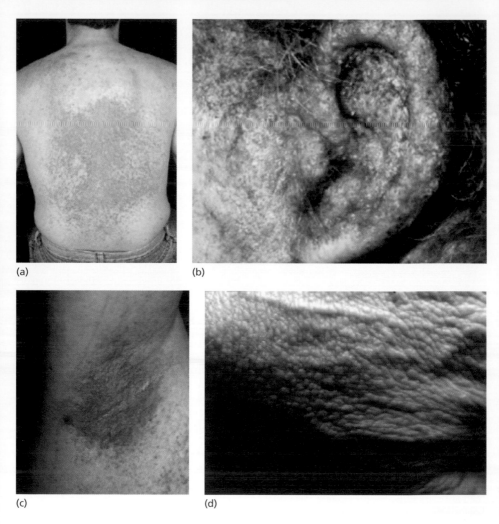

(a)

(b)

(c)

(d)

Figure 30.9 Darier disease. (a) Profuse keratotic papules in the seborrhoeic areas. (b) Confluent lesions on the ear of a 57-year-old man. (c) Confluent papules forming irregular, warty, fissured plaques in the axilla. (d) Multiple acrokeratosis verruciformis lesions on the dorsum of the hand highlighted with oblique illumination in a 45-year-old man.

and natal cleft, may form irregular, warty, fissured plaques (Figure 30.9c), sometimes becoming vegetating and malodorous. Acrokeratosis verruciformis plane wart-like lesions, best seen by transverse illumination, are commonest on the dorsal hands but can be detected in other sites (Figure 30.9d).

Hands, including nails, may show the earliest signs of disease. Nail fragility, painful longitudinal splits or distinctive red and white longitudinal bands terminating in V-shaped nicks are typical (Figure 30.10a,b). Over time nails may become severely dystrophic. Focal palmoplantar lesions, pits (Figure 30.10c) or keratoses are common, occasionally causing a more diffuse keratoderma. Mucosal involvement presents with white umbilicated or cobblestone papules (Figure 30.10d).

The disease usually runs a chronic relapsing course, although spontaneous remissions can

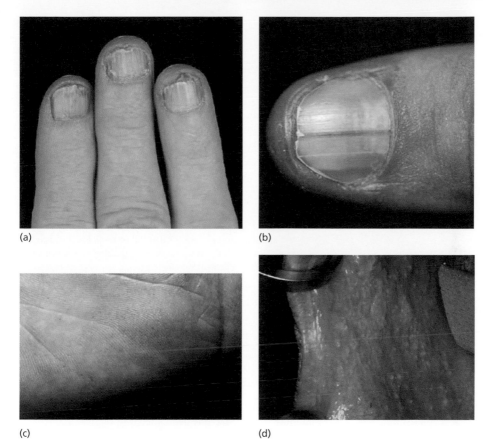

Figure 30.10 Darier disease. (a) Fragile nails with longitudinal splitting and terminal notching. (b) Early nail changes in a 28-year-old woman showing a fine white band and a longitudinal red band terminating in a notch. (c) Pitting on the palms of a 15-year-old boy. (d) Confluent oral buccal lesions in a 51-year-old man.

occur. Aggravating factors include friction, heat, sweating and sunlight or phototherapy. Malodorous and painful skin in DD impacts on social interaction and work or school, with corresponding reductions in health-related quality of life.

Mosaic presentation of DD can occur, following the lines of Blaschko. Impetiginisation and eczematisation are common, and patients have an increased susceptibility to infection with herpes simplex, herpes zoster or cowpox.

Differential diagnosis
Seborrhoeic dermatitis, Hailey–Hailey disease, Dowling–Degos disease.

Investigations
The disorder is usually diagnosed clinically, with histological confirmation. In disease flares there should be a high index of suspicion for superinfection, with samples sent for bacterial, viral and fungal investigations.

Management
First line: Emollients, topical antiseptics, avoid excess heat and UVB, treat infective flares.

Second line: Topical corticosteroids, topical retinoids.

Third line: Oral acitretin 0.25–0.5 mg/kg/day, isotretinoin 0.5 mg/kg/day.

Fourth line: 5-fluorouracil cream, tacrolimus ointment, oral alitretinoin, photodynamic therapy, botulinum toxin for flexural disease.

Hailey–Hailey disease

Hailey–Hailey disease (HHD) is an autosomal dominant genodermatosis characterised by erosions and blistering, most prominently in the flexures and sites of friction or trauma.

Epidemiology

An incidence of 1:50 000 has been reported, although HHD is probably under-recognised.

Pathophysiology

HHD is a disorder of keratinocyte adhesion. Histology of lesional skin demonstrates widespread partial loss of cohesion between suprabasal keratinocytes, or acantholysis, said to resemble a 'dilapidated brick wall'. Acantholytic clefts and bullae form suprabasally and may contain floating clusters of loosely coherent cells.

HHD is due to mutations in *ATP2C1*, a gene which encodes the calcium pump of the Golgi apparatus membrane. The disease is likely to be due to haploinsufficiency: most mutations are predicted to result in reduced or absent expression of the functional calcium pump. In HHD keratinocytes, trafficking of the adhesion molecules desmoplakin and desmoglein 3 to the cell membrane is reduced, interfering with normal intercellular keratinocyte adhesion.

Clinical features

Presents between the second and fourth decade with painful, pruritic and often malodorous lesions of flexures or other sites of friction. HHD may be localised or generalised, occasionally causing erythroderma. In the axilla, inframammary or abdominal folds, groin or perineum, lesions show fissuring and erosion with macerated epidermis (Figure 30.11), progressing in more severe cases to vegetations. Less occluded areas, such as truncal or neck lesions, are more likely to show vesicopustules or flaccid bullae. There may be crusted erosions resembling nummular eczema, or annular plaques with peripheral scales, often with post-inflammatory hyperpigmentation.

Common precipitating factors include heat, sweating, friction and infection. Lesions may localise at the sites of inflammatory dermatoses such as psoriasis and seborrhoeic dermatitis. Linear white bands (longitudinal leukonychia) are present in the nails of some patients, but without the nail fragility of DD. Even mild disease has been shown to reduce quality of life, and flexural or groin involvement can be particularly disabling.

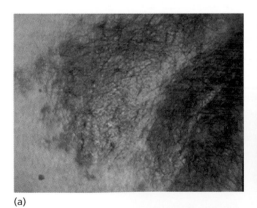
(a)

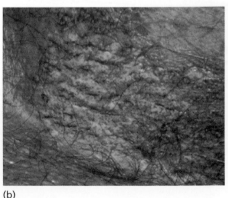
(b)

Figure 30.11 Lesions of Hailey–Hailey disease. (a) Typical fissured plaque in the axilla. (b) Inflamed, macerated and fissured lesions of the groin in a 40-year-old man.

Differential diagnosis

Flexural psoriasis, seborrhoeic dermatitis, nummular eczema, tinea corporis.

Investigations

Skin biopsy demonstrates the characteristic histology. Swabs for bacterial, fungal and viral investigations if indicated.

Management

First line: Loose clothing, absorbent pads in flexures, emollients, topical antiseptics, treat infective flares, weight loss in obese patients.

Second line: Topical corticosteroids.

Third line: Short course of oral prednisolone 20–30 mg/day for acute flares, oral retinoids.

Fourth line: Surgical ablation or excision, botulinum toxin.

31 Acquired and inherited hair disorders

Hair follicles undergo a repetitive sequence of growth and rest known as the hair cycle (Figure 31.1).

- *Anagen:* Period of active hair growth. The duration of this phase is responsible for determining the final length of the hair. Under normal circumstances, 80–90% of hair follicles on the human scalp are in anagen at any one time.
- *Catagen:* At the end of anagen, epithelial cell division declines and ceases, and the follicle enters an involutionary phase. The proximal end of the hair shaft keratinises to form a club-shaped structure and the lower part of the follicle involutes by apoptosis.
- *Telogen:* The period between the completion of follicular regression and the onset of the next anagen phase. The club hair is eventually shed through an active process termed *exogen.*

General investigation and management of hair disorders

Clinical photography
A photographic record is an important part of managing patients and assists objective assessment over a period of time.

Microscopy
Light microscopy should be used for the investigation of possible hair shaft disorders.

Scalp biopsy
Histology is helpful to investigate hair disorders in certain circumstances. Important considerations when taking a biopsy include the biopsy technique, selection of biopsy sites, processing of the biopsies and access to a dermatopathologist skilled in the interpretation of hair pathology.

Current practice is to take two 4 mm punch biopsies. Biopsies should be orientated in the direction of hair growth to minimise transection of follicles and should extend into the subcutaneous fat. Biopsies can be processed horizontally or vertically; Processing a scalp biopsy in a horizontal fashion allows all the follicles in a given biopsy to be seen, typically 30–40 hairs per 4 mm punch.

- *Suspected scarring alopecia:* One biopsy is sectioned vertically, and the second horizontally (Figure 31.2). Direct immunofluorescence can be requested if indicated.
- *Suspected non-scarring alopecia:* In non-scarring conditions it is more useful for both biopsies to be sectioned horizontally (Figure 31.3).

Rook's Dermatology Handbook, First Edition. Edited by Christopher E. M. Griffiths, Tanya O. Bleiker, Daniel Creamer, John R. Ingram and Rosalind C. Simpson.
© 2022 John Wiley & Sons Ltd. Published 2022 by John Wiley & Sons Ltd.

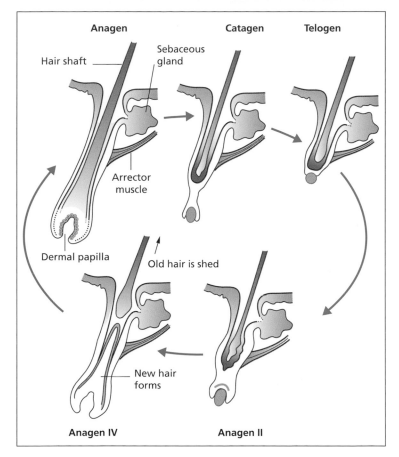

Figure 31.1 The hair cycle. (Source: Olsen EA. Androgenetic alopecia. In: Olsen EA, ed. Disorders of Hair Growth. New York: McGraw-Hill, 1994, 257–283. Courtesy of Elise Olsen. Reproduced with permission of McGraw-Hill.)

- *Wigs and hair pieces:* These can be made from either synthetic or real hair. They can be prescribed to manage the cosmetic/psychological impact of hair loss.

ACQUIRED HAIR DISORDERS

These are acquired disorders causing loss of hair. They may be diffuse or localised, scarring or non-scarring (see Chapter 87 for differential diagnosis of scalp hair loss in adults).

NON-SCARRING ALOPECIAS

Androgenetic alopecia and pattern hair loss

(Syn. Male pattern balding, male pattern hair loss, female pattern hair loss)

Hair loss due to a combination of genetic factors and the effects of androgens is referred to androgenetic alopecia (AGA) in men and female pattern hair loss (FPHL) in females.

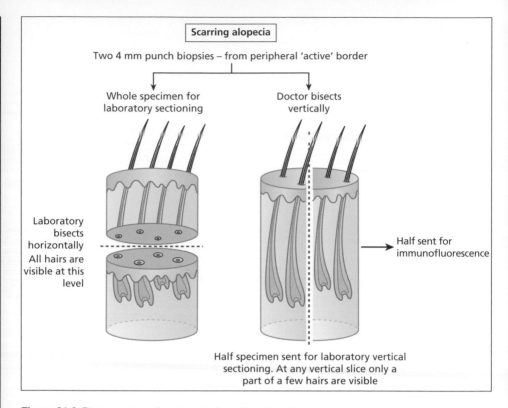

Figure 31.2 Biopsy process for suspected scarring alopecia.

Epidemiology

Almost all white males develop some recession of frontal hairline; 50–60% of men have a bald scalp by the age of 70 years. AGA is less common in East Asian men, reported frequencies vary.

The prevalence of FPHL in white women is reported as 3–6% in women aged under 30 years, increasing to 29–42% in women over age 70. It is less common in Asian females.

Pathophysiology

Androgens, particularly dihydrotestosterone, play a key role in AGA. Their role is less certain in FPHL. The mechanism of pattern hair loss is multifactorial, with the following factors contributing: genetic predisposition, follicular regression, shortened duration of anagen and follicular miniaturisation.

Histopathology shows a reduction in terminal hairs, an increase in secondary vellus hair, a vari-able increase in telogen and catagen hairs and a mild/moderate perifollicular lymphohistiocytic infiltrate.

Clinical features

Patterned hair loss occurs over the crown in both sexes. Terminal hairs are progressively replaced by shorter, finer hairs which may also appear less pigmented. See Figures 31.4 and 31.5 for recognised scales of AGA and FPHL.

Differential diagnosis

Chronic telogen effluvium.

Investigations

See Table 31.1.

Management

Without therapy, pattern hair loss is progressive at a variable rate. If sought for cosmetic reasons,

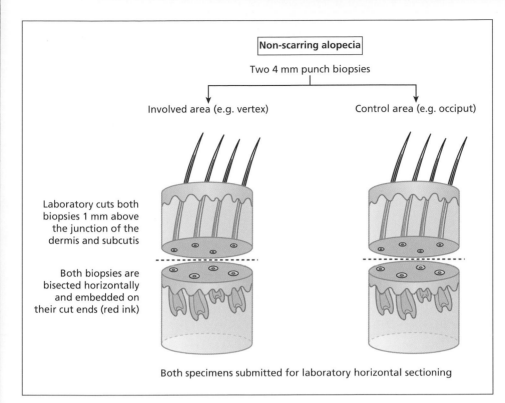

Non-scarring alopecia

Two 4 mm punch biopsies

Involved area (e.g. vertex)   Control area (e.g. occiput)

Laboratory cuts both biopsies 1 mm above the junction of the dermis and subcutis

Both biopsies are bisected horizontally and embedded on their cut ends (red ink)

Both specimens submitted for laboratory horizontal sectioning

Figure 31.3 Biopsy process for suspected non-scarring alopecia.

management strategies are outlined in Table 31.1. Any medical treatments commenced have to be continued to maintain clinical response.

Telogen effluvium

An increase in the shedding of telogen club hairs due to premature termination of the anagen phase of the hair cycle.

Pathophysiology

There are different functional types of telogen effluvium:

1. *Immediate anagen release*: Common after physiological stress and starting new medications. Follicles are stimulated to leave anagen and enter telogen prematurely, increased hair shedding occurs approximately 2–3 months later.
2. *Delayed anagen release*: Occurs in postpartum hair loss. During pregnancy, anagen duration is prolonged and hair cycling into telogen is reduced. Postpartum, a large number of follicles cycle into telogen together and increased shedding is noticed several months later.
3. *Short anagen syndrome*: Shortening of the duration of anagen can cause a persistent telogen hair shedding in some individuals.
4. *Immediate telogen release*: Results from premature exogen. May occur in AGA and 4–6 weeks after commencing minoxidil.
5. *Delayed telogen release*: occurs after prolonged telogen followed by transition to anagen. May occur seasonally in some humans.

Clinical features

Acute telogen effluvium occurs 2–3 months after a triggering physiological event. Daily hair loss ranges from under 100 to over 1000 hairs. It does not produce total baldness. Spontaneous complete regrowth occurs within 3–6 months.

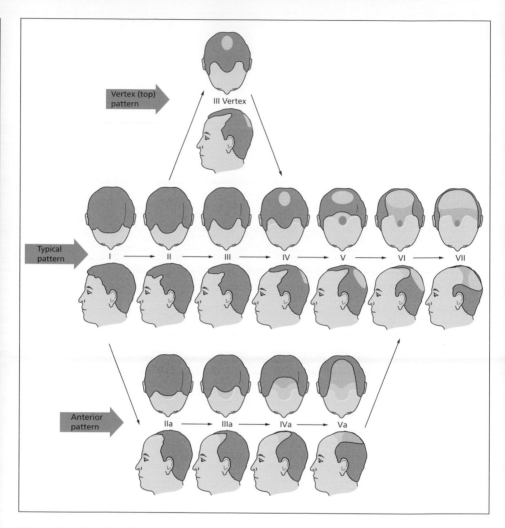

Figure 31.4 Hamilton–Norwood scale for grading male pattern hair loss. (Source: Based on Norwood OT. Male pattern baldness: classification and incidence. South Med J 1975, 68, 1359–1365.)

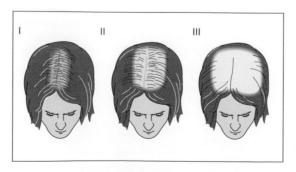

Figure 31.5 Ludwig scale for grading female pattern hair loss. (Source: Based on Ludwig E. Classification of the types of androgenetic alopecia (common baldness) occurring in the female sex. *Br J Dermatol* 1977, 97, 247–254.)

Table 31.1 Investigations and management of acquired non-scarring hair disorders

Condition	Hair-pull test	Dermoscopy	Blood tests, microbiology	Scalp biopsy	Management
AGA	Investigations are unnecessary unless there is diagnostic uncertainty				Minoxidil lotion (may cause local irritation) 5α-reductase inhibitors, either finasteride or dutasteride Surgery (hair transplantation)
FPHL	May have increase in telogen hairs	Contrasting hair density between the mid-frontal and occipital scalp No scarring seen	Full blood count, ferritin, thyroid function test, fasting lipids, fasting glucose If there are signs of virilisation/ hirsutism: serum testosterone, DHEAS 17-hydroxyprogesterone androstenedione, ovarian ultrasound, adrenal imaging	Terminal:vellus hair ratio <4:1 in FPHL	Minoxidil lotion Antiandrogens: cyproterone acetate, spironolactone, finasteride or flutamide
Acute telogen effluvium	Positive hair-pull test, with normal club hairs	No specific features	no specific blood tests or microbiology, unless alternative diagnoses suspected	No abnormality other than an increase in the proportion of follicles in telogen	Spontaneous complete regrowth occurs within 3–6 months
Chronic telogen effluvium	Positive hair-pull test, with normal club hairs	No specific features	Full blood count thyroid function tests. If clinically warranted: syphilis serology, antinuclear antibody titre, serum zinc levels and other investigations of nutritional status	Terminal:vellus hair ratio >8:1 in chronic telogen effluvium	Withdrawal of trigger (if relevant); full recovery of hair density may take 6 months May progress into FPHL, natural history unclear Minoxidil can reduce hair shedding
Alopecia areata	Increase in telogen hairs or dystrophic anagen hairs from affected areas	Exclamation mark hairs	If clinically indicated diagnostic tests may include fungal culture, serology for lupus erythematosus, serology for syphilis	Not usually indicated; may be helpful in diffuse alopecia and possible early scarring alopecia	Treatment not always required, especially if limited patchy loss <1 year duration Limited patchy alopecia: very potent topical steroid for at least 3 months, intralesional steroid injection Extensive/rapidly progressive alopecia: oral corticosteroids Contact immunotherapy

AGA, androgenetic alopecia; FPHL, female pattern hair loss; DHEAS, dehydroepiandrosterone sulphate.

Telogen gravidarum refers to the telogen hair loss seen 2–3 months after childbirth. Most resolve but a small proportion of women experience persistent episodic shedding that may be diffuse or localised.

Chronic telogen effluvium is hair shedding persisting for longer than 6 months. It may be primary (due to a change in hair cycle dynamics) or secondary (due to a variety of causes, including hormonal or metabolic disorders) (Figure 31.6).

Drug-induced diffuse telogen hair loss usually starts 6–12 weeks after instigation of treatment and is progressive while the drug is continued.

Differential diagnosis

Drug-induced telogen must be differentiated from chronic telogen effluvium.

An important differential for all of the telogens is androgenetic alopecia.

Investigations

See Table 31.1.

Management

See Table 31.1.

Alopecia areata

(Inc. Alopecia totalis, alopecia universalis)
A common, chronic, autoimmune, inflammatory disease that causes non-scarring hair loss.

Epidemiology

The incidence is 0.1–0.2% with a projected lifetime risk of 1.7%. It occurs in all ethnic groups. The age of onset is usually <40 years and there is equal sex distribution. It is associated with other autoimmune disorders; positive family history in 10–20% of affected individuals.

Pathophysiology

Alopecia areata is a T-cell mediated autoimmune disorder in genetically predisposed individuals. Associated with major histocompatibility complex genes, which control the activation and proliferation of T-regulatory lymphocytes and some genes expressed in the hair follicle. The role of

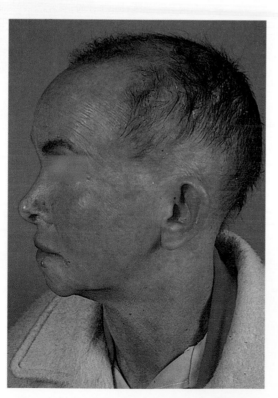

Figure 31.6 Chronic telogen effluvium resulting from acquired zinc deficiency resulting from prolonged parenteral feeding and inadequate zinc supplementation.

environmental factors is unclear. An inflammatory attack on anagen follicles precipitates follicles into telogen. Follicles re-enter anagen but development is halted in anagen and follicles return to telogen prematurely. Histology shows a predominantly lymphocytic infiltrate concentrated around the hair bulb at the edge of a patch of alopecia.

Clinical features

The characteristic initial lesion is a circumscribed, hairless, smooth patch (Figure 31.7a). The skin within the bald patch appears normal or slightly reddened. Short, easily extractable broken hairs (exclamation mark hairs) are often seen at the margins of the bald patches (Figure 31.7b). The subsequent progress is unpredictable; regrowth may occur within a few months or further patches may appear after varying intervals. Coalescing of patches can lead to a total loss of scalp hair (alopecia totalis) or a loss of all hair on the body (alopecia universalis). Regrowth is initially fine and non-pigmented, but usually the hairs gradually resume their normal calibre and colour.

In men, patches in the beard are conspicuous (Figure 31.7c). The eyebrows and eyelashes are lost in many cases of alopecia areata and may be the only sites affected. Alopecia along the back of the scalp hairline is known as ophiasis (Figure 31.7d). The disease process appears preferentially to affect pigmented hair. Alopecia areata causes fine stippled pitting of the nails (Figure 31.8).

Alopecia areata is classified as patchy alopecia, alopecia totalis (Figure 31.9) and alopecia universalis. Description of the pattern should include the presence of ophiasis, the involvement of sites on the trunk and limbs and the presence of nail disease.

Differential diagnosis

All causes of hair loss need to be considered, particularly tinea capitis, trichotillomania, systemic lupus erythematosus and secondary syphilis.

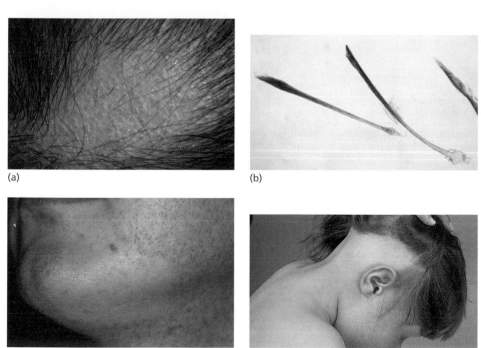

(a)　　　　(b)

(c)　　　　(d)

Figure 31.7 Alopecia areata. (a) Patch of alopecia areata showing broken 'exclamation mark hairs' towards the margins. (b) Close-up of exclamation mark hairs. (c) Alopecia areata affecting the beard. (d) The ophiasis pattern of alopecia areata.

PART 4: GENETIC DISORDERS INVOLVING THE SKIN

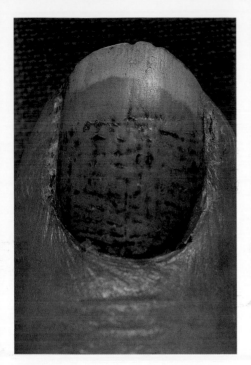

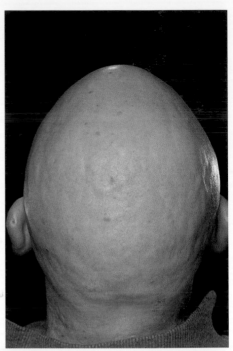

Figure 31.8 An organised pattern of pitting present on all fingernails 8 months prior to the onset of alopecia areata. The pits are highlighted with mascara.

Figure 31.9 Alopecia totalis. (Source: Courtesy of Dr J Ingram, University of Cardiff; Reproduced with permission of Cardiff and Vale University Health Board.)

Investigations
See Table 31.1.

Management
See Table 31.1. 34–50% of patients will recover within 1 year, although almost all will experience more than one episode of the disease. 14–25% progress to alopecia totalis or alopecia universalis, from which full recovery is unusual. Poor prognostic indicators are childhood onset and ophiasis pattern.

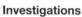

SCARRING ALOPECIAS

(Syn. Cicatricial alopecia)
Cicatricial alopecia is patchy hair loss, most commonly on the scalp, that follows the permanent destruction of hair follicles. It may be primary or secondary. Any hair-bearing skin may be affected. Approximately 7% of patients seen in specialist hair-loss clinics have scarring alopecia.

Follicular lichen planus

(See also chapter 12. Follicular lichen planus refers to lichen planus affecting the hair follicles. Three variants are recognised:

- Lichen planopilaris (LPP) is the commonest form and causes progressive scarring alopecia of the scalp.
- Frontal fibrosing alopecia (FFA) causes scarring alopecia of the frontal hairline typically in postmenopausal women.
- Graham–Little syndrome.

Epidemiology
FFA typically occurs in postmenopausal women, although it can occur earlier and in men. May be familial. Graham–Little syndrome mainly affects women between the ages of 30 and 70 years.

Pathophysiology

In LPP and FFA infiltration of inflammatory cells destroys the pilosebaceous unit. Basal cell damage by lymphocyte infiltration causes colloid body formation. Hairs are replaced by keratin plugs. The follicles are ultimately totally destroyed.

In Graham–Little syndrome the underlying follicle is progressively destroyed and eventually an atrophic epidermis covers sclerotic dermis. In the axillae and pubic region, the follicles are also destroyed but the skin does not appear clinically to be atrophic.

Clinical features

In LPP active areas show violaceous papules, erythema and scaling. The papules are replaced by follicular plugs and scarring (Figure 31.10). Eventually, the plugs are shed from the scarred area, which remains white, smooth and atrophic. Follicular orifices are absent within the area of alopecia. Other sites of predilection include the axillae, inguinal folds, sacrum and limb flexures.

In FFA recession of the frontal hairline is the cardinal feature (Figure 31.11), in contrast to AGA. The frontal hairline recedes in a straight line rather than bitemporally. Itch and pain are variable. Loss of eyebrows is a near universal finding. Body hair loss may also occur. Small papules on the cheeks and temples due to involvement of vellus follicles are seen in some patients.

In Graham–Little syndrome, progressive cicatricial alopecia of the scalp, loss of pubic and axillary hair without scarring and the rapid development of keratosis pilaris occur.

Differential diagnosis

Other causes of scarring alopecia.

Investigations

See Table 31.2.

Management

See Table 31.2. In some patients with LPP the disease course is slow and only causes a few bald patches, in others it causes extensive baldness. In FFA the natural history of frontal fibrosing alopecia is one of slow progression over many years. Recession of the hairline eventually stops in most cases.

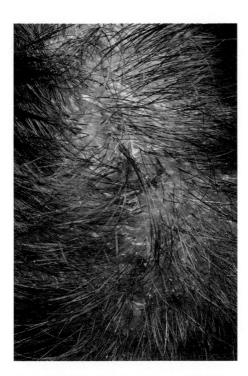

Figure 31.10 Scarring alopecia caused by lichen planus showing follicular plugs and scarring. (Source: Image courtesy of John Ingram, Cardiff University Archive; Reproduced with permission of Cardiff and Vale University Health Board.)

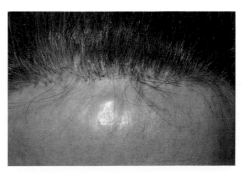

Figure 31.11 Frontal fibrosing alopecia showing scarring alopecia affecting the frontal hairline with follicular erythema and scale.

PART 4: GENETIC DISORDERS INVOLVING THE SKIN

Table 31.2 Investigations and management of acquired scarring hair disorders

Condition	Hair-pull test	Dermoscopy	Blood tests, microbiology	Scalp biopsy	Management
Follicular lichen planus	Positive at the margins, with twisted anagen hairs easily extracted	Loss of follicular orifices, and perifollicular erythema/ hyperkeratosis in active areas	–	As for non-specific cicatricial alopecia	Potent topical steroid scalp application Short course of oral corticosteroid may be used initially to stabilise the disease Hydroxychloroquine, acitretin and ciclosporin may be tried Evidence for treatments is poor
Pseudopelade of brocq	–	–	–	Absence of inflammation, scarring present, follicular plugging Decreased sebaceous glands, normal epidermis Direct immunofluorescence: negative	The alopecia is irreversible and does not respond to topical or intralesional corticosteroids The course is extremely variable, progression is often very slow and the entire process can burn out spontaneously at any stage, leaving behind only relatively small areas of alopecia
CCCA	–	Smooth shiny surface, some hairs left within area of alopecia	Culture for occult tinea capitis	Superficial perivascular and perifollicular lymphocytic infiltrate without interface change	Minimal hair grooming is recommended Potent topical corticosteroids may help Doxycycline or minocycline is useful in inflammatory cases with pustules Eventually burns-out spontaneously

Folliculitis decalvans	–	Inflammation and tufting can be seen without dermatoscope	Bacterial swabs from pustules Pluck hairs for fungal culture	PAS stain to rule out fungal infection	Mild cases: antiseptic shampoos and topical clindamycin Moderate/severe cases: flucloxacillin/ dicloxacillin/tetracyclines to induce remission but recurrence usually occurs when stopped Clindamycin 300 mg b.d. + rifampicin 300 mg; BD can induce prolonged remission Keratolytics and tar shampoos may reduce tufting Oral dapsone, laser depilation and surgical excision may be tried
Non-specific cicatricial alopecia	–	Loss of follicular ostia Hairs at the edge of a patch are often irregularly twisted	–	Histology variable and non-specific	No effective treatment known Prognosis is variable and unpredictable

CCCA, central centrifugal cicatricial alopecia; PAS, periodic acid Schiff.

PART 4: GENETIC DISORDERS INVOLVING THE SKIN

Chronic cutaneous lupus erythematosus

(Syn. Discoid lupus erythematosus)
See Chapter 23.

Pseudopelade of Brocq

An idiopathic, chronic, slowly progressive, patchy cicatricial alopecia that occurs without any evidence of inflammation.

Epidemiology
Women over 40 years are most commonly affected. Childhood cases are rare.

Pathophysiology
Aetiology and pathogenesis are unknown. It is almost always sporadic. Early lesions may have a light lymphocytic infiltrate around the upper two-thirds of the hair follicle. This infiltrate invades the walls of the follicles and sebaceous glands, and eventually destroys the pilosebaceous unit. Later patches show a thin atrophic epidermis overlying a sclerotic without inflammatory changes. Lichen planus can produce a very similar clinical picture and some believe that most cases of 'pseudopelade' are caused by lichen planus.

Clinical features
The alopecia is asymptomatic and always remains confined to the scalp. The initial patch is often on the vertex but may occur anywhere (Figure 31.12). The affected patches are smooth, soft and slightly depressed. Diagnostic criteria should be fulfilled before this specific diagnosis is made (Box 31.1).

Differential diagnosis
Lichen planopilaris, other causes of scarring alopecia.

Investigations
See Table 31.2.

Management
See Table 31.2.

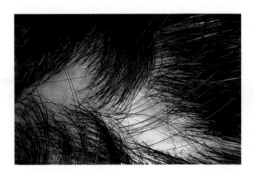

Figure 31.12 Pseudopelade of Brocq.

Box 31.1 Diagnostic criteria for pseudopelade of Brocq

Clinical criteria

- Irregularly defined and confluent patches of alopecia
- Moderate atrophy (late stage)
- Mild perifollicular erythema (early stage)
- Female:male ratio 3:1
- Long course (more than 2 years)
- Slow progression with spontaneous termination possible

Histological criteria

- Absence of marked inflammation
- Absence of widespread scarring (best seen with elastin stain)

- Absence of significant follicular plugging
- Absence, or at least a decrease, of sebaceous glands
- Presence of normal epidermis (only occasional atrophy)
- Fibrotic streams into the dermis

Direct immunofluorescence

- Negative (or only weak IgM on sun-exposed skin)

Central centrifugal cicatricial alopecia

(Syn. Hot comb alopecia)
Central centrifugal cicatricial alopecia (CCCA) is a scarring alopecia that mainly affects women of African ethnicity.

Epidemiology
The F:M ratio is approximately 3:1.

Pathophysiology
Pathogenesis is unknown, but likely to be multifactorial. Traumatic hair care practices have been implicated. A superficial perivascular and perifollicular lymphocytic infiltrate without interface change is seen in active areas. Sebaceous glands are lost; eccrine glands are spared. Hair follicle destruction is severe and widespread, and leaves prominent concentric lamellar fibrosis. Release of hair fragments into the dermis causes granulomatous inflammation.

Clinical features
Asymptomatic, slowly progressive and symmetrical alopecia predominately occurs centred on the crown with forward progression. There may be inflammation seen at the advancing margin but generally the skin is smooth, shiny and non-inflamed. The alopecia is incomplete, with a number of hairs remaining within the area of scarring.

Investigations
See Table 31.2.

Management
See Table 31.2.

Folliculitis decalvans and tufted folliculitis

An uncommon, progressive purulent folliculitis that may involve any hair-bearing site, although it is most common on the vertex of the scalp.

Epidemiology
Men may be affected from adolescence onwards, whereas women tend not to develop this condition until their 30s.

Pathophysiology
The cause of folliculitis decalvans is still not fully understood. Staphylococcus aureus may be grown from the pustules. The majority of people with bacterial pustular folliculitis of the scalp respond to antibiotics and heal without scarring. In folliculitis decalvans the folliculitis is more persistent, penetrates more deeply, tends to recur in the same site after apparently successful treatment with antibiotics and produces a scarring alopecia. Spread tends to be limited to neighbouring follicles so it is commonly unifocal.

Clinical features
Characterised initially by painful follicular pustules that become crusted. A patch of alopecia then develops from an expanding zone of folliculitis, eventually resulting in a central area of scarring. The scar is indurated and boggy rather than atrophic. Multiple hair tufts may be found emerging from a common dilated follicular opening, giving the appearance of doll's hair.

In advanced cases there is usually one, but occasionally more, rounded patches of alopecia over the vertex of the scalp surrounded by crusting and a few follicular pustules. Successive crops of pustules appear and are followed by progressive destruction of the affected follicles and lateral expansion of the alopecia (Figure 31.13).

Tufted folliculitis is a variant of folliculitis decalvans where circumscribed areas of scalp inflammation heal with scarring characterised by tufts of up to 30 hairs emerging from a single orifice (Figure 31.14).

Investigations
See Table 31.2.

Management
Treatment is mainly aimed at eradicating S. aureus from the scalp. See Table 31.2.

PART 4: GENETIC DISORDERS INVOLVING THE SKIN

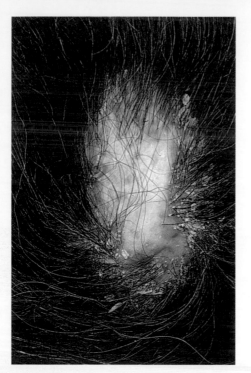

Figure 31.13 Folliculitis decalvans showing active pustulation and scarring.

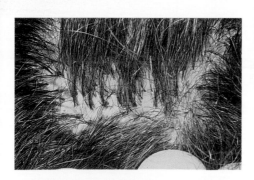

Figure 31.14 Tufted folliculitis.

Cosmetic alopecia

Cosmetic practices which result in damage to the hair shaft or the scalp. These include the application of heat, chemicals and traction.

Epidemiology

Traction alopecia is particularly common in African women.

Pathophysiology

The application of heat (e.g. from heated tongs) to damp hair may cause breakage due to the formation of bubbles in the hair shaft. Fracture of hair shafts may be caused by overuse of chemical treatments such as permanent waves and relaxers. Traction alopecia is brought about by hairstyles that impose sustained pulling on the hair roots, for example braiding (Figure 31.15), ponytails (Figure 31.16) and tight scarf styles.

Clinical features

Traction alopecia has many variants and clinical features include folliculitis, hair casts, reduction in hair density with vellus hairs and sometimes broken hairs in the affected areas. Scarring alopecia eventually occurs. It can be associated with headache, relieved when the hair is loosened.

Investigations

Perform bacterial swab or mycology if superadded infection is suspected, otherwise investigations not indicated.

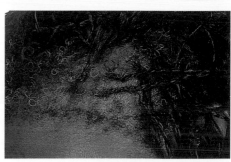

Figure 31.15 Traction alopecia from braiding.

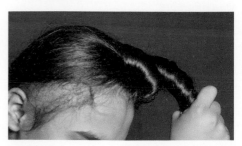

Figure 31.16 Traction alopecia in a Sikh boy.

Management

Avoidance of causative hair care practices. In its early stages traction alopecia may be reversible. Hairstyles that do not pull the hair tight must be adopted. Mild topical steroids can be helpful if inflammation is present, but this is not a substitute for a non-traction hairstyle. Once traction alopecia is established and follicles are lost, the hair loss is permanent.

Non-specific cicatricial alopecia

This causes an irregular area of cicatricial hair loss of the scalp with no distinguishing clinical or histological features.

Epidemiology

This is the most common diagnosis made among patients presenting with cicatricial alopecia; approximately one-third do not have an underlying cause diagnosed.

Pathophysiology

Damage to the bulge area of the hair follicle destroys any potential for hair regrowth. Histology is variable and non-specific. Scalp biopsies from the edge of a scarred patch may be either completely normal or show a non-specific lymphocytic infiltrate around the follicular infundibulum.

Clinical features

The initial patch often occurs over the crown. There is usually no erythema and the patches are smooth, shiny and slightly depressed.

Differential diagnosis

Other causes of scarring alopecia.

Investigations

See Table 31.2.

Management

See Table 31.2.

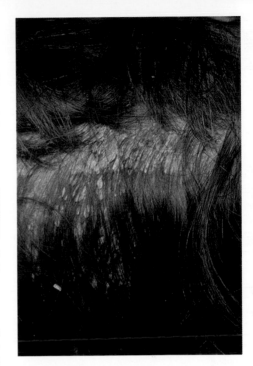

Fig 31.17 Pityriasis amiantacea secondary to psoriasis. (Source: Image courtesy of Dr J Ingram, Cardiff University archive.)

ACQUIRED DERMATOSES OF THE SCALP

Pityriasis amiantacea

Scaling on the scalp where matted scale progresses distally along the hair shaft (Figure 31.17).

Pathophysiology

Some believe pityriasis amiantacea is a form of severe psoriasis, others believe it is secondary to a range of causes (see Differential diagnosis). Scaling is caused by diffuse hyperkeratosis, parakeratosis and follicular keratosis, which surrounds each hair with a sheath of horn.

Clinical features

May be localised and confined to a small patch, or widespread. Lifting up the scale often results in hairs coming away, revealing a moist erythematous scalp. Hairs usually regrow if the underlying condition is treated.

Differential diagnosis

Seborrhoeic dermatitis, eczema, lichen simplex, psoriasis.

Investigations

The diagnosis is usually clinical, but scalp biopsy can be taken if there is any clinical doubt.

Management

Scale should be gently removed as described in the treatment of scalp psoriasis. Attention should then turn to treating the underlying condition, which typically involves the use of topical corticosteroids in an appropriate vehicle.

Dissecting cellulitis of the scalp

(Syn. Dissecting folliculitis, perifolliculitis capitis abscedens)

Dissecting cellulitis manifests with perifolliculitis of the scalp, deep and superficial dermal abscesses, sinus tracts formation and extensive scarring.

Epidemiology

Rare and occurs predominantly in dark-skinned males aged 18–40 years.

Pathophysiology

Aetiology unknown. No specific causative organism has been isolated. Associated with hidradenitis suppurativa and acne conglobata. Histology shows perifolliculitis, heavy mixed inflammatory infiltrate, abscess formation and destruction of pilosebaceous follicles and other appendageal structures.

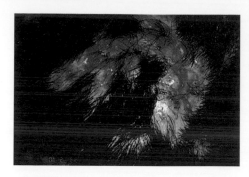

Figure 31.18 Dissecting cellulitis of the scalp. (Source: From Dyall-Smith D. Signs, syndromes and diagnoses in dermatology. Dissecting cellulitis of the scalp. Australas J Dermatol 1993, 34, 81–82, quiz 83–84.

Clinical features

Painful, firm, skin-coloured nodules develop near the vertex of the scalp, and later become softer and fluctuant (Figure 31.18). Confluent nodules form an irregular cerebriform pattern. There is often an exudate of blood-stained pus. Pressure on one region of the scalp may cause discharge of pus from a neighbouring intercommunicating ridge. Progressive scarring and permanent alopecia occur. The condition is chronic, with frequent acute exacerbations.

Other disorders of the follicular occlusion triad may be present and there may be an associated pilonidal sinus (the follicular occlusion tetrad) or spondyloarthropathy. An asymmetrical peripheral and axial arthritis occurs with sacroiliitis in 73%. Activity of the arthritis parallels activity of the skin.

Differential diagnosis

Kerion, pyoderma gangrenosum, erosive pustular dermatosis.

Investigations

Bacterial swab may show staphylococci, streptococci or *Pseudomonas*. Fungal scrape is negative.

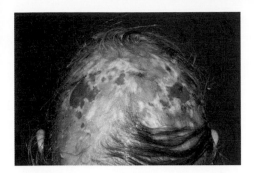

Figure 31.19 Erosive pustular dermatosis of the scalp.

Scalp biopsy will differentiate from other scarring alopecias. Direct immunofluorescence is negative.

Management

First line: Combination therapy with isotretinoin (1 mg/kg daily for minimum 6 months), prednisolone (0.5–1 mg/kg daily on a reducing course) and erythromycin (500 mg q.d.s. for 4 weeks)
Second line: For severe recalcitrant cases consider antitumour necrosis factor biological agents or excision and grafting.

Erosive pustular dermatosis of the scalp

Clinical entity affecting the elderly in association with advanced pattern hair loss.

Pathophysiology

There is a suggestion that local trauma and sun damage are important factors. Histology shows epidermal erosion, a dermal chronic inflammatory cell infiltration consisting of lymphocytes and plasma cells, and sometimes small foci of foreign body giant cells where the hair follicles have been destroyed.

Clinical features

Crusting and superficial pustulation overlies a moist, eroded surface (Figure 31.19). As the condition extends, areas of activity coexist with areas of scarring. Squamous carcinoma has been reported to develop in the scars.

Investigations

Biopsy if clinical diagnosis not clear.

Differential diagnosis

Pyogenic and yeast infection, pustular psoriasis, cicatricial pemphigoid, 'irritated' solar keratosis or squamous cell carcinoma.

Management

Potent topical corticosteroids. Maintenance therapy with sun protection and intermittent moderate-potency steroid can provide long-term relief.

INHERITED HAIR DISORDERS

Hair shaft defects

These are inherited conditions that usually result in hypotrichosis. May occur in isolation or part of a disorder.

Family history, neonatal or early onset and associated clinical features favour inherited hair diseases. Once it is clear that a patient is affected by an inherited form of hair defect it is important to establish (i) the mode of inheritance, (ii) extracutaneous manifestations and (iii) the absence or presence of microscopic structural hair shaft abnormalities. Correct genetic diagnosis is needed for proper genetic counselling and prenatal diagnosis, when indicated.

Table 31.3 summarises inherited hair-shaft structural abnormalities.

PART 4: GENETIC DISORDERS INVOLVING THE SKIN

PART 4: GENETIC DISORDERS INVOLVING THE SKIN

Table 31.3 Inherited hair-shaft structural abnormalities

Condition	Monilethrix (Syn. Beaded hair)	Pili torti (Syn. Twisted hair)	Trichorrhexis nodosa	Trichothiodystrophy	Pili annulati	Netherton syndrome (Syn. Bamboo hair)
Pathophysiology	Usually autosomal dominant Mechanism not known Note: pseudomonilethrix is an artefact produced by tweezers or compressing overlapping hairs	Mechanism not known A number of inherited conditions have pili torti	Believed to be a distinctive response of the hair shaft to injury, e.g. hairdressing practices Also part of inherited syndromes	Autosomal recessive, rare condition Disorder of DNA repair (see Chapter 37)	Autosomal dominant	Rare autosomal recessive disorder
Clinical features / hair findings	Beaded, fragile scalp hair (Figure 31.20) Gradually improves with age, may appear normal by puberty or early adulthood. Body/eyelash/eyebrow hairs are less frequently involved	Hairs show 180° twists under the microscope (Figure 31.22b) Scalp and body hairs are breakable, short and sparse (Figure 31.22a)	Irregularly spaced swellings along the hair shaft which are prone to fracture	Brittle and fragile hair; tiger tail on polarised microscopy (Figure 31.23) Hypotrichosis of scalp, eyebrows and eyelashes	Air-filled cavities are present within the hair shaft, causing alternating dark and light bands under the microscope	Hair is short, dry, lustreless and brittle Light microscopy shows 'bamboo hairs' (Figure 31.24) Eyebrows and lashes are sparse or absent
Associated features		Follicular papules in the nape area (Figure 31.21), keratosis pilaris and nail dystrophy	Found as part of complex syndromes	Found as part of complex syndromes	Nail dystrophy, short stature, progeroid facies with loss of adipose tissue, microcephaly, ocular manifestations, joint contractures, asthma	Generalised scaling and erythema present from birth Atopy, recurrent skin infections and a predisposition to skin malignancy

Differential diagnosis	Pili torti Pseudomonilethrix	Menkes disease (see Chapter 39), Björnstad syndrome, Netherton syndrome, Bazex syndrome	Usually a feature of conditions manifesting with hair fragility, e.g. Netherton syndrome, Menkes syndrome and trichothiodystrophy	Pili pseudoannulati (normal variant resulting from reflection of the light over flattened or twisted surfaces of the hair shaft)
Management	Minoxidil; oral retinoids successful in uncontrolled studies	Treat underlying condition	Treat underlying condition / There is no cure Overall median age of death is reported as 3 years	None specific - severity of the defect does not increase with age' / Avoidance of physical and chemical trauma

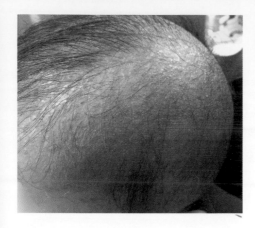

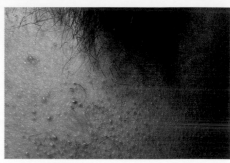

Figure 31.21 Monilethrix on the nape of the neck showing follicular keratoses and short, broken hairs.

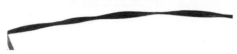

Figure 31.20 Short and sparse hair associated with follicular papules in a patient with monilethrix; hair beading typical of monilethrix on microscopy.

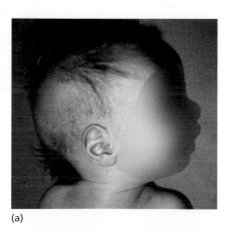

(a)

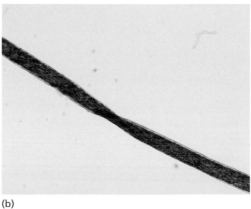

(b)

Figure 31.22 (a) Pale and sparse hair in a child with Menkes disease. (Source: Courtesy of Professor Rudolf Happle.) (b) Hair twisting along its axis, typical of pili torti. (Source: Courtesy of Professor Reuven Bergman.)

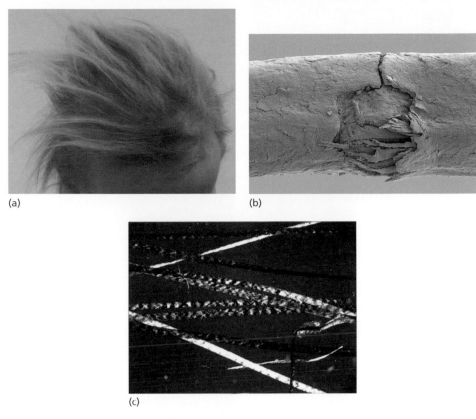

(a)   (b)

(c)

Figure 31.23 (a) Light-coloured and coarse hair in a patient with trichothiodystrophy. (Source: Courtesy of Professor Peter Itin.) (b) Defective cuticle visualised by scanning electron microscopy. (Source: Courtesy of Professor Peter Itin.) (c) Tiger tail banding under polarising light microscopy. (Source: Courtesy of Professor Reuven Bergman.)

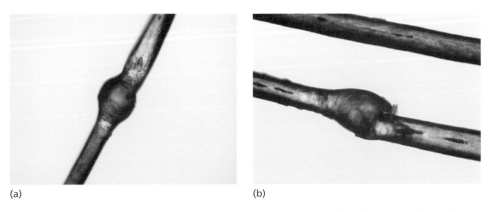

(a)   (b)

Figure 31.24 Netherton syndrome. (a) An invaginate node showing partial twisting of the hair at the upper pole. (b) An invaginate node acting as a point of weakness in the hair shaft.

EXCESSIVE GROWTH OF HAIR

Congenital generalised hypertrichosis

(Syn. Hypertrichosis lanuginose)
Fetal hair is not replaced by vellus and terminal hair but persists, grows excessively and is constantly renewed throughout life (Figure 31.25). Associated with other hereditary conditions: Hurler syndrome and other mucopolysaccharidoses (Chapter 39), Cornelia de Lange syndrome, Winchester syndrome, Berardinelli syndrome, fetal alcohol syndrome.

Other causes of hypertrichosis

- *Congenital localised hypertrichosis (Syn. Naevoid hypertrichosis)*: Excess hair present at birth and hamartomas that may have a delayed clinical presentation. They may occur in isolation as an area of increased hair density or in association with congenital melanocytic naevi, Becker naevi, spinal dysraphism ('faun tail', Figure 31.26) or neurofibromas.
- *Malignant acquired generalised hypertrichosis*: Sudden and generalised development of lanugo or non-androgen-dependent hair in adult life. A rare sign of underlying malignancy (gastrointestinal tract, lung or breast) but can also be due to other factors, including drugs.
- *Non-malignant acquired generalised hypertrichosis*: Can occur as the consequence of systemic disease and medications. Generally, the hair is coarser and less profuse than the lanugo hair associated with malignancy. Associated with drugs (e.g. ciclosporin, phenytoin, minoxidil, steroids), hypothyroidism, eating disorders and dermatomyositis.
- *Acquired localised hypertrichosis*: Associated with porphyria, topical medications (e.g. steroids, latanoprost/bimatoprost) and Graves disease.

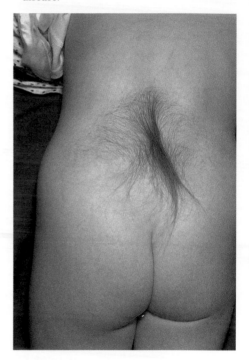

Figure 31.26 Lumbosacral hypertrichosis ('faun tail').

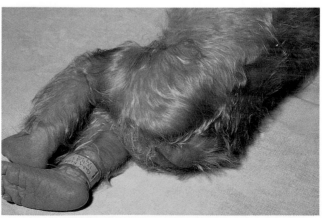

Figure 31.25 Congenital hypertrichosis lanuginosa. (Source: Courtesy of Dr Partridge, Leamington, UK.)

Acquired and inherited disorders of pigmentation

32

ACQUIRED HYPERPIGMENTATION

Physiological hyperpigmentation (tanning in response to UV radiation)

The tanning response to UV radiation varies between individuals, as summarised in Table 32.1, which lists the six common skin types.

Melasma

(Syn. Chloasma)

Melasma is the most common cause of facial melanosis and is manifested by hyperpigmented macules on the face which become more pronounced after sun exposure.

Epidemiology

Common. Increased pigmentation is almost invariable in pregnancy and is most marked in women with brown hair. Melasma is frequently seen in women on oral contraceptives and mostly starts between the ages of 20 and 40 years. More than 90% of cases are women and melasma is more common in light brown skin types, particularly Latin Americans and those from the Middle East or Asia.

Pathophysiology

UV exposure and hormonal factors, in particular pregnancy and oral contraceptives, are strongly linked with melasma. There is a family history in about 30% of those affected but no specific genes have been identified as yet.

Clinical features

Hyperpigmentation affects the upper lip, the malar regions, forehead and chin (Figure 32.1) and may be associated with darkening of the nipples and anogenital skin. Affected skin is brown in colour. The pigmentary changes are usually bilateral and are frequently symmetrical.

Wood's lamp examination can be helpful to identify the depth of the melanin pigmentation

Table 32.1 Classification of sun-reactive skin types

Skin type	Sun sensitivity	Pigmentary response
I	Very sensitive, always burn easily	Little or no tan
II	Very sensitive, always burn	Minimal tan
III	Sensitive, burn moderately	Tan gradually (light brown)
IV	Moderately sensitive, burn minimally	Tan easily (brown)
V	Minimally sensitive, rarely burn	Tan darkly (dark brown)
VI	Insensitive, never burn	Deeply pigmented (black)

Rook's Dermatology Handbook, First Edition. Edited by Christopher E. M. Griffiths, Tanya O. Bleiker, Daniel Creamer, John R. Ingram and Rosalind C. Simpson.
© 2022 John Wiley & Sons Ltd. Published 2022 by John Wiley & Sons Ltd.

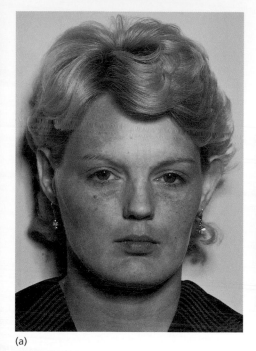

(a)

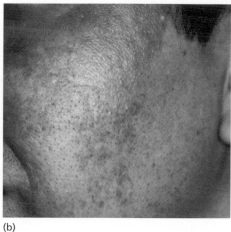

(b)

Figure 32.1 Melasma in (a) a Caucasian female and (b) an adult male from the Indian subcontinent.

and determine the type of melasma (epidermal, dermal or mixed). Epidermal melasma appears light brown and shows enhanced colour contrast with Wood's lamp examination. Dermal melasma appears slightly grey or bluish on gross examination and shows less colour contrast with Wood's lamp.

Differential diagnosis
Post-inflammatory hyperpigmentation from facial eczema, erythromelanosis follicularis faciei et colli, poikiloderma of Civatte, exogenous ochronosis.

Investigations
None needed.

Management
First line: Sun protection, change oral contraceptive to low-oestrogen, cosmetic camouflage.

Second line: Topical hydroquinone, tretinoin and corticosteroid compound cream.

Third line: Chemical peels, topical azelaic acid, laser therapy, dermabrasion.

Dermal melasma is generally less responsive to therapy, especially to topical modalities.

Poikiloderma of Civatte

Poikiloderma (telangiectasia, atrophy and dyspigmentation) which typically appears on the sides of the face and neck and on the upper anterior chest after years of repeated UV exposure.

Epidemiology
Incidence and prevalence are unclear. However fair-skinned women aged 30–50 are predominantly affected.

Pathophysiology
Exposure to light and photodynamic substances in cosmetics are likely to be environmental factors. Histology is similar to any case of poikiloderma.

Clinical features
Poikilodermatous changes develop symmetrically on the sides of the face, neck and upper aspect of the chest with hyperpigmentation, telangiectasia and dermal atrophy (Figure 32.2). The submandibular and submental areas are spared.

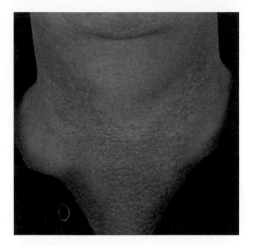

Figure 32.2 Poikiloderma of Civatte, showing submental and submandibular sparing on the neck of a 43-year-old man.

Differential diagnosis
Erythromelanosis follicularis faciei et colli, melasma.

Investigations
Patch testing can be useful if induction by allergen is suspected.

Management
First line: Sun protection, avoid perfumes.
Second line: Pulse dye laser, intense pulsed light.

Hypermelanosis due to endocrine disorders

There are a number of disorders causing hyperpigmentation (see Table 32.2).

Hypermelanosis in other systemic disorders

See below for a list of systemic causes of hypermelanosis.

- Neoplastic diseases
  - Oat cell carcinoma of the bronchus
  - Carcinoid tumours
  - Lymphoma
  - Phaeochromocytoma
- Rheumatic diseases
  - Systemic sclerosis and morphoea
  - Dermatomyositis
  - Lupus erythematosus
- Renal failure
- Primary biliary cirrhosis
- Haemochromatosis
- Cutaneous amyloidosis
- Nutritional deficiencies
  - Deficiencies of vitamins A, B12 and B3 and folate
- POEMS syndrome (*p*olyneuropathy, *o*rgano-megaly, *e*ndocrinopathy, *m*onoclonal gam-mopathy and *s*kin changes)

DRUG-INDUCED HYPERPIGMENTATION

Table 32.3 outlines the drugs that can cause hyperpigmentation.

Post-inflammatory hyperpigmentation

(Syn. Post-inflammatory hypermelanosis)
Residual macular pigmentation resulting from prior skin inflammation.

Epidemiology
Common, occurring more often in those with darker skin types. No sex or gender predisposition.

Pathophysiology
Occurs most often in conditions where inflammation affects the basal skin layer such as in lichen planus, lupus erythematosus and fixed drug eruption.

Clinical features
The pattern and distribution of the pigmentation will sometimes allow a retrospective diagnosis, as in lichen planus, herpes zoster, dermatitis herpetiformis and papular urticaria. Pigmentation is often prominent after lichenoid drug eruptions (Figure 32.5).

Investigations
None usually required because the diagnosis is obtained from history and examination.

PART 4: GENETIC DISORDERS INVOLVING THE SKIN

Table 32.2 Endocrine disorders causing hyperpigmentation

Condition	Addison disease	Acromegaly	Cushing syndrome	Hyperthyroidism
Pathophysiology	Increased secretion of pituitary melanotrophic hormones	Excessive growth hormone production	Overproduction of adrenocorticotropic hormone by pituitary corticotrophic adenoma or an ectopic non-pituitary tumour	Excessive production of thyroid gland hormones
Clinical features	Hyperpigmentation is diffuse and accentuated in sun-exposed areas, flexures and buccal mucosa (Figure 32.3)	Acquired diffuse hyperpigmentation	Marked hypermelanosis, mucous membranes often involved	Diffuse hyperpigmentation, involvement of mucous membranes uncommon

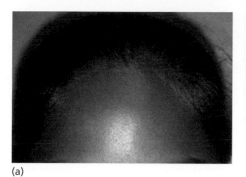

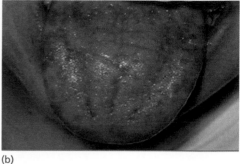

(a)   (b)

Figure 32.3 Addison disease: diffuse hypermelanosis of (a) the skin and (b) the tongue. (Source: Reproduced by permission of the copyright holder John Wiley and Son, Burk et al. Addison's disease, diffuse skin, and mucosal hyperpigmenation with subtle "flu-like" symptoms – a report of two cases. Pediatr Dermatol 2008, 25, 215–218.)

Table 32.3 Drugs causing hyperpigmentation

Drug	Description
Amiodarone	May cause photosensitive and phototoxic reactions in more than 50% of patients. Slate-gray or purple discoloration of mainly the sun-exposed skin, especially the face, in less than 5% (Figure 32.4). Higher risk with greater cumulative dose.
Anticonvulsants	Phenytoin, hydantoin and barbiturates may induce skin pigmentation.
Antimalarials	Bluish-grey pigmentation mainly on sun-exposed areas, including the face, neck and anterior legs and forearms may occur with chloroquine, quinine and quinidine. A yellowish pigmentation of the skin is common with mepacrine.
Clofazimine	Leprosy drug produces an initial redness of the skin due to drug accumulation. With prolonged treatment, a violaceous brown colour develops that is most noticeable in lesional skin.
Cytotoxic drugs	Onset of hyperpigmentation following antitumour agents is very variable, ranging from a week to several months and it can be either localised or diffuse. Pigmentation of the nails can be caused by many cytotoxic agents.
Psychotropic drugs	Trifluoperazine and imipramine can cause hyperpigmentation, and a small percentage of patients receiving high doses of chlorpromazine are also affected.
Tetracyclines	Tetracycline-induced skin discoloration, composed of well-circumscribed blue-grey macules, is mainly reported with minocycline and only rarely with other tetracyclines.

Management

Conservative management is usually recommended because spontaneous resolution generally occurs.

First line: Conservative. Resolution usually after 6–12 months but can be slower, particularly on lower legs.

Second line: Topical therapy, including retinoids, hydroquinone, azelaic acid.

Third line: Lasers. Q-switched ruby, alexandrite, Nd:YAG.

Exogenous ochronosis

Endogenous ochronosis is the term used to describe the pigmentary changes that occur in connective tissue in patients with alkaptonuria and is not discussed here. Exogenous ochronosis

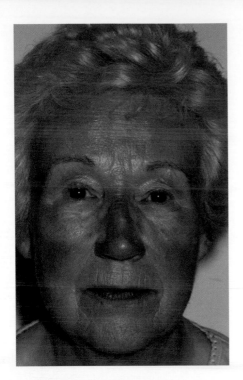

Figure 32.4 Slate-gray pigmentation from amiodarone.

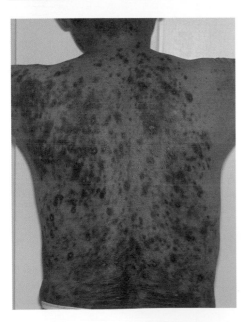

Figure 32.5 Post-inflammatory hyperpigmentation on the back following propranolol-provoked lichenoid drug reaction.

is discoloration of the skin after topical use primarily of hydroquinone, but may also be caused by phenol or resorcinol.

Epidemiology

The exact incidence is unknown and there are geographical variations depending on local use of skin-lightening cosmetics containing hydroquinone.

Pathophysiology

Histopathological examination is characterised by comma- or banana-shaped ochronotic collagen bundles. Deposition of ochre-coloured pigment can be seen.

Clinical features

Grey-brown or blue-black macules occur in the skin in contact with hydroquinone, normally the face, neck, back and the extensor surfaces of the limbs.

Differential diagnosis

Endocrinopathies: Addison disease, Cushing syndrome, hyperthyroidism.

Metabolic conditions: Porphyria cutanea tarda, haemochromatosis.
   Poikiloderma of Civatte.

Postinflammatory hyperpigmentation: Toxin- and drug-induced hyperpigmentation or discoloration (e.g. amiodarone, minocycline).

Investigations

Exogenous ochronosis is identified by the patient history. A skin biopsy provides helpful confirmation.

Management

First-line treatment is discontinuation of hydroquinone use and careful sun protection. Second-line treatment with superficial dermabrasion using carbon dioxide laser, glycolic acid peelings or Q-switched laser may improve the skin discoloration.

ACQUIRED HYPOPIGMENTATION

There are a number of causes of partial loss of normal pigmentation (hypopigmentation) and complete loss of pigmentation (depigmentation), as outlined in Figure 32.6.

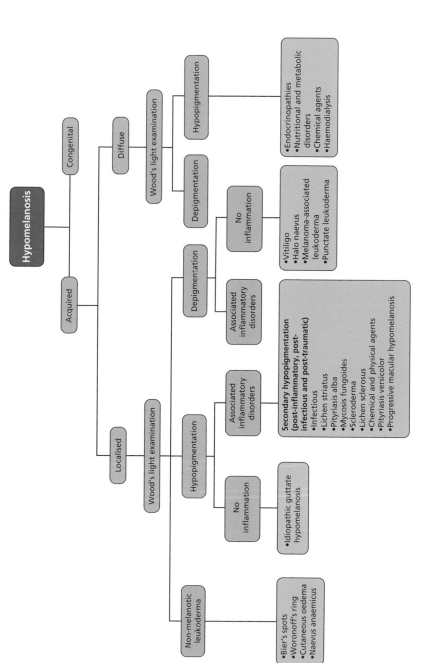

Figure 32.6 Algorithm for the differential diagnosis of hypomelanosis.

PART 4: GENETIC DISORDERS INVOLVING THE SKIN

Vitiligo

Vitiligo is a common form of localised depigmentation. It is an acquired condition resulting from the progressive loss of melanocytes.

Epidemiology

Global prevalence is 0.5–1% and there is probably no gender or ethnic variation. Onset can be at any age but in the majority of cases it becomes apparent in the third decade of life. Several conditions are associated with vitiligo, particularly autoimmune diseases, as listed in Box 32.1.

> **Box 32.1 Disorders associated with vitiligo**
> - Thyroid diseasea (hyperthyroidism and hypothyroidism)
> - Pernicious anaemia
> - Addison disease
> - Diabetes
> - Hypoparathyroidism
> - Myasthenia gravis
> - Alopecia areata
> - Morphoea and lichen sclerosus
> - Halo naevus
> - Malignant melanoma

Pathophysiology

Histochemical studies show only occasional melanocytes in the basal layer of the epidermis of affected skin areas. The exact pathophysiology of vitiligo is not understood. There is a genetic component because 30% of patients have a positive family history and vitiligo has been reported in monozygotic twins.

Clinical features

The amelanotic macules and patches of vitiligo are found particularly in acrofacial regions (Figure 32.7), as well as affecting areas of repeated friction such as the elbows, knees and ankles. Most commonly, the distribution of lesions is symmetrical. Segmental vitiligo is a clinical variant with typically unilateral involvement in a segmental/band-shaped distribution. Rarely, there is complete vitiligo (universalis). Hairs in the patches can remain normally pigmented, but can also depigment over time (poliosis/leukotrichia). Lesions are prone to sunburn due to loss of protective pigmentation. The Koebner phenomenon is observed in some cases, with occurrence of vitiligo in areas of skin trauma, such as surgery.

Differential diagnosis

Post-inflammatory hypopigmentation (e.g. pityriasis alba, lichen sclerosus, morphoea), post-infectious hypomelanosis (e.g. pityriasis versicolor, leprosy).

Investigations

Examination with the aid of a Wood's light is helpful to confirm the diagnosis and delineate extent of disease.

Management

Progression of vitiligo is unpredictable; it is usually gradually progressive but may extend rapidly over a period of several months and then remain quiescent for many years. Treatment is often unsatisfactory, particularly for acral lesions. Sun protection should be advised for affected sun-exposed areas and cosmetic camouflage should be offered.

First line: Topical therapy, including a trial of topical corticosteroid or topical calcineurin inhibitors for face/neck.

Second line: Phototherapy, either nbUVB or PUVA.

In those patients with extensive vitiligo and only a few residual areas of pigmentation, skin bleaching with laser therapy (e.g. Q-switched alexandrite 755 nm, Q-switched ruby 694 nm) or creams (e.g. 20% monobenzylether of hydroquinone) is sometimes considered.

Halo naevus

A halo naevus is a halo of hypopigmentation around a central cutaneous tumour. The tumour is usually a benign melanocytic naevus but

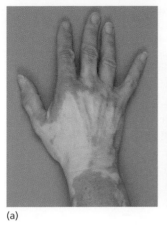
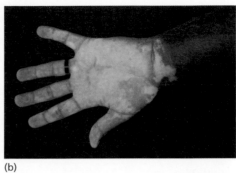

(a) (b)

Figure 32.7 Typical distribution of vitiligo on the hands under (a) natural light and (b) Wood's light.

may be a neuroid naevus, blue naevus, neurofibroma, or primary or secondary melanoma.

Epidemiology

The prevalence of halo naevi has been estimated to be approximately 1% in the white population. They occur at any age, but most frequently in younger people. There is an association with vitiligo and also Turner's syndrome.

Pathophysiology

Most halo naevi are compound naevi but junctional and dermal naevi are also affected. The naevi may be congenital or acquired. In the depigmented halo, there is an absence of melanocytes and there is frequently a lymphocytic infiltration of the naevus.

Clinical features

Circular areas of hypomelanosis 0.5–2.0 cm wide occur around pigmented naevi, particularly on the trunk, less commonly on the head and rarely on the limbs. Multiple lesions are common (Figure 32.8).

Investigation and management

The associated naevus should be assessed as for any other pigmented lesion. Most naevi will be benign and so conservative management is indicated. If melanoma is suspected then excision is required.

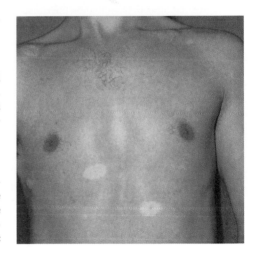

Figure 32.8 Multiple halo naevi in a young man who also had vitiligo.

Post-inflammatory hypopigmentation

(Syn. Post-inflammatory hypomelanosis)
Hypopigmentation occurring after the resolution of cutaneous inflammation.

Epidemiology

A common condition affecting males and females equally.

Pathophysiology

Box 32.2 lists the conditions that are the commonest causes. Mycosis fungoides is a rare additional cause.

Box 32.2 Commonest causes of post-inflammatory hypopigmentation

- Pityriasis versicolor
- Eczema
  - Pityriasis alba affecting the face of infants and children (Figure 32.9)
- Psoriasis
- Pityriasis lichenoides

Clinical features

Post-inflammatory hypopigmentation usually presents as moderately to well-demarcated areas of pigment loss. The distribution of the hypopigmentation is determined by the causative inflammatory dermatosis.

Investigations

If pityriasis versicolor is suspected: Wood's lamp examination to check for yellow-green fluorescence, skin scrapings for microscopic examination.

If mycosis fungoides is suspected: skin biopsy.

Management

In most cases post-inflammatory hypopigmentation resolves once the underlying cause is treated.

Progressive macular hypomelanosis

Progressive macular hypomelanosis (PMH) is a relatively common acquired dermatosis characterised by ill-defined nummular macules, mainly affecting the trunk.

Epidemiology

Adolescents and young adults are most often affected. The exact prevalence is unknown because PMH is often misdiagnosed.

Pathophysiology

It has been suggested that different subtypes of propionibacterium species might be responsible but the cause remains unproven.

Clinical features

PMH typically affects the trunk with ill-defined nummular hypopigmented non-scaly macules. The lesions are often more numerous around the midline (Figure 32.10).

Differential diagnosis

Pityriasis versicolor, post inflammatory hypopigmentation.

Investigations

Wood's light examination: orange-red fluorescence.

Management

PMH may regress spontaneously within a few years. Management strategies include topical antimicrobials and phototherapy.

Idiopathic guttate hypomelanosis

Idiopathic guttate hypomelanosis (IGH) is an acquired leukoderma with discrete round to oval porcelain-white macules approximately 2–6 mm diameter increasing in number with age.

Epidemiology

A common condition, seen in up to 80% of patients over the age of 70 years. There is probably no gender bias, but more women may seek a medical opinion. The condition particularly affects those of lighter skin types.

Pathophysiology

Histologically, IGH lesions are characterised by slight basket-weave hyperkeratosis with epidermal atrophy and flattening of the rete pegs; there is a decrease in melanocytes.

Clinical features

Clinically, the lesions are porcelain-white macules, usually 2–6 mm in size but sometimes larger (Figure 32.11). The borders are sharply

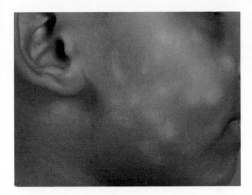

Figure 32.9 Pityriasis alba.

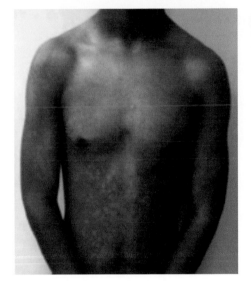

Figure 32.10 Progressive macular hypomelanosis in an 18-year-old man. (Source: Reproduced with permission from the copyright holder Springer Publishing Company, from Relyveld et al. Progressive macular hypomelanosis: an overview. Am J Clin Dermatol 2007, 8, 13–19.)

defined, often angular and irregular. Typical locations include the pretibial side of the legs and the forearms, as well as other chronic sun-exposed sites, including the face, neck and shoulders.

Management
Reassurance.

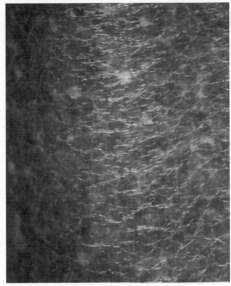

Figure 32.11 Idiopathic guttate hypomelanosis on the shins of a 57-year-old Afro-Caribbean woman.

INHERITED HYPERPIGMENTATION DISORDERS

Incontinentia pigmenti

Incontinentia pigmenti (IP) is a rare X-linked dominant multisystemic ectodermal dysplasia that is usually lethal in males and that presents classically in females with skin lesions, teeth abnormalities, alopecia, nail dystrophy and ocular and neurological findings.

Epidemiology
Birth prevalence is 0.6–0.7/1 000 000. F:M ratio is 20:1.

Pathophysiology
IP is caused by mutations of the IKBKG gene encoding the nuclear factor (NF)-κB essential modulator (NEMO). The mutation can be inherited from an affected mother or occur *de novo*. When the mother of an affected female carries the mutant *IKBKG*, the risk to siblings

of inheriting the mutant *IKBKG* allele at conception is 50%; most male conceptuses with loss-of-function mutation of *IKBKG* are miscarried.

Clinical features

IP cutaneous findings typically present perinatally with an erythematous vesicular rash (bullous stage I, Figure 00.10a) following Blaschko's lines. Stage I evolves within a few months to a verrucous stage II, occurring mainly on the limbs (Figure 32.12b). Stage III hyperpigmented streaks and whorls along Blaschko's lines begin within months and fade in adolescence (Figure 32.12c). Stage I rash can recur during febrile illness. Stage IV patients have pale, hairless, atrophic linear streaks or patches mostly on the lower extremities at adolescence (Figure 32.12d). Extracutaneous abnormalities observed in IP include delayed dentition and missing or malformed cone-shaped teeth (Figure 32.13). Other manifestations include onychodystrophy, alopecia and a wide range of ophthalmological abnormalities with retinal neovascularisation. Central nervous system

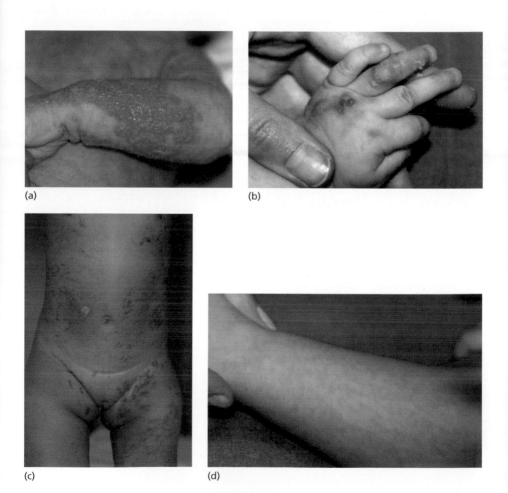

(a)   (b)

(c)   (d)

Figure 32.12 (a) Incontinentia pigmenti, vesiculobullous stage, frequently wrongly diagnosed as bullous impetigo. (b) Verrucous stage. (c) Pigmentary stage, with an obvious linear pattern following Blaschko's lines. (d) Hypopigmented stage with hair loss.

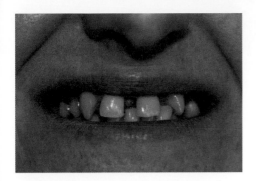

Figure 32.13 Dystrophic teeth in the carrier mother of a child with incontinentia pigmenti.

abnormalities may comprise microcephaly, seizures and neurocognitive and motor impairments. The majority (>60%) of patients are neurologically normal.

Differential diagnosis
Stage I lesions have to be distinguished from other bullous dermatoses (bullous impetigo, epidermolysis bullosa, herpes or varicella). Differential diagnosis of stage II includes warts or epidermal naevus syndrome. Any condition with 'linear and swirled' pigmentation overlaps with stage III. Stage IV resembles scarring, Ito's hypomelanosis or other hypopigmentary disorders with localised alopecia.

Management
No specific treatment is available for IP. Symptomatic treatment includes standard management of blisters. Ophthalmological follow-up is required for retinal neovascularisation monitoring and treatment (cryotherapy and laser photocoagulation) and treatment of retinal detachment if it occurs. Dental abnormalities should be managed by a paediatric orthodontist in combination with speech therapy and a paediatric nutrition programme. Patients should be referred to a paediatric neurologist for evaluation if microcephaly, seizures, spasticity or focal deficits are present. Brain magnetic resonance imaging is indicated in any child with functional neurological abnormalities or retinal neovascularisation.

INHERITED HYPOPIGMENTATION DISORDERS

Piebaldism

Piebaldism is a rare autosomal dominant trait characterised by well-demarcated irregular hypopigmented macules.

Epidemiology
The incidence of piebaldism is estimated at less than 1 in 20 000. Both sexes are affected equally and there is no ethnic predisposition.

Pathophysiology
The disease results from heterozygous mutations in *KIT*, encoding c-KIT, a membranal tyrosine kinase receptor responsible for triggering cell proliferation and migration. Dominant mutations in *KIT* result in impaired migration of melanocytes to the skin, as reflected by the absence of melanocytes and melanin in hypopigmented patches.

Clinical features
The commonest clinical feature of the disease is a white forelock (poliosis), often associated with a V-shaped area of leukoderma on the mid-forehead. The hypopigmented lesions of piebaldism have a predilection for the anterior part of the body and the mid-portion of the limbs (Figure 32.14). Often, white patches occur on the upper chest, abdomen and limbs, bilaterally but not necessarily symmetrically. The hands and feet, as well as the back, remain normally pigmented. The extent of the areas of depigmentation is variable and, rarely, the white forelock may be the only lesion. Piebaldism is usually not associated with extracutaneous manifestations.

Differential diagnosis
Vitiligo, alopecia areata, Waardenburg syndrome.

Management
The evolution of piebaldism is benign. Sun protection is recommended to protect the amelanotic areas from burning.

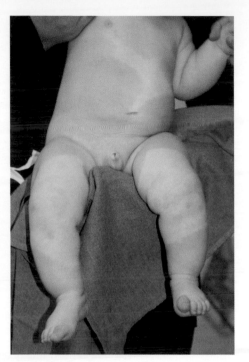

Figure 32.14 Typical body and limb pattern of hypopigmentation in piebaldism.

Waardenburg syndrome

Waardenburg syndrome (WS) is an autosomal dominant genetic disorder characterised by piebaldism and sensorineural deafness. A molecular classification is used (WS1–4) based on the mutant gene. It is an autosomal dominant condition except for the recessive WS4.

Epidemiology
Estimated incidence is 1 in 20 000–40 000.

Pathophysiology
All abnormalities seen in WS involve the neural crest lineage. Type 1 and type 3 result from loss-of-function mutations in the *PAX3* gene. Mutations in several different genes result in WS type 2 and type 4.

Clinical features
WS features congenital leukoderma reminiscent of piebald pattern in association with sensorineural deafness of varying severity. Areas of hypopigmentation may diminish in size or even disappear with time.

Management
Management of the hearing loss associated with WS1 depends on its severity. The hearing loss in WS1 is typically non-progressive. Hence, repeating the audiogram is usually unnecessary.

Oculocutaneous albinism

Oculocutaneous albinism (OCA) is a rare genetic disorder characterised by generalised depigmentation of the skin, hair and eyes, and by ophthalmological anomalies caused by a deficiency in melanin biosynthesis. A molecular classification is used (OCA1–7) derived from the mutant genes responsible.

Epidemiology
OCA is the most frequent form of diffuse hypopigmentation worldwide with a prevalence estimated around 1/20 000. The prevalence of the various OCA subtypes varies considerably from one continent to another, but OCA1 is the most frequent form worldwide. OCA2 is the most frequent form among African patients with a prevalence that reaches 1/1000 in some populations in Western Africa.

Pathophysiology
OCA is due to a deficiency of melanin biosynthesis but melanocytes are normally present and distributed. The reduction of the amount of melanin is responsible for an increased sensitivity to UV radiation and for a predisposition to skin cancers. The ophthalmological anomalies associated with albinism are not only a consequence of a lack of melanin but also of a lack of L-DOPA, an early intermediate of the synthesis of melanin, which has been shown to be required for normal retinal and visual development.

Clinical features
The pigmentation of the skin, hair and eyes is in general reduced but its degree varies with the

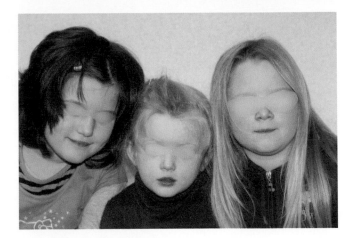

Figure 32.15 Oculocutaneous albinism type 1B (OCA1B) and siblings. The children in the centre and on the right are affected; the child on the left is unaffected.

type of albinism. It is important to check pigmentary characteristics in siblings and parents to consider the diagnosis of albinism in its subtle variants (see Figure 32.15).

All types of OCA and ocular albinism have similar ocular findings, including various degrees of congenital nystagmus, hypopigmentation of the iris leading to iris translucency, reduced pigmentation of the retinal pigment epithelium, foveal hypoplasia, reduced visual acuity usually in the range 20/60 to 20/400 and refractive errors, and sometimes a degree of colour vision impairment. Photophobia may also be prominent.

Differential diagnosis

Histidinaemia, homocystinuria, phenylketonuria, Hermansky–Pudlak syndrome, Chediak–Higashi syndrome.

Investigations

The diagnosis of OCA is based on clinical findings of hypopigmentation of the skin and hair. Ophthalmological examination should include an examination with optical coherence tomography of the retina showing characteristic foveal hypoplasia. Electrophysiological testing can demonstrate misrouting of the optic nerves, resulting in strabismus and impaired stereoscopic vision.

Due to clinical overlap between the OCA subtypes, molecular diagnosis is necessary to establish a correct diagnosis and subsequently provide patients and their families with prognostic information and genetic counselling.

Management

Sun protection is vital to avoid skin sunburns and skin cancers, with a special emphasis in patients living in high UV risk environments. Early referral to an ophthalmologist is mandatory. Decreased visual acuity is usually managed with corrective lenses while strabismus requires eye patching or surgical correction. Dark glasses are important to protect the eyes and prevent photophobia.

Hypomelanosis of Ito

Hypomelanosis of Ito is a rare neuroectodermal disorder often associated with mental retardation and epilepsy.

Epidemiology

Prevalence is unknown but incidence has been estimated between 1/10 000 and 1/8500.

Pathophysiology

Nearly all cases are sporadic, suggesting a postzygotic mutation, which is assumed to be lethal when transmitted to offspring. Various chromosomal anomalies have been identified and the current consensus is that the phenotype is the result of cutaneous mosaicism, either for a monogenic or a chromosomal disorder, rather than being a distinct disease.

Clinical features

The skin abnormalities are characterised by unusual unilateral or bilateral cutaneous macular hypopigmented whorls, streaks and patches, corresponding to the lines of Blaschko (Figure 32.16). Extracutaneous findings include neurological, ophthalmological and skeletal defects.

Differential diagnosis

Other mosaic depigmented lesions, focal dermal hypoplasia.

Management

Referral for neurology and/or ophthalmological opinions may be needed.

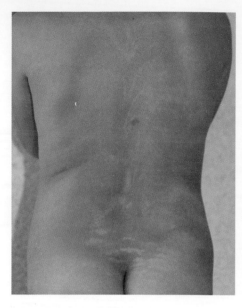

Figure 32.16 Hypomelanosis of Ito.

Epidermolysis bullosa

33

Epidermolysis bullosa (EB) describes a group of uncommon inherited (genetic) disorders characterised by blistering of the skin and mucosae following mild mechanical trauma. There are four major types of EB based upon the site of split where the blister occurs (Table 33.1 and Figure 33.1).

Epidemiology

The incidence and prevalence of EB are estimated to be 19.60 per million live births and 8.22 per million population, respectively. The incidence and prevalence rates for EB simplex are 10.75 and 4.60, for junctional EB are 2.04 and 0.44, for dominant dystrophic EB are 2.86 and 0.99 and for recessive dystrophic EB are 2.04 and 0.92, respectively. These rates are probably underestimated. There is no gender, racial, ethnic or geographical predilection.

Pathophysiology

Eighteen different genes have mutations relevant to the pathogenesis of EB (Figure 33.2). These genes encode proteins involved in the structural adhesion of cell–cell and cell–matrix junctions as well as keratinocyte integrity and differentiation. Changes in the target proteins lead to splitting of the skin at different sites (depending on the location of the affected protein).

EB simplex (Table 33.2)

The cleavage lies within the basal cells of the epidermis. Most are autosomal dominant, two-thirds have underlying mutations in KRT5 (keratin 5) or KRT14 (keratin 14).

Table 33.1 The major forms of EB (see Clinical features for further details)

Level of skin cleavage	EB type	EB subtype	Defective protein(s)
Intraepidermal	EB simplex	Suprabasal EB simplex	Transglutaminase-5, plakophilin-1, desmoplakin, plakoglobin
		Basal EB simplex	Keratins 5 and 14, plectin, exophilin-5, bullous pemphigoid antigen 1/dystonin
Intralamina lucida	Junctional EB	Junctional EB generalised	Laminin-332, type XVII collagen α6, β4, α3 integrin subunits
		Junctional EB localised	Type XVII collagen, laminin-332 α6, β4 integrin subunits
Sublamina densa	Dystrophic EB	Dominant dystrophic EB	Type VII collagen
		Recessive dystrophic EB	Type VII collagen
Mixed	Kindler syndrome		Kindlin-1 (fermitin family homologue-1)

Rook's Dermatology Handbook, First Edition. Edited by Christopher E. M. Griffiths, Tanya O. Bleiker, Daniel Creamer, John R. Ingram and Rosalind C. Simpson.
© 2022 John Wiley & Sons Ltd. Published 2022 by John Wiley & Sons Ltd.

Table 33.2 Different subtypes and clinical features of EB simplex

EB simplex type	EB simplex subtype	Targeted protein(s)	Clinical features
Suprabasal	Acral peeling skin syndrome, autosomal recessive	Transglutaminase-5	Resembles localised EB simplex but blisters occur on sides of feet
	EB simplex superficialis	Unknown	Very rare Superficial erosions rather than intact blisters
	Ectodermal dysplasia-skin fragility syndrome	Plakophilin-1	Widespread erosions present at birth Loss of scalp hair and eyebrows, perioral cracking
	Severe acantholytic EB	Desmoplakin[a], Plakoglobin[a]	Very severe blistering and erosions Abnormal nails, teeth, intraoral lesions and alopecia
Basal	EB simplex, localised	Keratins 5 and 14	Usually childhood onset Painful blistering on palms and soles, not on sides of feet (Figure 33.3)
	EB simplex, generalised severe ~30% sporadic	Keratins 5 and 14	Previously called Dowling–Meara EB simplex Severe blistering in early infancy, including mucous membranes, nail shedding, milia formation Later characterised by spontaneous herpetiform, annular or arcuate blistering on the trunk, limbs and neck (Figure 33.4) Blistering and hyperkeratosis of the palms and soles
	EB simplex, generalised intermediate	Keratins 5 and 14	Blisters within the first year of life Usually mild but scarring and milia seen in 60% of patients Palms and soles rarely affected
	EB simplex, mottled pigmentation	Keratin 5	Reticulate pattern of small, tan-coloured macules, often fade with age May be present at birth or appear during infancy Palmoplantar punctate keratosis, sometimes keratoderma Mild localised skin atrophy and nail dystrophy
	EB simplex, migratory circinate	Keratin 5	Very rare

EB simplex, autosomal recessive (K14)	Keratin 14	Scattered blisters, minor palmoplantar keratoderma and varying degrees of nail dystrophy, atrophic scarring, hyperpigmentation and mucosal blistering (Figure 33.5)
EB simplex, autosomal recessive (BP230)	230 kDa bullous pemphigoid antigen	Mild, generalised blisters, heal without scarring (Figure 33.6) Mucosae unaffected
EB simplex – autosomal recessive (exophilin-5)	Exophilin-5	Mild, scattered, trauma-induced skin fragility
EB simplex – muscular dystrophy	Plectin	Skin and mucosal fragility/blistering associated with neuromuscular disorder
EB simplex – Ogna	Plectin	Rare Seasonal blistering of the hands and feet Generalised bruising tendency, haemorrhagic bullae, and onychogryphotic great toenails

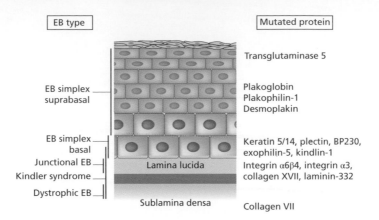

Figure 33.1 Epidermis and basement membrane illustrating the different levels where blisters occur in subtypes of EB as well as the location of the targeted proteins.

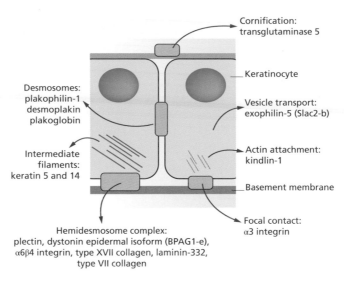

Figure 33.2 The collection of proteins involved in the pathogenesis of EB. Clinical features are detailed in Tables 33.2–33.4.

Junctional EB (Table 33.3)

The cleavage lies within the basement membrane (lamina lucida). Autosomal recessive inheritance. Eight genes have been identified in the pathology of this subtype.

Dystrophic EB (Table 33.4)

The cleavage is subepidermal. May be autosomal dominant or recessive. All result from *COL7A1*mutations, which encodes type VII collagen.

Kindler syndrome

Site of cleavage is variable. Autosomal recessive. Loss-of-function mutations on the KIND1/FERMT1 gene.

Clinical features

EB simplex

Can be categorised as 'suprabasal' or 'basal', with several different subtypes under these categories. Clinical features are shown in Table 33.2.

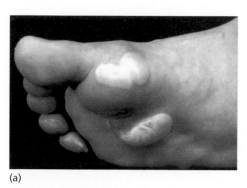

(a)

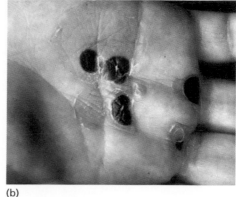

(b)

Figure 33.3 Localised EB simplex: (a) blisters on the foot and (b) blisters (some haemorrhagic) and erosions on the palm.

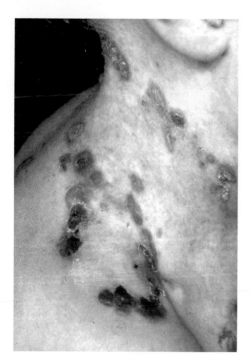

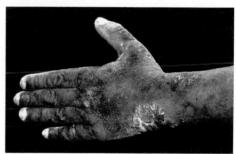

Figure 33.5 Acral blistering in a patient with autosomal recessive EB simplex with loss of keratin 14 expression in the skin.

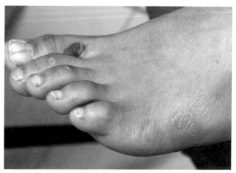

Figure 33.4 Grouped blisters on an erythematous base in generalised severe EB simplex.

Junjctional EB

Can be classified as generalised or localised with several different subtypes under these categories. Clinical features are shown in Table 33.3.

Figure 33.6 Localised blistering on the foot in a patient with autosomal recessive EB simplex due to autosomal recessive mutations in BP230. (Source: Courtesy of Dr A. Nanda, Kuwait.)

Table 33.3 Different subtypes and clinical features of junctional EB

Junctional EB type	Junctional EB subtype	Targeted protein(s)	Clinical features
Generalised	Severe	Laminin-332	Severe blisters/erosions at birth (Figure 33.7) Skin fragile, extensive epidermal loss on minimal skin handling Oropharyngeal involvement frequent High mortality in early infancy
	Intermediate	Laminin-332, type XVII collagen	Less severe, most survive to adulthood (Figure 33.8)
	Late onset	Type XVII collagen	Rare, symptoms present between 5 and 8 years of age
Localised	Localised	Laminin-332, type XVII collagen, α6 and β4 integrin subunits	Nail dystrophy, dental enamel changes, blistering of lower legs and feet only
	Inversa	Laminin-332	Lesions mainly in groin, perineal and axillary areas
	Laryngo-onycho-cutaneous syndrome	Laminin α3a	Lesions mainly affect the face and nails Associated with hoarseness of voice

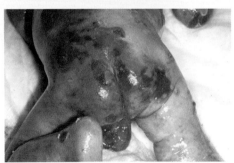

Figure 33.7 Extensive erosions over the buttocks in an infant with severe generalised junctional EB.

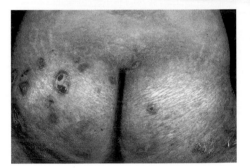

Figure 33.8 Erosions, scarring and atrophy on the buttocks of a patient with generalised intermediate junctional EB.

Dystrophic EB

Can be classified as dominant or recessive (Table 33.4). Characterised by skin fragility, blistering, scarring, nail dystrophy and milia formation. Mucosal involvement is common, and erosions and scarring can affect the mouth, oesophagus, genitalia and anus.

Kindler syndrome

Can initially resemble generalised or localised forms of dystrophic EB. Skin blistering lessens during childhood and instead signs of a progressive poikiloderma develop (Figure 33.13). Skin changes are worse in sun-exposed individuals.

Differential diagnosis

In the neonatal period differential diagnoses to consider include bullous congenital ichthyosiform erythroderma, staphyloccocal scalded skin syndrome, bullous impetigo, incontinentia pigmenti, neonatal herpes simplex, autoimmune bullous disease, aplasia cutis, focal dermal hipoplasia, Gunther disease.

Table 33.4 Different subtypes and clinical features of dystrophic EB

Dystrophic EB type[a]	Dystrophic EB subtype	Clinical features
Dominant	Generalised	Blisters following trauma overlying bony prominences Localised scarring, milia, dystrophic nails (Figure 33.9)
	Acral	Trauma-induced blistering, scarring and milia in acral skin
	Pretibial	Blisters, atrophy and scarring on the shins Dystrophic nails May mimic lichen planus Onset may be delayed
	Pruriginosa	Overlap with pretibial variant but with intense pruritus
	Nails only	Nail dystrophy but no history of blisters
	Bullous dermolysis of the newborn	Blistering in neonates spontaneously improves over the first few weeks or months of life
Recessive	Generalised severe	Very fragile skin, blisters on minimal trauma, occurs from birth Atrophic scars, milia, sloughy erosions, extreme pain, severe oral lesions Repeated blistering and scarring causes fusion of digits and 'mitten' deformity (Figures 33.10 and 33.11) Complications are growth retardation, anaemia and risk of squamous cell carcinoma at young age Death in middle-age
	Generalised intermediate	Much milder version of generalised severe recessive dystrophic EB
	Inversa	Blistering and scarring in the groins, axillae, neck and lumbar area (Figure 33.12) Risk of developing squamous cell carcinoma
	Localised	Usually mild, skin fragility, scarring and milia are mostly confined to hands, feet and nails
	Pretibial, pruriginosa and bullous dermolysis of the newborn	Can occur as a dominant or recessive trait See dominant section for clinical features

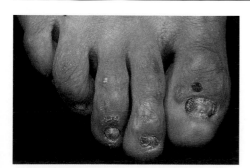

Figure 33.9 Nail changes and scarring of skin on the toes in dominant dystrophic EB. (Source: Courtesy of Professor R.A.J. Eady, St John's Institute of Dermatology, London, UK.)

In infants/older children/adults differential diagnoses to consider are acquired autoimmune bullous diseases, e.g. bullous pemphigoid, mucous membrane pemphigoid or linear IgA disease.

Kindler syndrome may mimic dyskeratosis congenita and Rothmund–Thomson syndrome.

Investigations

Shave biopsy of blister less than 12 h old is required. Ideally, non-involved skin should be rubbed to cause mild erythema and biopsy from this area should be taken. Biopsy should be sent for histology, electron microscopy and direct immunofluorescence. Level of split is established through electron microscopy.

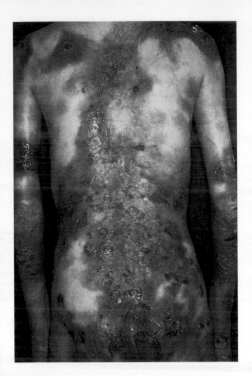

Figure 33.10 Extensive lesions on the back in severe generalised recessive dystrophic EB. (Source: Courtesy of Professor R.A.J. Eady, St John's Institute of Dermatology, London, UK.)

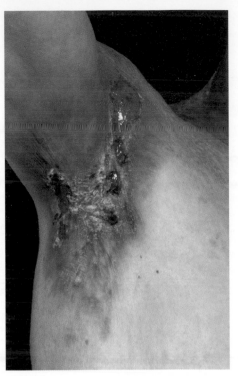

Figure 33.12 Scarring and erosions affecting the axilla and neck in the inversa form of recessive dystrophic EB. (Source: Courtesy of Professor R.A.J. Eady, St John's Institute of Dermatology, London, UK.)

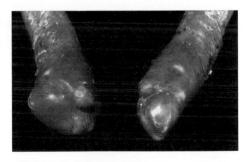

Figure 33.11 Mitten hand deformity in severe generalised recessive dystrophic EB. (Source: Courtesy of Professor R.A.J. Eady, St John's Institute of Dermatology, London, UK.)

Antigen mapping using immunohistochemical staining will establish the affected protein and DNA analysis of blood or saliva samples will establish the affected gene.

Management

There is no curative treatment for any form of EB. The mainstay of management is based on multidisciplinary input, protection of skin and avoidance of provoking factors. Paediatric nurse specialists should ideally coordinate and lead the management of neonates/infants with blistering skin disorders. Specialist services for the management of patients with EB are available. Early involvement of these services is paramount.

Protection of skin:

- Nurse neonates/infants on foam pads.
- Clean erosions with sterile normal saline, cover with non-adherent dressings.
- Consider topical antiseptics to reduce risk of infection.
- Identify and treat infection early.

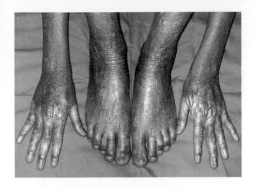

Figure 33.13 Poikiloderma in a 12-year-old Indian patient with Kindler syndrome.

Considerations for specific conditions:

- EB simplex: reduce heat/humidity as blisters worsen under these conditions, e.g. specialised footwear, Botox for hyperhidrosis.

- Generalised severe recessive dystrophic EB: 6-monthly review in multidisciplinary clinic, oral/dental care from dentist with experience in EB, monitor for oesophageal structures, artificial tears and urgent attention to any corneal abrasions, monitoring and management of anaemia, provide calcium and vitamin D replacement, monitor for osteoporosis, monitor for genito-urinary and renal complications, regular physiotherapy to aid with contractures, pain relief, monitor for squamous cell carcinoma development (6-monthly review).
- Split thickness skin grafts may be considered for chronic ulcers in patients with generalised recessive dystrophic EB or pretibial EB.

Genetic disorders of collagen, elastin and dermal matrix

34

INHERITED DISORDERS OF COLLAGEN

Ehlers–Danlos syndrome

Ehlers–Danlos syndrome (EDS) is a heterogeneous group of inherited disorders of connective tissue that variably impair the structure and function of the skin, joints, internal organs, eyes and blood vessels. It is characterised by joint hypermobility, skin hyperextensibililty and tissue fragility.

Epidemiology

The overall prevalence of EDS is 1/5000–10 000. The hypermobility type is the most common. Clinical features may be present at birth, but most patients present later in childhood as walking starts. There is no observed sex or racial variation.

Pathology

Defects in fibrillar collagens and more recently in intracellular trafficking, secretion and assembly of extracellular matrix (ECM) molecules, including proteoglycans and tenascin-X, have been found to be causal in different types of EDS. Skin histology is variable and often within normal limits. Typically, there is a loose, disordered dermal collagen network. Elastic fibres are usually increased and orientated irregularly. The 'pseudotumours' seen in classical EDS (type I) consist of fat and mucoid material in fibrous capsules; they may be calcified.

Clinical features

A diagnosis of EDS should be considered in anyone with the cardinal manifestations of skin hyperextensibility, skin fragility, easy bruising and joint laxity. Further features will depend on the subtype of EDS (Table 34.1). In classical EDS, the skin is soft, velvety and hyperextensible (Figure 34.1a) but retains its normal recoil. The skin on the palms and soles may be hyperlinear and loose. The skin is not usually otherwise lax until later in life, when redundant folds occur on the eyelids (blepharochalasis), face and limbs. Trivial lacerations form gaping wounds that heal very slowly to leave broad, atrophic 'cigarette paper' scars (Figure 34.1b,c). In the periodontitis type, the features are similar to classical EDS, with premature periodontal recession as a distinguishing feature (Figure 34.1d).

Differential Diagnosis

Cutis laxa, Turner syndrome and cartilage-hair hypoplasia syndrome are differentials for classical EDS. Vascular EDS overlaps clinically with Loeys–Dietz syndrome. Marfan syndrome should be considered if the presenting vascular complication is an aortic aneurysm or dissection.

Rook's Dermatology Handbook, First Edition. Edited by Christopher E. M. Griffiths, Tanya O. Bleiker, Daniel Creamer, John R. Ingram and Rosalind C. Simpson.
© 2022 John Wiley & Sons Ltd. Published 2022 by John Wiley & Sons Ltd.

Table 34.1 Clinical and molecular subtypes of EDS

EDS type	Synonym	Villefranche classification	Mode of inheritance	Clinical features	Ultrastructural findings	Molecular defect
I	Gravis	Classical	AD	Soft velvety hyperextensible skin, easy bruising, atrophic scars, hypermobile joints, pseudotumours	'Cauliflower' fibrils	*COL5A1* and *COL5A2* mutations identified in up to 90%
II	Mitis					
III	Hypermobile	Hypermobility	AD	Hypermobile joints, minimal skin abnormality	As above, but less pronounced	Haploinsufficiency of TNXB in some female patients
IV	Acrogeric or ecchymotic	Vascular	AD	Thin skin, easy bruising, small joint hypermobility, vascular/bowel rupture	Small variable fibrils	*COL3A1* mutations
V	X-linked	Other form	XLR	Resembles mild classical type, bruising more pronounced	–	?
VIA	Oculoscoliotic	Kyphoscoliosis	AR	Soft hyperextensible skin, hypermobile joints, scoliosis, ocular fragility, keratoconus	Small collagen bundles	Lysyl hydroxylase (*PLOD 1*) mutations
VIIA, B	Arthrochalasis multiplex congenita	Arthrochalasis	AD	Floppy infant, congenital hip dislocation, hypermobile joints, soft skin, normal scarring, short stature	Angular fibrils	A and B: *COL1A1* and *COL1A2* mutations reduces cross-link formation in collagen 1
VIIC	Dermatosparaxis	Dermatosparaxis	AR	Markedly hypermobile joints, soft and extremely fragile skin, easy bruising	Hieroglyphic fibrils	Procollagen *N*-proteinase (*ADAMTS2*) mutations
VIII	Periodontal	Other form	AD	Severe periodontitis, pigmented pretibial plaques and scarring	Small fibrils in some patients	Occasionally collagen III deficient
X	Fibronectin	Other form	AR	Similar to mild classical type with prominent easy bruising	Large, irregular fibrils	Fibronectin deficiency abnormality

AD, autosomal dominant; AR, autosomal recessive; CNS, central nervous system; ER, endoplasmic reticulum; XLR, X-linked recessive. Rare forms of EDS described after the Villefranche classification not shown.

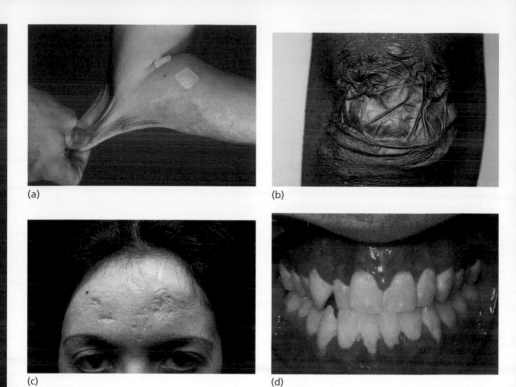

Figure 34.1 Clinical images of EDS. (a) Cutaneous hyperextensibililty in classical EDS. (b) Atrophic scarring of the elbow in classical EDS. (c) Scarring of the forehead in classical EDS. (d) Premature periodontal recession in periodontitis type EDS (type VIII).

Investigations

Molecular characterisation should be sought whenever possible (see Table 34.1). In vascular EDS, and to a much lesser extent classical and hypermobility EDS, there is an increased risk of cardiac valve prolapse, aortic dilatation and arterial aneurysm and rupture. An echocardiogram enables screening for valvular prolapse and aortic dilatation.

Management

A multidisciplinary approach is required with involvement of appropriate specialists (see below). Patients should receive genetic counselling.

Skin

Avoid contact sports, sun protection, care with skin suturing.

Joints

Avoid excessive activity, physiotherapy.

Pregnancy

High risk of obstetric problems, maternal mortality increased.

Vascular EDS

Celiprolol reduces risk of arterial dissection.

INHERITED DISORDERS OF ELASTIC FIBRES

Inherited generalised cutis laxa

Cutis laxa is characterised clinically by lax pendulous skin that only slowly recoils when pulled. The inherited forms include autosomal dominant, several autosomal recessive types and an X-linked type.

Epidemiology

Generalised cutis laxa is rare, with prevalence at birth estimated at 1/1 000 000. Both sexes are affected equally in autosomal dominant and recessive forms. X-linked cutis laxa affects males only.

Pathology

Cutis laxa is caused by disruption to normal elastic tissue function. Histopathologically, the skin is of normal thickness but the elastic fibres are sparse, short, fragmented and clumped, particularly in the upper dermis, and they show granular degeneration.

Clinical features

In autosomal dominant cutis laxa, the skin changes may develop at any age, but tend to present later than in the recessive form (Figure 34.2a).

The skin is soft and variably hyperextensible. Facial dysmorphism is mild but a beaked nose is common. Other organ involvement includes inguinal hernias, which are common, and lung, cardiac valve and large blood vessel complications ranging from mild to severe.

In autosomal recessive cutis laxa, typical facies comprise downward slanting palpebral fissures, a broad flat nose, sagging cheeks and large ears (Figure 34.2b). There are prominent skin folds around the knees, abdomen and thighs. Death due to respiratory complications is common in the first few years of life.

The X-linked recessive form is also known as occipital horn syndrome and is characterised by development of bladder diverticula during childhood, inguinal herniae, mild laxity of the skin and skeletal defects such as short humeri and clavicles. Bony occipital horns appear during adolescence.

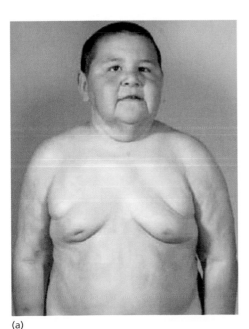

(a)

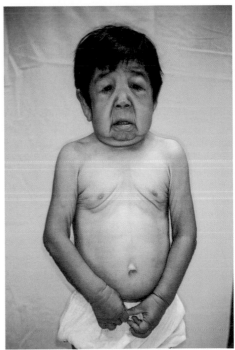

(b)

Figure 34.2 Clinical images of inherited generalised cutis laxa. (a) Autosomal dominant cutis laxa in a 13-year-old male. (Source: Berk DR, Bentley DD, Bayliss SJ, et al. Cutis laxa; A review. J Am Acad Dermatol 2012;66:842.e1–17. Reproduced with permission of Elsevier.) (b) Autosomal recessive type IA cutis laxa in a 4-year-old girl. (Source: Reproduced with permission of Dr Nik Kantaputra, Chiang Mai University, Chiang Mai, Thailand.)

Differential diagnosis
Wrinkly skin syndrome, acquired cutis laxa, EDS.

Investigations
Skin biopsy, chest X-ray, lung function tests and echocardiogram.

Management
Treatment is limited and is directed towards alleviating complications. Surgical removal of lax skin can be undertaken as patients generally heal well, although the benefits are not long term.

Williams–Beuren syndrome

Epidemiology
Williams–Beuren syndrome (WBS) is rare, affecting 1/10 000 persons. A cluster of WBS was reported in the UK following the administration of excessive doses of vitamin D to prevent rickets in pregnant women.

Pathology
The syndrome is sporadic in nearly all cases and is caused by deletion of part of one copy of chromosome 7, which contains at least 28 genes.

Clinical features
The syndrome is characterised by premature laxity of the skin, congenital heart disease (notably supravalvular aortic stenosis) and metabolic abnormalities. Dysmorphic facial features include a flat nasal bridge, short upturned nose and baggy connective tissue around the eyes.

Investigations and Management
Echocardiography surveillance for aortic stenosis is recommended and, if detected, surgery is the preferred treatment choice.

Infantile stiff skin syndromes

Four main types of infantile stiff skin syndromes are recognised: hyaline fibromatosis syndrome, stiff skin syndrome, Winchester syndrome and restrictive dermopathy. They are very rare syndromes characterised by hard stiff skin and joint contractures early in life.

Hyaline fibromatosis syndrome incorporates infantile systemic hyalinosis (ISH) and juvenile hyaline fibromatosis (JHF), the latter being reported more often. In ISH, skin becomes diffusely thickened and hard in first few weeks of life, while this process is delayed until 3 months to 4 years in JHF.

There are only 40 cases of stiff skin syndrome reported in the literature; diffuse firm thick skin leads to reduced joint mobility and causes flexion contractures. In Winchester syndrome, mutations in matrix metalloproteinase 14 cause thickened stiff skin, osteolysis, joint contractures, gingival hypertrophy and dwarfism. In restrictive dermopathy, there is intrauterine growth retardation, skin is tight, red and shiny with flexural erosions, there are enlarged fontanelles and clavicular dysplasia and death usually occurs within weeks after birth.

Premature ageing syndromes

Premature aging syndromes are described in Table 34.2.

DISORDERS OF ECTOPIC CALCIFICATION AND ABNORMAL MINERALISATION

Pseudoxanthoma elasticum

Pseudoxanthoma elasticum (PXE) is an autosomal recessive multisystem disorder characterised by disruption to and progressive calcification of elastic tissue predominantly in the dermis, blood vessels and Bruch membrane of the eye.

Epidemiology
Prevalence is approximately 1/50 000. F > M, which may reflect more skin involvement in women and more frequent presentation to dermatology due to impact on cosmesis.

Table 34.2 Premature aging syndromes

Condition	Progeria (Syn. Hutchinson–Gilford syndrome)	Werner syndrome (Syn. Pangeria)	Acrogeria	Familial mandibuloacral dysplasia	Mulvihill–Smith syndrome	Neonatal progeroid syndrome
Epidemiology	Very rare, affects 1 in 4 million newborns	Prevalence in Japan 1/20 000–1/40 000, in USA 1/200 000	Extremely rare with only about 40 cases described	Very rare, incidence less than 1/1 000 000	Only 11 cases have been described in the literature	Very rare with only about 30 cases reported
Pathology	Mutations in *LMNA* produce abnormal Lamin A	Autosomal recessive transmission of mutations in RECQL2 gene	Unclear if single or a group of conditions Reduction in subcutaneous fat	Mutations in LMNA or ZMPSTE24 genes produce abnormal Lamin A	Genetic cause is unknown	Autosomal recessive. May involve DNA repair defects
Clinical features	Infant failure to thrive Taut skin of face Hair loss Prominent joints	Premature greying of hair and alopecia Small stature High risk of cancer, diabetes and CV disease	Skin dry, thin, transparent, especially hands and feet Face appears 'pinched'	Mandibular hypoplasia, dysplastic clavicles, club-shaped terminal phalanges	Short stature, developmental delay, multiple pigmented naevi, microcephaly	Frontal and lateral bossing of skull, long fingers and atrophic nails, death usually in first year due to respiratory infections
Differential diagnoses	Mandibuloacral dysplasia, Mulvihill–Smith syndrome	Progeria, Rothmund–Thomson syndrome, systemic sclerosis	Distinguished from progeria and pangeria by no other organ problems	Progeria, acrogeria, Werner syndrome	Cockayne syndrome, multiple lentigines syndrome	Other syndromes that exhibit a progeroid phenotype at birth
Investigations	Molecular diagnostic confirmation Monitor for CV disease	Monitor for diabetes, CV disease and hypogonadism	Molecular diagnostic analysis	Molecular diagnostic analysis	No specific investigations	No specific investigations
Management	Support nutrition, physiotherapy, lonafarnib therapy	Supportive measures	No specific treatment	Treatment aimed at reducing metabolic complications	No specific treatment	Monitor for respiratory tract infections

CV, cardiovascular.

PART 4: GENETIC DISORDERS INVOLVING THE SKIN

Pathology

Mutations in the ABCC6 gene are causative, encoding a transmembrane transporter primarily expressed in the liver and kidneys. In the skin, elastic fibres in the mid-dermis are clumped, degenerate, fragmented and swollen, and the abnormal fibres stain positively for calcium. Similar changes occur in the media and intima of blood vessels, the Bruch membrane of the eye and in the endocardium and pericardium.

Clinical features

The complete syndrome consists of asymptomatic flexural skin lesions, visual disturbances and cardiovascular manifestations due to calcification. The features are late onset and slowly progressive. Skin changes including 'chicken skin' appearance of the lateral neck are usually noticed in patients' teens. Diagnostic criteria are shown in Table 34.3.

Table 34.3 Major and minor diagnostic criteria for PXE

Major criteria	
Skin	Yellowish papules/plaques on lateral neck and/or flexural areas of the body (Figure 34.3a)
	Biopsy from affected skin shows elastin fragmentation, clumping and calcification
Eye	Peau d'orange of retina (Figure 34.3b)
	One or more angioid streaks, each at least one disk diameter in length (Figure 34.3b)
Genetics	Pathogenic mutation of both alleles of the ABCC6 gene
	First-degree relative who meets diagnostic criteria for pseudoxanthoma elasticum
Minor criteria	
Eye	One angioid streak shorter than one disk diameter
	At least one 'comet' in the retina
	At least one 'wing sign' in the retina
Genetics	Pathogenic mutation of one allele of the ABCC6 gene

Definitive diagnosis requires the presence of at least two major criteria not belonging to the same (skin, eye, genetic) category.

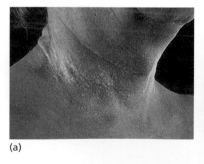 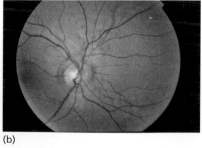

(a) (b)

Figure 34.3 Clinical signs of pseudoxanthoma elasticum. (a) Typical 'chicken skin' appearance involving the neck. (b) Angioid streaks radiating from the optic nerve. (Source: Courtesy of Miss L. Allen, Cambridge University Hospitals NHS Foundation Trust, Cambridge, UK.)

PART 4: GENETIC DISORDERS INVOLVING THE SKIN

Table 34.4 Additional dermal disorders

Condition	Adermatoglyphia	Lipoid proteinosis	Pterygium syndromes
Synonyms	'Immigration delay disease' due to absence of fingerprints	Urbach–Wiethe disease, hyalinosis cutis et mucosae, lipoglycoproteinosis	Multiple pterygium syndromes, popliteal pterygium syndromes
Epidemiology	Very rare	Rare	Rare
Pathology	Autosomal dominant Mutation of SMARCAD1	Autosomal recessive Infiltration of hyaline material into skin, oral cavity, larynx	Mutation in IRF6/RIPK4/CHRNG/ CHRNA1/CHRND.
Clinical features	Absence of epidermal ridges	Presents in infancy with hoarseness Waxy papules, hyperkeratosis or warty plaques of skin Characteristic 'beaded' papules along eyelid margins (Figure 34.4)	Webbing (pterygium) involves the neck, antecubital and popliteal fossae Muscle weakness leads to joint contractures (arthrogryposis).
Differential diagnoses	Adermatoglyphia is a feature of several complex ectodermal dysplasias	Erythropoietic protoporphyria, xanthomatosis, amyloidosis	–
Investigations	Molecular diagnostic analysis	Biopsy of affected skin, histochemical diagnosis using antibody to ECM1	Molecular diagnostic analysis
Management	Nil specific	Microlaryngoscopy and dissection of the vocal cords may be needed	Supportive

ECM1, extracellular matrix protein 1.

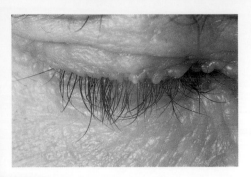

Figure 34.4 Lipoid proteinosis. Typical 'beaded' papules present along the margins of the upper eyelids. (Source: Courtesy of Dr R.C.D. Staughton, Chelsea and Westminster Hospital, London, UK.)

Differential diagnosis

Disseminated form of dermatofibrosis lenticularis (Buschke–Ollendorff), papular elastorrhexis.

Acquired syndromes that have PXE-like features (pseudo-PXE) include adverse effect of penicillamine, eosinophilia-myalgia syndrome, amyloidosis and several haemoglobinopathies such as congenital anaemia, sickle cell disease and thalassaemia.

Investigations

Calcium and phosphate levels, skin biopsy from lateral neck, echocardiogram, molecular analysis of the ABCC6 gene.

Management

No specific treatment for PXE exists. Annual ophthalmology and cardiovascular assessments are often recommended. Patients and their families should also receive genetic counselling.

Miscellaneous dermal disorders

Table 34.4 summarises some additional dermal disorders.

Disorders affecting cutaneous vasculature

35

Capillary malformation

(Syn. Port wine stain)
Capillary malformation (CM) is a sporadic, homogenous, pink, red or purple macule or patch present at birth.

Epidemiology
CM is the most common vascular malformation, found in approximately three of 1000 newborns, and the M:F ratio is 1:1.

Pathophysiology
A CM is characterised by the dilatation of normal numbers of capillaries of the papillary and upper reticular dermis combined with areas of increased numbers of normal-looking capillaries.

Clinical features
CMs are of variable size. They are usually located on the head and neck (Figure 35.1), but can also be seen on the trunk or limbs. A CM grows proportionately with the child and persists throughout life.

Sturge–Weber syndrome
A CM located on the territory of the ophthalmic division (V1) of the trigeminal nerve associated with ipsilateral leptomeningeal capillary–venous anomaly and/or ocular involvement. The CM can be bilateral and/or more extensive, covering the territory of the maxillary (V2) and mandibular (V3) branches of the trigeminal nerve, and sometimes the trunk and the limbs (Figure 35.2). About 75% of children with intracranial vascular anomaly develop seizures, most often before the age of 2 years, with a risk of contralateral neurological deficit and learning difficulties. Gyral calcifications can be observed. The major ocular complication is glaucoma, occurring in more than 50% of patients.

Klippel-Trenaunay syndrome (KTS)
A CM of the skin associated with a soft-tissue and bone overgrowth and hypertrophy in combination with varicose veins, with or without deep venous and lymphatic abnormalities. KTS is sporadic and congenital, characterised by asymmetrical overgrowth in girth and length of an extremity with a vascular lesion consisting of combined capillary, lymphatic and venous malformation (see Figure 35.3). There is often persistence of the embryonic vein of the lateral thigh (vein of Servelle) and anomalies of the deep venous system (stenosis, hypoplasia, aplasia). KTS is often associated with localised intravascular coagulopathy. There is a high risk for thromboembolism and subsequent pulmonary arterial hypertension.

Investigations
Most CMs do not require any investigation, unless there is an associated syndrome. Segmental lower extremity CMs need limb growth discrepancy check at about 8 years old. Rare syndromic forms should be considered for large and/or multifocal CMs.

Management
CMs are asymptomatic but occurrence in cosmetically sensitive areas can generate important psychosocial problems. Pulse dye laser is the treatment of choice and pain from the procedure may require general anaesthesia in

Rook's Dermatology Handbook, First Edition. Edited by Christopher E. M. Griffiths, Tanya O. Bleiker, Daniel Creamer, John R. Ingram and Rosalind C. Simpson.
© 2022 John Wiley & Sons Ltd. Published 2022 by John Wiley & Sons Ltd.

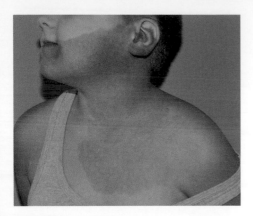

Figure 35.1 A 10-year-old boy with extensive CM involving the territory of the mandibular division of the trigeminal nerve, the neck and thorax.

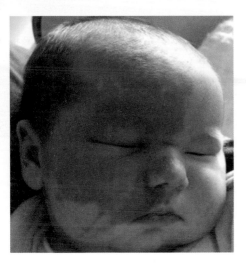

Figure 35.2 Sturge–Weber syndrome showing an 8-month-old boy with CM involving left V1, V2 and V3 and right V3 territories of the trigeminal nerve.

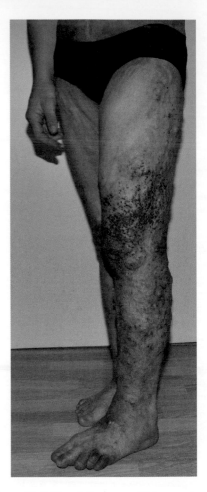

Figure 35.3 Klippel–Trenaunay–Weber syndrome with a capillarolymphatico VM on the left lower extremity with overgrowth.

children. Eyelid involvement should prompt an ophthalmological referral.

Arteriovenous malformation

Arteriovenous malformations (AVMs) are congenital, destructive, fast-flow vascular malformations that tend to worsen with time (Figure 35.4).

Epidemiology

The incidence of AVMs is largely unknown. The M:F ratio is 1:1.

Pathophysiology

AVMs consist of distorted arteries and veins with thickened muscle walls due to arteriovenous shunting and fibrosis. In AVM, the normal capillary bed is replaced by a nidus via which blood shunts from feeding arteries into draining veins (distinct from an arteriovenous fistula in which there is direct communication between an artery and a vein, usually iatrogenic or due to trauma).

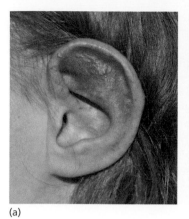
(a)

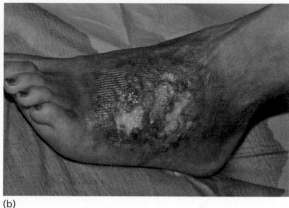
(b)

Figure 35.4 AVM spectrum. (a) A 4-year-old girl with stage 2 AVM of the left ear. (b) Extensive ulcerated stage 3 AVM of the left foot.

Clinical features

At birth, an AVM involving the skin can appear as a capillary blush, which can be misdiagnosed as a CM. The presence of increased warmth, thrill or bruit suggests a fast-flow component. AVMs expand slowly, but can worsen rapidly at puberty, during pregnancy, after trauma and, particularly, after incomplete treatment.

Differential diagnosis

Hereditary haemorrhagic telangiectasia (Rendu–Osler–Weber syndrome), mucocutaneous and gastrointestinal telangiectases, associated with AVMs/arteriovenous fistula in the lungs, liver or brain.

PTEN hamartoma tumour syndrome

Fast-flowing vascular anomalies are one element of this rare syndrome

Investigation

Doppler ultrasound shows high-velocity arterial and pulsatile venous flow with low resistance. T2-weighted MRI shows dilated veins and arteries within normal or hypertrophied tissue. Arteriography as a pretreatment examination identifies the feeding arteries and localises the nidus.

Management

Management depends on lesion type, location and symptoms. A multidisciplinary approach is needed, including a dermatologist, general physician or paediatrician, surgeon and interventional radiologist. An interventional approach requires care to avoid worsening the AVM.

Conservative: Antihypertensives, analgesia, compression garment, wound management.

Interventional (if failure of conservative therapy): Embolisation, surgical resection.

Venous malformation

(Syn. Venous angioma)

Venous malformations (VMs) are congenital vascular lesions characterised by localised light-to-dark blue masses consisting of malformed veins.

Epidemiology

Estimated incidence is 1:10 000 and the M:F ratio is 1:1. They are the most frequent vascular malformations referred to specialised centres. There is an association with localised intravascular coagulopathy.

Pathophysiology

Somatic, sporadic mutations in *TEK* encoding the endothelial cell tyrosine kinase receptor TIE2 are present in about 50% of VMs. Histologically, VMs are characterised by enlarged, convoluted, venous channels lined by a single flattened layer of endothelial cells surrounded by irregularly distributed smooth muscle cells.

Clinical features

VMs are usually solitary, light-to-dark blue masses that can be emptied by compression (Figure 35.5). There is no thrill or bruit.

Differential diagnosis

Mucocutaneous VM: Usually multifocal and <5 cm².

Blue rubber bleb naevus syndrome: Numerous cutaneous VMs, including palmoplantar, and internal VMs, including gastrointestinal.

Glomuvenous malformation: <5 cm² bluish purple lesions mainly on extremities. Histology shows smooth muscle 'glomus' cells surrounding enlarged venous channels.

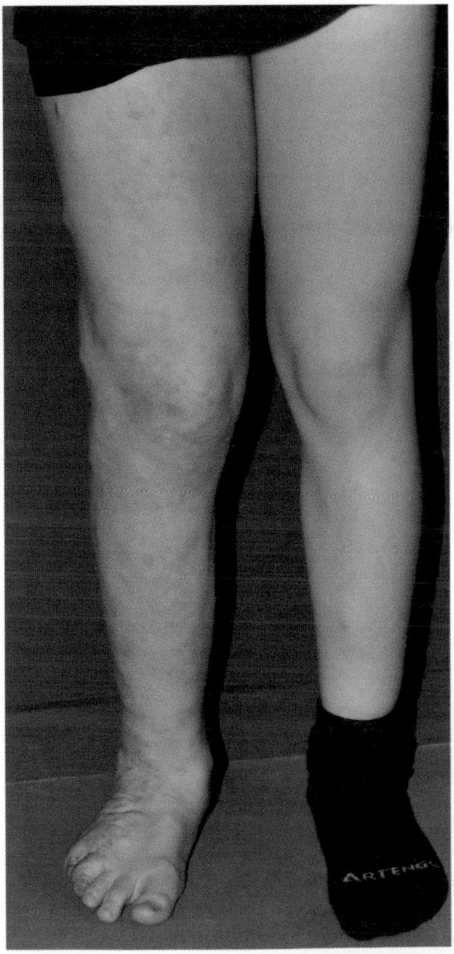

Investigations

Clotting screen (elevated D-dimer levels reflect increased fibrinolysis due to localised intravascular coagulopathy, doppler ultrasound, MRI.

Management

Limb involvement: Compression garment.
   Small lesion: Pulse dye laser.
   Larger lesion: Sclerotherapy, then surgical resection.

Lymphatic malformation

(Syn. Lymphangioma circumscriptum)
Lymphatic malformations (LMs) are focal lesions composed of dilated lymphatic channels disconnected from the lymphatic system. LMs can be macrocystic, microcystic or combined (Figure 35.6).

Epidemiology

LMs are rare and exact prevalence is unknown. The M:F ratio is 1:1.

Pathophysiology

Macrocystic LMs are composed of a single or multiple lymphatic cysts surrounded by a thick fibrous membrane. Microcystic LMs are characterised by dilated lymphatic channels with variable thickness of the walls.

Clinical features

Macrocystic LMs can be diagnosed in utero as early as the first trimester of pregnancy. They are often located on the neck, chest wall and axilla. They manifest as multilobulated, well-defined lesions that are translucent, soft, but only slightly compressible on palpation. Microcystic LMs are mostly located on the head and neck. They are ill-defined vesicular plaques, which often invade adjacent structures. Skin can be normal in colour, but becomes blue or purple when intracystic bleeding occurs (Figure 35.6b).

   LMs may cause asymmetry with bone overgrowth, especially on the face. They can suddenly

Figure 35.5 VM affecting the right leg.

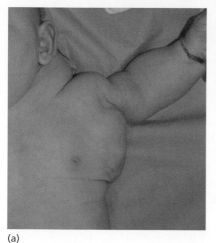

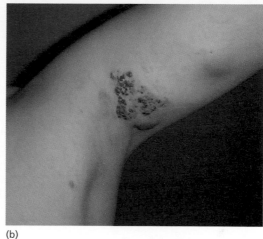

(a)   (b)

Figure 35.6 LM spectrum. (a) A 10-month-old girl with extensive macrocystic/microcystic LMs of the neck, thorax and axilla. (b) Microcystic dermal and subcutaneous LM of the left arm with intracystic bleeding.

become painful and enlarge due to intralesional bleeding or infection.

Differential diagnosis
LM with intracystic bleeding can resemble VM.

Investigations
Doppler ultrasound (in contrast to VMs, macrocystic LMs cannot be completely emptied by compression and often contain echogenic debris), MRI, clotting, including D-dimer and fibrinogen levels (extensive LMs, combined with VMs, can be associated with coagulation abnormalities).

Management
Complications: Systemic antibiotics for bacterial infection.

Macrocytic LMs: Fluid aspiration then percutaneous intralesional sclerosant.

Microcytic LMs: Multi-injection sclerotherapy.

36

Congenital naevi

The understanding of congenital naevi has changed over the last few years, with the discovery of the genetic basis of many lesions.

CLASSIFICATION OF CONGENITAL NAEVI

Clinical phenotypic classification

1. Congenital epidermal naevi.
2. Congenital pigment cell naevi.
3. Congenital connective tissue naevi.

These can each be divided into:

- Cutaneous involvement only: single or multiple lesions.
- Syndromic: associated with non-cutaneous features.

Histological classification

Within congenital epidermal naevi there are subclassifications based on the predominant cell type seen on histology:

- Keratinocytic naevi.
- Sebaceous naevi.
- Follicular naevi.
- Eccrine/apocrine naevi.

Within congenital pigment cell naevi there are subclassifications based on the histology of the pigment cells:

- Melanocytic naevus.
- Blue naevus.
- Spitz naevus.
- Naevus spilus.

Within congenital connective tissue naevi there are subclassifications based on the predominant cell type seen on histology:

- Collagen naevi.
- Elastic tissue naevi.
- Mucinous naevi.
- Fat naevi.

Genetic classification

For congenital naevi there are also subclassifications based on the causative genetic mutation, where known, for example mutations in *HRAS* and *KRAS* (e.g. sebaceous naevi), *AKT1* (e.g. Proteus syndrome) and *PIK3CA* (e.g. CLOVES syndrome).

A clinical diagnosis may therefore be initially of a congenital epidermal naevus syndrome, which with histological and genetic investigation becomes *AKT1*-mutated keratinocytic congenital epidermal naevus syndrome. Where this systematic classification leads to a clear diagnosis of a clinically well-defined syndrome (such as Proteus syndrome in this case), then the eponymous name should be used if preferred.

CONGENITAL EPIDERMAL NAEVI

Congenital epidermal naevi (CEN) is a descriptive term for congenital hamartomas of epidermal structures. This encompasses a wide range of clinical and histological phenotypes, which can occur as isolated cutaneous lesions or in association with extracutaneous features as part of diverse syndromes.

CEN syndromes are the association of CEN with extracutaneous features, with a predilec-

Rook's Dermatology Handbook, First Edition. Edited by Christopher E. M. Griffiths, Tanya O. Bleiker, Daniel Creamer, John R. Ingram and Rosalind C. Simpson.
© 2022 John Wiley & Sons Ltd. Published 2022 by John Wiley & Sons Ltd.

tion for neurological, ophthalmological, skeletal and endocrinological abnormalities.

Epidemiology

Sebaceous naevi have a prevalence of 1–3 in 1000. The birth prevalence of CEN syndromes is unknown; they are extremely rare, with Proteus syndrome occurring in less than one in 1 million births. CEN are usually present at birth; some types can appear in the first few years of life.

Pathophysiology

Most CEN are caused by single postzygotic mutations in an epidermal precursor cell, leading to epidermal mosaicism, with or without mosaicism in other organs. As a result the same mutation is found in all affected tissues in an individual with a CEN syndrome.

Epidermal naevi are localised hamartomatous processes of the epidermis that may show varying histopathological changes, most of which include hyperkeratosis, thickened epidermis and papillomatosis. The lesions are classified histologically based on the predominant epidermal component (sebaceous, keratinocytic, follicular, eccrine/apocrine) and whether or not there is an inflammatory component. In inflammatory linear verrucous epidermal naevus (ILVEN) there is usually a marked inflammatory component, including a psoriasiform appearance with epidermal hyperplasia and a dense associated superficial dermal inflammatory infiltrate. An important aspect of histopathological examination of keratinocytic naevi is the presence or absence of epidermolysis, as when present there is a possibility of transmitting the trait as a germline heterozygous dominant mutation if there is gonosomal mosaicism.

Clinical features

Single CEN lesions can be either round or linear, but larger or multiple lesions are Blaschko linear in distribution.

Epidermal naevi are superficial, raised and can have the appearance of being 'stuck on' to the surface of the skin rather than intrinsic to it; surface characteristics depend on the cell type that predominates.

Keratinocytic naevi: Vary from pale brown and nearly macular with a soft velvety feel, to brown or red, verrucous or hyperkeratotic, and can have a prominent inflammatory component.

ILVEN: Commonly appears in the first few years of life rather than at birth, and spreads gradually until stabilising in a classic Blaschko-linear distribution. It is characterised clinically by inflamed and hyperkeratotic skin that can be pruritic. It is usually confined to a single limb, but can be more extensive (Figure 36.1). Clinically and histologically, there is a significant overlap between ILVEN and psoriasis.

Sebaceous naevi: Have a greasy feel and appearance, are often yellowish or pink (Figure 36.2) but can sometimes be deeply pigmented.

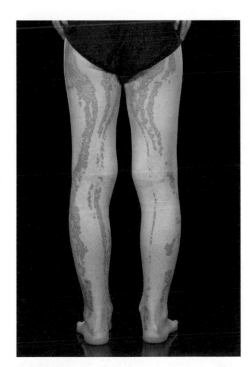

Figure 36.1 Extensive inflammatory linear verrucous epidermal naevus on the lower limbs in a Blaschko-linear distribution.

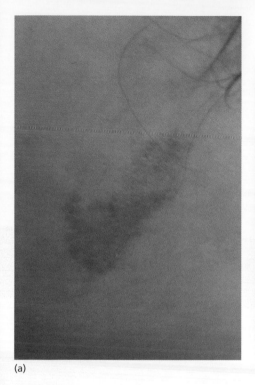

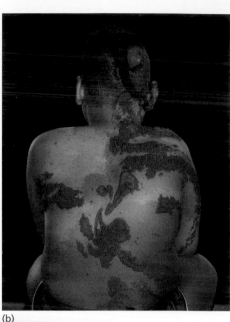

(a)   (b)

Figure 36.2 (a) Single sebaceous naevus on the cheek, with a yellowish hue and characteristic greasy texture. (b) Multiple pigmented sebaceous epidermal naevi on the trunk and scalp in a Blaschko-linear distribution, accompanied by large areas of café-au-lait macular pigmentation with superimposed melanocytic lesions.

Follicular naevi (naevus comedonicus or acne naevus): Characteristic in appearance, skin-coloured, with a high density of multiple, comedo-like lesions.

Congenital eccrine or apocrine naevi: Particularly rare, but are recognisable by localised hyperhidrosis, with porokeratotic variants of eccrine naevi exhibiting the classic signs of porokeratosis. Although syringocystadenoma papilliferum is thought to be a hamartoma of eccrine/apocrine glands, it frequently arises from a sebaceous naevus.

There are several clearly delineated CEN syndromes. Examples of these are outlined below (refer to main parent textbook for more detail).

Proteus syndrome (AKT1 mutations): Proteus syndrome is a mosaic disorder of overgrowth. Diagnostic criteria are well established and cutaneous lesions include keratinocytic epidermal naevi, connective tissue naevi, lipomas, vascular naevi and patchy lipohypoplasia or dermal hypoplasia.

PIK3CA-related overgrowth spectrum: This newly coined term reflects the common genetic basis of a wide variety of different clinical phenotypes, including CLOVES syndrome. This acronym is the description of associated congenital lipomatous overgrowth, vascular malformation, epidermal naevi (keratinocytic type) and skeletal abnormalities. It can be associated with neurological abnormalities.

Follicular naevus/naevus comedonicus syndrome: Naevus comedonicus has been described in association with cataracts, skeletal abnormalities and neurological abnormalities. The genetic basis is thus far unknown, although the genetic basis of isolated naevus comedonicus is known to be mutations in *FGFR2*.

Make sure distinct paragraph from previous syndrome Some CEN have an increased risk of superimposed benign tumour development; risk of malignant transformation is rare. For single isolated sebaceous naevi benign tumours with a risk of malignant transformation occur at a rate of ~1% (syringocystadenoma papilliferum being the commonest), whereas basal cell carcinoma occurs in less than 1% and squamous cell carcinoma is rarer.

Investigation

Varies with the type of naevus, clinical presentation and the known associations of that particular CEN (e.g. dental, ophthalmological, neurological, orthopaedic or metabolic assessment). The association of multiple keratinocytic or sebaceous epidermal naevi with hypophosphataemia merits routine investigation with a single baseline electrolyte and calcium/phosphate/alkaline phosphatase measurement. MRI of the central nervous system (CNS) should be performed if there are any concerns from neurological assessment.

Management

History, examination and relevant investigations for non-cutaneous associations are essential to distinguish isolated from syndromic CEN. Biopsy of the epidermal naevus is required to make an exact diagnosis, particularly for keratinocytic CEN of any size, to look for epidermolysis. Should the biopsy reveal epidermolytic CEN, referral should be made to a clinical geneticist for counselling at an appropriate age. Similarly, CEN that have an inherited dimension (e.g. CHILD syndrome, Cowden syndrome) should trigger a referral to clinical genetics.

Surgical excision can be suitable for small, single, epidermal naevi. Keratinocytic and sebaceous naevi are candidates for ablative laser therapy to reduce thickness and/or hyperkeratosis of the lesion, and smaller verrucous lesions can be treated with cryotherapy. ILVEN have been treated with CO_2 laser therapy with variable response, and case reports describe treatment with therapies for psoriasis such as topical calcipotriol, etanercept and oral retinoids. Treatment of extensive epidermolytic, hyperkeratotic and epidermal naevi is often with systemic retinoids; topical vitamin D analogues can be helpful.

CONGENITAL PIGMENT CELL NAEVI

Congenital melanocytic naevi

(Syn. Naevocellular naevus, naevus spilus-type CMN, neurocutaneous melanosis, Multiple CMN, CMN syndrome, *NRAS* mosaicism, Mosaic RASopathy)

Congenital melanocytic naevi (CMN) are benign, pigmented, melanocytic naevi present at birth.

Epidemiology

The prevalence at birth of small, single CMN is 1–2% of new births. F:M is 1.2:1.

Pathophysiology

Melanocytic naevi of congenital type are almost always compound naevi with junctional and predominant dermal components, composed of bland melanocytes that characteristically extend around adnexal structures and often into the underlying muscle and fat. There is no cytological atypia. Nodules may arise within CMN that are almost always proliferative nodules rather than melanoma.

CMN are caused by a somatic mutation *in utero*. Multiple CMN and CMN syndrome are usually caused by mutations in the gene *NRAS*. Single CMN have been found to carry *NRAS* (more commonly) or *BRAF* mutations.

Clinical features

Single or multiple lesions; commonly brown or black but can be purplish or red, particularly at birth. Frequently heterogeneous in colour and/or texture (Figure 36.3). Apart

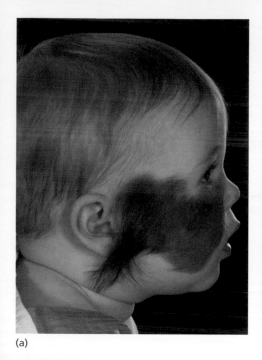

(a)

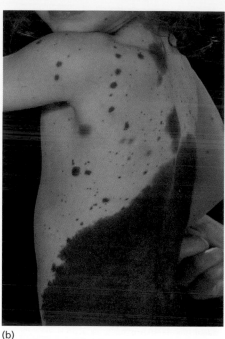

(b)

Figure 36.3 Congenital melanocytic naevi. (a) Single CMN on the face showing marked hypertrichosis. (b) Multiple CMN of different sizes on the trunk.

from the smallest lesions they are usually palpable, with increased surface markings. Lesions are darkest at birth and usually lighten to some degree over the first few years of life, occasionally dramatically.

For non-scalp CMN, overlying hair is often not apparent at birth and may develop in the first year. Scalp CMN often have thick luxuriant or wiry hair at birth, which grows at a significantly greater rate than the surrounding hair. The colour of the hair usually approximates to the scalp colour over time, but may remain of a different texture. Occasionally, CMN even on the scalp are not hair-bearing. CMN on the scalp can produce white hairs, and patchy hair loss within the CMN is not uncommon.

Two commonly arising benign proliferative lesions within CMN are proliferative nodules and diffuse neuroid proliferations.

- Classic proliferative nodules are often present at birth, are well circumscribed, symmetrical, round or oval, soft to firm and of any uniform colour (Figure 36.4). They are usually half to a

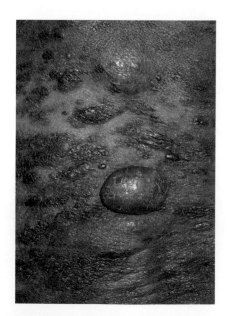

Figure 36.4 Benign proliferative nodule in a large congenital melanocytic naevus, present from birth and stable in behaviour.

few centimetres in diameter. These nodules can usually be resected if required.

- Diffuse neuroid proliferations are usually not present at birth, but can develop at any point during childhood, and often continue to grow slowly over time and can become more active around puberty. They have less well-defined edges, can be a few centimetres to many centimetres in diameter, are firm and often become pendulous when larger (Figure 36.5). They tend to recur after resection.

CMN syndrome: Encompasses anyone with CMN and non-cutaneous features. Neurological abnormalities are the commonest, with intraparenchymal melanosis in ~20% of cases with more than one CMN. 50% of cases are asymptomatic, 50% associated with neurodevelopmental delay, attention deficit hyperactivity disorder and autistic spectrum disorder or seizures.

The lifetime risk of melanoma in all sizes of CMN is 0.1–2%. The risk is very low for small

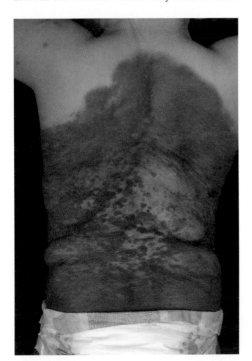

Figure 36.5 Multiple neuroid-type proliferations in a congenital melanocytic naevus.

single lesions, increasing to 10–14% in individuals with naevi of >60 cm. The median age for developing melanoma is ~7 years. Primary melanoma arises within the CNS in 50% of cases.

The characteristic facial features of children with CMN are wide or prominent forehead, hypertelorism, eyebrow variants, periorbital fullness, small/short nose, narrow nasal ridge, broad nasal tip, broad or round face, full cheeks, prominent premaxilla, prominent/long philtrum and everted lower lip.

Investigations

The diagnosis of CMN is usually a clinical one. Neurological investigations and monitoring for cutaneous or extracutaneous melanoma should be undertaken as in Figure 36.6.

Management

See Figure 36.6 for neurological monitoring.

Acute neurological symptoms should trigger urgent MRI of the whole CNS with contrast. A clinically diagnosed benign proliferative nodule should be photographed; if there is local lymphadenopathy the nodule should be removed, if no lymphadenopathy then review at 4 weeks and biopsy nodule if changing, otherwise clinical monitoring.

Prognosis of melanoma in patients with multiple CMN is poor, and death usually occurs within 6–12 months of diagnosis. Surgical removal of multiple CMN does not reduce the risk of malignancy in an affected individual.

Cosmetic management should be discussed with the family and patient, including hair removal methods. Lesions treated by superficial removal techniques such as dermabrasion, curettage or laser therapy may repigment or scar. Serial excision of single or cosmetically prominent lesions can produce very good results, although it will leave a scar.

Congenital Spitz naevus and congenital blue naevus

These are rare with histological features the same as the acquired naevi.

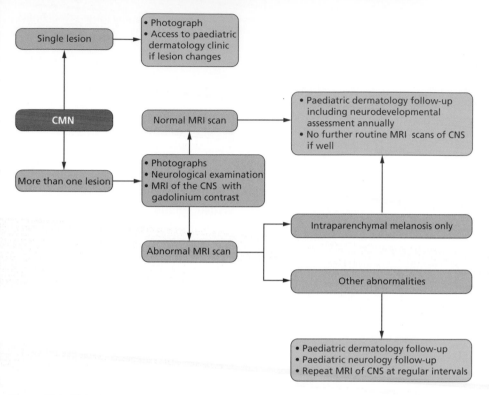

Figure 36.6 Clinical management algorithm for neurological investigation and follow-up of patients with CMN. CNS, central nervous system; MRI, magnetic resonance imaging.

Congenital naevus spilus

(Syn. Speckled lentiginous naevi)
Prevalence 1–2% at birth or early childhood. Not a major risk factor for melanoma. Histologically banal naevi arising in a macular lentigo with a subtle increase in melanocyte number. Clinically multiple darkly pigmented macules or papules (representing junctional and compound naevi) arising on a lentiginous macule (Figure 36.7), predominantly on the trunk and upper and lower extremities. Larger lesions can form part of phakomatosis pigmentokeratotica.

CONGENITAL CONNECTIVE TISSUE NAEVI AND FAT NAEVI

Benign cutaneous hamartomas of connective tissue components present at birth, named by the predominant cell type.

Epidemiology
Rare. The average age for presentation is 2 years.

Pathophysiology
Hamartomatous lesions of the dermis usually with a mixed histological composition but in which a predominant component is present, giving the lesion its name, or by the absence of a component, as in naevus anelasticus. Lesions are poorly circumscribed and non-encapsulated, and show thickening of the dermis with replacement of the normal dermis or subcutis with lesional tissue.

Clinical features
Can be single or multiple, and can be associated with extracutaneous features.

Isolated, congenital collagenomas are soft to firm, skin-coloured, brownish or yellowish nodules or plaques (Figure 36.8).

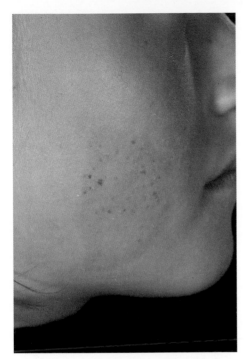

Figure 36.7 Single naevus spilus on the face showing a café-au-lait macule background with superimposed darker areas.

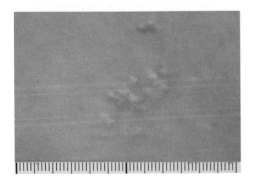

Figure 36.8 Collagenoma-type connective tissue naevus on the lower abdomen.

Congenital elastomas are firm, skin-coloured or creamy/yellowish papules or nodules, size ranging from millimetres to a centimetre, which often coalesce to form plaques or clusters.

Congenital lipomas present as localised, skin-coloured, soft proliferations with indistinct edges. The 'Michelin-tyre' baby phenotype has been associated with both fat naevus and diffuse smooth muscle hamartoma. In this phenotype the infant has generalised thickening of the skin with pronounced folds.

Elastomas (and occasionally collagenomas) can be the presenting feature of Buschke–Ollendorff syndrome, an autosomal dominant disorder caused by germline loss-of-function mutations in *LEMD3*. Lesions classically present in groups or plaques on the lower abdominal wall, trunk, arms and buttocks. Suspected cases should have limited plain radiographs to look for the characteristic findings of osteopoikilosis and melorheostosis.

Plantar collagenomas are seen in both Proteus syndrome and PIK3CA overgrowth syndromes; characteristic cerebriform appearance in Proteus syndrome.

Fibrous connective tissue naevi are a frequent feature of tuberous sclerosis (Chapter 38), but these lesions would not usually be present congenitally.

The principal importance of congenital lipomas in paediatric dermatology lies in the association of lumbosacral lesions and underlying spinal defects, which should be sought using appropriate imaging techniques.

Investigations
Diagnostic biopsy.

Management
Family history, examination and follow-up for any associated non-cutaneous or syndromic features are important. In the absence of these, single lesions can be followed up until deemed to be isolated and stable.

UNCLASSIFIABLE NAEVI

Becker naevus

The genetic basis of these naevi is not yet known. It is a relatively common hyperpigmented, generally non-linear lesion with an incidence of around 0.25%, commoner in males.

Histologically, there are features of lentiginous melanocytic hyperplasia, epidermal hyperplasia and smooth muscle hyperplasia.

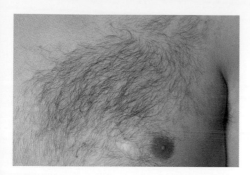

Figure 36.9 Becker naevus over left side of chest. (Source: Reproduced with permission of Cardiff and Vale University Health Board.)

The majority of lesions appear in the first two decades, classically at puberty. It is frequently but not always hypertrichotic and is commonest on the upper trunk (Figure 36.9). It can be associated with extracutaneous abnormalities, then termed Becker naevus syndrome, with aplasia or hypoplasia of the underlying breast tissue, or pectoralis major muscle (or sometimes shoulder muscles) or lipoatrophy. Other extracutaneous associations described are ipsilateral limb growth disturbance, supernumerary nipples and scoliosis. There is no effective treatment; lasers may improve the colour and reduce the hair.

DNA repair disorders with cutaneous features

37

DNA is continually being damaged by a variety of endogenous and exogenous sources. Defects in DNA repair pathways result in a number of disorders, many with skin involvement, commonly photosensitivity, cancer and premature ageing. Figure 37.1 summarises the two pathways involved in nucleotide excision repair (NER).

Xeroderma pigmentosum

Xeroderma pigmentosum (XP) presents clinically with progressive pigmentary abnormalities and an increased incidence of UV radiation-induced skin and mucous membrane cancers at sun-exposed sites. There are eight variants depending upon the affected DNA repair gene (XP-A to XP-G and XP variant).

Epidemiology

Incidence in the USA is estimated at 1:250 000, in Japan at 1:80 000, in Indian/Middle Eastern regions at 1:10 000–30 000 and at approximately 2.3 per million live births in Western Europe.

The incidence of XP in Japan is significantly higher than in Western countries, with the majority of XP patients in Japan belonging to the XP-A complementation group.

XP affects males and females equally and it occurs in all ethnic groups.

Pathophysiology

XP is an autosomal recessive disorder resulting from mutations in any one of eight genes. The products of seven of these genes (XP-A to XP-G) are involved in the recognition and repair of UVR-induced photoproducts in DNA by NER (Figure 37.1).

In the XP-variant (approximately 20% of XP patients), the problem is in replicating DNA containing UVR-induced damage.

Clinical features

XP has wide variability in clinical features; there are several clinical variants. In XP, the skin is normal at birth. Severity is dependent on the amount of sun exposure and the degree of UVR protection. 50% of XP patients suffer from severe and prolonged sunburn on minimal sun exposure. The remainder present with lentigines and hypopigmented macules at sun-exposed sites (Figure 37.2). XP patients have an over 10 000-fold increased risk of developing non-melanoma skin cancer and a 2000-fold increased risk of melanoma skin cancer under 20 years old. UVR exposure to the oral cavity results in mucocutaneous malignancy.

Patients are at increased risk of:

- Neurodegeneration (30%) in specific subtypes (cerebellar signs, ataxia/areflexia, progressive microcephaly, sensorineural deafness).
- Smoking-induced lung cancers.
- Cancers of the brain.
- Ocular manifestations (dry eye, conjunctiva inflammation, premature pyterigia, corneal scarring, visual impairment).
- Psychological morbidity due to social isolation.

Xeroderma pigmentosum variant (XP-V)

Caused by mutation in gene encoding enzyme for replication past UVR-damaged

Rook's Dermatology Handbook, First Edition. Edited by Christopher E. M. Griffiths, Tanya O. Bleiker, Daniel Creamer, John R. Ingram and Rosalind C. Simpson.
© 2022 John Wiley & Sons Ltd. Published 2022 by John Wiley & Sons Ltd.

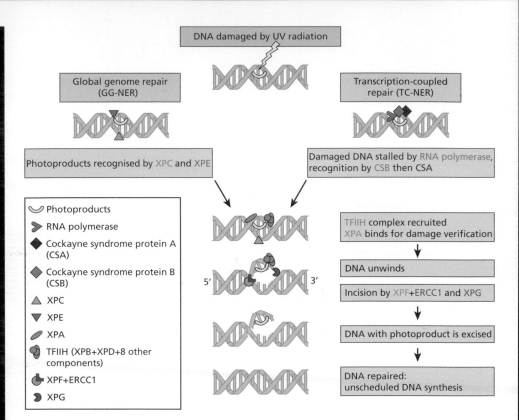

Figure 37.1 In global genome nucleotide excision repair (GG-NER), XPE (with its partner protein DDB1) binds to the photoproduct and recruits another protein, XPC, which recognises and binds to the strand opposite the photoproduct. In transcription-coupled NER (TC-NER), RNA polymerase II stalls at the site of the photoproduct. This then leads to the recruitment of CSA and CSB protein (defective in Cockayne syndrome and not XP). The two pathways then converge. TFIIH (a complex containing 10 peptides, including the helicases XPB and XPD) then opens up the DNA and subsequently XPA binds to verify the correct positioning of all the proteins. The heterodimeric nucleases ERCC1/XPF and XPG then cleave the damaged DNA strand at the 5' to 3' ends on either side of the photoproduct. The gap is filled in by using the undamaged DNA strand as template. This process is referred to as unscheduled DNA synthesis. (Source: Based on Sethi M, Lehmann AR, Fawcett H, et al. Patients with xeroderma pigmentosum complementation groups C, E and V do not have abnormal sunburn reactions. *Br J Dermatol* 2013, 169, 1279–1287.)

sites. Constitutes 20% of XP patients and is diagnosed after age 30. Manifests with multiple skin cancers without neurological involvement.

Xeroderma pigmentosum/Cockayne syndrome complex (XP/CS)

Very rare, autosomal recessive disorder. Manifests with cutaneous features of XP with systemic and neurological features of CS.

Xeroderma pigmentosum/trichothiodystrophy (XP/TTD) syndrome

Phenotypic features of TTD with clinical and cellular findings of XP.

Differential diagnosis

Trichothiodystrophy (Chapter 31), Cockayne syndrome and its variants, erythropoietic protoporphyria (Chapter 28) and Rothmund–Thomson syndrome.

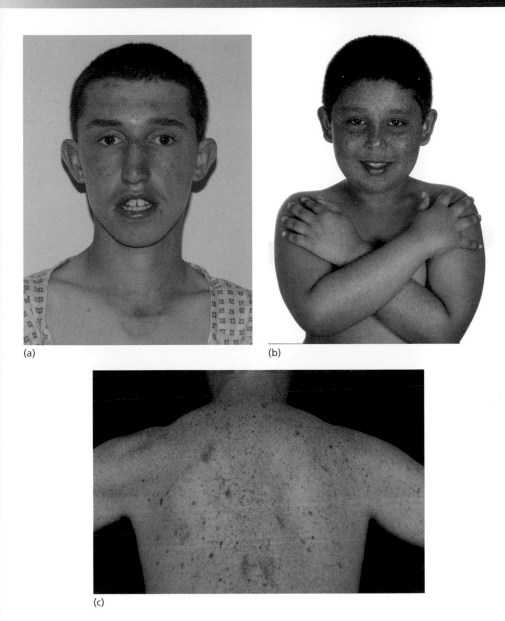

(a)

(b)

(c)

Figure 37.2 Xeroderma pigmentosum. (a) Severe and exaggerated sunburn on minimal sun exposure. (b) Lentigines and hypopigmented macules (seen on the forearms) at sun-exposed sites. (c) Pigmentary change and multiple surgical scars at sites of previous skin cancers.

Investigations

Skin fibroblast culture from a 4-mm punch biopsy taken from an unexposed area of the skin. DNA extracted from a blood sample can then identify the defective gene which gives further information about the XP subtype.

Management

There is no cure. Overall median age of death is 32 years. Skin cancer and neurodegeneration are the main causes of death. Neurological abnormalities are progressive and the median age at death in those with neurological involvement is significantly younger than in XP patients without.

General measures:

- Avoidance of UVR: high-factor sunscreen, UVR protective clothing/hats/gloves/sunglasses, UVR-blocking window films (including cars and fluorescent light sources).
- Vitamin D supplementation.
- Prohibit smoking.
- Multidisciplinary approach: dermatology, ophthalmology, genetic counselling, psychological support.

Management of skin lesions:

- Treat premalignant lesions early with topical therapy (e.g. 5-fluorouracil and imiquimod), avoid photodynamic therapy (irradiation involved may cause further skin damage).
- Early management of any cancers is essential.
- Retinoids may have a role in the prevention of skin cancer.

Cockayne syndrome

Cockayne syndrome (CS) is a rare autosomal recessive disorder of DNA repair. There are three types based on severity of disease.

Epidemiology

Very rare; annual incidence of 1:200 000 in European countries. CS affects males and females equally and it occurs in all ethnic groups.

Pathophysiology

Skin fibroblasts of patients with CS are abnormally sensitive to UVR due to a defective sub-pathway of nucleotide excision repair. This means that cells fail to restore normal levels of RNA synthesis after UVR exposure. May occur in combination with XP.

Clinical features

CS is characterised by cutaneous photosensitivity (from birth), progressive postnatal growth failure, microcephaly, characteristic bird-like facies (Figure 37.3) (prognathism, enophthalmia, a prominent thin nose, large ears and loss of subcutaneous fat), disproportionately large hands and feet, cachexia, premature ageing and dental caries. The skin is dry and thin, and the hair is often sparse.

There is no increased incidence of skin cancer.

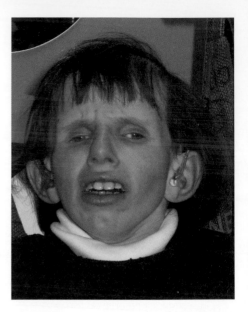

Figure 37.3 Cockayne syndrome demonstrating the characteristic bird-like facies with prominent enophthalmia.

Differential diagnosis

Progeria, XP, Rothmund–Thomson syndrome, Werner syndrome, Bloom syndrome, Hartnup disease.

Investigations

Skin fibroblast culture from a 4-mm punch biopsy taken from an unexposed area of the skin to test for defective DNA repair. Subsequently, analysis of DNA extracted from the blood can identify the defective gene and the causative mutation(s) in patients.

Management

As for XP: supportive care, multidisciplinary input, UV avoidance due to photosensitivity and vitamin D supplementation.

Trichothiodystrophy

See Chapter 31.

Muir–Torre syndrome

(**Syn. Hereditary non-polyposis colorectal cancer, Lynch II syndrome**)
Disorder of DNA repair characterised by sebaceous gland neoplasms and/or

keratoacanthomas associated with one or more visceral malignancies.

Epidemiology

Rare disorder; the majority are familial but sporadic cases have been described.

Pathophysiology

Caused by a mutation in one of the DNA mismatch repair genes. In about 90%, the mutation occurs in the MutS homologue 2 (MSH2) gene, which maps to chromosome 2p, similar to findings in Lynch syndrome. In less than 10% of cases, the mutation is found in the MutL homolog 1 (MLH1) gene, which maps to chromosome 3p. This results in micro-satellite instability in tumour tissue found in 46–100% of tumours associated with Muir–Torre syndrome.

Clinical features

Clinical variation exists but the condition is characterised by:

- Sebaceous gland neoplasms.
- Keratoacanthomas.
- One or more visceral malignancies, particularly gastrointestinal or genito-urinary. Malignancies are often multiple, behave less aggressively and are often low grade.

The majority of patients have a family history of cutaneous tumours and/or internal malignancy. Cutaneous tumours start to arise in the second/third decade. These can be before internal malignancy (22–32% of cases), concomitantly (6–12%) or after internal malignancy has been diagnosed (56–59%). Sebaceous adenomas are found in 25–68% of patients, sebaceous epitheliomas in 31–86% and sebaceous carcinomas in 66–100%. Keratoacanthoma may occur in about 20% of patients with Muir–Torre syndrome and may be multiple.

Most patients develop colorectal carcinoma and nearly 50% have two or more visceral carcinomas. Other internal malignancies include carcinoma of the endometrium, stomach, small bowel, genitourinary tract, breast, ovary, pancreas, liver and kidney.

Visceral tumours in Muir–Torre syndrome are usually low-grade malignancies. The sebaceous carcinomas in this syndrome, like the visceral malignancies, are less aggressive than their counterparts that occur independently.

Differential diagnosis

In familial adenomatous polyposis, patients develop colon carcinoma, colon polyps and other features not usually seen in Muir–Torre syndrome, including hepatoblastoma, thyroid, pancreatic, adrenal and bile duct tumours, along with osteomas, unerupted or extra teeth, congenital hypertrophy of the retinal pigment epithelium, desmoid tumours and benign skin lesions, epidermoid cyst and fibromas.

Gardner syndrome is a subtype of familial adenomatous polyposis with a higher risk of colon carcinoma and multiple colon polyps. However, patients may also develop sebaceous cysts, epidermoid cysts, fibromas, desmoid tumours and osteomas, not features of Muir–Torre syndrome.

Investigations

The diagnosis is generally made on clinical grounds; genetic screening to look for MLH1 and MSH2 gene mutations may be helpful.

Management

Multidisciplinary approach, mainly gastroenterologists and dermatologists. Although evidence for screening is relatively poor, the general recommendations are for patients to have an annual clinical examination, chest radiography and urine cytology. The frequency of performing colonoscopy varies from once every 3 years to every 1–2 years, particularly in higher risk patients. Female patients require an annual cervical smear and carcinoembryonic antigen testing, along with mammography every 1–2 years up to age 50 and then annually thereafter. Endometrial biopsy has also been recommended every 3–5 years.

Surgical clearance of internal tumours and sebaceous carcinoma should be performed where possible. For patients with solitary or few cutaneous lesions, surgery in the form of excision or curettage and cautery would be appropriate.

For patients with multiple benign cutaneous lesions, isotretinoin has been reported to prevent new tumour development.

Patients and their family members should receive genetic screening and counselling.

38 Hamartoneoplastic syndromes

Neurofibromatosis Type 1

Neurofibromatosis type 1 (NF1) is characterised by multiple café-au-lait macules and the occurrence of neurofibromas along peripheral nerves. Neurofibromatosis type 2 (NF2) is characterised by usually bilateral vestibular schwannomas (acoustic neuromas), as well as meningiomas; it does not have significant cutaneous manifestations and is not covered here.

Epidemiology

The prevalence of NF1 has been estimated at about 1 in 2500–3300 births.

Pathophysiology

NF1 is an inherited neuroectodermal abnormality with autosomal dominant inheritance and almost 100% penetrance by the age of 5 years. Up to 50% are sporadic cases. The *NF1* gene on chromosome 17 encodes neurofibromin, a suppressor of tumour activity. The cutaneous neurofibromas of NF1 are derived from peripheral nerves and their supporting structures, including neurilemmal cells.

Clinical features

See Box 38.1. The diagnosis requires the presence of at least two of the seven criteria.

Investigations and management

See Figure 38.2.

Tuberous sclerosis complex

Tuberous sclerosis complex (TSC) represents a genetic disorder of hamartoma formation in

Box 38.1 Diagnostic criteria for NF1

- Six or more café-au-lait macules (sharply defined, light brown patches) of >5 mm in greatest diameter in prepubertal individuals and >15 mm in greatest diameter in postpubertal individuals
- Two or more neurofibromas (Figure 38.1a) of any type or one plexiform neurofibroma
- Freckling in the axillary (Figure 38.1b) or inguinal regions
- Optic glioma
- Two or more Lisch nodules (Figure 38.1c)
- A distinctive osseous lesion such as sphenoid dysplasia or thinning of the long bone cortex with or without pseudoarthrosis
- A first-degree relative (parent, sibling, offspring) with NF1 by the above criteria

many organs, particularly the skin, brain, eye, kidney and heart.

Epidemiology

Incidence is approximately 1 in 10 000.

Pathophysiology

Inheritance of TSC is determined by a single autosomal dominant gene, showing great variability of expression, even within a single family. Approximately 60–70% of TSC cases are due to new mutations.

Clinical features

The syndrome involves skin lesions (in 60–70%), intellectual impairment and epilepsy, but these

Rook's Dermatology Handbook, First Edition. Edited by Christopher E. M. Griffiths, Tanya O. Bleiker, Daniel Creamer, John R. Ingram and Rosalind C. Simpson.
© 2022 John Wiley & Sons Ltd. Published 2022 by John Wiley & Sons Ltd.

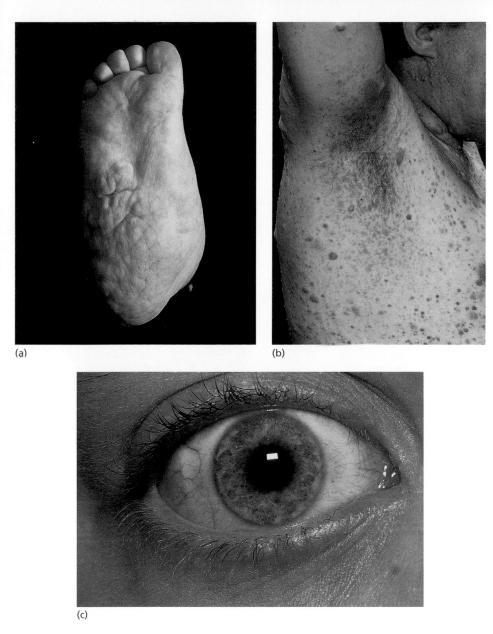

(a)

(b)

(c)

Figure 38.1 Neurofibromatosis type 1. (a) Extensive neurofibroma of the foot. (b) Axillary freckling and multiple neurofibromas. (c) Lisch nodules (pigmented iris hamartomas). (Source: All courtesy of Professor J. Harper, Great Ormond Street Hospital, London, UK.)

Neurofibromatosis type 1
Review guidelines

Annual Review Recommended

At time of diagnosis, or possible diagnosis, ALL patients should be seen in a genetics department.
Those with significant complications will be followed up as appropriate through the nationally funded Complex Nf1 Service.
Annual review should be undertaken by a community/district paediatrician and GP throughout childhood, and by a GP in adulthood. Patients, paediatricians and GPs have telephone access to the NF Service in Genetic Medicine for NF-related concerns.

Age	Genetics appointment	NF1 reviews carried out by	Vision checks
<6 and 50% risk	In first year and then at 2 and 5*¹	Care coordinated by genetics	Symptom check at Nf1 review
<8 affected	Confirmation of diagnosis and assessment. Genetic counselling for family	GP and community/district paediatrician. Liaison with NF service for complex cases	At least annual with paediatric ophthalmologist
8–15 affected	On request		Annual with optician/orthoptist
16–18 affected	Appointment for counselling re: adult complications and genetics	Care coordinated by GP	Symptom check at Nf1 review
>16 affected *²	On request		

*¹If no café-au-lait spots by 5 years, NF1 can be excluded in the majority of NF1 families.

*²Women aged 40–50 should be referred for annual mammography as per 'moderate risk' NICE guidelines.

Review checklist—children (0–16)
Record **height, weight** and **head circumference**. Take **blood pressure** as soon as feasible.
If raised, see the Adult review checklist (Figure 80.4b) for info.

	WHAT TO LOOK FOR	WHEN TO REFER
SKIN	Neurofibromas – can be itchy, and sometimes tender. May be cutaneous or subcutaneous. Plexiform neurofibromas – note location, appearance, size and hardness. Monitor large areas of café-au-lait pigmentation and/or excessive hair growth for development of a plexiform	Rapidly growing, painful or changing lesions: URGENT REFERRAL to Complex NF1 Service or specialist sarcoma team
SKELETON	Scoliosis – look for signs during entire growth period, and especially at puberty and during adolescent growth spurts. **Pseudarthrosis** – tibia most commonly affected but radius and ulna may be involved	Any curvature or bowing – REFER to orthopaedic surgeon
EYES	Have regular ophthalmic reviews taken place for those aged 0–7 years? Is there any evidence of a **squint, proptosis** or **reduced visual acuity**?	URGENT REFERRAL to ophthalmologist if there are concerns about the eye or visual symptoms
NEUROLOGICAL	Neurological symptom review, particularly **ataxia, headaches, loss of consciousness** and **visual disturbance**	REFER to Complex NF1 Service or neurologist if increase in frequency and/or severity of headaches or onset of other symptoms
DEVELOPMENT	Review development – noting in particular **coordination** and **speech difficulties**. There may be short stature and macrocephaly. **Precocious** or **late puberty** should be investigated	Consider REFERRAL to paediatric specialist
EDUCATION & BEHAVIOUR	There is an increased incidence of **learning** and **behaviour** (particularly attention difficulties, **ADD, ADHD and ASD**) problems. Identify possible special needs and appropriate resources to assess them	Consider REFERRAL for professional assessment of educational needs.

UNSURE? Do not hesitate to contact the NF1 team if you have any queries.

Figure 38.2 Management of NF1. Manchester checklist for screening for neurofibromatosis. (Source: Courtesy of Dr Sue Huson.)

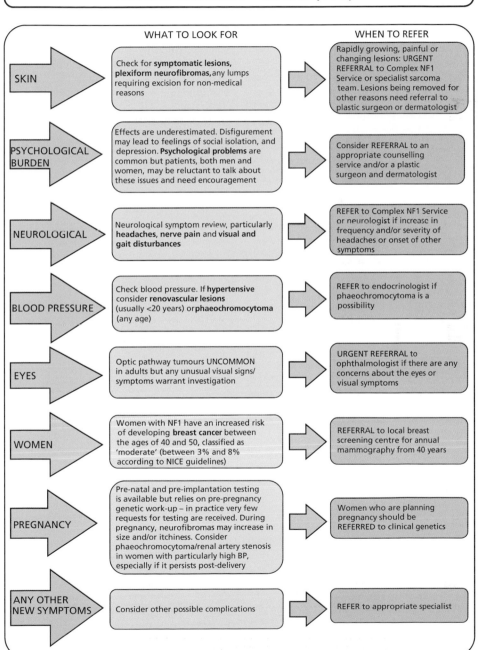

Figure 38.2 (Continued)

PART 4: GENETIC DISORDERS INVOLVING THE SKIN

show very wide variation in age of onset and severity. Four types of skin lesion are pathognomonic (Box 38.2).

> ### Box 38.2 Pathognomonic skin lesions of TSC
>
> * Angiofibromas (Figure 38.3) usually appear between the ages of 3 and 10 years. Firm, discrete, red brown, telangiectatic papules, 1–10 mm in diameter, extend from the naso-labial folds to the cheeks and chin.
> * Periungual fibromas appear at or after puberty as smooth, firm, flesh-coloured excrescences emerging from the nail folds. They are usually 5–10 mm in length.
> * The shagreen patch is an irregularly thickened, slightly elevated, soft, skin-coloured plaque, usually in the lumbosacral region.
> * White ovoid or ash-leaf-shaped macules, 1–3 cm in length, most easily detectable by examination under Wood's light, are frequently present on the trunk or limbs.

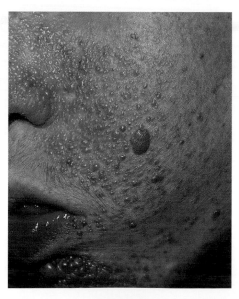

Figure 38.3 Tuberous sclerosis: angiofibromas. (Source: Courtesy of Professor J. Harper, Great Ormond Street Hospital, London, UK.)

Investigations
MRI or CT scanning of the brain is used to detect intracranial lesions.

Management
The cosmetic appearance of angiofibromas may be improved by pulsed dye vascular laser to reduce redness. More papular/nodular lesions are best treated with a carbon dioxide laser or other debriding interventions. Topical rapamycin at 1% or 2% concentration may be beneficial for cutaneous angiofibromas and systemic rapamycin may be useful for visceral tumours and neurological complications, including epilepsy. Neurosurgery should be considered when epilepsy is uncontrolled by drugs and there is a fixed, circumscribed, electroencephalographic focus.

Family screening and genetic counselling should be carried out by referral to a clinical genetics service. DNA testing is possible in 85% of cases.

Gardner syndrome

The term Gardner syndrome is given to the complex phenotype comprising multiple epidermoid cysts, fibrous tissue tumours, osteomas and polyposis of the colon.

Pathophysiology
Gardner syndrome is one of the *APC*-associated polyposis conditions, a group of disorders with familial polyposis as a central feature.

Clinical features
Epidermoid cysts, which may be numerous, are usually irregularly distributed on the face, scalp and extremities, and are less frequent on the trunk. They may first appear between the ages of 4 and 10 years, but often considerably later, and are ultimately present in almost all cases.

Polyposis of the colon or rectum usually arises during the second decade, but may occur in early childhood. It is present in about 50% of patients by the age of 20 years. Malignant change develops 15–20 years later in over 40% of reported cases.

Investigations
Multiple epidermoid cysts may be inherited as an isolated abnormality and have no sinister significance. However, they are an important indicator of possible asymptomatic polyposis. A detailed family history of malignancy should

be sought, and clinical and radiological examination of the skull is indicated to check for osteomas, another feature of Gardner syndrome. Molecular diagnosis is now possible by direct sequencing and duplication/insertion analysis.

Management
The mainstay of management is surveillance for somatic cancers, ideally under the direction of a cancer geneticist.

Cowden syndrome

In Cowden syndrome, multiple hamartomatous lesions of ectodermal, endodermal and meso-dermal origins are associated with a predisposition to malignant tumours, particularly of the breast.

Pathophysiology
Mutations in the PTEN (phosphatase and tensin homolog) gene underpin some, but not all cases.

Clinical features
Skin-coloured trichilemmomas are lichenoid papules up to 4 mm in diameter, which tend to coalesce to give a cobblestone appearance, distributed on and around the eyes and mouth. There are small translucent keratoses on the palms and soles, and on the palmar and plantar aspects of the fingers and toes. Verrucous and papillomatous lesions are seen in some patients on the labial and buccal mucosa, fauces and oro-pharynx, and may extend to the larynx.

Approximately 30% of reported female cases developed breast cancer. Fibrocystic disease of the breast sometimes leads to massive hyperplasia. Goitre or thyroid adenoma is present in many cases and thyroid carcinoma has been reported.

Differential diagnosis
Juvenile polyposis coli, Peutz–Jeghers syndrome.

Management
Once the diagnosis is confirmed, management is mainly focused on screening for relevant malignancies in conjunction with a medical genetics service: baseline thyroid ultrasound examination in adults, breast screening in women aged 30 years or more, colonoscopy in men and women over 35 years old, renal MRI in men and women over 40 years.

Skin manifestations should be managed as they would in any other circumstances. Locally destructive therapies such as cryotherapy or curettage and cautery are appropriate. Laser ablation and 5-fluorouracil can be helpful.

PART 4: GENETIC DISORDERS INVOLVING THE SKIN

39

Inherited metabolic disorders

These are inborn errors of metabolism caused by deficiencies of enzymes or transport proteins.

LYSOSOMAL STORAGE DISORDERS

Fabry disease

(syn Anderson–Fabry disease)
Rare X-linked lysosomal storage disorder, characterised by angiokeratomas and multisystem complications.

Epidemiology
Incidence is 1/40 000–60 000 male births.

Pathophysiology
X-linked recessive. Deficiency of α-galactosidase A leading to globotriaosylceramide accumulation in vascular endothelial, perithelial and smooth muscle cells. This causes aneurysmal dilatation of blood vessels, ischaemia and infarction. Histology of angiokeratomas shows dilated vessels in the upper dermis beneath a thinned epidermis. Vacuolated cells in the media and intima of small blood vessels present. It exhibits positive birefringence (accumulated glycosphingolipids).

Clinical features
Affected males present in childhood with burning pain in the extremities, followed by the diffuse appearance of angiokeratomas (Figure 39.1). Most adult males develop renal failure, and cardiac and cerebrovascular disease.

Heterozygous females are carriers and also develop later onset symptoms.

Other features are mucosal telangiectases, anhidrosis/hypohidrosis and lymphedema. Cardiac involvement occurs in almost all adult males; most men have proteinuria, hypertension and deteriorating renal function. Cerebrovascular disease leads to early strokes or transient ischaemic attacks. Some patients develop neurological problems without obvious thrombotic episodes.

Differential diagnosis
Angiokeratoma corporis diffusum occurs in several other lysosomal disorders (Table 39.1).

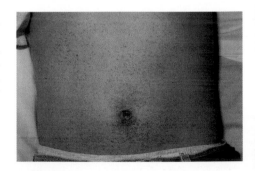

Figure 39.1 Angiokeratoma corporis diffusum around the umbilicus in a man with Fabry disease.

Rook's Dermatology Handbook, First Edition. Edited by Christopher E. M. Griffiths, Tanya O. Bleiker, Daniel Creamer, John R. Ingram and Rosalind C. Simpson.
© 2022 John Wiley & Sons Ltd. Published 2022 by John Wiley & Sons Ltd.

Table 39.1 Summary of the rarer lysosomal storage disorders

	Mucopoly-saccharidoses (seven different types)	Glycoprotein degradation disorders (several different types)	Mucolipidoses types II and III	Sphingolipidoses
Epidemiology	Affects 1:25 000	Very rare	–	Gaucher disease, 1:50 000
Patho-physiology	All autosomal recessive except Hunter syndrome (X-linked recessive) Degradation products of GAGs accumulate within lysosomes to cause disease	All autosomal recessive Glycoproteins on cell surfaces are degraded, leading to storage of oligosaccharides and/or glycopeptides	Autosomal recessive Multiple lysosomal enzymes fail to enter their organelle	All are autosomal recessive, except Fabry disease, which is X-linked Sphingolipids on cell membranes are degraded 'Foam cells' are found in the bone marrow and in the skin
Clinical features	Presentation in early childhood Range of severity between the different disorders: ivory white papules/nodules on the back (Hunter syndrome), widespread Mongolian blue spots, coarse facial appearance, deafness, upper airways problems, generalised hypertrichosis, hepatosplenomegaly, bone dysplasia, developmental regression	Range of clinical presentations depending on the condition, including angiokeratomas occur in fucosidosis, skeletal dysplasia, developmental delay	Gum hypertrophy, coarse facial features, severe neurological involvement, skeletal dysplasia, cardiomyopathy	Gaucher disease: Type 1 easy tanning, yellow/brown pigmentation, hepatosplenomegaly, thrombocytopenia; Type II causes neurological problems and may present with collodian baby phenotype; Type III causes hepatosplenomegaly Niemann–Pick disease: waxy indurated skin, brown/yellow pigmentation, papular lesions, Mongolian spots Farber disease: subcutaneous nodules. presents early infancy, hoarse cry, painful swollen joints
Investigations	Analysis of urine GAGs	Leukocyte lysosomal enzyme assay (many laboratories offer this for screening patients with relevant clinical features)	Raised plasma levels of the mistargeted lysosomal enzymes	Leukocytes enzyme assay
Management	Multidisciplinary input required and symptomatic management Specific therapies: • Haematopoietic stem cell transplantation for Hurler and Maroteaux–Lamy syndromes • Enzyme replacement therapy is available for MPS I, II, IV and VI	Only symptomatic treatment is currently available	Only symptomatic treatment is currently available	Gaucher disease type 1: Enzyme replacement therapy Haematopoietic stem cell transplantation for Gaucher disease with neurological involvement Miglustat (oral drug which reduces accumulation of glucocerebroside) for Niemann–Pick (type C) and Gaucher disease type 1 if unable to receive enzyme replacement therapy

GAGs, glycosaminoglycans; MPS, mucopolysaccharidoses.

Investigations

Skin biopsy. Plasma enzyme assay in males shows α-galactosidase A deficiency (females may have normal enzyme activity). Slit-lamp examination shows corneal dystrophy.

Management

Enzyme replacement therapy is indicated for all males and for female patients with cardiac, renal or neurological disease. Multidisciplinary input is required for pain management, and cardiac and renal involvement. Early diagnosis improves prognosis; genetic counseling and testing of individuals with a suspected or confirmed diagnosis of Fabry disease, with a family history of Fabry disease and those identified as female carriers of Fabry disease should be offered. Median survival is 50 years in males and 70 years in females.

DISORDERS OF AMINO ACID METABOLISM AND TRANSPORT

Multisystem disorders resulting from the deficiency of an amino acid or from the toxic accumulation of an amino acid or a related chemical (Table 39.2). Management of these conditions is

Table 39.2 Summary of amino acid metabolism and transport disorders which have cutaneous features

	Phenylketonuria (Syn. Phenylalanine hydroxylase deficiency)	Argininosuccinic aciduria	Hartnup disease
Epidemiology	Incidence approx. 1:12 000	Incidence 1:70 000	Incidence on newborn screening ranges from 1:14 000 to 1:45 000
Pathophysiology	Defects of phenylalanine hydroxylase prevents conversion of phenylalanine to tyrosine	Autosomal recessive urea cycle disorder	Autosomal recessive Impaired intestinal absorption of tryptophan (a neutral amino acid) causes reduced synthesis of nicotinamide
Clinical features	Increased incidence of eczema, reduced pigmentation of skin, hair and iris, psychomotor retardation, behavioral problems, seizures	Some present later with dry, brittle hair consistent with trichorrhexis nodosa Acute presentation with vomiting, confusion or coma due to acute hyperammonaemia in newborns	Dry, scaly patches occur on sun-exposed skin (Figure 39.2) Sun exposure causes erythema, sometimes with blistering Cerebellar ataxia
Investigations	Detected by newborn screening Plasma amino acid analysis in those who have not been screened	Urine amino acid analysis demonstrates argininosuccinic acid	Increased neutral amino acids in urine with low or low–normal concentrations in plasma
Management	Restriction of dietary phenylalanine	Dietary protein restriction L-arginine corrects the amino acid deficiency	Oral nicotinamide in conjunction with high-protein diet

multidisciplinary, led by paediatricians. Vary rare disorders are not discussed, e.g. tyrosinaemia type 2, alkaptonuria, prolidase deficiency.

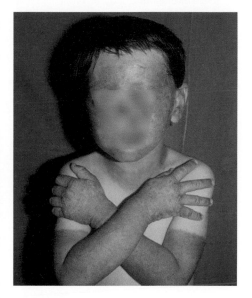

Figure 39.2 Hartnup disease: erythema and scaling on sun-exposed skin. (From Irvine AD, Hoeger PH, Yan AC (eds) Harper's Textbook of Dermatology, 3rd edn, 2011. Oxford: Wiley Blackwell.)

DISORDERS OF CHOLESTEROL SYNTHESIS

There are a number of inborn errors affecting cholesterol synthesis:

- Sterol $\Delta 8$-$\Delta 7$ isomerase deficiency (X-linked dominant chondrodysplasia punctata or Conradi–Hünermann syndrome) causes ichthyosis.
- 3β-hydroxysteroid C-4 dehydrogenase deficiency (congenital hemidysplasia with ichthyosiform erythroderma and limb defects, CHILD syndrome).
- Smith-Lemli-Opitz syndrome is the commonest disorder of cholesterol synthesis (incidence 1:15 000-1:60 000). It is an autosomal recessive disorder caused by 7-dehydrocholesterol reductase deficiency. There is a wide

range of severity. Cutaneous features include photosensitivity (which is severe), hypopigmented hair, hyperhidrosis of the palms, eczema and cutis marmorata.

OTHER METABOLIC DISORDERS

Other notable inherited disorders of metabolism include the following:

- *Mitochondrial respiratory chain disorders*: These have varied patterns of inheritance. Mitochondrial DNA is inherited exclusively from the mother. These disorders can affect any tissue due to their effect on adenosine triphosphate (ATP); neuromuscular problems are commonest. There is a multisystem presentation, and cutaneous features comprise multiple symmetrical lipomatosis on back/shoulders, acrocyanosis, palmoplantar keratoderma and hypertrichosis.
- *Congenital disorders of glycosylation*: Phosphomannomutase 2 deficiency (PMM2-CDG) is the commonest of these disorders. Autosomal recessive inheritance. Incidence is estimated at 1:40 000 in Sweden. Multisystem disorders are caused by defects in the glycosylation of proteins or lipids. It presents in neonates with a spectrum of severity. Cutaneous features comprise subcutaneous fat pads over the iliac crests with lipodystrophy of the rest of buttocks, Peau d'orange and lipoatrophy of the legs occur when older. Low PMM2 leucocyte activity. There is no effective treatment; mortality is about 20% in the first few years.
- *Disorders of biotin metabolism*: These include holocarboxylase synthetase deficiency and biotinidase deficiency (incidence 1:100 000). Autosomal recessive inheritance. Holocarboxylase synthetase deficiency when mild causes widespread, scaly, erythematous rash in nappy area. Severe disease causes significant metabolic complications. Biotinidase deficiency causes a perioral rash, skin infections, sparse hair/alopecia and psychomotor retardation. Holocarboxylase synthetase deficiency is diagnosed by excretion of characteristic organic acids, mutation analysis or fibroblast carboxylase activity. Biotinidase deficiency is detected by measuring plasma

biotinidase activity. Treatment is with oral biotin. If untreated the metabolic complications lead to death.

- *Menkes disease*: Very rare (approximately 1:250 000) X-linked recessive disorder causing mutation in copper transport gene which leads to copper deficiency. Clinical features are sparse, brittle hair (pili torti, trichorrhexis nodosa), lax skin and joints, developmental regression and mild learning difficulty. Low serum copper and caeruloplasmin concentrations are only diagnostic after 3 months of age; mutation analysis is the main method of detection. Treat with subcutaneous copper histidine; untreated leads to death by age 3.

- *Wilson disease (Syn. Hepatolenticular degeneration)*: Incidence is 1:30 000 to 1:100 000. Autosomal recessive deficiency of copper-transporting ATPase causes reduced excretion of copper which accumulates in organs. Skin changes are blue lunulae of nails, xeroderma, grey-brown and hyperpigmentation. Other features are corneal Kayser–Fleischer ring, and liver and neurological effects. Diagnosis is by low serum copper and caeruloplasmin concentrations; raised 24-h urine copper excretion. Treatment is with chelating agents or zinc increases copper excretion.

- *Familial tumoral calcinosis*: This includes hyperphosphataemic familial tumoral calcinosis (HFTC) and normophosphataemic familial tumoral calcinosis (NFTC). HFTC causes large painful calcified masses form over large joints. NFTC causes a vasculitis-like rash when young, which leads to calcified masses in the cutaneous and subcutaneous tissues when older. Surgery can be performed for symptomatic lesions.

Part 5
Psychological and Neurological Disorders and the Skin

Pruritus and prurigo

40

Chronic pruritus

(Syn. Itch)

Chronic pruritus (CP) is a sensation leading to the desire to scratch lasting for at least 6 weeks. It is a symptom of many dermatological diseases, as well as being a feature of certain systemic, neurological or psychiatric disorders.

Epidemiology

The prevalence of CP in the general population is 7%; with age the incidence of CP increases. M = F.

Pathophysiology

Pruritus is a symptom, not a disease, occurring in a large variety of underlying disorders, listed in Table 40.1. The pathophysiology of itch in each entity is also outlined in Table 40.1.

Clinical features

The important details in history taking are listed in Box 40.1 and the clinical features of itch in different disorders is displayed in Table 40.1. CP may occur on non-diseased skin or with a dermatosis. A full examination is needed to identify a causative dermatosis or exclude a dermatological source of the itch. Dermographism must be tested in all patients. Some itchy skin disorders evoke scratching and excoriation (e.g. scabies), whereas others prompt rubbing (e.g. lichen planus and urticaria). The mechanical trauma from scratching can produce excoriations, papules, nodules (nodular prurigo), lichenification (lichen simplex chronicus), scars and hyper/hypopigmentation. A general physical examination should include palpation of the liver, spleen and lymph nodes. CP can lead to psychological impairment.

Investigations

Investigations should be guided by the examination findings; in many cases no tests are necessary. If the cause is unclear some or all of the investigations in Box 40.2 should be undertaken.

Management

Treatment should be directed to managing the underlying cause. Standard pruritus-relieving measures are use of an emollient soap substitute, lukewarm showers/baths, daily application of a moisturiser and cotton clothing.
First line: Therapy directed to the cause of pruritus, if known. Non-sedating antihistamines, topical corticosteroids.
Second line: In pruritus of unknown origin, or in cases which are refractory to first-line measures, consider the following: topical capsaicin, topical calcineurin inhibitors, gabapentin, pregabalin, UV phototherapy (narrow band UVB or psoralen and UVA [PUVA]), immunosuppressants (e.g. ciclosporin), naltrexone.

Prurigo nodularis

(Syn. Nodular prurigo)

Prurigo nodularis (PN) is a reaction pattern due to chronic scratching. It is characterised by symmetrically distributed hyperkeratotic or eroded nodules.

Rook's Dermatology Handbook, First Edition. Edited by Christopher E. M. Griffiths, Tanya O. Bleiker, Daniel Creamer, John R. Ingram and Rosalind C. Simpson.
© 2022 John Wiley & Sons Ltd. Published 2022 by John Wiley & Sons Ltd.

Table 40.1 Conditions associated with pruritus

Disorder	Pathophysiology of pruritus	Clinical features of itch	Treatment of itch
Atopic eczema	Itch in atopic skin disease is multifactorial: dryness, inflammation, hyperplasia of skin nerves all contribute	Itch is an intrinsic part of atopic eczema Worse at night and aggravated by sweating and contact with wool Compounded by infection with *Staph aureus*	Emollients Treatment of eczema Habit reversal therapy to control scratching
Psoriasis	Itch mediated by T cells, cytokines (IL-17 & IL-31) and neuropeptides	Itch is common in psoriasis and may affect non-lesional as well as lesional skin	Emollients Treatment of psoriasis
Chronic kidney disease	Proposed pathogenic explanations: secondary hyperparathyroidism, raised IL-6 and Th1 lymphocyte-mediated inflammation	Persistent, generalised itching occurs in 10–80% of patients with chronic renal failure More common in haemodialysis than continuous ambulatory peritoneal dialysis Rare in children or in acute renal failure Secondary skin changes due to scratching are common	Emollients and management of secondary eczema UVB phototherapy often useful Gabapentin helpful in some patients Dialysis not especially effective Renal transplantation is only reliably effective treatment
Hepatobiliary disease	Autotoxin, bile acid receptor TGR5 and dysregulation of central opioid peptides are involved Primary biliary cholangitis and hepatitis C are common causes of cholestatic pruritus	Itch is an early symptom of hepatobiliary disease and is frequently debilitating Itch is generalised, or localised to the hands and feet	Bile salt sequestrants, rifampicin, phototherapy, naloxone or naltrexone
Polycythaemia vera and iron deficiency	Proposed pathogenic explanations: histamine release, platelet aggregation and iron deficiency	50% of PV patients with JAK2V617 mutation develop aquagenic pruritus within minutes of water contact Aquagenic itch may precede development of PV by years	Antihistamines are effective in 30% PUVA and UVB can help Interferon-α 2b, paroxetine, pregabalin and aspirin have been used Correction of iron deficiency in PV can improve itch

Thyroid disease	Thyrotoxicosis: vasodilatation causes increased skin temperature and lowered itch threshold	Generalised itch Dry skin of myxedema can also cause widespread pruritus	Correction of thyroid dysfunction
Diabetes mellitus	Pruritus may be associated with diabetic neuropathy	Itch is generalised but especially affects torso	Correction of blood sugar, emollients, phototherapy
Malignancy	Pathophysiology unknown	Premonitory pruritus may precede onset of Hodgkin's disease, myelodysplasia and polycythaemia vera by several years Solid tumours less likely to cause itch	Treat underlying malignancy SSRIs (e.g. paroxetine) or pregabalin can help
Drug-induced	Common culprits include opiates, chloroquine, imatinib Multiple mechanisms account for drug mediated itch	Generalised pruritus usually occurring with clear temporal relation to culprit drug	Stop culprit medication
Senescence	Predominantly from skin dryness	50% of individuals of 60 years and older have chronic itch	Emollients, modify ambient temperature
Notalgia parasthetica	Nerve root entrapment or sensory neuropathy of spinal nerves T2–T6	Burning itch at mid-scapular area of back	Capsaicin cream
Brachoradial pruritus	Cervical radiculopathy	F > M 60 years and older Itch at elbow and adjacent arm skin Worsened by sunlight	Gabapentin

PV, polycythaemia vera; SSRI, selective serotonin re-uptake inhibitors.

> **Box 40.1 Important details in history taking in CP patients**
>
> **Pruritus-specific history**
>
> Time point of start of CP and total duration
> Localisation (start, spreading)
> Quality, e.g. burning itch, pricking itch, tingling itch, itch resembling insects crawling on skin (formication)
> Course: variations during the day, continuous CP, attacks of itch, spontaneous improvement/deterioration
> Triggering factors, ameliorating factors
> Behavioural response to itch: scratching, rubbing or, rarely, slapping
> Temporal association with previous illnesses, surgeries, medication intake, other events
> Previous therapies: successful/unsuccessful
> Patient's own theory about the cause of CP
> Psychogenic stress factors
> Impairments in quality of life, burden, sleep disturbances
>
> **General history**
>
> Previous illnesses, including dermatoses
> Drug intake, infusions, blood transfusions
> Previous surgeries
> Allergies: type I/type IV allergies
> Atopic predisposition
> Clinical signs for malignancy (weight loss, fever, night sweats)
> Pregnancy

> **Box 40.2 Investigations in a patient presenting with CP**
>
> FBC
> U&E
> Liver function tests
> Lactate dehydrogenase (LDH)
> Tryptase
> Blood film
> ESR
> Glucose
> Ferritin
> Autoantibodies (including antimitochondrial antibodies)
> Skin biopsy (histopathology and direct immunofluorescence)
> Protein electrophoresis
> Hepatitis B & C antibodies
> Chest radiograph

Epidemiology

Estimated that the prevalence of PN is 1–2.5 per 10 000 persons. F > M. More common in older patients.

Pathophysiology

It is a reaction pattern occurring in CP. All factors which induce chronic scratching may lead to PN: an atopic predisposition is the commonest predisposing factor. Histologically, epidermal hyperplasia is prominent. Cutaneous neuropathy may occur with a thickening of myelinated dermal nerves, neuroma formation (Pautrier neuroma) and an increase in the number of subepidermal and dermal nerve fibres (neuronal hyperplasia). There is a significant decrease of sensory C fibres in the nodules and in non-lesional skin.

Clinical features

Patients tend to have a long history of itch and uncontrollable scratching. The typical lesion of PN is a pink nodule with a hyperkeratotic or eroded surface and a hyperpigmented border. PN lesions may be dome-shaped or plaque-like. Patients may have hundreds of lesions disseminated widely or a few confined to a localised area of itching (Figure 40.1 and 40.2). Sites of predilection are the dorsal arms and legs, the upper chest, back and buttocks. There is a relationship between emotional tension and bouts of scratching. Reactions to stress may be relieved by habitual, ritualised skin scratching.

Investigations

The aim of investigations is to identify any underlying dermatosis or systemic cause of pruritus (Table 40.1). The laboratory investigations are similar to those in the diagnostic work-up of CP (see Box 40.2).

Management

The general principles of PN management are the same as in CP. Treatment should be directed to management of the underlying cause and symptomatic therapy of itchy, traumatised skin. Standard pruritus-relieving measures are use of an emollient soap substitute, lukewarm showers/baths, daily application of a moisturiser and cotton clothing.
First line: Non-sedating antihistamines, topical corticosteroids, intralesional corticosteroid, topical calcineurin inhibitors, topical antipruritics (e.g. menthol in aqueous cream), bandages and occlusion.

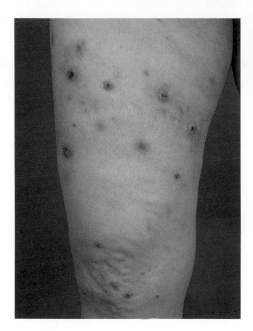

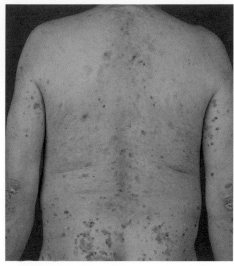

Figure 40.2 Patient with chronic pruritus on inflamed skin (psoriasis).

Figure 40.1 A 64-year-old patient with nodular prurigo of multiple aetiologies.

Second line: In pruritus of unknown origin, or in therapy refractory cases, consider the following: topical capsaicin, oral gabapentin, pregabalin, doxepin, amitriptyline. UV phototherapy (narrow band UVB or PUVA) can be helpful. If there is underlying inflammation consider a systemic immunosuppressant (e.g. ciclosporin).

Third line: Habit reversal therapy, other talk therapies, selective serotonin re-uptake inhibitors, thalidomide, naltrexone.

Lichen simplex chronicus

Lichen simplex chronicus (LSC) is a highly pruritic, circumscribed plaque caused by incessant scratching. (see also Chapter 14).

Epidemiology
Peak incidence is between 30 and 50 years. F > M.

Pathophysiology
Patients often have an atopic background. Histologically there is epidermal hyperplasia and hyperkeratosis, and the dermis contains a chronic inflammatory cell infiltrate.

Clinical features
Irresistible itching is the major complaint, accompanied by scratching and rubbing. The urge to scratch may be exacerbated by anxiety. Mechanical skin trauma is carried out using the fingernails, knuckles, or sometimes an instrument such as a pen. Scratching may be subconscious, but more often patients engage in it consciously until the pruritus is relieved. LSC is usually a solitary plaque 2–10 cm in diameter. In the early stages the skin is red; with time the affected skin becomes pigmented, thickened, slightly scaly and with accentuation of normal skin markings. Usual sites are neck, ankles, scalp, vulva and scrotum.

Investigations
Usually a clinical diagnosis, but a biopsy can distinguish LSC from lichen planus, lichen amyloidosis and psoriasis.

Management
Treatment is aimed at breaking the itch–scratch cycle and suppression of pruritus, usually by topical or intralesional corticosteroids. The application of an occlusive dressing/bandage will increase the effect of topical steroids. The management algorithm is the same as for PN.

41

Mucocutaneous pain syndromes

The dysaesthetic Syndromes

The mucocutaneous pain and genital dysaesthetic syndromes comprise a heterogeneous group of disorders in which there is abnormal sensation of the skin, generally in a specific site. A demonstrable cause for the abnormal sensations may or may not be present. There may be little, or nothing, to see by way of cutaneous clinical signs, or there may be evidence of excoriation, rubbing or skin traumatisation. The disorders may be divided into those with no demonstrable neurological cause and those with a believed or demonstrable neurological cause (Table 41.1).

Table 41.1 The dysaesthetic syndromes

With (usually) demonstrable neurological deficit	Without demonstrable neurological deficit
Sensory mononeuropathies	Scalp dysaesthesia
Notalgia parasthetica	Vulvodynia
Meralgia parasthetica	Penodynia/ scrotodynia
Post-herpetic neuralgia	Atypical trigeminal trophic syndrome
Trigeminal trophic syndrome	Trigeminal neuropathic pain syndrome
Erythromelalgia	Burning mouth syndrome

Post-herpetic neuralgia

Post-herpetic neuralgia (PHN) is a neuropathic pain which develops in the distribution of a sensory nerve involved in shingles.

Epidemiology
3.4 per 1000 patients per year. The risk for developing PHN 1 month after acute herpes zoster infection is 6.5%. It is more common in adults aged over 55 years.

Pathophysiology
PHN occurs in the 3-6 months following an episode of shingles. In the affected dermatome there is degeneration of small-fibre afferents. The virus itself may cause normally silent neurons to produce spontaneous action potentials. Ectopic impulses, provoked by mechanical or thermal stimuli, can occur at the site of dorsal root ganglion damage.

Clinical features
PHN presents with a persistent burning, stabbing or itching pain with sharp exacerbations. Sometimes pain is provoked by non-noxious stimuli, such as contact with clothing or changes in temperature. Some patients have sensory loss in the painful area (anaesthesia dolorosa), others have allodynia with minimal sensory loss.

Investigations
The diagnosis is made clinically.

Rook's Dermatology Handbook, First Edition. Edited by Christopher E. M. Griffiths, Tanya O. Bleiker, Daniel Creamer, John R. Ingram and Rosalind C. Simpson.
© 2022 John Wiley & Sons Ltd. Published 2022 by John Wiley & Sons Ltd.

Management

There is a gradual improvement in pain over time, but the sensory changes take longer to recover.
First line: Topical 5% lidocaine gel or lidocaine patch. Capsaicin cream can be helpful.
Second line: Amitriptyline (starting dose 10 mg at night, increase dose over time) or nortriptyline. Gabapentin or pregabalin as alternatives (again, start at low dose and increase over time).
Third line: Opioid analgesics and tramadol for short periods.

Vulvodynia, peno-scrotodynia

(Syn. Vestibulodynia, penile dysaesthetic syndrome)
These are pain syndromes of the anogenital skin.

Epidemiology

Vulvodynia occurs in 8% of women, peno-scrotodynia occurs in 2% of men. It usually affects younger adults in their 30s to 40s.

Pathophysiology

Probably involves dysfunction of the peripheral and/or central sensory nerve pathways which innervate the genital areas.

Clinical features

Severe burning, stabbing pain, sometimes described as 'rawness', affects either the whole genital skin or a specific zone. The pain may be provoked (e.g. by sexual contact) or it may be present all the time. There are few, if any, physical signs. Localised or generalised erythema may be seen, but this is often within the normal range and should not be over-interpreted. Point tenderness is more common in women than men. Sexual dysfunction (dyspareunia, erectile and ejaculatory disturbance) is common. While the condition is associated with psychosocial co-morbidities, it is not a primary psychiatric disorder.

Management

Treatment may take some time to achieve remission or symptom amelioration.

First line: Topical lidocaine gel.

Second line: Amitriptyline (starting dose 10 mg at night, increase dose over time), or other tricyclics (e.g. doxepin). Selective serotonin re-uptake inhibitors (SSRIs), gabapentin or pregabalin can be used as alternatives (start at low dose and increase over time).

Third line: Consider cognitive behavioural therapy (CBT), especially if there are psycho-sexual or psychosocial co-morbidities.

Trigeminal trophic syndrome

In trigeminal trophic syndrome (TTS) abnormal sensations in the distribution of the trigeminal nerve are associated with an irresistible desire to pick at the involved skin.

Epidemiology

TTS is rare. It occurs in middle-aged individuals. M:F is 2:1.

Pathophysiology

There are demonstrable defects in the trigeminal nerve pathways (peripheral or central) with, most probably, destruction of fibres conveying pain and temperature sensation. Causes of TTS include central sensory neuronal damage, herpes zoster- or herpes simplex-related neuritis, syringobulbia, posterior fossa tumour or occlusion of the posterior inferior cerebellar artery. It may follow iatrogenic damage to the trigeminal nerve by attempts to relieve intractable trigeminal neuralgia.

Clinical features

The patient complains of itching and burning pain or paraesthesiae in an area innervated by the trigeminal nerve. This is then picked, rubbed or scratched. Affected skin may be relatively anaesthetic so that the patient is not aware of the damage caused. Erosions increase in size and may destroy the nasal cartilage. Characteristically, the alar rim is involved but the tip of the nose spared. Ulcers may spread to the cheek and chin (Figure 41.1). Involvement of the upper lip and subsequent scarring can lead to lip elevation. Patients freely admit to traumatising the area in an attempt to relieve the sensation. Neurological examination may reveal decreased perception

PART 5: PSYCHOLOGICAL AND NEUROLOGICAL DISORDERS AND THE SKIN

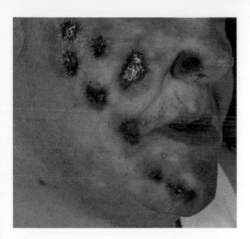

Figure 41.1 Trigeminal trophic syndrome with extensive erosions on the nose, cheek and chin.

of light touch and pain over the area, and sometimes an absent corneal reflex.

Atypical trigeminal trophic syndrome

In this variant the distribution is unusual, often involving the neck, or two regions of the trigeminal nerve There is no demonstrable trigeminal neuropathy or disease of the trigeminal nerve or central nervous system. The ulceration may be bilateral (Figure 41.2).

Differential diagnosis

Chronic skin picking disorder, dermatitis artefacta (however, the patient denies inducing the lesions in dermatitis artefacta).

Investigations

Imaging and neurophysiological tests can be used to investigate trigeminal nerve dysfunction.

Management

Therapy is aimed at reducing the dysaesthesia whilst treating the skin changes.

First line: Emollients and, if necessary, antibiotics. Protect the eroded areas with appropriate dressings. Neurological treatment: gabapentin, pregabalin, amitriptyline, or SSRIs.

Second line: Habit reversal. CBT may be helpful.

Erythromelalgia

Erythromelalgia is an intense burning sensation of the extremities, usually feet, associated with persistent fixed erythema.

Epidemiology

Incidence is 1.3 per 100 000 persons per year. The average age of presentation is 60 years. F > M.

Pathophysiology

There is a distal cutaneous small-fibre neuropathy with diminished sudomotor function (sweating). The neuropathy reduces sympathetic vasoconstrictive response, resulting in increased acral blood flow. Secondary erythromelalgia is usually due to an underlying haematological disorder: leukaemia, thrombocytosis or poly-

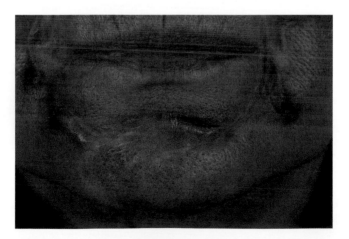

Figure 41.2 Patient with atypical trigeminal trophic syndrome in which lesions are bilateral.

cythemia vera. Raised microvascular viscosity is thought to be causative in these cases.

Clinical features

Feet are most commonly affected, but the disorder can affect the legs, hands, ears, neck and face. Patients experience an intense burning sensation with fixed erythema of involved skin. Usually there is a persistent background dysaesthesia with painful flares occurring at night. Exacerbating factors include heat and exercise; relief often comes with cooling the extremities. Between attacks, the extremities may feel normal or may be mildly cool, cyanotic, or uncomfortable. Patients will often lie in bed with their feet facing an open window, or immersed in bowls of cold water, or lying on cooling ice packs.

Differential diagnosis

Peripheral neuropathy, Raynaud phenomenon, acrocyanosis, peripheral vascular disease.

Investigations

The diagnosis is established clinically.

Management

Treatment is difficult.

First line: Skin treatment: lidocaine patches or doxepin cream. Calcium channel antagonists (e.g. nifedipine) can be helpful. Aspirin and other prostaglandin antagonists may relieve symptoms in some patients. Neurological treatments are also used: gabapentin, pregabalin, amitriptyline, SSRIs.

Second line: Sympathetic blockade, sympathectomy, or dorsal cord stimulation may be considered.

Secondary erythromelalgia

Treatment of the underlying myeloproliferative disorder is essential to control the skin problem.

Other management considerations

Patients should be educated to avoid provoking factors, such as warmth, dependent positioning and alcohol. Behaviour which exacerbates the condition, such as immersion of the affected body parts in cold water, should be discouraged.

PART 5: PSYCHOLOGICAL AND NEUROLOGICAL DISORDERS AND THE SKIN

42

Psychodermatology

A link between the mind and the skin is well recognised. Psychodermatology is the interface between dermatology, psychology and psychiatry. Skin–psyche interactions may be any of the following:

1. Skin disorders which can be influenced by psychological factors, e.g. psoriasis.
2. Primary psychiatric disease presenting to dermatology, e.g. delusional infestation.
3. Psychiatric illness developing as a result of skin disease, e.g. depression.
4. Co-morbidity of skin disease with another psychiatric disorder, e.g. alcoholism.

The complex biopsychosocial realities of living with chronic skin disease are clear. Psychosocial issues of mixing in peer groups and making personal relationships may be blighted by feelings of stigmatisation and disfigurement. While psychological factors may be prominent at the onset of a skin disease, anxiety, depression and suicidal ideation are not uncommon in patients living with chronic skin disease. Therefore psychological co-morbidities must be treated concomitantly with the skin condition. Psychodermatology specialist clinics have dermatologists, psychiatrists and psychologists working together.

DELUSIONAL BELIEFS

A primary delusion is a false, unshakeable belief that arises from internal processes which are not amenable to logic and are out of keeping with the patient's educational and cultural background. Primary delusions can be an isolated phenomenon (e.g. a monosymptomatic hypochondriacal psychosis) or part of a broader psychosis (e.g. schizophrenia).

Delusional infestation

(Syn. Delusional parasitosis, parasitophobia) In delusional infestation (DI) the patient is convinced that s/he is infested with a mite, parasite, insect or other pathogen. The patient will hold this belief unshakeably (delusional disorder).

Epidemiology
Prevalence is estimated at 17 cases per million people per year. Peak incidence is in middle-age; it is rare in children. M:F is 1:2.5. DI is found in all ethnicities.

Pathophysiology
DI may be primary (no underlying cause is found) or secondary to concomitant organic or psychiatric disease, or to substance/alcohol/drug misuse. Altered reasoning leads the patient to believe there is a true infestation. Functional MRI in DI patients indicates that there may be abnormalities in the cortical and mid-brain areas associated with the *interpretation* of perceptions.

Clinical features
Patients present with a belief that they are infested and will describe sensations of itching, biting or crawling. Most patients can 'see' the infestation. On examination, patients may have excoriations and erosions, skin signs which reflect attempts to

Rook's Dermatology Handbook, First Edition. Edited by Christopher E. M. Griffiths, Tanya O. Bleiker, Daniel Creamer, John R. Ingram and Rosalind C. Simpson.
© 2022 John Wiley & Sons Ltd. Published 2022 by John Wiley & Sons Ltd.

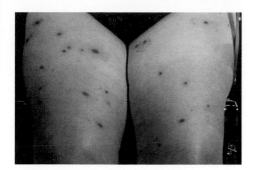

Figure 42.1 Excoriations in delusions of parasitosis in an amphetamine addict.

extricate the organism (Figure 42.1). Careful examination of the skin is needed to (i) exclude a genuine infestation, (ii) exclude organic causes of pruritus and (iii) reassure the patient that his/her symptoms are being addressed.

Differential diagnosis
Scabies, insect bite reactions, atopic eczema, pruritus of any cause.

Investigations
Many patients bring along specimens of the 'infesting' organisms. Specimens should be reviewed by a clinician and by microscopy. Blood tests (pruritus screen) and skin biopsy may be undertaken according to the clinical picture. Assessment of coexistent affective disease and suicidality is imperative; assessment of recreational drug and alcohol usage is also important.

Management
Patients with DI will usually present to dermatologists. They are often reticent about seeing psychiatrists. Recommendations for the management of DI are outlined in Figure 42.2.

Olfactory reference syndrome

(syn. Olfactory delusional syndrome, phantosmia) Olfactory reference syndrome (ORS) is the association of a smell hallucination and a 'contrite' reaction. In the contrite reaction patients wash themselves excessively, change clothing frequently and become socially withdrawn.

Epidemiology
ORS is rare. It is more common in young male adults. M:F is 4.5:1.

Pathophysiology
ORS can present at the onset of dementia; some cases can be precipitated by dopaminergic medication for Parkinson disease. ORS can also present as part of other psychiatric diseases.

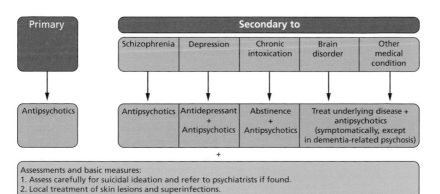

Figure 42.2 Management algorithm for delusional infestation. (Source: Lepping P, Freundenmann RW, Heuber M. Delusional infestation. In: Bewley A, Taylor RE, Reichenberg JS, Magid M, eds. Practical Psychodermatology. Oxford: Wiley, 2014, pp. 117–126. © 2014 John Wiley & Sons.)

PART 5: PSYCHOLOGICAL AND NEUROLOGICAL DISORDERS AND THE SKIN

Clinical features

Patients present with a history of experiencing an unpleasant smell from a specific part or from all over their body. The smell is unpleasant and may be faecal, putrific, sweaty, metallic or acrid. Patients go to great lengths to cleanse themselves of the smell (contrite reaction). The patient will reject any suggestion that the smell is not experienced by other people. Patients may present with a true delusional and hallucinatory illness, but some present as part of a body dysmorphic disease. The behaviour which describes the contrite reaction is common in obsessive–compulsive disorder (OCD).

Differential diagnosis

Trimethylaminuria (fish odour syndrome: a genetic metabolic disorder leading to a build-up of trimethylamine in body fluids), temporal lobe epilepsy (olfactory hallucinations are common).

Investigations

Urinalysis should be used to exclude trimethylaminuria.

Management

First line: Antidepressants (usually SSRIs).

Second line: Atypical antipsychotics in low doses, cognitive behavioural therapy.

OBSESSIVE AND COMPULSIVE BEHAVIOURS

Obsessive–compulsive behaviour in dermatology patients is common and manifests in a number of disorders, including body dysmorphic disorder, lichen simplex chronicus, nodular prurigo, skin-picking disorder, acné excoriée and trichotillosis.

Body dysmorphic disorder

(Syn. Dysmorphophobia)

Body dysmorphic disorder (BDD) is a preoccupation with a real or imagined defect in physical appearance. If a slight physical anomaly is present, the patient's concern is out of proportion to the anomaly.

Epidemiology

BDD occurs in 1–2% of the general population. F:M is 2:1. BDD often starts in adolescence, but may affect any age group. It is more common in patients seeking cosmetic surgery.

Pathophysiology

There is a spectrum from patients with overvalued ideas to those whose beliefs are held with delusional conviction. Theories suggest that sufferers from BDD have self-defeating thoughts, cognitive distortions and destructive beliefs about themselves and their appearance. The development of selective processing of emotional information about body image and physical appearance may be related to anxiety disorders and social phobia.

Clinical features

Women usually present with a focus on the skin of the face, breasts, nose and stomach, whereas men may present with concerns about hair (usually thinning), nose, ears, genitals and body build. Patients will often have intrusive thoughts about their perceived 'defect'. They may try to hide their 'defect' and may repeatedly attend for cosmetic surgery. There is a high degree of comorbidity with mood disorders, OCD, suicidal ideation and social phobia.

Investigations

BDD is a clinical diagnosis. Assess for underlying psychiatric disease and potential suicide risk.

Management

From the outset it is important to treat the psychological disease whilst addressing the perceived skin disease.

First line: SSRIs and cognitive behavioural therapy are the treatments of choice. Higher dosing regimens of SSRI than those used for depression are usually required.

Second line: Antipsychotics may be needed if there is delusional BDD.

Skin-picking disorder

(Syn. Compulsive skin picking)

Patients with skin-picking disorder admit to an urge to pick and gouge at their skin.

Epidemiology

Occurs in 2% of dermatology patients. F > M. The majority have pathological picking associated with atopic and other cutaneous diseases. There are two peaks of occurrence: (i) adolescence/early adult life and (ii) middle-aged women.

Clinical features

Patients can spend up to 3 h per day picking, thinking about picking, or resisting the urge to pick. Bouts can be ritualised to a set time and place, often the bathroom, frequently at bedtime. Any area may be affected but are commonly distributed within reach of the dominant hand. Lesions are excoriated erosions and deeper ulcers; older lesions become scarred (Figure 42.3). Chronic lesions may be atrophic, eventually seen as linear, coalescent areas. Lesions appear at all stages of development. Pre existing skin disease (e.g. atopic eczema or acne) is common, as are psychosocial co-morbidities. Depression and/or anxiety are often found.

Differential diagnosis
Trigeminal trophic syndrome (see Chapter 41)

Abnormal sensations in the distribution of the trigeminal nerve are associated with an irresistible desire to pick at the involved skin. In dermatitis artefacta (see below) patients deny that the skin lesions are self-inflicted.

Management

Of the skin: Appropriate treatment of the dermatosis (e.g. antibiotics if there is a clinical infection), treatment of pruritus (e.g. antihistamines).

Of the picking habit and co-morbidities: Habit reversal therapy, other talk therapies, SSRIs (usually in higher doses).

Trichotillosis

(Syn. Trichotillomania)

Trichotillosis is an OCD spectrum disorder. There is recurrent pulling out of the hair resulting in alopecia. A sense of tension before pulling the hair is relieved once the hair is pulled out.

Epidemiology

There are two peaks of occurrence: (i) childhood, mainly between the ages of 5 and 12 years, and (ii) adults who start hair-pulling in adolescence or early adult life. F:M is 15:1.

Pathophysiology

The aetiology of trichotillosis is not fully understood but seems to be related to underlying psychosocial problems: anxiety, depression, BDD and, commonly, family dysfunction.

Clinical features

Most patients relate that the trichotillosis is a compulsion that is irresistible and leads to a short-lived sense of relief when the hair has been pulled out. Some describe pulling hair in a hypnogogic (dream-like) state and having no control over the action. Hair-pulling is commonest from the scalp, mostly the vertex, but temporal, occipital and frontal hair loss is seen. On examination, there are areas of hair loss together with areas of hair regrowth demonstrated as stubble and longer hairs (Figure 42.4).

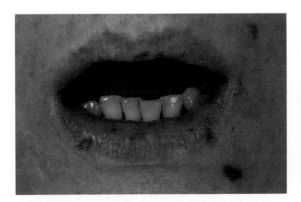

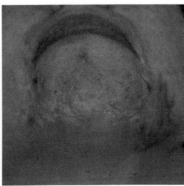

Figure 42.3 Skin-picking disorder.

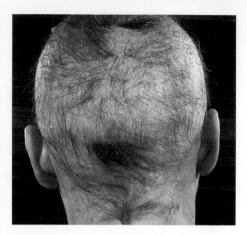

Figure 42.4 Adult trichotillomania. Extensive hair loss with a preserved tuft over the occiput.

The hair loss may range from a solitary patch to virtual total depilation. Dermoscopy reveals broken hair shafts and hairs of different lengths.

Differential diagnosis

Alopecia areata; causes of scarring alopecia.

Investigations

The diagnosis is usually clinical. Scalp biopsy can be used to distinguish trichotillosis from scarring alopecia. Histology shows curling of the hair bulb and perifollicular damage.

Management

Habit reversal therapy.

FACTITIOUS SKIN DISEASE

In factitious skin disease the dermatosis is caused by the fully aware patient who chooses to hide the cause from their doctors. For all factitious skin disease it is crucial to ensure that organic skin disease is excluded, and to ascertain *why* the patient is presenting with the disease, rather than *how*.

Dermatitis artefacta

(Syn. Dermatitis factitia)
Dermatitis artefacta (DA) is a skin disease caused by the actions of the fully aware patient

on his/her skin. These patients hide the responsibility for their actions from their doctors.

Epidemiology

The majority of cases begin in adolescence and in adults under 30 years of age. In adults there is a female preponderance with F:M ratio varying from 4:1 to 20:1. In prepubertal children F:M is 1:1.

Pathophysiology

The patient appears to want the sickness role. There are complex underlying drivers, e.g. self-hate, guilt, conflict with authority figures. An illness allows avoidance of adult responsibilities. The development of DA is more common in those with a memorable early experience of illness or in those who have a family member who is (or has been) unwell.

Clinical features

There is a history of not knowing how the lesions occurred (the 'hollow history'). Lesions appear at an identical stage in development, in crops or groups, sometimes symmetrically. Established lesions undergo deterioration at the same time as new lesions appear. The commonest site of involvement is the face, particularly the cheeks, then dorsa of the hands and forearms (Figure 42.5). Lesions can occur on covered skin: breasts, abdomen and genitalia. Lesions are usually linear or angulated or with patterns which do not conform to recognised skin diseases (Figures 42.6 and 42.7). They are caused by thermal, chemical or instrumental injury. Excoriations may be made with nail files, cheese graters or wire brushes. Blisters can be

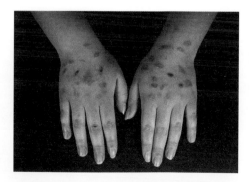

Figure 42.5 Dermatitis artefacta. Symmetrical and predominantly monomorphic lesions on the hands.

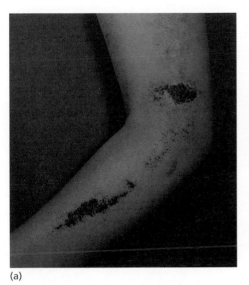

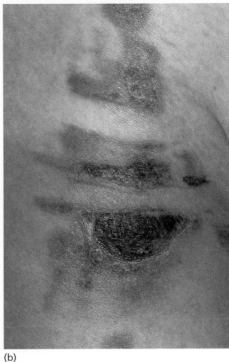

(a)   (b)

Figure 42.6 Dermatitis artefacta. (a) Crude, linear, angulated and destructive factitious dermatitis. (b) Note the straight edges and sharp angulation of some of the lesions.

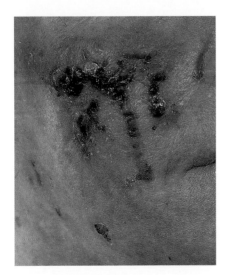

Figure 42.7 Dermatitis artefacta showing the 'drip sign' caused by the downward passage of a corrosive liquid on the skin.

induced by corrosive liquids or by extreme cold induced by aerosol sprays. Patients are often passive despite widespread disfigurement. Anger is usual from parents or partners.

Differential diagnosis
Skin-picking disorder
Patients admit to picking and gouging their skin.

Trigeminal trophic syndrome
Abnormal sensations in the distribution of the trigeminal nerve are associated with an irresistible desire to pick at the involved skin.

Investigations
DA is a clinical diagnosis. A skin biopsy may provide essential supportive information and help to exclude organic disease.

Management

Treat the skin damage appropriately; occlusive bandaging will allow lesions to heal (except for those of the most determined patients). Do not confront the patient with knowledge of their fabrication: usually a cause will be revealed as soon as the patient feels safe with the clinician. Adult patients may respond to a non-confrontational 'face-saving' strategy. This mechanism works by suggesting that the patient does some 'personal homework' to find a solution to their illness.

Part 6
Skin Disorders Associated with Specific Cutaneous Structure

Acquired disorders of epidermal keratinisation

43

Acquired ichthyosis

Acquired ichthyosis (AI) is usually associated with a systemic disorder or a reaction to medication.

Epidemiology

AI is a rare condition occurring mainly in adulthood but has been reported in children. Box 43.1 lists the disorders, particularly malignancy, endocrinopathy, drug reactions, some infections and autoimmune conditions, that have been associated with AI. Severe xerosis mimicking AI can be observed in atopic individuals who migrate from very humid atmospheres such as South-East Asia to Europe.

Pathophysiology

The pathogenesis of AI is not fully understood and differs according to the entity with which it is associated. Histologically, the epidermis shows compact hyperkeratosis with a thinned or absent granular cell layer.

Clinical features

The onset of AI is typically sudden with initial involvement of the lower limbs followed by more widespread skin involvement. Pruritus can be severe. The scalp shows abundant fine scales and there may be palmoplantar hyperkeratosis. The flexures and face are typically spared due to higher humidity and the size and number of sebaceous glands, respectively.

Box 43.1 Disorders associated with AI

- Neoplasia: particularly Hodgkin disease, mycosis fungoides, multiple myeloma, Kaposi and other sarcomas and carcinomas (lung, breast, ovary, cervix)
- Drug reactions: statins, nicotinic acid, cimetidine and clofazimine
- Endocrinopathies: diabetes, thyroid disease, hyperparathyroidism and hypopituitarism
- Infections: leprosy, tuberculosis, HIV and HTLV-1 associated myelopathy
- Autoimmune conditions: dermatomyositis, systemic lupus erythematosus and scleroderma/lupus overlap syndrome
- Chronic metabolic derangements: malnutrition, malabsorption syndromes, essential fatty acid deficiency and pancreatic insufficiency (Shwachman syndrome)
- Anorexia nervosa
- Miscellaneous: sarcoidosis, bone marrow transplantation and chronic renal failure

---

Differential diagnosis

Xeroderma, asteatotic eczema, atopic eczema, drug eruptions, hereditary ichthyoses.

Investigations

The diagnosis of AI is made clinically. However, a search for an underlying cause should be undertaken, with particular care not to overlook

---

Rook's Dermatology Handbook, First Edition. Edited by Christopher E. M. Griffiths, Tanya O. Bleiker, Daniel Creamer, John R. Ingram and Rosalind C. Simpson.
© 2022 John Wiley & Sons Ltd. Published 2022 by John Wiley & Sons Ltd.

the possibility of occult malignancy, especially lymphoma.

Management

The primary aim is to identify the underlying cause of the disorder. Its treatment can lead to improvement of the dermatosis. Other treatment is similar to the management of hereditary ichthyosis involving emollients, particularly those containing urea.

Acanthosis nigricans

Acanthosis nigricans (AN) may present as an isolated skin condition or may be associated with a wide range of conditions, including obesity, endocrinopathies and internal neoplasms.

Epidemiology

AN secondary to non-malignant conditions is very common, with a prevalence of up to 20% of adults and 7% of children (20% of obese children). AN secondary to malignancy is rare. Prevalence increases with greater skin pigmentation. Box 43.2 lists the conditions and medications associated with AN. Obesity is the commonest cause.

Pathophysiology

Flexural involvement and an association with obesity suggest that perspiration and/or friction are contributing factors. Despite its name, AN shows no or minimal acanthosis or hyperpigmentation microscopically. Histology shows hyperkeratosis and papillomatosis with finger-

---

Box 43.2 Disorders and medications associated with acanthosis nigricans

- Obesity
- Polycystic ovary syndrome
- Endocrinopathies, including diabetes
- Autoimmune conditions, including lupus erythematosus
- Internal malignancy, particularly gastric cancer
- Drug-induced: insulin, systemic corticosteroids, testosterone, exogenous oestrogens, including oral contraceptives

---

like upward projections of dermal papillae. Pigmentation is due to the hyperkeratosis; there is no increase in melanocyte numbers or in melanin production.

Clinical features

AN presents as asymptomatic, symmetrical velvety dark patches which are most commonly seen in the axillae, groins and on the back and sides of the neck (Figure 43.1). The posterior neck is the most common site in children. Skin tags (acrochordons) may be present in affected areas. AN may become widespread, with delicate velvety furrowing of mucosal surfaces and involvement of the eyelids and conjunctivae. Associated nail changes include leukonychia and subungual hyperkeratosis.

Differential diagnosis

Addison disease, pellagra, haemochromatosis.

Investigations

The diagnosis of AN is made clinically. Screening for diabetes mellitus is recommended. Screening for other underlying endocrinopathies or malignancy may be necessary, depending on any abnormalities picked up on functional enquiry.

Management

Weight loss if relevant and management of any underlying condition.

Keratosis pilaris

Keratosis pilaris (KP) is a common skin condition characterised by follicular keratotic papules and perifollicular erythema. It can be considered a variant of normal rather than a disease.

Epidemiology

KP is a very common condition, affecting 50–80% of adolescents and about 40% of adults. It often presents in the first decade of life and may worsen around puberty. In some patients, the disorder improves with age. Females are probably more frequently affected than males. It may be associated with ichthyosis vulgaris and atopic

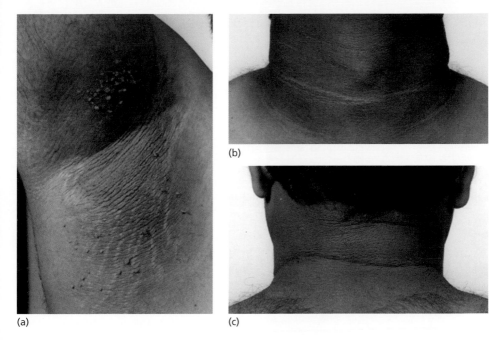

Figure 43.1 Typical acanthosis nigricans in an obese 41-year-old man of South Asian descent with type 2 diabetes. Note associated striae and skin tags in the axilla (a) and darkening and velvety thickening of the skin around the root and nape of the neck (b) and (c).

eczema, but all three conditions are common and so the association may be coincidental.

Pathophysiology

KP is inherited as an autosomal dominant trait with variable penetrance. Histology of KP shows hyperkeratosis, hypergranulosis and plugging of hair follicles. The hair can become ingrown, resulting in an inflammatory response. KP may show seasonal variation, improving in the summer.

Clinical features

There are small, keratotic papules on the lateral aspects of the limbs, particularly the upper arms (Figure 43.2) and thighs. The buttocks and the lumbar areas are also frequently affected. These areas acquire a 'goose-bump' appearance and rough texture. Lesions can become pustular, with superficial pustules developing in affected follicles, precipitated by rubbing on clothing. On the buttock, deeper inflammatory lesions and nodules may develop.

KP atrophicans faciei. also called ulerythema ophryogenes or keratosis rubra pilaris faciei atrophicans, affects the cheeks and lateral eyebrows (madarosis). Fixed erythema, follicular plugging and pitted scarring occur, progressing to alopecia in some cases.

Erythromelanosis follicularis faciei et colli. is a condition that has been described as a subtype of KP and is seen in India and other countries in the Far and Middle East. It manifests as follicular hyperkeratosis accompanied by erythema and hyperpigmentation and affects, as the name indicates, the face, particularly the cheeks and neck (Figure 43.3).

Differential diagnosis

Darier disease, pityriasis rubra pilaris, atopic eczema, lichen nitidus, eruptive vellous hair cysts, acne/folliculitis (if lesions become inflamed), rosacea (keratosis pilaris atrophicans faciei).

Investigations

KP is a clinical diagnosis.

PART 6: SKIN DISORDERS ASSOCIATED WITH SPECIFIC CUTANEOUS STRUCTURE

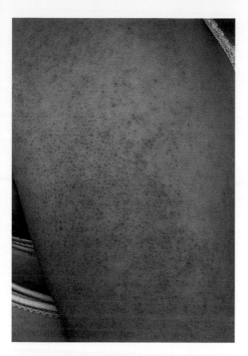

Figure 43.2 Keratosis pilaris on the extensor aspect of the upper arm.

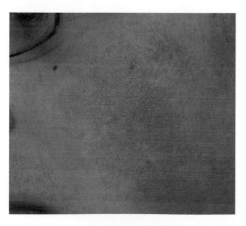

Figure 43.3 Erythromelanosis follicularis faciei et colli in a young Asian man.

Management

In many mild cases, KP does not require treatment. If needed, emollients containing urea are first-line therapy and topical keratolytics, e.g. salicyclic acid, may be considered in addition.

Porokeratoses

A porokeratosis is a clonal expansion of keratinocytes which differentiate abnormally but are not truly neoplastic. Clinical subtypes may be localised or disseminated (Box 43.3). Squamous cell carcinomas may develop within lesions.

Epidemiology

Porokeratosis is a rare disease. Disseminated superficial actinic porokeratosis (DSAP) is the most common form, representing more than half of all cases. Porokeratosis of Mibelli and linear porokeratosis typically appear during infancy or childhood. Punctate palmoplantar porokeratosis and disseminated palmoplantar porokeratosis usually appear in adolescence while DSAP generally first manifests in adult life. Porokeratosis of Mibelli, genital porokeratosis and punctate porokeratosis are more common in males whereas DSAP is more common in women. Linear porokeratosis has an equal sex ratio. All forms of porokeratosis are seen predominantly in Caucasian ethnic groups.

Pathophysiology

All forms of porokeratosis have been reported to have familial clusters with autosomal dominant patterns of inheritance but with variable penetration. Exposure to UV radiation is a factor in the induction of superficial actinic porokeratosis and porokeratosis of Mibelli.

Box 43.3 Clinical classification of porokeratoses

Localised forms

- Porokeratosis of Mibelli
- Linear porokeratosis
- Punctate palmoplantar porokeratosis
- Genital porokeratosis
- Perianal porokeratosis

Disseminated forms

- Disseminated superficial actinic porokeratosis
- Disseminated superficial porokeratosis
- Systematised linear porokeratosis
- Disseminated palmoplantar porokeratosis

Histologically, porokeratoses are characterised by a cornoid lamella, which is a thin column of tightly packed parakeratotic keratinocytes within a keratin-filled invagination of the epidermis through the stratum corneum.

Clinical features

Porokeratoses are usually asymptomatic but may be pruritic and, if verrucous, may cause discomfort from pressure. They present with single or multiple papules or plaques which develop into annular lesions with a well-defined ridge-like hyperkeratotic border, the cornoid lamella.

Localised forms

Porokeratosis of Mibelli. Starts as a single or small group of keratotic papules which may be pigmented. These gradually grow over years to form one or more irregular plaques with a thin, keratotic and well-demarcated border. The central area may be atrophic, either hyper- or hypopigmented, hairless and anhidrotic (Figure 43.4a). Lesions are generally distributed on the extremities but can occur anywhere on the body. Occasionally, giant and verrucous forms of the disease may occur.

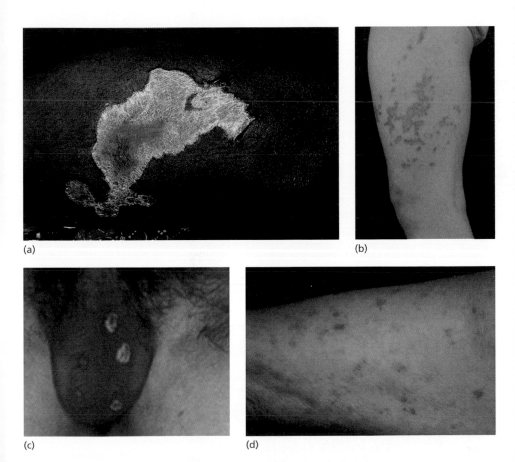

(a)　　　　　　　　　　　　　　　　(b)

(c)　　　　　　　　　　　(d)

Figure 43.4 Clinical images of porokeratoses. (a) Porokeratosis of Mibelli. (b) Linear porokeratosis. (c) Genital porokeratosis: multiple lesions limited to the scrotum. (Source: Chen TJ, Chou YC, Chen CH, Kuo TT, Hong HS. Genital porokeratosis: a series of 10 patients and review of the literature. Br J Dermatol 2006, 155, 325–329.) (d) Disseminated superficial actinic porokeratosis: view of upper arm.

PART 6: SKIN DISORDERS ASSOCIATED WITH SPECIFIC CUTANEOUS STRUCTURE

Linear porokeratosis. Generally occurs in infancy as unilateral streaks or plaques of reddish-brown papules along limbs or the side of the trunk, head or neck following Blaschko lines, indicating underlying somatic mosaicism (Figure 43.4b). There is a higher risk of malignant change in linear porokeratosis than in other forms of porokeratosis.

Punctate palmoplantar porokeratosis. A rare type of porokeratosis in which seed-like punctate keratoses form on the palms and soles during adulthood.

Genital porokeratosis. A rare localised type which it is important to be aware of as it is frequently misdiagnosed clinically. It occurs almost exclusively in men, more often affecting the scrotum than the penis (Figure 43.4c).

Perianal porokeratosis (Syn. Porokeratosis ptychotropica). Very rare, requiring histology to confirm.

Disseminated forms

Disseminated superficial actinic porokeratosis (DSAP) (Chapter 80). Presents with few or multiple flesh-coloured, pink or reddish-brown finely scaling macules with a thin but well-defined raised border (Figure 43.4d).

Disseminated superficial porokeratosis. Not necessarily related to sun exposure and presents in both sun-exposed and sun-protected sites, including sometimes oral mucosa and genitalia. It may be associated with immunodeficiency (e.g. organ transplantation, malignancy, HIV infection) or may develop sporadically during childhood.

Systematised linear porokeratosis. A disseminated variant of linear porokeratosis which may be unilateral or generalised and follows the lines of Blaschko.

Disseminated palmoplantar porokeratosis (Syn. Porokeratosis palmaris, plantaris disseminata). A rare generalised form of punctate palmoplantar porokeratosis. Palmoplantar lesions are followed by multiple widely disseminated wart-like keratoses in both sun-exposed and sun-protected areas.

Differential diagnosis
See Table 43.1.

Table 43.1 Differential diagnosis of porokeratoses

Condition	Differential diagnosis
Porokeratosis of Mibelli	Psoriasis
Disseminated palmoplantar porokeratosis	Psoriasis
DSAP	Actinic keratosis, stucco keratosis
Linear porokeratosis	Linear verrucous epidermal naevus, lichen striatus and incontinentia pigmenti
Punctate palmoplantar porokeratosis	Viral warts

Investigations
Where there is diagnostic doubt, biopsy of the border of a lesion has greatest diagnostic value, demonstrating the cornoid lamella. Patients presenting with sudden onset of porokeratosis should be investigated for causes of immunosuppression, including HIV and haematological malignancies.

Management
In patients with immunosuppression or in linear porokeratosis where the malignancy rate is increased, screening for skin cancer is advised. Localised treatment for porokeratoses includes cryotherapy, topical 5-fluorouracil, topical imiquimod, curettage and cautery, photodynamic therapy, topical retinoids and topical vitamin D analogues. Systemic retinoids are used as second-line therapy, namely isotretinoin and acitretin.

Transient acantholytic dermatosis

(Syn. Grover disease)
Transient acantholytic dermatosis (TAD) is a relatively common transient or persistent monomorphous, papulovesicular eruption mainly affecting the trunk, which may be pruritic or asymptomatic.

Epidemiology

TAD is a relatively common inflammatory dermatosis with an approximate incidence of 0.1% and is likely to be underdiagnosed. TAD is a disease of older patients with a mean age at diagnosis of 61 years but may manifest throughout adult life. The disease has a male predominance and is commonest in white populations.

Pathophysiology

The cause of TAD is unknown. TAD has been associated with exposure to natural UV radiation, heat and sweating. The primary histological feature is the presence of small foci of acantholysis with dyskeratosis, intraepidermal clefting and sometimes vesicle formation.

Clinical features

The commonest presentation is of a papulovesicular erythematous eruption on the trunk of a middle-aged or elderly white male. It starts with small papules and vesicles that quickly crust and develop keratotic erosions (Figure 43.5). The eruption is usually very itchy and the patient presents with multiple excoriations, although in some patients there is no pruritus. The distribution may extend to cover the proximal limbs. In many patients, TAD may be transient as its name suggests, lasting 2–4 weeks, but in some it may persist for months or years or follow a chronic relapsing course.

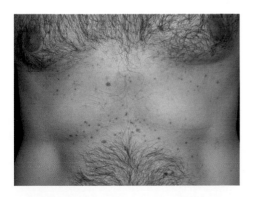

Figure 43.5 Transient acantholytic dermatosis: typical appearance on the abdomen. (Source: Reproduced by courtesy and with permission of Professor Luis Requena, Universidad Autónoma de Madrid, Spain.)

Differential diagnosis

Folliculitis, papular urticaria, scabies.

Investigations

Skin biopsy if diagnostic doubt.

Management

First line: Avoid sunlight exposure, strenuous exercise and heat.
Second line: Topical therapy, including potent corticosteroid, vitamin D analogues and calcineurin inhibitors.
Third line: Oral, including antihistamines, short course of corticosteroid, retinoid and methotrexate.

Keratolysis exfoliativa

(Syn. Focal palmar peeling)
Keratolysis exfoliativa (KE) is a common disease of young adults in which discrete areas of superficial skin peeling occur on the palms.

Epidemiology

KE is common. It typically affects young adults and there is no known ethnic or sex predilection. KE often presents during warmer weather. It can be aggravated by detergents, solvents and other irritants.

Pathophysiology

The cause is unknown. Histology and electron microscopy show cleavage and partially degraded corneodesmosomes within the stratum corneum.

Clinical features

KE presents initially as small superficial blister-like air-filled pockets on the palms and palmar aspects of the fingers or occasionally the feet. This may be associated with localised hyperhidrosis. The roofs of the pockets rupture centrally as they expand centrifugally, leaving a ragged rim of residual scale surrounding an irregular superficial dry erosion (Figure 43.6). There is no or minimal pruritus and vesicles are not present. Peeled areas of skin lack normal barrier function and may become dry and fissured, particularly on the fingertips.

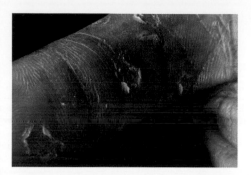

Figure 43.6 Keratolysis exfoliativa: close-up view of right index finger.

Differential diagnosis

Pompholyx eczema, psoriasis, tinea manuum, epidermolysis bullosa simplex, acral skin peeling syndrome.

Investigations

Usually none needed.

Management

KE is usually a self-limiting condition and treatment may not always be needed.

First line: Avoid contact with irritants.

Second line: Emollients (containing urea).

Third line: Topical salicylic acid.

Xerosis and asteatosis

Xerosis cutis (dry skin) and asteatosis (lacking in fat) are alternative terms used to describe an acquired abnormality of the skin which has lost its normal soft smooth surface and feels dry and rough to the touch. This may be the result of a range of endogenous and exogenous factors, especially ageing and low ambient humidity and is associated with impaired epidermal barrier function.

Epidemiology

Xerosis is very common particularly after the seventh decade. It appears to be slightly more common in men and more prevalent in younger people in sub-Saharan Africa. In younger people it is associated with marasmus, malnutrition, diabetes, renal failure and renal dialysis.

Pathophysiology

There is a deficiency of all stratum corneum lipids as well as premature expression of involucrin and persistence of corneodesmosomes. Xerosis is more common in winter when humidity is low due to central heating.

Clinical features

Xerosis most often affects the shins. It may become widespread but spares the face, neck, palms and soles. In elderly immobile hospitalised patients, it will frequently affect the abdomen and, in women, the anterior surfaces of the breasts, but spares the back and the under-surfaces of the breasts.

Affected skin looks dull, dry and covered with fine scale which sheds readily. The surface may become crazed with criss-cross superficial cracks in the stratum corneum giving the skin a crazy-paving appearance (Figure 43.7). Xerosis may progress to an eczematous inflammation known as asteatotic eczema (eczéma craquelé, Chapter 14).

Differential diagnosis

Atopic eczema, ichthyosis.

Management

First line: Avoid contact with irritants, increase local humidity.

Second line: Emollients.

Third line (if eczema develops): Topical corticosteroid, topical calcineurin inhibitors.

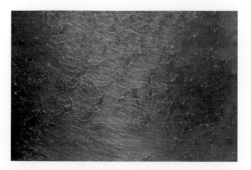

Figure 43.7 Xerosis cutis eczéma craquelé.

Acne

44

Acne vulgaris

(Syn. Acne vulgaris)
A chronic inflammatory disease of the pilosebaceous unit.

Epidemiology

One of the commonest skin diseases; highest prevalence is in adolescence, occurring in 80% of teenagers. Approximately 25% of women aged 31–40 years and 10% aged 41–50 years have acne.

It most commonly presents between the ages of 10 and 13 years in both sexes but at a younger age in girls aligning with earlier puberty. Nowadays it is presenting earlier and lasting longer; this has been linked with earlier onset of puberty, which may also relate to diet/obesity and other lifestyle factors.

Comedonal acne can be detected in some children before any overt signs of puberty, Early development of comedonal acne in girls may be a predictor of more severe disease in later life.

F > M in post-adolescent acne. Severe acne in late adolescence M > F. Table 44.1 summarises medical conditions that may predispose to or protect against acne. Most acne patients have no underlying endocrinological abnormalities. A number of lifestyle and environmental factors which predispose to acne or modulate its course have been reported, although data are frequently contradictory.

Pathophysiology

Inherited factors influence the acne phenotype in monozygotic and to a lesser extent dizygotic twins. The risk of acne in a first-degree relative of someone with acne is four to five times higher than in relatives of unaffected individuals. The risk of adult (persistent or late-onset) acne in first-degree relatives of patients with acne aged 25 years or over is similar. Susceptibility to adolescent acne seems to be more strongly linked to the maternal than the paternal line. Acne occurs earlier in patients with a positive family history and may affect clinical presentation and treatment outcomes (Table 44.2). Canadian Inuit only began to develop acne and other diseases of Western civilisation following the urbanisation of their communities.

Studies to date suggest the risk of having acne and the severity appear to increase with age-adjusted body mass index in adolescents.

70% of women have a flare of acne 2–7 days before the onset of menstruation.

There is seasonal variation, with fewer patients seeking treatment in the summer months. Workers in a hot, humid environment have an increased prevalence of acne, hence high temperatures and humidity may negate any beneficial effects of sunlight. An acne variant, acne aestivalis or Mallorcan acne, has been reported in people exposed to sunshine on vacation. Small follicular papules appear, especially on the upper trunk, during or after a holiday in a hot humid environment.

Acne results from the combination of increased sebaceous gland activity with seborrhoea, abnormal follicular differentiation with increased keratinisation, microbial hypercolonisation of the follicular canal and increased inflammation primarily through activation of the adaptive immune system. Along with a genetic predisposition, other major factors include androgens and pro-inflammatory lipids.

The Th17 pathway is activated and may play a pivotal role in the disease process.

Propionibacterium acnes

P. acnes strains modulate the expression of immune markers differently both at gene and protein levels.

Rook's Dermatology Handbook, First Edition. Edited by Christopher E. M. Griffiths, Tanya O. Bleiker, Daniel Creamer, John R. Ingram and Rosalind C. Simpson.
© 2022 John Wiley & Sons Ltd. Published 2022 by John Wiley & Sons Ltd.

Table 44.1 Medical conditions that may predispose to acne or in which acne prevalence is reduced

Condition	Abnormalities associated with this condition and relevant to acne	Effect/comments
PCOS	Raised serum DHEAS, total and/or free testosterone and androstenedione, reduced SHBG. Also raised luteinising hormone, insulin, IGFBP-1 and IGF-1	Predisposes and/or worsens; effect on acne modified by BMI
SAHA syndrome: subtype of PCOS (Figure 44.1)	Serum androgens often but not always elevated	Predisposes
HAIR-AN syndrome: subtype of PCOS	Pronounced insulin resistance, with markedly raised serum insulin	Predisposes Insulin resistance is proportional to BMI Onset usually during puberty/adolescence
Premature adrenarche	Raised serum DHEA, DHEAS and androstenedione; often accompanied by insulin resistance	Girls > boys Predisposes to earlier onset of acne and to PCOS
Insulin resistance	Reduced IGF-1 and IGFBP-1	Predisposes
Hyperinsulinaemia	Raised serum insulin, IGF-1 and reduced IGFBP-3	Predisposes
Non-classical congenital adrenal hyperplasia associated with 21-hydroxylase deficiency	Elevated serum 17-OHP, progesterone, androstenedione, corticotrophin-releasing hormone, and ACTH	Predisposes to early onset
Anorexia nervosa	Serum growth hormone raised, concomitantly IGF-1 is low	Predisposes
Turner syndrome	45,X Rudimentary ovaries with reduced androgen synthesis leading to reduced serum levels of testosterone and androstenedione during puberty in affected girls	Protects via reduced sebum production Only affects girls
Laron syndrome	Congenital deficiency of IGF-1	Protects
Mayer–Rokitansky–Küster–Hauser syndrome without WNT4 mutation	Serum androgens are normal	Protects Lower prevalence of acne and PCOS but ovaries intact
Mayer–Rokitansky–Küster–Hauser syndrome with WNT4 mutation	Raised serum testosterone	Predisposes via inability to repress ovarian androgen synthesis

Table 44.1 (Continued)

Condition	Abnormalities associated with this condition and relevant to acne	Effect/comments
Cushing syndrome (iatrogenic and endogenous)	Elevated serum cortisol, ACTH and corticotrophin-releasing hormone	Predisposes Can cause acne in pre-adrenarchal children
Ectopic ACTH syndrome	Elevated serum ACTH	Predisposes Acne in pre-adrenarchal children
PAPA syndrome	Mutations in *PSTPIP1* IL-1β and circulating neutrophil granule enzyme levels in serum are raised Impaired production of IL-10 and increased production of GM-CSF	Acne is one of three diagnostics, pyogenic sterile arthritis and pyoderma gangrenosum being the others
PASH syndrome	Raised IL-1β (systemically or locally) or aberrant regulation of the function of this cytokine	Acne one of three diagnostic features, suppurative hidradenitis and pyoderma gangrenosum being the others
PASS syndrome	Raised TNF-α (systemically or locally) or aberrant regulation of the function of this cytokine	As PASH but with axial spondyloarthritis
SAPHO syndrome	*P. acnes* sometimes recovered from bone samples	Acne one of five diagnostic features, synovitis, pustulosis, hyperostosis and osteitis being the others
Adrenal and ovarian tumours	Elevated serum androgens exclusively or with other raised hormones	Predisposes
Male pseudohermaphroditism	17β-hydroxysteroid dehydrogenase type 3 deficiency 5α-reductase type 2 deficiency	Normal pubertal development, normal levels of sebum and no altered risk of acne
Complete androgen insensitivity syndrome	Mutation in the androgen receptor	Protects These patients produce no sebum and do not get acne
Exaggerated adrenarche	Specific elevation of adrenal hormones produced by the zona reticularis in adults; exaggerated DHEAS and androstenedione responses to ACTH stimulation test	Predisposes

ACTH, adrenocorticotrophic hormone; BMI, body mass index; HAIR-AN, hyperandrogenism, insulin resistance and acanthosis nigricans; DHEAS, dehydroepiandrosterone sulphate; IGF, insulin-like growth factor; IGFBP, IGF binding protein; PAPA, pyogenic arthritis, pyoderma gangrenosum and acne; PASH, pyoderma gangrenosum, acne and suppurative hidradenitis; PASS, pyoderma gangrenosum, acne and spondyloarthritis; PCOS, polycystic ovary syndrome; SAHA, seborrhoea, acne, hirsutism and alopecia; SAPHO, synovitis, acne, pustulosis, hyperostosis and osteitis.

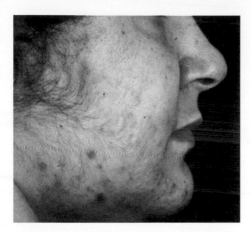

Figure 44.1 Seborrhoea, acne, hirsutism and/or androgenic alopecia (SAHA) syndrome.

Table 44.2 Lifestyle and environmental factors that may predispose to acne

Factor	Strength of evidence
Diet	Moderate for glycaemic index and milk/milk products, low for other foodstuffs
Body mass index	Low
Smoking	High for comedonal acne in mature women with a history of chronic smoking; otherwise low
Alcohol consumption	Low
Psychological stress	Low
Cosmetics	Low
Prescription medicines	High for some drugs, low for others
Anabolic and androgenic steroids	High
Seasonal factors	High
Sunlight	Low
Lack of sleep/insomnia	Low

Clinical features

Acne is a polymorphic inflammatory disease of the skin which occurs most commonly on the face (in 99% of cases; Figure 44.2) and to a lesser extent on the back (60%) and chest (15%). (Figure 44.3). Characterised by open and closed comedones (Figure 44.4) papules, pustules and nodules of varying degree of inflammation and depth (Figure 44.5). The face, back and/or chest are the most frequently affected sites. Post-inflammatory macules, pigment changes (Figure 44.6) and scarring commonly occur (Figure 44.7). Seborrhoea along with scarring and post-inflammatory erythema and/or pigment changes are common features. These may all contribute to significant physical and psychosocial impact.

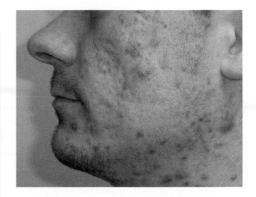

Figure 44.2 Moderate to severe inflammatory acne on the face.

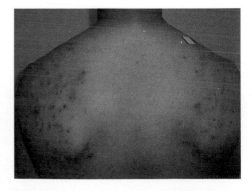

Figure 44.3 Acne on the back showing sparing of the central back.

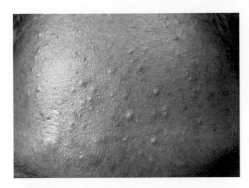

Figure 44.4 Predominantly comedonal acne. (Source: Courtesy of Dr S. Chow, KL Skin Centre, Malaysia.)

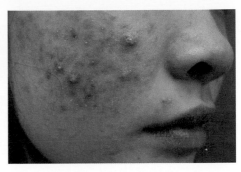

Figure 44.6 Post-inflammatory macules and pigment changes interspersed with inflammatory acne. (Courtesy of Dr S. Chow, KL Skin Centre, Malaysia.)

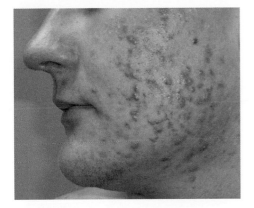

Figure 44.5 Moderate to severe inflammatory acne including a mixture of non-inflammatory and inflammatory lesions with seborrhoea.

The clinical picture varies from very mild comedonal acne, with or without sparse inflammatory lesions, to aggressive fulminant disease with associated systemic upset. Non-inflamed lesions are the earliest lesions to develop in younger patients with both open comedones (blackheads) and closed comedones (whiteheads). Open comedones frequently appear in a mid-facial distribution and when evident early they indicate poor prognosis. Closed comedones are generally 1 mm in diameter, skin coloured and have no visible follicular opening. These lesions are often inconspicuous and require adequate lighting and stretching of the skin to be seen. Most patients have a mixture of lesions.

Several subtypes of comedones have been described.

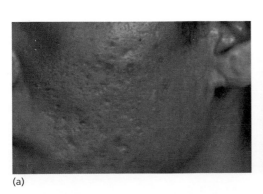
(a)

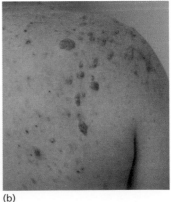
(b)

Figure 44.7 Acne scarring. (a) Atrophic scarring on the cheeks. (Courtesy of Dr C.L. Goh, National Skin Centre, Singapore.) (b) Hypertrophic keloid scarring of the trunk.

PART 6: SKIN DISORDERS ASSOCIATED WITH SPECIFIC CUTANEOUS STRUCTURE

- 'Sandpaper' comedones consist of multiple very small whiteheads, frequently distributed on the forehead (Figure 44.8), which produce a roughened, gritty feel to the skin.
- 'Macrocomedones' (Figure 44.9) are large whiteheads greater than 1 mm in diameter.
- 'Submarine' comedones (Figure 44.10) are large comedonal structures greater than 0.5 cm in diameter that reside more deeply in the skin. They are frequently associated with recurrent inflammatory nodular lesions.

Lesions include papules and pustules (≤5 mm) and can be extensively distributed on the face and/or back (Figure 44.11). Deep-seated pustules and nodules (>5 mm) may also occur (Figure 44.12). Sinus tracts may develop between nodules and/or deep pustules, leading to scarring (Figure 44.13).

Itch is a rare symptom.

Inflammatory macules represent regressing lesions that may persist for many weeks (Figure 44.14). Scarring is commonly seen as a consequence of acne and can present as atrophic scarring (Figure 44.15) or hypertrophic or keloid scarring (Figure 44.16).

Differential diagnosis
Active acne
Includes milia, syringomas, fibrofolliculomas, ectopic sebaceous glands (Fordyce spots), pilosebaceous naevoid disorders, acneiform naevi, adenoma sebaceum sebaceous (epidermoid) cysts and steatocystoma multiplex, granulomatous rosacea, keratosis pilaris, pyoderma faciale, perioral dermatitis, folliculitis decalvans, dissecting

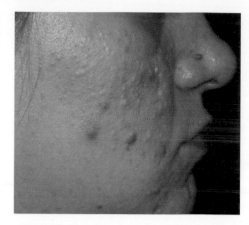

Figure 44.9 Multiple macrocomedones interspersed with some inflammatory lesions on the cheeks of a female patient with acne. (Source: Courtesy of Professor M. Jackson, University of Louisville, Kentucky, USA.)

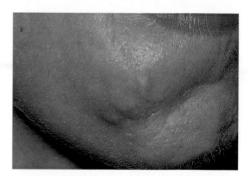

Figure 44.10 Submarine comedones. This patient required stretching of the skin in order for them to be seen.

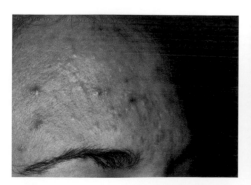

Figure 44.8 Sandpaper comedones on the forehead.

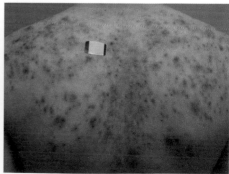

Figure 44.11 Severe acne of the back with many inflammatory papules and pustules.

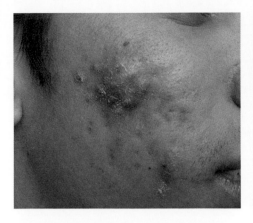

Figure 44.12 Nodular acne of the right cheek with scars. (Source: Courtesy of Dr S. Chow, KL Skin Centre, Malaysia.)

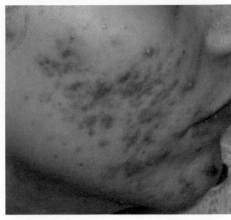

Figure 44.14 Inflammatory macules contribute to the erythema seen in acne.

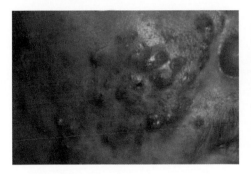

Figure 44.13 Nodular/conglobate acne with sinus tracts. (Source: Courtesy of Dr C.L. Goh, National Skin Centre, Singapore.)

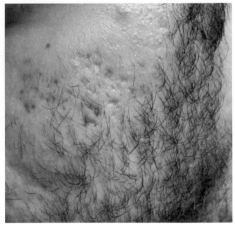

Figure 44.15 Atrophic scarring with associated inflammatory change. (Source: Courtesy of J. Del Rosso Las Vegas Skin & Cancer Clinic, Las Vegas, Nevada, USA.)

cellulitis of the scalp, hidradenitis suppurativa, Malassezia folliculitis, keloidal folliculitis, scalp folliculitis, Favre Racouchot syndrome and Gram-negative folliculitis.

Acne scarring

Scarring due to hydroa vacciniforme, ulery-thema oophryogenes, folliculitis keloidalis, varioliform atrophy and porphyria cutanea tarda. Acne necrotica varioliformis is associated with itching and smallpox-like scars, particu-larly around the scalp margin.

Investigations

Severity is assessed visually according to the extent of disease and number of lesions and frequently described as mild, moderate or severe. The Leeds photometric grading scale is the most commonly used global grading system.

Acne scarring should also be included in the assessment of acne severity.

Investigations may be required to exclude an underlying endocrinopathy (Box 44.1). Table 44.3 outlines hormonal investigations required to identify an endocrine problem.

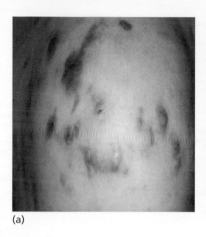
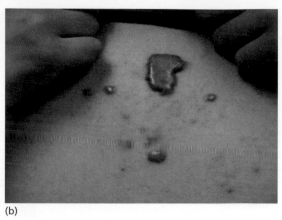

(a)   (b)

Figure 44.16 (a) Hypertrophic scarring of the shoulders in the context of moderate to severe acne. (b) Keloid scarring on the trunk associated with mild acne. (Source: Courtesy of Dr S. Chow, KL Skin Centre, Malaysia.)

Box 44.1 Signs and symptoms that may indicate an underlying endocrinopathy suggesting the need for investigation

1. Signs of hyperandrogenism alongside acne
   - Seborrhoea
   - Hirsutism
   - Androgenic alopecia
   - Cushingoid features
   - Increased libido
   - Deepening of voice
   - Clitoromegaly
   - Acanthosis nigricans
2. Acne reported to be
   - Therapy-resistant acne
   - Rapidly relapsing
   - Very severe
   - Marked seborrhoea
   - Sudden onset particularly in the context of other signs of hyperandrogenism

---

Table 44.3 Hormonal investigations required to identify endocrine problems

Suspected clinical diagnosis	Hormonal evaluation
PCOS	Luteinising hormone
	FSH
PCOS	Total free testosterone
PCOS	Prolactin
CAH	DHEAS
CAH	17-hydroxyl progesterone
CAH	ACTH stimulation test
NCAH	TSH
Ovarian tumour	Free testosterone
Adrenal tumour	DHEAS

ACTH, adrenocorticotrophic hormone; CAH, congenital adrenal hyperplasia; DHEAS, dehydroepiandrosterone sulphate; FSH, follicle-stimulating hormone; NCAH, non-classical congenital adrenal hyperplasia; PCOS, polycystic ovary syndrome; TSH, thyroid- stimulating hormone.

Psychosocial complications

Severe acne may be related to increased anger and anxiety. When compared to other serious organic diseases, acne patients describe levels of social, psychological and emotional problems as great as those reported with chronic disabling diseases such as asthma, epilepsy, back pain, arthritis and diabetes Clinical depression has been demonstrated in acne patients; this does not necessarily correlate with the clinical severity of disease. Suicide in acne patients has been reported and the depressed acne patient should be assessed for suicide risk.

Solid facial oedema (Morbihan disease)
A rare and disfiguring complication of acne.

Osteoma cutis
Represents focal ossifications in the subcutaneous and dermal tissue. This uncommon complication of acne is described more commonly in women with longstanding inflammatory acne and usually needs no treatment. The calcification presents as small 2–4 mm persistent papules which are firm to the touch.

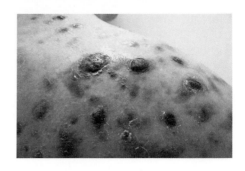

Figure 44.17 Pyogenic granulomas in severe acne.

Pyogenic granulomas
Occasionally seen on the trunk in patients with very severe acne (Figure 44.17).

Management
The aims of acne management are summarised in Box 44.2.

Certain factors link to severity of acne and risk of relapse (Table 44.4).

> **Box 44.2 Aims of acne management**
> - Alleviate symptoms
> - Clear existing lesions
> - Limit disease activity by preventing new lesions forming as well as scars developing
> - Avoid negative impact on quality of life

Table 44.4 Summary of factors associated with acne severity and relapse

Specific factor	Impact
Positive family history	Linked to
	• Earlier occurrence of acne
	• Increased retentional lesions
	• Increased relapses
Early onset	Infantile acne shown to link to
	• Resurgence of acne in teenage years
	• More severe acne in teenage years
	• More frequent relapse in teenage years, mid-facial comedonal lesions prepuberty linked to more severe disease
	• Earlier onset of acne relative to menarche related to more severe disease
Duration of acne	Prolonged duration of disease associated with reduced efficacy
	A family history of acne >25 years associated with more adult acne in relatives
Seborrhoea	High sebum production correlates with more severe acne
	High sebum production relates to reduced response to systemic antibiotics
Extent, location and nature of lesions	Truncal acne associated with reduced response to systemic therapy when compared to acne on the face

Therapy is determined by severity and extent of disease but should be guided by other factors such as duration, response to previous treatments, predisposition to scarring, post-inflammatory erythema and pigmentation, as well as patient preference, lifestyle and treatment cost.

Figures 44.18–44.20 outline first-, second- and third-line management. Oral isotretinoin

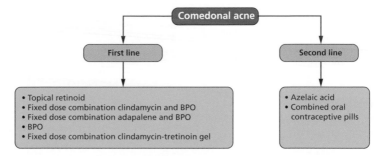

Figure 44.18 Treatment algorithm for comedonal acne. BPO, benzoyl peroxide.

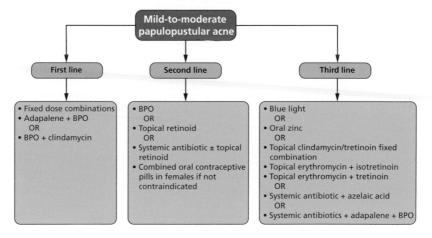

Figure 44.19 Treatment algorithm for mild to moderate inflammatory acne. BPO, benzoyl peroxide.

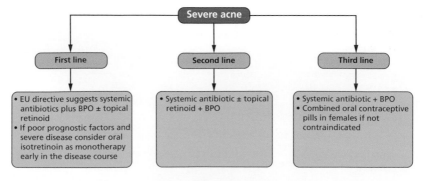

Figure 44.20 Treatment algorithm for severe acne. BPO, benzoyl peroxide.

Table 44.5 Defining the severity of acne according to lesion type and extent

Type of acne	Descriptive of clinical lesions
Comedonal acne	Both open (blackheads) and closed (whiteheads) comedones
Mild acne	Mixed but fairly localised inflamed and non-inflamed lesions Superficial inflammatory lesions usually <5 mm in diameter
Mild to moderate papulopustular acne	More extensive papulopustular lesions frequently in association with non-inflammatory lesion
Severe acne	Inflammatory lesions frequently deep seated and may evolve into nodules and deep pustules Small nodules are defined as firm inflammatory lesions >5 mm; large nodules are >1 cm
	Large nodules extend over large areas and frequently result in painful lesions, exudative sinus tracts and disfiguring tissue destruction and scarring
	Acne conglobata includes multiple grouped comedones, interspersed with papules, which are tender inflammatory nodules of varying sizes, some of which are suppurative and coalesce to form sinus tracts Extensive scarring is a frequent outcome

should be considered earlier in patients demonstrating poor prognostic factors, as outlined in Table 44.5,

Topical therapy should be applied to all areas of affected skin as histology of normal-looking skin from an acne-prone site demonstrates microcomedones as the precursors of all clinical lesions.

Isotretinoin

National regulatory authorities have approved a pregnancy prevention programme. This programme includes advice on education, therapy management and control of the distribution of oral isotretinoin. Both patients and prescribers must be fully aware of teratogenicity. The patient should acknowledge the problem by signing a consent form and should accept detailed counselling by the clinician prior to and during treatment.

Therapy management includes medically supervised pregnancy testing before, during and 5 weeks after a course of therapy and provides advice on contraception.

Mood changes including depression are common among adolescents and have been reported in acne patients treated with isotretinoin.

An acute flare of acne early in a course of isotretinoin is a recognised problem in about 6% of cases and is clinically significant in half of these. If the acne is very inflammatory, a lower dose of isotretinoin alongside oral corticosteroids may be required. Vitamin supplements containing vitamin A should be avoided alongside isotretinoin, as additive toxic effects could ensue.

Other treatments

Light cautery or hyfrecation has been shown to help patients with multiple macrocomedones; these are usually whiteheads but occasionally blackheads (up to 1.5 mm in diameter) and chloracne can be improved. A topical anaesthetic preparation is applied beneath an occlusive dressing. The cautery or hyfrecation should be set as low as possible to produce little or no pain. The aim is to produce very low-grade thermal damage.

Visible light

Blue light has been given a low-strength recommendation in the management of mild to moderate papulopustular acne.

Lasers and photodynamic therapy

Surgical ablative therapy is most effective; techniques reported include combined dermabrasion and punch biopsy, scalpel incisions and curettage, extirpation of the small bone fragments after microdissection and laser therapies. The erbium:YAG laser is said to be associated with minimal thermal injury, with better cosmetic results than the carbon dioxide laser.

Chemical peels

Light chemical peels can be used to remove comedones as well as superficial scarring and hyperpigmentation.

ACNE VARIANTS: ACNE ASSOCIATED WITH PSYCHOLOGICAL PROBLEMS

Acné excoriée

(Syn. Excoriated acne, picker's acne)
Mainly occurs in adolescent girls (Figure 44.21); incidence is increasing in mature females and is frequently associated with stress. It is self-inflicted due to compulsive picking of real or imagined acne lesions on the face. Obsessive compulsive disorder and body dysmorphic disorder (BDD) may be associated. The persistent trauma frequently results in significant scarring.

Treatment is challenging. Some patients may just need to break the habit of picking whilst others may have a compulsive skin picking disorder which may require psychological therapy or psychotropic drugs. 585-nm pulsed dye laser along with cognitive psychotherapy can be us for facial scarring and ulceration resulting from acné excoriée

A small number of patients with BDD have acne as their prime symptom. The perceived acne is out of proportion to physical signs. Patients require significant support; they are often depressed or have obsessional compulsive behaviours or anxiety. A significant risk of suicide has been reported. Patients with BDD require dermatological and psychiatric management as many have global mental disorders.

Granulomatous acne

The clinical picture is usually that of deep, well-demarcated lesion(s), especially on the cheeks (Figure 44.22). Response to therapy is slow and often unsatisfactory; antibiotics and isotretinoin are of limited benefit; oral steroids are often required.

Mechanical acne
(Syn. Acne mechanica)
Acne that occurs at the site of repeated mechanical trauma and/or frictional obstruction of the pilosebaceous outlet, resulting in comedo formation.

Examples include 'fiddler's neck', which may occur on the neck of violin players and is characterised by well-defined plaques with the presence of comedones, lichenification and pigmentation. Tight clothing may cause localised acne in the frictional sites.

Drug-induced acne

Some drugs may cause acneiform reactions; these account for about 1% of all drug-induced skin eruptions. Table 44.6 identifies drugs that have been implicated in acneiform eruptions.

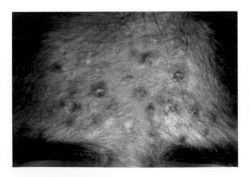

Figure 44.21 Acné excoriée on the forehead of a female. (Source: Courtesy of Dr C.L. Goh, National Skin Centre, Singapore.)

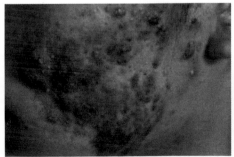

Figure 44.22 Granulomatous acne of the face. (Source: Courtesy of Dr C.L. Goh, National Skin Centre, Singapore.)

Table 44.6 Drug classes and types of medication that may exacerbate or cause acne

Drug class or type	Examples
Corticosteroid	
Topical	Betamethasone
Oral	Prednisolone
Inhaled	Budesonide
ACTH	ACTH, synthetic ACTH
Anabolic steroid/synthetic androgen (Figure 44.23)	Danazol, nandrolone, stanozolol
Anticonvulsant	Carbamazepine, phenytoin, phenobarbitone, troxidone, gabapentin, topiramate
Antidepressant	Lithium, sertraline
Other neuroleptic/antipsychotic	Pimozide, risperidone
Antitubercular	Isoniazid, pyrazinamide
Antineoplastic/EGFR antagonists	Dactinomycin, pentostatin, cetuximab
Antiviral	Ritonavir, ganciclovir
Calcium antagonist	Nilvadipine, nimodipine
Halogen	Sodium fluoride, potassium iodine
Human growth hormone	Genetically engineered human growth hormone
Vitamins	Vitamin B_{12}, possibly other B vitamins

ACTH, adrenocorticotropic hormone; EGFR, epidermal growth factor receptor.

Acne cosmetica

Represents an acne variant associated with chronic use of cosmetics containing potentially comedogenic substances. Cited agents include lanolin, petrolatum, certain vegetable oils, butylstearate, lauryl alcohol and oleic acid. Skin-bleaching agents containing steroids can cause or exacerbate acne in dark-skinned women.

Pomade acne

Pomades are greasy preparations used to defrizz curly hair. They can trigger non-inflammatory acne.

Detergent acne

This uncommon form develops in patients who wash many times each day in the mistaken hope of improving their existing acne. Trauma and the alkalinity of soap are likely to be involved in the mechanism

Occupational acne

(**Syn. Chemically induced acne, chloracne**)
A group of disorders characterised by the formation of acne-like lesions in patients previously not prone to acne after exposure to occupational agents, in most cases chemical compounds. It can be induced by diverse environmental agents.

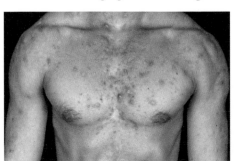

Figure 44.23 Severe acne vulgaris in a male body builder.

Chloracne is caused by certain polyhalogenated organic (aromatic) compounds containing naphthalenes, biphenyls and phenols (herbicides and herbicide intermediates) and is considered to be one of the most sensitive indicators of systemic poisoning by these compounds.

Dioxins, a large family of halogenated aromatic hydrocarbons, are the most potent environmental chloracnegen. The most potent environmental chloracnegen of this group is 2,3,7,8-tetrachlorodibenzo-p-dioxin.

Epidemiology

Most cases have resulted from occupational and non-occupational exposures. Non-occupational chloracne mainly resulted from contaminated industrial wastes and contaminated food products.

The production of polychlorinated biphenyls has been prohibited by the Stockholm Treaty on Persistent Organic Pollutants made effective from 2004.

Clinical features

A history of exposure to chloracnegens, progressively emerging comedones, papules, nodules and cysts followed by scars, skin xerosis and decreased sebogenesis and high serum concentration of chloracnegens (Figure 44.24) differentiates chloracne from acne vulgaris.

Investigations

The assessment of chloracnegens in serum can only be carried out in specialised laboratories. Histopathological changes also offer important clues in the diagnosis of chloracne as follows.

Pathophysiology

- Epidermal hyperplasia.
- Follicular hyperplasia: Replacement by keratinising epidermal cells.
- Sebaceous glands disappear and are replaced by keratinising epidermal cells.
- Sebaceous gland involution after a complete loss of structure. The remaining sebocytes appear normal. Sebaceous gland involution is due to cessation of sebocyte replenishment.

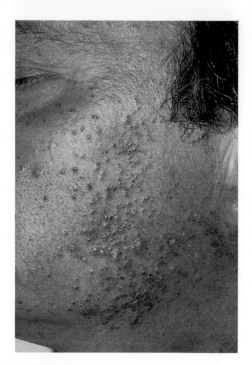

Figure 44.24 Chloracne: multiple comedonal lesions on the face.

Management

The aim of treatment is to lower or to eliminate the accumulated dioxins in the body at the very beginning of intoxication, e.g. by using dioxin-chelating substances such as synthetic dietary fat substitutes.

Topical tretinoin for at least 1 year.

Acne fulminans

A rare and severe destructive form of acne presenting primarily in adolescent males.

Epidemiology

A rare form of acne and incidence appears to be diminishing, possibly due to more effective and earlier use of treatments. It is predominantly seen in young white males aged between 13 and 22 years. Frequency and severity are much greater in patients of northern European descent compared with those from East Asian origin.

Pathophysiology

Possibly an autoimmune complex disease. Immune complexes are found predominantly in patients with musculoskeletal problems. Elevated blood levels of testosterone may play a role. The increase in physiological levels of testosterone in males at puberty may explain this predisposition.

The susceptibility gene is the CD2-binding protein 1 (*CD2BP1*).

Clinical features

Most patients describe mild to moderate acne for 0.5–5 years before a sudden onset of febrile ulcerative necrotic acne lesions alongside arthralgia, fever and various systemic inflammatory signs and symptoms. Patients typically fail to respond to antibiotic therapy.

Patients present with numerous, inflammatory tender and ulcerative nodules covered with haemorrhagic crusts (Figures 44.25 and 44.26). These are predominantly distributed on the upper chest, back and shoulders and pyogenic granulomatous-like lesions may be present. The face may also be involved and the lesions undergo rapid degeneration resulting in ulcerations filled with necrotic debris. Comedonal lesions are rare.

Systemic signs and symptoms are present in the majority of patients and include malaise, arthralgia, joint swellings, polyarthritis, myalgia, fever and anorexia and weight loss. A marked leucocytosis which may be leukaemoid is frequent; patients may also demonstrate anaemia. A subset

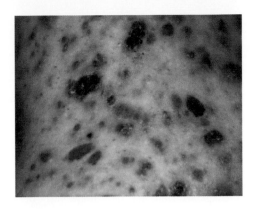

Figure 44.26 Erosive crusting lesions on the back of a young male with acne fulminans.

of patients with no systemic symptoms but with severe acne comparable to that seen in acne fulminans has been described as 'sine fulminans'.

Painful splenomegaly, erythema nodosum and bone pain due to aseptic osteolysis have also been reported. Bone involvement is common, including lytic bone lesions and destructive lesions resembling osteomyelitis.

Acne fulminans may occur in the context of synovitis, acne, pustulosis, hyperostosis and osteitis (SAPHO) syndrome and is considered by some as a spectrum of this autoinflammatory disorder. Pyogenic arthritis, pyoderma gangrenosum and acne (PAPA) syndrome affects mainly the skin and joints and may present with either acne fulminans or conglobata.

Differential diagnosis

The main differential diagnosis is severe acne conglobata in which comedonal lesions are generally much more florid.

Investigations

Abnormal laboratory findings may include an increased erythrocyte sedimentation rate (ESR), elevated C-reactive protein and thrombocytosis, together with a normochromic and normocytic anaemia. Characteristically, a leucocytosis is found sometimes with an associated leukaemoid reaction. Elevated liver enzymes and microscopic haematuria, proteinuria and other kidney abnormalities may be

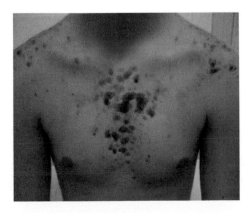

Figure 44.25 Acne fulminans in a young male.

identified. Patients with osteolytic lesions may have elevated serum alkaline phosphatase.

Management

The acute myalgia, arthralgia and fever can be treated with oral salicylates or non-steroidal anti-inflammatory drugs and graduated physical exercise. Crusts should be removed by soaking the skin with emollient oil followed by the use of a potent steroid/antimicrobial cream for 2–3 weeks.

Oral prednisolone therapy should be commenced first line and decreased slowly over 2–3 months. Low-dose oral isotretinoin (0.2 mg/kg) should be cautiously introduced either after 3–4 weeks of systemic steroid therapy or in parallel with oral corticosteroids and then gradually increased as tolerated and according to clinical response.

The prognosis for patients treated effectively with corticosteroids and isotretinoin is extremely good. Recurrent acne fulminans is very rare. Relapse may occur as corticosteroid therapy is reduced but the risk reduces over time and is unusual after a year. The most common complication is significant and disfiguring scarring.

Acne conglobata

This is a rare and severe form of acne characterised by multiple and extensive inflammatory papules, tender nodules and abscesses, which commonly coalesce to form malodorous draining sinus tracts.

Epidemiology

A rare disease presenting in the second to third decade and may persist into the 40s and 50s. M > F.

It may occur in the context of a number of inflammatory disorders, including hidradenitis suppurativa, pyoderma gangrenosum, arthritis, SAPHO syndrome, PAPA syndrome, pyoderma gangrenosum, acne and suppurative hidradenitis (PASH) syndrome and pyoderma gangrenosum, acne and spondyloarthritis syndrome (PASS).

Pathophysiology

The primary cause remains unknown.

May be triggered by testosterone, anabolic steroid abuse, withdrawal of testosterone and androgen-secreting tumour and has been described following exposure to aromatic hydrocarbons or ingestion of halogens.

Familial cases have been reported with linkage to chromosome 15q24-26 in the region of IL-16 and *CRABPI* genes.

Clinical features

May develop in the setting of acne vulgaris that has been quiescent for a number of years but frequently the onset is insidious with a chronic and unremitting course. Active inflammatory lesions may persist for many years and typically continue until the fourth decade of life. The healing of lesions is slow and associated with significant discomfort and scarring.

Patients present with multiple comedones, often in groups and demonstrate highly inflammatory papules, pustules, tender nodules, interconnecting abscesses and draining sinus tracts (Figure 44.27). The nodules characteristically increase in size and deep ulcers may develop beneath the nodules which interconnect and produce draining sinus tracts

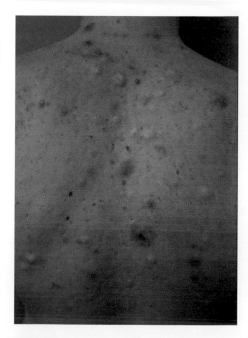

Figure 44.27 Acne conglobata of the back with multiple inflammatory lesions, grouped comedones, cysts and scarring.

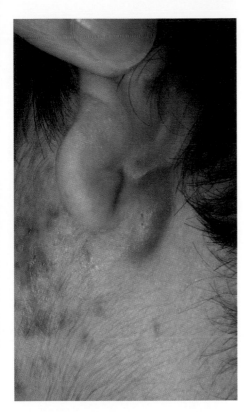

Figure 44.28 Patient with acne conglobata present with abscesses and cysts, causing interconnecting sinus tracts.

(Figure 44.28). Hypertrophic and atrophic scars are frequently present.

Differential diagnosis

Severe inflammatory acne or acne fulminans.

Management

There is significant scarring resulting, in most cases, in disfigurement and psychosocial sequelae.

Therapy is challenging and aims to reduce the morbidity associated with discomfort and malodour with the use of appropriate analgesia alongside antiseptic washes and antibiotics.
First line: Oral isotretinoin for 4–6 months is the treatment of choice. Isotretinoin may need to be combined with oral antibiotics such as erythromycin or trimethoprim. Concomitant use of systemic steroids such as prednisolone for 2–4 weeks may also provide benefit to control the inflammatory component of the disease at initial

onset and intermittently during acute exacerbations. Large nodules can be aspirated and injection with intralesional triamcinolone or cryotherapy may be beneficial. Surgery may be required to lay open abscesses and sinus tracts. Resultant scarring has been improved with the use of fractional laser postsurgical intervention.

Acne in childhood

Preadolescent acne is uncommon. Descriptive terms used for acne in pre-adolescent children are generally based on age and include neonatal, infantile, mid-childhood and prepubertal acne.

Epidemiology
Neonatal acne

Defined as the presence of even a small number of comedones may affect up to 20% of neonates. The best recognised is neonatal cephalic pustulosis, an acneiform eruption thought to be caused by *Malassezia* (Figure 44.29). Presents at birth through to the age of 4–6 weeks. M:F is 5:1.

Infantile and mid-childhood

Infantile acne is less common than neonatal acne and mid-childhood acne is very rare. Typically presents between 3 and 12 months but may occur as late as 16 months. M > F. Mid-childhood acne occurs from age 1 to 7 years.

Prepubertal acne

Prepubertal acne is defined as acne that commences before the onset of puberty. Acne has been reported in 60–71.3% of premenarchal

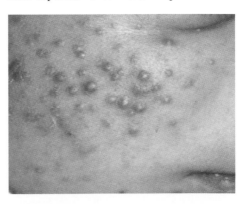

Figure 44.29 Neonatal cephalic pustulosis.

females. A mid-facial comedonal distribution is associated with poor prognosis. It presents before true puberty and may occur from age 7 to 11 years. Girls may present with acne as young as 8 years of age. It may be associated with underlying endocrinopathies and virilising tumours. SAPHO syndrome has been reported in childhood.

Pathophysiology

The underlying pathogenesis of neonatal acne is thought to relate to hyperactivity of the sebaceous glands stimulated by neonatal androgens from the testes in boys and adrenals in girls and boys.

The aetiology of infantile acne also remains poorly understood. Similar to neonatal acne, it may be associated with increased levels of androgens produced by adrenal glands in both sexes and by the testes in boys.

The onset of sebum production triggers the expansion of *P. acnes* and this occurs earlier in children who develop acne than in those who do not.

In the case of neonatal cephalic pustulosis, a relationship has been suggested between the clinical presentation and *Malasezzia furfur*, *Malasezzia sympodialis* and other species

Certain medications may be implicated in prepubertal acne as identified in the section on drug-induced acne. Maternal ingestion of phenytoin has been implicated.

Clinical features
Neonatal acne
Presents with erythematous papulopustular lesions commonly distributed on the cheeks, chin and forehead (Figure 44.30). Occasionally, these extend to the neck, scalp and upper trunk.

Neonatal cephalic pustulosis
Also referred to as neonatal acne. This usually presents in the first 3 weeks of life and prevalence varies between 10 and 66% of newborns. It is characterised by erythematous papular/pustular lesions especially on the cheeks but also on the chin, eyelids, neck and upper chest. Comedonal lesions are not usually seen.

Infantile acne
The central cheeks are frequently affected with a combination of inflamed papules and

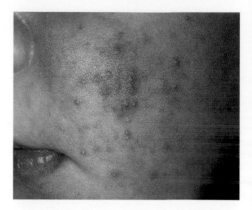

Figure 44.30 Neonatal acne presenting in the first few weeks of life.

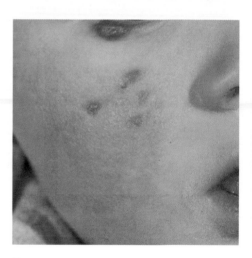

Figure 44.31 Infantile acne may involve cystic lesions and scarring. (Source: Courtesy of Dr J. Ravenscroft, Queens Medical Centre, University of Nottingham, UK.)

vpustules with open and closed comedones (Figure 44.32). The presentation is usually more widespread than neonatal acne.

Acne conglobata can present in infants, resulting in severe inflammatory cystic lesions, sinus tract formation and significant scarring (Figure 44.31).

Mid-childhood acne
Acne developing at an early age should always raise the suspicion of androgen excess.

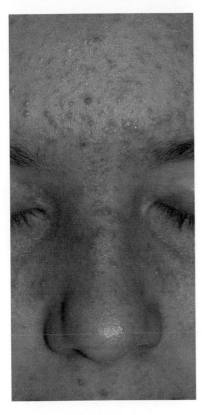

Figure 44.32 Mid-facial comedones are associated with poor prognosis.

Prepubertal acne

Acne in prepubertal children usually presents with comedonal lesions with or without some inflammatory papules. Lesions are frequently located in a mid-facial distribution and may precede any other signs of maturation. Mid-facial comedonal acne (see Figure 44.32) can be the first sign of pubertal maturation in females, preceding areolar development, pubic hair and the menarche.

Differential diagnosis
Infantile acne

Includes neonatal acne, acne venenata infantum, chloracne and hyperandrogenism.

Mid-childhood acne

Includes keratosis pilaris and milia alongside endocrinopathies and conditions relating to hyperandrogenism.

Prepubertal acne

Includes childhood granulomatous periorificial dermatitis, lupus miliaris disseminatus faciei and childhood granulomatous rosacea alongside endocrinopathies and disorders associated with an androgen excess.

Investigations

It is important to consider underlying endocrinopathies and investigate accordingly with the support of a paediatric endocrinologist.

Management

The principles of treating acne in children involve adopting simple regimens that target the clinical lesions and pathophysiological factors implicated in acne whilst avoiding adverse effects. See the algorithm in Table 44.7.

Table 44.7 Therapeutic options for childhood acne

Treatment options
Gentle cleansers, oil-free emollients
If marked pustules then use topical azole cream
First line
Benzoyl peroxide or topical retinoid (if primarily comedonal)
Fixed combination products if mixed lesions all indicated from 12 years with the exception of 0.1% adapalene/2.5% BPO, which is indicated from 9 years
Second line for more severe disease
Oral erythromycin (oral trimethoprim if allergic to macrolides) combined with BPO to avoid emergence of antibiotic-resistant *P. acnes* ± topical retinoid Tetracyclines are not to be used in children <12 years of age
Third line
Severe recalcitrant scarring acne, exclude underlying hyperandrogenism
Consider oral isotretinoin

BPO, benzoyl peroxide.

45

Rosacea, flushing and blushing

ROSACEA

Rosacea is a chronic disorder with fluctuating severity that encompasses a spectrum of changes that occur mainly in the facial skin but may also involve the eyes.

A common feature in the majority of patients is the presence of facial erythema variably associated with the following:

- Facial vascular changes: subtype 1 (erythematotelangiectatic rosacea, ETTR).
- Inflammatory lesions: subtype 2 (papulopustular rosacea PPR).
- Hypertrophic changes: subtype 3 (phymatous rosacea, PR).
- Ocular involvement: subtype 4 (ocular rosacea, OR).

Epidemiology

Rosacea is a disorder that predominantly affects fair, pale-skinned, sun-sensitive individuals, reflected in the much higher frequency in northern Europe as opposed to those countries with darker skin-type populations. Onset is in middle-age, 30–50 years. Females present at an earlier age whilst males develop more severe rosacea, including rhinophyma.

Prevalence of rosacea is difficult to estimate accurately due to the lack of a commonly accepted clear definition of rosacea and its subtypes. ETTR is the commonest subtype and is about four times more prevalent than PPR. ETTR was found in 14% of the Irish population. PPR has a prevalence of 2% in northern

European populations and constitutes about 1% of all rosacea patients. The prevalence of OR is unknown because of the lack of specificity of the clinical features.

Up to 25% of patients with rosacea have a family history and may develop rosacea at an earlier age than those without a family history.

Pathophysiology

It is unlikely that a single pathophysiological pathway is responsible for the diverse clinical features seen in rosacea. In ETTR ultraviolet radiation may be an aetiological factor.

The potential role of microorganisms in the pathogenesis of rosacea is supported by the up-regulation of Toll-like receptor 2 (TLR2) receptors in PPR and increased cathelicidin expression and leukocyte activity. Microorganisms that might potentially induce rosacea include *Staphylococcus epidermidis*, *Chlamydophila pneumoniae* and the *Demodex*-associated bacterium *Bacillus oleronius*. Alterations in the cutaneous microenvironment in patients with rosacea such as changes in lipid profile, cutaneous pH or skin barrier function may facilitate an overgrowth of commensal organisms. These organisms may then trigger a host immune reaction once a critical level is reached.

Demodex mite proliferation (Figure 45.1) in the pilosebaceous follicles of the face is a possible aetiological factor in the cutaneous and ocular inflammation in PPR. These mites may also play a role in the modulation of the host innate immune system.

Rook's Dermatology Handbook, First Edition. Edited by Christopher E. M. Griffiths, Tanya O. Bleiker, Daniel Creamer, John R. Ingram and Rosalind C. Simpson.
© 2022 John Wiley & Sons Ltd. Published 2022 by John Wiley & Sons Ltd.

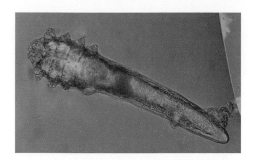

Figure 45.1 *Demodex folliculorum* mite showing its elongated worm-like posterior body (opistostoma) and four sets of short legs on the upper body (podostoma). The mouth parts (gnathostoma) are at the front of the podostoma. Magnification 100×.

It has been suggested that the phymatous changes of PR may be brought about by the upregulation of fibrosis-promoting matrix metalloproteinases as a result of increased mast cell numbers and keratinocyte and macrophage activation.

The pathogenesis of OR seems to be closely associated with meibomian gland dysfunction. A reduced tear break-up time in patients with rosacea is found as a result of inadequate lipid components of the tear film. Meibomian cysts (usually painless), representing chronic inflammation of the meibomian glands, may appear in crops. *Demodex* mite infestation may play a role in the initiation of inflammatory ocular changes that occur in these modified sebaceous glands of the eyelid.

Increased environmental temperature and dietary factors (ingesting hot liquids, spicy foods, large meals, alcohol, etc.) are often cited as potentially exacerbating rosacea. These elements may cause a transient increase in facial erythema and exacerbate a flushing tendency (predominantly in ETTR), but there is no evidence that they worsen the inflammatory lesions of PPR or the phymatous or ocular changes of PR and OR, respectively.

The histopathology of ETTR is characterised by the presence of enlarged and dilated bizarre-shaped capillaries and venules in the upper part of the dermis. A mild perivascular and interstitial lymphocytic infiltrate with frequent plasma cells is commonly seen in this subtype.

Occasional *Demodex* mites may be present within the follicles. Solar elastosis is a prominent finding in ETTR patients.

The inflammatory infiltrate is much more conspicuous in PPR. While there is often a perivascular infiltrate of lymphocytes, the most marked changes involve the follicles, with numerous neutrophils, plasma cells and less commonly eosinophils. Ruptured follicles with granulomatous changes may be present in florid cases. Sometimes *Demodex* mite remnants are seen within these granulomas or abscesses.

Sebaceous gland hyperplasia (which is marked in severe rhinophyma) with striking dermal fibrotic changes and a variable degree of perivascular lymphocytic/neutrophilic infiltration are the histological features of PR.

The histological findings of OR are non-specific (see Chapter 60).

Some degree of granulomatous inflammation may be seen in biopsies from all forms of rosacea. In this condition, sarcoidal or tuberculoid granulomas with or without abscess formation are seen.

Clinical features
Rosacea can have a significant social impact, particularly in patients with flushing, in female patients and in patients with rhinophyma. Seborrhoeic dermatitis may coexist.

The clinical features and grading of the subtypes are listed in Table 45.1. In clinical practice there is an overlap of clinical features between the different subtypes and individual patients may have more than one subtype.

Granulomatous rosacea (acne agminate, lupus miliaris disseminatus faciei)
An uncommon entity in which persistent, firm, non-tender, red to brown papules or nodules arise on otherwise normal-appearing skin around the mouth and eyes and on the cheeks (Figure 45.7). They resolve without significant scarring. It can resemble cutaneous sarcoid clinically and histologically.

Differential diagnosis
The differential diagnosis of the different rosacea subtypes is outlined in Table 45.2.

Table 45.1 Rosacea subtypes: clinical features and severity grading

Subtype	Clinical features

Subtype 1: Erythematotelangiectatic rosacea
Mild (grade 1):
  Occasional flushing
  Mild erythema
Moderate (grade 2):
  Frequent flushing
  Moderate erythema
  Telangiectases present
Severe (grade 3):
  Severe flushing
  Marked erythema
  Many telangiectases
	Figure 45.2
	
	• Individuals usually have skin type 1 or 2
	• Facial erythema present usually with tolangiectases
	• Facial vascular hyperreactivity and a tendency to flushing with environmental temperature change and some dietary components (hot liquids, etc.)
	• Skin sensitivity and dryness, easily irritated skin, frequent burning and stinging sensation
	• Intolerance of sunlight/harsh winds
	• Associated actinic damage common

Subtype 2: Papulopustular rosacea
Mild (grade 1):
  Few papules/pustules (<5)
  Mild perilesional erythema
  Little tendency to flush
Moderate (grade 2):
  Several papules/pustules (>5 but <10)
  Significant coalescing erythema around lesions
  Tendency to temperature intolerance and flushing
Severe (grade 3):
  Many papules/pustules (>10)
  Plaques of coalescing erythema
  Oedema may be present
  Scaling and dermatitic changes may be present
  Marked intolerance of temperature change (cold to heat) with resultant flushing
	Figures 45.3 and 45.4
	• Erythema (mainly centrofacial) mostly related to inflammatory lesions (perilesional erythema)
	• Telangiectases may be present
	• Dome-shaped erythematous papules and papulopustules (small areas of apical pustulation is usual) mainly on the central face but can occur elsewhere (scalp/behind ears) and be asymmetrical
	• Flushing and skin sensitivity may be present but not as prominent as in ETTR
	• Dryness/dermatitis or mild facial oedema may be present in severe cases
	• Lesions heal without scarring

Subtype 3: Phymatous rosacea
For rhinophyma (the commonest form of this subtype)
Mild (grade 1):
  Puffiness of nose
  Prominent follicular openings (patulous follicles)
  No change in nasal contour
Moderate (grade 2):
  Bulbous nasal swelling
  Change in nasal contour without nodular distortion
Severe (grade 3):
  Marked nasal swelling
  Nasal distortion with nodular component
	Figure 45.5
	
	• Thickened, nodular skin
	• Patulous follicles (early disease)
	• Bulbous, distorted features (advanced disease)
	• Most commonly affects the nose but can also affect the chin, forehead (frontophyma), ears (otophyma) and eyelids
	• May be associated with other features of rosacea, occur in isolation or be due to other causes (e.g. actinic damage)
	• Perinasal telangiectases sometimes prominent
	• Flushing not a common association

Table 45.1 (Continued)

Subtype	Clinical features
Subtype 4: Ocular rosacea	Figure 45.6
Mild (grade1):	• Usually bilateral but severity in each eye may vary
Mild itch/gritty feeling	• Dry, gritty sensation, sometimes itch
Mild scaling/erythema of lid margins	• Limits use of contact lenses
Mild conjunctival injection	• Watering of eyes
Moderate (grade 2):	• Conjunctival telangiectasia
Burning/stinging sensation	• Collarettes of scale around base of the eyelashes
Crusting/marked erythema of lid margins	• Blepharitis with crusting
Collarettes and sleeves of keratin on the lash shafts	• Swelling and erythema of eyelids
Conjunctival injection	• Chalazia (painless) and hordeola (painful)
Hordeolum/chalazion formation	• Conjunctivitis/keratitis, episcleritis, scleritis, iritis (rare)
Severe (grade3):	
Pain/photosensitivity	
Blurred vision	
Loss of eyelashes (madarosis)	
Corneal changes	
Scleral involvement	

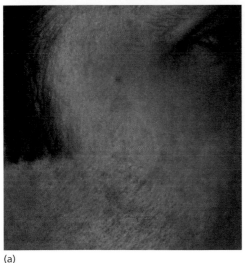
(a)

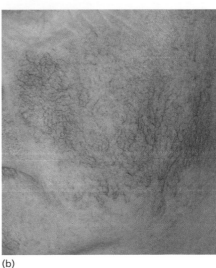
(b)

Figure 45.2 Erythematotelangiectatic rosacea. (a) Facial erythema in moderate ETTR. (b) Prominent telangiectatic vessels on the lateral cheeks.

Investigations

Diagnostic biopsy only required in atypical presentations.

Management

The approach to the management of rosacea differs according to the principal subtype.

General skin measures include sun protection, emollients and soap.

The use of topical corticosteroids should be avoided. Patients with a tendency to flushing (mainly those with ETTR) should avoid agents that provoke flushing such as hot drinks, spicy foods, alcohol and some drugs.

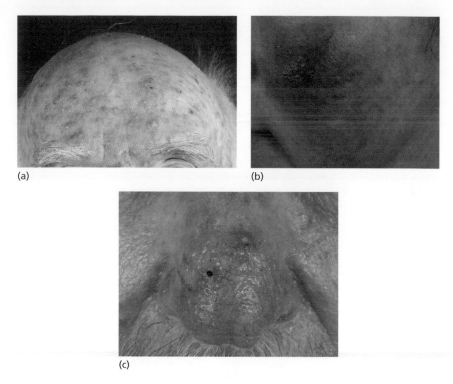

(a) (b)

(c)

Figure 45.3 Papulopustular rosacea. (a) Papules and pustules on the forehead of a patient with PPR. (b) Erythema of the medial cheek area in a patient with grade 3 PPR who had several inflammatory lesions coalescing into a plaque in this area. (c) Small areas of pustulation are visible on the apex of some papules in this patient with grade 2 PPR on the bridge of his nose.

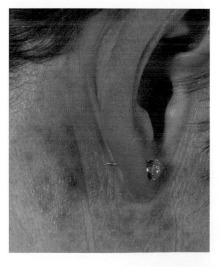

Figure 45.4 Grouped papules behind the ear of a patient with moderate papulopustular rosacea. This is a commonly overlooked location of inflammatory lesions.

Erythematotelangiectatic rosacea. *First line:* Topical α-receptor agonists such as brimonidine or oxymetazoline.

Second line: Laser therapy for facial erythema and telangiectasia. Low-dose β-blocking medications (propranolol, nadolol, carvedilol) or clonidine for flushing. Psychological counselling and group therapy sessions.

Third line: Botulinum toxin. Highly selective sympathectomy in disabling cases.

Papulopustular rosacea. *First line:* Topical metronidazole, azelaic acid or ivermectin for active inflammatory lesions.

Second line: Systemic antibiotic therapy with tetracyclines, erythromycin or trimethoprim.

Third line: Systemic metronidazole. Isotretinoin low dose.

Phymatous rosacea. *First line:* As for PPR for accompanying inflammatory lesions. Topical skin-peeling agent if there are large occluded follicles. Electrocautery or laser for telangiectases.

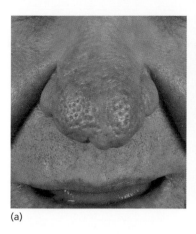
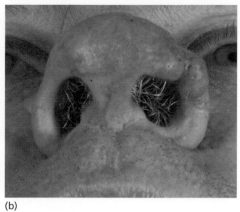

(a)   (b)

Figure 45.5 (a) Moderate to severe rhinophyma showing nasal distortion with a peau d'orange appearance of the prominent nasal follicles. (b) Swelling and distortion of the left nasal alar due to rhinophyma. Sometimes these changes are best visualised (as in this case) by viewing the nose from below.

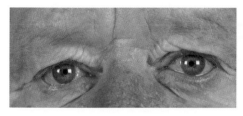

Figure 45.6 Ocular rosacea. Moderate (grade 2) OR with bilateral involvement, particularly of the lower eyelids.

Second line: Low-dose isotretinoin therapy for 2–6 months (Figure 45.10).
Third line: Ablation of phymatous tissue with carbon dioxide laser. Surgical remodelling of nose.

Ocular rosacea See Chapter 60.

FACIAL DERMATOSES WITH AN UNCERTAIN NOSOLOGICAL RELATIONSHIP TO ROSACEA

There is a range of facial dermatoses that share some features with rosacea but for which there is currently no consensus as to their nosological relationship. These are described below.

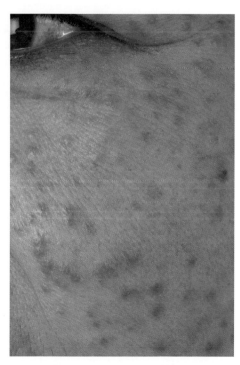

Figure 45.7 Granulomatous rosacea in a 55-year-old woman with a sudden onset of asymptomatic facial rash 4 months earlier. There is a profuse eruption of small, firm, monomorphic, plum-red, dome-shaped papules on the chin and cheeks and around the eyes. Histology showed multiple dermal granulomas.

Table 45.2 Differential diagnosis of rosacea subtypes

Subtype	Differential diagnosis
Subtype 1: Erythematotelangiectatic rosacea	• Chronic photodamage (difficult to distinguish) • Seborrhoeic dermatitis (characteristic distribution and scale) and may accompany several subtypes of rosacea • Facial contact dermatitis (demarcation and history) • Flushing/blushing due to other causes • Lupus erythematosus (both systemic and subacute) • Dermatomyositis (systemic symptoms and serology) • Ulerythema ophryogenes (presence of follicular keratoses) • Trichostasis spinulosa
Subtype 2: Papulopustular rosacea	• Acne vulgaris • Granulomatous rosacea (lupus miliaris disseminatus faciei) Perioral dermatitis (distribution and morphology differ) • Tinea faciei (skin scrapings) • Jessner's lymphocytic infiltrate (skin biopsy necessary for diagnosis) (see Chapter 73) • Pityriasis folliculorum (demodicosis: characteristic follicular scale; multiple *Demodex* mites on skin scraping)
	• Rosacea-like dermatoses due to medications (topical calcineurin inhibitors, epidermal growth factor receptor inhibitors, topical or systemic steroids) (Figure 45.8) • Granuloma faciale (may mimic rhinophyma) • Lymphocytoma cutis (biopsy necessary for diagnosis)
Subtype 3: Phymatous rosacea	• Solid facial lymphoedema (Figure 45.9) • Infection (cutaneous tuberculosis) • Sarcoid (lupus pernio) • Chronic cutaneous lupus erythematosus of the nose • Granuloma faciale (may mimic rhinophyma) • Malignancy (squamous carcinoma/lymphoma/other)
Subtype 4: Ocular rosacea	• Other causes of chronic blepharitis, dry eye syndrome, etc. (Chapter 60)

Idiopathic facial aseptic granuloma

Idiopathic facial aseptic granuloma (IFAG) typically presents between 8 months and 13 years of age as a solitary inflammatory nodule on the cheek or eyelid superficially resembling an insect bite (Figure 45.11). The nodules are asymptomatic, usually red or purple in colour and soft to palpation. They may attain a diameter of 2–3 cm before spontaneously involuting after several months.

Pyoderma faciale

(Syn. Rosacea conglobata, rosacea fulminans)

A rare rosacea-like eruption that has a gradual onset, mainly in young women with oily skin, often during or immediately following pregnancy (Figure 45.12). It may arise *de novo* but may also develop in patients with pre-existing rosacea. It is characterised by marked facial erythema with nodular abscesses and indurated haemorrhagic plaques that can result in significant scarring.

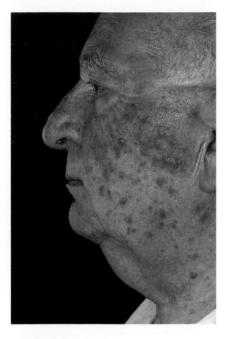

Figure 45.8 Corticosteroid-induced rosacea-like facial dermatosis.

Unlike acne conglobata, comedones are not a feature and the trunk is spared.

Solid facial lymphoedema

(Syn. Lymphoedematous rosacea, solid facial oedema)

Persistent erythema and firm non-pitting oedema of the upper two-thirds of the face, affecting especially the eyelids, cheeks, nose,

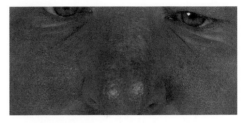

Figure 45.9 Solid facial lymphoedema is characterised by the presence of persistent, non-tender, firm, upper facial swelling. Note the creases under the eyes in this patient indicating the presence of this unusual type of facial erythema and swelling.

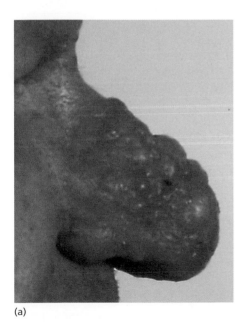

(a)

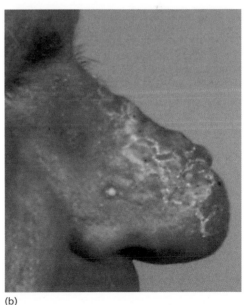

(b)

Figure 45.10 Rhinophyma before (a) and after (b) 4 months of treatment with isotretinoin.

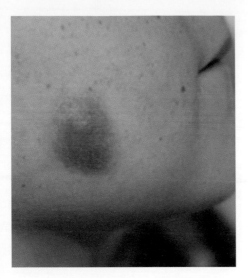

Figure 45.11 Idiopathic facial aseptic granuloma showing a well-defined plum-coloured nodule on the face of a 7-year-old boy. (Source: From González Rodríguez AJ, Jordá Cuevas E. Idiopathic facial aseptic granuloma. Clin Exp Dermatol 2015, 40, 298–300.)

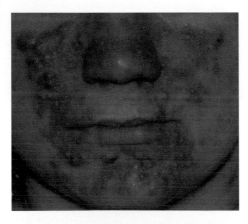

Figure 45.12 Pyoderma faciale showing an abrupt onset of severe inflammation with extensive pustule formation in a young woman.

and glabella (Figure 45.9). It is not preceded by rosacea.

It has been hypothesised that recurrent inflammation results in structural damage to the draining lymphatic vessels. Characterised histologically by dermal oedema, perifollicular fibrosis and perivascular and perifollicular infiltration of lymphocytes, and mast cells.

Management is difficult. Long-term, low-dose isotretinoin for up to 24 months in combination with manual lymphatic drainage may be helpful.

Corticosteroid-induced rosacea-like facial dermatosis

A papulopustular eruption accompanied by erythema that may closely resemble rosacea (Figure 45.8) due to the use of potent topical corticosteroids on the face. More common in females.

Patients experience marked sensitivity of the involved skin to the slightest irritant, itching, burning and intense redness. Whenever the topical coticosteroid is discontinued, the eruption flares, leading to a state of dependence.

The most important intervention is withdrawal of the topical corticosteroid. Patients must be advised to anticipate a flare of the rosacea. To reduce the severity of flare a less potent steroid or topical calcineurin inhibitor may be used initially. Topical or systemic antibiotic therapy as used for idiopathic rosacea may help suppress flares in the early stages of steroid withdrawal. The eruption may take several weeks or months to subside but clears completely if topical corticosteroids are avoided.

Periorificial dermatitis

(**Syn. Perioral dermatitis, periocular dermatitis**)
An erythematous, papulopustular facial dermatosis.

Epidemiology
F > M.

Pathophysiology
The cause is not known although in some cases there is a link with topical or inhaled steroid use. As with corticosteroid-induced rosacea-like dermatosis it is likely that perturbation of the skin microbiome is relevant.

There is a mild spongiotic dermatitis with perifollicular inflammation and pustules.

Granulomas and *Demodex* mites are not normally found.

Clinical features

Symmetrical (occasionally unilateral) papules and pustules on an erythematous and/or scaling base in a perioral (Figure 45.13), perinasal or periocular distribution (Figure 45.14); no comedones are seen. Normally there is a small border of unaffected skin around the mouth. The patient may describe burning irritation or itch.

Differential diagnosis

The clinical picture is distinctive; important differential diagnoses include rosacea, acne, seborrheic dermatitis and allergic contact dermatitis.

Management

It is important to discontinue any topical corticosteroids. Treat with a 4-week course of an oral tetracycline, topical erythromycin or topical metronidazole.

Childhood granulomatous periorificial dermatitis

(Syn. Facial Afro-Caribbean childhood eruption)
A rare dermatosis of childhood, of unknown aetiology, principally in prepubertal children of African descent. Asymptomatic, flesh-coloured, dome-shaped papules (Figure 45.15) in the perioral and periocular skin but can affect other parts of the head and neck. Its granulomatous nature can be confirmed by diascopy.

Biopsy shows non-caseating epithelioid granulomas and a perivascular inflammatory infiltrate.

It resolves spontaneously within a few months to about 3 years without treatment but may leave milia or small pitted scars.

FLUSHING AND BLUSHING

Flushing and blushing are the result of transient cutaneous vasodilatation that is usually physiological in nature.

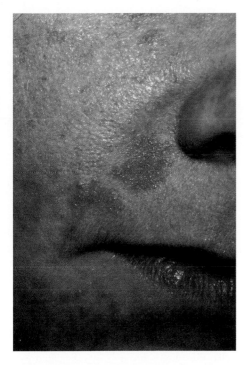

Figure 45.13 Perioral dermatitis.

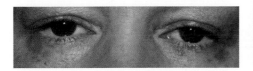

Figure 45.14 Periocular dermatitis, cluster of inflammatory papules occurring on the lateral aspect of lower eyelids, abutting on to the outer canthus.

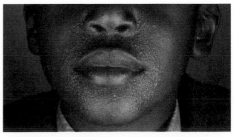

Figure 45.15 Childhood granulomatous periorificial dermatitis. (Source: Courtesy of Professor Hywel Williams, University of Nottingham, UK.)

PART 6: SKIN DISORDERS ASSOCIATED WITH SPECIFIC CUTANEOUS STRUCTURE

A blush signifies a psychosocial response to an experienced emotion, whereas a flush is a thermoregulatory response to increased body temperature.

CAUSES OF FLUSHING

Vasoactive mediators of flushing can be external due to food or drugs (Box 45.1) or internal disorders (Box 45.2).

Neurally activated flushing may be associated with sweating ('wet flushing') whereas flushing due to circulating vasoactive mediators does not usually involve sweating and is referred to as 'dry flushing.

Box 45.1 External causes of flushing

Drugs

- 5-hydroxytryptamine 3 receptor antagonists: ondansetron, ramosetron, tropisetron
- Angiotensin-converting enzyme inhibitors: captopril, enalapril, lisinopril, perindopril, ramipril
- β_3 adrenoceptor agonists: fluvoxamine, mirtazapine
- Calcium-channel blockers: nifedipine, verapamil
- Metronidazole
- Nitrates: isosorbine mononitrate/dinitrate, glyceryl trinitrate
- Sildenafil, tadalafil, vardenafil, mirodenafil (phosphodiesterase inhibitors)
- Tamsulosin
- Venlafaxine
- Morphine and other opiates
- Tamoxifen
- Contrast media
- Certain drugs cause flushing when taken with alcohol, e.g. antimalarials, disulfiram, metronidazole, tacrolimus ointment

Foods

- Spicy food (especially chilli pepper)
- Caffeine
- Alcohol (especially if alcohol dehydrogenase deficient)
- Fruit (lemons, tomato)
- Vegetables (spinach)
- Cheese (histamine rich, e.g. Roquefort)
- Sodium nitrite rich meats (e.g. salami)
- Fish (scombroid poisoning/ciguatoxin)

Box 45.2 Internal causes of flushing

- Thermoregulatory: heat exposure, exercise, fever
- Menopause
- Rosacea
- Carcinoid
- Phaeochromocytoma
- Mastocytosis
- Anaphylaxis
- Polycythaemia
- Cholinergic urticaria
- Neurological disorders, e.g. Parkinson disease, migraine, Frey syndrome
- Renal cell carcinoma
- Medullary carcinoma of the thyroid
- Thyrotoxicosis
- Pancreatic cell tumour
- Dumping syndrome
- POEMS (polyneuropathy, organomegaly, endocrinopathy, monoclonal gammopathy and skin changes) syndrome

---

Clinical presentation

When assessing a patient, it is important to assess the environmental setting, the extent and pattern of cutaneous involvement and whether sweating or other systemic symptoms accompany the vasodilatation.

Patients with excessive blushing complain of an involuntary and prolonged reddening primarily of the facial skin, which is often precipitated by anxiety, emotion or psychological upset. Frequently, 'skip' areas of pallor can be observed within the blush, with sparing of the area around the mouth giving the impression of 'circumoral pallor' (Figure 45.16). The ears characteristically develop an intense erythema, involving primarily the helix and antihelix. Blushing is not usually associated with facial sweating, but there may be accompanying palmar hyperhidrosis and tremor.

Patients with frequent flushing complain of sudden intense reddening of the face, neck and chest, representing an exaggeration of the normal response to vigorous exercise or temperature change. A flush may evolve in a similar manner to a blush, but often has a more widespread distribution extending to the anterior chest and sometimes the abdomen, particularly the epigastric region. Localised facial sweating may be a feature of flushing. Patients with carcinoid syndrome can

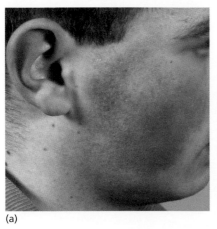
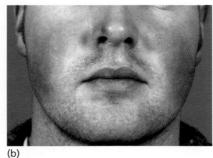

(a)   (b)

Figure 45.16 These images demonstrate the typical distribution of the blush, as seen in two young men who presented for the management of frequent blushing. Note the 'skip areas' of pallor on the upper lateral cheek in (a). Sparing of the skin around the mouth suggestive of 'circumoral pallor' is evident in both cases (a,b). The ears reddened with blushing in both men.

experience associated diarrhoea and wheezing. Flushing associated with itch can be seen in patients with mastocytosis. Exertional flushing can sometimes be seen in patients with cholinergic urticaria. Flushing after a warm bath is occasionally reported in patients with polycythaemia. Flushing localised to the nose has been reported as a prodrome to migraine attacks. Flushing characteristics associated with certain disorders are listed in Table 45.3.

Table 45.3 Disorders associated with flushing

Disease	Characteristics of flush
Menopause	Rising feeling of intense heat, profuse sweating and diffuse facial flushing, lasting from 3 to 5 min up to 20 times/day.
Rosacea	Subgroup have frequent flushing with specific triggers such as spicy food, moving from a cold to warm environment. Not all patients with rosacea flush.
Carcinoid syndrome (Chapter 85)	The flush associated with classic carcinoid syndrome (due to midgut carcinoids) begins suddenly and lasts from 30 s up to 30 min. The face, neck and upper chest may flush red to violaceous, with a mild burning sensation. Severe flushes are accompanied by hypotension and tachycardia. The flushes associated with gastric carcinoid tumours are atypical and tend to be red-brown, patchy, sharply demarcated, with bizarre gyrate or serpiginous patterns that may resolve centrally; usually with an intense pruritus.
	In patients with the bronchial carcinoid variant, the flushes can be very severe and prolonged, lasting hours to days. Most flushing episodes occur spontaneously, but they may be provoked by eating, drinking alcohol, defaecation, emotional events, palpation of the liver and anaesthesia.
Mastocytosis (Chapter 18)	Sudden onset; features may be similar to that of an allergic or anaphylactic reaction, often with identifiable triggers such as narcotics, opioids, non-steroidal anti-inflammatory drugs, systemic anaesthesia, exercise, massage, alcohol, infection, *Hymenoptera* stings
Phaeochromocytoma (Chapter 85)	Flushing of the face, neck, chest and trunk. Paroxysmal attacks last 15 min to hours. Usually occur spontaneously but may be triggered by deep abdominal palpation, diagnostic procedures (e.g. colonoscopy), induction of anaesthesia, surgery, with certain foods or beverages containing tyramine or with certain drugs (e.g. monoamine oxidase inhibitors).

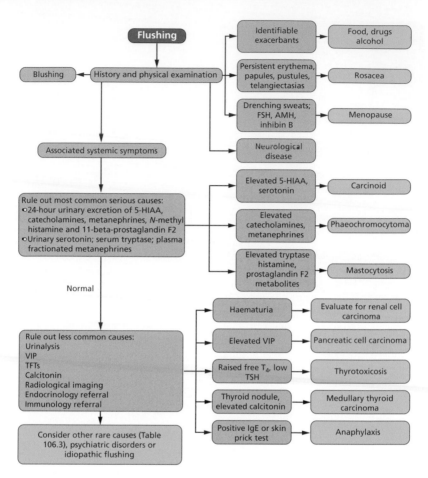

Figure 45.17 Flushing and blushing: investigations algorithm. (Source: Modified from Izikson L, English JC 3rd, Zirwas MJ. The flushing patient: differential diagnosis, workup, and treatment. *J Am Acad Dermatol* 2006, 55(2), 193–208.)

Investigations

A thorough history, with particular emphasis on precipitating or exacerbating factors, drug usage and food intake and a detailed review of systemic symptoms including queries relating to anxiety and stress, is essential in the evaluation of an individual who presents with a complaint of excessive flushing (see Figure 45.17).

Management

See Figure 45.18.

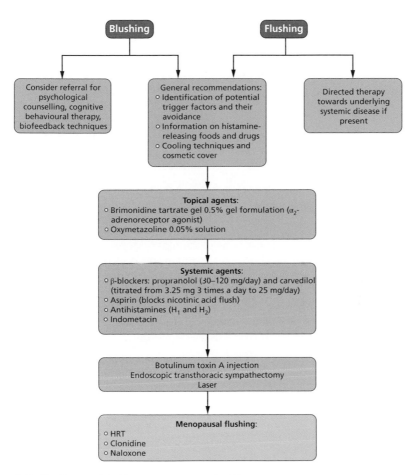

Figure 45.18 Flushing and blushing: management algorithm.

PART 6: SKIN DISORDERS ASSOCIATED WITH SPECIFIC CUTANEOUS STRUCTURE

46 Hidradenitis suppurativa

(Syn. Acne inversa)

Hidradenitis suppurativa (HS) is a chronic, inflammatory, painful, follicular disease of apocrine gland-bearing skin that usually presents after puberty and may have a large impact on quality of life.

Epidemiology

Overall prevalence estimates vary from 0.1% in US insurance datasets to more than 1% in self-completed questionnaires in European populations. Usual age of onset is between the second and fourth decades and women are affected more than men in a ratio of 3:1. There is an association with smoking and obesity, as well as Crohn disease. HS is part of the 'follicular occlusion tetrad' which also includes pilonidal sinus, acne conglobate and dissecting cellulitis of the scalp. There are elevated rates of type 2 diabetes, hyperlipidaemia and hypertension which, along with smoking, contribute to increased risks of cardiovascular disease. There are also higher rates of depression.

Pathophysiology

Histologically, follicular occlusion leading to rupture of the follicular unit is an important early event and exposure of hair shafts to the immune system may result in subsequent chronic inflammation. See Table 46.1 for pathogenic hypotheses.

Clinical features

The diagnosis of HS is clinical and all three diagnostic criteria described in Table 46.2 are required.

Table 46.1 Pathogenic hypotheses in HS and associated evidence

Genetic	About one-third of patients have an affected first-degree relative. Rarely, pathogenic mutations in γ-secretase, a protein involved in keratinocyte differentiation, are present. Genetic testing is not routinely offered.
Environmental	Smoking and obesity are strong risk factors but HS can develop in non-smokers of normal BMI.
Endocrine	Suggested by onset soon after puberty, female preponderance and menstrual exacerbations in some patients.
Microbiological/immune dysregulation	Skin bacteria are present in subcutaneous HS biopsies but this may be due to non-sterile skin tunnels. Pro-inflammatory cytokines are increased in HS lesions.

Rook's Dermatology Handbook, First Edition. Edited by Christopher E. M. Griffiths, Tanya O. Bleiker, Daniel Creamer, John R. Ingram and Rosalind C. Simpson.
© 2022 John Wiley & Sons Ltd. Published 2022 by John Wiley & Sons Ltd.

Table 46.2 Diagnostic criteria for HS

Typical lesions	Some of: deep-seated painful nodules, abscesses, draining skin tunnels, rope-like scars and multiheaded open pseudocomedones (see Figure 46.1)
Predominantly flexural location	Axillae, groins, perineal, natal cleft, buttocks, infra- and intermammary folds
Chronicity and recurrence	Multiple and/or recurrent lesions occurring over time

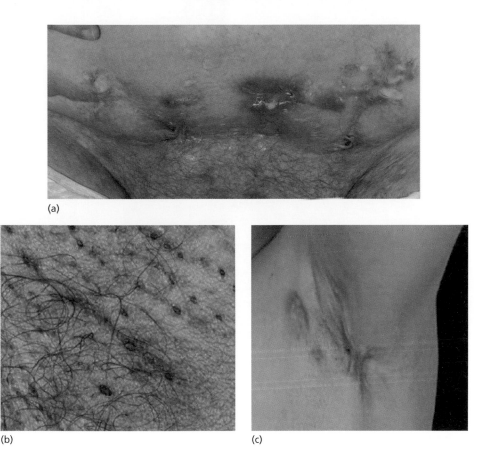

(a)

(b)　　　　(c)

Figure 46.1 Lesion types found in HS. (a) Inflamed nodules and draining skin tunnels. (b) Tombstone comedones in the axilla. (c) Rope-like scar.

Disease severity (staging)

Baseline severity of HS can be defined by the Hurley staging system (Figure 46.2). One of the treatment aims in HS is to prevent disease progression to avoid irreversible scarring.

Outcome measures

The Hurley system is not suitable for monitoring response to treatment because it is insufficiently sensitive to change. Patient-reported instruments such as a pain score and quality of

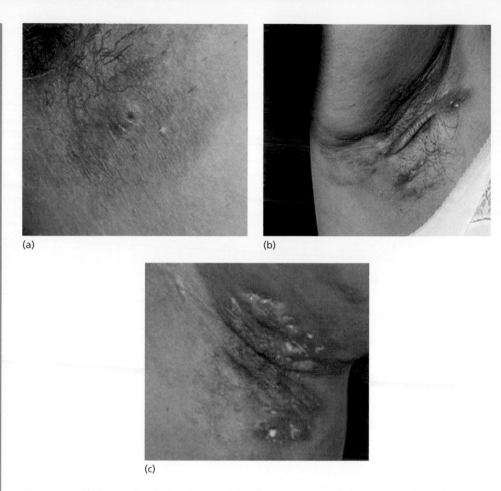

(a)

(b)

(c)

Figure 46.2 Hurley staging system. In stage 1 (mild) there is recurrent abscess formation but without skin tunnels or scarring, in stage 2 (moderate) there are widely separated skin tunnels and scarring, while in stage 3 (severe) there are multiple interconnected abscesses, skin tunnels and scarring which form diffuse plaques. (a) Stage 1 (mild), (b) stage 2 (moderate) and (c) stage 3 (severe).

life scale can be used. Physician-reported instruments include lesion count systems such as the HiSCR endpoint, which defines treatment success as a 50% reduction in baseline inflammatory nodules and abscesses, with no increase in draining skin tunnels.

Differential diagnosis

For solitary abscesses, secondary infection of epidermoid or other cysts should be considered, while predominantly anogenital involvement raises the possibility of Crohn disease.

Investigations

Investigations have a limited role in HS. Cellulitis is uncommon, but microbiological samples should be sent if superinfection is suspected. Ultrasound can be used to define subclinical extension of skin tunnels, and magnetic resonance imaging may be helpful in severe perineal disease to check for bowel fistulae and to plan surgical procedures.

Management

Multidisciplinary team management is ideal to coordinate medical and surgical treatment options and support lifestyle changes. Weight management and smoking cessation should be encouraged where relevant. Analgesia, such as non-steroidal anti-inflammatory drugs, may be required for acute flares and chronic pain.

Treatment is generally approached in a step-wise manner (see below) based on disease severity and lack of response to previous treatment. Medical and surgical treatment options can be offered in parallel.

Medical treatment

First line: Topical antimicrobials and oral tetracyclines.

Second line: Clindamycin and rifampicin given together, both 300 mg twice daily, for 10 weeks; other oral systemics, including acitretin or dapsone.

Third line: TNFi therapy.

Surgical treatment

First line: Incision and drainage or deroofing of skin tunnels (laying open skin tunnels).

Second line: Narrow margin excision or ablative lasers.

Third line: Extensive excision followed by secondary intention healing, skin flap or skin grafting.

PART 6: SKIN DISORDERS ASSOCIATED WITH SPECIFIC CUTANEOUS STRUCTURE

47 Disorders of the sweat glands

Eccrine sweat glands are distributed over the whole skin surface, including the glans penis and foreskin, but not on the lips, external ear canal, clitoris or labia minora. Apocrine sweat glands in the adult are localised to the axillae, perianal region and areolae of the breasts. Apocrine glands enlarge during puberty and their activity is androgen dependent.

DISORDERS OF ECCRINE SWEAT GLANDS

Hyperhidrosis

Hyperhidrosis is defined as excessive production of sweat, more than is required for thermoregulation.

Epidemiology

Self-reported prevalence in young adults is 16% but less than half of these have excess sweat secretion rates when measured objectively. There is no gender or racial preponderance.

Pathophysiology

Most cases of generalised hyperhidrosis are idiopathic, but there are some specific causes, listed in Box 47.1.

Clinical features

Box 47.2 lists the subclassification of hyperhidrosis.

> **Box 47.1 Causes of generalised hyperhidrosis**
>
> - Febrile infective illnesses: tuberculosis, malaria, endocarditis, etc.
> - Metabolic diseases: hyperthyroidism, hyperpituitarism, hypoglycaemia, phaeochromocytoma
> - Menopause
> - Underlying solid malignancy including lymphoma
> - Congestive heart failure
> - Central nervous system: Parkinson disease, episodic hypothermia with hyperhidrosis, generalised hyperhidrosis without hypothermia
> - Peripheral neuropathies: familial dysautonomia (Riley–Day), congenital autonomic dysfunction with universal pain loss, cold-induced sweating syndrome
> - Drugs: selective serotonin reuptake inhibitors such as fluoxetine

Palmoplantar hyperhidrosis (Figure 47.1a)
Commonly begins in childhood or around puberty. Excessive sweating can be continuous, when it is usually worse in summer, or phasic, when it is precipitated by minor emotional or mental activity. It predisposes to pompholyx eczema, pitted keratolysis of the feet and allergic sensitisation to footwear constituents.

Rook's Dermatology Handbook, First Edition. Edited by Christopher E. M. Griffiths, Tanya O. Bleiker, Daniel Creamer, John R. Ingram and Rosalind C. Simpson.
© 2022 John Wiley & Sons Ltd. Published 2022 by John Wiley & Sons Ltd.

> **Box 47.2 Types of hyperhidrosis**
> - Generalised
> - Focal: palmar, plantar, axillary and cranio-facial
> - Localised circumscribed and asymmetrical hyperhidrosis
> - Compensatory
> - Gustatory

Axillary hyperhidrosis (Figure 47.1b)
Usually phasic but may be continuous. It usually occurs after puberty and can be precipitated by undressing.

Cranio-facial hyperhidrosis (Figure 47.1c)
Typically occurs in middle age and is generally phasic, precipitated by heat, exercise and eating.

Localised hyperhidrosis
Causes are outlined in Box 47.3. Excessive sweating may be due to neurological lesions involving any part of the sympathetic pathway from the brain to the nerve ending.

Compensatory hyperhidrosis
Occurs in normal sweat glands when those elsewhere are not functioning because of neurological or skin disease, diabetes mellitus or after sympathectomy. It is also a component of Ross syndrome.

Gustatory hyperhidrosis
Precipitated by eating specific foods, such as spicy foods, occurs physiologically in many people. It also occurs in pathological conditions involving the autonomic nervous system (Box 47.4).

Investigations
In generalised hyperhidrosis, any investigations are influenced by the duration of the problem and by a functional enquiry of general health. Thyroid function tests should be considered. Gravimetric determination of sweat rate is seldom performed now.

Management
Localised hyperhidrosis of the axillae can be treated topically with aluminium chloride, applied to dry skin to avoid irritation. Iontophoresis is second-line therapy and may use either tap water or anticholinergic drugs such as 0.05% glycopyrronium bromide solution. Botulinum toxin injections for the axilla, hands or feet typically last about 6 months before repeat treatment is required and multiple injections are needed to treat an involved region.

Third-line therapy and therapy for *generalised hyperhidrosis* involves oral anticholinergic drugs such as propantheline bromide and oxybutynin. Use of these drugs may be limited by adverse effects of generalised anticholinergic blockade, including dry mouth, constipation and blurred vision. Sympathectomy, usually endoscopic, is now performed relatively rarely because complications, including compensatory hyperhidrosis, are common.

Miliaria

(Syn. Prickly heat)
A common acute or subacute skin condition that arises due to the occlusion or disruption of eccrine sweat ducts in hot humid conditions, resulting in a leakage of sweat into the epidermis (miliaria crystallina and miliaria rubra) or dermis (miliaria profunda).

Epidemiology
Miliaria crystallina occurs commonly in infants (Chapter 64). The incidence of miliaria profunda is highest in hot, humid conditions; it nearly always follows repeated attacks of miliaria rubra and is uncommon except in the tropics.

Pathophysiology
Miliaria rubra is common on the trunk in hospitalised patients who have to be nursed on their backs on bedding that has waterproof occlusive membranes below the sheets.

The level of occlusion or disruption of the eccrine duct varies between the three subtypes. In miliaria crystallina, the obstruction is very superficial, within the stratum corneum. In miliaria rubra, later changes include keratinisation of the intraepidermal part of the sweat duct. In miliaria profunda, there is rupture of the duct at the level of or below the dermal–epidermal junction.

Clinical features
Miliaria crystallina
Clear, thin-walled vesicles, 1–2 mm in diameter without an inflammatory areola, usually symptomless and develop in crops, mainly on the trunk.

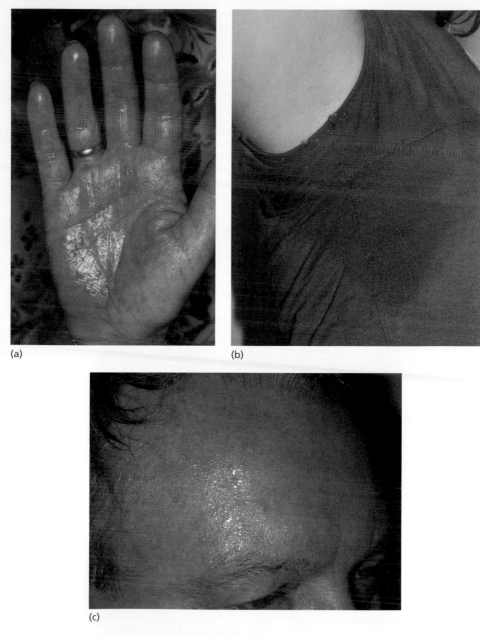

(a)

(b)

(c)

Figure 47.1 Focal hyperhidrosis. (a) Palmar hyperhidrosis. (b) Axillary hyperhidrosis: patients often wear white or black clothing as the wetness is not as visibly obvious as with coloured clothes. (c) Cranio-facial hyperhidrosis. It may be sufficiently profuse to drip off the face and wet the hair.

> **Box 47.3 Causes of localised hyperhidrosis**
>
> - Spinal cord injury
> - Intrathoracic neoplasia
> - Frey syndrome
> - Granulosis rubra nasi
> - Functional and true sweat gland naevi
> - Sweating associated with local skin disorders: glomangioma, blue rubber bleb naevi, pachydermoperiostosis, pretibial myxoedema, POEMS syndrome, burning feet syndrome
> - Idiopathic unilateral circumscribed hyperhidrosis
>
> POEMS, polyneuropathy, organomegaly, endocrinopathy, monoclonal protein and skin changes.

> **Box 47.4 Classification of gustatory hyperhidrosis**
>
> - Idiopathic
> - Central
> - Post-herpetic
> - Post-peripheral nerve injury: auriculotemporal, chorda tympani, greater auricular, cervical plexus
> - Peripheral autonomic neuropathy: diabetes mellitus

Miliaria rubra

Typical lesions develop on the body, especially in areas of friction with clothing and in flexures. The lesions are uniformly minute erythematous papules, which may be present in very large numbers. In infants, lesions commonly appear on the occluded skin of the neck, groins and axillae (Figure 47.2).

Miliaria profunda

The affected skin is covered with asymptomatic pale, firm papules 1–3 mm across, especially on the body.

Management

Management includes cooling measures and topical therapy such as 0.05% menthol or a mild potency corticosteroid.

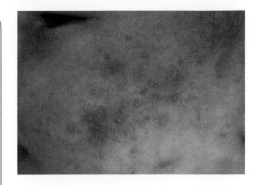

Figure 47.2 Miliaria rubra affecting the cheeks of an infant. (Source: Courtesy of Dr Richard Logan, Bridgend, UK.)

Neutrophilic eccrine hidradenitis

(Syn. Chemotherapy-associated eccrine hidradenitis)

Acute inflammation of the eccrine sweat glands may be seen in several clinical situations, in particular secondary to cytotoxic chemotherapy.

Epidemiology

Overall, the condition is rare.

Pathophysiology

Histologically there is necrosis of the eccrine epithelium in association with a dense neutrophilic infiltrate. Chemotherapy for haematological malignancy (such as cytarabine) is the commonest cause.

Clinical features

Chemotherapy-associated neutrophilic eccrine hidradenitis typically occurs 8–10 days after starting treatment. Painful erythematous papules and plaques develop on the limbs, neck and face. The condition typically resolves within 2 weeks of treatment ending and may recur with subsequent courses of chemotherapy.

A childhood variant affects children without malignancy.

Differential diagnosis

Other neutrophilic dermatoses such as Sweet's syndrome; cutaneous infections.

Management

A potent topical corticosteroid can be used prior to spontaneous resolution.

Disorders of apocrine sweat glands

See Table 47.1

Table 47.1 Disorders of apocrine sweat glands

Condition	Bromhidrosis	Trimethylaminuria (Syn. Fish odour syndrome)	Chromhidrosis	Apocrine miliaria (Syn. Fox–Fordyce disease)
Synonyms	Abnormal sweat odour Osmidrosis		–	
Epidemiology	Malodour usually develops around puberty	Found in 7% of self-reported malodour	True chromhidrosis is rare	Uncommon, F > M
Pathophysiology	Corynebacteria transform apocrine gland fatty acids	Inability to oxidise trimethylamine into odourless trimethylamine oxide	Caused by secretion of lipofuscins in apocrine sweat	Apocrine sweat duct occlusion by aggregates of epithelial cells
Clinical features	Odour noticed by patient or others drives presentation	Unpleasant odour, often worse after eating seafood, eggs, beans	Striking yellow, green or blue hue to apocrine sweat	Skin-coloured, dome-shaped follicular papules in apocrine regions, preceded by itch
Investigations	–	Measure urinary trimethylamine	Wood's light fluorescence of clothing, fluorescence microscopy of skin biopsy	–
Management	Deodorants, topical antibacterials, botulinum toxin A	Low carnitine and choline diet, short courses of metronidazole/neomycin, oral charcoal	Topical capsaicin, botulinum toxin A	*First line*: Topical steroids, clindamycin, retinoids *Second line*: Oral retinoids

Acquired and inherited nail disorders

48

The component parts of the nail apparatus are shown in Figure 48.1. The nail is firmly attached to the nail bed; it is less adherent proximally, apart from the posterolateral corners. Approximately one-quarter of the nail is covered by the proximal nail fold, and a narrow margin of the sides of the nail plate is often occluded by the lateral nail folds.

NAIL SIGNS AND THEIR SIGNIFICANCE

A number of nail signs (abnormalities of shape, attachment, nail surface, colour) can be seen, some are a variation of normal and some represent underlying pathology. Table 48.1 details structural abnormalities of the nail (including shape, attachment and nail surface changes). Table 48.2 details colour changes that may occur.

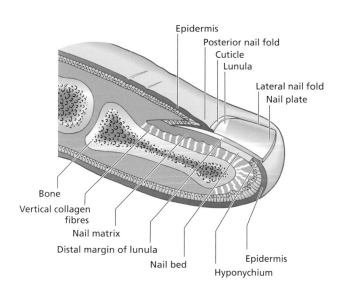

Epidermis
Posterior nail fold
Cuticle
Lunula
Lateral nail fold
Nail plate
Bone
Vertical collagen fibres
Nail matrix
Distal margin of lunula
Nail bed
Epidermis
Hyponychium

Figure 48.1 Longitudinal section of a digit showing the dorsal nail apparatus.

Rook's Dermatology Handbook, First Edition. Edited by Christopher E. M. Griffiths, Tanya O. Bleiker, Daniel Creamer, John R. Ingram and Rosalind C. Simpson.
© 2022 John Wiley & Sons Ltd. Published 2022 by John Wiley & Sons Ltd.

Table 48.1 Structural abnormalities of the nail

Sign	Description	Cause/associations
Anonychia (Figure 48.2)	Absence of all or part of one or several nails	Congenital Acquired due to scarring of nail matrix (burns, trauma, inflammatory dermatoses) Transient after intense physiological or local inflammatory process
Beading and ridging	Minor nail surface abnormalities	More prominent with age, not associated with underlying cause
Clubbing (Syn. Acropachy)	Increased transverse and longitudinal nail curvature with hypertrophy of the soft-tissue components of the digit pulp	Cardiopulmonary disease Liver disease Malignancy
Koilonychia (Figure 48.3)	Reverse curvature in the transverse and longitudinal axes, giving a concave appearance	Iron deficiency Haemochromatosis May be familial (autosomal dominant) Common in infancy on great toenail
Longitudinal grooves (Figure 48.4)	Full or partial thickness grooves in the longitudinal axis	Median canaliform dystrophy of Heller (Figure 48.5) most distinctive form due to unknown cause Similar appearance can occur as part of a habit tic deformity (Figure 48.6) Tumours pressing on the matrix can cause longitudinal groove
Nail shedding	Loss of nails	Complete loss of the nail plate (onychomadesis) due to local or systemic disease Dermatoses, e.g. bullous disorders, toxic epidermal necrolysis, rapid onset pustular psoriasis, epidermolysis bullosa Trauma Medication, e.g. retinoids
Onycholysis (Figure 48.7)	Distal and/or lateral separation of the nail from the nail bed	Idiopathic Secondary to psoriasis, fungal infection, eczema, medication, photo-onycholysis
Onychoschizia (lamellar nail dystrophy) (Figure 48.8)	Transverse splitting into layers at or near the free edge	Common in infants Not usually associated with underlying cause
Pincer nail (Figure 48.9)	Increased transverse curvature, nail growth is towards the midline Can be painful	Psoriasis (>1 nail involved) Inherited (>1 nail involved) Nail matrix lesion (1 nail involved)
Pitting	Punctate erosions in the nail surface	Psoriasis (less regular) Alopecia areata (regular)
Pterygium (Figure 48.10)	'Winged appearance' caused by a central fibrotic band which divides the nail proximally in two	Caused by inflammatory destructive process, commonly trauma, lichen planus, graft-versus-host disease
Trachyonychia (Figure 48.11)	Rough surface affecting all of the nail plate	Associated with alopecia areata, psoriasis and lichen planus May be idiopathic Appearance seen in 20-nail dystrophy
Transverse grooves (Syn. Beau lines) (Figure 48.12)	Full or partial thickness transverse lines through the nail, occur several weeks after precipitating event Changes grow out	Localised: trauma, inflammation or neurological events Generalised: secondary to acute systemic event (Beau lines)

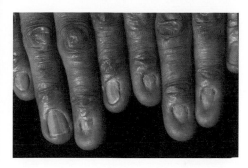

Figure 48.2 Anonychia.

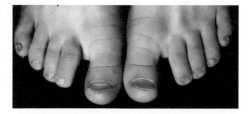

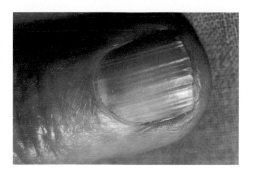

Figure 48.3 Koilonychia.

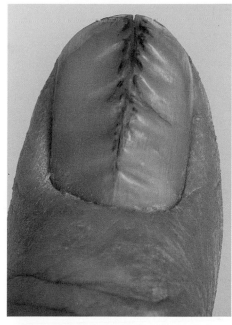

Figure 48.5 Median canaliform dystrophy of Heller.

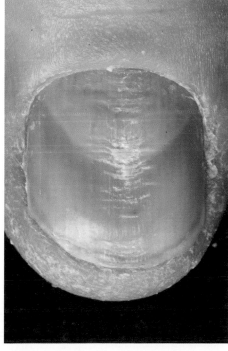

Figure 48.4 Longitudinal ridging of the nail.

Yellow nail syndrome

Yellowing occurs due to thickening. The lunula is obscured and there is increased transverse and longitudinal curvature of the nail plate with loss of cuticle (Figure 48.13). Usually presents in adults. Nail changes are usually accompanied by lymphedema. Recurrent pleural effusions, chronic bronchitis and bronchiectasis are associated. Nail growth is greatly reduced. Itraconazole or fluconazole combined with oral vitamin E may be of use to treat.

Figure 48.6 Transverse ridges resulting from habit tic.

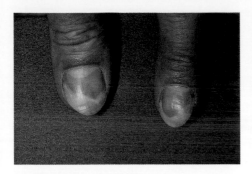

Figure 48.7 Onycholysis.

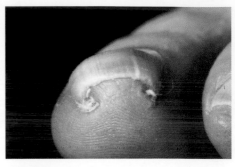

Figure 48.9 Pincer nail.

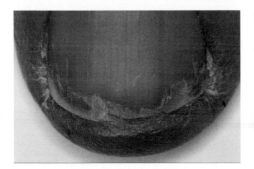

Figure 48.8 Onychoschizia (transverse splitting).

BENIGN TUMOURS OF THE NAIL

The following are commonly encountered benign nail tumours.

Glomus tumour

See Chapter 75. A benign tumour of the myoarterial glomus arising mainly in the pulp or nail bed or matrix of the distal phalanx. There are two main clinical presentations: a small reddish or bluish spot (<1 cm) seen through the nail plate (Figure 48.14) or longitudinal erythronychia with distal notching or overlying longitudinal fissure. MRI is best to investigate this lesion. Treatment consists of surgical removal of the tumour.

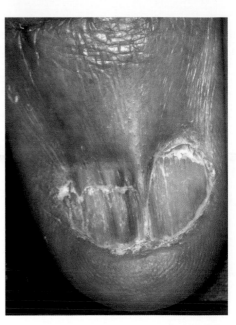

Figure 48.10 Nail pterygium due to lichen planus.

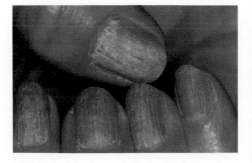

Figure 48.11 Trachyonychia.

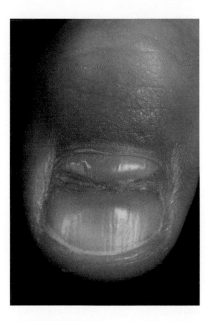

Figure 48.12 Beau's lines present as transverse grooves in the nail matching the proximal margin of the nail matrix and lunula.

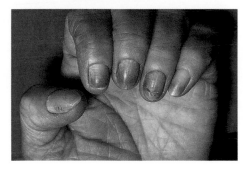

Figure 48.13 Yellow nail syndrome.

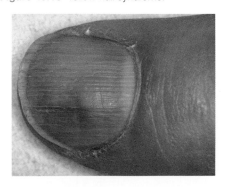

Figure 48.14 Painful glomus tumour of the nail bed. Note the bluish hue.

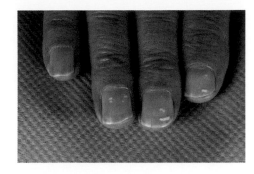

Figure 48.15 Punctate leukonychia.

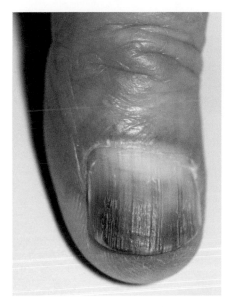

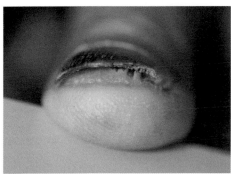

Figure 48.16 Green pigmentation of onycholytic fingernail due to *Pseudomonas*.

Table 48.2 Colour changes of the nail

Sign	Description	Cause/associations
Leukonychia	White discoloration of the nail	Hereditary: rare, all nails milky white Transverse leukonychia: reflects a systemic disorder Punctate leukonychia: occurs in areas of minor trauma or in alopecia areata (Figure 48.15) Terry's nail: white proximally and normal distally secondary to cirrhosis, congestive cardiac failure or diabetes Half-and-half nails: proximal white zone and distal brownish sharp demarcation; occurs in chemotherapy and chronic renal failure Paired white bands parallel to the lunula are associated with hypoalbuminaemia
Longitudinal erythronychia	Longitudinal red streak	Lichen planus, Darier disease, acrokeratosis verruciformis of Hopf
Nail pigmentation	Dark or coloured pigmentation of the nail	Common causes of surface pigment changes: nicotine, henna Pseudomonas infection often causes green pigmentation in association with onycholysis (Figure 48.16) Cytotoxic drugs Brown longitudinal streak (linear melanonychia): common variant in darker skinned people, abnormal in white skinned people, Hutchinson sign is suspicious for melanoma
Red lunulae	Erythema of all or part of the lunula	Associated with cardiac failure (multiple nails), myxoid cyst, glomus tumour (isolated nails)
Splinter haemorrhages	Longitudinal haemorrhages in the nail bed	Trauma, associated with psoriasis, dermatitis and fungal infection Large numbers may indicate a systemic cause, e.g. bacterial endocarditis, antiphospholipid syndrome or medication
Other colour changes		Yellowing: prolonged tetracycline therapy, topical 5-flurouracil Yellow-orange discolouration: staining from use of nail polish Blue discolouration: secondary to mepacrine, antimalarials

Subungual exostosis

An isolated slow-growing benign osteochondral outgrowth from the distal phalanx (Figure 48.17). Confirm by X-ray to demonstrate exostosis.

Digital myxoid pseudocyst

The second most common benign tumours of the digits. They originate from two sources: the ganglion type derives from joint fluid and synovial cells while the myxomatous type derives from dermal-based fibroblasts. Different clinical subtypes are as follows:

- Type A: a nodule between the distal interphalangeal joint and the proximal nail fold (Figure 48.18).
- Type B: in the proximal nail fold and pressing on the underlying matrix, resulting in a longitudinal groove in the nail plate (Figure 48.19).
- Type C: the digital myxoid pseudocyst exerts pressure from under the matrix, giving rise to a reddish or bluish lunula (Figure 48.20).

Cryotherapy should be attempted at least twice for type A. Surgical excision may be attempted but relapse is common. Other treatments include aspiration, infrared coagulation and sclerosant injection. There is generally a high recurrence rate. It is reasonable not to offer treatment at all.

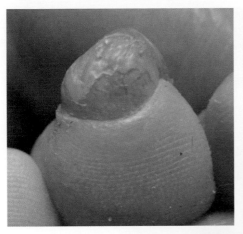
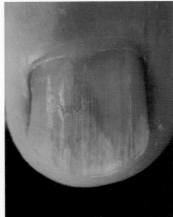
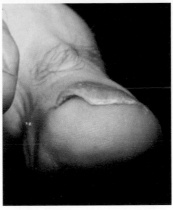

Figure 48.17 Subungual exostosis: exophytic growth of bone emerging from under the nail plate through collarette of skin (note the telangiectases).

Acquired ungual fibrokeratoma

A solitary benign asymptomatic nodule with a hyperkeratotic tip that forms in the periungual area or, rarely, within or under the nail plate (Figure 48.21). Trauma is thought to be the major causative factor.

Pyogenic granuloma

See Chapter 75. A common acquired benign vascular tumour frequently encountered at the nail apparatus (nail bed and folds). Usually due to trauma. Histological examination should always be undertaken to rule out amelanotic melanoma or squamous cell carcinoma (SCC) when faced with a single pyogenic granuloma without a clear aetiology. First-line treatment is with potent topical steroid under occlusion for up to 6 weeks. Second-line treatment is curettage.

MALIGNANT TUMOURS OF THE NAIL

Squamous cell carcinoma

See Chapter 80. The most frequent malignant tumour of the nail apparatus, where presentation as *in situ* SCC (Bowen disease, Figure 48.22) is more common than invasive SCC (Figure 48.23).

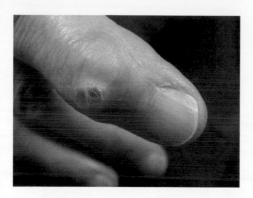

Figure 48.18 Digital myxoid pseudocyst type A.

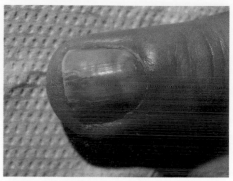

Figure 48.20 Digital myxoid pseudocyst type C. Note the red macule within the lunula.

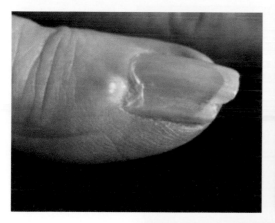

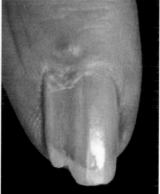

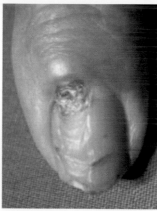

Figure 48.19 Digital myxoid pseudocyst type B. Note the longitudinal groove arising from underneath the proximal nail fold where the matrix is compressed by the overlying pseudocyst and extending to the free edge of the nail.

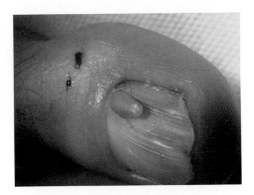

Figure 48.21 Submatricial fibrokeratoma pressing onto the underlying matrix with subsequent longitudinal smooth groove.

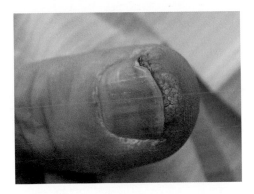

Figure 48.22 Bowen disease: warty lesion of the distal bed and hyponychium. The lesion was treated for several years as a wart.

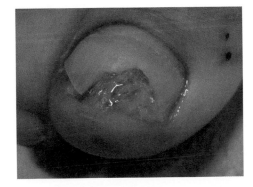

Figure 48.23 Onycholysis and oozing of the great toenail bed due to invasive SCC.

Associated with human papillomavirus-associated genital disease. The most common clinical findings are subungual hyperkeratosis, onycholysis, oozing and nail plate destruction. Keratoacanthoma-like SCC is a rare but aggressive variant that is usually situated in the most distal portion of the nail bed. Surgical excision is required for all of these lesions.

Melanoma

See Chapter 81 for information and images of melanoma affecting the nail.

NAIL FOLD INFECTIONS

Infections of the nail fold are represented by inflammation, swelling and abscess formation.

Acute paronychia

Commonly due to staphylococcal infection but may be of fungal or viral origin. Most patients are children and adolescents. Usually results from local injuries, e.g. from a thorn or splinter, torn hangnails or nail biting. May complicate chronic paronychia. Acute paronychia presents as a painful red swelling of the lateral paronychial area (Figure 48.24). Superficial lesions can be drained by incision with a pointed scalpel without anaesthesia. Deeper lesions should be treated with appropriate antibiotics as guided by local microbiology. If there is no clear sign of response within 2 days, surgical intervention under local anaesthesia is required, particularly in children.

Herpetic paronychia

(Syn. Herpetic whitlow)
Primary inoculation of the herpes simplex virus. Uncommon, occurs mostly in children under 2 years. Very painful, single or grouped blisters close to the nail ± honeycomb appearance. The blisters become purulent and may rupture to be replaced by crusts (Figure 48.25). Takes about 3 weeks to resolve. Transmission to contacts may occur, which is particularly important for

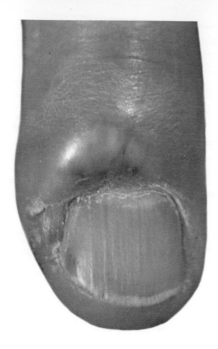

Figure 48.24 Acute bacterial paronychia (whitlow).

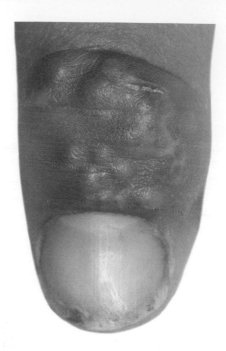

Figure 48.25 Herpetic whitlow.

dental workers and nurses as they may come into contact with herpes labialis. Treatment probably does little to shorten the course of the disorder, but cleaning with chlorhexidine followed by application of a bland cream is recommended. Long-term prophylaxis with oral aciclovir, famciclovir or valaciclovir may be useful if frequent recurrences.

Chronic paronychia

See Table 48.3 and Figure 48.26. An inflammatory dermatosis of the nail folds causing retraction of the periungual tissues with secondary effects on the nail matrix, nail growth and soft-tissue attachments (Figure 48.26a–c). Predominantly occurs in those who perform wet-work. Sometimes seen in children as a result of finger or thumb sucking. Chronic

inflammation probably arises from an irritant reaction to material sequestered beneath the proximal nail fold. The loss of the cuticle means that detergent and other solvents may gain access to this tight space and act like a prolonged irritant patch test. It begins as a slight erythematous swelling of the paronychia. The cuticle is lost and pus may form below the nail fold. Inflammation adjacent to the nail matrix disturbs nail growth, resulting in irregular transverse ridges and other surface irregularities, which may be combined with discoloration. *Candida* or *Pseudomonas* infection can coexist. Treatment includes avoidance of precipitants, keeping the hands dry, effective hand care and topical therapy with a steroid/antimicrobial combination. Surgical intervention for severe, treatment-resistant disease can be offered.

Table 48.3 Differential diagnosis between four common nail disorders: fungal infections, psoriasis, chronic paronychia and dermatitis

	Fungal infections	Psoriasis	Chronic paronychia	Dermatitis
Colour	Often yellow or brown; part or whole of nail	May be normal or yellow or brown	Edge of nail often discoloured brown or black	May be normal
Onycholysis	Frequent	Frequent	Usually absent	Confined to tip or absent
Pitting	Infrequent	Often present and fine	Uncommon	Coarse pits frequent
Filaments or spores in potash preparations	Filaments, usually abundant	Absent	May be spores in edge of nail; filaments and spores in scrapings from nail fold	Absent
Cross-ridging	Absent	Uncommon	Frequent	Frequent
Other	Associated fungal infections elsewhere	Associated psoriasis elsewhere or family history of psoriasis	Predominantly women; wet work and cold hands cause predisposition	Recent history of dermatitis on hands

DERMATOSES AFFECTING THE NAILS

Nail psoriasis

See Chapter 10 and Table 48.3. Up to 50% of psoriatics have nail involvement. Nail signs of psoriasis include pits (Figure 48.27), onycholysis (Figure 48.28), subungual hyperkeratosis (Figure 48.29), nail plate discoloration (oil spots), uneven nail surface, splinter haemorrhages, acute and chronic paronychia and transverse midline depressions in the thumbnails. The Nail Psoriasis Severity Index (NAPSI) is an instrument for precise documentation of nail abnormalities for use in trials and, more generally, for assessing response to interventions.

Acropustulosis
A clinical variant which involves destructive pustulation of the nail unit (Figure 48.30). It may present as a component of pustular psoriasis, palmoplantar pustulosis, acrodermatitis continua of Hallopeau or, on isolated digits, as parakeratosis pustulosa.

Management of nail psoriasis is with general hand care, local potent topical corticosteroids (short-term use to proximal nail fold), triamcinolone injection under local anaesthetic (no more than two or three times), topical vitamin D analogues and local PUVA to the nail unit. Systemic treatment in severe intractable disease which is functionally disabling may warrant systemic treatment (Table 48.3), e.g. acitretin, methotrexate, apremilast and biologics. Nail signs often improve when a patient is given systemic therapy to treat more widespread psoriasis.

Darier disease of the nails

See Chapter 30. 96% of patients with Darier disease are reported to have acral changes of which nail changes are the most common. Features include red and/or white longitudinal streaks,

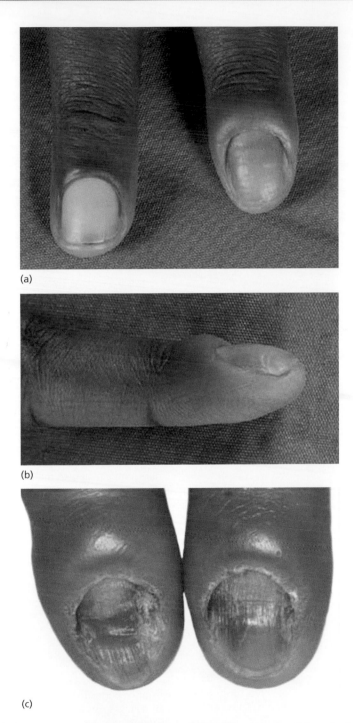

Figure 48.26 Chronic paronychia: (a) and (b) paronychial swelling, loss of cuticle and mildly dystrophic nail in early disease; (c) severe nail dystrophy in more advanced disease.

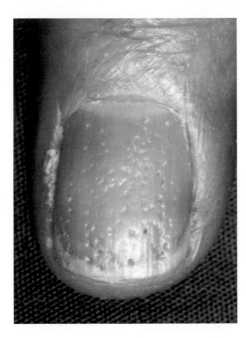

Figure 40.27 Psoriasis: pitting.

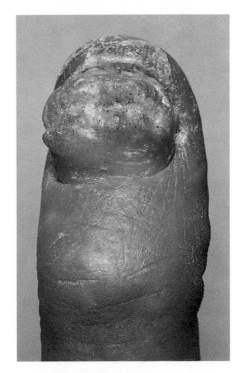

Figure 48.29 Psoriasis: subungual hyperkeratosis.

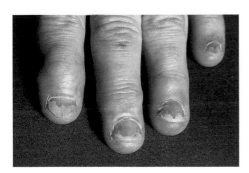

Figure 48.28 Psoriasis: distal onycholysis.

V-shaped nick (Figure 48.31), subungual hyperkeratotic papules, excess ridging and a rough nail surface and total leukonychia.

Eczema involving the nails

See Chapters 16 and 69, and Table 48.3. Nail changes in eczema may be seen in the context of eczema elsewhere, with hand eczema, or as

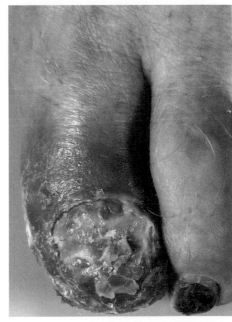

Figure 48.30 Acropustulosis: nail plate has been destroyed by intense pustular inflammation.

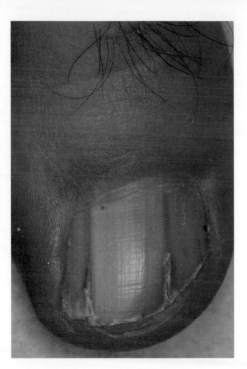

Figure 48.31 Darier disease: white and red longitudinal lines and distal notching.

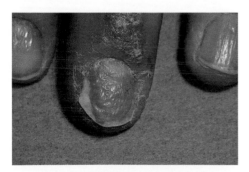

Figure 48.32 Nail involvement in atopic eczema in childhood.

an isolated finding with periungual and subungual features (Figure 48.32). A combination of atopy and an exogenous irritant or allergic contact reaction is common. Clinical features are listed in Table 48.3. Nails may also be smooth and shiny secondary to rubbing. Management

consists of general hand care, barrier preparations, potent topical steroids (short-term use especially in young children) and PUVA.

Lichen planus of the nails and related conditions

See also Chapter 12. Nails are involved in about 10% of cases of disseminated lichen planus.

Pathophysiology

Histology of 20 nail dystrophy shows hypergranulosis due to disordered keratinisation that causes both subungual hyperkeratosis and poor nail plate formation. In other forms of nail lichen planus, in addition to hypergranulosis, there is occasionally saw-toothing of the rete pattern, but rarely are colloid bodies seen.

Clinical features

Nail plate changes include thinning or thickening, onychorrhexis, brittleness, crumbling or fragmentation and accentuation of surface longitudinal ridging (Figure 48.33). Transient or permanent longitudinal melanonychia, longitudinal erythronychia or leukonychia are sometimes seen as a post-inflammatory phenomenon. When inflammation is intense and widespread nails may be shed (Figure 48.34). Pterygium can occur.

Clinical variants are:

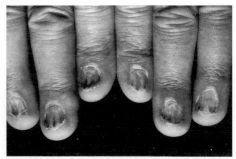

Figure 48.33 Severe onychatrophy with longitudinal melanoychia, from juvenile onset lichen planus of nails.

Table 48.4 Systemic therapies in common dermatological diseases affecting the nail

	Ciclosporin	Methotrexate	Prednisolone	Acitretin	Fumaric acid esters	Azathioprine	Biologicals	Small molecules
Psoriasis	++	+	−	+	+	−	++	+
Lichen planus	+	−	++	+	−	+	−	−
20-nail dystrophy	+	−	++	−	−	−	−	−
Eczema	++	+	+	−	−	+	−	−

Justification for all systemic treatments in nail disease may be based on the combined presentation of skin and nails. It is less common to prescribe on the basis of nail disease alone. Course duration can usually be limited to pulses of 3 months in a 9–12 month period, repeated if needed. Doses are as for the cutaneous disease.
++ Good choice, with moderate evidence supporting its use.
+ Reasonable choice, with case reports or small series supporting use.
− Little or no published evidence.

PART 6: SKIN DISORDERS ASSOCIATED WITH SPECIFIC CUTANEOUS STRUCTURE

- *20-nail dystrophy:* Trachyonychia may involve all 20 nails but may affect as few as four or five. Seen in autoimmune diseases and is also a recognised variant of lichen planus.
- *Keratosis lichenoides chronica (variant of chronic lichen planus)*: 30% have nail involvement, with hyperkeratotic hypertrophy of periungual tissues.
- Lichen planus nail changes are seen in *graft-versus-host disease*.

Management

Early treatment is required to ensure that the disease does not progress and to minimise irreversible scarring (Table 48.4).

Mild disease: Potent topical corticosteroids to proximal nail fold, triamcinolone acetonide injection under local anaesthetic.

Severe disease: See Table 48.4.

GENETIC DISORDERS OF NAILS

Pachyonychia congenita

Autosomal dominant group of disorders caused by mutations in one of five genes encoding nail keratins. Characterised by toenail dystrophy, plantar keratoderma and plantar pain (see Chapter 30).

Nail–patella syndrome

(Syn. Hereditary onycho-osteodysplasia)
A rare disorder characterised by nail changes and dystrophy of the patella and iliac horns.

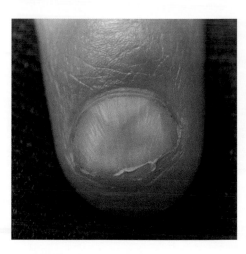

Figure 48.35 Nail dystrophy with triangular lunula of the nail–patella syndrome. (Source: Courtesy of Dr Mark Holzberg.)

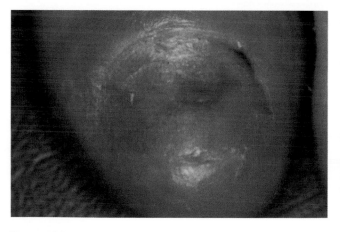
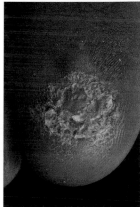

Figure 48.34 Anonychia following lichen planus.

Autosomal dominant inheritance in the majority causes mutations in the LMX1B gene. Nail dysplasia with the characteristic triangular lunula instead of the crescent-shaped lunula occurs in most affected individuals and may be the only feature (Figure 48.35). Flexion of the distal interphalangeal joints and hyperextension of the proximal interphalangeal joints leads to 'swan-necking'. Patellar involvement (74% of patients) is often asymmetrical and commonly characterised by small irregularly shaped or absent patella with recurrent dislocation or subluxation. A smaller proportion of patients have elbow, renal or ocular abnormalities. Management is multidisciplinary with appropriate analgesia, physiotherapy and orthopaedic input.

49 Acquired disorders of dermal connective tissue

CHANGES IN DERMAL CONNECTIVE TISSUE DUE TO AGEING AND PHOTODAMAGE

Both intrinsic ageing and UV exposure result in dermal connective tissue changes which affect the skin's appearance in old age. Elastic fibres deteriorate from age 30 years onwards, regardless of sun exposure.

There are three types of wrinkles:

1. *Crinkles*: Deterioration of elastin causes very fine wrinkling, even in areas not exposed to sunlight.
2. *Glyphic wrinkles*: Accentuation of normal skin markings on skin prematurely aged by elastotic degeneration caused by sunlight.
3. *Linear furrows*: Long, straight or slightly curved grooves, including horizontal frown lines along the forehead, the 'crows' feet' radiating from the lateral canthus of the eye and the creases from the nose to the corners of the mouth.

Solar elastosis

(Syn. Actinic elastosis)
A component of hypertrophic skin photodamage.

Epidemiology
Related to the cumulative lifetime exposure to UV radiation; more common in outdoor workers and in those living in sunny climates. Usually presents in >40s but cumulative sun exposure is more important than age. Fair-skinned people are most affected.

May occur in photosensitised skin, e.g. porphyria cutanea tarda.

Pathophysiology
Usually results from prolonged exposure to sunlight, infrared radiation may be causative. Reduced collagen and accumulation of amorphous masses of degenerate elastic fibres in the papillary and upper reticular dermis occur.

Clinical features
Changes develop gradually over years. Characterised by yellowish discoloration and skin thickening (Figure 49.1). The forehead, scalp and posterior neck are most affected. On the neck it may be divided by well-defined furrows into an irregular rhomboidal pattern (cutis

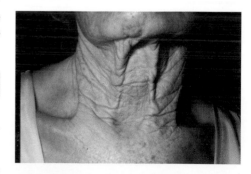

Figure 49.1 Actinic elastosis on the neck of an elderly female patient.

Rook's Dermatology Handbook, First Edition. Edited by Christopher E. M. Griffiths, Tanya O. Bleiker, Daniel Creamer, John R. Ingram and Rosalind C. Simpson.
© 2022 John Wiley & Sons Ltd. Published 2022 by John Wiley & Sons Ltd.

rhomboidalis nuchae). There may be more sharply marginated, thickened plaques on the face or neck. Actinic elastosis may be complicated by actinic granuloma.

Clinical variants include the following:

Actinic comedonal plaque (Syn. Favre–Racouchot syndrome)
Confluent plaques studded with comedones; usually periorbital skin (Figure 49.2).

Elastotic nodules of the ear (Syn. Weathering nodules)
Single or multiple firm papules on the anterior crus of the antihelix, usually in middle-aged or elderly males. May minic basal cell carcinoma.

Collagenous and elastotic marginal plaques of the hands
Papules and plaques on the dominant hand along the radial aspect of the index finger, the first web space and the ulnar aspect of the thumb.

Differential diagnosis
Plane xanthoma, pseudoxanthoma elasticum (PXE) and colloid milium may sometimes cause confusion.

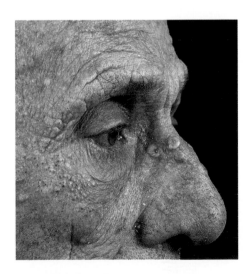

Figure 49.2 Favre-Racouchot syndrome: Nodular actinic elastosis with comedones and cysts in an elderly man (Source: Courtesy of Professor R. Marks, St Vincent's Hospital, Melbourne, Australia.)

Investigations
Skin biopsy if diagnostic doubt.

Management
First line: Prevention by photoprotection.

Second line: Topical retinoids.

Adult colloid milium and colloid degeneration of the skin

A rare but probably underdiagnosed dermatosis defined histologically by the presence of colloid in dermal papillae.

Epidemiology
Rare, usually affects fair-skinned outdoor workers living in sunny climates.

Pathophysiology
Cause unclear; UV exposure is strongly implicated. Occupational exposure to mineral oils has also been implicated. Cases have been reported in association with ochronosis after the long-term application of strong hydroquinone bleaching creams.

Clinical features
Small dermal papules 1–5 mm in diameter, yellowish-brown, sometimes translucent, symmetrically distributed in irregular groups in sun-exposed areas (Figure 49.3). Most frequently on the face, periorbital region, dorsa of the hands, neck and ears. Most cases reach peak development within 3 years then remain unchanged. Nodular colloid degeneration is a variant presenting as a single nodule up to 5 cm in diameter.

Differential diagnosis
The rare juvenile form manifests before puberty and is often familial.

Investigations
Biopsy required for definitive diagnosis.

Management
Dermabrasion and long-pulsed Er:YAG laser may be helpful.

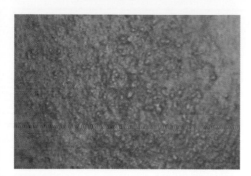

Figure 49.3 Adult colloid milia with multiple tiny yellowish translucent papules (Source: From Mehregan D, Hooten J. Adult colloid milium: a case report and literature review. Int J Dermatol 2011, 50, 1531–1534.)

CUTANEOUS ATROPHY

Skin atrophy describes clinical changes produced by decreased dermal connective tissue, characterised by thinning and loss of elasticity. Atrophy of the skin occurs to a varying degree in a large number of conditions (Box 49.1).

Atrophy due to corticosteroids

Systemic, topical, intralesional or inhaled corticosteroids can produce dose-related cutaneous atrophy. The effect is most marked from potent topical steroids under occlusion.

Pathophysiology

Suppression of dermal hyaluran synthase 2 causes alteration of dermal collagen. Inhibition of enzyme activity involved in collagen biosynthesis leads to suppression of types I and III collagen synthesis. Collagen turnover rate is probably decreased. Steroid-induced vasoconstriction leads to prolonged superficial ischaemia, which may contribute to atrophy development.

Clinical features

The skin becomes thin and fragile with easy bruising often after trivial and striae may develop (Figure 49.4). Changes are generalised in patients on systemic corticosteroids (more marked at sites of photodamage and trauma). Thinning due to topical corticosteroids may be localised to the site(s) of application. Severe dermal atrophy can follow injection of intralesional steroids.

Box 49.1 Acquired forms of cutaneous atrophy

Generalised cutaneous thinning

- Ageing (see above)
- Rheumatoid disease
- Glucocorticoids (exogenous or endogenous)

Acquired poikiloderma

Striae

Atrophic scars

- Stellate pseudoscars
- Infections, e.g. varicella, certain tuberculides, some deep mycoses, e.g.sporotrichosis, onchocerciasis
- Cutaneous lupus erythematosus
- Lupus vulgaris
- Intralesional steroid injections
- Diabetic dermopathy
- Exposure to ionising radiation

- Ehlers–Danlos syndrome
- Mild trauma in older patients

Spontaneous atrophic scarring of the cheeks

Acrodermatitis chronica atrophicans (Lyme borreliosis)

Atrophodermas

- Follicular atrophoderma
- Linear atrophoderma (Moulin)
- Atrophoderma of Pasini and Pierini

Paroxysmal haematoma of the finger (Achenbach syndrome)

Panatrophy

- Local panatrophy
- Facial hemiatrophy

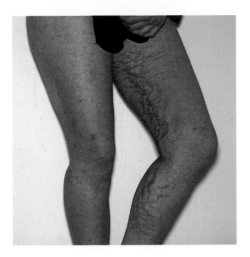

Figure 49.4 Striae of the legs due to long-term application of a potent topical steroid in a young woman with psoriasis.

Differential diagnosis

See Box 49.1.

Investigations

Blood glucose and bone density if systemic steroid toxicity is suspected.

Management

Prevention: Use steroid-sparing systemic drugs and topical agents such as calcineurin inhibitors.

Specific treatments: Vitamin C therapy might help restore normal skin thickness; concurrent application of retinoic acid may partially prevent the epidermal atrophy due to steroids; intralesional saline injections can restore surface contour.

Striae

(Syn. Stretch marks)
Visible linear scars which form in areas of dermal damage produced by stretching of the skin.

Epidemiology

Very common, especially in adult women; associated with growth spurts, e.g. puberty, body building and pregnancy. May reflect structural abnormalities of connective tissue, e.g. Marfan syndrome.

Pathophysiology

Cause unclear, likely genetic susceptibility. Histology of early disease shows oedematous dermis and perivascular lymphocytic cuffing. Late disease shows thinning of the epidermis with flattened dermal papillae.

Clinical features

Commonest sites are the outer aspect of the thighs and the lumbosacral region in boys (Figure 49.5), and the thighs, buttocks and breasts in girls. Pubertal growth striae are concentrated symmetrically over and on either side of the spine. Early lesions may be raised and irritable, but subsequently become flat, smooth and red or bluish in colour. They are irregularly linear, several centimetres long and 1–10 mm wide. They eventually fade and generally become paler than the surrounding skin.

Striae secondary to Cushing syndrome or steroids may be larger and more widely distributed. Pregnancy-induced striae are most conspicuous on the abdominal wall and later on the breasts.

Differential diagnosis

Cushing syndrome; linear focal elastosis.

Investigations

Exclude Cushing syndrome if suspected.

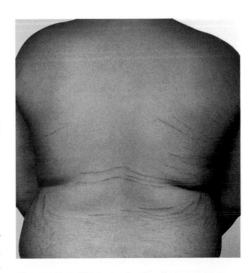

Figure 49.5 Striae due to obesity in a young man.

Management

There is no evidence to recommend any specific therapy. Striae gravidarum generally improve after delivery; adolescent striae have an excellent prognosis; corticosteroid-induced striae may disappear or become less conspicuous on cessation of treatment.

Poikiloderma

Poikiloderma is a descriptive term comprising atrophy, macular or reticulate pigmentation and telangiectasia. There may be associated scaling, hypopigmentation, petechiae and signs of inflammation such as lichenoid papules.

Pathophysiology

Can be acquired or congenital.

May be a pattern of cutaneous response to injury by cold, heat or ionising radiation. Poikiloderma of civatte (see Chapter 32) is a similar reaction mediated by photosensitising chemicals in cosmetics. Inflammatory dermatoses, such as lichen planus, may give rise to poikilodermatous changes.

Poikiloderma is seen in some systemic autoimmune diseases: dermatomyositis, lupus erythematosus and rarely systemic sclerosis. Poikiloderma atrophicans vasculare is an early presenting feature of cutaneous T-cell lymphoma.

Congenital poikiloderma is a feature of several inherited disorders, including Kindler syndrome (see Chapter 33), dyskeratosis congenita, Rothmund–Thomson and Weary syndromes and erythrokeratoderma variabilis.

Investigations

Investigate for underlying systemic condition if suspected.

Management

Treat any underlying condition.

Spontaneous atrophic scarring of the cheeks

(Syn. Varioliform atrophy)
Spontaneous scars developing on the cheeks.

Epidemiology

Probably autosomal dominant. Occurs in young adults or children. Rarely reported but probably underdiagnosed.

Pathophysiology

Mild loss of collagen or elastic fibres; there may be thickening of the stratum corneum on histology.

Clinical features

Shallow atrophic lesions with sharp margins. May be linear, rectangular or varioliform (Figure 49.6). Slight erythema and scaling sometimes precede lesions.

Differential diagnosis

Atrophoderma vermiculatum, chickenpox scars and artefact.

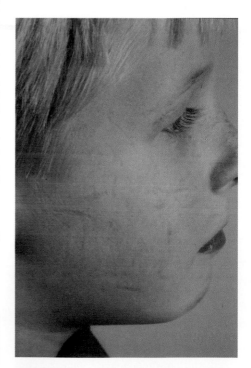

Figure 49.6 Spontaneous atrophic scarring of the cheeks.

Acrodermatitis chronica atrophicans

Late skin manifestation of Lyme borreliosis (see Chapter 4).

Atrophodermas

There are three variants of atrophodermas:

Follicular atrophoderma
Dimple-like depressions at the follicular orifices usually involving the dorsum of the hands and feet. Associated with Conradi–Hünermann–Happle syndrome, Bazex–Dupré–Christol syndrome, hyperkeratosis palmoplantaris, follicular keratosis or palmoplantar hyperhidrosis.

Linear atrophoderma
Probable atrophic variant of morphoea. Presents with linear atrophic hyperpigmented plaques in the distribution of Blaschko's lines.

Atrophoderma of Pasini and Pierini
Also probably an atrophic variant of morphoea. Presents in childhood or adolescence with one or more patches of skin which become bluish and sharply depressed, usually on the back, chest and abdomen (Figure 49.7). Psoralen and UVA (PUVA) or hydroxychloroquine may be helpful.

Paroxysmal haematoma of the finger

(Syn. Achenbach syndrome)
Benign, spontaneous onset of one or more painful haematomas in the fingers (Figure 49.8).

Epidemiology
Usually affects middle age; F > M.

Pathophysiology
Cause unknown but potentially due to localised acquired fragility of vascular connective tissue.

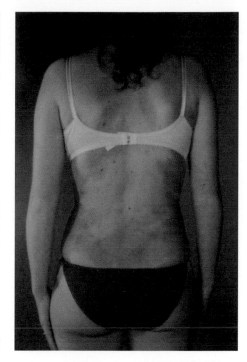

Figure 49.7 Atrophoderma of Pasini and Pierini.

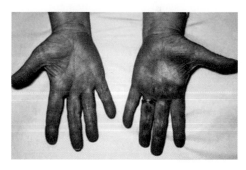

Figure 49.8 Paroxysmal haematoma of the finger. (Source: Courtesy of Dr J. Verbov, Royal Liverpool University Hospitals, Liverpool, UK.)

Clinical features
Sudden bruising occurs spontaneously or after minor trauma; the patient is asymptomatic between flares.

Differential diagnosis
It may be mistaken for easy bruising due to steroid atrophy. The absence of ischaemic features

and rapid improvement exclude occlusive vascular disease.

Investigations
Clinical diagnosis.

Management
Spontaneously resolves within days.

DISORDERS OF ELASTIC FIBRE DEGRADATION

Classification and causes of lax skin are listed in Box 49.2.

Acquired cutis laxa

(Syn. Generalised elastolysis)
Lax skin occurring in association with other disorders. May be acquired following inflammatory skin disease or following exposure *in utero* to drugs.

Epidemiology
Associated with urticarial eruptions, nephrotic syndrome, complement deficiency, sarcoidosis, syphilis, primary amyloidosis, multiple myeloma, drug hypersensitivity and Klippel–Trenaunay syndrome. Focal elastolysis can also occur in association with lupus erythematosus, severe rheumatoid arthritis and coeliac disease. d-penicillamine may cause cutis laxa, elastosis perforans serpiginosa and pseudoxanthoma-like changes.

Pathophysiology
Dermal elastic tissue is markedly reduced, collagen is normal. Fibroblasts express increased elastolytic activity; serum α_1-antitrypsin and elastase inhibition are decreased. Histology shows confirmation reduction in elastic fibres.

Clinical features
May rarely develop at any age following episodes of urticaria or angio-oedema, extensive inflammatory skin disease (such as systemic lupus erythematosus or erythema multiforme) or febrile illness (Figure 49.9). Changes may be mild and confined to a limited area, or widespread causing massive folds of lax skin. Purpura

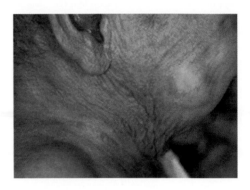

Figure 49.9 Acquired cutis laxa following a generalised inflammatory dermatitis in an 18-month-old child. (Source: From Haider M, Alfadley A, Kadry R, *et al*. Acquired cutis laxa type II (Marshall syndrome) in an 18-month-old child: a case report. Pediatr Dermatol 2010, 27, 89–91.)

Box 49.2 Classification and causes of lax skin

Lax skin

Common causes

Photoageing
Marked weight loss
recovery from severe oedema.

Less common causes

Generalised elastolysis (cutis laxa):
(a) congenital (see Chapter 34)
(b) acquired (see below)

Localised elastolysis:
(a) anetoderma (see below)
(b) blepharochalasis
(c) chronic atrophic acrodermatitis
(d) granulomatous slack skin (due to lymphoma)
(e) other localised lesions, including dermal elastolysis, post-inflammatory elastolysis and cutis laxa, elastic tissue naevi.

may follow slight trauma and fibrotic nodules form over bony prominences. Internal organs may be involved.

Post-inflammatory elastolysis and cutis laxa (Marshall syndrome)

A clinical variant preceded by neutrophilic inflammation. The inflammatory lesions are urticarial-like or multiple red papules, which slowly enlarge to form rings 2–10 cm in diameter. Associated with α_1-antitryspin deficiency.

Differential diagnosis

Congenital causes: Ehlers–Danlos syndrome (skin is hyperextensible but not lax); PXE (yellowish skin with facial sparing).

Investigations

Clinical features: loose skin that recoils slowly after stretching.
Skin biopsy.
Investigations and referral to appropriate speciality if internal organ involvement suspected.

Management

Plastic surgery if indicated to reduce cosmetic disability.

Anetoderma

(Syn. Macular atrophy)

A circumscribed area of slack skin associated with loss of dermal substance on palpation and a loss of elastic tissue on histological examination. It can be primary or secondary in nature.

Epidemiology

Rare, usually occurs in women aged 20–40. More frequent in central Europe. Primary anetoderma is strongly associated with antiphospholipid syndrome. Secondary anetoderma has been reported in association with tuberculosis and leprosy, urticaria pigmentosa, pityriasis versicolor, granuloma annulare, Stevens–Johnson syndrome, B- and T-cell lymphoma as well as others.

Pathophysiology

Inflammatory cells release elastase, which causes focal elastolysis. A perivascular infiltrate with prominent plasma cells is seen. Metalloproteinases are increased in lesional skin.

Clinical features

Possible history of a previous inflammatory, perhaps urticated, lesion at the site.

Primary anetoderma

0.5–1.0 cm round/oval pink macules typically develop on the trunk, thighs and upper arms, may reach 2–3 cm size. Sometimes there are larger plaques of erythema. Each lesion fades and flattens to leave an atrophic macule (Figure 49.10) of varying colour (skin colour, grey, white or blue). May be few or very numerous lesions. New lesions often continue to develop for many years.

Secondary anetoderma

Atrophic areas do not always develop at the sites of the known inflammatory lesions. They are soft, round or oval areas which occur mainly on the trunk. 'Confetti-like macular atrophy' may be a clinical variant with hypopigmented shiny atrophic patches occurring on the upper limbs and trunk.

Differential diagnosis

Extragenital lichen sclerosus, focal dermal hypoplasia, atrophic scars, aquired cutis laxa (may represent different forms of the same condition).

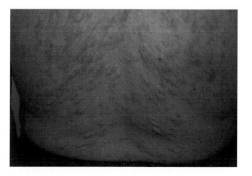

Figure 49.10 Primary anetoderma associated with antiphospholipid antibodies. (Source: From Eungdamrong J, Fischer M, Patel R, Meehan S, Sanchez M. Anetoderma secondary to antiphospholipid antibodies. Dermatol Online J 2012, 18(12), 26.)

Investigations

Primary anetoderma: test for antiphospholipid syndrome.

Management

No specific treatment. Treat underlying phospholipid syndrome if identified; treat underlying disease or infections causing secondary anetoderma.

Dermal elastolysis

Idiopathic loss of the elastic fibres in the mid-dermis (mid-dermal elastolysis) or upper dermis (upper-dermal elastolysis) leads to widespread wrinkling.

Epidemiology

Mid-dermal elastolysis affects young to middle-aged females. Possibly associated with a pro-thrombotic state. Upper dermal elastolysis affects young African girls.

Pathophysiology

May follow granuloma annulare or other inflammatory conditions (post-inflammatory elastolysis). There is increased elastolytic activity and reduced elastin mRNA compared with normal skin. The perifollicular variant shows non-inflammatory perifollicular loss of elastin fibres.

Clinical features

Mid-dermal elastolysis has three clinical variants, all asymptomatic:

- *Type 1*: Cigarette paper-like fine wrinkling affecting the trunk and upper arms.
- *Type 2*: Perifollicular papules, small, grey–white, finely wrinkled, round or oval areas, each with a central hair follicle.
- *Type 3*: Reticular variant; orange-red inflammatory papules precede net-like areas of atrophy, mainly affects arms.

Upper dermal elastolysis: Lesions are preceded by inflammatory lesions.

Differential diagnosis

PXE.

Management

No definitive treatment exists. Topical retinoic acid may be helpful.

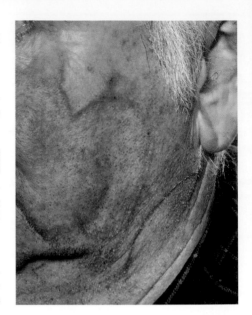

Figure 49.11 Typical actinic granulomas on the face and neck of an elderly man.

Actinic granuloma
(Syn. Annular elastolytic giant cell granuloma)
Uncommon condition affecting actinic-damaged skin that results from a low-grade reactive inflammatory process. Abnormal elastic fibres are progressively destroyed by an expanding ring of elastolysis and granulomatous inflammation. Asymptomatic lesions, single or multiple, affect sun-exposed skin. Small pink papules slowly extend to form a ring of firm superficial dermal thickening with an atrophic centre (Figure 49.11). No treatment is of proven benefit. May improve with photoprotection.

Linear focal elastosis

(Syn. Elastotic striae)
An acquired disorder of elastic tissue deposition that may represent a keloidal reaction to striae distensae.

Epidemiology

Incidence and prevalence unknown. Predominantly affects adolescent males of all ethnicities.

Pathophysiology

Lesions may be associated with a growth spurt, familial cases are reported. Elastogenesis may occur in response to local trauma, UV light or perhaps following the development of striae distensae. Intrinsic defects of elastic fibre metabolism may play a role.

Clinical features

Characterised by asymptomatic yellow linear bands arranged horizontally on the lower back. In contrast to striae densae, lesions are palpable. Striae often coexist.

Investigations

None needed.

Managenent

None needed, of cosmetic significance only.

FIBROMATOSES

Fibromatosis is fibrous overgrowth of dermal and subcutaneous connective tissue; the commonest cause is knuckle pads. These are circumscribed thickenings overlying the finger joints. True prevalence is uncertain but probably common. Onset between 15 and 30 years. Strong association with other fibromatoses (e.g. palmar and plantar fibromatosis). Aetiology is unclear. Trauma probably more relevant in 'pseudo knuckle pads'. Knuckle pads are smooth, circumscribed nodules, slow growing up to 0.5–1.5 cm. Most

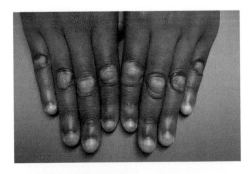

Figure 49.12 Knuckle pads. (Source: From Hyman CH, Cohen PR. Report of a family with idiopathic knuckle pads and review of idiopathic and disease-associated knuckle pads. Dermatol Online J 2013, 19(5), 18177.)

commonly dorsa of the proximal interphalangeal joints (Figure 49.12). Management is conservative; consider intralesional 5-fluorouracil if symptoms. For pseudo knuckle pads minimise trauma ± topical keratolytics.

ABNORMAL FIBROTIC RESPONSES TO SKIN INJURY

Keloids and hypertrophic scars

Excessive connective tissue response to injury. Preceding trauma may be trivial. A keloid extends beyond the original boundaries of a defect whereas a hypertrophic scar is confined to the original defect and usually resolves after several months (Figure 49.13).

Epidemiology

Most common in African, Hispanic or Asian ethnic groups with a prevalence of 4.5–16.0%. Positive family history in 5–10% of Europeans with keloids,

Usually occurs between puberty and age 30 years. F > M. Associated with other fibromatoses.

Pathophysiology

Trauma, often minor, in susceptible individuals leads to increased type I and type III collagen. Greater dermal expression of extracellular matrix proteins including fibronectin, versican, elastin, and tenascin. Endothelial proliferation, increased fibroblasts, forming irregular nodules or whorls of hyalinised collagen is seen on histology of early lesions. Late lesions are acellular with thick, poorly vascularised bands of immature collagen.

Clinical features

Three to four weeks after trauma scars become raised and thickened. They are firm skin-coloured, pink or red plaques; hypertrophic scars remain within the boundaries of the initial wound, whereas keloids become smoother and rounder and extend outside the wound boundary (Figures 49.13–49.16).

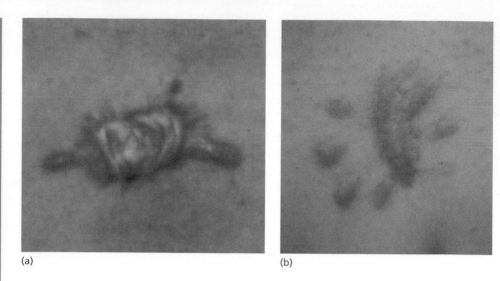

(a) (b)

Figure 49.13 Contrast between two scars from the presternal area: (a) spontaneous keloid and (b) hypertrophic scar following excision of benign mole. The former shows partial involution after injection of triamcinolone.

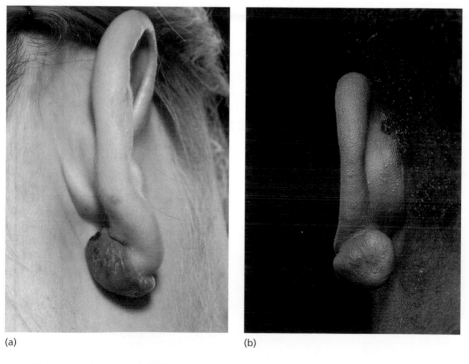

(a) (b)

Figure 49.14 a and b 'earlobe keloid scars'.

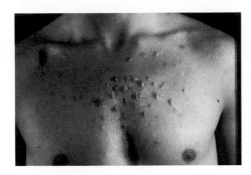

Figure 49.15 Keloid nodules secondary to acne.

Differential diagnosis

Usually straightforward diagnosis. Other differential diagnoses include fibrosarcoma and dermatofibrosarcoma protuberans, a malignancy developing in a scar or scar sarcoid.

Investigations

Biopsy if diagnostic doubt.

Management

Avoid non-essential surgery.
First line: Intralesional corticosteroids repeated monthly.
Second line: Silicone gel sheeting.
Third line: Mechanical pressure, surgical excision, 5-flurouracil, photodynamic therapy have all been tried but evidence level poor.

PERFORATING DERMATOSES

Skin disorders whereby material is eliminated from the dermis by extrusion through the epidermis to the skin surface by a process of transepidermal (transepithelial) elimination.

Acquired perforating dermatosis

(Syn. Acquired reactive perforating dermatosis)

An acquired disorder of transepidermal elimination of degenerate collagen, elastin and other connective tissue components.

Epidemiology

Prevalence 4–11% of patients on haemodialysis. Usually occurs age 50–60, F:M = 3:1. Strong association with chronic kidney disease and diabetes.

Pathophysiology

Lysosomal enzymes derived from leukocytes might be responsible for the altered staining of collagen fibres, the degradation of elastic fibres and the impairment of keratinocyte adhesion, which allows trans epidermal elimination of dermal components.

Histology shows cup-shaped invagination of the epidermis, which is plugged with necrotic inflammatory debris. Collagen bundles are arranged vertically at the base of the lesion and there is transepidermal elimination of collagen fibres.

Clinical features

Pruritus is common. Keratotic dome-shaped papules develop primarily on extensor aspects of the limbs and trunk (Figure 49.17).

Clinical variants include the following:

Familial reactive perforating collagenosis

Rare inherited form usually precipitated by environmental cold or trauma. Usually starts in early childhood, lesions regress spontaneously leaving a slight scar, but new lesions may appear.

Verrucous perforating collagenoma

Rare reaction to the traumatic introduction of foreign materials, e.g. fiberglass.

Perforating disease due to exogenous agents

Occasionally, a chemical which has been applied to the skin topically or by intradermal injection can be eliminated by the transepidermal route.

Differential diagnosis

Molluscum contagiosum, papular urticaria or other perforating disorders.

Investigations

Biopsy findings are characteristic.

Management

Spontaneous improvement may occur if renal function improves. No good evidence

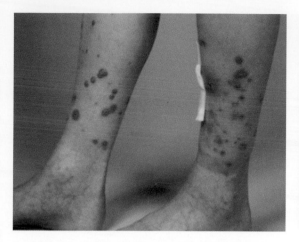
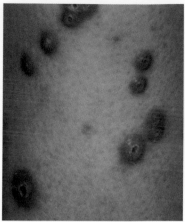

Figure 49.16 Acquired perforating dermatosis: a 48-year-old woman with a 25-year history of type 1 diabetes with retinopathy and renal failure, and a 12-year history of skin ulceration with multiple tender crusted sores which were slow to heal.

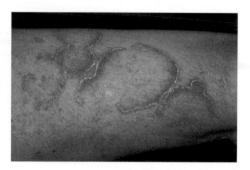

Figure 49.17 Elastosis perforans serpiginosa in a patient with vascular Ehlers–Danlos syndrome.

for treatment, topical retinoids, oral isotretinoin, methotrexate, rifampicin, emollients, intralesional steroids and topical steroids under occlusion. Narrow-band UVB, PUVA and photodynamic therapy have all been used.

Elastosis perforans serpiginosa

(Syn. Perforating elastoma)
Extruded material is derived from elastic fibres in the upper dermis.

Epidemiology
Rare, usually presents between 5 and 20 years, M > F. Closely associated with heritable connective tissue disorders and Down syndrome.

Pathophysiology
Probable primary abnormality in the dermal elastin provokes a cellular response that leads to extrusion of the abnormal elastic tissue. Lesions are commonly seen in areas subjected to wear and tear. Histology shows papule with a well-circumscribed area of epidermal hyperplasia communicating directly with the dermis with a horny plug containing debris derived from elastin.

Clinical features
Usually asymptomatic. Small, horny or umbilicated papules are arranged in lines, circles or segments of circles in a serpiginous pattern (Figure 49.18). May enlarge to 15–20 cm. The back and sides of the neck are most commonly affected.

Differential diagnosis
Porokeratosis of Mibelli, familial reactive perforating collagenosis and perforating granuloma annulare.

Investigations

Skin biopsy is diagnostic, but biopsy scars readily become keloidal.

Management

Usually self-limiting, no good evidence for treatment.

First line: Conservative management.

Second line: Trial of cryotherapy initially to test site.

Third line: Curettage (excision is not recommended).

50 Sarcoidosis and granulomatous skin disorders

Sarcoidosis

Sarcoidosis is a multisystem granulomatous disease of unknown aetiology that mainly involves the lungs, mediastinal and peripheral lymph nodes, eyes and skin. Cutaneous involvement may be the presenting sign of systemic sarcoidosis.

Epidemiology

Most prevalent in developed countries, ranging from 10 to 40 per 100 000 in the US and Europe. Peak incidence is between 20 and 40 years, with a second peak around the age of 60. Prevalence is slightly higher in women for systemic sarcoidosis and is 2:1 F:M for cutaneous sarcoidosis. In the USA, sarcoidosis is commoner and more severe in African Americans than in Caucasians.

Pathophysiology

The histopathological changes are similar in all organs affected by sarcoidosis. The main feature is the sarcoid granuloma, defined as aggregates of epithelioid cells with a sparse lymphocytic component, called a 'naked granuloma.' Caseous necrosis is typically absent. In skin, sarcoid granulomas are usually observed in the dermis but can also extend to subcutaneous tissue. CD4 positive helper T lymphocytes are present at the centre of granulomas with a smaller population of CD8 positive cytotoxic T lymphocytes at the periphery.

Clinical features

Clinical features of cutaneous sarcoidosis are shown in Table 50.1 and Figure 50.1.

In systemic sarcoidosis, clinical onset may be acute or insidious. Acute or subacute sarcoidosis develops over a period of weeks and usually has a good prognosis. It is characterised by mild constitutional symptoms such as fatigue, malaise, anorexia, weight loss, low-grade fever, arthralgia and respiratory symptoms. Insidious onset of respiratory or other organ problems over several months without constitutional symptoms correlates with a chronic course and permanent organ damage (Table 50.2).

Differential diagnosis

See Table 50.1 for differential diagnosis of cutaneous lesions, depending on subtype.

Investigations

Consider: skin biopsy (also culture for mycobacteria), chest radiograph, serum angiotensin-converting enzyme level, haematological and biochemical profiles, including calcium level, TB testing (tuberculin test or interferon-γ release assay), pulmonary function tests, slit-lamp and ophthalmoscopic examination, electrocardiogram.

Management

Treatment options for mild to moderate cutaneous sarcoidosis include a potent topical steroid, intralesional corticosteroids, or

Rook's Dermatology Handbook, First Edition. Edited by Christopher E. M. Griffiths, Tanya O. Bleiker, Daniel Creamer, John R. Ingram and Rosalind C. Simpson.
© 2022 John Wiley & Sons Ltd. Published 2022 by John Wiley & Sons Ltd.

Table 50.1 Cutaneous sarcoidosis

Subtype	Description	Differential diagnosis
Maculopapular	Yellow-brown or red/brown colour No overt epidermal changes Often transient at disease onset (Figure 50.1a)	Xanthelasmata, rosacea, secondary syphilis, DLE, trichoepitheliomata, sebaceous adenoma, granuloma annulare, syringomata
Nodular and plaque	Multiple round or oval, infiltrated reddish-brown plaques >10 mm in diameter Located on the face, scalp, back, buttocks and extremities (Figure 50.1b)	Lupus vulgaris, necrobiosis lipoidica, morphoea, leprosy, leishmaniasis, DLE, granuloma annulare
Lupus pernio	Red-purple asymptomatic plaques on nose, cheeks, ears, lips, forehead and fingers On cheeks, a prominent telangiectatic component is characteristic (Figure 50.1c)	Rosacea, lupus vulgaris, DLE
Scar-sarcoidosis	Can involve scar from any cause, including surgery, trauma, acne, venepuncture and vaccination (Figure 50.1d) Includes tattoo sarcoidosis	Tattoo sarcoidosis should be differentiated from foreign-body reactions to tattoo pigment
Subcutaneous	Multiple indurated asymptomatic subcutaneous nodules with no epidermal involvement located mainly on extremities Fingers may develop asymptomatic firm fusiform swelling, sarcoid dactylitis (Figure 50.1e)	Epidermal cysts, multiple lipomata, calcinosis, rheumatoid nodules, morphoea, cutaneous metastases, TB, deep mycoses
Non-specific: erythema nodosum	Frequently initial manifestation (Figure 50.1f) Marker of acute and benign sarcoidosis, affecting younger people In association with bilateral hilar and right paratracheal adenopathies, known as Löfgren syndrome	TB should be excluded

DLE, discoid lupus erythematosus.

systemic hydroxychloroquine/chloroquine or methotrexate. Oral tetracyclines, such as minocycline 100 mg twice daily, can also be used in parallel.

For severe disfigurement or lupus pernio, oral prednisolone is used to establish remission, followed by the introduction of corticosteroid-sparing agents such as hydroxychloroquine/chloroquine or methotrexate. anti-tumour necrosis factor alpha therapies such as infliximab or adalimumab are considered for treatment-resistant disease.

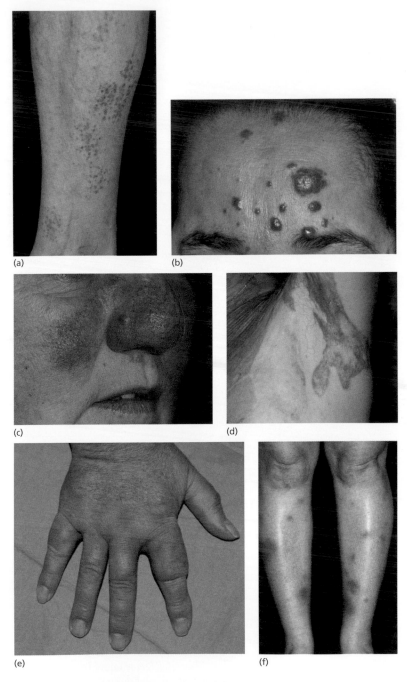

Figure 50.1 Clinical images of subtypes of cutaneous sarcoidosis. (a) Maculopapular sarcoidosis on the arm. (b) Dermal plaque and nodules on the forehead. (c) Classical lupus pernio affecting the nose and cheeks. (d) Scar sarcoidosis in a burn in the axilla. (e) Sarcoid dactylitis. (f) Erythema nodosum in a patient with Löfgren syndrome.

Table 50.2 Features of systemic sarcoidosis

Organ	Description	Proportion of all patients with sarcoidosis (%)
Lungs and mediastinum (pulmonary)	Patients may be asymptomatic or present with dry cough and dyspnoea on exercise CXR shows bilateral hilar lymphadenopathy (stage I), pulmonary involvement (stage III), or both (stage II) (Figure 50.2)	90
Reticuloendothelial	Intrathoracic and/or peripheral lymphadenopathy, including cervical, supraclavicular, epitrochlear, axillary and inguinal Splenomegaly in 5–10%	>80
Liver	Non-caseating granulomas are present in up to 75% of liver biopsies, but macroscopic signs are less common	20–30
Eye	May be asymptomatic Findings include anterior or posterior uveitis, chorioretinitis, periphlebitis, papilloedema and retinal haemorrhage	15–20
Neurosarcoidosis	Cranial nerve involvement, particularly facial paralysis, is commonest Other problems include aseptic meningitis and seizures	5–10
Heart	Supraventricular and ventricular arrhythmias, complete heart block, cor pulmonale secondary to pulmonary fibrosis	5
Others	Parotid enlargement, hypercalcaemia and hypercalciuria	

CXR, chest radiograph.

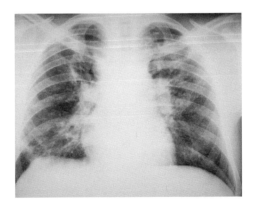

Figure 50.2 Chest radiograph showing stage II pulmonary sarcoidosis (bilateral and right paratracheal lympadenopathy and pulmonary infiltrates with upper and middle lobe predominance).

Granuloma annulare

Granuloma annulare (GA) is a disease of the skin and subcutaneous tissue characterised by granulomatous annular plaques, nodules or papules containing foci of altered collagen surrounded by histiocytes and lymphocytes.

Epidemiology

More common in women, with F:M ratio of 2:1. Localised GA is most common in children and young adults but can occur at any age. Generalised GA occurs more commonly in adults, with a mean age of onset around 50 years. There is a possible association between disseminated GA and diabetes mellitus, although high-quality evidence is lacking.

Pathophysiology

The aetiology and pathogenesis of GA are unknown, but it appears likely that GA represents a reaction pattern to a variety of triggering factors, such as infections and trauma.

Histologically, the most characteristic feature is necrobiotic palisading granulomas, situated in the superficial and mid-dermis, characterised by foci of necrobiosis surrounded by histiocytes and lymphocytes, with the histiocytes commonly forming a palisaded pattern.

Clinical features

See Table 50.3.

Differential diagnosis

See Table 50.3 for differentials based on subtype of GA.

Investigations

Localised and generalised GA is usually a clinical diagnosis. A biopsy may be needed to confirm subcutaneous or perforating GA. Consider diabetes mellitus screening in disseminated disease.

Management

In most cases, particularly in children, reassurance of eventual resolution is all that is needed. Resolution typically takes months to years and recurrence, often at the original site, is common.

In persistent localised GA, a trial of topical steroid or tacrolimus/pimecrolimus may be considered. For generalised GA, phototherapy in the form of psoralen and UVA (PUVA), narrow band UVB, or UVA1 can be considered. Systemic therapies include dapsone, methotrexate and ciclosporin.

Table 50.3 Clinical features divided by subtype

Subtype	Description	Proportion of cases (%)	Differential diagnosis
Localised	Solitary or multiple annular lesions composed of smooth, skin-coloured or erythematous papules may enlarge centrifugally before eventually clearing Acral sites are commonest (Figure 50.3a)	>75	Annular lichen planus, erythema migrans of Lyme disease; psoriasis and tinea corporis would be scaly
Generalised (disseminated)	Multiple annular, ill-defined lesions on trunk and limbs, often with faintly violaceous central area (Figure 50.3b,c)	15	Erythema annulare centrifugum, tuberculides, tertiary syphilis, mycosis fungoides
Subcutaneous	Occurs mainly in children Nodular lesions on scalp and legs, especially pre-tibial region	<5	Trauma, infection, tumours, sarcoidosis, rheumatoid nodules
Perforating	Localised or generalised papules develop yellowish centres with clear, viscous fluid that dries to form a crust	<5	Molluscum contagiosum, other perforating disorders, sarcoidosis, papulonecrotic tuberculide

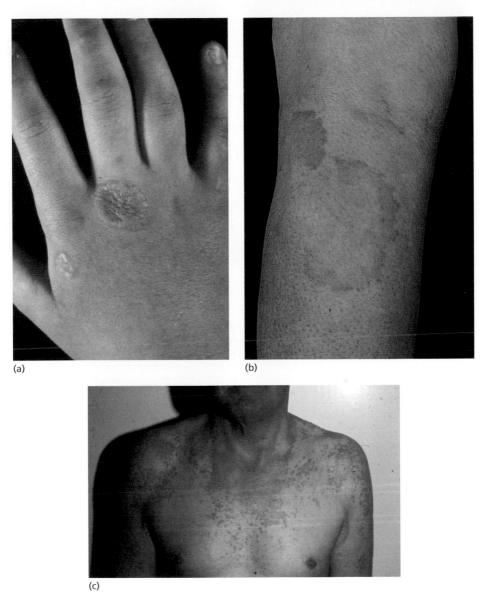

Figure 50.3 Granuloma annulare. (a) Localised GA over the knuckles. (b) Generalised GA on lower limb. (c) Generalised GA showing a photo-distribution over the 'V' of the neck and shoulders.

Necrobiosis lipoidica

(Syn. Necrobiosis lipoidica diabeticorum)
Necrobiosis lipoidica usually occurs on the legs, in some cases associated with diabetes mellitus (DM) or glucose intolerance.

Epidemiology
Necrobiosis lipoidica is relatively uncommon. It is associated with DM but only about 1% of people with DM develop the condition and concomitant DM in those with the condition varies from 15% to 67% in case series. Can affect those

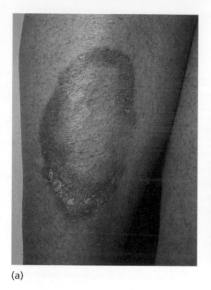
(a)

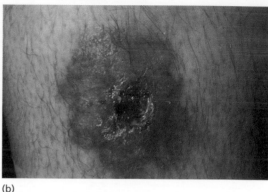
(b)

Figure 50.4 Necrobiosis lipoidica. (a) Lesion on shin. (b) Ulcerated lesion.

with type 1 or type 2 DM. Women are affected more often, with a 3:1 F:M ratio.

Pathophysiology

Pathogenesis remains unknown. Histological appearances are similar to granuloma annulare, but areas of necrobiosis are usually more extensive and less well defined, and there is also a perivascular inflammatory infiltrate including plasma cells.

Clinical features

Characterised by well-defined red-brown indurated plaques with an atrophic yellow centre (Figure 50.4a). It is most commonly seen on the legs, typically the pretibial skin, and may ulcerate in up to one third of patients (Figure 50.4b), causing considerable pain. Lesions are often bilateral.

Differential diagnosis

Lesions with marked fatty infiltration, particularly when not on the legs, may be mistaken for xanthomas. Necrobiotic xanthogranuloma is a rare Langerhans cell histiocytosis with a similar appearance.

Investigations

Skin biopsy is not usually necessary except in atypical cases. Consider annual screening for diabetes.

Management

Evidence is sparse and treatment efficacy is often limited.

First line: No treatment, topical corticosteroid, intralesional corticosteroid.

Second line: PUVA, photodynamic therapy, pulsed dye laser.

Cutaneous Crohn disease

This is a granulomatous inflammation of the skin in patients with underlying Crohn disease.

Clinical features

Granulomatous involvement of the skin may occur by extension of Crohn disease, particularly in the lips, perineum, umbilicus and at the sites of surgery or around a stoma. It is characterised by sinuses, abscesses and induration (Figure 50.5). It is usually seen in the presence of active underlying Crohn disease but may predate its diagnosis, particularly in children.

Oro-facial granulomatosis (Figure 50.6) may be associated with sarcoidosis or food allergy or be part of Melkersson–Rosenthal syndrome. When isolated, it is regarded by some as a localised form of Crohn disease. It may predate intestinal Crohn disease by many years.

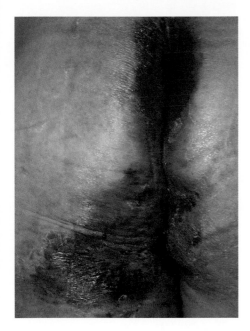

Figure 50.5 Severe perianal Crohn disease.

The skin may also rarely be involved at distant sites, sometimes called metastatic Crohn disease. The presentation is variable with ulcers, nodules, plaques, papules, pustules or abscesses.

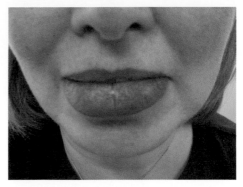

Figure 50.6 Lip swelling due to oro-facial granulomatosis. (Source: Courtesy of Dr E.P. Burova, Bedford Hospital, UK.)

Management

Treatment of active gastrointestinal Crohn disease may improve cutaneous involvement. For localised disease, topical corticosteroids or topical tacrolimus may be beneficial. Systemic treatment with oral corticosteroids and/or azathioprine should be considered when topical therapy is insufficient.

51

Panniculitis

Inflammation of the subcutaneous fat can be due to a range of inflammatory diseases. Panniculitis is classified as either septal or lobular; the presence of vasculitis, nature of inflammatory infiltrate, type of adipocyte necrosis, and any other histological features are needed to make a final diagnosis. Table 51.1 summarises classification of the panniculitides and Tables 51.2–51.5 summarise the key features of the main disorders encountered.

Panniculitis can occur due to numerous different underlying conditions. Adipocytes have excellent vascular supply; interference with arterial supply results in necrotic changes within the fat lobule (predominantly lobular panniculitis), while venous disorders manifest by alterations in septal and paraseptal areas (predominantly septal panniculitis). Large vessel vasculitis involving the septal vessels is not usually associated with substantial inflammation of the fat lobules, whereas vasculitis involving small blood vessels of the lobule usually causes extensive necrosis of adipocytes. By definition, panniculitis is difficult to characterise by clinical examination alone. Deep skin biopsy is often required to make a diagnosis. Histology can be helpful to differentiate between different types of panniculitis (see Box 51.1 and Table 51.1).

Panniculitis has been reported to be associated with several other systemic conditions (Box 51.2).

Box 51.1 Type of adipocyte necrosis providing diagnostic clues in panniculitis

- *Lipophagic necrosis*: Necrotic adipocytes are replaced by foamy macrophages. Usually seen in lipodermatosclerosis and traumatic panniculitis.
- *Liquefactive fat necrosis*: Seen in α_1-antitrypsin deficiency panniculitis and in pancreatic panniculitis.
- *Hyalinising fat necrosis*: Necrotic adipocytes appear as mummified anucleated cells. Seen in lupus panniculitis and panniculitis associated with dermatomyositis.

- *Membranous fat necrosis*: A late-stage type of adipocyte necrosis. Seen in lipodermatosclerosis, but also non-specific and seen in other late-stage panniculitidies.
- *Ischaemic fat necrosis*: Centre of fat lobules may show lipophagic granulomata. Occurs in erythema induratum of Bazin, calciphylaxis, infectious panniculitis and cutaneous polyarteritis nodosa.
- *Basophilic fat necrosis*: Results from aggregations of bacteria, characteristically seen in infectious panniculitis.

Box 51.2 Other conditions with which panniculitis has been associated

- Dermatomyositis
- Subcutaneous Sweet syndrome
- Behçet disease
- Rheumatoid arthritis

- Bowel-associated dermatosis-arthritis syndrome
- Sarcoidosis

Rook's Dermatology Handbook, First Edition. Edited by Christopher E. M. Griffiths, Tanya O. Bleiker, Daniel Creamer,
John R. Ingram and Rosalind C. Simpson.
© 2022 John Wiley & Sons Ltd. Published 2022 by John Wiley & Sons Ltd.

Table 51.1 Summary of classification of the panniculitides

	Examples
Predominantly septal panniculitides	
With vasculitis (see Table 51.2)	
Veins	Superficial migratory thrombophlebitis
Arteries	Cutaneous polyarteritis nodosa
No vasculitis (see Table 51.3)	
Lymphocytes and plasma cells predominantly	
With granulomatous infiltrate in septa	Necrobiosis lipoidica
No granulomatous infiltrate in septa	Deep morphoea
Histiocytes predominantly (granulomatous)	
With mucin in centre of palisaded granulomas	Subcutaneous granuloma annulare
With fibrin in centre of palisaded granulomas	Rheumatoid nodule
With large areas of degenerate collagen, foamy histiocytes and cholesterol clefts	Necrobiotic xanthogranuloma
Without mucin, fibrin or degeneration of collagen, but with radial granulomas in septa	Erythema nodosum
Predominantly lobular panniculitides	
With vasculitis (see Table 51.4)	
Small vessels: venules	Erythema nodosum leprosum
	Erythema induratum of Bazin
Large vessels: arteries	Erythema induratum of Bazin (less common)
No vasculitis (see Tables 51.5a and b)	
Few or no inflammatory cells	Sclerosing panniculitis
Necrosis at the centre of the lobule with vascular calcification	Calcific uraemic arteriolopathy (calciphylaxis)
Lymphocytes predominant	
With superficial and deep perivascular dermal infiltrate	Cold panniculitis
With lymphoid follicles, plasma cells and nuclear dust of lymphocytes	Lupus panniculitis
	Panniculitis associated with dermatomyositis
Neutrophils predominant	
Extensive fat necrosis with saponification of adipocytes	Pancreatic panniculitis
With neutrophils between collagen bundles of deep reticular dermis	α_1-antitrypsin deficiency panniculitis
With bacteria, fungi or protozoa	Infective panniculitis
With foreign bodies	Factitious panniculitis
Neutrophilic lobular panniculitis	Subcutaneous Sweet syndrome
Histiocytes predominant (granulomatous)	
No crystals in adipocytes	Subcutaneous sarcoidosis
With crystals in histiocytes or adipocytes	Traumatic panniculitis
	Subcutaneous fat necrosis of the newborn
	Poststeroid panniculitis
	Sclerema neonatorum
	Gouty panniculitis
	Fungal panniculitis due to zygomycosis, mucormycosis and aspergillosis
With cytophagic histiocytes	Cytophagic histiocytic panniculitis and subcutaneous panniculitis-like T-cell lymphoma[a]
With sclerosis of the septa	Sclerosing post-irradiation panniculitis

[a] Although these disorders are characterised by a neoplastic proliferation of cytotoxic T lymphocytes rather than an authentic panniculitic process, they are included in the classification of the panniculitides because they may mimic panniculitis both clinically and histopathologically.

PART 6: SKIN DISORDERS ASSOCIATED WITH SPECIFIC CUTANEOUS STRUCTURE

Table 51.2 Predominantly septal panniculitides with vasculitis

Condition	Superficial migratory thrombophlebitis (Chapter 55)	Cutaneous polyarteritis nodosa (Chapter 54)
Description	Inflammation and thrombosis of superficial veins	Medium-sized vessel vasculitis
Pathophysiology	Caused by a hypercoagulable state; large septal veins affected Most common cause is chronic venous insufficiency	Associated with p-ANCA Medium-sized arteries/arterioles involved at the septa of the upper subcutis
Clinical features	Painful induration with erythema, vessels form cord-like structures (Figure 51.1)	Livedo reticularis/livedo racemosa, ulcerated nodules on lower limbs (Figure 51.2)
Differential diagnosis	Cutaneous polyarteritis nodosa	Superficial migratory thrombophlebitis
Investigations	Rule out hypercoagulable states, paraneoplastic processes (Trousseau sign) and Behçet disease	Direct immunofluorescence Serum ANCA
Management	Treat underlying cause	Tapering high-dose oral corticosteroids, oral steroid sparing agents if required long term

ANCA, anti-neutrophil cytoplasm antibodies.

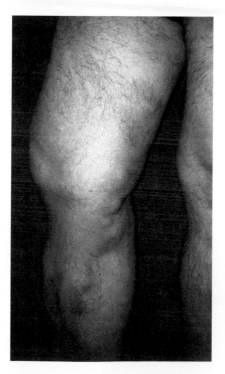

Figure 51.1 Superficial thrombophlebitis. Varicosities and erythematous nodules with linear arrangement involving the right lower extremity.

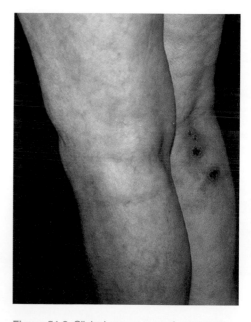

Figure 51.2 Clinical appearance of cutaneous polyarteritis nodosa showing livedo reticularis of the lower extremities with ulcerated nodules on the right calf of a middle-aged woman.

Table 51.3 Predominantly septal panniculitides without vasculitis

	Erythema nodosum	Deep morphoea (Chapter 25)	Subcutaneous granuloma annulare
Description	Most common panniculitis	Group of related diseases, including morphoea profunda, eosinophilic fasciitis and disabling pansclerotic morphoea of children	Rare variant of granuloma annulare affecting children and young adults
Pathophysiology	Common triggers: bacterial infections, sarcoidosis, inflammatory bowel disease Less common: malignancy and medications Miescher radial granulomas are histological hallmark	Characterised by variable fibrosis, sclerosis and atrophy May be an entirely panniculitic process with no involvement of the epidermis or dermis	True panniculitis without dermal involvement, palisading granulomas with mucin in the centre
Clinical features	Peak age 20–30 years F > M Acute onset, erythematous, tender, non-ulcerating nodules/plaques, on lower legs (Figure 51.3) Bruise-like resolution occurs Fever and malaise common	Indurated, hyperpigmented and slightly depressed plaques (Figure 51.4)	Subcutaneous nodules may also have classical granuloma annulare papular lesions Rarely lesions extend to produce destructive arthritis and limb deformity
Differential diagnosis	Behçet disease	Lipoatrophy	Epithelioid sarcoma
Investigations	FBC, ESR, anti-streptolysin O titre, urinalysis, throat swab, CXR (or tuberculin test) Clinical diagnosis can be made without biopsy	Biopsy	Biopsy
Management	Treat underlying cause Usually self-resolving in 3–4 weeks Bed rest, analgesia	No high-quality evidence: methotrexate + intravenous or oral corticosteroids, mycophenolate mofetil	Leave to resolve spontaneously

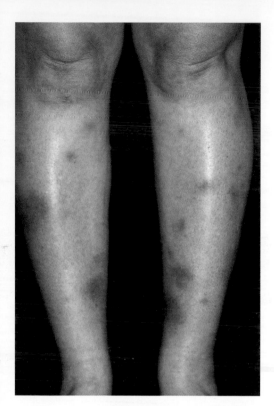

Figure 51.3 Characteristic eruption of erythema nodosum with lesions in different stages of evolution involving the anterior aspect of the legs of an adult woman. Some early lesions consist of bilateral erythematous nodules and plaques, whereas later stage lesions show a bruise-like appearance. Lesions are typically tender.

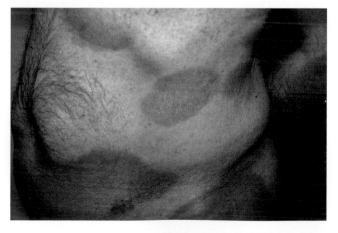

Figure 51.4 Morphoea profunda. The lesions consist of indurated, hyperpigmented and slightly depressed plaques.

Table 51.4 Predominantly lobular panniculitis with vasculitis

Condition	Erythema nodosum leprosum (Chapter 5)	Erythema induratum of Bazin (Chapter 5)
Description	Type II leprosy reaction characterised by a necrotising vasculitis involving small to medium-sized vessels of the deep dermis and subcutis	Chronic recurrent reactive disorder linked to infection with *M. tuberculosis* Commonest form of cutaneous tuberculosis 'Nodular vasculitis' is the term used to differentiate erythema induratum *not* linked to *M. tuberculosis*
Pathophysiology	Immune complex-mediated response to the release of mycobacterial antigen patients with multibacillary leprosy, usually after initiation of treatment Inflammation is predominantly in the dermis with necrotising vasculitis but may extend to subcutis causing panniculitis	Type IV, cell-mediated response hypersensitivity reaction to fragments of tuberculous bacilli There are multiple aetiological associations for cases not associated with tuberculosis Small venules of fat lobules most typically affected, but larger veins of connective tissue less frequently involved
Clinical features	Acute onset of erythematous nodules which may ulcerate	Erythematous nodules/plaques typically on the posterior aspect of the legs of an adult woman (Figure 51.5) Lesions may ulcerate, precipitated by cold weather or venous stasis
Investigations	Nectorising vasculitis on histology See Chapter 5 for investigation of leprosy	Combination of clinical morphology, a positive tuberculin test and evidence of tuberculosis elsewhere in the body, ± biopsy Screen for subclinical active tuberculosis infection Note: Mycobacteria are not cultured from the cutaneous lesions
Management	See Chapter 5 Treat underlying cause, symptomatic management of symptoms	Full specific antituberculous therapy according to current recommended guidelines for systemic tuberculosis Response takes 1–6 months Rest, non-steroidal anti-inflammatory drugs and compression bandaging may be helpful

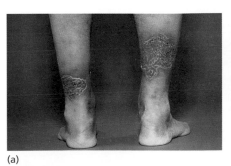
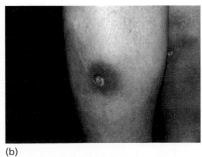

(a)   (b)

Figure 51.5 Clinical features of erythema induratum. (a) Erythematous nodules and plaques on the posterior aspect of the legs of an adult woman. (b) Some of the lesions are ulcerated.

Table **51.5a** Predominantly lobular panniculitis without vasculitis

Condition	Lipodermatosclerosis (Chapter 55)	Calcific uraemic arteriolopathy	Cold panniculitis	Lupus panniculitis (Chapter 23)	Pancreatic panniculitis
Description	Long-term chronic panniculitis associated with chronic venous insufficiency	Life-threatening vasculopathy	Injury to subcutaneous fat induced by cold exposure	Destructive inflammation of subcutaneous fat caused by systemic lupus erythematosus	Panniculitis occurring in association with pancreatitis
Synonyms and inclusions	Sclerosing panniculitis	Calciphylaxis	Equestrian cold panniculitis	Lupus erythematosus profundus; subcutaneous lupus erythematosus	Enzymatic fat necrosis
Epidemiology	Common	1% of patients with chronic renal failure, usually middle aged or elderly, F:M = 4:1	Most common in children	3–5% of patients with discoid lupus erythematosus	2–3% of patients with pancreatic disease; commoner in alcoholic males
Pathophysiology	Venous hypertension increases capillary permeability, causing leakage of fibrinogen and formation of fibrin rings around vessels, with impedance of oxygen exchange and tissue anoxia	Uncertain Calcium deposition in small vessel walls of skin and subcutis Associated with end-stage kidney disease, renal transplantation, diabetes Rarer associations: obesity, warfarin, corticosteroids, connective tissue disease	Exposure to cold causes fat necrosis, Diet high in saturated fatty acids may predispose to the condition as they have a higher freezing point than unsaturated fatty acids	Cutaneous infiltrate primarily in deeper portions of the skin	Pancreatic enzymes probably cause panniculitis with liquefactive necrosis (saponification) of adipocytes Associated with pancreatitis, malignancy, postprocedural, pancreatic anatomical abnormalities

Condition	Lipodermatosclerosis (Chapter 55)	Calcific uraemic arteriolopathy	Cold panniculitis	Lupus panniculitis (Chapter 23)	Pancreatic panniculitis
Clinical features	Diffuse sclerosis and pigmentation of the skin and subcutaneous tissue (lipodermatosclerosis) affecting the lower extremities of middle-aged or elderly women (see Chapter 55)	Irregular tender purpura progresses to full-thickness skin infarction and ulceration Commonly lower extremities and abdomen	Neonates and infants: erythematous/violaceous indurated plaque/nodules, usually cheeks and chin; no systemic symptoms Adults: usually overweight females, lesions occur in thighs and buttocks Also described in horseriders in winter (Figure 51.6)	Indurated sharply defined nodules/ plaques which resolve with localised lipoatrophy Most commonly face, upper arms (Figure 51.7), upper trunk, breasts, buttocks and thighs May see other signs of chronic lupus	Tender, erythematous/ red-brown nodules that spontaneously ulcerate, discharging oily brown liquid (Figure 51.8); commonly affects ankles or lower limbs, arthritis may occur
Differential diagnosis	Bacterial cellulitis/ erysipelas, erythema nodosum	Pyoderma gangrenosum, metastatic cutaneous calcification	Subcutaneous fat necrosis of the newborn, sclerema neonatorum, lupus panniculitis, poststeroid panniculitis, perniosis, frostbite	Dermatomyositis, deep morphoea, panniculitis at the injection sites, subcutaneous panniculitis-like T-cell lymphoma	Erythema induratum, α₁-antitrypsin deficiency and infectious panniculitis
Investigations	Clinical diagnosis unless diagnostic doubt	Full biochemical workup Rule out malignancy	Skin biopsy	Skin biopsy Lupus band on direct immunofluorescence	Skin biopsy; amylase, lipase or trypsin often raised Investigate for other causes, e.g pancreatic carcinoma if indicated
Management	Compression therapy, skin care	Correct biochemical abnormalities, debride necrotic tissue, optimise renal function No universally accepted specific treatment, IV sodium thiosulphate most promising treatment	Usually resolves spontaneously; avoid cold exposure, recommend avoidance of tight-fitting clothes	Treat underlying systemic lupus erythematosus	Treat underlying pancreatic disease

PART 6: SKIN DISORDERS ASSOCIATED WITH SPECIFIC CUTANEOUS STRUCTURE

Table 51.5b Predominantly lobular panniculitis without vasculitis

Condition	α_1-antitrypsin deficiency panniculitis	Infective panniculitis	Factitious (artefactual) panniculitis	Traumatic panniculitis
Description	A genetic disorder characterised by low serum levels of α_1-antitrypsin	Several bacterial and fungal infections may cause panniculitis as their main clinical manifestation	Panniculitis that results from external injury to subcutaneous fat	Damage of subcutaneous tissue induced by physical and chemical agents
Epidemiology	Homozygous PiZZ phenotype 1:3500 in northern Europe		Associated with psychiatric disorders	
Pathophysiology	α_1-antitrypsin is the main protease inhibitor in serum Panniculitis is most severe in patients with homozygous Z allele (PiZZ variant); subcutaneous fat is susceptible to proteolytic degradation when not protected by α_1-antitrypsin	Usually in the immunosuppressed. *Bacterial panniculitis* may occur secondary to septicaemia, direct inoculation or direct spread from underlying infection *Mycobacterial panniculitis* can be caused by haematogenous spread *Fungal panniculitis* may occur secondary to disseminated fungal infection or by direct inoculation following trauma	Vasoconstriction with ischaemia at injection sites and the local inflammatory response probably cause panniculitis May be iatrogenic from injections, cosmetic fillers which biodegrade slowly or are nonresorbable, extravasation of antineoplastic chemotherapy (severe panniculitis) Cupping and acupuncture Factitious occurs secondary to injection of a wide range of substances by patients who are psychiatrically ill	Physical injuries may be from trauma, cold, electricity or chemicals Traumatic separation and devascularisation of subcutaneous fat from its blood supply Causes fat necrosis, which becomes encapsulated

Condition	α₁-antitrypsin deficiency panniculitis	Infective panniculitis	Factitious (artefactual) panniculitis	Traumatic panniculitis
Clinical features	Erythematous nodules and plaques mainly trunk/shoulders/hips May resemble cellulitis, may ulcerate (Figure 51.9) Heals with atrophic scars Chronic relapsing course	*Bacterial*: solitary or multiple nodules due to dissemination of bacteria *Mycobacterial*: may be widespread or show sporotrichoid spread, especially in immunosuppressed (Figure 51.10) *Fungal*: solitary painless nodule that spreads slowly, localised mostly to exposed areas of the skin	Variable, depending on the causative age If factitious: often bizarre appearance, lesions distributed in areas easily accessible to patient's hands If iatrogenic: due to medication injection panniculitis will occur at site of injection of drug	Specific variants: breast masses in women with pendulous breasts; semicircular lipoatrophy on thighs (especially women) Post-traumatic panniculitis may present as a solitary or as multiple subcutaneous nodules Severity of the injury and panniculitis severity usually unrelated
Differential diagnosis	Erythema induratum, pancreatic panniculitis, factitial panniculitis; infective panniculitis	May resemble subcutaneous panniculitis-like T-cell lymphoma	–	–
Investigations	Skin biopsy; reduced α₁-antitrypsin levels	Gram stain, PAS, Ziehl–Neelsen and methenamine–silver, as well as cultures should be performed on skin biopsy sample	Skin biopsy shows intense inflammatory infiltrate and may demonstrate foreign material	Skin biopsy
Management	Avoid surgical debridement (may worsen) Tetracycline antibiotics or dapsone may be helpful for mild cases α₁-antitrypsin replacement in severe cases	Treat underlying infective cause	Wide-spectrum antibiotics may be needed If artefact suspected: occlude area with bandage Intralesional steroid for panniculitis due to cosmetic fillers ± surgical removal of the implanted material Supportive care or withdrawl of responsible injectable drug	Usually self-limiting

PAS, periodic acid-Schiff.

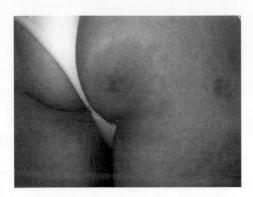

Figure 51.6 Erythematous nodule on gluteal region of a woman with equestrian cold panniculitis.

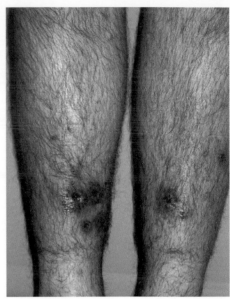

Figure 51.8 Pancreatic panniculitis in an alcoholic male. Nodular lesions, many of them ulcerated around the ankles.

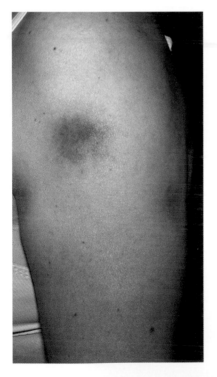

Figure 51.7 Clinical features of lupus panniculitis showing an active erythematous subcutaneous nodule and areas of hyperpigmented lipoatrophy secondary to regressed lesions.

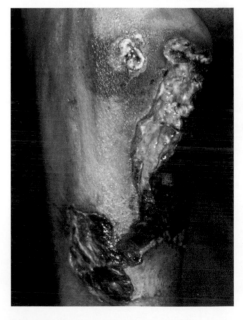

Figure 51.9 Panniculitis associated with α_1-antitrypsin deficiency. Necrotic ulcers exudate oily material that results from necrotic adipocytes.

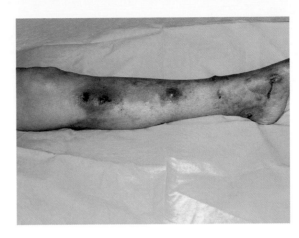

Figure 51.10 Sporotrichoid arrangement of subcutaneous nodules, several of them ulcerated and draining serous or oily discharge in an immunocompromised patient. Cultures isolated *M. chelonae*.

PART 6: SKIN DISORDERS ASSOCIATED WITH SPECIFIC CUTANEOUS STRUCTURE

52

Lipodystrophies and other acquired disorders of subcutaneous fat

Acquired lipodystrophy

Acquired lipodystrophy refers to a heterogeneous group of disorders in which there is generalised, partial or localised loss of subcutaneous fat (Table 52.1).

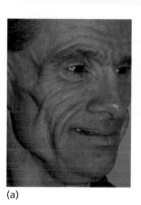
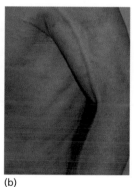
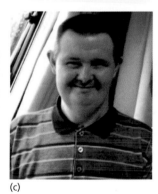

(a)   (b)   (c)

Figure 52.1 Acquired generalised lipodystrophy. (a) Lipoatrophy of the face. (b) Lipoatrophy of the torso and arms. (c) A photograph of the patient taken 5 years earlier, before disease onset. (Source: Aslam A, Savage DB, Coulson IH. Acquired generalised lipodystrophy associated with peripheral T cell lymphoma with cutaneous infiltration. Int J Dermatol 2015, 54, 827–829.)

Rook's Dermatology Handbook, First Edition. Edited by Christopher E. M. Griffiths, Tanya O. Bleiker, Daniel Creamer, John R. Ingram and Rosalind C. Simpson.
© 2022 John Wiley & Sons Ltd. Published 2022 by John Wiley & Sons Ltd.

Table 52.1 Acquired lipodystrophies

	Acquired generalised lipodystrophy	Acquired partial lipodystrophy (Syn. Barraquer-Simons syndrome)	Semicircular lipoatrophy
Epidemiology	Rare Mostly presents in childhood F:M = 3:1	Rare Mostly presents in childhood F:M = 3:1	Rare Presents in the third to fourth decade F > M
Pathophysiology	Mechanism of fat loss is unknown Associated with insulin resistance and impairment of pancreatic β-cell response to glucose	Autoimmune destruction of adipocytes Most patients have C3 nephritic factor C3 levels are low	Repeated mechanical pressure on affected sites causes loss of subcutaneous fat
Clinical features	Generalised loss of fat from face, torso and limbs occurring in childhood Diabetes, acanthosis nigricans and hepatic fibrosis are common (Figure 52.1)	Insidious fat loss starting at face and progressing to torso and arms Legs unaffected One-third of patients develop mesangiocapillary glomerulonephritis ± SLE (Figure 52.2)	Typically localised, transverse, semicircular depressions occur on anterolateral thighs following prolonged leaning against hard surface (e.g. desk edge)
Management	Facial fillers or autologous fat transfer to replace lost volume.	IVIg to treat C3 nephritic factor and mesangiocapillary glomerulonephritis	Remove mechanical pressure

SLE, systemic lupus erythematosus; IVIg, intravenous immunoglobulin.

PART 6: SKIN DISORDERS ASSOCIATED WITH SPECIFIC CUTANEOUS STRUCTURE

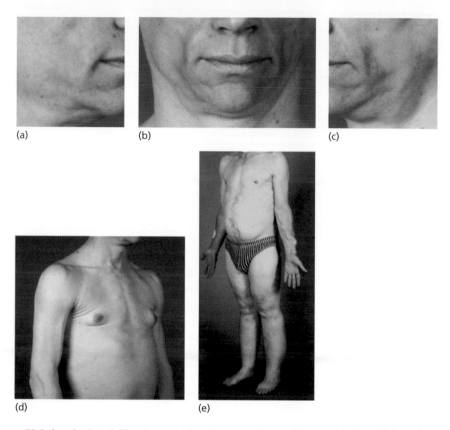

Figure 52.2 Acquired partial lipodystrophy in a 31-year-old man with associated renal failure. (a)–(c) Marked loss of facial fat. (d) Prominence of arm veins and breast tissue resulting from subcutaneous fat loss. (e) Preservation of subcutaneous fat in the lower half of the body.

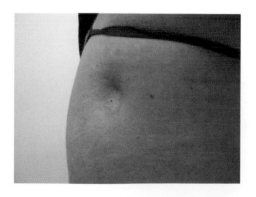

Figure 52.3 Delling of the skin over the right hip due to subcutaneous fat atrophy at the site of depot corticosteroid injection.

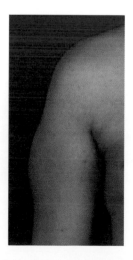

Figure 52.4 Insulin-induced fat hypertrophy of the lateral aspect of the upper arm.

Drug-induced lipodystrophy

Certain drugs are associated with non-inflammatory acquired disorders of subcutaneous fat, as outlined in Table 52.2.

Table 52.2 Drug-induced lipodystrophies

	Corticosteroid-induced localised lipoatrophy	Insulin-induced localised lipoatrophy	Insulin-induced localised fat hypertrophy	HIV-associated lipodystrophy
Epidemiology	A fairly common complication of intralesional corticosteroid injection	Common prior to the introduction of purified human insulin Now rare	Occurs in up to 30% of patients with type 1 diabetes	Prevalence of ~40% HIV-infected individuals
Pathophysiology	Direct traumatic and hormonally-destructive effect of corticosteroid on fat	Impurities in certain insulins can cause local allergic reaction against adipocytes	Caused by anabolic and lipogenic effects of insulin	Protease inhibitors and nucleoside reverse transcriptor inhibitors act by inhibiting lipogenesis and mitochondrial enzymes
Clinical features	Circular depressed plaque which develops weeks to months after injection Overlying erythema and hypopigmentation (Figure 52.3)	Surface contour depression due to loss of subcutaneous fat	Subcutaneous swellings at site of insulin injections (Figure 52.4)	Loss of fat from face, arms and legs Fat gain occurs on breasts, waist and upper back (Figure 52.5)
Management	Infiltration of affected area with normal saline may help	Rotation of insulin injection sites Change to purified human insulin	Change injection sites Change to infusion pump which will reduce insulin requirements	Facial fillers or autologous fat transfer to replace lost volume Liposuction to remove excess fat

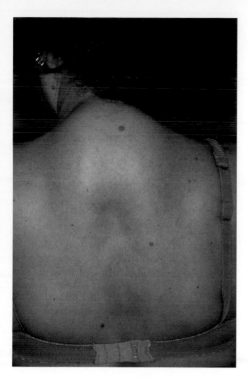

Figure 52.5 Buffalo hump appearance in an HIV patient with lipodystrophy. (Source: Courtesy of Professor L. Requena, Universidad Autónoma de Madrid, Spain.)

Disorders of fat accumulation

A number of disorders are characterised by adipocyte hyperplasia and overgrowth of subcutaneous fat, as outlined in Table 52.3.

Table 52.3 Disorders of fat accumulation

	Benign symmetrical lipomatosis (Syn. Madelung disease)	Dercum disease	Lipoedema
Epidemiology	Rare M > F	Rare Fourth to fifth decade F > M	Occurs at puberty Exclusively in women
Pathophysiology	Adipose tissue in lipomas is indistinguishable from mature fat Lipomas are not encapsulated and have increased vascular and fibrous elements	Differing metabolic activity between painful adipose tissue and unaffected sites may be relevant	Hormonally driven enlargement of the subcutaneous fat compartment Oedema is minimal
Clinical features	Multiple, symmetrical, unencapsulated fat deposits develop on the neck, shoulder girdle and proximal upper and lower extremities (Figure 52.6)	Pain in adipose tissue of limbs, trunk and buttocks in obese individuals Lipomas may be present Pain usually in the medial aspect of affected limbs (Figure 52.7)	Symmetrical enlargement of the legs with sparing of feet Associated with pain, tenderness and easy bruising Lymphoedema may develop
Management	Surgical excision of excess fat	NSAIDs ± intralesional lidocaine or corticosteroid	Manual lymphatic drainage and compression therapy

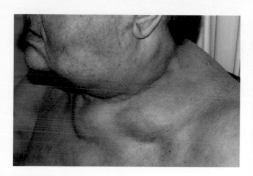

Figure 52.6 Benign symmetrical lipomatosis. Non-tender, fatty deposits around the neck. (Source: Courtesy of Professor L. Requena, Universidad Autónoma de Madrid, Spain.)

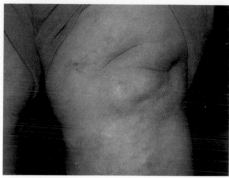

Figure 52.7 Dercum disease. Painful lipomas on the thighs (Source: Courtesy of Professor L. Requena, Universidad Autónoma de Madrid, Spain.)

NORMAL VARIANTS OF FAT ACCUMULATION

Cellulite

Cellulite is an architectural disorder of human adipose tissue characterised by a dimpled and nodular appearance of the skin.

Epidemiology
It is estimated that between 85% and 98% of post-pubertal females display some degree of cellulite. White women are affected more frequently.

Pathophysiology
A genetic predisposition is proposed since most women with cellulite report its occurrence in other family members. Topographically there are herniations of subcutaneous fat through the fibrous connective tissue support matrix. Affected women have a higher percentage of thinner, perpendicularly orientated dermal septa which facilitates herniation of adipose tissue into the reticular dermis. Histopathological specimens demonstrate indentations of subcutaneous fat into the dermis.

Clinical features
There is dimpling and nodularity of the skin of the pelvic region, lower limbs and abdomen. The surface irregularity is especially apparent when the skin is pinched. Cellulite can affect individuals with both high and low body mass index (BMI).

Differential diagnosis
Obesity is characterised by hypertrophy and hyperplasia of adipose tissue that is not necessarily limited to the pelvis, thighs and abdomen. The skin is not dimpled in obesity.

Management
Treatments proposed for cellulite lack substantial proof of efficacy.

First line: Cellulite severity decreases following weight loss in those with higher BMI.

Second line: Topical application of 0.3% retinol for 6 months or more.

Third line: Subcision may temporarily improve cellulite appearance. Liposuction performed superficially (the site of cellulite adipose tissue) carries a risk of necrosis and poor cosmetic outcome. Laser-assisted liposuction and/or laser-assisted lipoplasty are less invasive modalities than traditional liposuction and may be the preferred treatment.

Obesity

As well as metabolic and cardiovascular consequences, obesity exposes people to significant effects on other body systems, including the skin.

Epidemiology

Rates of people being overweight and obese (BMI > 25 kg/m^2) have risen in many countries. In 2013, 62.1% of adults in England were overweight or obese, while 10% of all children entering school (aged 4–5 years) were classified as obese (weight ≥95th centile for age).

Pathophysiology

The hyperinsulinaemia associated with obesity increases androgen production from adipose tissue and reduces the production of sex-hormone-binding globulin, thus increasing circulating free androgen levels. This manifests as an increased incidence of acne, hirsutism, androgenetic alopecia and polycystic ovary syndrome in the obese. Altered adipocytokine secretion in the obese may have an effect on inflammation: delayed-type hypersensitivity responses and psoriasis activity both decline with weight reduction.

Clinical features

Obese patients are susceptible to numerous skin disorders:

- *Hyperhidrosis*: Dissipation of body heat is impaired, which increases the reliance on sweating for thermoregulation.
- *Intertrigo*: Friction, sweating and maceration in body folds can lead to a painful, erosive intertriginous dermatitis with secondary candidosis.
- *Venous insufficiency*: High intra-abdominal pressures will cause lower limb venous hypertension and increase the risk of venous eczema and venous ulceration.
- *Lymphoedema*: The mechanical effects of obesity may impede lymphatic drainage from the lower legs and abdominal apron folds resulting in lymphoedema (Figure 52.8).
- *Keratoderma*: The chronic high pressure exerted on the skin of the soles of the feet may result in plantar hyperkeratosis.
- *Cutaneous infections*: There is an increased prevalence of candidosis, dermatophytosis, erythrasma, folliculitis and furunculosis.

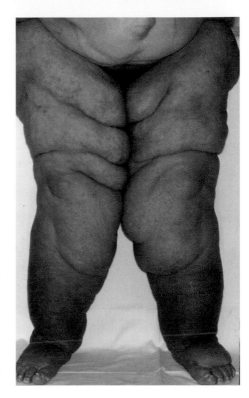

Figure 52.8 Gross obesity with bilateral lymphoedema of lower legs.

Lymphoedema in the obese is commonly complicated by streptococcal cellulitis. Obesity also increases the risk of surgical wound infection and of necrotising fasciitis.

- *Other skin disorders*: Dercum disease (see earlier in this chapter) is strongly associated with obesity. Obesity aggravates a variety of other skin disorders, including hidradenitis suppurativa and pilonidal sinus.

Management

Weight loss will reverse many of the cutaneous sequelae of obesity. Severe obesity-induced skin disorders can be an indication for bariatric surgery.

PART 6: SKIN DISORDERS ASSOCIATED WITH SPECIFIC CUTANEOUS STRUCTURE

Part 7
Vascular Disorders Involving the Skin

Purpura

53

Purpura (bruising) is defined as discoloration of the skin or mucous membranes due to extravasation of red blood cells. Petechiae are small, 1–2 mm, purpuric lesions. Ecchymoses are larger extravasations of blood. Overall causes of purpura are listed in Table 53.1.

Platelet disorders

Specific platelet disorders causing purpura are detailed in Table 53.2.

Pigmented purpuric dermatoses

(Syn. Capillaritis)

Epidemiology
Adults are mainly affected. The commonest subtype, Schamberg disease, affects mainly middle-aged to older men. Purpura annularis telangiectodes occurs in adolescents and young adults, especially women.

Pathophysiology
Inflammation and haemorrhage of capillaries and other superficial papillary dermal vessels are the cause of these diseases.

Clinical features
Table 53.3 details the relevant clinical features.

Investigations
Usually a clinical diagnosis. If there is diagnostic doubt, skin biopsy can be performed for histological confirmation.

Management
First line: Reassurance, no active treatment.

Second line: Support hosiery if lower limbs involved.
Third line: Phototherapy, topical steroid/topical calcineurin inhibitor.

Cryogobulinaemia (see Chapter 54)

Cryoglobulins are immunoglobulins that reversibly precipitate (gel) in the cold, resulting in vascular occlusive syndromes in the skin. Occlusion syndromes triggered by cold exposure are suggested by an acral distribution of lesions of necrosis or purpura, often with retiform features, and sometimes associated with acral livedo reticularis. Other reported cutaneous findings include acral cyanosis, Raynaud phenomenon, urticarial lesions, involvement of ears or nose and ulceration. There may be associated arthritis or arthralgia. For more details see the cryogobulinaemic vasculitis section of Chapter 54.

Livedoid vasculopathy/ atrophie blanche

Epidemiology
This syndrome is common as either an idiopathic or secondary syndrome, particularly affecting young to middle-aged women. It can occur in association with chronic venous hypertension and varicosities. Antiphospholipid syndrome (APLS), with or without a lupus association, can produce the clinical syndrome.

Pathophysiology
The pathogenesis of livedoid vasculopathy is unknown in the absence of APLS. Skin biopsy

Rook's Dermatology Handbook, First Edition. Edited by Christopher E. M. Griffiths, Tanya O. Bleiker, Daniel Creamer, John R. Ingram and Rosalind C. Simpson.
© 2022 John Wiley & Sons Ltd. Published 2022 by John Wiley & Sons Ltd.

Table 53.1 Causes of purpura and ecchymosis

Platelet disorders	Coagulation disorders	Microvascular occlusion	Mechanical	Inflammation	External/other causes
Thrombocytopenia	Inherited, e.g. haemophilia or acquired factor deficiency	Dysproteinaemias, e.g. hypergammaglobulinaemic purpura	Raised intravascular pressure, e.g. gravitational purpura (lower leg), tourniquet stasis	Vasculitis, e.g. Henoch–Schönlein purpura	Physical, e.g. exercise-induced
Abnormal platelet function	Drugs, e.g. anticoagulants	Cryoproteinaemias	Decreased support, e.g. actinic or corticosteroid purpura, scurvy, amyloidosis	Capillaritis: idiopathic, drug-induced, pre-mycotic	Artefactual causes (including possible child abuse)
Thrombocytosis	Localised, e.g. heparin injection sites/some insect bites	Emboli: crystal, fat, myxoma, infective	Inherited disorders of connective tissue, e.g. pseudoxanthoma elasticum	Non-thrombocytopenic toxin- and drug-induced purpura	Easy bruising syndrome and purpura simplex
	Metabolic, e.g. vitamin K deficiency		Abnormal vasculature	Purpura associated with infections	Paroxysmal finger haematoma (Achenbach syndrome)
	Thrombophilias, e.g. protein C deficiency		Purpura around vascular lesions, e.g. tufted angioma	Contact purpura	Painful bruising (autoerythrocyte sensitisation)
	Disseminated intravascular coagulopathy and purpura fulminans			Actinic purpura	
	Secondary to systemic disease				

Table 53.2 Platelet disorders causing purpura

Thrombocytopaenia (decreased platelet numbers)	Abnormal platelet function	Thrombocytosis (increased platelet numbers)
Defective platelet production due to bone marrow aplasia (toxic, immunological, idiopathic), neoplasia (leukaemia, myeloma, carcinomatosis) or replacement (myelofibrosis, radiation damage, sarcoidosis)	Inherited and congenital, e.g. Von Willebrand disease, hereditary haemorrhagic telangiectasia, Wiskott–Aldrich syndrome (δ-granule abnormality)	Essential thrombocythaemia, including polycythaemia vera
Other impaired production: Wiskott–Aldrich syndrome, vitamin B12 or folate deficiency	Drug-induced	Other myeloproliferative syndromes
Metabolic: uraemia, alcohol, drugs	Uraemia	Blood loss, trauma, burns
Infections, sepsis syndrome	Cardiac bypass	Post-splenectomy
Diminished platelet survival due to antibodies: neonatal/post-transfusion/intravenous immunoglobulin; autoantibodies in idiopathic thrombocytopenic purpura, marrow transplant, antiphospholipid syndrome, systemic lupus erythematosus	Dysproteinaemias (especially IgA myeloma and macroglobulinaemia)	Malignant disease
Mechanical: prosthetic heart valves	Myeloproliferative disorders	Tuberculosis
Drugs, including heparin necrosis, and vaccines	Cold-stored (blood bank) platelets	Sarcoidosis
Excessive platelet consumption: disseminated intravascular coagulation, haemangioma, haemolytic–uraemic syndrome, thrombotic thrombocytopenic purpura		
Sequestration: splenomegaly, hypothermia		

demonstrates hyaline changes in the walls of superficial dermal vessels and luminal fibrin deposition; intraluminal thrombus is usually found.

Clinical features

Persistent, very painful and often punched-out ulcerations of the legs, especially around the malleoli, in women are typical features and the disease is bilateral in most cases. Healing results in a porcelain-white scar (atrophie blanche), frequently surrounded by telangiectasia.

Differential diagnosis

Venous and arterial insufficiency, rheumatoid arthritis, cutaneous vasculitides and malignant atrophic papulosis.

Table 53.3 Presentation of different pigmented purpuric dermatoses

Syndrome	Clinical features	Location
Schamberg disease	Orange-red flat patches with 'cayenne pepper' spots on the borders Old lesions become yellow-brown patches (Figure 53.1) Oval or irregular outline pinpoint petechiae inside patches Successive crops	Usually lower legs; also involves trunk, arms, thighs and buttocks Irregularly distributed on both sides with few or many patches
Itching purpura	Pruritic, scaly petechial or purpuric macules, papules and patches Appears similar to Schamberg disease	Usually lower extremities
Pigmented purpuric lichenoid dermatosis of Gougerot and Blum	Combination of Schamberg-like and purpuric red-brown lichenoid thickened papules Chronic, can be pruritic	Usually lower extremities
Lichen aureus	Isolated, persistent patch Varying colour, purple-brown to golden or rust	Usually lower extremities Commonly overlies a varicose vein
Purpura annularis telangiectodes (Majocchi disease)	Annular brown plaques, 1–3 cm in size. Plaques gradually spread outwards Punctuate telangiectases and petechiae inside border	Trunk, lower extremities (proximal)
Contact allergy		Only affects skin in contact with material responsible (e.g. clothing dye, rubber)
Exercise-induced	Crops of small red spots following prolonged or vigorous exercise Fade to brown and disappear within days Possible burning sensation accompanies new lesions	Commonly on ankles

Investigations

Lividoid vasculopathy is primarily a clinical diagnosis. If there is diagnostic doubt, consider skin biopsy and direct immunofluorescence, as well as blood tests for lupus anticoagulant, anticardiolipin antibodies and rheumatoid factor.

Management

First line: Stop smoking (if relevant), compression hosiery.

Second line: Aspirin.

Third line: Fibrinolytic agents, anticoagulants.

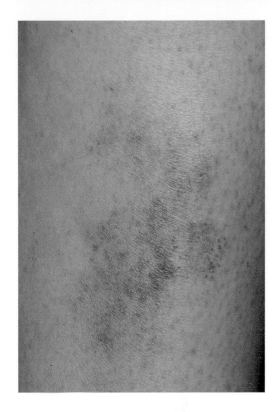

Figure 53.1 Schamberg disease on the shin, showing yellow-brown patches. (Source: Courtesy of Dr Richard Motley, Cardiff & Vale University Health Board.)

Calcific uraemic arteriolopathy

(Syn. Cutaneous calciphylaxis)

Calcific uraemic arteriolopathy is a complication of renal failure and dialysis, associated with high mortality rates and characterised by painful skin ulceration.

Epidemiology

The condition is rare. Highest prevalence is in the sixth decade and there is a F:M ratio of 4:1. While nearly all patients have renal failure, there are also very rare independent associations with alcoholic liver disease and chemotherapy.

Pathophysiology

Most patients have secondary or tertiary hyperparathyroidism. Additional risk factors include obesity, liver disease, corticosteroid use and elevated calcium–phosphate product. Histopathologically, there is calcification in the medial layer of the wall of small subcutaneous vessels, with necrosis of overlying tissue.

Clinical features

Early lesions tend to present as painful purpuric plaques, often with a retiform or stellate pattern, and may show central necrosis. Some may become semi-confluent as a 'broken' livedo. The abdomen, anterior thighs and hips are typical sites but the breasts may be involved, and in some patients the disease is mainly acral. Mineral-hard induration with extending ulcer and eschar formation typically develops.

Investigations

Deep skin biopsy, blood tests for renal function, liver function, calcium, phosphate and parathyroid hormone; plain radiograph typically shows extensive vascular calcification.

Differential diagnosis

Skin lesions may resemble the lesions of hyperoxaluria, cryoglobulinaemia, antiphospholipid syndrome and cutaneous vasculitides.

Management

The prognosis is generally considered poor, with a mortality of 50–80%.

First line: Good wound care, low-calcium dialysate fluids and non-calcium oral phosphate binders.

Second line: Sodium thiosulphate, cinacalcet hydrochloride.

Third line: Parathyroidectomy.

Vasculitis

54

The vasculitides are classified according to the size of vessel which is involved: small, medium, or large. Cutaneous vasculitis often results in painful, palpable purpura in which leakage of blood from the vasculature into the interstitium causes petechiae or purpura (failure to blanch on diascopy). The other skin sign which occurs commonly in vasculitis is livedo reticularis, either a completely reticulate livedo or a broken livedo (incomplete net).

Some or all of the investigations in Table 54.1 should be undertaken if vasculitis is suspected. The purpose of investigation is twofold: first to look for evidence of vasculitis in other organ systems, and second to identify an underlying disorder which predisposes towards vasculitis.

Table 54.1 Investigations to be undertaken if vasculitis is suspected

Investigation	Notes
Blood and urine tests	
Urinalysis	Haematuria and proteinuria in renal involvement
Urea and electrolytes	Raised creatinine and urea in renal involvement
Full blood count	Raised white cells in infection/cryoglobulinaemia Thrombocytopenia may cause purpura
Liver function	Low albumin in renal disease
Erythrocyte sedimentation rate	May be raised in systemic vasculitis, infection and malignancy
C-reactive protein	May be raised in infections
ANCA	May be present in systemic vasculitides (see text)
Antinuclear antibodies Complement C3 and C4	May be present in autoimmune connective tissue disease May be reduced in active vasculitis Low C4 level with normal C3 is typical in cryoglobulinaemic vasculitis
Specialist haematological tests for thromboembolic disease, such as lupus anticoagulant and anticardiolipin antibodies	If thrombo-occlusive disease is possible from the history, examination or histology
Cryoglobulins	If there is skin, kidney and joint vasculitis Not necessarily triggered by cold See section on cryoglobulinaemic vasculitis for method of transporting blood for cryoglobulin analysis

(Continued)

Rook's Dermatology Handbook, First Edition. Edited by Christopher E. M. Griffiths, Tanya O. Bleiker, Daniel Creamer, John R. Ingram and Rosalind C. Simpson.

Table 54.1 (Continued)

Investigation	Notes
Tissue tests	
Skin biopsy from early lesion (less than 48 h old) for histopathology Biopsy lesional skin	Indicates if rash is vasculitis or a thromboembolic disorder Histology also indicates size of blood vessel involvement, predominant inflammatory cell type and presence of granulomas
Skin biopsy from early lesion for direct immunofluorescence	Indicates if IgA vasculitis
Skin biopsy for culture	May be useful for chronic infections, e.g. TB
Infection	
Infection screen: cultures, serology and radiology HIV, hepatitis B and C	Depends on age, history of travel and country of residence, history and examination Screen for acute and/or chronic infections Should be excluded in all patients with vasculitis
Malignancy	
Malignancy screen: blood tests and radiology for malignancy	Relevant tests depend on the age of patient, history and examination
Inflammatory disease	
Investigations for other systemic inflammatory disease	If diseases (e.g. inflammatory bowel disease, rheumatoid arthritis) are suspected from history and examination

ANCA, antineutrophil cytoplasmic antibody.

SMALL VESSEL VASCULITIDES

Cutaneous small-vessel vasculitis

(Syn. Leucocytoclastic vasculitis)

Epidemiology
Incidence is 15–30 cases/million/year. Age of onset: second to eighth decades.

Pathophysiology
In 50% of cases cutaneous small-vessel vasculitis (CSVV) is triggered by an infectious pathogen or a medication (culprits in drug-induced cases include the penicillins and propylthiouracil). The other 50% of cases are idiopathic. Immune complexes are deposited in the walls of small cutaneous vessels leading to activation of complement (C3a and C5a), which attracts neutrophils. Histopathology shows leukocytoclastic vasculitis: swelling of the endothelium, fibrinoid necrosis of vessel walls, extravasation of erythrocytes and an infiltrate of neutrophils with leukocytoclasia.

Clinical features
The major skin manifestation is palpable purpura, ranging from 1 mm to several centimetres in size. Crops of purpura arise simultaneously on areas prone to stasis, commonly the lower legs (Figure 54.1), and are sometimes associated with ankle oedema. CSVV is often asymptomatic, although pruritus, pain or burning may occur, as well as fever, arthralgia and myalgia. Usually macular in the early stages, the purpura or petechiae may progress to papules, nodules, vesicles, plaques, bullae or pustules (Figure 54.2). Necrosis and ulceration may

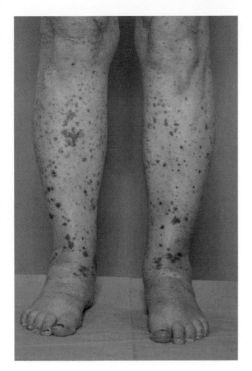

Figure 54.1 Cutaneous small-vessel vasculitis producing palpable purpura. (Source: Courtesy of Andrew Carmichael.)

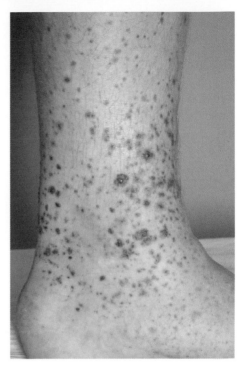

Figure 54.2 Cutaneous small vessel vasculitis demonstrating a haemorrhagic vesicle. (Source: Courtesy of Andrew Carmichael.)

follow. Lesions resolve within weeks to months. 10% of patients have recurrent disease.

Investigations
See above, including skin biopsy.

Management
First line: Remove or treat a triggering agent (e.g. drug or infection). Minimise venous stasis with the elevation of dependent areas and use of compression hosiery. If modest skin involvement, manage with supportive care only. In more severe cases, use oral prednisolone 0.5 mg/kg/day for 2 weeks, tapering over a further 2 weeks.

Second line: Colchicine or dapsone. Alternatively, immunosuppressant agents, such as azathioprine or methotrexate.

IgA vasculitis

(Syn. Henoch–Schönlein purpura)

Epidemiology
Annual incidence is 10–20/100 000/year in children, and about 1–1.5/100 000/year in adults. The peak incidence is between the ages of 4 and 6 years. Adult-onset immunoglobulin A (IgA) vasculitis can occur at any age.

Pathophysiology
IgA vasculitis is an immune complex vasculitis characterised by IgA1-dominant immune deposits affecting small vessels of the skin, kidney and other organs. There are increased levels of IgA in the serum and circulating IgA-containing immune complexes.

Clinical features
IgA vasculitis manifests at the outset with purpura, arthralgia and abdominal pain. The presentation may be identical to CSVV. It typically involves the extensor aspects of the legs, buttocks and arms (Figure 54.3) in a symmetrical fashion. Dusky urticarial papules, vesicles,

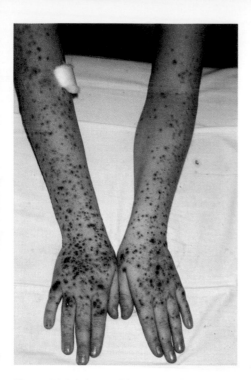

Figure 54.3 IgA vasculitis on upper limbs.

bullae and necrotic ulcers may also develop. Renal involvement occurs in 40–50% of patients (haematuria and proteinuria), gastrointestinal involvement in 65% (30% develop gastrointestinal bleeding) and painful arthritis in 75% (most frequently knees and ankles). Individual skin lesions usually fade within 5–7 days but crops of lesions can recur for a few weeks to several months.

Investigations
See above. Biopsy the involved skin of a fresh lesion. A sample should be sent for direct immunofluorescence as well as routine histology. Although perivascular IgA deposits are characteristic this finding is not specific for IgA vasculitis.

Management
The condition is usually self-limiting. Systemic corticosteroid treatment may be effective in the treatment of abdominal pain, arthritis and nephritis. As in all forms of vasculitis with systemic involvement refer to the appropriate internal physician.

First line: Prednisolone 0.5 mg/kg/day for 2 weeks, tapering over a further 2 weeks.
Second line: If needed consider pulsed intravenous methylprednisolone, ciclosporin A, cyclophosphamide, azathioprine, mycophenolate mofetil.

Cryoglobulinaemic vasculitis

Epidemiology
A rare form of vasculitis. About 80% of cryoglobulinaemic vasculitis cases are secondary to hepatitis C infection.

Pathophysiology
Cryoglobulins are immunoglobulins that precipitate spontaneously when serum is cooled to a temperature below 37°C. In cryoglobulinaemic vasculitis cryoglobulins are deposited as immune complexes in small vessels of the skin, joints, peripheral nerves and kidneys. As well as hepatitis C infection, other causes include B-cell lymphoproliferative disorders, autoimmune diseases (e.g. Sjögren syndrome), other viral disorders (hepatitis B, HIV) and essential mixed cryoglobulinaemia. Cryoglobulins may be divided into three main subtypes:

1. Monoclonal immunoglobulin, usually IgG or IgM, accounts for about 10–25% of cases and is usually associated with lymphoproliferative disease, especially multiple myeloma or Waldenström macroglobulinaemia.
2. Mixed polyclonal (usually IgG) immunoglobulin and monoclonal (usually IgM-κ) immunoglobulin, the latter having rheumatoid factor activity, accounts for about 25% of cases.
3. Polyclonal IgM with rheumatoid factor activity and polyclonal IgG with antigenic activity account for about 50–65% of cases.

Histologically there is a leucocytoclastic vasculitis of arteries and veins that may extend into the subcutis.

Clinical features
Palpable purpura is universal (Figure 54.4). Bullae, necrotic ulcers and retiform purpura may also develop. Myalgia, headache, fever, weight loss, sensorimotor neuropathy and

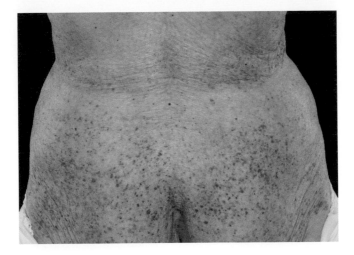

Figure 54.4 Cryoglobulinaemic vasculitis.

ononeuritis multiplex are common. Renal involvement is usually in the form of membranoproliferative glomerulonephritis, and presents with nephrotic range proteinuria.

Investigations
See above, including skin biopsy. For the assay of serum cryoglobulins, care should be taken to ensure that the patient's blood is transported to the laboratory at 37°C. A low complement C4 level with a near normal C3 is typical in cryoglobulinaemic vasculitis. Rheumatoid factor is positive in high titres. Check for hepatitis B and C serology.

Management
First line: Prednisolone 0.5 mg/kg/day for 2 weeks, and tapering with response. In patients with hepatitis C infection, treat with combination of glucocorticoids, antiviral therapy and immunomodulatory agents.
Second line: Rituximab.

Hypocomplementaemic urticarial vasculitis

(Syn. Anti-C1q vasculitis)

Epidemiology
A very rare form of vasculitis. F > M. Most commonly presents in fourth decade, but childhood cases have been described.

Pathophysiology
In hypocomplementaemic urticarial vasculitis (HUV) small-vessel vasculitis is accompanied by urticaria and hypocomplementaemia. It is associated with anti-C1q antibodies. The serum of patients with HUV contains polyclonal IgG with C1q precipitin activity within the Fab fragments. These IgG antibodies are directed against the collagen-like region of C1q, resulting in a reduction of C1q in the serum and subsequent activation of the complement pathway. Lesions of urticarial vasculitis typically show leukocytoclastic vasculitis.

Clinical features
Characterised by indurated weals containing purpuric foci which are painful, itchy and persist for more than 24 h (Figure 54.5). HUV weals resolve with areas of discoloration, bruising or pigmentation. Angio-oedema is common and may be a presenting feature. Glomerulonephritis, arthritis, obstructive pulmonary disease and ocular inflammation are common.

Investigations
See above, including skin biopsy. Check C3, C4, antinuclear antibody and antibodies to double-stranded DNA.

Management
First line: Antihistamine + prednisolone (0.5 mg/kg/day for 2 weeks, tapering over a further 2 weeks).

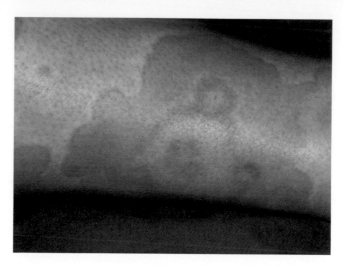

Figure 54.5 Urticarial vasculitis.

Second line: Dapsone or colchicine or hydroxychloroquine.

ANCA-associated vasculitides

The antineutrophil cytoplasmic antibody (ANCA)-associated vasculitides (AAVs) are a group of conditions characterised by their association with the presence of antibodies directed against proteinase 3 (PR3) and myeloperoxidase (MPO) (Table 54.2). PR3 and MPO are proteins that serve as antigens inside the azurophilic granules in the cytoplasm of a neutrophil.

MEDIUM VESSEL VASCULITIDES

Polyarteritis nodosa and cutaneous polyarteritis nodosa

Polyarteritis nodosa (PAN) is a rare necrotising arteritis of medium or small arteries. Cutaneous PAN (cPAN) is a single-organ vasculitis which can be considered a limited expression of PAN and does not exhibit systemic involvement.

Epidemiology
The peak age is between 40 and 60 years of age.

Pathophysiology
PAN can be the first manifestation of hepatitis B and occurs in most cases within 6 months of infection. Histologically there is a neutrophilic inflammatory infiltrate in the walls of medium-sized arteries and arterioles. Involved vessels demonstrate a target-like appearance from an eosinophilic ring of fibrinoid necrosis.

Clinical features
Painful dermal or subcutaneous nodules are located on the lower legs near the malleoli, but can extend proximally to the thighs, buttocks, arms or hands. The nodules may ulcerate (Figure 54.9). Livedo reticularis is common (Figure 54.9); broken livedo is typical in cutaneous PAN. In severe cases of systemic PAN reti-form purpura may develop. Gangrene of the digits can also occur.

Systemic features
Systemic PAN
Headache, fever, arthralgia, myalgia, weight loss, hypertension, myocardial infarction, abdominal pain, intestinal infarction, arterial

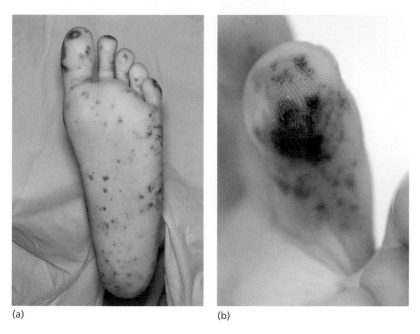

(a)   (b)

Figure 54.6 Granulomatosis with polyangiitis. (a) Acral purpura (b) Cutaneous infarction at tip of digit.

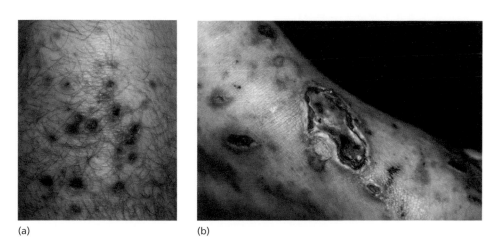

(a)   (b)

Figure 54.7 Granulomatosis with polyangiitis. (a) Ulcerated lesions of cutaneous small-vessel vasculitis. (b) Larger ulcerated lesions with background vasculitis.

PART 7: VASCULAR DISORDERS INVOLVING THE SKIN

Table 54.2 The ANCA-associated vasculitides

	Microscopic polyangiitis	Granulomatosis with polyangiitis (Syn. Wegener granulomatosis)	Eosinophilic granulomatosis with polyangiitis (Syn. Churg–Strauss syndrome)
Epidemiology	Incidence 2.5–10/million/year, rising to 45/million/year in 65+ years age group	Incidence 3–10/million/year May be a latitudinal divide: GPA more common in northern than southern latitudes In children, median age of onset is 14 years; in adulthood 50–59 years	Incidence 1–2.5 per million/year In known asthma sufferers incidence may be 67/million/year Peak incidence around the age of 50; very rare in children
Pathophysiology	ANCA has a prime role in the pathogenesis Necrotising vasculitis of small vessels causes glomerulonephritis, pulmonary vasculitis and skin signs	ANCA has a prime role in the pathogenesis Necrotising vasculitis of small to medium vessels with granulomatous inflammation of upper and lower respiratory tract accompanies glomerulonephritis and skin signs	Allergy probably plays a central role with the inflammatory response being primarily Th2 As with MPA and GPA, ANCA also has a pathogenetic role Necrotising vasculitis of small to medium vessels with extravascular granulomas occurs in conjunction with asthma and eosinophilia Also causes glomerulonephritis
Clinical features	Fever, weight loss, myalgia, arthralgia, palpable purpura, digital infarcts, splinter haemorrhages, oral ulcers, livedo reticularis Also pulmonary involvement (pulmonary haemorrhage) and renal involvement	Palpable purpura, papulo-necrotic lesions and ulcers on limbs and extremities (Figures 54.6 and 54.7) Oral ulcers can occur and pyoderma gangrenosum-like lesions URT: otitis, epistaxis, rhinorrhoea, sinusitis, nasal mucosal inflammation (leading to saddle nose deformity) LRT: cough, dyspnoea, haemoptysis Also renal involvement	Palpable purpura, nodules on limbs and scalp, livedo reticularis, retiform purpura, necrotic ulcers (Figure 54.8), Raynaud phenomenon, migratory erythema URT: allergic rhinitis and nasal polyps LRT: asthma Also renal, cardiac, neurological involvement

Investigations	See above for vasculitis investigations ANCA: PR3 or MPO Skin biopsy: leucocytoclastic vasculitis Chest X-ray ± high-resolution chest CT scan	See above for vasculitis investigations ANCA: PR3 or MPO Skin biopsy: leucocytoclastic vasculitis ± granulomatous inflammation Chest X-ray ± high-resolution chest CT scan	See above for vasculitis investigations ANCA: PR3 or MPO Skin biopsy: leucocytoclastic vasculitis of both arteries and veins, extravascular granulomas, tissue eosinophilia Blood: eosinophilia (a requisite for diagnosis) Chest X-ray ± high-resolution chest CT scan
Management	Systemic corticosteroid ± cyclophosphamide	Systemic corticosteroid + methotrexate or cyclophosphamide	Systemic corticosteroid or cyclophosphamide

ANCA, antineutrophil cytoplasmic antibody; GPA, granulomatosis with polyangiitis; LRT: lower respiratory tract; MPA, microscopic polyangiitis; MPO, myeloperoxidase; PR3, proteinase 3; URT: upper respiratory tract.

aneurysms, renal impairment, cerebrovascular ischaemia, peripheral neuropathy.

Cutaneous PAN

Mild constitutional symptoms. Occasionally can be associated with extra-cutaneous complications, e.g. mononeuritis multiplex.

Differential diagnosis

ANCA-associated vasculitis, non-vasculitic vascular occlusion (e.g. antiphospholipid syndrome), panniculitis, nodular vasculitis, erythema induratum.

Investigations

See above, including a deep skin biopsy. Diagnosis of PAN requires histological evidence of medium-sized artery vasculitis. ANCA is negative. Screening for potential infective triggers should be undertaken. Biopsies can be taken from other symptomatic organs. If biopsies are unsupportive, visceral angiography may identify multiple microaneurysms suggesting systemic PAN.

Management

Systemic PAN. Combination of cyclophosphamide and systemic corticosteroids. For patients with hepatitis B-associated PAN: high-dose corticosteroids for 2 weeks, followed by antiviral treatment and plasma exchange.

Cutaneous PAN. *First line:* Non-steroidal anti-inflammatory drugs and compression hosiery. Prednisolone 0.5 mg/kg/day for 2 weeks, and tapering with response.
Second line: Methotrexate.

OTHER SKIN DISORDERS CHARACTERISED BY VASCULITIS

Kawasaki disease

(Syn. Mucocutaneous lymph node syndrome)

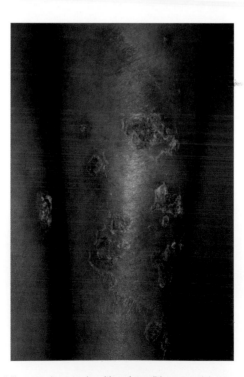

Figure 54.8 Esosinophilic granulomatosis with polyangiitis: necrotising vasculitis with ulceration.

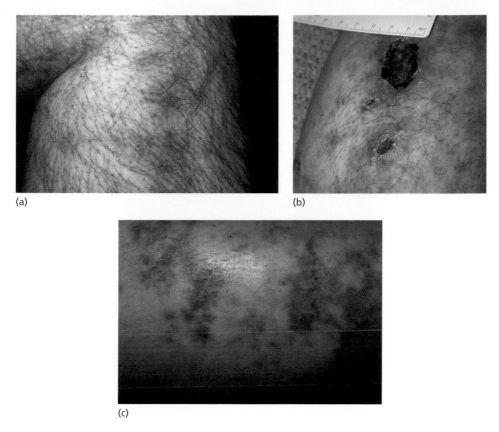

(a)

(b)

(c)

Figure 54.9 Cutaneous polyarteritis nodosa. (a) Erythematous nodules on the lower leg. (b) Vasculitic ulcers. (c) Necrotising livedo of the leg.

The 2012 Chapel Hill Consensus defined Kawasaki disease as an arteritis associated with the mucocutaneous lymph node syndrome and predominantly affecting medium and small arteries.

Epidemiology

The disease almost always occurs in children. There is a mild male predilection. The disease is much more common in Asia, particularly in Japan. In 2010 the incidence in Japan was 240/100,000/year for children aged less than 5 years. UK incidence for the same age group is 8.4/100,000/year.

Pathophysiology

Thought to be due to an inflammatory response to an unidentified infectious agent in genetically susceptible hosts. The angiitis affects nearly all organs, with a high frequency of cardiac involvement. Predominantly a vasculitis of medium-sized arteries, but can involve smaller and larger calibre blood vessels. The inflammatory process results in breakdown of internal and external elastic laminae resulting in aneurysms, thrombosis, scarring and stenosis of the affected blood vessel. A functional polymorphism of the *ITPKC* (inositol-1,4,5-trisphosphate 3-kinase C) gene on chromosome 19q13.2 is significantly associated with a susceptibility to Kawasaki disease and coronary artery aneurysms.

Clinical features

Occurs typically in infants and children less than 5 years of age. Patients present with at least 5 days of fever, irritability, vomiting, anorexia, cough, diarrhoea, runny nose, weakness and abdominal and joint pain. The initial acute phase is characterised by acral and perianal erythema and acral oedema. The dermatosis is particularly prominent in the nappy area, where there is marked erythema and early desquamation. Cheilitis causes the lips to be fissured. There is a strawberry tongue and cervical lymphadenopathy, typically a single large cervical node. Eye involvement leads to conjunctivitis and anterior uveitis. The fever is spiking and unresponsive to paracetamol. The febrile stage lasts up to 2 weeks and is followed by a second phase lasting 4–6 weeks when the risk of death from coronary aneurysms is greatest. In the convalescent stage a distinctive pattern of desquamation occurs, beginning at the tips of the fingers and progressing proximally. Convalescence takes up to 3 months and is characterised by a normalisation of the ESR and CRP levels. Larger aneurysms may expand, leading to myocardial infarction in the convalescent phase. Those with established heart disease may enter a chronic phase with a risk of late aneurysm rupture even in adult life.

Deaths may occur due to myocarditis, dysrhythmias, pericarditis, rupture of aneurysms and occlusion of coronary arteries. Coronary aneurysms are demonstrated in around 20% of patients (and in 90% of those who die); some will regress (potentially with stenosis) but giant aneurysms (>80 mm) may require bypass surgery.

Differential diagnosis

Scarlet fever, systemic-onset juvenile idiopathic arthritis and erythema multiforme can mimic Kawasaki disease, as can other localised and systemic infections. The diagnosis should be suspected in a child with prolonged fever.

Investigations

There are no diagnostic tests and Kawasaki disease remains a clinical diagnosis.

Management

Patients should be treated in a specialist paediatric unit. Aspirin and intravenous immunoglobulin (IVIg) are the mainstay of treatment.

First line: IVIg and aspirin should be given early. Early IVIg reduces the coronary aneurysm risk from around 25% to less than 5%. Delaying IVIg beyond day 10 of fever increases the risk of death, particularly in boys under 1 year old. IVIg is given as a single dose of 2 g/kg over 12 h. Aspirin 100 mg/kg/day is given initially until the fever has settled and is then reduced to 3–5 mg/kg/day for 6–8 weeks in those with no cardiac abnormality, but longer in those with coronary aneurysms.

Second line: For children who remain febrile 36 h after the first dose of IVIg, a further dose of 2 g/kg can be given. Patients who are unresponsive to IVIg can be treated with high-dose prednisolone 2 mg/kg/day, which should be tapered after normalisation of the CRP.

Erythema elevatum diutinum

Erythema elevatum diutinum (EED) is a rare, chronic, cutaneous eruption which has the histological features of CSVV.

Epidemiology

Occurs most commonly in adults, fourth to seventh decades.

Pathophysiology

EED has been associated with autoimmune diseases, multiple myeloma, myelodysplasia, pyoderma gangrenosum and relapsing polychondritis. Histologically, acute lesions are characterised by leukocytoclastic vasculitis with tissue eosinophilia. Chronic lesions demonstrate angiocentric eosinophilic fibrosis, capillary proliferation and infiltration of macrophages, plasma cells and lymphocytes.

Clinical features

Lesions of EED are red-blue or red-brown papules, plaques and nodules occurring most commonly over the dorsa of the hands, knees, buttocks and Achilles tendons (Figure 54.10). Initially, the lesions are soft, but eventually

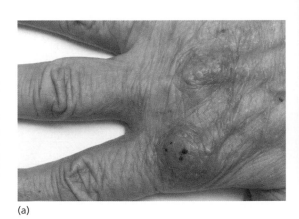

(a)

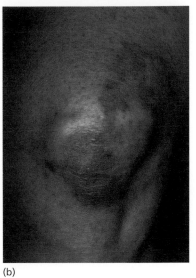

(b)

Figure 54.10 Erythema elevatum diutinum. (a) On the hands. (b) On the knee.

fibrose to leave atrophic scars. Lesions of EED may be painful.

Differential diagnosis
Sweet's syndrome, sarcoidosis, rheumatoid nodules.

Investigations
Skin biopsy.

Management
High potency topical corticosteroid or intralesional corticosteroid. Dapsone is often effective.

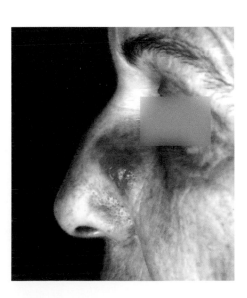

Figure 54.11 Granuloma faciale. Reddish brown plaque on the nose (Source: Courtesy of Dr G. Dawn, Monklands Hospital, UK).

Granuloma faciale

Granuloma faciale (GF) is an inflammatory condition of facial skin with the histological features of CSVV.

Epidemiology
Rare. Most common in 40–60-year-olds. M > F.

Pathophysiology
GF is a histological variant of leukocytoclastic vasculitis accompanied by a prominent eosinophilic infiltrate. The vascular changes may be mild (perivascular distribution of inflammatory cells) or florid (leucocytoclastic vasculitis with fibrinoid necrosis).

Clinical features
Soft, smooth, red-brown nodules or plaques occur at any facial site (Figure 54.11). They are usually asymptomatic. Multiple lesions are present in one-third of cases. The surface demonstrates prominent follicular orifices and telangiectases. Occasionally lesions will occur on extra-facial skin.

Differential diagnosis
Granulomatous rosacea, sarcoidosis, cutaneous lupus erythematosus, cutaneous tuberculosis.

Investigations
Skin biopsy.

Management
First line: Topical tacrolimus 0.1% or topical or intralesional corticosteroids.

Second line: Excision or cryosurgery has been used in refractory cases.

Dermatoses resulting from disorders of the arteries and veins

55

Arterial disease and peripheral ischaemia

Atherosclerosis of the lower limb is a condition most frequently managed by vascular surgeons, but patients may present to dermatologists when peripheral ischaemia leads to infarction and ulceration of the skin (ulceration is described in Chapter 56).

Epidemiology

Atherosclerosis affects 5% of men over the age of 50 years. Of this group, 20% develop critical limb ischaemia if they have concomitant diabetes. Tobacco smoking, a family history of arterial disease and hyperlipidaemia are additional risk factors.

Pathophysiology

Cardiovascular risk factors induce endothelial injury and endothelial dysfunction. Monocytes recruited to the inflamed endothelium produce foam cells that result in atherosclerotic plaques. Platelets adhere to ulcerated plaques and platelet aggregates may embolise distally or initiate local thrombosis.

Clinical features

There is often a history of claudication, which is cramping pain on walking, usually in the posterior calf, relieved with rest. There may also be a history of skin ulceration. Critical ischaemia is indicated by rest pain at night usually in the foot.

Clinical signs include an erythematous or dusky mottled hue to legs, while elevation of the leg leads to a white foot. Trophic changes encompass dry skin, fissures, loss of hair and thickened nails (Figure 55.1a). Platelet emboli can lodge in the vasculature, causing areas of discoloration in the toes and sole of the foot, and can appear 'vasculitic-like' (Figure 55.1b). Ulceration of skin may occur at pressure points and on the dorsum of the foot (Chapter 56).

Differential diagnosis

Buerger disease, embolism leading to acute ischaemia, external arterial compression (popliteal entrapment or cervical rib), dissecting aneurysms, coagulation disorders (polycythaemia, thrombocytosis), vasculitis.

Rook's Dermatology Handbook, First Edition. Edited by Christopher E. M. Griffiths, Tanya O. Bleiker, Daniel Creamer, John R. Ingram and Rosalind C. Simpson.
© 2022 John Wiley & Sons Ltd. Published 2022 by John Wiley & Sons Ltd.

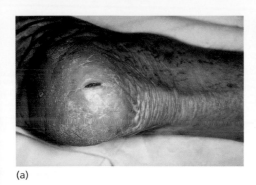
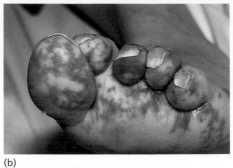

(a) (b)

Figure 55.1 (a) Trophic changes, including dry skin and fissures. (b) Platelet emboli can lodge in the vasculature, causing areas of discoloration in the toes and sole of the foot, and can appear 'vasculitic-like'.

Table 55.1 Investigations for patients with suspected peripheral vascular disease

Doppler ultrasound to measure the ankle–brachial Doppler pressure index Normal result = 1 Ratio 0.71–0.9 = mild peripheral vascular disease Ratio 0.41–0.7 = moderate Ratio <0.41 = severe Ratio <0.2 associated with gangrene	After the Doppler ultrasound probe has been used to locate the dorsalis pedis or posterior tibial vessel, a sphygmomanometer cuff is placed around the limb above the ankle and inflated (Figure 55.2). The red cells flowing past the tip of the ultrasound probe create an audible noise. As the cuff is inflated above systolic pressure, flow in the artery ceases and the noise disappears. This ankle–brachial systolic gradient is normally 1.0. A fall in ankle pressure results in a reduction of the pressure index. Falsely high indices may be obtained if the vessels are calcified and fail to compress at systolic pressure. This is especially true for diabetic limbs. In such circumstances a more accurate means of assessment is to measure the Doppler pressures at the toe.
Duplex ultrasound scanning	Duplex ultrasound scanning is often the initial investigation and is used as a screening test to confirm the major sites of stenosis or occlusion in the vascular tree. A duplex ultrasound scan provides both a B-mode image of the artery and a measurement of blood velocity; these can be combined to provide a map of stenoses and occlusions within the arterial tree from the aorta to the crural (calf) vessels. The greater the velocity, the tighter the stenosis.
Arteriography: guided by vascular surgeons and interventional radiologists	There are several techniques available. Contrast-enhanced magnetic resonance angiography is favoured but in patients in whom it is contraindicated or not tolerated then computed tomography angiography is used.

Investigations

See Table 55.1.

Management

Once the diagnosis of peripheral vascular disease is made, the patient is best managed by a vascular surgeon who can address the underlying cause.

Telangiectases

Telangiectases are chronically dilated capillaries or venules. They represent dilatations (expansion, stretching) of pre-existing vessels without any apparently new vessel growth (angiogenesis) occurring (Table 55.2).

Table 55.2 Causes of telangiectases

Primary telangiectases	Secondary telangiectases
Generalised essential telangiectasia	Prolonged vasodilatation (rosacea, venous
Hereditary benign telangiectasia	disease, calcium-channel blocking drugs,
Hereditary haemorrhagic telangiectasia	smoking)
Unilateral naevoid telangiectasia	Chronic UV exposure (ageing skin) and
Ataxia-telangiectasia	post-irradiation
Bloom syndrome	Post-traumatic
Vascular naevi (naevus flammeus)	Atrophy (poikiloderma and steroid induced)
Angiomas and angiokeratomas	Raynaud phenomenon, CREST syndrome,
Angioma serpiginomum	scleroderma, morphoea, lupus erythematosus
Mycosis fungoides and angiotrophic lymphoma	Dermatomyositis
Spider naevi	Mastocytosis: telangiectasia macularis eruptiva
Naevus anaemicus with telangiectatic vessels	perstans
Cutis marmorata telangiectatica	
Solitary plaque-like telangiectatic glomangioma	

CREST, calcinosis, Raynaud phenomenon, oesophageal dysmotility, sclerodactyly and telangiectasia.

Spider telangiectases

(Syn. Spider naevus)

These are common small vascular lesions found on the skin of the upper body which are benign. They have a characteristic appearance which can resemble a spider.

Epidemiology

Prevalence is up to 15% of the normal population, particularly in children and in women who are pregnant or taking the oral contraceptive pill. No difference in racial groups has been reported but the lesions are much more visible in patients with less pigmented skin. There is an association with liver disease and also thyrotoxicosis.

Pathophysiology

The main vessel of the spider telangiectasis is an arteriole. The blood flows from this to the periphery, and then passes into a capillary network.

Clinical features

Lesions appear suddenly. They are asymptomatic but can be a cosmetic issue. Spider telangiectases can be single or multiple and present as 1–1.5 mm red papules surrounded by arborising telangectases (Figure 55.3). The central

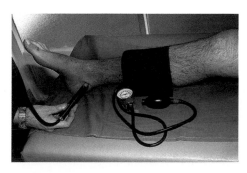

Figure 55.2 Doppler ultrasound to measure the ankle–brachial Doppler pressure index.

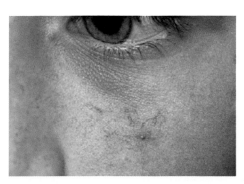

Figure 55.3 Spider telangiectasia.

body is usually pulsatile on diascopy. Classically, when the central arteriole is compressed, the skin blanches and the lesion temporarily vanishes but rapidly returns when the pressure is released. They are found on the upper body, in the territory of the superior vena cava, sometimes at sites of trauma and on the hands and fingers in children.

Differential diagnosis
Hereditary haemorrhagic telangiectasia
Lesions are typically macular, punctate or linear, without pulsation.

Investigations
No investigations needed in healthy children and adults with single lesions or only a few typical lesions. Identify and treat underlying disease.

Multiple lesions
Pregnancy test, blood tests to check for underlying liver disease or thyrotoxicosis.

Management
Spider telangiectases are asymptomatic and may resolve spontaneously. When on the face, they can be a cosmetic issue and management is outlined below.
First line: Conservative approach, cosmetic camouflage.
Second line: Electrodessication, laser including 585-nm pulsed dye laser or KTP 532-nm laser.

Cherry angiomas

(Syn. Campbell de Morgan spots)
These are very common cherry-red papules seen in the skin due to abnormal vascular proliferations.

Epidemiology
The commonest angiomas seen in the skin. Prevalence increases with age and they are found in 5% of adolescents and 75% of adults older than 75 years; F = M. Exposure to chemicals such as bromides, solvents and mustard gas has been associated with the development of cherry angiomas and there are reports linked

to ciclosporin therapy and also onset during pregnancy.

Pathophysiology
Cherry angiomas are true capillary haemangiomas formed by numerous, newly formed capillaries with narrow lumens and prominent endothelial cells arranged in a lobular pattern in the papillary dermis.

Clinical features
They appear as small asymptomatic red dots on the skin usually in the third and fourth decade of life. They often start as pin prick sized lesions which gradually grow. Cherry angiomas may be single or multiple lesions predominantly on the upper trunk and arms. They can arise anywhere on the skin, although rarely on the hands and feet and not on the mucous membranes. Typically, they appear as round to oval, bright red, dome-shaped papules and pinpoint macules varying from less than 1 mm in diameter to up to several millimetres in diameter. The larger lesions may be purple in colour. If traumatised cherry angiomas may bleed.

Differential diagnosis
Angiokeratoma, infantile haemangioma, bacillary angiomatosis, blue rubber bleb naevus syndrome.

Investigations
Usually a clinical diagnosis but a biopsy is confirmatory if there is any diagnostic doubt.

Management
No treatment is needed in most cases. For lesions that are bleeding or for cosmetic reasons treatment options include shave excision, hyfrecation, cryotherapy, pulsed dye laser and intense pulsed light.

Angiokeratomas

These are small benign cutaneous vascular lesions which present as red/blue or purple papules.

Epidemiology

The lesions may be congenital or acquired and therefore can be present at birth. They are more frequently seen in childhood and early adulthood. Overall incidence and prevalence is unknown but they are much rarer than other telangiectases such as cherry angiomas and spider naevi. They are commoner in females, with a F:M ratio of 3:1.

Pathophysiology

Angiokeratomas are not true angiomas but occur in existing vessels and are characterised by superficial vascular ectasia and overlying acanthosis or hyperkeratosis. Angiokeratoma circumscriptum has no genetic basis, unlike angiokeratoma corporis diffusum seen in Fabry disease (Chapter 39).

Clinical features

Angiokeratomas are usually red/blue or purple in colour, sometimes with a slightly rough surface. They may appear black if they have thrombosed or if they have been traumatised and bled. Lesions vary from small papules to larger plaques. Dermoscopy can be helpful in revealing blood-filled vascular spaces (Figure 55.4).

Angiokeratoma of Mibelli is a clinical variant involving acral skin, while Angiokeratoma of Fordyce involves scrotal skin (see Chapter 61). Angiokeratoma corporis diffusum is seen in Fabry disease (see Chapter 39. Angiokeratoma circumscriptum is usually congenital and associated with naevus flammeus or cavernous haemangioma.

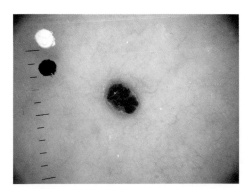

Figure 55.4 Dermoscopic view of angiokeratoma.

Differential diagnosis

Melanoma, cherry angioma.

Investigations

No investigations are needed for isolated lesions. For multiple lesions, Fabry disease should be considered and genetic testing undertaken.

Management

No treatment needed in most cases. Surgical excision is considered if there is diagnostic doubt. Other treatments include hyfrecation and laser, in particular KTP or 800-nm diode laser.

Venous lakes (Chapter 59)

Venous lakes are composed of dilated venules. They are dark purple/blue papules that appear on the face, lips and ears of elderly patients.

Epidemiology

The overall incidence of venous lakes is unknown, but the mean age at presentation is in the seventh and eighth decades of life. They are commoner in men, with a range of M:F ratios in the literature.

Pathophysiology

Venous lakes are dilated venules. The lesions consist of a single layer of flattened endothelial cells and a thick wall of fibrous tissue. There is often elastosis in the surrounding tissue, which may be due to background sun exposure.

Clinical features

The patient usually presents with a painless dark purple/blue papule often on the lip (Figure 55.5), which bleeds if traumatised. The papule is soft and compressible. Venous lakes are usually single but multiple lesions can occur.

Differential diagnosis

Melanoma: cannot be emptied by compression, cherry angioma, angiokeratoma.

Investigations

None are necessary but biopsy can be confirmatory if the diagnosis is in doubt.

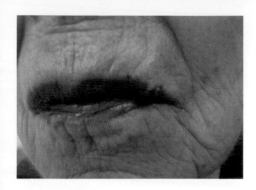

Figure 55.5 Venous lake on upper lip.

Management

No treatment needed in most cases. Treatments include excision, cryotherapy, laser (pulsed dye, KTP, argon, carbon dioxide).

Venous insufficiency

This is a state which occurs when the blood no longer flows in the correct path from the superficial system into the deep venous system and thence back to the heart. This results in venous congestion and impairment of the venous system of the lower limbs. If untreated venous insufficiency in either the deep or superficial system causes the progressive syndrome of chronic venous insufficiency.

Epidemiology

One large study in 30 000 subjects found a prevalence of 7% for varicose veins and 0.86% for 'symptomatic' chronic venous insufficiency. Prevalence increases with age. In the USA, it is thought that approximately 2.5 million people have chronic venous insufficiency. There is no consensus in the literature regarding any difference in prevalence between the sexes. No ethnic predilection is known, but prevalence rates are higher in more developed countries, which may reflect more sedentary/ standing occupations, higher rates of obesity and lower levels of physical activity.

Pathophysiology

Venous reflux is regarded as the major cause of venous disorders. Reflux is the presence of retrograde flow in a vein in response to a stimulus such as a calf squeeze. It occurs during standing when the valves are incompetent. It can occur in the superficial, deep and perforating veins of the lower extremity. Underlying causes are shown in Table 55.3.

> **Box 55.1 Mechanisms involved in the pathogenesis of chronic venous disease**
> - Accumulation of leukocytes, which are activated by plasminogen activator.
> - Leukocytes start their migration out of the vasculature and undergo degranulation.
> - Proteolytic enzyme release leads to breakdown of extracellular matrix, causing reduced healing and promoting ulceration.
> - Capillary proliferation and increased permeability occurs in response to vascular endothelial growth factor.
> - Dermal tissue fibrosis ensues.

Table 55.3 Causes of chronic venous insufficiency

Venous disease	Superficial venous incompetence (varicose veins)
	Deep venous incompetence
	Primary deep venous obstruction (rare)
	Previous deep vein thrombosis
	External compression
Impaired calf muscle pump function	Immobility
	Joint disease
	Paralysis
	Obesity (immobility, femoral vein compression, high abdominal pressures)
Congestive cardiac failure	–

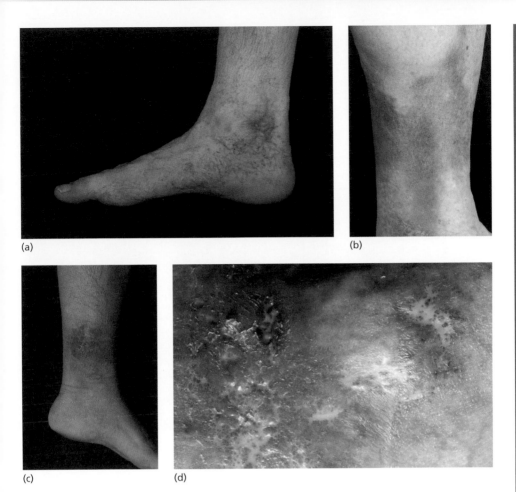

(a)

(b)

(c)

(d)

Figure 55.6 Clinical images of venous insufficiency. (a) Ankle flare. (b) Hyperpigmentation. (c) Venous eczema. (d) Atrophie blanche adjacent to venous ulceration.

Venous reflux leads onto a chronic inflammatory process at the microvascular level which produces the skin changes seen in chronic venous insufficiency. Potential mechanisms are summarised in Box 55.1.

Clinical features

Patients with superficial venous insufficiency may complain of burning, swelling, throbbing, aching, cramping and heaviness in the legs (Figure 55.6). Those with deep venous insufficiency almost always have pain. The symptoms are often improved by elevation and rest of the legs. The clinical signs are summarised in Table 55.4.

Differential diagnosis

These depend on the presenting features:

- *Swelling:* deep vein thrombosis, cellulitis, drug adverse effects, e.g. calcium channel antagonists.
- *Venous eczema:* other forms of eczema, including allergic contact dermatitis.
- *Ulceration:* arterial/ mixed aetiology.
- Lymphoedema of another cause.

Table 55.4 Clinical features of chronic venous insufficiency

Feature	Description	Pathology
Swelling (oedema)	Pitting oedema (especially around the ankle) Worst at the end of the day Usually disappears at night Night cramps	Capillary filtration rate increases as a consequence of increased ambulatory venous (and consequently capillary) pressure and overwhelms lymph drainage This oedema always has a low protein content
Ankle flare (see Figure 55.6a)	Presence of abnormally visible cutaneous blood vessels at the ankle with several components: 'venous cups', blue and red telangiectases and capillary 'stasis spots'	A direct consequence of increased capillary pressure, which causes these vessels to expand
Hyperpigmentation (see Figure 55.6b)	Pigmentation in the 'gaiter area' of distal lower leg Pinpoint or patchy pigmentation may be minimal but may also extend over large indurated skin region	Haemosiderin accumulates from extravasation of red cells Melanin deposited due to post-inflammatory hyperpigmentation
Pressure erythema	Grouped, confluent, very small telangiectasiae develop Often found near incompetent perforating veins Pressure erythema is one of the first signs of evolving venous insufficiency	Direct result of increased venous pressure causing vascular dilatation
Venous eczema (see Figure 55.6c and Chapter 14)	Starts around varicosities at the medial ankle Relatively sharply demarcated Papules and vesicles, which may extend beyond the main area of eczematous skin Scaling and itching develops Chronic lichenified eczema may develop with time May lead to secondary spread onto adjacent and distant sites	Histopathological features of eczema Aetiology not fully understood but involves homing of activated T lymphocytes
Lipodermatosclerosis May be due to venous insufficiency and also secondary lymphatic failure (see Chapter 57)	Often found just above the medial malleolus, at the level of the Cockett perforating veins, which are usually incompetent, as is the great saphenous vein When the small saphenous vein is incompetent, the lipodermatosclerosis often affects the lateral side of the calf Early stage lipodermatosclerosis may feel a little indurated and often has an inflamed erythematosus appearance In longstanding disease, there is a 'woody' hardness to the skin and subcutaneous tissues with pigmentation	Increased matrix turnover is caused by a chronic inflammatory reaction The most characteristic histological findings are dermal and subcutaneous fibrosis, with fat degeneration

Atrophie blanche	Atrophic ivory-white depressed skin lesion often located on the lower legs Usually multiple lesions (diameter 0.5–15 cm) Contains many centrally enlarged capillaries that are visible as red dots Often asymptomatic, but associated ulceration can be very painful (see Figure 55.6d) Not unique to venous insufficiency (also seen in, e.g., lupus erythematosus, scleroderma, vasculitides, cryoglobulinaemia, polycythaemia and leukaemia)	The result of decreased capillary density caused by microthrombi and matrix degradation causing hypoxia There is an atrophic epidermis and a thickened, scleroderma-like dermis with proliferative dilated capillaries One or more capillaries are often occluded with fibrinoid material
Varicosities	Dilated and tortuous veins May be primary varicosities May be secondary, following deep venous thrombosis	
Lymphoedema	Develops when the previously healthy local lymphatic system fails in the face of an overwhelming filtration load, with eventual structural obliteration of lymphatic routes	
Ulceration (see Chapter 56)		End stage of chronic venous insufficiency

PART 7: VASCULAR DISORDERS INVOLVING THE SKIN

Investigations

Duplex ultrasonography is the initial investigation of choice and allows the communications between deep and superficial veins to be directly assessed. MRI venography can be undertaken by specialist units.

Management

Graduated compression stockings are the standard treatment (class 2, 30–40 mmHg; or class 3, >40 mmHg). They improve venous dynamics during the day and can be removed when lying down. A Cochrane meta-analysis showed that compression stockings are more effective than no compression in healing venous ulcers and higher compression pressures are more effective than lower ones; multilayer compression bandaging was superior to single-layer bandaging. Compliance may be an issue due to difficulty getting the stockings on and off.

Correction of the major reflux pathways may be possible via vascular surgeons or interventional radiologists. This may involve endothermal ablation and endovenous laser treatment of long saphenous vein, ultrasound-guided foam sclerotherapy or conventional surgery.

Ulceration resulting from disorders of the veins and arteries

56

Venous leg ulcer

Venous leg ulcers (VLUs) are chronic skin ulcers at the gaiter area that result from chronic peripheral venous hypertension. They represent the most advanced grade of chronic venous insufficiency (CVI) (see Chapter 55).

Epidemiology
The lifetime risk of a VLU is 0.5% and the point prevalence is 0.05%. VLUs primarily affect individuals aged over 65 years. There are higher rates of VLUs in more developed countries due to higher levels of obesity and standing occupations.

Pathophysiology
VLUs represent the end stage of CVI (see Chapter 55). There are some other disorders associated with VLUs, as listed in Box 56.1.

Clinical features
VLUs are common at the gaiter area (Figure 56.1), embedded in trophic skin changes attributed to CVI (venous eczema, lipodermatosclerosis, pigmentation, see chapter disorders of arteries and veins). VLUs are less commonly located in the lateral retromalleolar area or the lateral dorsum of the foot and the dorsum of the toes, related to deep and short saphenous vein reflux.

> **Box 56.1 Disorders associated with venous leg ulcers**
>
> - Chronic venous insufficiency
> - Venous thromboembolism
> - Obesity
> - Superficial venous thrombophlebitis
> - Varicose veins
> - Stasis dermatitis
> - Lipodermatosclerosis
> - Acroangiodermatitis
> - Ankle joint ankylosis
> - Rheumatoid arthritis
> - Neuromuscular diseases with impact on venous calf pump ejection

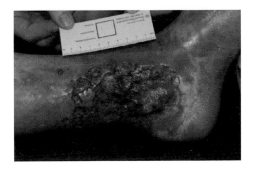

Figure 56.1 Venous leg ulcer. A 77-year-old patient with chronic venous insufficiency following recurrent venous thromboembolism.

Rook's Dermatology Handbook, First Edition. Edited by Christopher E. M. Griffiths, Tanya O. Bleiker, Daniel Creamer, John R. Ingram and Rosalind C. Simpson.

Differential diagnosis

Mixed leg ulcer or arterial leg ulcer, hypertensive ischaemic leg ulcer, vasculitic leg ulcer, pyoderma gangrenosum, skin neoplasm (basal cell carcinoma and squamous cell carcinoma).

Investigations

Ankle brachial pressure index (see Chapter 55), photography to document velocity of healing, microbiological culture and antibiotic sensitivities if clinical evidence of secondary infection, elliptical skin biopsy of ulcer margin if malignancy is suspected, blood tests to assess nutritional status, including total protein and albumin levels.

Management

Management of a VLU is summarised in Figure 56.2.

Mixed leg ulcer

Mixed leg ulcers (MLUs) are VLUs in a leg with peripheral arterial disease (PAD).

Epidemiology

The lifetime incidence of MLUs is estimated to be 0.2% with a point prevalence of 0.02%.

Pathophysiology

Pathophysiology combines the aetiologies of VLU and PAD, hence the predisposing factors include family history, obesity, standing occupation, venous thromboembolism, varicose veins, smoking, diabetes, hyperlipidaemia, hypertension, coronary heart disease and stroke.

Clinical features

Mixed leg ulcers cannot be clinically distinguished from VLUs, although a bimalleolar location (both medial and lateral skin ulcers on the same leg) occurs more frequently in MLUs, see Figure 56.3).

Differential diagnosis

See VLUs above.

Investigations

See VLUs above.

Management

Summarised in Figure 56.4.

Arterial leg ulcer

Arterial leg ulcers (ALUs) are chronic skin ulceration primarily caused by skin ischaemia due to advanced PAD.

Epidemiology

The lifetime incidence of ALUs is estimated to be 0.1% with a point prevalence of 0.01% and incidence increases with age.

Pathophysiology

PAD leads to tissue ischaemia. Occlusion of one or several branches of an atherosclerotic calf artery prevents the circulation reaching a well-circumscribed area of skin, which becomes cyanotic and then necrotic, resulting in ulcer formation.

Clinical features

ALUs begin as areas of painful skin necrosis, generally at the lateral or pretibial aspect of the leg. Typically, an ALU develops within normal-looking skin. Severe pain is a characteristic feature. The ulcer surface area tends to grow progressively. Clinically, there is a well-delineated zone of skin necrosis covered with eschar or remnants of necrotic wound border. Steep ulcer margins are usual, with a white or black wound base, exhibiting virtually no granulation tissue (Figure 56.5). Smaller ALUs are round in shape and have a 'punched-out' appearance. Larger ALUs are polycyclic and figurate.

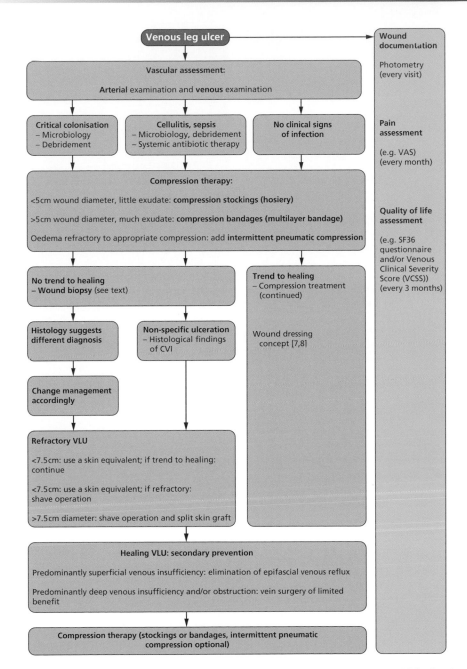

Figure 56.2 Algorithm for the management of VLUs. CVI, chronic venous insufficiency; VAS, visual analogue scale; VLU, venous leg ulcer.

PART 7: VASCULAR DISORDERS INVOLVING THE SKIN

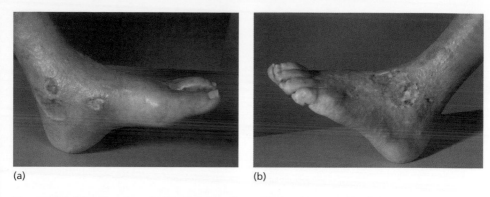

(a)   (b)

Figure 56.3 Mixed leg ulcer. An 80-year-old patient with chronic venous insufficiency as well as peripheral arterial disease resulting in bimalleolar leg ulcers. (a) Chronic leg ulceration of the medial ankle. (b) The same patient with a chronic leg ulcer of the lateral ankle region.

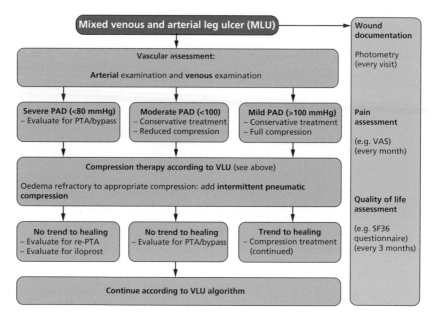

Figure 56.4 Algorithm for the management of MLUs. PAD, peripheral arterial disease; PTA, percutaneous transluminal angioplasty; VAS, visual analogue scale; VLU, venous leg ulcer.

Differential diagnosis
See VLUs above.

Investigations
See VLUs above.

Management
Summarised in Figure 56.6.

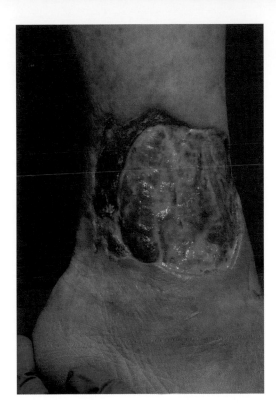

Figure 56.5 Arterial leg ulcer. An 80-year-old patient with spontaneous and rapidly progressive, painful skin ulceration of the right lateral ankle region. Vascular assessment showed advanced peripheral arterial disease.

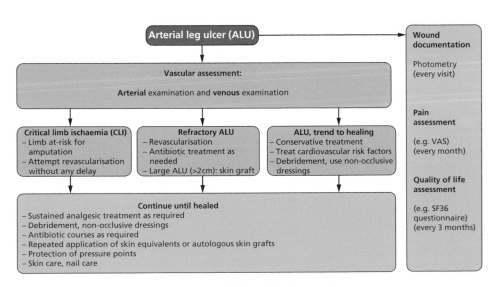

Figure 56.6 Algorithm for the management of ALUs. VAS, visual analogue scale.

57

Disorders of the lymphatic vessels

Lymphatic dysfunction interferes with fluid homeostasis, tissue immunity and peripheral fat mobilisation. Most chronic oedemas arise from increased microvascular filtration overwhelming the lymph drainage (relative lymphatic failure; Table 57.1). Examples are heart failure, venous disease and nephrotic syndrome. Oedema arising principally from a failure in lymph drainage is lymphoedema (absolute lymphatic failure).

Chronically swollen leg

Swelling of the lower limb, due to oedema, is caused by increased microvascular fluid filtration overwhelming lymph drainage. Causes of increased filtration such as increased venous pressure, low amount of plasma proteins and inflammatory states need to be considered as well as reasons for impaired lymph drainage.

Epidemiology
Chronic leg swelling is common but data are few.

Pathophysiology
Mixed lymphovenous disease, also known as phlebolymphoedema, is a mixed aetiology swelling of the lower limb due to chronic venous insufficiency and lymphatic insufficiency. Mixed lymphovenous disease refers to chronic oedema arising from chronic venous hypertension causing increased microvascular fluid filtration overwhelming lymph drainage. Over time established lymphoedema results from the compromised lymphatics. The pathophysiology of this process is summarised in Figure 57.1.

Obesity is a common underlying contributory factor in lower limb lymphoedema. Box 57.1 summarises the mechanisms involved in obesity-related lower limb lymphoedema.

Clinical features
Lymphoedema characteristically produces skin thickening. Increasing chronicity and severity produce hyperkeratosis (Figure 57.2) and papillomatosis (elephantiasis). A failure to pinch a fold of skin at the base of the second toe (Kaposi–Stemmer sign, Figure 57.3) is pathognomonic of lymphoedema. In more advanced cases fat deposition and fibrosis lead to a more indurated or 'brawny' swelling that results in bulging folds of skin and subcutaneous tissue.

The chronically swollen red leg usually indicates lipodermatosclerosis (LDS; Figure 57.4). LDS is an inflammatory condition of the skin and subcutaneous tissues affecting the lower third of the leg. It is caused by sustained high interstitial fluid and venous pressure due to chronic venous disease or due to lymphoedema without venous reflux. Pain and tenderness are characteristic. Over time, the erythema changes to brown pigmentation and the leg contour takes on an 'inverted champagne bottle' shape (Figure 57.4).

Rook's Dermatology Handbook, First Edition. Edited by Christopher E. M. Griffiths, Tanya O. Bleiker, Daniel Creamer, John R. Ingram and Rosalind C. Simpson.

Table 57.1 Causes of chronic oedema

Increased capillary filtration			Reduced lymph drainage	
↑Capillary pressure	↓Plasma proteins	↑Capillary permeability	Primary lymphatic insufficiency	Secondary lymphatic insufficiency
↑Venous pressure: Right heart failure Deep-vein thrombosis Venous obstruction Calcium channel antagonists Dependency Overtransfusion: Salt and water overload Advanced renal failure ↑Blood flow: Inflammation Arteriovenous fistula	↑Loss: Nephrotic syndrome Protein-losing enteropathy ↓Synthesis: Cirrhosis Advanced cancer Malabsorption Malnutrition	Inflammation: Varicose eczema Psoriasis Chronic infection Urticaria and angio-oedema Drugs	Germline mutation: Genes known (Milroy disease, lymphoedema-distichiasis syn.) Genes unknown (Meige disease) Mosaic mutation: Lymphatic malformation Overgrowth spectrum	Iatrogenic Surgery Radiotherapy Cancer Infection Filariasis Cellulitis Accidental trauma Obesity Immobility Sustained lymph load: Venous disease Heart failure Venous obstruction Deep-vein thrombosis

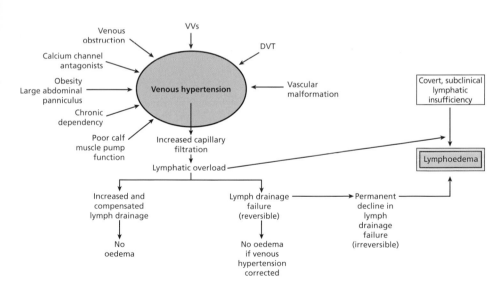

Figure 57.1 Causes of mixed lymphovenous disease. VVs, varicose veins; DVT, deep vein thrombosis.

Box 57.1 Contributing factors to obesity-related lower limb lymphoedema

- Poor mobility (to stimulate lymph drainage)
- Venous hypertension:
  - Dependency (armchair legs)
  - Abdominal girth/pendulous abdomen obstructing venous drainage in thighs
- Sleep apnoea syndrome
- Drug therapy, e.g. calcium-channel antagonists
- Co-morbidities, e.g. heart failure or post-thrombotic syndrome

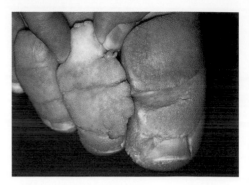

Figure 57.3 The Kaposi–Stemmer sign: an inability to pinch or pick up a fold of skin at the base of the second toe indicates lymphoedema.

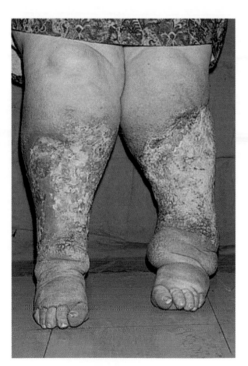

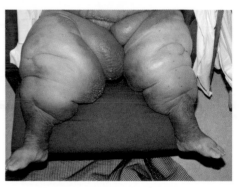

Figure 57.4 Acute and chronic lipodermatosclerosis; the bright red skin (acute) could be mistaken for bacterial cellulitis but it is an inflammatory response to the skin fluid congestion. The treatment is decongestive lymphatic therapy with or without antibiotic cover.

Figure 57.2 Lymphoedema associated with chronic venous disease causing hyperkeratosis of the lower legs.

Differential diagnosis

See Table 57.2.

Investigations

See Box 57.2.

Management

Treat cause: heart failure, malignancy etc.

Minimise secondary infection: regular emollient, treat tinea pedis, prophylactic antibiotic for recurrent cellulitis (low-dose prophylactic penicillin, oral phenoxymethylpenicillin 250 mg twice daily, given for a period of 12 months almost halves the risk of cellulitis recurrence during the intervention period compared with placebo).

Table 57.2 Causes of a swollen leg

Genetic			Acquired				
Vascular	Lymphatic	Other	Vascular	Lymphatic	Inflammatory	Musculoskeletal	Tumours
Vascular malformation Diffuse phlebectasia Klippel–Trenaunay syndrome Parkes–Weber syndrome Maffucci syndrome	Lymphoedema Lymphatic malformation Lymphangiomatosis	Overgrowth spectrum: Fat hypertrophy Lipomatosis Lipoedema Proteus syndrome Muscle hamartoma/overgrowth Gigantism/hemihypertrophy	Deep vein thrombosis Post-thrombotic syndrome Chronic venous reflux Venous outflow obstruction Dependency syndrome Thrombophlebitis Venous injury, e.g. intravenous drug abuse Acute arterial ischaemia Idiopathic/cyclical oedema of women Drugs, e.g. calcium channel antagonists	Obesity Lymphoedema: Cancer surgery Radiotherapy Filariasis Podoconiosis Trauma Reconstructive surgery Vein harvesting/vein stripping Immobility/armchair legs Factitial Chronic regional pain syndrome	Cellulitis Pretibial myxoedema Varicose eczema Psoriasis Pompholyx Sarcoidosis Herpes simplex	Rheumatoid arthritis Ruptured Baker's cyst Joint effusion Haematoma Torn muscle Pathological fracture Achilles tendonitis Myositis ossificans	Lymphoma Sarcoma Metastases

> **Box 57.2 Investigations for lymphoedema**
>
> - Plasma albumin to exclude hypoproteinaemia
> - B-type natriuretic peptide (BNP): normal level excludes acute heart failure
> - Venous duplex ultrasound to determine contribution from venous reflux
> - For suspected venous/lymphatic obstruction: ilioinguinal ultrasound/CT/MRI
> - Lymphoscintigraphy (isotope lymphography) if a primary lymphatic aetiology is suspected, which involves an intradermal/subcutaneous injection of a radiolabelled tracer protein, exclusively cleared by lymphatics
> - Skin biopsy if malignancy or pretibial myxoedema suspected

External compression: bandage, hosiery, pneumatic compression.

Physical therapy: exercise if possible, massage (manual lymphatic drainage).

Chronically swollen arm

Swelling of the upper limb is usually due to oedema from lymphatic insufficiency, in particular breast cancer treatment, or from venous obstruction.

Epidemiology

The commonest reason for upper limb swelling is lymphoedema following breast cancer treatment. More than one in five women who survive breast cancer will develop arm lymphoedema.

Pathophysiology

The causes of a swollen arm are in Table 57.3. Breast cancer treatments causing lymphoedema include either axillary lymphadenectomy or radiation therapy. Venous outflow obstruction may be due to axillary/subclavian vein compression, or stenosis or occlusion from thrombosis. Subclavian vein thrombosis may occur in cancer patients receiving chemotherapy through central lines or due to pacemaker insertion, trauma, surgery immobilisation, oral contraceptive pill use, pregnancy or malignancy.

Clinical features

Breast cancer related lymphoedema (BCRL) may exhibit pitting oedema but in more advanced cases fat and fibrosis contribute more to the swelling, so the consistency of the swelling may be fatty or firm. The distribution of swelling along the arm varies between patients and swelling may be confined to a specific region of the upper limb. In some patients the hand may be swollen, whilst in others the hand may be spared despite more proximal swelling of the forearm or upper arm.

Differential diagnoses

See Table 57.3.

Investigations

See list for swollen lower limb section.

Management

See strategies outlined in swollen lower limb section.

The usual treatment for primary subclavian vein thrombosis is oral anticoagulation. Venous compression or stenosis may benefit from stenting.

Swollen face, head and neck

Facial swelling may be generalised or localised, e.g. to the eyelid(s), lips or one cheek. It may extend beyond the face to involve the head and neck. To be defined as chronic it should persist for more than 3 months. Chronic swelling of the face is most often due to fluid oedema but can arise due to an increase in other tissue components, such as blood vessels in a capillary malformation (port wine stain), acromegaly, overgrowth spectrum (hemihypertrophy) or tumours.

Table 57.3 Causes of a swollen arm

Congenital/genetic			Acquired			
Vascular	**Lymphatic**	**Other**	**Vascular**	**Lymphatic**	**Musculoskeletal**	**Tumours**
Vascular malformation	Lymphoedema	Overgrowth spectrum:	Subclavian vein thrombosis:	Lymphoedema:	Rheumatoid arthritis	Lymphoma
Diffuse phlebectasia	Lymphatic malformation	Proteus syndrome	Effort thrombosis	Axillary surgery	Haematoma	Sarcoma
Klippel–Trenaunay syn	Lymphangiomatosis	Fat hypertrophy	Venous catheterisation	Radiotherapy	Torn muscle	Metastases
Arteriovenous malformation		Muscle hamartoma	Chemotherapy ports	Cancer	Pathological fracture	
		Gigantism/ hemihypertrophy	Chest radiotherapy	Neurological deficit	Myositis ossificans	
		Lipoedema	Thoracic outlet syndrome	Chronic regional pain syndrome	Osteomyelitis	
		Dercum disease	Superior vena cava obstruction	Lymphangitis: (bacterial infection lymphangitis:	Septic arthritis	
		Madelung disease (benign symmetrical lipomatosis)	Intravenous drug abuse	herpes simplex, psoriasis, rheumatoid arthritis)		
				Yellow-nail syndrome		

Epidemiology

There are no data for facial lymphoedema due to inflammatory disorders. About half of patients develop secondary lymphoedema as a late effect of head and neck cancer treatment.

Pathophysiology

Gravitational factors contributing to increased microvascular filtration do not play a part except overnight when the patient is lying down, hence facial swelling is often at its worst in the morning.

The causes of head and neck swelling are given in Table 57.4. In any head and neck location, a single severe attack of cellulitis may cause enough damage to the lymphatics to result in chronic lymphoedema. Other potential underlying disease processes vary depending on the exact location affected.

Clinical features

The clinical features of facial lymphoedema depend on the underlying aetiology. Swelling usually affects the central forehead (Figure 57.5a), periocular skin and cheeks (Figure 57.5b) and may be asymmetrical.

Oedema of the upper or lower lip (or both)

May be from a vascular anomaly or result from recurrent angio-oedema, oro-facial granulomatosis (OFG), sarcoidosis, infective cheilitis or from the administration of lip fillers for cosmetic purposes. OFG starts with intermittent bouts of swelling resembling angio-oedema affecting the lips or cheeks, but over time the condition may become persistent. An extension of the oedema within the mouth is common and manifests as rugose changes on the buccal mucosal and tongue (scrotal tongue).

Chronic oedema of the eyelids

Common. Conditions that need to be considered include dermatomyositis, Graves disease and particularly rosacea/acne. Eyelid swelling may be due to acquired lax skin from photoageing and other processes that have undermined tissue compliance, such as blepharochalasis. Contact allergy or angioedema, if persistent or recurrent, may slowly compromise lymphatic function. Angiosarcoma or Kaposi sarcoma may infiltrate local lymph drainage and manifest with eyelid oedema. Medical conditions to be considered with periocular oedema are dermatomyositis, Cushing syndrome (moon face) and thyroid disease, particularly Graves disease.

Lymphoedematous enlargement of the ear

May be caused by chronic inflammatory disorders such as rosacea (otophyma), psoriasis and eczema. Other causes include pediculosis, trauma and primary (congenital) lymphoedema.

Differential diagnosis

See Table 57.4.

Investigations

Skin biopsy if granulomatous disease, rosacea, dermatomyositis, angiosarcoma or Kaposi sarcoma is suspected. MRI or CT imaging may be useful if an underlying pathology such as cancer, sinusitis or dental root infection is suspected. Lymphoscintigraphy can be performed on the head and neck but is difficult to interpret.

Management

Treatment of facial lymphoedema will depend on the cause. Any inflammation will need to be treated to reduce the higher lymphatic load arising from increased vascular permeability and blood flow. In rosaceous lymphoedema, antibiotic therapy is relatively ineffective in reducing swelling; low-dose isotretinoin may provide more benefit but treatment may need to be continued for 1–2 years. General management strategies include raising the head of the bed during overnight sleep and massage techniques and facial exercises.

Swollen genitalia

Genital lymphoedema may affect the shaft of penis and/or scrotum in men or the mons pubis in women.

Epidemiology

The commonest cause of genital lymphoedema and hydrocele worldwide is filariasis. Genital lymphoedema M > F, probably because of anat-

Table 57.4 Causes of head and neck swelling

Congenital/genetic		Acquired		
Vascular	**Lymphatic**	**Overgrowth**	**Tumours**	**Inflammatory**	**Miscellaneous**
Vascular malformation	Syndrome (neck webbing): Turner Noonan Generalised lymphatic dysplasia Mosaic with segmental lymphoedema Lymphangioma/lymphatic malformation	Macrocephaly, e.g. macrocephaly capillary malformation syndrome	Metastatic head and neck cancer Angiosarcoma Radical neck lymphadenectomy Radiotherapy	Rosacea/acne Cellulitis/erysipelas Oro-facial granulomatosis Tuberculosis Sarcoidosis Dental abscess Sinusitis Dermatomyositis Dermatitis/eczema, psoriasis, contact allergy Blepharochalasis Pediculosis Angioedema	Acromegaly Accidental trauma (cauliflower ear) Cushing syndrome Graves disease

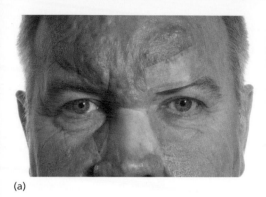
(a)

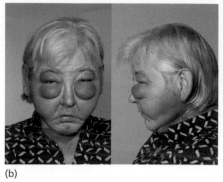
(b)

Figure 57.5 Clinical features of facial lymphoedema. (a) Solid 'brawny' facial oedema. (b) Facial lymphoedema following treatment for carcinoma of the tongue.

Table 57.5 Causes of lymphoedema of the genitalia and mons pubis

Primary (congenital/genetic)	Secondary
Noonan syndrome	Cancer (advanced primary, inflammatory cancer,
Hennekam syndrome	pelvic relapse, skin infiltration)
Generalised lymphatic dysplasia	Lymphadenectomy (pelvic, bilateral, ilio-inguinal)
Chylous reflux	Radiotherapy
Emberger syndrome	Accidental trauma
Lymphoedema distichiasis	Obesity
Yellow-nail syndrome	Crohn disease/anogenital granulomatosis
	Hidradenitis suppurativa
	Infections:
	Filariasis
	Cellulitis
	Lymphogranuloma venereum
	Donovanosis
	Systemic causes (heart failure, nephrotic syndrome)

omy and the dependent nature of male external genitalia.

Pathophysiology

Genital lymphoedema may be primary or secondary (Table 57.5). The genitalia have bilateral lymph node drainage. For swelling to occur, drainage pathways to both inguinal regions must be insufficient or local genital lymphatics must become occluded bilaterally.

Clinical features

In primary lymphoedema swelling may be present at birth or develop later in life, invariably one or both lower limbs are swollen at the time of onset of genital lymphoedema.

Longstanding lymphoedema causes thickening and hyperkeratosis of the overlying skin with the production of papillomas. These probably arise from lymph congestion within the dermal lymphatics, which, in the early stages, can appear as 'lymph blisters' on the skin surface before the tissues become organised and fibrotic. This expansion of congested dermal lymphatics due to backpressure (dermal backflow) is called lymphangiectasia (Figure 57.6). The 'lymph blisters' will rupture on occasion, resulting in a copious release of lymph (lymphorrhoea), mimicking incontinence or excessive sweating. Secondary consequences are an increased risk of contact dermatitis and cellulitis.

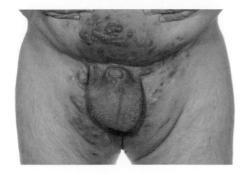

Figure 57.6 Genital lymphoedema secondary to hidradenitis suppurativa. Note the cutaneous lymphangiectasia that predisposes to lymphorrhoea. (Source: Thomas CL, Gordon KD, Mortimer PS. Rapid resolution of hidradenitis suppurativa after bariatric surgical intervention. Clin Exp Dermatol 2014, 39(3), 315–317.)

Differential diagnosis
See Table 57.5.

Investigations
If active filarial infection is likely, consider complement fixation test or night-time blood smears. Skin biopsy to diagnose granulomatous disease or cancer infiltrating dermal lymphatics. CT or MRI imaging to detect lymphatic obstruction within the pelvis or ilioinguinal glands from cancer or other pathologies.

Management
Treat cause: Cancer, hidradenitis suppurativa, infection.

Minimise secondary infection: Good skin care, prophylactic antibiotic for recurrent cellulitis, massage/compression.

Surgery: Hyfrecation/diathermy for lymphangiectasia, circumcision in men.

Primary lymphoedema

Primary lymphoedema arises due to an intrinsic abnormality involving a genetically determined aplasia, hypoplasia, malformation or dysfunction of the lymphatic vessels. It may occur as a non-syndromic Mendelian condition or less commonly as part of a complex syndromic disorder.

Epidemiology
Primary lymphoedema is rare.

Pathophysiology
Mutations in several genes are known to cause primary lymphoedema (Figure 57.7).

Lymphoedema is also an associated feature of several syndromes, as listed in Table 57.6.

Clinical features
Primary lymphoedema, or lymphoedema due to an underlying genetic abnormality, should always be suspected in a patient presenting with swelling and no obvious underlying medical cause. Primary lymphoedema may be present at birth or develop later in life. The body site(s) involved, ranging from one limb to whole body swelling, depends on the subtype of lymphoedema.

The clinical signs of primary lymphoedema can range from mild swelling to that of severe enlargement. Protein-rich materials, lipids and debris accumulate in addition to interstitial fluid. This results in 'solid' and 'fluid' components to the swelling, giving rise to the 'brawny' nature of chronic oedema that resists pitting.

Historically, all cases of congenital lower limb lymphoedema were classified as Milroy disease. However, several different subtypes are now recognised based on phenotypic and genotypic variation (Figure 57.7).

Differential diagnosis
See Figure 57.7 and Table 57.6.

Investigations
As for other causes of lymphoedema dealt with in this chapter. Lymphoscintigraphy may have particular value where lymphatic aplasia, hypoplasia or malformation is suspected.

Management
See management sections earlier in this chapter.

Lipoedema
Lipoedema is a condition characterised by abnormal adipose deposition within the lower

PART 7: VASCULAR DISORDERS INVOLVING THE SKIN

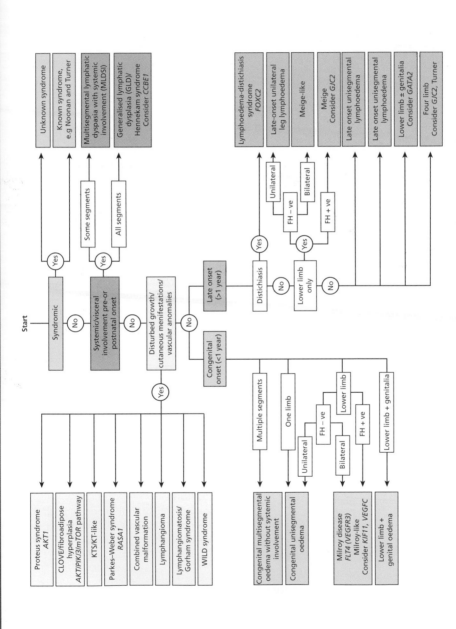

Figure 57.7 Classification pathway for primary lymphoedema. Text in red indicates the suggested genetic test for the subgroup. FH, family history: +ve, positive; -ve, negative; KT, Klippel–Trenaunay; KTS, Klippel–Trenaunay syndrome. (Source: From Connell F, Gordon K, Brice G, et al. The classification and diagnostic algorithm for primary lymphatic dysplasia: an update from 2010 to include molecular findings. Clin Genet 2013, 84(4), 303–314, and Mortimer PS, Rockson SG. New developments in clinical aspects of lymphatic disease. *J Clin Invest* 2014, 124(3), 915–921.)

Table 57.6 List of known syndromes associated with lymphoedema and the causative gene (or chromosomal abnormality) if known

Syndrome	Chromosome/gene
Aagenaes syndrome	Not known
Carbohydrate-deficient glycoprotein types 1a, 1b, 1h	*PMM2*, *PM1*, *ALG8*
Cardio-facio-cutaneous syndrome	RAS-MAP kinase pathway, including *KRAS*, *BRAF*, *MAP2K1*, *MAP2K2*
CHARGE syndrome	*CDH7*
Choanal atresia-lymphoedema	*PTPN14*
Ectodermal dysplasia, anhidrotic, immunodeficiency, osteopetrosis and lymphoedema (OLEDAID syndrome)	*IKBKG (NEMO)*
Fabry disease	*GLA*
Hennekam syndrome	*CCBE1*, *FAT4*
Hypotrichosis-lymphoedema-telangiectasia	*SOX18*
Irons–Bianchi syndrome	Not known
Lymphoedema-distichiasis syndrome	*FOXC2*
Lymphoedema-myelodysplasia (Emberger syndrome)	*GATA2*
Macrocephaly-capillary malformation	*PIK3CA*
Microcephaly with or without chorioretinopathy, lymphoedema and mental retardation	*KIF11*
Milroy disease	Some cases due to *FLT4* mutations encoding VEGFR-3
Mucke syndrome	Not known
Noonan syndrome	RAS-MAP kinase pathway *PTPN11*, *KRAS*, *SOS1* and others
Oculo-dento-digital syndrome	*GJA1*
Progressive encephalopathy, hypsarrhythmia and optic atrophy	Not known
Phelan–McDermid syndrome	22q terminal deletion or ring chromosome 22
Prader–Willi syndrome	15q11 microdeletion or maternal uniparental disomy 15
Thrombocytopenia with absent radius	1q21.1 microdeletion and *RBM8A*
Turner syndrome	45, X0
Velo-cardio-facial syndrome	22q11 microdeletion
Yellow-nail syndrome	Not known

PART 7: VASCULAR DISORDERS INVOLVING THE SKIN

limbs. It occurs almost exclusively in females, usually at a time of hormonal change, and is thought to be an inherited disorder.

Epidemiology
Prevalence is unknown and lipoedema may be misdiagnosed as obesity or lymphoedema. Onset is typically at puberty or other times of hormonal change such as pregnancy or commencement of the oral contraceptive pill. No ethnic differences have been reported.

Pathophysiology
The aetiology of lipoedema is unknown. It is uncertain whether the condition results from adipocyte hypertrophy or hyperplasia, or a combination of both. Histological examination of tissue biopsies and liposuction aspirates show oedema of the adipocytes and/or interstitium, but no other abnormalities. Patterns of inheritance of the condition with frequent mother to daughter transmission are consistent with either X-linked dominant inheritance or autosomal dominant inheritance with sex limitation.

Clinical features
Affected individuals develop bilateral and symmetrical 'fatty' non-pitting swelling, usually confined to the legs and hips. The feet are spared, giving rise to an 'inverse shouldering' or 'bracelet' effect at the ankles (Figure 57.8). Patients frequently experience pain, tenderness and easy bruising of the affected areas. Over time, the patient may develop similar clinical signs in their upper arms.

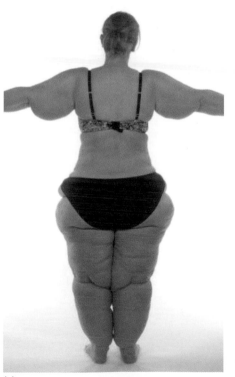
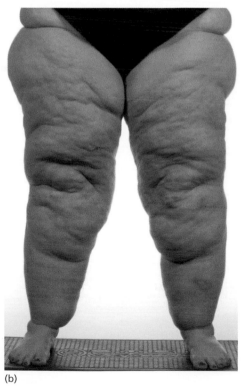

(a)   (b)

Figure 57.8 A patient with classic lipoedema. (a) Symmetrical fatty swelling of both lower limbs with sparing of the trunk. Increased adipose deposition of the upper arms is present. (b) Lipoedema features include sparing of the feet with 'inverse shouldering' of the ankles. Fat pads are developing on the medial aspect of both knees.

Differential diagnosis

Lymphoedema, obesity, Dercum disease (see Chapter 52) (multiple, painful, diffuse or nodular lipomas with generalised obesity).

Investigations

The diagnosis of lipoedema is currently clinical with no absolute phenotypic features or confirmatory test.

Management

No curative therapies are available for lipoedema. Management goals are aimed at the improvement of symptoms, particularly pain, prevention of lipoedema progression and prevention of lipo-lymphoedema. Management strategies are below.

Weight loss: Exercise, dietary advice.

Physical therapies: Compression and manual lymph drainage if coexistent lymphoedema.

Liposuction: Probably more effective at earlier stages of the disease.

Podoconiosis

(Syn. Endemic non-filarial elephantiasis, mossy foot)
Podoconiosis refers to the development of bilateral lower limb lymphoedema, thought to occur as a result of prolonged exposure to irritant mineral-rich soils.

Epidemiology

It is estimated that 4 million people are affected by podoconiosis, mainly in tropical Africa, Central and South America and South-East Asia. Ethiopia is the country with the highest reported prevalence, with an estimated 1 million people living with the disease. Estimated prevalence is 4% in Ethiopia, 8% in Cameroon and 4.5% in Uganda. Onset is typically in the first or second decade of life, but may occur later. Occupations involving prolonged contact with soil, especially farming without footwear, are associated with a higher risk.

Pathophysiology

Current evidence suggests a pivotal role of mineral particles within the soil in a genetically susceptible individual.

Clinical features

Presents with a prodromal phase of pruritus of the forefoot skin and a burning sensation of the feet. Early changes are similar to that of any other cause of lower limb lymphoedema. The affected individual develops bilateral lymphoedema of the foot and ankle regions. Lymphorrhoea, hyperkeratosis, papillomatosis, fibrosis and gross disfigurement of the below-knee regions develop if the condition is untreated. The toes develop a characteristic macerated and 'mossy' appearance (Figure 57.9). Recurrent lower limb cellulitis is a frequent complication.

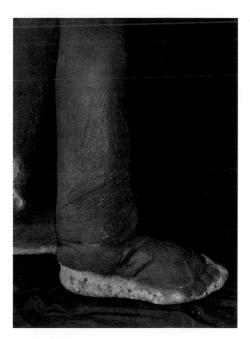

Figure 57.9 Lower limb lymphoedema due to podoconiosis. Note the presence of toe maceration and typical 'mossy' appearance of the foot. (Source: Reproduced with permission from D. Markos.)

PART 7: VASCULAR DISORDERS INVOLVING THE SKIN

Differential diagnosis
Filariasis: Unilateral lower limb swelling that extends above the knee.

Leprotic lower limb lymphoedema: Loss of sensation, thickened palpable nerves, trophic ulceration.

Investigations
To exclude active filarial infection, consider complement fixation test or night-time blood smears. A skin biopsy may be needed to check for leprosy/Kaposi sarcoma.

Management
Primary prevention: Good footwear (especially in high risk occupations).

Good foot care: Careful washing, topical antiseptics.

Physical therapies: Compression bandaging.

Part 8
Skin Disorders Associated with Specific Sites, Sex and Age

Dermatoses of the external ear

58

The external ear consists of the auricle (or pinna), the external auditory canal and the outer layer of the tympanic membrane. The auricle is a convoluted, elastic and cartilaginous plate covered by skin which is continuous medially with the lining of the external auditory canal (Figure 58.1).

Chondrodermatitis nodularis

(Syn. Chondrodermatitis nodularis helicis)
Chondrodermatitis nodularis (CN) is a benign, painful, inflammatory condition involving cartilage and overlying skin of the ear.

Epidemiology
CN is common in older persons. 10M:1F. It occurs mainly in fair-skinned individuals.

Pathophysiology
Pressure, such as sleeping predominantly on one side, is a common precipitating factor. Arteriolar narrowing in the perichondrium may be the pathological trigger. Histologically there is a nodule of degenerate collagen surrounded by granulation tissue with an overlying acanthotic epidermis. There is inflammation of the underlying perichondrium.

Clinical features
The lesion is a painful nodule with surrounding erythema. The surface may be scaly or crusted, concealing a small ulcer. In men ~90% of nodules are situated on the helix, usually at the upper pole and more frequently on the right (Figure 58.2), but may occur on the antihelix, tragus, concha and antitragus, in order of decreasing frequency. In women, the left and right ears are affected equally. The pain, which is sometimes severe, is initiated by pressure and occasionally by cold. Typically the pain of CN interferes with sleep.

Differential diagnosis
Basal cell carcinoma, squamous cell carcinoma, weathering nodules (asymptomatic nodules on the free edge of the helix in older men).

Investigations
Biopsy should be performed if there is any doubt about the diagnosis.

Management
First line: Pressure relief during sleep: doughnut-shaped pillow or protective hollowed-out foam.

Second line: Intralesional corticosteroid injection or liquid nitrogen cryotherapy.

Third line: Surgery: remove the focus of abnormal cartilage and retain as much as possible of the overlying skin.

Otitis externa

(Syn. Swimmer's ear)
Otitis externa (OE) is an inflammatory and infective condition of the skin of the auditory

Rook's Dermatology Handbook, First Edition. Edited by Christopher E. M. Griffiths, Tanya O. Bleiker, Daniel Creamer, John R. Ingram and Rosalind C. Simpson.
© 2022 John Wiley & Sons Ltd. Published 2022 by John Wiley & Sons Ltd.

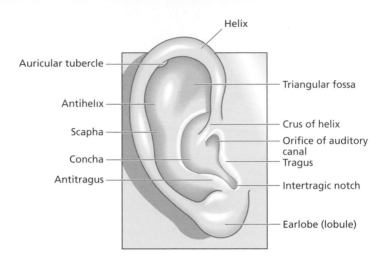

Helix

Auricular tubercle

Antihelix

Scapha

Concha

Antitragus

Triangular fossa

Crus of helix

Orifice of auditory canal

Tragus

Intertragic notch

Earlobe (lobule)

Figure 58.1 Anatomical landmarks of the auricle.

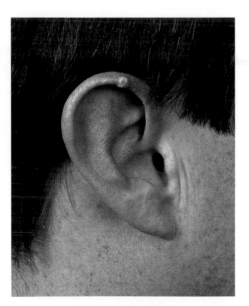

Figure 58.2 Chondrodermatitis nodularis of the helix. A superficially ulcerated, exquisitely tender nodule.

canal and adjacent pinna. Acute and chronic forms are recognised.

Epidemiology
Acute diffuse OE has an annual incidence of about 1:250. It is commoner in the summer months due to higher temperatures, increased humidity and engagement in water sports.

Pathophysiology
High temperature and humidity encourages maceration and secondary infection of the ear canal skin, while trauma to the ear canal (e.g. from fingernails), water retention and over-zealous cleansing all contribute. *Pseudomonas aeruginosa* infection is typical in swimmers and in hot humid environments. *Staphylococcus aureus* is also often isolated. In the tropics fungal infections (otomycosis) are relatively common: *Aspergillus*, *Candida*, *Penicillium* and *Mucor* spp.

Clinical features
In acute OE there is itching of the external auditory meatus, pain, hearing loss and purulent discharge. Erythema, swelling and scaling spreads from the meatus to the concha (Figure 58.3). There may be associated low-grade fever, malaise and regional lymphadenopathy. In chronic OE the symptoms persist for more than 2 months and the infective/inflammatory condition is often complicated by a concurrent dermatological disorder, e.g. atopic eczema, seborrhoeic dermatitis or psoriasis. In necrotising OE skin infection by *Pseudomonas aeruginosa* spreads to deeper structures and causes necrosis.

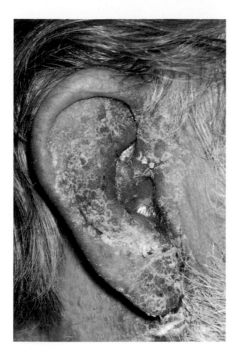

Figure 58.3 Otitis externa. The pinna and skin nearby is erythematous with crusting and scaling. The entrance to the canal is narrowed.

Differential diagnosis
Psoriasis, seborrhoeic dermatitis, allergic contact dermatitis, cutaneous lupus erythematosus.

Investigations
Swabs for bacteriology and mycology.

Management
Topical antibiotic–steroid ear drops (e.g. flumetasone–clioquinol). If the ear canal is swollen, use an ear wick. Ibuprofen and/or paracetamol for pain relief. Consider a systemic antibiotic if there is low-grade pyrexia and/or cellulitis. In chronic OE, treat any concomitant dermatosis: atopic eczema, psoriasis and seborrhoeic dermatitis.

Skin manifestations of the ear in systemic diseases

Some systemic diseases are accompanied by signs occurring on the ears (Box 58.1).

Box 58.1 Skin manifestations of the ear in systemic diseases

Disease	Clinical features in ears
Acromegaly	There may be enlargement of the auricular cartilage and coarsening of the overlying skin.
Addison disease	Pigmentary changes may involve the ear. Ossification of the auricular cartilage.
Bazex syndrome (acrokeratosis paraneoplastica) (see Chapter 84)	Hyperkeratosis commonly affects the ears in Basex syndrome – a marker for internal malignancy.
Gout	Gouty tophi frequently involve the pinna and can precede or follow the onset of joint disease.
Leprosy (see Chapter 5)	In lepromatous leprosy the earlobe skin becomes thickened and is a valuable site for smears.
Lupus erythematosus (LE) (see Chapter 23)	All forms of LE can involve the ears. The concha is a characteristic site for discoid LE.
Relapsing polychondritis	Redness, tenderness and swelling of the ear, but with sparing of the lobe.
Rheumatoid disease	Rheumatoid nodules can occur on the ears.
Sarcoidosis (see Chapter 50)	Cutaneous sarcoidosis can involve the ear, especially the lupus pernio variety.

59 Disorders of the lips and mouth

BENIGN LESIONS IN THE MOUTH AND ON THE LIPS

Benign lesions occurring on the skin of the lips or mucosal surfaces of the oral cavity need to be distinguished from malignant tumours (Table 59.1).

PIGMENTATION IN THE MOUTH AND ON THE LIPS

Hyperpigmentation occurring on the lips will be apparent to the patient and may have important clinical implications. Examination of buccal mucosae is necessary to identify intra-oral pigmentation which may also be clinically significant (Box 59.1).

INFECTIONS OF THE MOUTH AND LIPS

Viral and yeast infections of the skin and mucous membranes commonly involve the mouth (see Chapters 3 and 7). The most frequent oral infective disorders are summarised in Table 59.2.

Mouth ulcers

Mouth ulcers occur frequently, are usually symptomatic and have a range of underlying causes (see Box 59.2).

Recurrent aphthous ulcers

Recurrent aphthous stomatitis (RAS) is characterised by recurring episodes of multiple mouth ulcers. There are three main sub-types of RAS (Table 59.3). Patients are usually healthy, but RAS can be associated with systemic disorders (Table 59.4).

Management of recurrent aphthous stomatitis

The natural history of RAS is one of eventual remission in most cases.

First line: Predisposing factors should be corrected, good oral hygiene (chlorhexidine or triclosan mouthwashes), topical minocycline and tetracycline mouth rinses may be of benefit, ulcer pain and healing time can be reduced with hydrocortisone hemisuccinate pellets 2.5 mg or triamcinolone acetonide in carboxymethylcellulose paste used four times daily.

Second line: Stronger topical corticosteroid (e.g. betamethasone, beclomethasone, fluticasone, mometasone, clobetasol), systemic corticosteroid (e.g. prednisolone).

Third line: Thalidomide, in doses from 50 mg up to 300 mg daily, can induce remission, but teratogenicity and neuropathy risks must be considered. Other therapies have been used, including carbenoxolone and dapsone. In severe cases biological agents may be indicated.

Rook's Dermatology Handbook, First Edition. Edited by Christopher E. M. Griffiths, Tanya O. Bleiker, Daniel Creamer, John R. Ingram and Rosalind C. Simpson.
© 2022 John Wiley & Sons Ltd. Published 2022 by John Wiley & Sons Ltd.

Table 59.1 Benign lesions in the mouth and on the lips

Disorder	Epidemiology	Pathophysiology	Clinical features	Management
Fordyce spots (Figure 59.1)	Extremely common: present in 80% of the population	Benign Enlarged sebaceous glands containing neutral lipids	Yellowish micropapules on buccal or labial mucosa, particularly inside commissures Not noticeable until after puberty	No treatment is indicated
Melanotic macule (Figure 59.2)	Occurs in up to 3% of normal persons, at any age Most often seen in white adults	Benign Increased pigmentation of the epithelial basal layer, accentuated at the tips of rete ridges (similar to freckle and lentigo)	Acquired, small, flat, brown to black, asymptomatic macule Usually solitary, especially on the vermilion of the lips, also on gingiva, buccal mucosa or palate Most occur near the midline on the lower lip vermilion	No treatment is needed, but can be excised to exclude melanoma Can be removed by laser for cosmetic reasons
Angina bullosa haemorrhagica (Figure 59.3)	Common Usually seen in the elderly	Subepithelial blisters containing blood No association with immunological or bleeding disorder	Blood blisters on soft palate which rupture to leave ulcers	Symptomatic treatment
Venous lake	Common Usually seen in the elderly	Venous dilatation lined by endothelium and a thick wall of fibrous tissue	Blue or purple soft swelling on lower lip	No treatment is needed, but lesion can be excised or ablated with electrodessication
Mucocoele (Syn. Mucous retention cyst) (Figure 59.4)	Common	Escaped mucous from damaged minor salivary gland duct into lamina propria	Solitary, painless, dome-shaped, white-blue nodule, especially on lower labial mucosa	Excision or cryotherapy
Papilloma	Common in HIV infection	Papillomatous lesion with acanthosis and koilocytosis HPV induced Some are dysplastic	Commonly at junction of hard and soft palate White or pink wart-like papilloma	Excision
White sponge naevus	Rare familial disorder, autosomal dominant	Hyperplastic acanthotic epithelium with oedema causes basket-weave appearance	First appears in childhood Non-painful white plaques involving buccal mucosae, gingiva and floor of the mouth	Benign condition with an excellent prognosis No treatment necessary

PART 8: SKIN DISORDERS ASSOCIATED WITH SPECIFIC SITES, SEX AND AGE

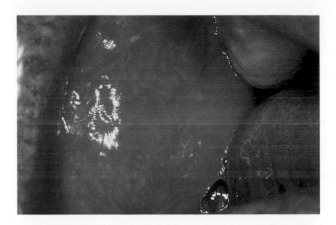

Figure 59.1 Fordyce spots on the buccal mucosa: enlarged sebaceous glands visible as yellowish micropapules.

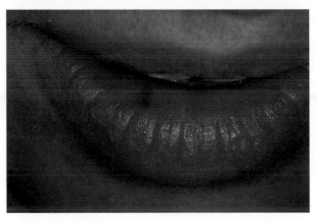

Figure 59.2 Melanotic macule of the lower lip.

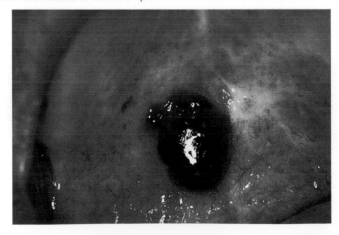

Figure 59.3 Angina bullosa haemorrhagica: a large blood blister in a typical site on the soft palate.

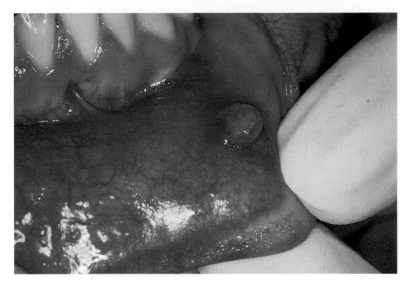

Figure 59.4 Superficial mucocoele on the labial mucosa.

> **Box 59.1 Causes of pigmentation in the mouth and on the lips**
>
> Localised:
>   Amalgam tattoo
>   Freckle (Syn. Ephelis)
>   Naevus
>   Melanotic macule
>   Malignant melanoma
>   Kaposi sarcoma (Figure 59.5)
>   Peutz–Jeghers syndrome (Figure 59.6)
>   Laugier–Hunziker syndrome
>
> Generalised:
>   Racial
>   Localised irritation (e.g. smoking)
>   Drugs (e.g. phenothiazines, antimalarials, minocycline, contraceptives, phenytoin)
>   Addison disease
>   Nelson syndrome
>   Ectopic adrenocorticotrophic hormone (e.g. bronchogenic carcinoma)
>   Heavy metals
>   Albright syndrome
>   Haemochromatosis

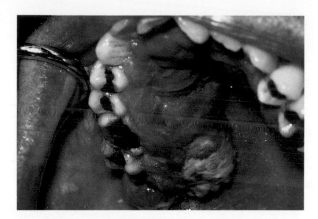

Figure 59.5 Intra-oral Kaposi sarcoma. (Source: Courtesy of Dr J.B. Epstein, Cancer Control Agency, Vancouver, Canada.)

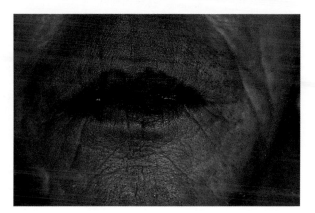

Figure 59.6 Peutz–Jeghers syndrome.

DISORDERS OF THE TONGUE

Inflammatory processes can involve the surface of the tongue, causing a range of appearances (Table 59.5).

DISORDERS OF THE LIPS

Cheilitis is the term used to describe an inflammatory or dysplastic process involving the lips. The major types of cheilitis are summarised in Table 59.6.

MOUTH INVOLVEMENT IN SKIN DISEASES

Many skin diseases involve the lips and buccal mucosae (Table 59.7). Definitive treatment of disease involvement at these sites is usually achieved through management of the underlying process. Local therapy to the mouth usually includes the use of topical chlorhexidine and benzydamine mouthwashes, and topical corticosteroid solutions.

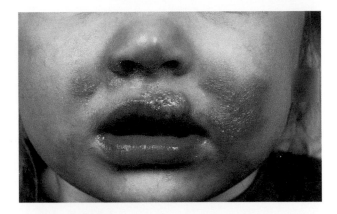

Figure 59.7 Primary herpetic stomatitis with extraoral lesions.

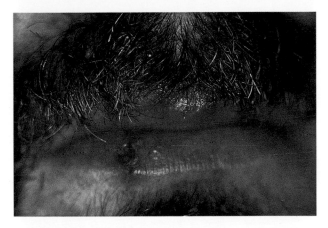

Figure 59.8 Herpes labialis (cold sore).

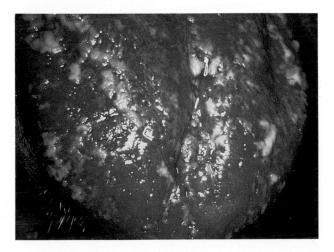

Figure 59.9 Acute pseudomembranous candidosis (thrush).

PART 8: SKIN DISORDERS ASSOCIATED WITH SPECIFIC SITES, SEX AND AGE

Table 59.2 Common infections of the mouth and lips

Disorder	HSV stomatitis (Figure 59.7)	Recurrent labial HSV (Syn. Herpes labialis) (Figure 59.8)	Acute pseudomembranous candidosis (Syn. Thrush) (Figure 59.9)	Chronic candidosis (Figure 59.10)
Pathophysiology	HSV is transmitted in saliva and can be shed in asymptomatic individuals 80% adults HSV-1 20% adults HSV-2 Incubation period is 3–7 days	Following primary herpes stomatitis, HSV remains latent in the trigeminal ganglion. 1/3 patients have recurrences (herpes labialis)	Infection by Candida albicans Healthy neonates may develop thrush Predisposing factors in other patients include antibiotics, steroids, xerostomia, immunosuppression and immunodeficiency (e.g. leukaemia or HIV infection)	Infection by Candida albicans and other Candida species Immune defects, denture wearing and smoking all predispose to chronic oral candidosis
Clinical features	Predominantly children and adolescents Primary herpetic stomatitis: malaise, anorexia, irritability, fever, tender cervical lymphadenopathy, diffuse gingivitis, multiple vesicles and ulcers	Itchy papules at the mucocutaneous junction of lip progress to vesicles, pustules and crusted erosion (cold sore) Lesions can become infected with Staph aureus	Soft, white patches/plaques on any intra-oral mucosal surface Lesions can be wiped off leaving an area of erythema	Chronic hyperplastic candidosis: typically tough adherent white patches Also seen is an erythematous form of oral candidosis, which can occur as an acute or chronic infection Denture candidosis: erythema and oedema of mucosa in contact with upper denture

Investigations	Usually a clinical diagnosis Viral swab: PCR detection of HSV DNA Conventional ELISA for serum antibodies has poor sensitivity and specificity	Usually a clinical diagnosis Viral swab: PCR detection of HSV DNA	Usually a clinical diagnosis Swab sent to microbiology	Usually a clinical diagnosis Swab sent to microbiology
Management	Herpetic stomatitis resolves spontaneously in 7–14 days but the HSV remains latent Supportive treatment: antipyretic analgesics, chlorhexidine and benzydamine mouthwashes Systemic antiviral agents (aciclovir, famciclovir) are useful in early stages of disease and in immunocompromised	5% aciclovir cream at first sign of cold sore Prevention of recurrent herpes labialis with prophylactic antivirals: oral aciclovir (800 mg daily) or valaciclovir (500 mg daily) for 4 months	Treat predisposing causes Topical polyenes (e.g. nystatin, amphotericin) or imidazoles (e.g. miconazole)	Treat predisposing causes Topical polyenes (e.g. nystatin, amphotericin) or imidazoles (e.g. miconazole) Chronic hyperplastic candidosis may respond only to systemic flucytosine, fluconazole, itraconazole, or caspofungin

HSV, herpes simplex virus.

PART 8: SKIN DISORDERS ASSOCIATED WITH SPECIFIC SITES, SEX AND AGE

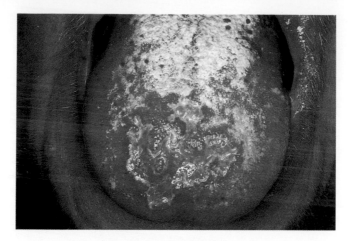

Figure 59.10 Chronic candidosis on the posterior portion of the tongue. There is also ulcerated herpes simplex virus infection anteriorly. The patient had leukaemia.

Box 59.2 Causes of mouth ulcers

Disorder	Example
Trauma	Friction from orthodontic appliance, thermal burn, cheek biting
Infection	Herpes simplex virus, herpes zoster virus, hand, foot and mouth disease, herpangina
Aphthous ulceration	Recurrent aphthous stomatitis (see Tables 59.3 and 59.4)
Malignancy	Squamous cell carcinoma
Systemic disease	Behcet's disease, Sweet's syndrome, lupus erythematosus
Drugs	Methotrexate, chemotherapy agents
Irradiation	Therapeutic irradiation for malignant disease, total body irradiation prior to haematopoietic stem cell transplantation

---

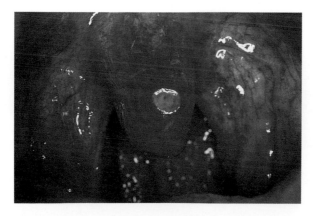

Figure 59.11 Recurrent aphthae.

Table 59.3 Recurrent aphthous ulcers

	Minor aphthae (80%) (Syn. Mikulicz ulcers) (Figure 59.11)	Major aphthae (10%) (Syn. Sutton ulcers) (Figure 59.12)	Herpetiform ulcers (10%) (Figure 59.13)
Age of onset	Childhood or adolescence	Childhood or adolescence	Young adult
Ulcer size/shape/symptoms	2–4 mm Round or oval Linear if on buccal mucosa Mild pain	May be 10 mm or larger Round or ovoid with an inflammatory halo Painful	Initially vesicles, which develop into tiny erosions coalescing to large ragged ulcers Extremely painful
Number of ulcers	1–6	1–6	10–100
Sites affected	Mainly vestibule, labial, buccal mucosa and floor of mouth; rarely on tongue, gingivae or palate	Any site, including the dorsum of the tongue or palate	Any site but often on the under surface of tongue
Duration of each ulcer	Up to 10 days	Up to 1 month Recur frequently	Up to 1 month
Other comments	Most common type of aphthae Heal without scarring	May heal with scarring May be associated with a raised ESR	Affects females predominantly Recurs so frequently that ulceration may be continuous HSV not involved aetiologically

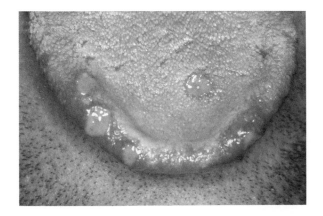

Figure 59.12 Major aphthous ulcers.

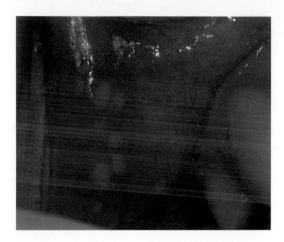

Figure 59.13 Herpetiform ulceration.

Table 59.4 Systemic disorders associated with recurrent aphthous stomatitis

	Comments
Autoinflammatory disorders	Association of recurrent mouth ulcers with fevers and serositis
Behçet syndrome	Association of recurrent mouth ulcers with ocular lesions, genital ulcers and multisystem disease
Endocrine factors	In some women, RAS can be related to a fall in progestogens in the luteal phase of the menstrual cycle
Gastrointestinal disease	Malabsorption states (pernicious anaemia, coeliac disease and Crohn disease) may precipitate RAS
Haematinic deficiency	In some studies 10–20% of patients with RAS have deficiencies of iron, folic acid or vitamin B12
Immunodeficiency	A few patients have an immune defect such as HIV disease
Other factors	Trauma, certain foods, stress and cessation of smoking may play a part in RAS

MOUTH INVOLVEMENT IN SYSTEMIC DISEASES

Many systemic diseases involve the mouth or are accompanied by signs occurring in the oral cavity (Box 59.3).

Table 59.5 Disorders affecting the surface of the tongue

Disorder	Deficiency glossitis (Syn. Atrophic glossitis) (Figure 59.14)	Coated tongue (Syn. Furred tongue; black hairy tongue) (Figure 59.15)	Fissured tongue (Syn. Plicated tongue; scrotal tongue) (Figure 59.16)	Benign migratory glossitis (Syn. Geographic tongue) (Figure 59.17)	Median rhomboid glossitis (Figure 59.18)
Pathophysiology	Caused by deficiency of iron, folate or vitamin B12	Edentulous adults, smokers, soft diet, poor oral hygiene, fasting Ill patients who cannot maintain oral hygiene or with hyposalivation	Common condition (5% population) Noted from childhood	Common problem Any age Histology: epithelial thinning at the centre of the lesion with an infiltrate of neutrophils	Uncommon, mainly older patients, smokers, diabetes Histology: irregular pseudoepitheliomatous hyperplasia
Clinical features	Tongue is red, sore and has a featureless smooth surface Can be associated with angular stomatitis and/or mouth ulcers	Affects mainly the posterior part of the dorsum of the tongue The filiform papillae are long and stained brown or black Coating consists of epithelial and microbial debris	Fissures occur on the dorsum of the tongue Often accompanied by benign migratory glossitis	Painful or asymptomatic Map-like red areas on the tongue with white margins Increased thickness of intervening papillae Patterns change within hours or days	Red central lesion of rhomboidal shape on dorsum of tongue Candidosis may coexist
Treatment	Replacement of the deficiency	Stop smoking, increase standards of oral hygiene, brush the tongue with a hard toothbrush	Reassurance	If sore, benzydamine hydrochloride 0.15% spray or mouthwash	May respond to cessation of smoking and to the use of antifungals

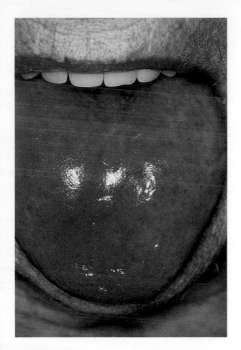

Figure 59.14 Deficiency glossitis from vitamin B12 deficiency.

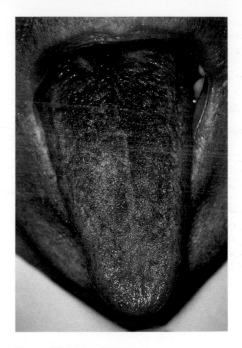

Figure 59.15 Coated tongue.

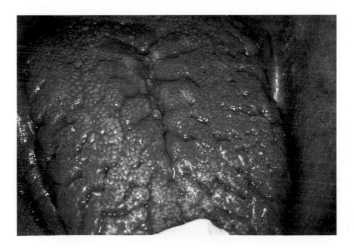

Figure 59.16 Fissured tongue.

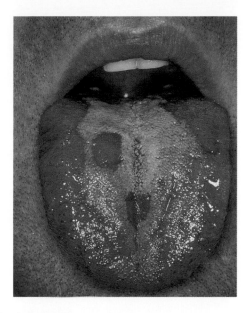

Figure 59.17 Benign migratory glossitis.

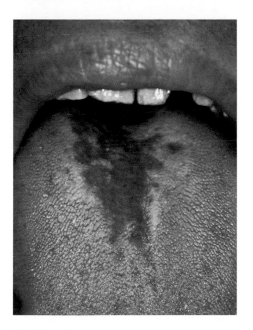

Figure 59.18 Median rhomboid glossitis.

PART 8: SKIN DISORDERS ASSOCIATED WITH SPECIFIC SITES, SEX AND AGE

Table 59.6 Types of cheilitis

Disorder	Actinic cheilitis	Angular cheilitis (Figure 59.19)	Lip lick dermatitis	Factitious cheilitis (Syn. Cheilitis artefacta) (Figure 59.20)	Granulomatous cheilitis (including Melkersson–Rosenthal syndrome) (Figure 59.21)
Epidemiology	Fair skinned adults, fourth to eight decades M > F	Older individuals, especially those with dentures	Children > adults	Rare Mostly seen in girls and young women	Rare M = F Onset usually in childhood, but may be delayed
Pathophysiology	Prolonged exposure to high-intensity sunlight affects vermillion of lower lip due to its anatomical orientation UV radiation causes inflammation and keratinocyte dysplasia	Multifactorial, including local candidosis, immunodeficiencies and nutritional deficiencies Also mechanical factors from oblique, curved fold at angle of mouth	Repeated lip licking causes saliva-induced irritant contact dermatitis and cheilitis Lip licking may be a compulsive disorder	Application of caustic agents, or sucking, biting, rubbing, licking of lips to cause inflammation. Occasionally presents, with disuse crusting from lack of cleansing	May be localised form of sarcoidosis, ectopic Crohn disease, orofacial granulomatosis Some cases are a reaction to cobalt or food additives (e.g. cinnamic aldehyde) Histologically: oedema, perivascular lymphocytic infiltration, small granulomas
Clinical features	Initially lower lip is red and swollen Over time lip becomes dry and scaly with white plaques	Triangular area of erythema ± scaling at angles of mouth	Redness of lips and eczema of adjacent skin in circumora distribution	Inflammation of lips with crusting which may be haemorrhagic Crusts can become very thick	Sudden diffuse swelling of lips (upper > lower) and sometimes cheeks Attacks may be accompanied by fever and constitutional symptoms Oedema initially subsides, but may persist with recurrent attacks A fissured tongue is seen in 20–40% of cases, lower motor neurone facial palsy occurs in 30%, mild regional lymphadenopathy in 50%
Management	5% fluorouracil cream, photodynamic therapy, laser ablation, vermillionectomy Monitor for potential development of squamous cell carcinoma	Treat local candidosis, treat dentures with candidacidal solution	Stop lip licking Greasy emollient	Appropriate psycho-dermatology management	Avoidance of any triggering antigens Intralesional triamcinolone, short courses of oral corticosteroids, clofazimine, anti-TNF biological agents

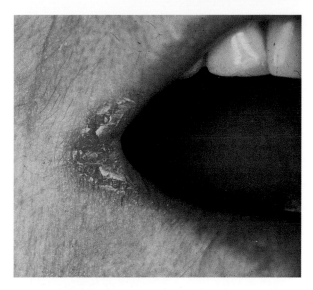

Figure 59.19 Angular cheilitis.

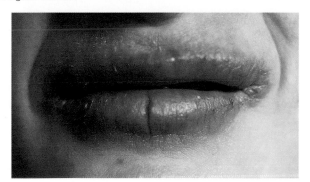

Figure 59.20 Factitious cheilitis due to repeated lip sucking.

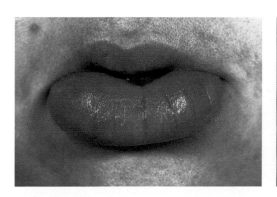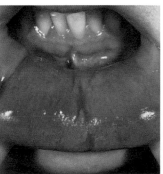

Figure 59.21 Granulomatous cheilitis of the lower lip. (Source: Courtesy of Addenbrooke's Hospital, Cambridge, UK.)

PART 8: SKIN DISORDERS ASSOCIATED WITH SPECIFIC SITES, SEX AND AGE

PART 8: SKIN DISORDERS ASSOCIATED WITH SPECIFIC SITES, SEX AND AGE

Table 59.7 Oral manifestations of skin diseases

Disease	Erythema multiforme (see Chapter 19)	Lichen planus (see Chapter 12) (Figures 59.22–59.24)	Mucous membrane pemphigoid (see Chapter 22)	Pemphigus vulgaris (see Chapter 22) (Figure 59.25)	Stevens–Johnson syndrome/toxic epidermal necrolysis (see Chapter 66) (Figure 59.26)
Relation to skin disease	Oral involvement may occur alone or in combination with skin disease	Oral involvement may occur alone or in combination with skin disease	Oral involvement in 1/3 of cases	Oral involvement is typical and commonly the presenting feature	Oral involvement is typical and commonly an early feature
Distribution of oral lesions	Typically affects labial mucosa	Buccal and/or lingual mucosae Also gingivae	Gingivae, soft palate	Any part of oral mucosa	All oral sites, including gingivae Lips usually involved
Lesion type in mouth	Painful, discrete red lesions which blister, leading to erosions with surrounding erythema and swelling	White reticular, papular, or plaque-like lesions Desquamative gingivitis	Desquamative gingivitis is typical Blisters on soft palate	Blisters readily rupture, leaving large irregular erosions which become secondarily infected	Blisters readily rupture, leaving widespread erosions Haemorrhagic cheilitis

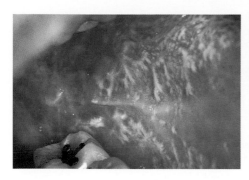

Figure 59.22 Lichen planus. White reticular lesions on the buccal mucosa.

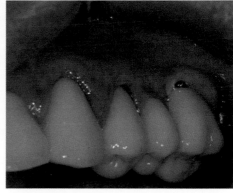

Figure 59.24 Lichen planus. Gingival involvement.

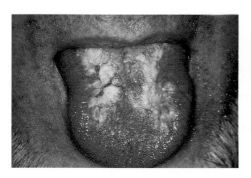

Figure 59.23 Lichen planus. White plaques on the tongue.

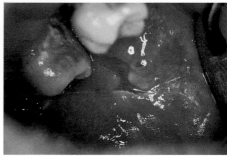

Figure 59.25 Pemphigus vulgaris. Irregular oral erosions.

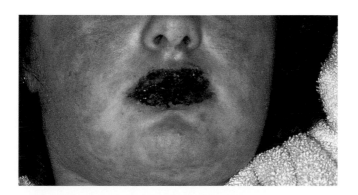

Figure 59.26 Stevens–Johnson syndrome. Haemorrhagic crusting of the lips.

Box 59.3 Oral manifestations of systemic disorders

Disorder	Oral manifestation
Acromegaly	Spaced teeth, mandibular prognathism, macroglossia
Addison disease	Mucosal hyperpigmentation
Amyloid	Macroglossia, purpura
Behcet syndrome	Aphthous-like ulcers
Crohn disease	Mucosal tags, gingival hyperplasia, cobblestoning of mucosa, ulcers, glossitis, angular cheilitis
Down syndrome	Macroglossia, fissured tongue, hypodontia
Gardner syndrome	Osteomas
Graft-versus-host disease	Acute: gingivitis, mucositis, erythema, pain
	Chronic: lichenoid changes, hyperkeratotic plaques, microstomia, xerostomia, dental decay, oral infections, mucocoeles, ulcers
Hepatitis C	Lichen planus, Sjogren syndrome
Hereditary haemorrhagic telangiectasia	Telangiectasiae, bleeding
Kawasaki disease	Sore tongue, cheilitis
Leukaemia	Infections, ulcers, purpura, bleeding tendency, gingival swelling in myelomonocytic leukaemia
Lupus erythematosus	Systemic lupus erythematosus: ulcers
	Discoid lupus erythematosus: lichenoid plaques on labial mucosae and vermillion, white patches with irradiating white striae on buccal mucosae ('sunburst patches')
Malabsorption	Aphthous ulcers, glossitis, angular cheilitis
Peutz–Jeghers syndrome	Melanosis
Polyarteritis nodosa	Ulcers
Primary biliary cholangitis	Lichen planus, Sjogren syndrome
Sarcoidosis	Gingival swelling
	Heerfordt syndrome: parotid gland swelling, lacrimal gland swelling, facial palsy
Scurvy (vitamin C deficiency)	Gingival swelling, purpura, ulcers
Sjogren syndrome	Xerostomia, dental decay, oral infections
Sweet syndrome	Aphthous-like ulcers
Syphilis	Chancre, mucous patches, ulcers, gumma
Systemic sclerosis	Microstomia, telangiectasiae
Tuberous sclerosis	Enamel defects, gingival fibromatosis

LEUKOPLAKIA

The white patches and plaques of leukoplakia can be benign or precancerous. Leukoplakia may also be a marker for cancer elsewhere in the upper aerodigestive tract

Epidemiology
Prevalence is 1% of adults, most cases in 50–70 years age group. M > F.

Pathophysiology
Risk factors for leukoplakia are as for carcinoma, mainly tobacco, alcohol and betel. Human papilloma virus can cause proliferative verrucous leukoplakia. Candida can also induce leukoplakia. Leukoplakias show increased keratin production, change in epithelial thickness and disordered epithelial maturation. The presence of severe epithelial dysplasia indicates a significant risk of malignant development.

Clinical features
Leukoplakia is a white patch or plaque on the mucosa that cannot be rubbed off and is not recognised as a specific disease entity (e.g. lichen planus, candidosis). There is a wide range of clinical presentations from homogeneous white plaques (Figure 59.27), which carry a low risk of malignant transformation, to nodular, speckled plaques (Figure 59.28). Verrucous white lesions have a high malignancy risk. High-risk sites for malignant transformation are the soft palate, ventrolateral tongue and floor of the mouth, referred to as sublingual keratosis (Figure 59.29). There is an overall annual malignant transformation rate of about 1–2% over 10 years.

Differential diagnosis
White sponge naevus, oral koilocytosis, hairy leukoplakia, squamous cell carcinoma (SCC) *in situ*, extramammary Paget disease of the oral mucosa.

Investigations
Biopsy.

Management
Excision. Surveillance of the patient to check for recurrence or new lesion(s).

ORAL SQUAMOUS CELL CARCINOMA

More than 90% of malignant neoplasms on the lips and in the mouth are SCCs.

Epidemiology
Worldwide, approximately 400 000 new cases of intraoral cancer are diagnosed annually. Mouth cancer is particularly common in people from the developing world. More common in people over 45. M > F.

Pathophysiology
Male preponderance attributable to risk-associated habits: tobacco, excess alcohol intake, betel use. Occupational exposure to strong sunlight is a risk factor for lip SCC. HPV infection is also implicated. HPV-related tumours tend to be seen in younger patients, occur in the fauces (mucosal arches at back of mouth cavity) and have a better prognosis.

Clinical features
Some oral SCCs arise in clinically apparently normal mucosa, others are preceded by potentially malignant disorders, such as erythroplakia (erythroplasia), leukoplakia, lichenoid lesions and actinic cheilitis. Cancers can develop on the lips (Figure 59.30), tongue (especially posterolateral border), floor of the mouth, buccal mucosae, palate, gingivae or oropharynx (Figure 59.31). The initial lesion is usually solitary and asymptomatic. In advanced SCCs there is often a red or red/white nodule or ulcer with irregular margins which are indurated. There may be pain, especially in tongue lesions and lesions on the floor of the mouth.

Investigations
Biopsy.
    CT scan of head and neck once SCC has been confirmed.

Management
The treatment of oral SCC requires a multispecialty approach. Surgery and radiation are the definitive treatment modalities for both early and locally advanced disease. Surgical resec-

PART 8: SKIN DISORDERS ASSOCIATED WITH SPECIFIC SITES, SEX AND AGE

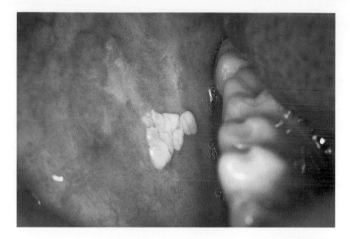

Figure 59.27 Homogeneous leukoplakia in the buccal mucosa.

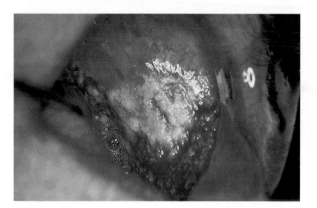

Figure 59.28 Speckled leukoplakia.

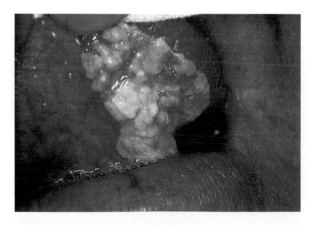

Figure 59.29 Sublingual keratosis.

tion can involve sacrificing critical structures. Radiation often produces significant acute and late toxicity. Chemotherapy alone is not a cura- tive therapeutic modality, but may improve out- comes when used in conjunction with radiation for locally advanced disease.

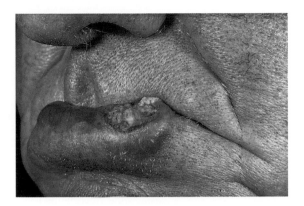

Figure 59.30 Squamous cell carcinoma of the lip.

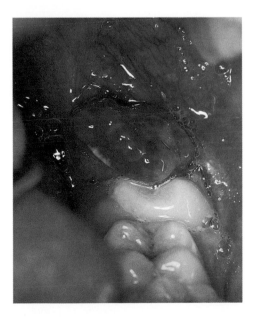

Figure 59.31 Oral squamous cell carcinoma.

60 Dermatoses of the eye and eyelids

There are a number of skin disorders which can involve the eyes and threaten visual acuity. An ophthalmic assessment is often necessary in the management of these patients.

Atopic eye disease

Ocular involvement in atopic patients ranges from 15 to 40% (see Chapter 16). The atopic eye diseases comprise a group of disorders which have variable involvement of the conjunctiva, cornea and lens. Seasonal/perennial allergic conjunctivitis is mild and occurs commonly (Figure 60.1). The other forms of atopic conjunctivitis are rare but can be severe: atopic keratoconjunctivitis, atopic blepharoconjunctivitis and vernal keratoconjunctivitis. Cataracts develop in up to 25% of patients with atopic eczema; typically they are anterior, subcapsular and occur in the pupillary area. Cataracts as a side effect of corticosteroids occur in a posterior, subcapsular position.

Management

Most cases of atopic eye disease are managed with topical ocular therapy. The risk of cataract and glaucoma with long-term application of potent topical steroids to eczema on the periocular skin favours the use of topical calcineurin inhibitors (tacrolimus, pimecrolimus) to these sites. Dupilumab, used to treat moderate-to-severe atopic eczema, can be associated with ocular side effects, notably dry eyes, conjunctivitis and keratitis. Because of the potential for sight-threatening complications, severe atopic eye disease is best managed by an ophthalmologist.

Chronic blepharitis

Blepharitis is a general term describing inflammation of the lid: anterior blepharitis refers to inflammation of the anterior lid margin and is concentrated around the lashes; posterior blepharitis describes inflammation of the posterior lid margin. In dermatological practice blepharitis is most commonly encountered in seborrhoeic dermatitis (seborrhoeic blepharitis) and rosacea (ocular rosacea). Approximately half of patients with seborrhoeic dermatitis and rosacea have signs of ocular involvement. Staphylococcal infection can also cause a chronic anterior blepharitis, whereas meibomian disorders can cause a posterior blepharitis. The clinical features of different forms of chronic blepharitis are presented in Table 60.1.

Management

The treatment of blepharitis is that of the underlying cause. Patients with blepharitis usually need to be managed jointly with ophthalmology. Generic treatments for the types of eyelid involvement are outlined in Table 60.2.

Cicatrising conjunctivitis

Cicatrising conjunctivitis is caused by a variety of immunobullous and other autoimmune mucocutaneous disorders. Disruption and destruction of the ocular surface in cicatrising conjunctivitis can lead to corneal blindness. The degree of conjunctival involvement varies between disorders, for example in pemphigus vulgaris the severity of conjunctivitis is generally mild, whereas in mucous membrane pemphigoid eye involvement can be

Rook's Dermatology Handbook, First Edition. Edited by Christopher E. M. Griffiths, Tanya O. Bleiker, Daniel Creamer, John R. Ingram and Rosalind C. Simpson.
© 2022 John Wiley & Sons Ltd. Published 2022 by John Wiley & Sons Ltd.

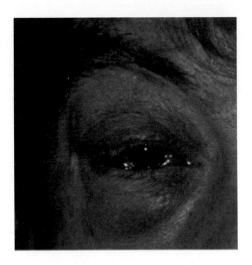

Figure 60.1 Seasonal allergic conjunctivitis. Erythema and oedema of the eyelid and redness of the conjunctiva.

sight-threatening. Consequently, cicatrising conjunctivitis must be managed by an ophthalmologist. The conditions which cause progressive conjunctival scarring are listed in Box 60.1.

Systemic diseases and ocular involvement

A number of systemic diseases with skin manifestations have important clinical features which involve the eyelids and/or eyes, as outlined in Table 60.3.

Tumours and Cysts of the Eyelid

The eyelid gives rise to a large number of cysts and tumours. Tumours can arise from the epidermis and dermis in addition to the adnexal structures, which include the meibomian and Zeis sebaceous glands eccrine glands, Moll apocrine sweat glands, and the specialised hair follicles of the eyelashes. Tumours and cysts occurring on eyelids are listed in Table 60.4.

Table 60.1 Clinical features of types of chronic blepharitis

Anterior blepharitis		Posterior blepharitis	
Staphylococcal blepharitis	**Seborrhoeic blepharitis**	**Ocular rosacea**	**Meibomian seborrhoea**
Symptoms			
Burning, itching, photophobia	Minimal	Foreign body sensation, burning, discomfort, photophobia	Foreign body sensation, burning, discomfort, photophobia
Lid signs			
Unilateral/patchy lid margin involvement, fibrinous scales, dilated vessels, styes (Figure 60.2)	Bilateral involvement, greasy scales	Chalazia, meibomitis, irregular lid margins	Plugged orifices without inflammation
Conjunctival and corneal signs			
Follicles, papillae and hyperaemia of lower tarsal conjunctiva Coarse punctate keratitis in lower third of cornea	Mild conjunctival injection Coarse punctate keratitis in lower third of cornea	Conjunctival hyperaemia, papillary conjunctivitis Marginal corneal infiltration and ulceration	Minimal injection Foamy tear film

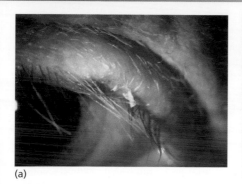
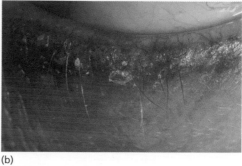

(a)   (b)

Figure 60.2 (a) *Staphylococcal blepharitis*: fibrinous scales on the anterior lid margin with madarosis (loss of lashes) and poliosis (white lashes). (b) Localised ulcerative *Staphylococcal blepharitis*. (Source: Courtesy of Mr J. Dart, Moorfields Eye Hospital, London, UK.)

Table 60.2 Treatment of chronic blepharitis

Aims of treatment	Therapeutic guidelines
For anterior lid margin disease	
Treat infection	Topical antibiotics (chloramphenicol or fucidic acid) 4 times daily to lid margins
	Oral oxytetracycline or erythromycin 500 mg twice daily for 10 days
Clean lid margins	'Lid scrubs': twice daily with a cotton wool bud dampened in boiled water
Lid hyperaemia and exudate	Topical chloramphenicol/hydrocortisone 0.5–1.0% lid margins twice daily for 1 month
For posterior lid margin disease	
Mechanically unblock meibomian glands	Hot compresses for 3–5 min to liquefy meibomian secretions Massage of tarsal plate with cotton wool bud (or finger) twice daily
Alter meibomian secretions	Oral tetracycline (e.g. doxycycline 100 mg or lymecycline 408 mg) once daily or erythromycin (250–500 mg) twice daily for 12 weeks minimum
For the tear film	
Restore tear film	Artificial tears drops 2–4 hourly
For associated conjunctivitis (papillary or mixed follicular and papillary)	
Reduce inflammation	Fluoromethalone 0.1% four times daily for 1 week, reducing to once daily over next 4 weeks
Treat associated skin disease	Seborrhoeic dermatitis (see Chapter 15)
	Rosacea (see Chapter 45)
For keratitis	
Punctate keratitis/marginal keratoconjunctivitis	Fluoromethalone 0.1% four times daily for 1 week, reducing to once daily over next 4 weeks

> **Box 60.1 Skin disorders associated with progressive conjunctival scarring**
>
> *Immunobullous diseases*
> Mucous membrane pemphigoid (MMP) (Figure 60.3)
> Linear IgA disease
> Epidermolysis bullosa acquisita
> Paraneoplastic MMP (anti-laminin-332)
> Paraneoplastic pemphigus
> Pemphigus vulgaris
>
> *Other mucocutaneous diseases*
> Stevens–Johnson syndrome/toxic epidermal necrolysis (Figure 60.4)
> Erythema multiforme
> Lichen planus
> Graft-versus-host disease

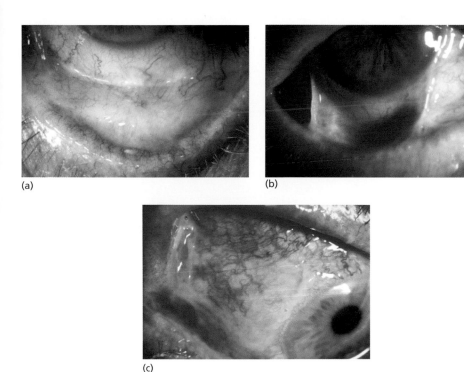

(a)

(b)

(c)

Figure 60.3 Ocular signs of MMP. (a) Inferior fornix shortening and subconjunctival scarring. (b) Conjunctival symblepharon tethering the globe to the lower lid. (c) Conjunctival ulceration in an acute exacerbation.

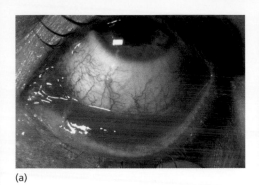
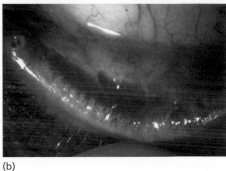

(a)   (b)

Figure 60.4 Ocular signs of Stevens–Johnson syndrome/toxic epidermal necrolysis (SJS/TEN). (a) Acute ocular SJS/TEN: hyperaemic conjunctiva with a papillary reaction and mucopurulent discharge. (b) Chronic ocular SJS/TEN: lower tarsal conjunctival scarring with squamous metaplasia and keratinisation. A punctal plug is *in situ* to conserve tears in a dry eye. (Source: Courtesy of Mr J. Dart, Moorfields Eye Hospital, London, UK.)

Table 60.3 Systemic diseases with skin and eye involvement

Systemic disease	Eye disease
Sarcoidosis	Papules on eyelids; proptosis from orbital sarcoid; granulomatous conjunctivitis; bilateral granulomatous uveitis; dry eye from lacrimal gland involvement
Systemic lupus erythematosus	Dry eye; peripheral corneal ulcers; episcleritis in 10%, scleritis rarer; retinal vasculitis common during exacerbations of systemic disease (associated with CNS vasculitis or lupus nephritis)
Sjögren syndrome	Lacrimal gland inflammation causing dry eye; conjunctivitis; punctate keratopathy
Behçet syndrome	Conjunctivitis; keratitis; episcleritis; uveitis (commonest ocular manifestation); retinal ischaemia
Granulomatosis with polyangiitis	Episcleritis (very common); retinal vasculitis; optic neuritis; orbital pseudotumour
Polyarteritis nodosa	Episcleritis; scleritis; keratitis

Table 60.4 Clinical features and treatment of tumours and cysts occurring on the eyelid

Lesion	Clinical features	Treatment
Xanthelasma	Yellow plaques on medial part of eyelids (Figure 60.5) Usually bilateral, mostly in elderly Associated with hypercholesterolaemia in 60% of patients	If treatment is warranted: topical trichloroacetic acid; surgical excision; CO_2 laser
Chalazion	A firm lump seen when lid is everted Caused by inflammatory reaction around a blocked sebaceous gland	Usually resolve spontaneously Can be removed by curettage

(Continued)

Table 60.4 Continued

Lesion	Clinical features	Treatment
Cyst of Moll	Small translucent nodule on anterior lid margin close to lacrimal punctum (Figure 60.6) Caused by blockage of Moll apocrine sweat gland	Excision
Cyst of Zeis	Small opaque nodule on anterior lid margin (Figure 60.7) Arises from sebaceous gland of Zeis	Excision
Eccrine hidrocystoma	Translucent blue cyst occurring on eyelids or cheeks Usually solitary, may be multiple	Local destruction (e.g. hyfrecation) or excision
Apocrine hidrocystoma	Solitary, translucent, dome-shaped nodule of peri-ocular skin, especially lateral to the outer canthus	Excision
Syringoma	Multiple, small, skin-coloured papules on cheeks and eyelids bilaterally	Local destruction (e.g. hyfrecation)
BCC	70% arise on the lower eyelid (Figure 60.8) Morphoeic BCCs can mimic a patch of dermatitis If a BCC penetrates the orbital septum it can threaten the orbit, particularly those near the medial canthus	Mohs micrographic surgery is treatment of choice Surgery at the medial canthus carries a risk of tear duct damage
SCC	Occurs on lower eyelid and lid margin Nodular, plaque-like or ulcerated lesions (Figure 60.9) SCCs >2 cm in diameter and with deep penetration have increased risk of metastasis	Mohs micrographic surgery is the treatment of choice
Sebaceous gland carcinoma	Very rare: <1–5% of malignant tumours of the eyelid Arises from the meibomian glands Occur on upper eyelid, resembles a chalazion (Figure 60.10)	Wide local excision is the treatment of choice The multicentric nature of the tumour may limit the use of Mohs micrographic surgery

BCC, basal cell carcinoma; SCC, squamous cell carcinoma.

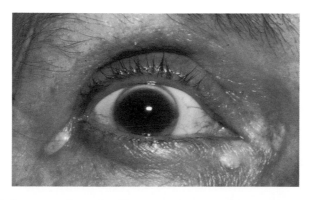

Figure 60.5 Xanthelasmata on the eyelids. The cornea shows arcus senilis, which is also associated with hypercholesterolaemia.

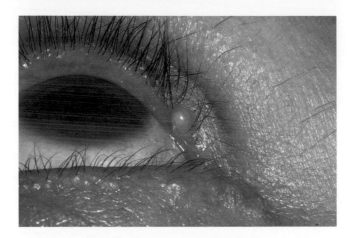

Figure 60.6 Cyst of Moll. (Source: Courtesy of Mr N. Joshi, Chelsea and Westminster Hospital/ Medical Illustration UK, London, UK.)

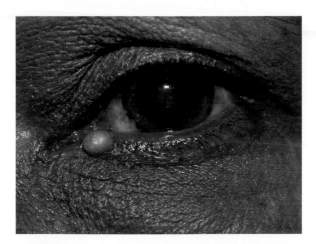

Figure 60.7 Cyst of Zeis.

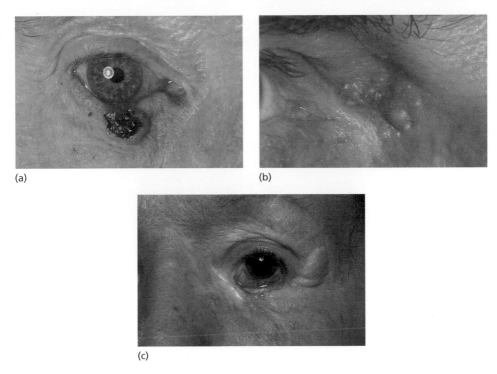

(a)

(b)

(c)

Figure 60.8 Basal cell carcinoma. (a) Ulcerated BCC on the lower lid. (b) Poorly defined BCC at medial canthus. (c) Morphoeic BCC along the lower lid. (Source: Courtesy of Mr N. Joshi, Chelsea and Westminster Hospital/Medical Illustration UK, London, UK.)

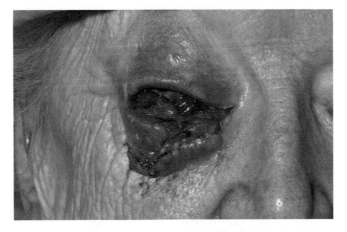

Figure 60.9 Squamous cell carcinoma. (Source: Courtesy of Mr N. Joshi, Chelsea and Westminster Hospital/Medical Illustration UK, London, UK.)

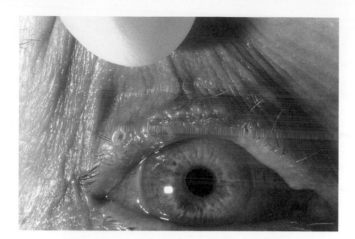

Figure 60.10 Sebaceous gland carcinoma. Infiltrating lesion on the upper lid. (Source: Courtesy of Mr N. Joshi, Chelsea and Westminster Hospital/Medical Illustration UK, London, UK.)

Dermatoses of anogenital skin

61

There are dermatoses and lesions which have either a predilection for anogenital skin or occur exclusively in this region. Common dermatoses that are easily recognised elsewhere may have a modified appearance on vulval, penile and perianal skin.

BENIGN LESIONS OF ANOGENITAL SKIN

See Tables 61.1, 61.2 and 61.3.

INFLAMMATORY DERMATOSES OF ANOGENITAL SKIN

The management of all inflammatory dermatoses of the anogenital skin requires a generic approach with use of a soap substitute (e.g. emulsifying ointment) and regular application of a bland moisturiser. The use of wet wipes should be discouraged.

Lichen sclerosus

(Syn. Lichen sclerosus et atrophicus)
Lichen sclerosus (LS) is a common inflammatory dermatosis with a predilection for anogenital skin.

Epidemiology

LS is 6–10 times more common in females than males. There are two peaks of incidence, in children and in older adults. It affects 1 in 30 postmenopausal women.

Pathophysiology

There is some evidence in women that LS is a genetically determined autoimmune disorder. In males LS appears to be due to chronic exposure of skin under the prepuce to urine. Dysfunction of the penile naviculomeatal valve leads to post—micturition micro-incontinence and release of urine onto susceptible skin. Histopathologically the epidermis in LS is atrophic with basal cell hydropic degeneration and flattening of the rete pegs. The superficial dermis is oedematous and hyalinised. Deep to the hyalinzed zone is a band-like lymphohistiocytic infiltrate. Telangiectatic vessels are common, as are extravasated red cells.

Clinical features

Vulva. The presenting symptom is usually itching. Vulval soreness and dyspareunia are common. The sites most commonly affected are the genito-crural folds, the inner aspects of the labia majora, labia minora, clitoris and clitoral hood. Vaginal lesions do not occur, as LS spares mucosal epithelium. Lesional skin is atrophic, whitened and extends around the vulva (Figure 61.8). Perianal involvement in a figure-of-eight configuration is common in female patients (Figure 61.9). There may also be oedema, purpura, bullae, erosions, fissures and ulceration. Scarring of the vulva can lead to introital narrowing, loss of the labia minora and sealing over of the clitoral hood with burying of the clitoris (Figure 61.8). There is an association between vulval squamous cell carcinoma (SCC) and LS, but the incidence is less than 4%. Extragenital LS occurs in 10% of women and is characterised by ivory white papules and plaques with follicular delling on the upper back, wrists, buttocks, and thighs.

Rook's Dermatology Handbook, First Edition. Edited by Christopher E. M. Griffiths, Tanya O. Bleiker, Daniel Creamer, John R. Ingram and Rosalind C. Simpson.
© 2022 John Wiley & Sons Ltd. Published 2022 by John Wiley & Sons Ltd.

PART 8: SKIN DISORDERS ASSOCIATED WITH SPECIFIC SITES, SEX AND AGE

Table 61.1 Benign lesions of the penis and scrotum

Lesion	Epidemiology	Clinical features	Pathophysiology	Management
Pearly penile papules (Figure 61.1)	Occur in up to 50% of boys/men	Pink or skin-coloured papules on coronal margin	Angiofibromas	Reassurance Can be excised if symptomatic
Median raphe cyst	Rare Congenital Often only apparent in adulthood	Midline cystic swelling of the ventral penis near the glans May become traumatised or infected	Histologically either dermoid or mucoid cyst, depending on their embryology	Surgery if symptomatic
Mucoid cyst	Rare Present at birth or develop in childhood	Small, flesh-coloured cystic papules/nodules Commonly on the ventral glans or foreskin Symptomatic if become infected Can interfere with intercourse	Arise from ectopic urethral tissue during embryological development	Surgery if symptomatic
Scrotal calcinosis (Figure 61.2)	Common Adult men	Solitary or multiple Hard, smooth, white papules or nodules on the scrotum, rarely the penis	Cutaneous calcinosis	Surgery if symptomatic
Angiokeratoma (Figure 61.3)	Common Adult men	Multiple, blue to purple, smooth, 2–5 mm papules on the scrotum; rarely on penile shaft and glans	Angiokeratoma	Reassurance Excision or electrodessication if symptomatic

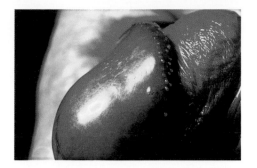

Figure 61.1 Pearly penile papules. (Source: Courtesy of Dr D.A. Burns, Leicester, UK.)

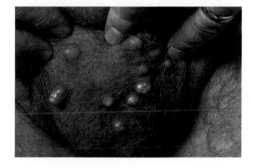

Figure 61.2 Scrotal calcinosis. (Source: Courtesy of Dr D.A. Burns, Leicester, UK.)

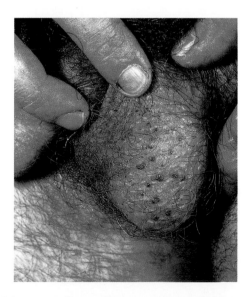

Figure 61.3 Scrotal angiokeratomas. (Source: Courtesy of Dr D.A. Burns, Leicester, UK.)

PART 8: SKIN DISORDERS ASSOCIATED WITH SPECIFIC SITES, SEX AND AGE

Table 61.2 Benign lesions of the vulva

Lesion	Epidemiology	Clinical features	Pathophysiology	Management
Fordyce spots (Figure 61.4)	Common	Numerous yellow papules on the inner aspects of the labia majora and labia minora	Hyperplastic, visible sebaceous glands	Reassurance
Bartholin's cyst	Common Adult women	1–3 cm swelling on lower third of the inner labium majus Mostly asymptomatic but may become infected	Obstruction of Bartholin gland duct Cyst lined by transitional epithelium	Surgical enucleation
Papillary hidradenoma	Occur mostly in middle-aged white women	1–2 cm nodule on labia majora, interlabial sulcus, or lateral surface of the labia minora If multiple, lesions occur on one side of the vulva Usually asymptomatic, may be painful	Sweat gland adenoma with apocrine differentiation	Surgery if symptomatic
Mucinous cyst	Adult women	Single or multiple lesions in vestibule	Cyst lined by a layer of mucinous epithelium	Surgical enucleation
Labial melanotic macule	Young women	Solitary, small, flat, brown to black macule	Benign increased pigmentation of the epithelial basal layer, accentuated at the tips of rete ridges	Reassurance
Vulval melanosis (Figure 61.5)	Young women	Multiple pigmented macules on inner labia minora and vestibule Individual lesions are often asymmetrical with an irregular outline	Basal layer hyperpigmentation, but no increase in melanocytes Also dermal melanophages	Reassurance
Angiokeratoma	Common Adult women	Small vascular papules on labia majora Can bleed if traumatised, especially in pregnancy	Angiokeratoma	Reassurance Excision or electrodessication if symptomatic

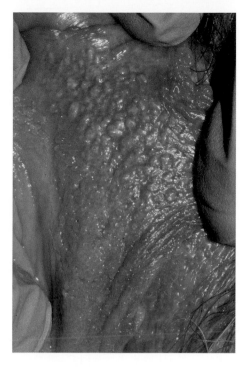

Figure 61.4 Fordyce spots.

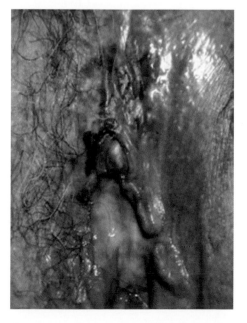

Figure 61.5 Vulval melanosis.

Table 61.3 Benign lesions of the perineum and perianal skin

Lesion	Epidemiology	Clinical features	Pathology	Management
Perianal skin tag (anal tag) (Figure 61.6)	Common Perianal skin tags can be a manifestation of Crohn disease	1-3 cm diameter, firm asymptomatic polyp at anal margin	Result from thrombosed external haemorrhoid	Surgical excision
Cutaneous endometriosis	Rare Adult women	Small bluish nodules on perineum Also umbilicus and episiotomy scar May be painful May increase in size with menstrual cycle and bleed at menstruation	Endometrial glands and stroma	Surgical excision
Pilonidal sinus (Figure 61.7)	26/100,000 Mostly second and third decades 2M:1F	Discharging nodule in midline of natal cleft, commonly sacrococcygeal region Can occur in association with hidradenitis suppurativa	Caused by entrapment of hairs in pilosebaceous unit	Surgical excision

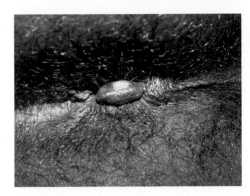

Figure 61.6 Perianal skin tag.

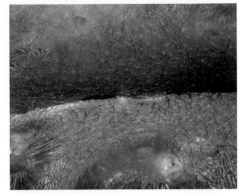

Figure 61.7 Pilonidal sinus in a natal cleft with buttock abscesses.

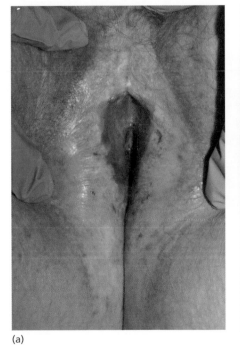

(a)

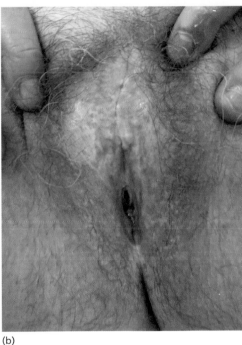

(b)

Figure 61.8 (a) Scarring in LS with ecchymosis. (b) Scarring in LS with loss of the labia minora and sealing of the clitoral hood.

Penis. Patients describe itching and burning of genital skin. Symptoms of sexual dysfunction are also common: bleeding, tearing and splitting. In both boys and men phimosis (non-retractile foreskin) may be the presenting feature of LS (Figure 61.10). Lesional skin presents as atrophic white patches or plaques, or lilac, slightly scaly patches with telangiectasia and purpura (Figure 61.11). Scarring changes can cause narrowing of the meatal orifice, adhesions in the coronal sulcus and effacement of the frenulum. Involvement of the foreskin will often cause prob-

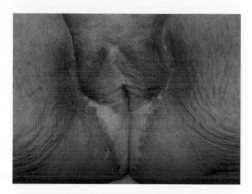

Figure 61.9 Anogenital LS in a typical figure-of-eight configuration.

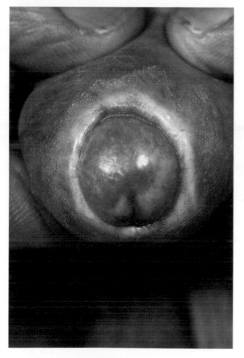

Figure 61.10 Lichen sclerosus causing phimosis. (Source: Courtesy of Dr D.A. Burns, Leicester, UK.)

lems with retraction due to a circumferential sclerotic band (Figure 61.12). The term balanitis xerotica obliterans (BXO) describes an inflammatory-scarring process of the glans penis caused by LS and other dermatoses, such as lichen planus and cicatricial pemphigoid. LS may also present with a foreskin fixed in retraction (paraphimosis), urinary retention (even renal failure) and chronic

penile oedema. Perianal or extragenital LS does not occur in men.

Differential diagnosis

Vitiligo, lichen planus, Zoon balanitis, mucous membrane pemphigoid.

In girls LS can be mistaken for sexual abuse. Sexual abuse may also be the initiating/exacerbating factor of LS.

Investigations

Skin biopsy, if there is diagnostic doubt.

Management

First line, penis and vulva: Soap substitute. Super-potent topical corticosteroid, e.g. clobetasol propionate 0.05%, applied once nightly for 4 weeks, then alternate nights for 4 weeks, and twice a week for a further month. Thereafter topical corticosteroid ointment can be used, as required, to control itching.

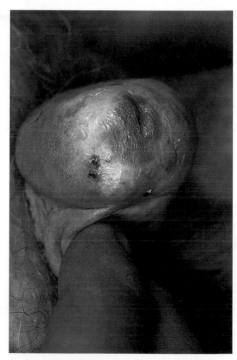

Figure 61.11 Lichen sclerosus. White plaques and haemorrhagic areas on the glans. (Source: Courtesy of Dr D.A. Burns, Leicester, UK.)

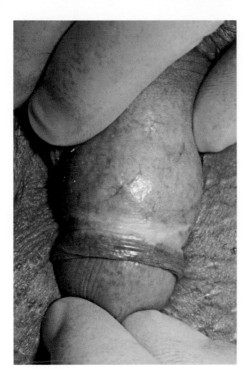

Figure 61.12 Lichen sclerosus. Sclerotic band of the prepuce causing 'waisting'. (Source: Courtesy of Professor C.B. Bunker, with permission from Medical Illustration UK, Chelsea & Westminster Hospital, London, UK.)

Second line, penis: Circumcision, frenuloplasty, and meatotomy can reverse the scarring damage of LS. In boys, complete circumcision is the treatment of choice because all affected tissue is removed and any secondary involvement of the glans probably resolves.

Second line, vulva: Surgery is only indicated for the management of functional problems caused by post-inflammatory scarring, premalignant lesions and malignancy.

Lichen planus

See Chapter 12.

Clinical features

Vulva. Three clinical forms of lichen planus (LP) are recognised.

Classic/papular lichen planus
The typical violaceous papules are seen on the outer labia majora, interlabial sulci and clitoral hood. These may coalesce into plaques or annular lesions. Wickham striae may be present (Figure 61.13).

Erosive lichen planus
Symmetrical erosions occur most commonly at the fourchette and vestibule. These may have an irregular edge with Wickham striae. The vulval mucosa is eroded with, in some cases, marked loss of architecture. Vaginal involvement is characterised by glazed erythema, which is friable and bleeds easily. Vaginal synechiae and adhesions may develop and can lead to vaginal stenosis. Vulvovaginal–gingival syndrome (Syn. Syndrome of Hewitt and Pelisse) is a distinctive erosive subtype of LP which principally affects the inner aspects of the labia minora, vestibule and vagina in association with a characteristic gingival erythema.

Hypertrophic lichen planus
The least common form of vulval LP. Thickened, intensely pruritic plaques, sometimes with a violaceous edge, occur on the labia majora, perineum and perianal skin. Vaginal lesions do not occur in classic or hypertrophic LP.

Penis. LP presents with itchy red-purple papules, patches, plaques and annular lesions on the glans and penile shaft (Figure 61.14). It may also present as phimosis. The male genitalia represent the commonest site for the annular subtype of LP. Occasionally, an erosive form of LP is encountered on the penis, including a form with chronic erosive gingival lesions.

Seborrhoeic dermatitis

See Chapter 15.

Clinical features

Vulva. The signs may be subtle, but scaling and erythema are seen on the inguinal folds, labia majora, perineum and perianal skin. Keratin debris may build up in the interlabial sulci and sometimes under the clitoral hood.

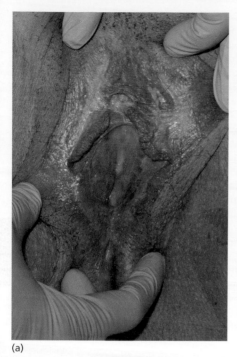
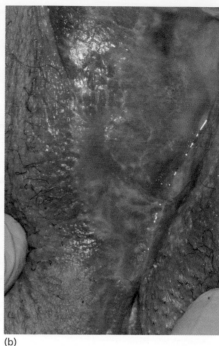

(a)

(b)

Figure 61.13 (a) Classic vulval lichen planus showing plaques in the interlabial sulci. (b) Classic vulval lichen planus with Wickham striae.

Penis. Demarcated or diffuse erythema of glans and prepuce is common. Extensive involvement causes erythema of penile shaft, scrotum and groins.

Perineum and perianal skin. Erythema involving the inguinal folds, perianal skin and natal cleft can occur in extensive seborrheic dermatitis (Figure 61.15).

Psoriasis

See Chapter 10.

Clinical features

Vulva. Well-demarcated red plaques occur on the labia majora extending to the mons pubis (Figure 61.16). Typical silvery scaling is lost on genital skin but may be seen on mons.

Penis. Erythema on the inner aspect of the foreskin and on the glans is typical. Lesions resemble extragenital psoriasis on the circumcised penis.

Perineum and perianal skin. Well-demarcated erythema involving the inguinal folds, perianal skin and natal cleft is typical of flexural psoriasis. A long fissure at the base of the natal cleft is common.

Hidradenitis suppurativa

See Chapter 46.

Clinical features

Vulva. Nodules, abscesses, sinuses and fistulae can involve the labia majora in severe cases.

Penis. Purulent discharge from abscesses and sinuses in the groins can lead to secondary inflammation of scrotal and penile skin.

Perineum and perianal skin. Men are more likely to have perineal and perianal involvement than women. Inflammation and scarring can extend widely over inguinal folds, perineum, perianal skin, buttocks and thighs (Figures 61.17 and 61.18). Persistent perineal sinuses are frequent. Deep-seated lesions can lead to anal fistulae.

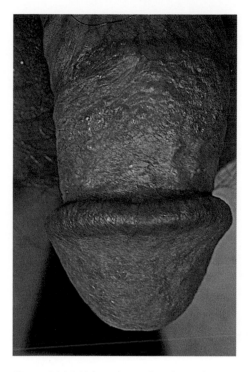

Figure 61.14 Lichen planus. Papules and annular lesions on the glans and shaft. (Source: Courtesy of Professor C.B. Bunker, with permission from Medical Illustration UK, Chelsea & Westminster Hospital, London, UK.)

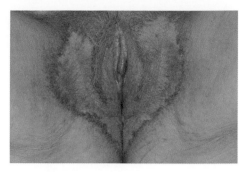

Figure 61.16 Vulval psoriasis.

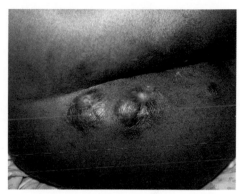

Figure 61.17 Hurley stage I hidradenitis suppurativa presenting as chronic furunculosis on the buttocks.

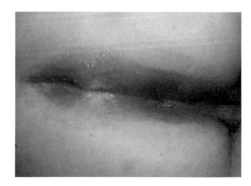

Figure 61.15 Seborrhoeic dermatitis affecting the natal cleft and perianal skin.

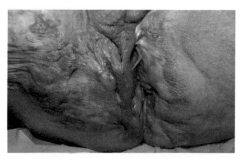

Figure 61.18 Hurley stage III severe hidradentitis suppurativa affecting the perineum and causing extensive keloid scar formation in a 75-year-old male patient.

Zoon balanitis

(Syn. Plasma cell balanitis)
Zoon balanitis (ZB) is an asymptomatic, inflammatory condition of the glans and mucosal prepuce.

Epidemiology
A disorder of the middle-aged and older uncircumcised male.

Pathophysiology
ZB is an irritant dermatosis caused by a dysfunctional prepuce. Retention of urine and squames between two apposed surfaces leads to a disturbed 'preputial ecology', frictional trauma and irritation by urine. Histologically there is epidermal attenuation with an absent granular layer, spongiosis and lozenge-shaped basal keratinocytes. There is a plasma cell dermal infiltrate with extravasated erythrocytes and haemosiderin,

Clinical features
Well-demarcated, glistening, moist, bright red or brown patches involve the glans and inner prepuce (Figure 61.19). Dark-red stippling ('cayenne pepper spots') can be seen on lesional skin. Lesions lie symmetrically across the coronal sulcus.

Differential diagnosis
LS, psoriasis, seborrhoeic dermatitis, non-specific balano-posthitis.

Investigations
The diagnosis is usually made clinically but may require biopsy.

Management
ZB can improve with the intermittent application of a mild-moderate topical corticosteroid, but it usually persists or relapses. Circumcision is curative.

Lipschutz ulcer

An acute ulcerative condition of the vulva.

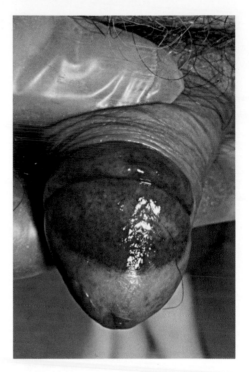

Figure 61.19 Zoon balanitis. Symmetrical moist erythema of the glans and prepuce. (Source: Courtesy of Professor C.B. Bunker, with permission from Medical Illustration UK, Chelsea & Westminster Hospital, London, UK.)

Epidemiology
Rare. Affects teenage and young adult women.

Pathophysiology
Thought to be reactive to an infection (e.g. Epstein–Barr virus).

Clinical features
Starts as haemorrhagic blisters which break down to form painful, rapidly expanding ulcers. Affects lower inner labia majora. Can be bilateral.

Differential diagnosis
Herpes simplex virus infection, Behçet disease, major aphthous ulcers.

Investigations

The diagnosis is usually made clinically.

Management

Moderately potent topical steroid ointment is helpful. 5% lidocaine ointment can be used for analgesia. If severe, a short course of oral prednisolone can accelerate healing.

INFECTIVE DERMATOSES OF ANOGENITAL SKIN

Human papilloma virus

See Chapter 3.

Clinical features

Vulva. Warty papules can affect any surface of the vulva (Figure 61.20). Extensive vegetating masses (condylomata acuminate) can cover the vulva, perineum and perianal skin.

Penis. Warty papules can affect any surface of the penis. Circumcised men are more likely to have genital warts than uncircumcised. In uncircumcised men, warts are more likely to be distal.

Perineum and perianal skin. Warty papules, plaques and nodules may be profuse and extend into the anal canal. Perianal warts may occur in infants and young children (Figure 61.21). Sexual abuse needs to be considered in all cases.

Candidiasis

See Chapter 7.

Clinical features

Vulva. Vaginal infection causes a heavy white discharge which may lead to candida vulvitis characterised by well demarcated erythema extending to perineum and genito-crural folds. There is a scaly or vesiculo-pustular edge with satellite pustules beyond the margin. The disorder is itchy.

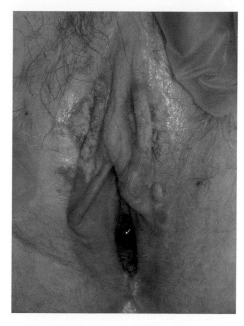

Figure 61.20 Vulval warts with plaques in the interlabial sulci.

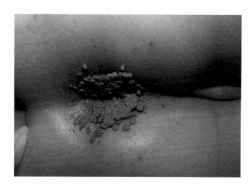

Figure 61.21 Florid perianal warts in a 5-year-old male.

Penis. Candidal infection of genital skin in men is considerably less common than in women and is often a secondary infection of a pre-existing dermatosis. Candidal balano-posthitis is characterised by glazed erythema with marginal scaling, micropapules, pustules and erosions.

Streptococcal infections

See Chapter 4.

Most streptococcal infections of the anogenital skin are caused by Group A β-haemolytic streptococcus.

Clinical features

Vulva. Vulval cellulitis most commonly follows trauma or surgery. There is erythema and oedema with systemic features. Streptococcal infection can also cause necrotising fasciitis of the vulva with painful, rapidly extending necrosis. It carries a high mortality.

Penis and scrotum. Streptococcal infection (and other organisms) of the male genital skin can cause Fournier gangrene (necrotising fasciitis). Typically it starts as a painful red swelling of scrotal skin developing into an area of superficial and deep necrosis accompanied by severe systemic toxicity.

Perineum and perianal skin. Streptococcal perianal dermatitis occurs in children between ages of 6 and 10 months. It causes itch and soreness, and is characterised by sharply demarcated boggy erythema of the perianal skin.

Malakoplakia

Malakoplakia results from an atypical inflammatory response to *Escherichia coli* or other pathogens.

Pathophysiology

Malakoplakia is due to macrophage dysfunction, and primary or acquired immunodeficiency is common. The organisms involved include *E. coli*, *Pseudomonas* and *Staphylococcus aureus*. Histology shows confluent sheets of histiocytes with eosinophilic granular cytoplasm and small eccentric nuclei. Round, laminated structures, known as Michaelis–Gutmann bodies, are found within these cells.

Clinical features

Malakoplakia most often affects the urinary or gastrointestinal tract, but cutaneous lesions may occur on the vagina, vulva and perineum. The lesions include persistent plaques, ulcers, nodules and sinuses.

Differential diagnosis

Crohn disease, hidradenitis suppurativa, malignancy.

Investigations

Bacteriology culture of lesions (swab and/or tissue) and skin biopsy.

Management

Long-term antibiotics are needed. Surgery may be required for the sinuses.

MALIGNANT AND PRE-MALIGNANT DERMATOSES

Vulval intraepithelial neoplasia (VIN), penile intraepithelial neoplasia (PeIN) and anal intraepithelial neoplasia (AIN) are non-invasive, premalignant diseases of the anogenital skin which may progress to squamous cell carcinoma.

Vulval intraepithelial neoplasia

There are two forms: undifferentiated VIN and differentiated VIN (Table 61.4).

Table 61.4 Forms of VIN

	Undifferentiated VIN	Differentiated VIN
Epidemiology	Younger women	Older women
Pathophysiology	Strong association with HPV types 16 and 18 Not generally associated with LS Causally related to smoking, immunosuppression	Not associated with HPV, but strongly associated with LS

(Continued)

Table 61.4 (Continued)

	Undifferentiated VIN	**Differentiated VIN**
Histopathology	Warty, basaloid or mixed variants There is 2/3 to full-thickness loss of cellular stratification in epidermis, with large hyperchromatic cells, dyskeratosis, multinucleated cells and typical or atypical mitoses	Histology may be mistaken for a benign dermatosis: subtle abnormalities in the basal layer with normal keratinocyte differentiation above this
Clinical features	Itchy or asymptomatic, solitary/multiple lesions Often multifocal Diverse morphology: smooth or warty plaques; skin-coloured, red or white (Figure 61.22)	Itchy or asymptomatic Usually unifocal Red, hyperkeratotic lesions on a background of LS
Progression to SCC	Low risk	High risk
Treatment	Responds to medical treatment (e.g. topical 5-fluorouracil cream, 5% imiquimod cream) or surgery for small isolated lesions	Surgical excision is treatment of choice

HPV, human papillomavirus; SCC, squamous cell carcinoma; LS, lichen sclerosus.

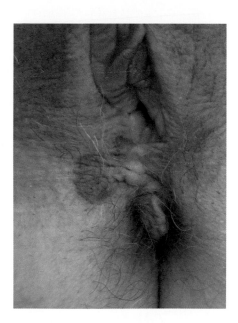

Figure 61.22 Vulval intraepithelial neoplasia (undifferentiated).

Penile intraepithelial neoplasia

See Table 61.5.

Anal intraepithelial neoplasia

See Table 61.6.

Table 61.5 Penile intraepithelial neoplasia

	PeIN
Epidemiology	Young men High prevalence of PeIN in sexual partners of women with CIN
Pathophysiology	Local carcinogenic influences: uncircumcised, chronic inflammation (especially LS), phimosis, immunosuppression, smoking. HPV is implicated in 70–100% of cases BP strongly associated with HPV-16 Two histopathological forms: undifferentiated PeIN and differentiated PeIN
Histopathology	Differentiated PeIN: basal and parabasal atypia of epithelium Undifferentiated PeIN: up to full thickness epithelial atypia with koilocytes
Clinical features	There are three clinical presentations. EQ: red shiny patches or plaques on the glans and prepuce BDP: red, slightly pigmented, scaly patches and plaques on the keratinised penis BP: warty papules, usually multiple and often pigmented (Figure 61.23)
Progression to SCC	10–33%
Treatment	Responds to medical treatment (eg topical 5-fluorouracil cream, or 5% imiquimod cream). Other treatments include cryotherapy, curettage and electrocautery, excisional surgery, glans resurfacing, Mohs micrographic surgery, laser and photodynamic therapy. Circumcision removes a major risk factor for cancer.

LS, lichen sclerosus; HPV, human papillomavirus; SCC, squamous cell carcinoma; EQ, erythroplasia of Queyrat; BDP, Bowen disease of the penis; BP, Bowenoid papulosis; CIN, cervical intra-epithelial neoplasia.

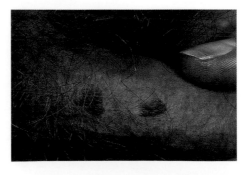

Figure 61.23 Bowenoid papulosis. (Source: Courtesy of Dr D.A. Burns, Leicester, UK.)

Table 61.6 Anal intraepithelial neoplasia

	AIN
Epidemiology	0.45 cases/100,000 Estimated to occur in 50% of MSM, 5% of renal transplant recipients
Pathophysiology	Local carcinogenic influences: immunosuppression, receptive anal sex, anogenital warts (strongly associated with HPV 16 and 18) Highest risk group is HIV+ MSM
Histopathology	Absent epithelial maturation with nuclear pleomorphism and numerous mitoses
Clinical features	Asymptomatic red, shiny or scaly plaque on perianal skin (Figure 61.24) May occur in continuity with lesion in anal canal Bowenoid papulosis (see PeIN) may occur on perianal and groin skin
Progression to SCC	Progression of high-grade AIN to SCC is ~10% at 5 years
Treatment	Multidisciplinary approach with colorectal surgery Often responds to medical treatment (e.g. topical 5-fluorouracil cream or 5% imiquimod cream) Other treatments include CO_2 laser, curettage, and electrocautery, excisional surgery

MSM, men having sex with men; HPV, human papillomavirus; SCC, squamous cell carcinoma.

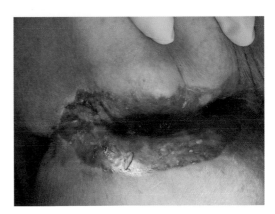

Figure 61.24 Patch of high-grade anal and perianal intra-epithelial neoplasia.

PART 8: SKIN DISORDERS ASSOCIATED WITH SPECIFIC SITES, SEX AND AGE

Table 61.7 Squamous cell carcinoma of the anogenital skin

	Penis	Vulva	Anus
Epidemiology	Highest incidence is in Africa, South America, and Asia: 2-4 cases/100 000 Lowest incidence is in the USA and Europe: 0.3–1/100 000	Incidence is 1-2 cases/100 000	1.5 cases/100 000 Incidence is 40–70× higher in HIV+ patients Highest in MSM who practice anoreceptive sex
Pathophysiology	Pre-cancerous penile dermatoses (see above) are risks for penile SCC, as are LS and conditions causing balanoposthitis and phimosis Oncogenic HPV, particularly types 16 and 18, have been implicated in up to 45% of penile SCC	Two types: 60% vulval SCCs occur in elderly women on a background of LS or LP 40% occur in younger women and are associated with oncogenic HPV	Almost all cases arise from AIN Oncogenic HPV, particularly types 16 and 18, have been implicated in up to 50% of anal SCC
Clinical features	Plaque or nodule, usually on the glans, which may be ulcerated. Often a long history of penile problems (balanoposthitis, phimosis) and a background dermatosis (LS, BP, BDP, EQ) The inguinal lymph glands must be examined. (Figures 61.25 and 61.26)	There is a plaque or nodule which causes soreness and itch Bleeding can occur if the tumour is ulcerated (Figure 61.27)	Hard mass, which may be polypoid or ulcerated at anal margin May arise from anal canal Symptoms include pruritus ani, pain, bleeding and tenesmus Regional lymph node involvement occurs in 30% at presentation (Figure 61.28)
Management	Surgical excision Penile surgery may need to be radical: total or partial penectomy, depending on location and extent	Surgical excision is determined by the site and size of the tumour	A multidisciplinary approach is needed, including involvement of anorectal surgeon, radiotherapist and medical oncologist

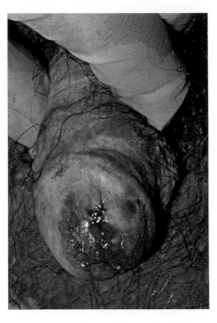

Figure 61.25 High-grade dysplasia and invasive SCC. (Source: Courtesy of Professor C.B. Bunker, with permission from Medical Illustration UK, Chelsea & Westminster Hospital, London, UK.)

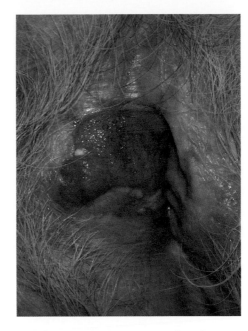

Figure 61.27 Vulval squamous cell carcinoma arising on a background of LS.

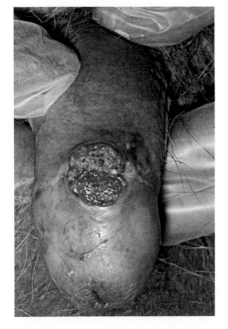

Figure 61.26 Squamous cell carcinoma. Severe background LS. (Source: Reproduced from Bunker CB. Skin conditions of the male genitalia. *Medicine* 2001, 29, 9–13.)

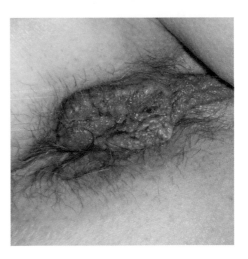

Figure 61.28 Large polypoid mass of perianal SCC.

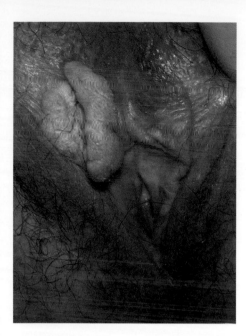

Figure 61.29 Verrucous carcinoma of the vulva on a background of LS.

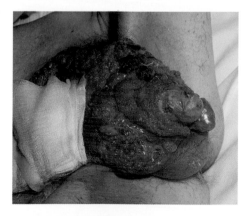

Figure 61.30 Verrucous carcinoma of the penis. (Source: Courtesy of Professor R.M. MacKie, Glasgow University, Glasgow, UK.)

Squamous cell carcinoma of the anogenital skin

See Table 61.7 and Chapter 80.

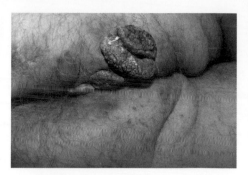

Figure 61.31 Verrucous carcinoma of the perianal skin of a male.

Verrucous carcinoma

(Syn. Buschke–Lowenstein tumour)
Verrucous carcinoma (VC) is a clinically distinctive, well-differentiated SCC arising on anogenital skin. It can be associated with LS or HPV infection. In women, VC presents as a warty, cauliflower-like tumour arising from the vulva (Figure 61.29). In men, it presents as an exophytic polypoid tumour of the glans penis (Figure 61.30). VC arising from the anus also occurs (Figure 61.31). VC can reach 4–7 cm in diameter and can ulcerate. Treatment is surgical excision.

Extramammary Paget disease

Extramammary Paget disease (EMPD) is a malignant skin condition occurring in sites rich in apocrine glands, such as the vulva and anogenital region.

Epidemiology
Rare. Occurs in the fifth decade or later. F > M.

Pathophysiology
In 75% of cases EMPD arises as a primary neoplasm from apocrine gland ductal cells, keratinocyte stem cells, or clear cells of Toker. 25% arise from an underlying adenocarcinoma. Histopathology shows intraepidermal infiltration by neoplastic cells showing glandular differentia-

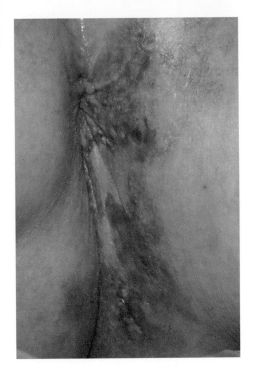

Figure 61.32 Extramammary Paget disease of the perianal skin.

tion. There are nests of large vacuolated cells with circular nuclei and foamy pale cytoplasm in the epidermis (Paget cells). GCDFP-15 (apocrine marker) is expressed in EMPD without underlying malignancy; cytokeratin 20 is positive in EMPD with an associated adenocarcinoma.

Clinical features
EMPD can occur anywhere in the anogenital area, including the glans penis. It is usually itchy. Clinically there is a unilateral pink patch or plaque with a well-demarcated rounded margin (Figure 61.32). Lesional skin may contain both red and white areas giving a so-called "strawberries and cream" appearance. It tends to progress slowly over a number of years so that a delay in diagnosis is not uncommon. The commonest area of involvement is the vulva, then perianal area (M > F), scrotum and penis. It can affect the axilla. Eventually one area within the plaque may become thickened and ulcerated. Lymph node metastasis can occur. It is important to examine for an underlying adenocarcinoma in the anus, rectum, cervix, bladder or prostate.

Differential diagnosis
Psoriasis, eczema, tinea cruris, Bowen disease.

Investigations
Diagnosis is by biopsy. A search for an underlying adenocarcinoma should be undertaken.

Management
Wide excisional surgery or Mohs micrographic surgery is the treatment of choice. Other treatments include topical 5% imiquimod cream, 5-fluorouracil cream, radiotherapy and photodynamic therapy. A combination of treatments is often required. Recurrence is common. An underlying neoplasm needs appropriate treatment.

62 Dermatoses occurring in pregnancy

During pregnancy there are marked changes in the levels of sex hormones, particularly oestrogen and progesterone, and this can lead to profound changes in the skin. These physiological skin changes must be distinguished from true skin disease (Table 62.1).

Pruritus gravidarum

(Syn. Obstetric cholestasis)
Pruritus gravidarum is itching secondary to a mild variant of intrahepatic cholestasis of pregnancy.

Epidemiology
Occurs in 0.02–2.4% of pregnancies.

Pathophysiology
Intrahepatic cholestasis of pregnancy is a reversible form of hormonally triggered cholestasis that develops in genetically predisposed women.

Clinical features
Itching begins in the second or third trimester and can be localised (abdomen, palms and soles) or widespread. About 10% of patients

Table 62.1 Physiological skin changes in pregnancy

Melasma (chloasma)	Symmetrical areas of pigmentation on forehead, temples, central face Occurs in 70% of women during second half of pregnancy
Linear nigra	Linear zone of pigmentation extending down from the umbilicus on the midline of the abdomen (Figure 62.1).
Breasts	Hyperpigmentation of the nipples and areolae
Naevi	Increase in size, number and pigmentation of naevi
Vascular	Palmar erythema, spider naevi, non-pitting oedema (face, hands, feet), pyogenic granuloma
Stretch marks	Striae distensae on thighs and abdomen (Figure 62.1)
Hair	Hypertrichosis followed by post-partum telogen effluvium
Nails	Distal onycholysis, transverse grooving and brittleness

Rook's Dermatology Handbook, First Edition. Edited by Christopher E. M. Griffiths, Tanya O. Bleiker, Daniel Creamer, John R. Ingram and Rosalind C. Simpson.
© 2022 John Wiley & Sons Ltd. Published 2022 by John Wiley & Sons Ltd.

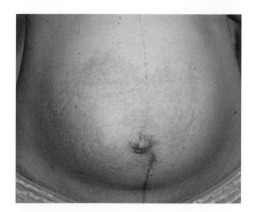

Figure 62.1 Physiological skin changes in pregnancy showing a prominent linea nigra and striae distensae at 28 weeks' gestation.

may be mildly jaundiced. Secondary skin lesions develop due to scratching. After delivery, pruritus disappears spontaneously within days to weeks, but may recur with subsequent pregnancies and oral contraception. Fetal prognosis can be impaired with an increased risk of prematurity, fetal distress and stillbirth.

Differential diagnosis

Atopic eruption of pregnancy. Other causes of pruritus.

Investigations

Serum bile acids are elevated. Alkaline phosphatase may be raised (which is normal for pregnancy due to placental production), liver transaminases are usually normal.

Management

First line: Topical emollients, such as aqueous cream + 1–2% menthol. Oral antihistamines: loratadine and cetirizine. Oral ursodeoxycholic acid 15 mg/kg/day (off licence).

Second line: S-adenosyl-L-methionine, dexamethasone, cholestyramine.

Other recommendations: Weekly fetal cardiotocography to monitor fetal heart rate and detect early signs of fetal distress. Maternal vitamin K replacement (if jaundice is present). Early delivery (36–37 weeks) may be necessary. Dexamethasone may be needed for fetal lung maturity.

Polymorphic eruption of pregnancy

(Syn. Pruritic urticarial papules and plaques of pregnancy)

Polymorphic eruption of pregnancy (PEP) is a benign, self-limiting pruritic inflammatory disorder that usually affects primigravidae in the last few weeks of pregnancy.

Epidemiology

The incidence is about 1:160 pregnancies.

Pathophysiology

Occurs within striae distensae at the time of greatest abdominal distension, suggesting that damage to connective tissue due to overstretching may play a central role. An increase in CD1a cells in the inflammatory infiltrate indicates that previously inert structures might develop antigenic character.

Clinical features

Typically starts on the abdomen, often within the striae distensae, with pruritic urticarial papules that coalesce into plaques, spreading to the buttocks and proximal thighs (Figure 62.2). It can become generalised in severe cases. In contrast to pemphigoid gestationis, umbilical sparing is a characteristic finding. Later on, the morphology may become more polymorphic: vesicles (never bullae), non-urticated erythema, atypical target lesions and eczematous lesions. PEP is associated with excessive maternal weight gain and multiple pregnancy. In most cases this condition is self-limiting and will get better towards the end of pregnancy or immediately following delivery. 15% of cases occur post-partum. Maternal and fetal prognosis is unimpaired by PEP.

Differential diagnosis

Atopic eruption of pregnancy. PEP can be mistaken for the pre-bullous stage of pemphigoid gestationis.

Investigations

Skin biopsy shows spongiosis and upper dermal oedema with a perivascular infiltrate of lymphocytes, eosinophils and histiocytes. Direct

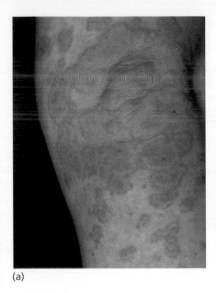

(a)

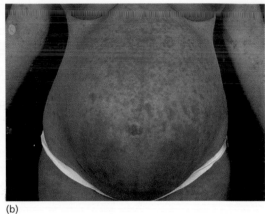

(b)

Figure 62.2 Typical lesions of polymorphic eruption of pregnancy on (a) the arm and (b) the abdomen. (Source: Courtesy of Dr D.A. Burns, Leicester Royal Infirmary, Leicester, UK.)

immunofluorescence is negative, distinguishing PEP from pemphigoid gestationis.

Management

First line: Topical emollients: aqueous cream + 1–2% menthol. Moderately potent or potent topical corticosteroid ointment. Oral antihistamines: loratadine and cetirizine.

Second line: Prednisolone 0.5 mg/kg/day and tapered with response.

Other recommendations: Consider early induction of labour if patient is close to term. Reassure patient that the rash is not serious for them or their baby, and that it will disappear at, or soon after, delivery.

Pemphigoid gestationis

(Syn. Herpes gestationis)
Pemphigoid gestationis (PG) is an autoimmune bullous disorder that presents mainly in late pregnancy or the immediate postpartum period.

Epidemiology

The incidence varies from 1:2000 to 1:50 000 pregnancies depending on the prevalence of the human leukocyte antigen haplotypes DR3 and DR4.

Pathophysiology

Circulating complement-fixing IgG antibodies of the subclass IgG1 bind to the NC16A domain of BP-180 (bullous pemphigoid antigen-2) in the hemidesmosomes of the dermo-epidermal junction, leading to blister formation. Antibodies also bind to the basement membrane zone of chorionic and amniotic epithelia. Aberrant expression of MHC class II molecules on the chorionic villi suggests an allogenic immune reaction to a placental matrix antigen, thought to be of paternal origin.

Clinical features

Presents with pruritus, which precedes skin lesions. The eruption usually starts as red urticated papules and plaques on the abdomen, characteristically involving the periumbilical skin (Figure 62.3a,b). Thereafter the dermatosis spreads onto the limbs and torso. Patches of urticated erythema, eczematous plaques, and atypical target lesions are common in the early stages and lead to difficulty in differentiating pre-bullous PG from PEP. Diagnosis becomes clear with the appearance of blisters (Figure 62.3c). Blisters are tense, like bullous pemphigoid and distributed

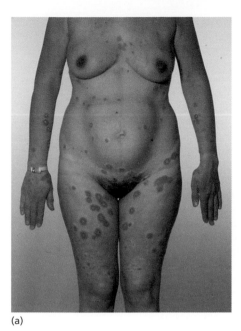

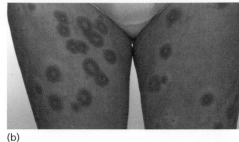

(b)

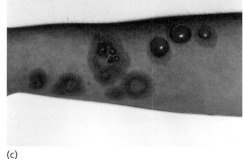

(a)   (c)

Figure 62.3 Pemphigoid gestationis that erupted 3 days postpartum showing (a) widespread erythematous urticated plaques on the trunk and limbs with early blistering. (b) Close-up view of urticated targetoid plaques on the upper thighs. (c) Close-up view showing tense intact blisters on the forearms on a background of urticated erythema.

widely. Mucous membranes are usually spared. It tends to wax and wane during pregnancy, with frequent improvement in late pregnancy followed by a flare-up at the time of delivery (75% of patients). After delivery, the lesions usually resolve within weeks to months but may recur with menstruation and hormonal contraception.

Fetal prognosis is generally good but there is an increase in prematurity and small-for-date babies: the risk correlates with disease severity, as represented by early onset and extensive blister formation. Passive transfer of antibodies from the mother to the foetus results in 10% of newborns developing mild skin lesions (neonatal PG) which resolve spontaneously within days to weeks.

PG can recur in subsequent pregnancies; further episodes present at an earlier gestation and with increased severity. However, 'skip' pregnancies can occur. Patients have an increased risk of developing other organ-specific autoimmune diseases, in particular Graves disease.

Differential diagnosis
In the pre-bullous stage it can be mistaken for PEP and atopic eruption of pregnancy.

Investigations
Skin biopsy of early lesions shows dermal oedema with a perivascular inflammatory infiltrate of lymphocytes, histiocytes and eosinophils. The bullous stage shows subepidermal blistering. Direct immunofluorescence of perilesional skin shows linear C3 deposition along the dermo-epidermal junction in 100% of cases and IgG deposition in 30% of cases. Circulating IgG antibodies can be detected by indirect immunofluorescence in 30–100% of cases, binding to the roof of the artificial split on salt-split skin. Antibody levels, showing correlation

with disease activity, may also be monitored using ELISA and immunoblot techniques.

Management

First line: Topical emollients: aqueous cream + 1–2% menthol. Moderately potent or potent topical corticosteroid ointment. Oral antihistamines: loratadine and cetirizine.

Second line: Prednisolone 0.5–1 mg/kg/day and tapered with response.

Third line: Azathioprine, plasma exchange, intravenous immunoglobulins.

Other recommendations: After delivery the full range of immunosuppressive treatment may be administered if necessary. For the affected newborn, conservative management is all that is required until maternal antibodies are cleared from the fetal circulation.

Atopic eruption of pregnancy

(Syn. Prurigo gestationis)
Atopic eruption of pregnancy (AEP) is a benign pruritic disorder of pregnancy characterised by eczematous papular lesions in patients with an atopic susceptibility.

Epidemiology

AEP is the most common dermatosis in pregnancy, accounting for 50% of cases of pregnancy-related dermatoses.

Pathophysiology

Predominance of the Th2 immune response in pregnancy (increased secretion of Th2 cytokines: IL-4, IL-10) explains the manifestation of atopic skin disease in AEP.

Clinical features

AEP usually starts in the first trimester. Most patients develop atopic skin changes for the first time (or after a long remission); fewer patients suffer an exacerbation of pre-existing eczema. Widespread eczema affecting typical atopic sites is the most usual presentation (Figure 62.4). A smaller proportion of patients develop papules on the torso and limbs, and prurigo nodules on the shins and arms. Recurrence in subsequent pregnancies is common.

Differential diagnosis

Pruritus gravidarum, PEP, pre-bullous PG.

Investigations

The diagnosis is usually made clinically without need for investigations.

Management

First line: Topical emollients. Moderately potent or potent topical corticosteroid ointment. Oral antihistamines: loratadine and cetirizine.

Second line: Narrow-band UVB phototherapy.

Third line: Prednisolone 0.5 mg/kg/day and tapered with response. Azathioprine is safe in pregnancy.

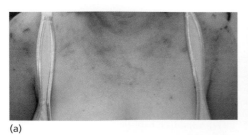

(a)

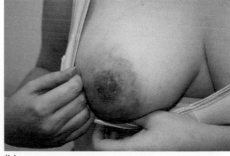

(b)

Figure 62.4 Atopic eruption of pregnancy (a) on the upper trunk and shoulders in the second trimester and (b) with nipple eczema.

Dermatoses of neonates

63

The commonly used terms in neonatology are defined in Box 63.1.

NEONATAL BARRIER FUNCTION OF SKIN

A normal full-term infant has a functional stratum corneum with an almost fully developed barrier function. Transepidermal water loss is high in the first few days of life but normalises quickly. Toxicity resulting from percutaneous absorption in the full-term neonate is related to three factors: the greatly increased ratio of surface area to volume, the presence of occlusive conditions (e.g. waterproof diapers) and high ambient temperatures/humidity.

In preterm infants there is impaired barrier function (especially <34 weeks' gestation), but barrier function in these babies will improve rapidly after birth and be normal by the end of the second or third week of life.

A topical agent should not be applied to the skin of any baby without careful consideration of the potential hazards of percutaneous absorption, particularly in those with skin diseases or in small, preterm neonates.

NORMAL CHANGES OCCURRING IN NEONATAL SKIN

Vernix caseosa

At birth the skin is covered with a whitish, greasy film, the vernix caseosa, which is secreted from the fetal sebaceous glands. The vernix may cover the entire skin surface or it may be present only in body folds. It dries rapidly and flakes off within a few hours of birth.

Peripheral cyanosis

Peripheral cyanosis (or acrocyanosis) is a feature of the newborn (particularly at full term) and is marked on the palms/soles and around the mouth.

Erythema neonatorum

A few hours after birth, many babies develop a generalised hyperaemia, known as erythema neonatorum, which fades within 24–48 h.

> **Box 63.1 Nomenclature of neonatology**
>
> Neonatal period: first 4 weeks of extrauterine life
> Infancy: first year of extrauterine life
> Premature (preterm): born before the 37th week of gestation
> Full term: born in weeks 37–42 of gestation
> Postmature: born after the 42nd week of gestation
> Low birth weight: <2500 g at birth
> Intrauterine growth retardation: birth weight low for gestational age (small-for-dates)

Rook's Dermatology Handbook, First Edition. Edited by Christopher E. M. Griffiths, Tanya O. Bleiker, Daniel Creamer, John R. Ingram and Rosalind C. Simpson.
© 2022 John Wiley & Sons Ltd. Published 2022 by John Wiley & Sons Ltd.

Harlequin colour change

Up to 15% of neonates show a colour difference along the midline during the first week of life when the baby is lying on its side. The upper half of the body becomes pale, the lower half develops a deep red colour. The duration of the episode lasts between 30 s and 20 min. If the baby is turned on the other side, the colour change may reverse.

Cutis marmorata

Neonates who are subjected to cooling will develop a reticulate blue 'marbling' of the skin. Although it mostly disappears on rewarming, many babies have a faint marbling even under optimal environmental conditions.

Desquamation

Superficial desquamation occurs in up to 75% of normal neonates. It appears at the ankles on the first day of life and reaches its maximum extent by the eighth day. It may remain localised to the hands and feet, or become widespread. It is more severe in neonates who are small-for-dates, whatever their gestational age.

Sucking blisters

One or two blisters or erosions on the fingers, lips or forearms are occasionally present at birth, believed to be caused by sucking *in utero*. These heal without sequelae.

Neonatal occipital alopecia

Fetal scalp hair enters a telogen (or shedding) phase at 12 weeks before term. The hair then enters an anagen (or growth) phase from front to back, but the occipital zone is still shedding at term. Thus there is occipital alopecia in the first weeks of life.

Hair shedding in infancy

There appear to be two waves of hair loss and regrowth from front to back during early infancy, but by the end of the first year the normal pattern of hair growth is established.

Sebaceous gland hypertrophy and milia

Sebaceous gland hyperplasia (SGH) is a physiological event in the newborn, reflecting the influence of maternal androgens. The lesions are pinpoint, yellowish papules, most prominent on the nose, cheeks, upper lip, and forehead, but also seen on the torso. SGH is associated in 40% of infants with milia (follicular epidermal cysts), which are also tiny papules, but white. Milia appear at the same sites as SGH and may be few in number or numerous.

Hyperpigmentary disorders

A linea nigra occurs in many babies and may persist for 2–3 months. Mongolian blue spots are common in babies of type IV–VI skin (up to 85%). Hyperpigmentation of the scrotum may occur in up to 30% of oriental babies. Linear or reticulate pigmentary anomalies can be seen in black newborns.

Oral findings

Epstein's pearls are 1–2 mm in diameter, yellowish white, keratinous cysts seen in the mouths of up to 85% of all neonates, along the alveolar ridges and/or in the midline at the junction of the hard and soft palate. These disappear within a few weeks. Succulent gums (or hypertrophic gingivitis) are common in neonates. A whitish hue to the oral mucosa ('leukoedema') is also common.

SKIN ABNORMALITIES ASSOCIATED WITH PRETERM AND POSTMATURE STATES

There are a number of cutaneous anomalies which occur in preterm and postmature neonates. In the preterm neonate the skin is translucent with visible vessels, lanugo hair covers the infant. In the small-for-dates and postmature infant there is a lack of subcutaneous fat, causing the infant to look thin or wrinkled. In these babies the vernix may be absent and the skin may be stained yellow-green by meconium. All the changes resolve spontaneously during the neonatal period.

SKIN LESIONS ARISING FROM PROCEDURES PERFORMED IN THE ANTENATAL AND NEONATAL PERIODS

Medical interventions in the antenatal period and during delivery are now commonplace. Some of these procedures can result in cutaneous sequelae, outlined in Table 63.1. Procedures undertaken in the neonatal period can also induce iatrogenic skin lesions (see Table 63.2).

NEONATAL RASHES

Neonatal rashes are common and can be accompanied by vesicles and pustules. The differential diagnosis of pustular eruptions in the neonate is outlined in Box 63.2.

Toxic erythema of the newborn

A common, transient rash seen in the first few days of life.

Table 63.1 Complications arising from antenatal procedures

Procedure	Complication or disorder
Amnioicentesis needles	Punctate scars and dimples
Antenatal biopsies (skin, liver, tumours)	
Intrauterine red cell transfusion (used in haemolytic disease/rhesus incompatibility)	Gangrene of the abdominal wall
Scalp electrodes (monitoring fetal heart rate)	Scarring alopecia/cephalohaematoma Neonatal HSV at the site of electrodes
Scalp blood sampling	Scalp abscess
Forceps delivery	Subcutaneous fat necrosis
Scalpel injury during Caesarean section	Lacerations/scars
Ventouse extraction	Annular scalp blisters, scarring alopecia

Table 63.2 Complications arising from neonatal medical procedures

Procedure	Cutaneous complication
Umbilical artery catheterisation	Aortic thrombosis/spasm, arterial embolism (lower limb ischaemia/gangrene)
Transcutaneous oxygen monitoring (heated electrode)	Superficial burn
Electrocardiograph electrodes	Traumatic purpura and, later, anetoderma
Trans-illumination	Blister at acral sites
Extravasation of intravenous medication	Cutaneous necrosis
Heel pricks	Cutaneous calcification (localised)
Needle insertions (repeated)	Punctate white scars (speckled scarring)
Chemical burns: antiseptics/cleansers	Cutaneous necrosis

> **Box 63.2 Pustular eruptions in the neonate**
>
> Congenital or neonatal candidiasis
> Congenital syphilis
> Eosinophilic pustulosis
> Herpes simplex virus infection
> Impetigo
> Infantile acne
> Infantile acropustulosis
> *Malassezia* pustulosis
> Miliaria
> Neonatal listeriosis
> Neonatal pustulosis of transient myeloprolif-
> erative disorder
> Pustular psoriasis
> Scabies
> Toxic erythema of the newborn
> Transient pustular melanosis

Epidemiology

Occurs in 30–50% of neonates. Incidence decreases with prematurity and smallness for dates.

Pathophysiology

Histologically, there is an inflammatory infiltrate comprising principally of eosinophils. Pustules are follicular, indicating that the inflammation may be elicited by neonatal sebum.

Clinical features

The usual onset is during the first 48 h after birth, but it can occur at any time until the fourth day. It is rarely present at birth. There is an eruption of erythematous blotches; the number of lesions varies widely. They are most profuse on the torso, particularly the anterior trunk, but can appear on the face and proximal limbs. Lesions do not occur on palms and soles. In severe cases there are papules and pustules. Spontaneous recovery occurs within 3 days.

Investigations

It is a clinical diagnosis. A smear of pustule contents will show eosinophils but no organisms.

Management

No treatment is needed.

Miliaria

(Inc. Miliaria crystallina, miliaria rubra)
A papulo-vesicular disorder due to blockage of eccrine sweat ducts.

Epidemiology

Occurs in about 5–8% of neonates.

Pathophysiology

Immature sweat ducts and high levels of heat and humidity are important factors. Miliaria crystallina is characterised by the presence of intracorneal or subcorneal vesicles in communication with the sweat ducts. In miliaria rubra, spongiosis and spongiotic vesicles occur adjacent to the blocked sweat dusts.

Clinical features

Miliaria crystallina arises during the first 2 weeks of life, presenting as crops of asymptomatic, clear vesicles without associated erythema, resembling drops of water. Typical sites are the forehead, scalp, neck and upper trunk (Figure 63.1). The vesicles rupture within 24 h, followed by desquamation. Miliaria rubra consists of itchy, red papules and papulo-vesicles on a background of macular erythema. Lesions arise in flexural areas, especially the neck, groins and axillae, or at occluded sites. Lesions subside within 3 days, but recurrences are common.

Investigations

Miliaria is a clinical diagnosis.

Management

Miliaria crystallina spontaneously improves as the sweat ducts mature. Remove the child from

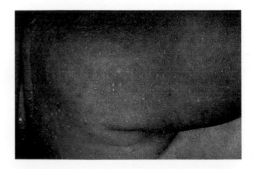

Figure 63.1 Miliaria crystallina on the upper arm of a 7-day-old infant.

conditions of high heat/humidity and from any occlusive clothing or bedding.

Transient pustular melanosis

A pigmented and pustular eruption present at birth.

Epidemiology
More common in black neonates.

Pathophysiology
The aetiology is unknown. A skin biopsy of a pustule shows intra- or subcorneal collections of neutrophils and a few eosinophils.

Clinical features
Flaccid, superficial, fragile pustules without surrounding erythema are present at birth. Favoured sites include the chin, neck, forehead, back. and buttocks. Ruptured pustules leave pigmented macules, which are more prominent in black than white infants. The pigmentation may persist for about 3 months.

Investigations
It is a clinical diagnosis. Smear of a pustule shows neutrophils. Bacterial culture is negative.

Management
No treatment is needed.

NEONATAL INFECTIONS

The clinical features of some of the more important infections affecting the skin during the neonatal period are summarised in Table 63.3.

NEONATAL INFLAMMATORY DISORDERS

Neonatal lupus erythematosus

Neonatal lupus erythematosus (NLE) is a disorder of transient skin lesions caused by transplacental passage of maternal autoantibodies to Ro-SSA or La-SSB.

Epidemiology
1–2% of Ro/La-positive mothers will have babies with NLE.

Pathophysiology
Ro and La antigens are found in fetal skin and cardiac conducting tissue. During mid to late fetal development maternal IgG anti-Ro antibodies (rarely anti-La or anti-U_1-RNP) can cross the placenta, bind to cardiac conduction cells and damage the atrioventricular node. Anti-Ro antibodies can also damage fetal skin. Skin biopsy demonstrates epidermal atrophy, basal vacuolar degeneration of keratinocytes, colloid bodies and a perivascular and periappendageal lymphohistiocytic inflammatory infiltrate. In 50% of cases direct immunofluorescence shows IgG, IgM and C3 deposition at the dermo-epidermal junction.

Clinical features
In two-thirds of cases skin lesions are present at birth. In the remainder lesions appear during the first 2–3 months. Well-defined circular lesions, which are frequently annular and sometimes scaly, occur on the forehead, temples and upper cheeks, and on the scalp and neck (Figure 63.3). A 'spectacle-like' distribution of lesions around the eyes is characteristic. Lesions can be provoked by sun exposure. Atrophy and telangiectasiae are frequent long-term sequelae. In most cases, skin lesions have resolved within the first year.

Congenital heart block due to fibrosis of the conducting tissue occurs in about 1–2% of Ro-positive pregnancies and can be detected as early as the 18th week of gestation by ultrasound or electrocardiography. A smaller proportion will have combinations of hepatomegaly, splenomegaly, pneumonitis, autoimmune haemolytic anaemia and thrombocytopenia.

Investigations
A skin biopsy for histology and direct immunofluorescence should be undertaken to look for findings of NLE. Ro and La autoantibodies should be assayed in both the mother and the child.

Management
The skin lesions of NLE often require no treatment, but a mild potency topical steroid can hasten resolution. Sun protection is essential.

Table 63.3 Neonatal infections

	Fetal varicella syndrome
Organism	Maternal primary infection with varicella zoster virus (chickenpox) will transmit to the fetus in 25% of cases Maternal varicella infection between 7th and 20th weeks of pregnancy can cause spontaneous abortion or FVS
Clinical features	Localised scarring, especially on limbs, sometimes with limb hypoplasia and cutis aplasia Mortality of up to 25% in infants with FVS
Management	Pregnant women exposed to varicella-zoster should be given varicella-zoster immune globulin
	Neonatal herpes simplex
Organism	Transmission of HSV type 1 and 2 through contact with infected genital tract during delivery Rarely infection from ascending infection
Clinical features	Isolated or grouped vesicles especially on face, scalp and in mouth Occasionally widespread erosions (Figure 63.2)
Management	Treat with IV aciclovir Mortality is low with skin-limited infection; mortality is high with HSV2, in premature infants and in disseminated infection
	Congenital rubella
Organism	Rubella contracted by fetus before 20th week of gestation may cause disseminated infection
Clinical features	Red/purpuric macules on face, scalp, neck and torso Intrauterine growth retardation, microcephaly, microphthalmia
Management	Supportive treatment Vaccination programmes should eradicate this problem
	Bullous impetigo
Organism	*Staphylococcus aureus,* phage group II strains
Clinical features	Perineum, perianal area and neck are main sites Blisters contain clear or turbid fluid with narrow pink areolae
Management	Topical antibiotic Systemic antibiotics if extensive impetigo and/or if baby is unwell
	Staphylococcal scalded skin syndrome
	See chapters 4 and 64.
	Congenital and neonatal candidiasis
Organism	Congenital: fetus infected via maternal candida chorioamnionitis Neonatal: infection during delivery from candida in mother's genital tract
Clinical features	Congenital: extensive eruption of pink-red macules which become pustular or bullous over 1–3 days; palmo-plantar lesions are characteristic Neonatal: erythema in napkin area, especially perianal skin, with moist erythema, peripheral pustules and satellite lesions; oral involvement
Management	Topical anticandidal cream for skin infection IV amphotericin B or fluconazole in systemic infection

(Continued)

Table 63.3 (Continued)

	Malassezia **pustulosis (neonatal cephalic pustulosis)**
Organism	*Malassezia furfur*
Clinical features	Red papulo-pustular eruption on the face and scalp
Management	2% ketoconazole cream

FVS, fetal varicella syndrome.

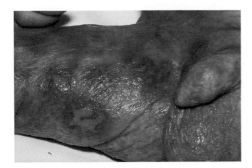

Figure 63.2 Neonatal herpes simplex virus infection, showing congenital ulceration and scarring.

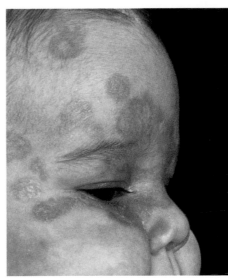

Figure 63.3 Neonatal lupus erythematosus showing fading facial lesions in a characteristic periorbital distribution, with residual atrophy, in a 4-month-old infant.

NLE antibodies disappear from the infant's serum within 6 months. Cardiac conduction defects tend to be permanent, up to 50% of affected infants require a pacemaker. The risk of recurrence in further pregnancies appears to be about 20–25%. The pregnancy of a woman who has Ro, La, or U_1-RNP antibodies should be monitored to detect a slow fetal heart rate.

'Blueberry muffin' baby (dermal erythropoiesis)

This term has been used to describe a characteristic eruption in neonates, often present at birth, comprising widespread, red-purple macules, papules and nodules of dermal erythropoiesis. Favoured sites are the trunk, head and neck. The lesions generally fade into light brown macules within a few weeks of birth. Dermal erythropoiesis occurs in a number of congenital infections and a variety of congenital haematological disorders (see Table 63.4). Recognition of this disorder necessitates immediate investigation by the neonatologists to identify an underlying cause. A skin biopsy may be needed.

Disorders of the subcutaneous fat

The clinical features of neonatal fat disorders are outlined in Table 63.5.

Table 63.4 Causes of blueberry muffin baby

Underlying disease process	Specific examples
Congenital infections	Rubella, cytomegalovirus, coxsackie B2, syphilis, toxoplasmosis
Haematological	Hereditary spherocytosis, Rhesus haemolytic anaemia, ABO blood group incompatibility, twin–twin transfusion syndrome
Drug induced	Erythropoietin
Neoplasia	Congenital leukaemia, neuroblastoma, congenital rhabdomyosarcoma, Langerhans cell histiocytosis
Inflammatory	Neonatal lupus erythematosus

Table 63.5 Neonatal disorders of subcutaneous fat

	Neonatal cold injury	Sclerema neonatorum	Subcutaneous fat necrosis of newborn
Frequency	Previously common, now rare	Rare, usually seen in neonatal intensive care units	Uncommon
Patient	Full-term neonates, often small for dates, born at home	Usually severely ill neonates Often preterm, or small-for-dates, or post-term	Healthy infants, usually full-term or post-term
Pathogenesis	Low environmental temperature causing hypothermia	Associated with severe illnesses, particularly hypothermia, infections, and congenital heart disease	Associated with local tissue hypoxia and cold injury
Histology	Thin panniculus	Thickened connective tissue trabeculae, radial needle-like clefts	Granulomatous inflammation, fat necrosis
Clinical features	Starts during the first week of life Affects extremities and spreads centrally Pitting oedema initially with erythema or cyanosis of face and extremities	Starts during the first week of life Affects lower limbs initially, becoming generalised Diffuse, yellow-white, woody induration with immobility of limbs	Starts in first 6 weeks of life Affects trunk, buttocks, thighs, arms, face Firm, violaceous subcutaneous nodules and plaques of varying sizes Overlying skin is bluish-red Lesions disappear within a few months Associated with hypercalcaemia
Outcome	Mortality around 25%	Mortality >50%	Generally excellent

DEVELOPMENTAL ABNORMALITIES

Collodion baby

Collodion baby describes a clinical entity present at birth where a child is born with an 'extra' skin resembling a shiny membrane or collodion (see Chapter 30).

Epidemiology
Approximately 1:100 000 deliveries.

Pathophysiology
Almost 90% of collodion babies will go on to develop a severe form of autosomal recessive ichthyosis in the first few weeks of life, most usually lamellar ichthyosis and non-bullous ichthyosiform erythroderma. In 10% of cases the collodion baby phase is followed by a mild ichthyosis of lamellar type, or indeed normal skin (self-healing ichthyosis). Histologically the collodion membrane is a compact, thickened orthokeratotic stratum corneum; the epidermis and dermis are both relatively normal.

Clinical features
The infant is bright red and encased in a taut, glistening, yellowish, translucent covering resembling collodion. The face is immobilised; tension on the skin results in ectropion, eversion of the lips (eclabion), and effacement of the nose and ears. The nostrils may be blocked. Fingers, hands, toes and feet may be immobilised. The collodion baby is at risk from the effects of skin barrier dysfunction: impaired temperature and fluid regulation, acute renal failure, septicaemia and respiratory failure. Within hours the membrane dries and cracks, and bleeding may occur along the resulting fissures. Within 2 days it starts to peel off but may reform several times. Shedding of the collodion membrane will be complete within 4 weeks. Subsequently, the typical features of ichthyosis emerge.

Investigations
Collodion baby is a clinical diagnosis. Genetic analysis can identify the underlying ichthyosis.

Management
Supportive care: the baby should be incubator nursed in a high-humidity atmosphere with careful monitoring of body temperature and fluid balance. Treat the skin with 50:50 white soft paraffin/liquid paraffin. Prevention of infection is imperative. Skin punctures should be kept to a minimum and vascular access should be avoided as far as possible.

Aplasia cutis congenita

Aplasia cutis congenita (ACC) is a congenital localised skin defect. In 85% of cases it is an isolated lesion near the vertex of the scalp, but ACC can involve skin at any body site and be associated with underlying defects in muscle, bone or dura.

At birth lesions can be healed (with a parchment-like scar) or be open (ulcerated). A ring of hair around the defect ('hair-collar' sign) is associated with an underlying defect. Prognosis for a single superficial lesion is excellent, causing a cosmetic problem only. Cases with underlying tissue defect carry a variable prognosis.

Congenital muscle hamartoma

A solitary, soft, skin-coloured or pink plaque a few centimetres in diameter, usually on the lumbo-sacral skin. Excess hair may develop over the lesion. Congenital muscle hamartomas demonstrate worm-like fasciculation when rubbed (pseudo-Darier sign). Rarely multiple lesions occur or diffuse smooth muscle hamartomas leading to the 'Michelin-tyre' baby phenotype.

HETEROTRIMERIC G-PROTEIN MOSAIC DISORDERS

G-protein is a heterotrimeric guanosine nucleotide-binding protein. Mosaicism for G-protein subunit mutations produces three syndromes: McCune-Albright syndrome, Sturge-Weber syndrome and phakomatosis pigmentovascularis.

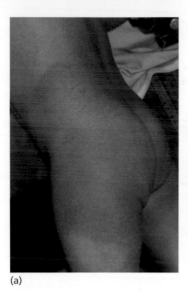
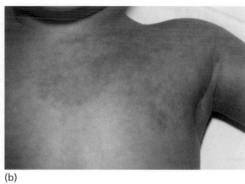

(a)   (b)

Figure 63.4 Phakomatosis pigmentovascularis showing the characteristic combination of (a) dermal melanocytosis (Mongolian blue spot) and (b) port-wine stain (capillary malformation).

McCune-Albright syndrome

Caused by mosaicism for activating mutations in the gene *GNAS*. McCune-Albright syndrome is a triad of:

- *Café-au-lait macules:* large, present at birth or in first few years of life, occur in a segmental distribution (respecting the midline) and have irregular margins.
- *Polyostotic fibrous dysplasia:* presents with pathological fractures or bone/joint pain; can be diagnosed from plain x-rays of skull, mandible, pelvis, long bones.
- *Endocrinopathies:* commonly gonadotrophin independent precocious puberty. Other endocrine disorders also occur.

Sturge–Weber syndrome

Caused by mosaicism for activating mutations in the gene *GNAQ*. Sturge–Weber syndrome consists of:

- *Port-wine stains (capillary malformations):* extensive facial and truncal lesions; the full syndrome is most strongly associated with port-wine stains affecting any part of the forehead and upper eyelid.
- *Brain abnormalities:* typically intracerebral vascular malformations which cause: seizures, neurodevelopmental delay, headache, stroke-like episodes, behavioural problems.
- *Glaucoma:* can be present at birth; caused by intraocular vascular malformations.

Phakomatosis pigmentovascularis

Caused by mosaicism for activating mutations in the genes *GNA11* or *GNAQ*. Phakomatosis pigmentovascularis is a descriptive term for a group of phenotypes unified by the coexistence of pigmentary and vascular cutaneous lesions. The commonest form consists of a port-wine stain (capillary malformation) and dermal melanocytosis (Mongolian blue spot) (Figure 63.4). Other subtypes include phenotypes with naevus spilus, linear epidermal naevus and cutis marmorata telangiectatica congenita.

The known associations of phakomatosis pigmentovascularis include naevus anaemicus, scleral or intraocular melanocytosis, glaucoma, intracerebral vascular malformations, hemihypertrophy of limbs and facial asymmetry, melanoma of the choroid and conjunctiva and melanocytoma of the optic disc.

Dermatoses of infants

64

INFLAMMATORY DERMATOSES

For the purposes of this chapter the infant period is regarded as from 4 weeks to 18 months, with emphasis on the first year of life.

Atopic eczema

See Chapter 16.

Atopic eczema (AE) is very common in developed countries and is the most frequent reason for infants to be referred to a dermatologist. A European cohort study has estimated that the cumulative prevalence of AE in the first 2 years of life is 21.5%, but prevalence peaks at 10% at 18 months, and slightly earlier for boys than girls. In infants, AE characteristically begins on the face in a balaclava-like distribution with subsequent spread to the torso and limbs (Figure 64.1). In some children a discoid pattern occurs, particularly on the back and legs, especially in toddlers, which may be mistaken for tinea corporis. Evidence of flexural involvement in infancy has the highest predictive value of AE persisting at age 3 years. AE in the majority of infants clears over time: 43.2% of children with early AE are in complete remission by age 3 years. The management of infantile AE for the most part is topical and aimed at restoring skin barrier function, reducing inflammation, treating secondary infection and providing parental education and support. Food allergy is reported in 10–30% of children with AE. In infants it is cow's milk, egg, peanut and soy that are the most prevalent. Although exclusive breast-feeding for the first 6 months appears protective, prolonged breast-feeding beyond this time does not appear to confer an advantage. There appears to be no benefit in delaying weaning onto solids beyond 4 months of age. Although dietary manipulation is popular with parents it needs to be undertaken in an informed and evidence-based manner to ensure that the infant's growth, development and nutrition are all maintained.

Pityriasis alba

See Chapter 16.

Pityriasis alba is common in slightly older children, but is also seen in infants. It is charac-

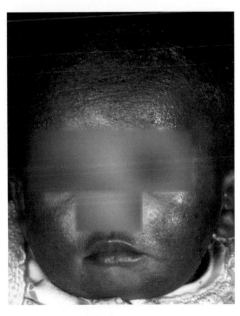

Figure 64.1 Atopic eczema showing facial involvement in the characteristic 'balaclava 'pattern in a 5-month-old.

Rook's Dermatology Handbook, First Edition. Edited by Christopher E. M. Griffiths, Tanya O. Bleiker, Daniel Creamer, John R. Ingram and Rosalind C. Simpson.
© 2022 John Wiley & Sons Ltd. Published 2022 by John Wiley & Sons Ltd.

terised by transient, hypopigmented, oval areas on the face, especially lower cheeks, associated in some cases with fine scale. The condition is most noticeable in children with darker skin types and may be a source of concern to parents. Individual lesions resolve over a few weeks but can recur. Pityriasis alba is considered to be part of the atopic diathesis. No specific treatment is needed, but emollients can help reduce the scale. Topical steroids should be avoided.

Cradle cap

Cradle cap is most common between the ages of 4 and 16 weeks, and affects approximately 40% of infants. Large flakes of yellow scale with minimal inflammation occur on the vertex and frontal regions of the scalp (Figure 64.2). Eyebrows may be involved. It can occur in isolation or in association with seborrhoeic dermatitis. The condition is asymptomatic and the infant is always well. It resolves spontaneously after a few weeks. In extensive cases, Langerhans cell histiocytosis (LCH) should be considered. An ointment-based emollient will help lift the scale.

Infantile seborrhoeic dermatitis

See Chapter 16.

Infantile seborrhoeic dermatitis (ISD) is distinct from seborrhoeic dermatitis in later life. ISD occurs most commonly before the age of 2 months, but can develop up to 4 months. There is macerated erythema in the skin folds of

neck and groins in addition to erythema and scale on the scalp and eyebrows (Figure 64.3). ISD is rarely symptomatic, but may cause great parental concern. Typically the inflammation resolves with transient hypopigmentation. Differential diagnosis includes irritant napkin dermatitis, atopic eczema and LCH. If the onset is acute or the infant is febrile or there is significant desquamation, Kawasaki disease should be considered. In mild cases, treatment with emollient alone is effective. In moderate to severe ISD cases a combination steroid–antifungal cream can be used for a short period. Some infants may go on to develop atopic eczema and the two conditions can merge.

Napkin dermatitis

Napkin (diaper) dermatitis is uncommon in the developed world since the advent of modern disposable nappies, which are highly absorbent

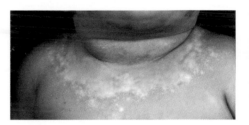

Figure 64.3 Seborrhoeic dermatitis showing macerated erythema in the neck folds of a 3-month-old girl, associated with some post-inflammatory hypopigmentation.

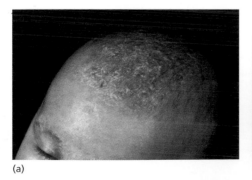

(a)

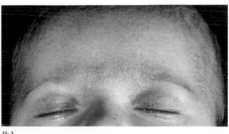

(b)

Figure 64.2 Cradle cap. (a) Scale over the vertex and frontal regions in a 6-week-old infant. (b) Adherent yellow scale in the eyebrows and on the forehead of an 8-week-old infant.

and reduce skin contact with urine. Urine is an irritant which will cause erythema and erosions following prolonged contact. Affected areas are the genital skin and the buttocks; the skin folds may be spared. Punched-out ulcers may occur in persistent cases of napkin dermatitis (known as Jacquet dermatitis). Overuse of potent steroids under occlusion in napkin dermatitis can lead to a granulomatous, nodular reaction on the buttocks, called infantile gluteal granuloma. The treatment of napkin dermatitis is aimed at keeping the skin dry and using barrier creams or emollients to restore normal epidermis.

Infantile psoriasis

See Chapter 10.

One-third of individuals with psoriasis develop the disease before the age of 15 years, and one-quarter of children affected present before the age of 2 years. All patterns of psoriasis have been described in children: guttate, chronic plaque, pustular and erythrodermic. In infants napkin psoriasis is the most common pattern (Figure 64.4). A mild topical steroid ointment and an emollient is usually effective treatment. Infantile psoriasis may be self-limiting.

Parakeratosis pustulosa

Parakeratosis pustulosa is a localised inflammatory condition involving the distal phalanx. Usually a solitary digit is involved, fingers more frequently than toes. Characteristically, the thumb, index finger or great toe is affected. There is sharply demarcated erythema and scaling of the skin adjacent to the nail fold, with accompanying nail dystrophy (Figure 64.5). Pustulation is seen in 25% of cases, but swabs are sterile and mycology is negative. The nail may be shed. The condition is fairly resistant to topical steroid, but usually resolves over the course of 12–18 months.

Infantile acropustulosis

An itchy vesiculo-pustular eruption of hands and feet. The onset is usually in the first year of life, particularly the first 6 months. It is more common in boys. Recurrent crops of intensely itchy vesiculo-pustules appear principally on the soles and sides of the feet, particularly around the heel (Figure 64.6). Lesions also occur on the palms, the dorsa of the feet, hands, ankles, wrists and forearms. Scattered lesions may also occur on the face, scalp, and trunk. Excoriation results in erosions and then crusting. Smear of a pustule shows neutrophils and eosinophils. Bacterial culture is negative. The differential diagnosis is scabies and sometimes the condition follows a genuine scabies infestation. Healing is succeeded by macular post-inflammatory hyperpigmentation. Each crop lasts for 7–14 days, occurring at intervals of 2–4 weeks, often more frequently in the summer months. Treatment is with potent topical

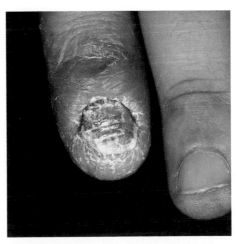

Figure 64.5 Parakeratosis pustulosa showing erythema of the index finger with associated nail dystrophy.

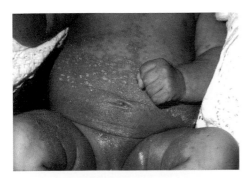

Figure 64.4 Infantile psoriasis.

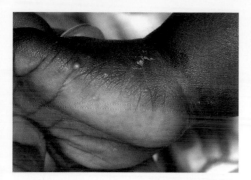

Figure 64.6 Infantile acropustulosis showing discrete pustules along medial border of the foot of an 11-month-old boy.

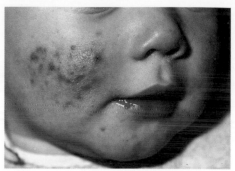

Figure 64.7 Infantile acne showing papules, pustules and comedones in a 6-month-old boy.

corticosteroids. Attacks gradually diminish in intensity until they cease altogether, usually within 2 years of the onset.

Infantile acne

See Chapter 44.

Infantile acne is rare, but is not associated with an endocrinopathy. The mean age of onset is 6 months: 3M:1F. The typical presentation is of inflammatory papules on the cheeks; one-quarter of patients get comedones (Figure 64.7). Topical treatment with benzoyl peroxide or erythromycin will help mild cases. More extensive disease should clear with oral erythromycin; prolonged treatment for 18–24 months may be required. In severe disease oral isotretinoin is safe and effective. Scarring can complicate infantile acne.

Urticaria

See Chapter 17.

One half of infants presenting with urticaria have a personal or family history of atopy. Viral infection is the trigger of acute urticaria in the majority of cases, but food allergy may be responsible in up to 10% of cases: the commonest allergens are cow's milk, eggs and wheat. Angio-oedema accompanies urticarial weals in 60% of cases, but anaphylaxis is rare. Chronic urticaria occurs in 30% of infant cases and is likely to be caused by physical factors. Cholinergic urticaria precipitated by exercise, emotion and heat is common. Urticaria in infancy may be a feature of systemic disease, including systemic lupus erythematosus, juvenile rheumatoid arthritis and mastocytosis.

VIRAL INFECTIONS

Viral exanthems

Viral exanthems account for the most common presentation to a paediatric emergency department. The most frequent exanthems seen in children are outlined in Table 64.1.

Molluscum contagiosum

This is an extremely common viral infection characterised by discrete, pearly, umbilicated papules 2–5 mm in diameter (Figure 64.9). Lesions usually occur in the axilla or groin, but may be widespread, especially in children with atopic eczema. It is readily spread between siblings. The eruption is usually self-limiting, but is often a source of parental concern. Ablative treatment with cryotherapy (if tolerated) or topical treatment with either hydrogen peroxide creams or potassium hydroxide solutions can speed resolution.

BACTERIAL INFECTIONS

Impetigo

Impetigo is a highly contagious cutaneous infection and is the commonest overall infection in children worldwide. It is usually caused by *Staphylococcus aureus*, less frequently

Table 64.1 Clinical features of the viral exanthems

Disease	Roseola (Syn. Exanthem subitum)	Fifth disease (Syn. Exanthem infantum)	Hand, foot and mouth disease	Varicella (Syn. Chicken pox)	Measles
Virus	HHV-6 (less commonly HHV-7)	Parvovirus B19	Coxsackie A16 and A6, enterovirus 71	Varicella zoster virus	Measles RNA paramyxovirus
Incubation period	5–14 days	7–14 days	7 days	14–21 days	7–14 days
Epidemiology	Very common 40% infected with HHV-6 by 12 months, 90% by 2 years	20% infected with parvovirus B19 by 3 years	Very common	Very common	The decline in uptake of MMR vaccination in the UK over recent years has been associated with a loss of herd immunity
History and exanthem	High fever for 3 days, then a fine, lacy, macular erythema with occipital lymphadenopathy Rash fades over 48 h	Onset with hot, bright red cheeks ('slapped cheeks'), followed by a reticulate rash on the torso and limbs with palmoplantar erythema Rash fades over 7 days	Painful vesicles (which may ulcerate) develop in the mouth, and small, and tense blisters with a red areola occur on the palms and soles (Figure 64.8) Lesions fade within 3 days	1–2-day prodrome of malaise and fever, then papulovesicles appear on the trunk, scalp or genital regions Lesions occur in crops, crusting over as they resolve Classically, lesions in different stages of evolution are seen Eruption becomes widespread but retains centripetal pattern	3-day prodrome of fever and coryza followed by small white Koplik spots on the buccal mucosa Rash on fourth day of illness, initially on the forehead, spreads onto the face, trunk and limbs

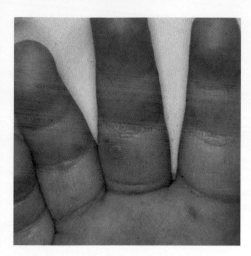

Figure 64.8 Hand, foot and mouth disease showing small vesicles with surrounding erythema on the palmar aspect of the fingers.

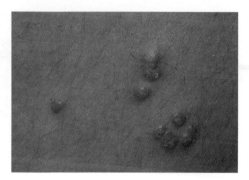

Figure 64.9 Typical umbilicated lesions of molluscum contagiosum. (Source: Courtesy of Addenbrooke's Hospital, Cambridge, UK.)

Strepococcus pyogenes. Honey-coloured crusts appear on a background of erythema (Figure 64.10). The child is well. Most frequently children aged 2–5 years are affected, but since the condition is so infectious spread within families, including to infants, is common. Non-bullous impetigo typically affects the face, whereas bullous impetigo occurs more commonly in intertriginous areas such as the napkin area, axillae or neck folds. In bullous impetigo the *Staphylococcus* produces exotoxins specific for desmoglein 1 and affected areas are painful and become eroded. Topical or oral antibiotics are given depending on severity.

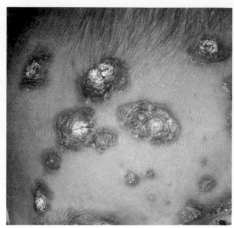

Figure 64.10 Impetigo showing multiple crusted lesions on the forehead of a 9-month-old.

Staphylococcal scalded skin syndrome

Staphylococcal scalded skin syndrome (SSSS) is a rare, desquamating dermatosis caused by staphylococcal toxins. Most cases are caused by *Staphylococcus aureus* phage gp II, strains 71 and 55. Primary infection is at a site distant from skin peeling, e.g. umbilicus, conjunctiva. This can cause difficulties in isolating the causal organism. SSSS has a median age of 2 years and an equal sex incidence. There is a seasonal peak in the autumn. Following a prodrome of fever, irritability and malaise, tender erythema appears at the flexures, perioral region and central face with subsequent development of superficial flaccid blisters, typically progressing to peeling and erosions (Figure 64.11). Blistering is mediated by epidermolytic toxin A and/or B, which cleaves the epidermis by damaging desmoglein 1. Pain is a prominent feature and affected infants resist movement or touch. Management is with intravenous antibiotics and supportive care with emollients, attention to fluid balance and adequate analgesia. Sparing of the mucous membranes helps differentiate SSSS from Stevens–Johnson syndrome/toxic epidermal necrolysis. Resolution of SSSS takes 2–3 weeks. Mortality is low in otherwise healthy infants.

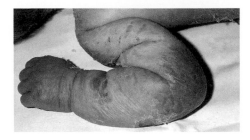

Figure 64.11 Staphylococcal scalded skin syndrome showing widespread peeling and erosion in a 3-month-old.

Blistering distal dactylitis

Blistering distal dactylitis is a *Staphylococcus aureus* infection of the fingertips. Occasionally a β-haemolytic *Streptococcus* can be implicated. Typically, large acral bullae 1–3 cm in diameter develop on the finger pulps. Blisters may also occur proximally on the digits and even on the palms. When multiple bullae are present, *Staphylococcus* is the more likely culprit organism, and the condition can be considered to be a localised bullous impetigo. The differential diagnosis includes epidermolysis bullosa simplex and sucking blisters, but the clinical signs are fairly diagnostic and swabs are confirmatory. Management is by deflating the blisters, dressing eroded areas and using appropriate antibiotics. Resolution is rapid.

Perianal dermatitis

A beefy erythema with oedema is seen in a well-demarcated distribution 2–3 cm around the anal margin in young infants (Figure 64.12). Pain can be severe and blood may be seen in the stool. The condition is due to β-haemolytic streptococcal infection. It responds rapidly to appropriate oral antibiotics.

FUNGAL INFECTIONS

Cutaneous candidiasis

See Chapter 7.

Transient oral candidiasis is not infrequent in infants: infection may have been acquired during delivery. Secondary colonisation of eroded

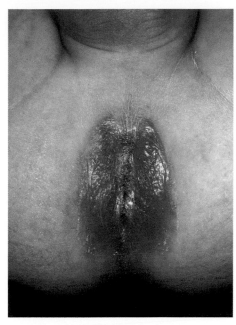

Figure 64.12 Perianal dermatitis showing well-circumscribed erythema and oedema in an 8-week-old baby.

or macerated skin in intertriginous areas, especially the napkin region, may occur. Satellite pustules are characteristic. Topical treatment will usually suffice. Recurrent or extensive infections should prompt investigation for an underlying immunodeficiency.

Tinea facei and tinea corporis

See Chapter 7.

Tinea infections remain rare in infants, but when they occur the diagnosis may be missed. In young infants, the face is the most common site of involvement. Infection with *Trichophyton tonsurans* now predominates, especially in urban areas and amongst children of African or Caribbean heritage. In cases of *T. tonsurans* tinea corporis the reservoir of infection is usually an infected scalp, either the child's own scalp or an older sibling. Annular, inflammatory lesions, which clear from the centre, occur on the face and body but most usually the cheek in infants (Figure 64.13). Lesions may be vesicular

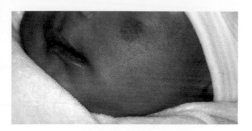

Figure 64.13 Tinea facei in a 4-week-old baby innoculated from an older sibling with tinea capitis.

and often resolve with post-inflammatory hyperpigmentation. Treatment for purely cutaneous lesions is a topical antifungal agent for 2 weeks, but if scalp involvement is suspected or proven, oral therapy will be required.

Tinea capitis

See Chapter 7.

Scalp ringworm infection remains rare in infants, but when it does occur in this age group the diagnosis may be missed and mistaken for seborrhoeic dermatitis. Presenting signs include patchy alopecia, diffuse scale and black dots due to broken-off hairs. Pustules, or a focal inflammatory kerion, may occur. Cervical lymphadenopathy is common. Oral therapy with terbinifine or itraconazole is preferable to griseofulvin. Both drugs are well tolerated in young children; itraconazole has the advantage of being available in a liquid formulation.

ANTHROPOD INFESTATIONS

Scabies

See Chapter 9.

Extreme pruritus characterises infestation with the mite *Sarcoptes scabei*. The condition is highly contagious. In infants, burrows may be seen on the palms and soles more characteristically than in the finger webs, and the wrists are also commonly involved. Burrows can appear quite inflammatory with surrounding secondary eczematous changes. Nodular lesions develop in the axillae and

genital region if the infestation is untreated. Eradication requires treatment of the individual and all close contacts using a topical scabecidal lotion or cream, applied in two applications 7 days apart. In recalcitrant cases ivermectin has been shown to be safe and well tolerated in infants. Post-scabetic pruritus may be prolonged and symptomatic treatment is usually required.

REACTIVE CONDITIONS

Acute haemorrhagic oedema in infancy

Acute haemorrhagic oedema is a benign, cutaneous, leucocytoclastic vasculitis arising after respiratory infection, medication administration or immunisation. The condition affects children between the ages of 4 months and 2 years, with males being affected twice as frequently as females. Fever is mild and systemic disturbance is minor. The limbs and face are the most commonly affected areas. Lesions are discrete or confluent with purpura often appearing in a targetoid or cockade (rosette) pattern (Figure 64.14). Oedema mainly affects the eyelids, face and extremities. Visceral and joint involvement is not typical. The differential diagnosis includes Henoch–Schönlein purpura, purpura fulminans, erythema multiforme, urticaria and Kawasaki disease. Resolution occurs within 3 weeks and recurrences are not a feature.

Kawasaki disease

See Chapter 54.

Kawasaki disease is a febrile illness with systemic vasculitis. It typically affects children aged 3–6 years, but can be seen in infants. High fever lasting up to 8 days, associated with conjunctival injection and red, cracked lips is followed by a generalised maculopapular rash with prominent swelling and erythema of the hands and feet, which then desquamate. Cervical lymphadenopathy may be pronounced. Leucocytosis, thrombocytosis and high ESR are characteristic. Recognition of the clinical signs is imperative, as early diagnosis and treatment are central to preventing complications, especially coronary artery

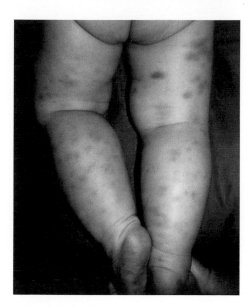

Figure 64.14 Multiple eccymotic and purpuric areas on the legs of a 10-month-old with acute haemorrhagic oedema in infancy.

aneurysms. Kawasaki disease in infants is more likely to be atypical (the rash and conjunctivitis may be much less prominent) and treatment instituted late. This results in a higher risk of complications and poorer outcome. Management comprises the early administration of intravenous immunoglobulin, as soon as the diagnosis is suspected, plus supportive measures.

Chronic bullous disease of childhood

(Syn. Childhood linear IgA bullous dermatosis)
See Chapter 22.

Chronic bullous disease of childhood (CBDC) is an autoimmune, blistering disease that occurs in prepubertal children. It is usually idiopathic but may be triggered by infections, drugs, or a vaccination. Children present with the abrupt onset of tense, clear or haemorrhagic vesicles and bullae on normal or erythematous skin. Lesions are often widespread and can involve the face (perioral pattern), trunk and extremities. There is a particular predilection for the lower trunk, genital area and medial thighs. New lesions arise

around resolving lesions, and these annular bullae surrounding a central crust are said to resemble a string of pearls or a cluster of jewels. Direct immunofluorescence reveals linear IgA staining of the basement membrane zone. CBDC usually requires systemic therapy: corticosteroids or erythromycin. Spontaneous resolution tends to occur after several months to a few years.

Gianotti–Crosti syndrome

(Syn. Infantile papular acrodermatitis)
Gianotti–Crosti syndrome (GCS) is a distinctive eruption affecting the face, buttocks and extremities. It is generally triggered by a viral infection; known culprits include hepatitis B virus, Epstein–Barr virus, human herpesvirus 6 and Coxsackie virus. GCS presents as an eruption of monomorphic, flat-topped, pink to red-brown papules or papulovesicles in a symmetrical distribution (Figure 64.15). It favours the cheeks and extensor surfaces of the limbs and buttocks. Lesions may sometimes be found on the trunk and flexor surfaces. The onset is often preceded by a viral illness, but constitutional symptoms are usually mild when the eruption appears. The rash lasts for a minimum of 10 days but may persist for up to 8 weeks. There is no specific treatment. Recurrences are unusual.

Papular urticaria

Papular urticaria arises as a result of a hypersensitivity reaction to insect bites, usually appearing as crops of more-or-less symmetrically distributed,

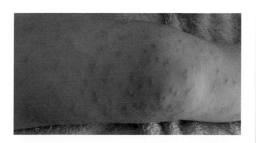

Figure 64.15 Gianotti–Crosti syndrome. Multiple monomorphic papules over the knees developed 2 weeks after an upper respiratory tract infection in this 1-year-old.

itchy papules and papulovesicles, most frequently on exposed areas of the limbs. Lesions are often heavily excoriated, secondary bacterial infection is common. It tends to occur more in the summer months, when blood-feeding insects are plentiful, but can it occur at any time of year, particularly if caused by insects that breed in a domestic environment, such as cat fleas. The clinical picture may be complicated by the reactivation of old lesions by new bites at a different site. Histopathology demonstrates papillary dermal oedema and perivascular lymphocytes, eosinophils and mast cells. Treatment includes topical steroids and systemic antihistamines, but response is usually limited. The condition will only be controlled if insect bites can be avoided. Children eventually outgrow this disorder.

Eosinophilic pustulosis

Eosinophilic pustulosis (Syn. Eosinophilic pustular folliculitis) is a rare condition, usually presenting before the age of 14 months and clearing by 3 years. As lesions are not always truly follicular, the term eosinophilic pustulosis is preferred. It is more common in males than females (M:F 4:1). Recurrent crops of itchy papulo-pustules on a red base develop on the scalp, and less commonly on the trunk and limbs, including hands and feet (Figure 64.16). The lesions resolve in 1 or 2 weeks, to be followed by further crops every few weeks. Spontaneous resolution usually occurs by 3 years of age. Affected infants are well. Histopathology of scalp lesions shows a perifollicular and periappendageal infiltrate of eosinophils, with neutrophils and mononuclear cells. The differential diagnosis

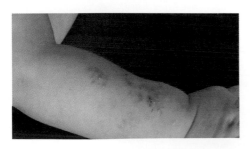

Figure 64.16 Eosinophilic pustulosis showing crops of small itchy pustules on the arm of a male infant.

includes staphylococcal folliculitis, scabies, herpes simplex, infantile acropustulosis and LCH. Because of the self-limiting nature of eosinophilic pustulosis specific treatment recommendations are lacking, but cetirizine and topical steroids have been used.

Acrodermatitis enteropathica

A rare autosomal recessive disorder (prevalence ~1:500 000) of intestinal absorption of zinc, caused by defects in ZIP4 the main intestinal zinc transporter. Zinc is a co-factor for many enzymes. The skin, intestine and immune system are affected. Symptoms start after weaning in breast-fed babies and at 4–10 weeks of age if they are formula-fed. An erosive dermatitis develops around the mouth and anus, and on the acral skin of the hands and feet (including paronychia). The affected skin is red, glazed and may be vesicular. Other features are alopecia, diarrhoea and failure to thrive. Serum zinc is low (copper levels may also be low). Treatment is with oral zinc.

DEVELOPMENTAL AND GENETIC CONDITIONS

Dermoid cysts

Dermoid cysts arise from skin trapped within embryonic fusion lines. They may contain adnexal structures such as hair and eccrine glands, or rarely bone and teeth. They occur most commonly on the head, presenting as firm subcutaneous nodules, particularly in the area of the anterolateral fronto-zygomatic suture (Figure 64.17), but also on the parieto-occipital scalp and the nose. Dermoid cysts may connect to underlying structures, including the central nervous system if lying over the midline.

Preauricular cysts and sinuses

Preauricular cysts and sinuses arise from a failure of fusion of the first two branchial arches and present as a tiny pit just anterior to the upper anterior helix.

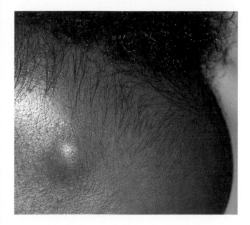

Figure 64.17 A dermoid cyst.

When bilateral they may be transmitted as an autosomal dominant trait. Usually asymptomatic in infancy, preauricular sinuses can become infected. Surgery entails complete excision of the sinus tract and associated cysts. They may be associated with deafness and with other anomalies, as in branchio-oto-renal syndrome and branchio-otic syndrome.

Pigmentary mosaicism

Pigmentary mosaicism presents as streaks and whorls of hypo- or hyperpigmentation which follow Blaschko's lines and which display midline demarcation (Figure 64.18). Pigmentary mosaicism may also manifest as patches, flag-like, leaf-like (phylloid) or chequerboard shapes, or as patchy variation without midline demarcation. It arises from a variety of cytogenetic abnormalities and can be associated with a range of other clinical features, frequently neurological and musculoskeletal.

MISCELLANEOUS CONDITIONS

Pedal papules of infancy

Symmetrical, painless, flesh-coloured nodules, characteristically on the medial aspect of the heels in infants, may be present at birth, but are usually not apparent until infancy. They occur in up to 40% of infants. They may be solitary,

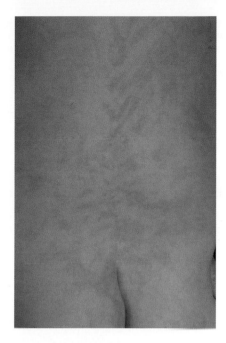

Figure 64.18 Whorls of hyperpigmentation following Blaschko's lines.

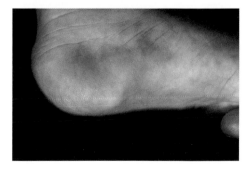

Figure 64.19 Pedal papule of infancy showing a soft swelling on the medial aspect of the heel.

but unlike piezogenic papules in adults tend to be larger and asymptomatic (Figure 64.19).

Calcified cutaneous nodules of the heels

Small, firm, calcified dermal lesions can occur on the heels of infants who have been on neonatal intensive care units and subjected to multiple heel pricks for venesection. Histologically, the lesions appear to have features of epidermal cysts and so are believed to arise from epidermal implantation through trauma, with subsequent calcification of the cyst, rather than dystrophic calcification per se. Natural resolution over the course of 18 months is the norm, but if slow to resolve they may cause pain on pressure when walking in older children.

Non-accidental injury

Non-accidental injury (NAI) is a widespread problem in infants and toddlers. In children with multiple attendances at A&E, or unexplained injuries, the concern of NAI should be raised. Subconjunctival haemorrhages in an infant should arouse suspicion that the child is a victim of shaken baby syndrome. Burns, signs of neglect or signs of sexual abuse may all form part of the spectrum. Human bites may produce bruising rather than puncture marks; bites inflicted by adults are indicative of NAI. A young child becoming withdrawn, or wary of adults, should arouse suspicion of NAI and appropriate measures taken.

Hair loss in infancy

Absent or diffusely sparse hair in infancy can arise from abnormalities of initiation of growth, hair shaft abnormalities and abnormal cycling. Alopecia areata is relatively rare in the first year of life and early onset tends to indicate a poor prognosis. Telogen effluvium is less common in infants than in adults, and is more likely to be related to a sudden and transient illness than to drugs or hormonal fluctuations. Loose anagen syndrome refers to a condition seen in children, usually girls, who have sparse hair with easily extracted anagen hairs, with misshapen bulbs, absent root sheaths and ruffled cuticles ('wrinkled socks').

Langerhans cell histiocytosis

See Chapter 74.

LCH is the commonest of the histiocytic disorders in childhood, most frequently presenting under the age of 1 year; boys are affected twice as often as girls. The types of LCH are divided into four groups (Box 64.1). Cutaneous features are variable, including seborrhoeic dermatitis-like erythema and scaling, papules, pustules, vesicles, nodules, petechiae and ulceration (Figure 64.20). Single-system disease has almost 100% survival. Up to 56% of infants

> **Box 64.1 Langerhans cell histiocytosis clinical groups**
> - Acute, disseminated LCH (Syn. Letterer–Siwe disease)
> - Chronic, localised LCH (Syn. Eosinophilic granuloma)
> - Progressive, multifocal, chronic LCH (Syn. Hand–Schüller–Christian disease)
> - Benign, self-healing LCH (Syn. Congenital self-healing reticulohistiocytosis, Hashimoto–Pritzker disease).

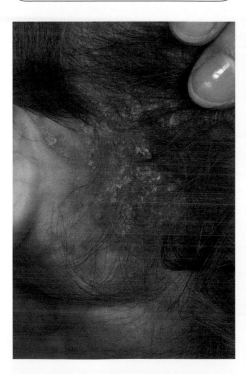

Figure 64.20 Langerhans cell histiocytosis. Crusted papules and erythema on the scalp.

presenting with skin-only disease may progress to multisystem disease.

Juvenile xanthogranuloma

Juvenile xanthogranuloma (JXG) often presents in the first year of life; it is more common in boys than girls. JXG starts as a red-brown papule which becomes orange (Figure 64.21). They occur most frequently on the face, scalp and upper torso. Localised cutaneous JXG heals spontaneously, sometimes leaving an atrophic scar. Benign cephalic histiocytosis has many similarities to JXG and may be the same disease. It usually presents in the first or second year of life as multiple, small, yellow-red macules and papules, initially on the head, but sometimes spreading to other sites. The lesions heal spontaneously without scarring.

Mastocytosis

See Chapter 18.

Mastocytosis in infancy is usually limited to the skin, with three distinct clinical presentations: (i) maculopapular (formerly urticaria pigmentosa), (ii) diffuse cutaneous mastocytosis (Figure 64.22) or (iii) solitary mastocytoma (Figure 64.23). Serum tryptase is a good marker for mast cell burden in infants. Parents of infants with extensive skin involvement should be given advice on the avoidance of mast cell degranulation factors, including aspirin, non-steroidal anti-inflammatory drugs, codeine, opiates, polymyxin B and contrast media. Therapy with an antihistamine should control symptoms. Children with a history of anaphylaxis should be supplied with an adrenaline autoinjector.

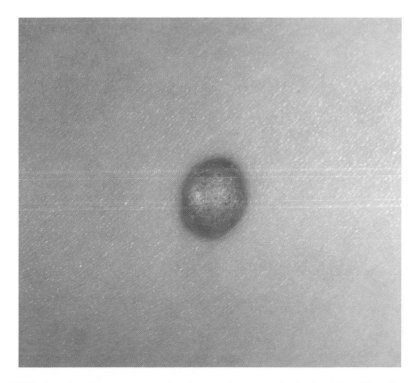

Figure 64.21 Juvenile xanthogranuloma showing a well-circumscribed yellowish nodule with an erythematous margin on the upper back of a 6-month-old.

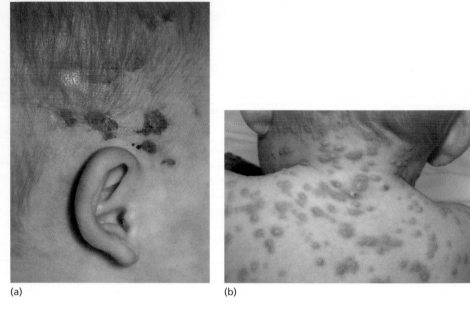

(a)   (b)

Figure 64.22 Mastocytosis. (a) Mast cell degranulation causing erythematous papules and crusts on the scalp. (b) Papules and plaques on the back of an infant with diffuse cutaneous mastocytosis.

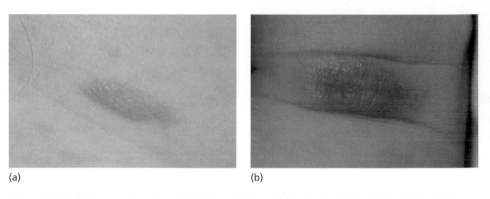

(a)   (b)

Figure 64.23 Solitary mastocytoma: (a) before rubbing and (b) urticated after rubbing (Darier sign).

Infantile and congenital haemangiomas

65

Infantile haemangiomas

(Syn. **Strawberry naevus, capillary haemangioma**)
Infantile haemangiomas (IHs) are common, benign, vascular tumours that develop in early infancy. The natural history is of proliferation in the first few months of life and thereafter spontaneous involution over a matter of years.

Epidemiology
Occur in approximately 4% of infants. F > M. Amniocentesis, *in vitro* fertilisation, breech presentation, being first born and low birth weight (<2500 g) are all associated with the development of IH.

Pathophysiology
Evidence for a genetic aetiology includes a two-fold increased relative risk among siblings of an affected proband in some families, and an autosomal dominant inheritance pattern with linkage to 5q in other families. It is likely that somatic mutations lead to uncontrolled proliferation of haemangioma cells. Mutations in the integrin-like receptor Tumour Endothelial Marker 8 (TEM8), and in *VEGFR2*, have been identified in a subpopulation of haemangioma-derived endothelial cells. Placental anomalies are an important risk factor.

The histopathology of IH varies with biological stage. During the growth phase there are solid groups of cells with few lumina; during the involution phase a lobular appearance develops. Immunohistochemistry is positive for factor VIII, CD31 and von Willebrand factor. Glucose transporter protein-1 (GLUT-1) positivity can be useful in differentiating IHs from other vascular lesions, such as congenital haemangiomas.

Clinical features
At presentation IHs need to be distinguished from vascular malformations (see Table 65.1). An IH is evident shortly after birth as a flat pink mark, or a telangiectatic patch, or an area of pallor. Superficial IHs undergo rapid growth in the first 2 months of life to produce a raised, cherry red plaque (Figure 65.1). Deep haemangiomas, which involve the deep dermis and sub-cutis, present later and continue to grow for longer (Figure 65.2). Mixed haemangiomas (features of superficial and deep type) are common (Figure 65.3). Most IHs reach 80% of their final size by 3 months of age and complete their growth by 9 months. Some show little proliferation and remain as a patch of telangiectatic vessels (abortive IH). 15% of IHs cause the infant complications and will prompt active intervention. The main complications of IHs are listed in Box 65.1.

During the proliferative phase IHs are firm, with involution they become softer and develop islands of grey within the redness. In most cases, involution is complete at a median age of 3 years. In some patients involution continues for a few more years. Permanent changes (telangiectases, atrophy and residual fibro-fatty tissue) occur in 25–60% of untreated haemangiomas.

Rook's Dermatology Handbook, First Edition. Edited by Christopher E. M. Griffiths, Tanya O. Bleiker, Daniel Creamer,
John R. Ingram and Rosalind C. Simpson.
© 2022 John Wiley & Sons Ltd. Published 2022 by John Wiley & Sons Ltd.

Table 65.1 Distinction between IHs and vascular malformations

	Infantile haemangioma	Vascular malformation
Clinical features	Usually becomes evident within the first week of life	Usually present at birth
	Proliferates rapidly	Proportionate growth
	Involutes over years	Does not involute
Epidemiology	More common in girls and low birth weight infants	No gender or birth-weight bias
Immunohistochemistry	GLUT-1 positive	GLUT-1 negative

GLUT-1, glucose transporter protein-1.

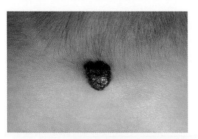

Figure 65.1 Superficial IH. A small haemangioma in the proliferative phase on the forehead of a 3-month-old infant.

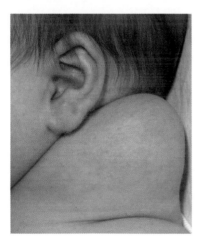

Figure 65.2 Deep IH. A deep-seated lesion involving the lateral neck in an 8-week-old infant.

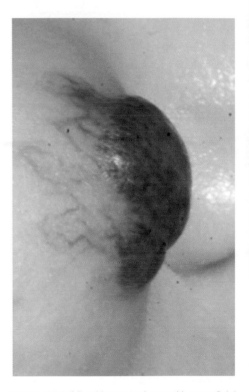

Figure 65.3 Mixed haemangioma with superficial and deep components on the face of a 7-week-old infant.

Segmental IH of the face and of the lumbosacral region may be associated with underlying structural anomalies (see Table 65.2). Multifocal haemangiomas are small, range from a few in number to myriads. They are histologically and immunohistochemically identical to solitary cutaneous haemangiomas. Most affected infants follow an uncomplicated course, but some children with multifocal haemangiomas have symptomatic visceral lesions, notably of the liver.

Box 65.1 Main complications of infantile haemangiomas

Ulceration (Figure 65.4)	Common, up to 20% of cases, especially at 4–6 months of age Most likely in large lesions; those present on neck, ano-genital skin or lip; segmental morphology Associated with bleeding and infection Ulceration results in scarring
Disfigurement	Permanent distortion can occur in haemangiomas on central face, lips and nose, particularly those with a dermal component
Functional impairment (Figure 65.5)	Peri-ocular haemangiomas: astigmatism, visual axis obstruction, strabismus, amblyopia, visual loss Airways and nose haemangiomas: breathing problems Lip haemangiomas: feeding problems Peri-anal haemangiomas: painful defaecation, bleeding

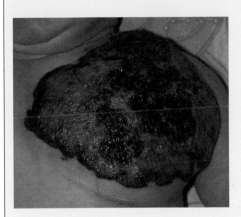

Figure 65.4 Ulcerated IH.

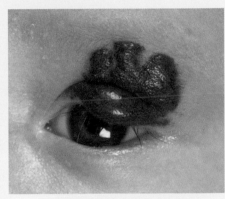

Figure 65.5 Eyelid haemangioma interfering with the line of vision.

Investigations

The diagnosis is usually clinical. Occasionally ultrasound may be required to distinguish IHs from other soft tissues masses or vascular malformations. Head and neck magnetic resonance angiography, echocardiogram and ophthalmological examination are recommended for patients with large facial segmental haemangiomas.

Management

Without treatment the prognosis is excellent for small IHs: most resolve spontaneously without sequelae. In the early stages parents are concerned about aesthetic issues and require detailed explanation of the natural history of IHs.

Propranolol is the first line treatment and is indicated for IHs causing functional impairment, disfigurement or ulceration. Propranolol treatment guidelines are summarised in Boxes 65.2–65.5. Contraindications to treatment with propranolol are listed in Box 65.2. Pre-treatment investigations are listed in Box 65.3. The propranolol treatment regimen is outlined in Box 65.4. Treatment regimen for pre-term infants, or those with co-morbidities, is outlined in Box 65.5.

In most infants the treatment can be safely stopped at 12–14 months. Treatment should extend beyond the proliferation phase: premature cessation of propranolol may lead to rebound growth of the IH.

Topical β-blockers can be effective for superficial haemangiomas, e.g. timolol maleate, usually as a gel-forming solution, one drop three times a day to non-ulcerated, non-mucosal lesions.

Table 65.2 Anomalies associated with segmental IHs

Facial segmental haemangioma	Lower body segmental haemangioma
Posterior fossa malformations, **h**aemangiomas, **a**rterial anomalies, **c**ardiac anomalies, **e**ye abnormalities, **s**ternal pit/supra-umbilical raphe (PHACES association)	**L**ower body haemangioma, **u**rogenital anomalies, **u**lceration, **m**yelopathy, **b**ony deformities, **a**no-rectal malformations, **a**rterial anomalies, **r**enal anomalies (LUMBAR association) (Figure 65.6)
	Spinal dysraphism, **a**nogenital anomalies, **c**utaneous anomalies, **r**enal and urological anomalies, **l**umbosacral haemangioma (SACRAL association)
	Perineal haemangioma, **e**xternal genitalia malformations, **l**ipomyelomeningocele, **v**esico-renal abnormalities, **i**mperforate anus (PELVIS association)

Source: Data from International Society for the Study of Vascular Anomalies (ISSVA). ISSVA classification for vascular anomalies 2014. http://www.issva.org (last accessed May 2015).

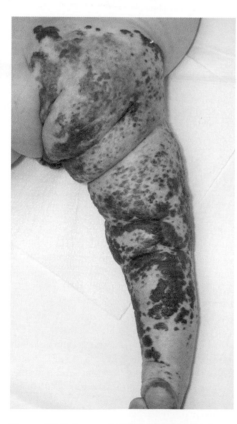

Figure 65.6 Segmental IH in an infant aged 6 weeks. It was associated with complex spinal dysraphism.

Pulsed dye laser can be helpful for the treatment of ulceration, and for telangiectases and erythema post-involution. Surgery may be necessary for IHs in the proliferative phase if functional impairment or ulceration cannot be managed medically. In the involution phase surgery may be indicated if there is abnormal contour due to a fibrofatty residuum or distortion of an important anatomical structure.

Congenital haemangiomas

Rapidly involuting congenital haemangiomas (RICHs), non-involuting congenital haemangiomas (NICHs) and partially involuting congenital haemangiomas (PICHs) are clinically distinct from IHs.

Epidemiology
M = F

Pathophysiology
Congenital haemangiomas are benign vascular tumours that proliferate *in utero* and do not grow postnatally. They may be evident at 12 weeks of gestation by prenatal ultrasound studies. RICH regress within 1–2 years, NICH do not regress. All types are GLUT-1 negative. Histology of RICH shows small lobules of capillaries with plump endothelium peripherally,

Box 65.2 Contraindications to the use of propranolol

Absolute: Hypoglycaemic episodes

Second/third-degree heart block

Hypersensitivity to propranolol

Relative: Frequent wheezing

Blood pressure outside normal range for age*

Heart rate outside normal range for age*

*Treatment to be initiated in conjunction with paediatrician.
Recommendations from British Society of Paediatric Dermatologists Guidelines 2018. Br J Dermatol 2018, 179, 582.

Box 65.3 Pre-treatment investigations needed prior to initiation of propranolol

Cardiovascular and respiratory examination

ECG: In infants with heart rate outside normal range, or with family history of arrhythmia, sudden death, sudden loss of consciousness, maternal connective tissue disease

Echo: In infants with heart rate outside normal range, or with murmur, or with segmental IH

Glucose: In infants born pre-term or small-for-dates, who are feeding poorly or have hypoglycaemic episodes

Recommendations from British Society of Paediatric Dermatologists Guidelines 2018. Br J Dermatol 2018, 179, 582.

Box 65.4 Propranolol treatment regimen

Clinical photographs must be taken at baseline

Recommended formulation is propranolol hydrochloride oral solution 5 mg/ml

Initial dose is 1 mg/kg daily in three divided doses*

After 24 h increase dose to 2 mg/kg daily in three divided doses*

Continue at this dose, or up to a maximum of 3 mg/kg daily in three divided doses*

Treatment should extend beyond proliferative period of IH

*Blood pressure and heart rate do not have to be monitored between visits for well infants.
Recommendations from British Society of Paediatric Dermatologists Guidelines 2018. Br J Dermatol 2018, 179, 582.

Box 65.5 Propranolol treatment regimen for pre-term infants, or those with cardiac, respiratory or metabolic co-morbidities

Admit these infants for 2–4 h on initiation and with dose increments

Initial dose is 0.5 mg/kg daily in three divided doses

Heart rate and blood pressure measurements before the first dose and every 30 min for 2–4 h

Glucose monitoring only for those at risk of hypoglycaemia (pre-term, low weight)

Infants with cervico-facial segmental IH need to be discussed with paediatricians

Recommendations from British Society of Paediatric Dermatologists Guidelines 2018. Br J Dermatol 2018, 179, 582.

and more thin-walled vessels with surrounding fibrous tissue centrally. Histology of NICH shows large lobules of small vessels in a stroma of fibrous tissue containing abnormal appearing arteries and veins.

Clinical features

Congenital haemangiomas usually arise on the head or the extremities. RICH typically present as blue or purple tumours, often with telangiectases and peripheral pallor (Figure 65.7). Sometimes there is a central ulcer, scar or depression. The rapid regression may leave pronounced atrophy. Large lesions may cause haemodynamic instability. NICH present as

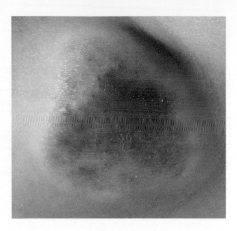

Figure 65.7 Rapidly involuting congenital haemangioma on the leg of a 6-week-old male, showing peripheral pallor.

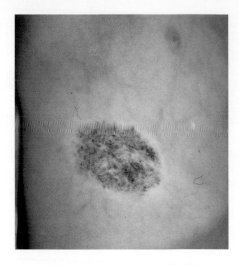

Figure 65.8 Non-involuting congenital haemangioma in an 11-year-old child.

violaceous plaques or tumours with coarse telangiectases and peripheral pallor (Figure 65.8). They grow in proportion with the affected individual, but never regress.

Investigations
Ultrasonography of RICH demonstrates a uniform hypoechoic mass with centrilobular draining channels. NICH often show prominent arterial flow on ultrasound. RICH may be associated with transient thrombocytopenia.

Management
Embolisation or excision may need to be considered for RICHs that are ulcerated, bleeding or causing haemodynamic instability. There is no convincing evidence that β-blockers accelerate involution of RICH. For NICH requiring treatment, surgery is the preferred option.

Part 9
Skin Disorders Caused by External Agents

Cutaneous adverse reactions to drugs and radiotherapy

66

BENIGN CUTANEOUS ADVERSE REACTIONS

Benign cutaneous adverse reactions (BCARs) represent a range of drug eruptions, each with a different clinical presentation (see Table 66.1). Many of these eruptions mimic other common dermatoses (e.g. exanthems, urticaria) but are triggered by an adverse reaction to a medication. The latency period, which is the time from onset of culprit drug to time of reaction onset, is different for each BCAR. Numerous drugs can act as the triggering agent in the BCAR dermatoses, but each entity has a relatively restricted list of common culprits (Table 66.2). Most patients developing a BCAR are unlikely to suffer serious morbidity.

SEVERE CUTANEOUS ADVERSE REACTIONS

The severe cutaneous adverse reactions (SCARs) are Stevens-Johnson syndrome/toxic epidermal necrolysis (SJS/TEN), acute generalised exanthematous pustulosis (AGEP) and drug reaction with eosinophilia and systemic symptoms (DRESS). The SCAR syndromes are all associated with serious morbidity and mortality. They are dermatological emergencies.

Stevens-Johnson syndrome/ toxic epidermal necrolysis

(Syn. Lyell syndrome)
SJS/TEN is a severe mucocutaneous reaction, usually to a drug, characterised by widespread epidermal/epithelial sloughing.

Epidemiology
Incidence: 1–6 cases/million/year. 2F:1M

Pathophysiology
Drug-induced cytotoxic T cells initiate widespread epithelial necrosis while soluble factors, notably granulysin, trigger keratinocyte apoptosis. Histopathological features of SJS/TEN range from individual keratinocyte necrosis to full-thickness epidermal death and subepidermal blistering. A culprit drug is demonstrated in 85% of cases: the common culprits are listed in Box 66.1. In 15% of patients a culprit drug is not identified and some of these

---

Rook's Dermatology Handbook, First Edition. Edited by Christopher E. M. Griffiths, Tanya O. Bleiker, Daniel Creamer, John R. Ingram and Rosalind C. Simpson.
© 2022 John Wiley & Sons Ltd. Published 2022 by John Wiley & Sons Ltd.

PART 9: SKIN DISORDERS CAUSED BY EXTERNAL AGENTS

Table 66.1 Benign cutaneous adverse reactions to drugs

	Drug-induced exanthem	Drug-induced urticaria (see Chapter 17)	Drug-induced subacute cutaneous lupus erythematosus (see Chapter 23)	Lichenoid drug eruption (see Chapter 12)	Fixed drug eruption
Epidemiology	Common	Common	Rare	Rare	Rare
Pathophysiology	Drug-specific cytotoxic T-cells	Drug-specific IgE Pseudo-allergy in some cases	Ro antibody- mediated keratinocyte cytotoxicity aggravated by drug	Autoreactive T cells against drug–MHC antigen complex	Delayed type hypersensitivity Activation of resident CD8+ T cells
Latency	7–10 days	24–36 h on first occasion A few minutes on re-challenge	Varies from a few weeks to several months	weeks to months	30 min to 8 h after exposure
Clinical features	Morbilliform eruption of pink macules on torso and limbs (Figure 66.1)	Urticaria and, sometimes, angio-oedema (Figure 66.2)	Red annular and polycyclic lesions on upper torso, proximal limbs Facial erythema	Papules, patches and plaques of lichenoid inflammation Eruption often photodistributed (Figure 66.3)	Solitary oval red patch Recurs on re-exposure at same site Continued exposure to culprit will induce multiple lesions (Figure 66.4)
Differential Diagnosis	Viral exanthem, DRESS (see below)	Acute idiopathic urticaria, chronic spontaneous urticaria	Erythema annulare centrifugum, polymorphic light eruption, other forms of cutaneous lupus erythematosus	Lichen planus, cutaneous lupus erythematosus	Herpes simplex, contact dermatitis, erythema dyschromicum perstans
Investigations	Usually clinical diagnosis Skin biopsy may help distinguish drug exanthem from infective exanthem	Drug-specific serum IgE Skin prick testing and intra-dermal testing	Skin biopsy Ro, La antibodies	Skin biopsy	Skin biopsy Patch testing with culprit drug on lesional skin

Management	Stop culprit drug Emollient, topical steroid if itchy	Stop culprit drug Oral/IV antihistamine ± oral or IV corticosteroid	Stop culprit drug Topical or systemic steroid Photoprotection	Stop culprit drug Potent topical steroid	Stop culprit drug Potent topical steroid
Complications	Exfoliative erythroderma may occur with continued exposure to culprit	Anaphylaxis may occur	Rarely associated with features of systemic lupus erythematosus	Erythroderma, secondary skin infection	Generalised bullous fixed drug eruption can develop with repeated exposure to culprit

DRESS, drug reaction eosinophilia and systemic symptoms; MHC, major histocompatibility complex.

PART 9: SKIN DISORDERS CAUSED BY EXTERNAL AGENTS

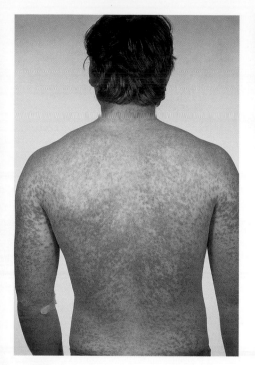

Figure 66.1 An exanthem caused by ampicillin.

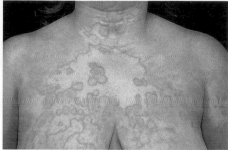

Figure 66.2 Urticaria induced by aspirin. (Source: Courtesy of St John's Institute of Dermatology, King's College London, UK.)

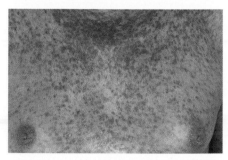

Figure 66.3 Lichenoid drug eruption caused by pravastatin.

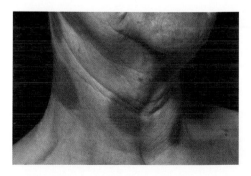

Figure 66.4 Multiple discrete lesions of fixed drug eruption induced by aspirin.

cases are triggered by infections, notably *Mycoplasma pneumoniae*. In Han Chinese people there is a strong genetic predisposition to carbamazepine-induced SJS/TEN in subjects with HLA-B*1502, and allopurinol-induced SJS/TEN with HLA-B*5801.

Clinical features

The latent period between initiation of the culprit drug and onset of SJS/TEN is typically 7–10 days. A prodrome of malaise, fever and upper respiratory tract symptoms precedes the rash, which develops on the face and chest initially and then disseminates widely. Pruritus and cutaneous pain are typical. An erosive, haemorrhagic mucositis of the eyes (Figure 66.5), mouth, nose (Figure 66.6) and genitalia (Figure 66.7) is an early feature. Skin lesions include atypical targets (Figure 66.8), purpuric macules (Figure 66.9), confluent erythema (Figure 66.10), vesicles and blisters (Figure 66.11). Nikolsky sign is positive. The end point is sloughing of necrotic epidermis leaving areas of denuded, exposed dermis (Figure 66.12). SJS is defined as epidermal detachment of <10% of the body surface area (BSA), TEN is detachment of >30% of BSA, overlap SJS-TEN is detachment of 10–30% of BSA. Ocular involvement (chemosis, conjunctivitis, pseudomembranes, conjunctival and corneal ulcers) causes ocular pain and visual impairment. Oral and oesophageal disease compromises

Table 66.2 Common culprit drugs in BCARs

Drug-induced exanthem	Drug-induced urticaria	Drug-induced subacute cutaneous lupus erythematosus	Lichenoid drug eruption	Fixed drug eruption
Carbamazepine	Cephalosporins	Thiazides	Antimalarials	Aspirin
Cephalosporins	NSAIDs	Diltiazem	β–blockers	NSAIDs
Cotrimoxazole	Penicillins	Verapamil	Furosemide	Oral
Carbopenems	Quinine	Terbinafine	Gold	contraceptive
NSAIDs	Rifampicin	Ranitidine	Phenothiazines	Penicillins
Penicillins	Sulphonamides	Leflunomide	Thiazides	Phenolphthalein
Phenytoin	Vancomycin	Omeprazole	Tolazamide	Phenytoin
		Hydroxychloroquine	Lithium	Quinine
			Statins	Sulphonamides
				Tetracyclines

NSAIDs, non-steroidal anti-inflammatory drugs.

Box 66.1 Commonest drugs causing SJS/TEN

Allopurinol
Carbamazepine
Lamotrigine
Nevirapine
Oxicam non-steroidal anti-inflammatory drugs (e.g. meloxicam)
Phenobarbital
Phenytoin
Sulfamethoxazole and other sulfa antibiotics
Sulfasalazine

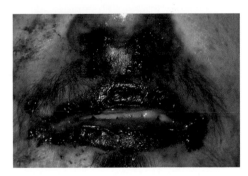

Figure 66.6 Stevens–Johnson syndrome/toxic epidermal necrolysis. Lip and nostril involvement. Severe cheilitis has produced thick haemorrhagic crusts. This SJS/TEN patient had a coagulopathy which resulted in bleeding from the involved mucosae of the mouth and nose.

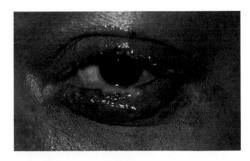

Figure 66.5 Stevens–Johnson syndrome/toxic epidermal necrolysis. Ocular involvement. There is eyelid oedema, conjunctivitis and keratitis: the green material is exudate stained by fluorescein dye used for ophthalmic examination.

drinking and eating. Urogenital involvement leads to dysuria and/or retention. Involvement of the respiratory tract presents with dyspnoea, increased respiratory rate, bronchial hypersecretion and hypoxia. A form of *Mycoplasma*-induced SJS usually occurring in children, is characterised by prominent mucous membrane involvement with only a few skin lesions; it has been termed *Mycoplasma pneumoniae*-associated mucositis.

Extensive epidermal detachment in SJS/TEN leads to a series of homeostatic dysfunctions, collectively contributing to acute skin failure (see Box 66.2).

Mortality in SJS is less than 10%, whereas mortality in TEN is approximately 30%. Overall SJS/TEN mortality is around 22%. The cause of death in SJS/TEN is usually septicaemia-induced multiorgan failure. SCORTEN (SCORe of TEN) is a seven-point prognostic scoring system used to predict mortality (Box 66.3).

Differential diagnosis

Although the full-blown syndrome of TEN is usually clinically obvious, it can be difficult to discriminate the early stages of SJS/TEN from other bullous dermatoses. The differential diagnosis of SJS/TEN is outlined in Box 66.4.

Investigations

Investigations are needed to substantiate the diagnosis, exclude other blistering dermatoses and identify systemic complications. Important tests are listed in Box 66.5.

Management

A multidisciplinary team should be convened to manage an SJS/TEN patient. The following clinical specialties need to be involved: dermatology ± burns plastic surgery, intensive care, ophthalmology, thoracic medicine, gastroenterology, gynaecology/urology, oral medicine, specialist dermatology nursing (or burns nursing), dietetics.

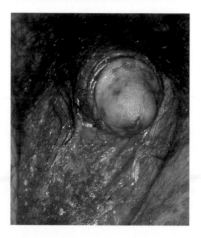

Figure 66.7 Stevens–Johnson syndrome/toxic epidermal necrolysis. Genital involvement. There is confluent erythema of the scrotum and discrete lesions on the glans penis. Redness at the meatus indicates that urethral involvement is likely.

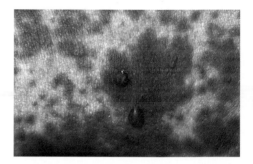

Figure 66.9 Stevens–Johnson syndrome/toxic epidermal necrolysis. Purpuric macules. The dusky, purpuric lesions on this patient's skin are coalescing and blistering.

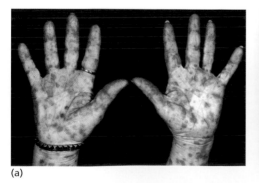

(a)

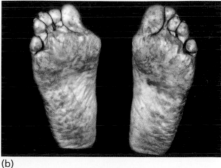

(b)

Figure 66.8 Stevens–Johnson syndrome toxic epidermal necrolysis. Palmoplantar involvement. Multiple circular lesions (atypical targets) are present on (a) the palms and (b) the soles. Blistering is occurring at both sites, but prominently on the feet.

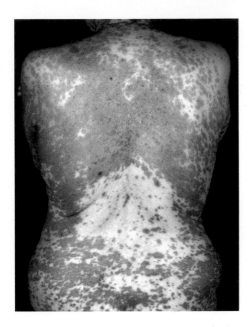

Figure 66.10 Stevens–Johnson syndrome/toxic epidermal necrolysis. Confluent erythema. Individual lesions may coalesce to form large areas of erythema, as seen on this patient's back. In her case, blistering/epidermal detachment was negligible.

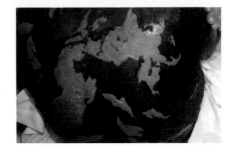

Figure 66.12 Stevens–Johnson syndrome/toxic epidermal necrolysis. Denuded skin. Extensive epidermal loss in TEN produces large areas of exposed dermis.

Box 66.2 Features of acute skin failure in SJS/TEN

- Deranged thermoregulation: hypothermia
- Excessive transcutaneous fluid loss: hypoperfusion and acute kidney injury
- Metabolic problems: hyperglycaemia, hypoalbuminaemia
- Haematological problems: anaemia and leucopenia
- Cutaneous infection: systemic sepsis and multi-organ failure

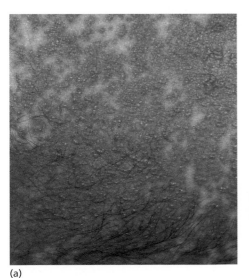

(a)

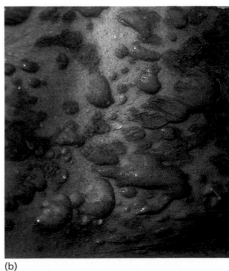

(b)

Figure 66.11 Stevens–Johnson syndrome/toxic epidermal necrolysis. Blistering. Lesional skin in SJS/TEN typically blisters forming both vesicles (a) and large flaccid bullae (b).

PART 9: SKIN DISORDERS CAUSED BY EXTERNAL AGENTS

Box 66.3 Parameters which constitute SCORTEN

Age greater than 40 years
Presence of malignancy
Heart rate >120 beats/min
Epidermal detachment >10% of BSA at admission
Serum urea >10 mmol/L
Serum glucose >14 mmol/L
Arterial bicarbonate level <20 mmol/L
Each parameter contributes one point to the score. Mortality worsens with increasing SCORTEN (Table 66.3).

Table 66.3 SCORTEN predicted mortality

Number of parameters	Predicted mortality (%)
0	1.2
1	3.9
2	12.2
3	32.4
4	62.2
5	85.0
6	95.1
7	98.5

Box 66.4 Differential diagnosis of SJS/TEN

Erythema multiforme major
Pemphigus vulgaris
Mucous membrane pemphigoid
Bullous pemphigoid
Paraneoplastic pemphigus
Bullous lupus erythematosus
Linear IgA bullous dermatosis
Generalised bullous fixed drug eruption
Acute bullous acute graft-versus-host disease
Staphylococcal scalded skin syndrome
Acute generalised exanthematous pustulosis

Box 66.5 Investigations needed in SJS/TEN

Biopsy of lesional skin through blister margin, for routine histopathology
Biopsy taken from peri-blister lesional skin, for direct IMF
Full blood count
Urea and electrolytes
Glucose, amylase, bicarbonate
Arterial blood gases
Liver function tests
Inflammatory markers (ESR, CRP)
Coagulation studies
Mycoplasma serology
ANA, ENA
dsDNA antibodies
Complement
Indirect immunofluorescence
Chest X-ray

The most important manoeuvre is to stop the culprit drug as soon as it has been identified.

First line: If epidermal loss is >10% BSA transfer to a specialist unit (intensive care unit or burns unit). Patient must be barrier nursed in a side room. Venous access for fluid replacement must be sited through non-lesional skin. A urinary catheter is needed. Oral fluid and oral food intake is often not tolerated, therefore a nasogastric tube for enteral feeding and fluids is usual. Specialist nursing is essential for the delivery of skin care, which includes topical therapy and dressings. The skin should be gently cleansed each day with a diluted solution of chlorhexidine. 50/50 white soft paraffin/liquid paraffin emollient should be applied to the whole skin every few hours. Exposed dermis should be covered with non-adhesive silicon dressings. The supportive care package should pay particular attention to:

- *Heated environment:* Heating the patient's room to 25–28°C will limit energy losses and reduce metabolic stresses.
- *Fluid replacement:* Extensive epidermal detachment will result in large insensible transcutaneous fluid losses, compounded by decreased oral intake due to disease involvement of the mouth. During the acute illness, replace fluids intravenously, using a crystalloid fluid at 2 mL/kg body weight/% of BSA epidermal detachment, or alternatively use urine output to guide fluid replacement.
- *Nutritional regimen:* Feeding must be initiated early to support metabolic disturbances, minimise protein losses and promote healing. Enteral nutrition is preferable to parenteral nutrition to reduce peptic ulceration and limit translocation of gut bacteria. If oral feeding is not tolerated, feed via nasogastric tube. During the early, catabolic phase of SJS/TEN 20–25 kcal/kg/day should be delivered, while requirements in the recovery, anabolic phase increase to 25–30 kcal/kg/day.
- *Analgesia:* Skin pain in SJS/TEN is severe. Patients should receive adequate background simple analgesia to ensure comfort at rest, with the addition of opiates, as required, delivered either by patient-controlled analgesia or infusion. Additional analgesia is often needed to address increased pain associated with patient handling, repositioning and dressing changes.
- *Preventing/treating infection:* Regular swabbing of skin for colonisation/infection is imperative. Signs of infection or a positive skin/blood culture should trigger immediate initiation of antibiotic therapy.
- *Eye care:* Regular examination by an ophthalmologist is essential. 2-hourly application of an ocular lubricant is required along with daily ocular hygiene to remove debris and clear conjunctival adhesions. Consider topical corticosteroid drops (with advice from ophthalmology). In the presence of corneal ulceration apply broad spectrum topical antibiotic. Amniotic membrane transplantation has an important role in the management of SJS/TEN eye disease if there is extensive loss of ocular surface epithelium.

Second line: The use of an active intervention in the early stages of SJS/TEN is controversial. National guidelines vary in the support given for systemic drug treatment, while some experts recommend that management should concentrate purely on intensive supportive care. Although evidence for unambiguous benefit from systemic treatments is currently lacking, there are three treatments which are commonly used in SJS/TEN:

1. Systemic corticosteroid, e.g. prednisolone 0.5–1 mg/kg daily for 7–10 days or IV methylprednisolone 500 mg on 3 consecutive days.
2. Intravenous immunoglobulin 0.5–1 g/kg daily for 3–4 consecutive days.
3. Ciclosporin 3 or 4 mg/kg/day in divided doses for 10 days, and tapered.

Chronic complications of SJS/TEN

Survivors from an acute episode of SJS/TEN may develop delayed sequelae which cause reduced quality of life, morbidity and even increased mortality (Box 66.6).

Box 66.6 Long-term complications of SJS/TEN

Eyes: Corneal and conjunctival ulceration and scarring, dry eye, distichiasis, entropion, trichiasis, ocular surface failure and permanent visual impairment

Skin and nails: Dyspigmentation, eruptive melanocytic naevi, onychomadesis

Pulmonary: Bronchiolitis obliterans

Gastrointestinal: Oesophageal stricture, small intestinal ulcers, vanishing bile duct syndrome

Urogenital: Phimosis, urethral strictures, vaginal and introital adhesions

Psychological: Post-traumatic stress disorder

Acute generalised exanthematous pustulosis

AGEP is a drug eruption characterised by the rapid appearance of erythema and sheets of pustules (toxic pustuloderma).

Epidemiology

Incidence estimated at 1–5 cases/million/year. Mostly adults. Slight female preponderance.

Pathophysiology

Drug-specific CD4+ and CD8+ cells in AGEP produce CXCL8 and IL-8, a neutrophil-attracting chemokine. Mutations in the *IL36RN* gene, which codes for the IL-36 receptor antagonist (IL-36Ra), occur in a subgroup of patients with AGEP. Histopathological features of AGEP are dermal oedema, epidermal spongiosis and intraepidermal or subcorneal neutrophil pustules. 90% of cases of AGEP are drug-induced, the commonest drugs causing AGEP are listed in Box 66.7. 10% of AGEP cases may be triggered by an infection, e.g. *Mycoplasma pneumoniae*, coxsackie virus, parvovirus B19 and cytomegalovirus.

Clinical features

The latent period between initiation of the culprit drug and onset of AGEP is typically 2–5 days. A prodrome of malaise, fever and a burning or itching sensation is common. The eruption usually starts with oedematous erythema in the major flexures (neck, axillae, inframammary and inguinal folds). Sheets of hundreds of sterile non-follicular pustules develop on lesional skin (Figure 66.13). Other signs include atypical

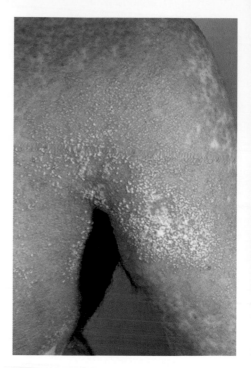

Figure 66.13 Acute generalised exanthematous pustulosis. Sheets of sterile non-follicular pustules on the arm of a patient who developed AGEP 3 days after starting amoxicillin.

targets and purpura. Skin involvement may become extensive and induce the systemic features of erythroderma: fever, heat loss, fluid loss, haemodynamic compromise, secondary infection. Even without erythroderma AGEP may be accompanied by hepatic, renal and pulmonary dysfunction.

Once the culprit drug has been stopped the eruption settles within a few days, resolving with post-pustular desquamation.

Acute localised exanthematous pustulosis is a localised form of AGEP, characterised by pustules confined to a single body area, most commonly the neck.

Differential diagnosis

Generalised pustular psoriasis (both the von Zumbusch and Lapiere variants), subcorneal pustular dermatosis (Sneddon–Wilkinson disease), IgA pemphigus, *Candida* infection, DRESS.

Box 66.7 Commonest drugs causing AGEP

Pristinamycin
Aminopenicillins
Quinolones
Chloroquine and hydroxychloroquine
Sulfonamides
Terbinafine
Diltiazem

Investigations

Skin biopsy.

Laboratory investigations: Blood count (looking for neutrophilia and eosinophilia), biochemical tests (looking for renal and liver dysfunction, and hypocalcaemia), C-reactive protein.

Management

First line: Stop culprit drug. Initiate skin-directed therapy with emollients and topical corticosteroids.

Second line: Systemic corticosteroids (e.g. prednisolone 0.5–1 mg/kg/day). If necessary: intravenous fluid replacement, critical care management and appropriate organ support.

Drug reaction with eosinophilia and systemic symptoms

(Syn. Drug-induced hypersensitivity syndrome)

DRESS is a severe drug hypersensitivity syndrome characterised by a rash and systemic upset consisting of haematological and solid-organ disturbances (e.g. hepatitis, acute kidney injury, pneumonitis, myocarditis).

Epidemiology

Rare. F > M. Mean age of onset is fifth decade.

Pathophysiology

Culprit drug binds directly to the major histocompatibility complex with subsequent presentation to the T-cell receptor provoking a T-cell response. The reaction of DRESS is mediated by drug-specific cytotoxic T-cells. The commonest drugs causing DRESS are listed in Box 66.8. Herpes virus reactivation (HHV6 and 7, Epstein Barr virus [EBV], cytomegalovirus [CMV]) may act synergistically with drug-induced immune responses. In the Han Chinese there is an increased risk of carbamazepine-induced DRESS in subjects carrying the HLA-B*1502 haplotype and allopurinol-induced DRESS with HLA-B*5801. Histopathological features of DRESS are spongiosis, a superficial infiltrate of eosinophils and lymphocytes, basal cell vacuolar change and necrotic keratinocytes.

> **Box 66.8 Commonest drugs causing DRESS**
>
> Allopurinol
> Antiepileptics: carbamazepine, phenytoin, lamotrigine
> Antibiotics: vancomycin, amoxicillin, minocycline, piperacillin-tazobactam
> Sulfa drugs: sulfasalazine, dapsone, sulfadiazine, sulfamethoxazole
> Omeprazole
> Ibuprofen

Clinical features

The latent period between initiation of the culprit drug and onset of DRESS is 2–8 weeks. Non-specific symptoms of the early phase are malaise and fatigue. Typical rashes of DRESS include an urticated papular exanthem (Figure 66.14), a morbilliform eruption, erythroderma (Figure 66.15) and an erythema multiforme-like dermatosis consisting of purpuric macules and atypical targets (Figure 66.16). The latter subtype may be associated with a more severe systemic phenotype. DRESS is usually accompanied by a high fever, facial oedema and widespread lymphadenopathy. The haematological abnormalities are eosinophilia and an atypical lymphocytosis. There is functional derangement of at least one internal organ, typically the liver. Severity of liver involvement varies from a mild hepatitis to fulminant hepatic failure, which is the primary cause of mortality in

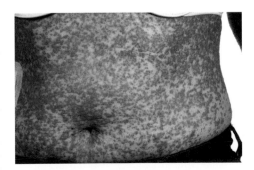

Figure 66.14 Drug reaction with eosinophilia and systemic symptoms. The most common clinical phenotype is a widespread, urticated, papular exanthem, seen here in a patient who developed DRESS to phenytoin.

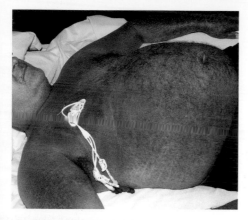

Figure 66.15 Drug reaction with eosinophilia and systemic symptoms. Exfoliative erythroderma seen in a patient with DRESS following allopurinol.

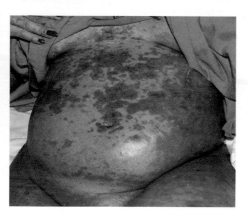

Figure 66.16 Drug reaction with eosinophilia and systemic symptoms. The erythema multiforme-like phenotype in DRESS is often accompanied by more severe liver dysfunction; this patient went on to develop acute liver failure.

DRESS (estimated at 5–10%). Renal involvement (interstitial nephritis), cardiac involvement (pericarditis, myocarditis), lung involvement (pleuritis, pneumonitis) and gastrointestinal involvement (oesophagitis, pancreatitis, colitis) are all recognised. DRESS is an acute illness, but the convalescent phase can be complicated by thyroid dysfunction and diabetes. A minority of patients enter a chronic phase of disease characterised by persistence of the cutaneous features and/or the systemic involvement.

Differential diagnosis

Sepsis caused by viral or bacterial infection, erythroderma (of any cause, including cutaneous T-cell lymphoma), AGEP, angioimmunoblastic T-cell lymphoma.

Investigations

Investigations are needed to substantiate the diagnosis and identify systemic complications. Important tests are listed in Box 66.9.

The international consortium for the study of severe cutaneous adverse reactions, RegiSCAR, has developed a scoring system which quantifies clinical signs and laboratory parameters to produce a value which supports the diagnosis of DRESS (Box 66.10).

Box 66.9 Investigations needed in DRESS

Biopsy of lesional skin for routine histopathology
Full blood count and blood film
Urea and electrolytes
Glucose, amylase
Liver function tests
Creatine kinase
Thyroid function tests
Inflammatory markers (ESR, CRP)
HHV 6&7, EBV, CMV
Chest X-ray
ECG, echocardiogram (if cardiac symptoms)

Box 66.10 RegiSCAR scoring system for DRESS

Lymphadenopathy	+1
Atypical lymphocytosis	+1
Eosinophilia	+1 or +2
Rash >50% BSA	+1
Rash consistent with DRESS	+1
Internal organ involvement	+1 or +2
Investigations excluding other diagnosis	+1
Fever <38.5°C	−1
Biopsy not suggesting DRESS	−1
Complete resolution <15 days	−1

A score of 4 or more indicates a probable or definite case of DRESS.

Management

First line: Stop culprit drug. Apply a highly potent topical steroid ointment to lesional skin. Systemic corticosteroid therapy: either oral prednisolone 0.5–1 mg/kg/day and tapering with response, or IV methylprednisolone 0.5–1 g/day for 3 consecutive days, followed by a tapering course of oral prednisolone

Second line: Consider ciclosporin if refractory to corticosteroid treatment.

DERMATOSES CAUSED BY CHEMOTHERAPEUTIC AGENTS

Chemotherapy agents often cause side effects. The skin is a site of major drug-induced toxicity.

Toxic erythema of chemotherapy

Toxic erythema of chemotherapy (TEC) is the term used to describe a variety of overlapping cutaneous reactions to chemotherapy agents.

Epidemiology

Common. Affects all ages. M = F.

Pathophysiology

TEC is caused by a direct toxicity of the chemotherapeutic agent following excretion through the eccrine duct, the acrosyringium and the epidermis. High density of eccrine glands in palmoplantar skin explains the predilection of TEC at these sites. The commonest drugs causing TEC are listed in Box 66.11. Histopathological features of TEC include hyperplastic eccrine ducts with necrotic duct cells, syringosquamous metaplasia and epidermal dysmaturation.

Box 66.11 Commonest drugs causing toxic erythema of chemotherapy

Cytarabine
Anthracyclines (e.g. doxorubicin)
5-Fluorouracil
Capecitabine
Taxanes (e.g. docetaxel)
Methotrexate

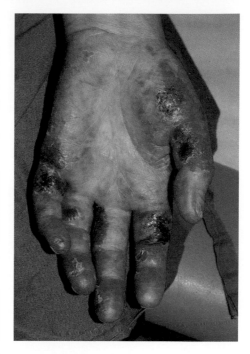

Figure 66.17 Severe palmar toxic erythema of chemotherapy (palmoplantar erythrodysaesthesia) secondary to docetaxol treatment, demonstrating erythema, desquamation, and erosions.

Clinical features

The latent period between initiation of the culprit chemotherapy agent and onset of TEC is 2 days to 3 weeks. Pain, pruritus and tenderness develop on the hands and feet and/or intertriginous areas. Red, oedematous patches, and plaques appear on acral skin and major flexures (Figure 66.17). The erythema may become dusky and blister. The clinical variants of TEC are described in Table 66.4.

Investigations

Usually a clinical diagnosis. Sometimes a skin biopsy is necessary to exclude other diagnoses, such as infective dermatoses.

Management

There is no need to stop the chemotherapy. Treatment is symptomatic. If the reaction is severe, lower chemotherapy dose or lengthen the interval between chemotherapy cycles.

Table 66.4 Clinical variants of toxic erythema of chemotherapy

Disorder	Palmoplantar erythrodysaesthesia	Intertriginous eruption associated with chemotherapy (eccrine squamous syringometaplasia)	Neutrophilic eccrine hidradenitis
Latent period after chemotherapy initiation	1 day to 3 weeks	1 day to 3 weeks	1 day to 3 weeks
Clinical features	Burning sensation precedes acral erythema with oedema. The reaction generally resolves 1–2 weeks after stopping chemotherapy	Dusky patches and plaques in axillary and inguinal folds and antecubital fossae	Red nodules or plaques on extremities, trunk, face and palms. Fever
Differential diagnosis	Palmoplantar psoriasis, acute pompholyx eczema	Intertrigo, flexural psoriasis, flexural seborrheic dermatitis	Erysipelas, Sweet syndrome, leukaemia cutis
Main culprits	Doxorubicin, cytarabine, docetaxel, fluorouracil, capecitabine. Reaction enhanced with combination of docetaxel + capecitabine	Cytarabine, doxorubicin, daunorubicin, gemcitabine	Cytarabine

Papulopustular eruption

Papulopustular eruptions (PPEs) are a side effect of many of the newer targeted agents used in cancer therapy, especially epidermal growth factor receptor (EGFR) inhibitors, tyrosine kinase inhibitors and mitogen-activated protein kinase inhibitors.

Epidemiology

PPE can occur in up to 90% of patients receiving an EGFR inhibitor. All ages are affected.

Pathophysiology

EGFR inhibitors interfere with EGFR-mediated signalling to cause growth arrest and premature differentiation of follicular keratinocytes. This induces a folliculocentric inflammatory response. The commonest drugs causing PPE are listed in Box 66.12. Histopathological features of PPE are a neutrophilic folliculitis and follicular rupture.

Box 66.12 Commonest drug triggers for PPE

EGFR-targeting monoclonal antibodies

Cetuximab (for treating colorectal cancer)
Panitumumab (for treating colorectal cancer)
Cetuximab (for treating head and neck cancers)

Tyrosine kinase inhibitors

Erlotinib (for treating lung and pancreatic cancer)
Gefitinib (for treating lung cancer)
Lapatinib (for treating breast cancer)

Mitogen-activated protein kinase inhibitors

Trametinib (for treating *BRAF* mutated melanoma)
Selumetinib (for treating lung cancer)

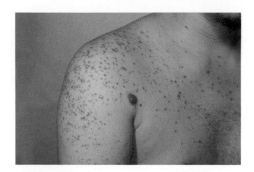

Figure 66.18 Papulopustular eruption, secondary to an EGFR inhibitor.

Clinical features

The latent period between initiation of culprit drug and onset of PPE is 1–2 weeks. Burning pain and pruritus precedes the development of sterile follicular pustules and papules (without comedones) on the scalp, face, chest and back (Figure 66.18). Abdomen, buttocks and extremities can be affected. Patients with fair skin are at particular risk of EGFR inhibitor-induced PPE. Evidence suggests that the presence and severity of PPE correlates with improved tumour response to the targeted agent.

Differential diagnosis

Drug-induced acne, *Malassezia* folliculitis, *Staphylococcus* folliculitis, eosinophilic folliculitis.

Investigations

Usually a clinical diagnosis. Sometimes a skin biopsy is necessary to exclude other diagnoses.

Management

There is no need to stop the targeted agent. Treatment is symptomatic. First-line treatment is 1% hydrocortisone cream and an oral tetracycline antibiotic, either doxycycline or lymecycline. Some patients require oral low-dose isotretinoin.

CHEMOTHERAPY-INDUCED HAIR CHANGES

Alopecia is a frequent side effect of cancer chemotherapy, hypertrichosis occurs less commonly.

Chemotherapy-induced alopecia

Chemotherapy-induced alopecia (CIA) is caused by cytostatic effects on follicular epidermis. It occurs in approximately 65% of all patients receiving cancer chemotherapy. Combination therapy consisting of two or more agents usually produces a greater incidence of more severe CIA compared with single-agent therapy. The drugs that are most commonly associated with CIA are listed in Box 66.13. On discontinuing therapy the alopecia is usually reversible and spontaneously recovers within 1–3 months and is fully recovered by 6 months. The management of CIA consists of careful explanation, psychological support and providing access to wigs. Methods of scalp cooling are thought to limit local drug induced cytotoxicity by reducing skin perfusion through vasoconstriction.

Chemotherapy-induced hypertrichosis

Excessive growth of scalp and body hair can be caused by certain chemotherapeutic agents (Box 66.14). The EGFR inhibitors are the commonest culprits. EGFR is expressed in the

> **Box 66.13 Cancer chemotherapy agents associated with alopecia**
>
> Antimicrotubule agents (e.g. paclitaxel, docetaxel)
> Topoisomerase inhibitors (e.g. etoposide, doxorubicin)
> Alkylators (e.g. cyclophosphamide, ifosfamide)
> Antimetabolites (e.g. 5-fluorouracil)

> **Box 66.14 Cancer chemotherapy agents associated with hypertrichosis**
>
> Interferon α
> Cetuximab
> Erlotinib
> Gefitinib

PART 9: SKIN DISORDERS CAUSED BY EXTERNAL AGENTS

outer root sheath of the hair follicle and functions as an on–off switch guarding entry to, and exit from, the anagen growth phase.

CHEMOTHERAPY-INDUCED NAIL CHANGES

Nail abnormalities are a common side effect of systemic chemotherapy. Damage from cytotoxic agents to the nail matrix epithelium causes defective nail plate production and disordered nail growth. The drugs most commonly implicated in causing nail changes, and the types of nail dystrophy caused, are listed in Box 66.15.

CHEMOTHERAPY-INDUCED PIGMENTATION CHANGES

Cancer chemotherapy agents can cause an increase or decrease in skin pigmentation. Bleomycin-induced flagellate hyperpigmentation, the most striking form of hyperpigmentation, appears to be induced by minor trauma to the skin causing increased blood flow and local accumulation of the drug (Figure 66.19). Chemotherapy-induced hypopigmentation is generally caused by destruction of melanocytes.

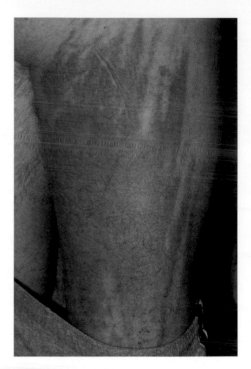

Figure 66.19 Flagellate hyperpigmented dermatosis on a patient's leg induced by bleomycin.

The commonest culprits causing hyperpigmentation are listed in Box 66.16; hypopigmentation culprits are listed in Box 66.17.

Box 66.15 Cancer chemotherapy agents associated with nail dystrophy

Bleomycin (onycholysis, dystrophy)
Cetuximab (onycholysis, paronychia)
Cyclophosphamide (Beau's lines, onycholysis)
Daunorubicin (transverse leuconychia [Mee's lines])
Docetaxol (onycholysis, Beau's lines, pigmentation, onychomadesis)
Doxorubicin (onycholyis, Beau's lines)
Fluorouracil (onycholysis, dystrophy, onychomadesis)
Melphalan (transverse leuconychia [Mee's lines])
Paclitaxel (onycholysis, Beau's lines, pigmentation, onychomadesis)
Sorafenib, sunitinib (subungual haemorrhage)

Box 66.16 Cancer chemotherapy agents associated with hyperpigmentation

Bleomycin
Busulfan
Capecitabine
Cyclophosphamide
Daunorubicin
Doxorubicin
5-Fluorouracil
Hydroxyurea
Methotrexate
Vinorelbine

Source: Data from Alley E, Green R, Schuchter L. Cutaneous toxicities of cancer therapy. *Curr Opin Oncol* 2002, 14, 212–216.

> **Box 66.17 Cancer chemotherapy agents associated with hypopigmentation**
>
> Doxorubicin
> Imatinib
> Dasatinib
> Gefitinib
> Vemurafenib
> Imiquimod
> Interferon α
> Interferon β
> Interleukin 2
> Interleukin 4
> Mitoxantrone

> **Box 66.18 Chemotherapy agents associated with phototoxicity**
>
> 5-Fluorouracil
> Methotrexate
> Dacarbazine
> Dactinomycin
> Hydroxyurea
> Thioguanine
> Mitomycin C
> Vinblastine
> Doxorubicin
> Vemurafenib

CHEMOTHERAPY-INDUCED PHOTOSENSITIVITY

Chemotherapy-induced photosensitivity reactions are mostly phototoxic and less commonly photoallergic. UV recall reactions are an unusual but striking side effect of chemotherapy.

Phototoxic reactions

See Chapter 68.

Phototoxic reactions are due to the damaging effects of photoactivated chemicals on cell membranes and DNA. A phototoxic reaction is characterised by a burning sensation occurring within 12–24 h of culprit drug exposure in light-exposed sites over the face, neck, anterior 'V' of the chest and forearms. It can present with painful, well-demarcated erythema and oedema progressing to blistering and desquamation. The reaction resolves with hyperpigmentation over several months. Chemotherapeutic agents associated with phototoxicity are listed in Box 66.18.

Recall reaction

Recall reaction is characterised by a drug-induced inflammatory eruption confined to an area of skin that has previously been irradiated or sunburnt. The recall reaction is initiated by a culprit medication given within 2 months of expo-

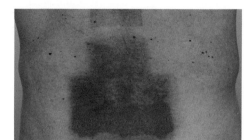

Figure 66.20 Radiation recall reaction secondary to vemurafenib confined to the previous irradiated site.

sure to radiation and is characterised by erythema and oedema confined to the field of irradiation (Figure 66.20). Anticancer agents, in particular cytotoxics, are the most common causes (Box 66.19), but other drugs such as antibiotics have been implicated.

> **Box 66.19 Chemotherapy agents associated with recall reactions**
>
> Gemcitabine
> Methotrexate
> Docetaxel
> Paclitaxel
> Hydroxyurea
> Etoposide
> Doxorubicin
> Capecitabine
> Tamoxifen
> Vemurafenib
>
> Source: Data from Choi JN. Chemotherapy induced iatrogenic injury of skin: new drugs and new concepts. *Clin Dermatol* 2011, 29, 587–601.

DERMATOSES CAUSED BY RADIOTHERAPY

In radiotherapy high-energy ionising radiation, usually X-rays, is used to kill cancer cells. Radiotherapy is associated with acute and chronic cutaneous side effects.

Acute radiation dermatitis

Acute radiation dermatitis occurs within 90 days of exposure to radiation. Radiation-induced keratinocyte damage induces DNA injury repair via activation of the p53 pathway and a simultaneous release of inflammatory cytokines. It is confined to areas of skin that have been irradiated, and the skin changes are usually sharply demarcated. As the cumulative dose of radiation increases, the transient erythema occurring during the first weeks of radiotherapy may evolve into persistent erythema and oedema. Further progression to desquamation and, in severe cases, skin necrosis and ulceration can also occur. Mucositis can develop if mucosal surfaces are included within the treatment zone.

Chronic radiation dermatitis

The onset of chronic radiation dermatitis may occur from 15 days to 10+ years after the beginning of radiation therapy. It is an extension of the acute process and involves further inflammatory changes in the skin. There is an increase in collagen and damage to elastic fibres which results in loss of follicular structures and destruction of the sweat and sebaceous glands. The skin appears hypopigmented, telangiectatic and atrophic. Ultimately lesional skin may become necrotic and ulcerate (Figure 66.21).

Post-irradiation morphoea is a potential complication after radiotherapy, particularly radiotherapy for breast cancer. It can occur months to years after treatment, and is associated with considerable morbidity and pain, as well as being cosmetically disfiguring (Figure 66.22).

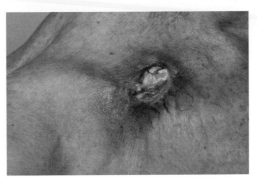

Figure 66.21 Radionecrosis causing ulceration over the clavicle occurring 20 years after radiotherapy treatment.

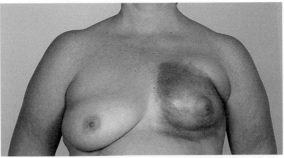

Figure 66.22 Morphoea affecting the left breast confined to the radiotherapy zone for breast cancer treatment.

Dermatoses caused by cold and heat

67

DERMATOSES CAUSED BY COLD

Cold-induced diseases can be divided into two groups: diseases of cold exposure and diseases of abnormal susceptibility to cold (Box 67.1).

Frostbite

Frostbite describes skin damage caused by freezing. Frostnip is a milder form of cutaneous cold damage.

Epidemiology

Frostbite occurs in individuals stranded in cold weather: skiers, climbers and homeless people.

Box 67.1 Dermatoses caused by cold

DISEASES OF COLD EXPOSURE

Frostbite
Trench foot

Diseases of abnormal susceptibility to cold

Raynaud phenomenon
Livedo reticularis
Cryoglobulinaemia
Cold agglutinins
Cold haemolysis
Cold urticaria
Perniosis
Acrocyanosis
Erythrocyanosis
Cold erythema
Cold panniculitis
Neonatal cold injury

Pathophysiology

Fast freezing produces intracellular ice, slow freezing causes extracellular ice. Slow rewarming causes the formation of larger, more destructive ice crystals. Reflex vasoconstriction in exposed extremities compounds tissue damage.

Clinical features

In frostnip there is painful erythema which reverses with rewarming. In superficial frostbite there is painful erythema, then a sense of warmth and finally white and waxy lesional skin. Deep frostbite extends to subcutis and involves nerves, major vessels, muscle and bone. Blistering, full-thickness skin necrosis and gangrene can be seen in severe cases. Damage to nerves and blood vessels causes parasthesiae, abnormal cold sensitivity and hyperhidrosis.

Investigations

A clinical diagnosis. Magnetic resonance angiography can help identify vascular occlusion and soft tissue injury.

Management

First line: Rapid rewarming by immersion in water at 37–39°C is recommended. NSAIDs, such as ibuprofen, may reduce vasoconstriction and reduce the pain of rewarming.
Second line: Intravenous infusion of vasodilatory prostaglandins (e.g. iloprost, a prostacyclin analogue). Intra-arterial infusion of tissue plasminogen activator may reduce need for digital amputation. Aspirin may also help.

Third line: Surgical removal of gangrenous tissue should be delayed until there is a distinct demarcation between viable and non-viable tissue, a process that usually takes several weeks.

Perniosis

(Syn. Chilblains)
An abnormal reaction to cold characterised by localised inflammation on acral skin.

Epidemiology
Occurs in susceptible individuals in climates which are both cold and damp. F:M 4:1

Pathophysiology
Aetiological factors include poor nutrition, anorexia nervosa and systemic diseases, most typically lupus erythematosus and haematological malignancies (especially acute myeloid leukaemia). Perniosis occurring on fingers and toes is a complication of Covid-19 infection ('Covid toes'). There is cold-induced vasoconstriction of the deep cutaneous arterioles with concomitant dilatation of the smaller, superficial vessels. Histopathology demonstrates perivascular inflammation and dermal oedema.

Clinical features
Perniosis affects areas of the skin vulnerable to cold exposure, such as the digits, nose and ears. Lesions are symmetrical, red-purple and can be macular, papular, nodular or plaque-like. Pruritus and burning pain are common. In severe cases blistering and ulceration may occur. Some lesions may be asymptomatic. Each lesion tends to undergo spontaneous resolution after 2–3 weeks.

Differential diagnosis
Granuloma annulare, peripheral arterial disease, vasculitis.

Investigations
Perniosis is a clinical diagnosis. Investigate any potential underlying disorder, such as lupus erythematosus and, if suspected, haematological malignancy.

Management
Warm clothing and central heating are preventative. Potent steroid ointment can help symptoms.

Acrocyanosis

A persistent cyanotic or erythrocyanotic mottled discoloration of acral skin.

Epidemiology
Occurs typically in adolescents. F > M.

Pathophysiology
There is vasospasm of peripheral arterioles, aggravated by cold, and dilatation of the subpapillary venous plexus. Acrocyanosis may be idiopathic or secondary to a number of systemic disorders (Box 67.2).

Clinical features
There is a painless mottled duskiness of the hands, feet and, sometimes, the face. The changes may be transient after cold exposure but usually persist during the winter and summer. Idiopathic acrocyanosis usually starts in adolescence and persists into adult life.

Differential diagnosis
Raynaud phenomenon.

Investigations
Acrocyanosis is a clinical diagnosis.

Management
There is no effective medical treatment for acrocyanosis, but an underlying condition often needs to be managed.

Box 67.2 Aetiology of acrocyanosis

- Idiopathic
- Secondary
  - Antiphospolipid antibody syndrome
  - Paraproteinaemias
  - Essential thrombocythaemia
  - Cold agglutinin disease
  - Cryoglobulinaemia
  - Anorexia nervosa
  - Postural orthostatic tachycardia syndrome
  - Brachial plexus neuropathy
  - Severe learning difficulties

Erythrocyanosis

A persistent, dusky erythema occurring on the thighs and lower legs.

Epidemiology
Most common in adolescent girls and middle-aged women.

Pathophysiology
Occurs at sites with a thick layer of subcutaneous fat, such as the thighs and lower legs. The subcutaneous fat insulates superficial vessels from the warmth of underlying vasculature rendering them susceptible to cold exposure.

Clinical features
Typically seen on the lower legs of adolescent girls, the thighs and buttocks of overweight boys and the thighs and lower legs of middle-aged women. It is characterised by dusky discoloration of the skin and may be accompanied by keratosis pilaris, angiokeratomas and telangiectases. It is exacerbated by cold and therefore usually more prominent during the winter. Oedema and fibrosis may be seen as chronic manifestations of erythrocyanosis.

Investigations
None are required.

Management
Warm clothing, exercise, weight reduction and elastic support hosiery may be helpful.

Livedo reticularis

A mottled, cyanotic discoloration of the skin with a characteristic network pattern.

Pathophysiology
The blood supply of the skin is arranged in cones, the bases of which measure 1–4 cm in diameter and lie on the skin's surface. Each cone is supplied by an arteriole, which passes through the dermis perpendicular to the surface. When blood flow through the feeding arterioles is diminished, deoxygenated blood at the anastamotic junctions produces a cyanotic

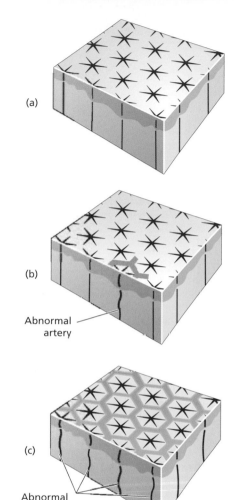

(a)

(b)

Abnormal artery

(c)

Abnormal arteries

Figure 67.1 (a) Normal vasculature. (b) Livedo racemosa due to patchy arterial pathology. (c) Livedo reticularis due to diffuse arterial pathology.

network pattern on the skin, which is livedo reticularis (Figure 67.1). Livedo reticularis may be physiological, idiopathic or secondary to intravascular obstruction or vessel wall disease (Box 67.3).

Clinical features
Livedo reticularis usually affects the legs but the arms and trunk may also be affected. Cold exacerbates the cyanotic discoloration. In the lower

---

Box 67.3 Classification of livedo reticularis

Physiological livedo reticularis
   Cutis marmorata
Idiopathic or primary livedo reticularis
   Congenital:
      Cutis marmorata telangiectatica congenita
   Acquired idiopathic:
      Uncomplicated
      With winter ulceration
      With summer ulceration
      With systemic vascular involvement
Secondary livedo reticularis
   Intravascular obstruction:
      Stasis:
         Paralysis
         Cardiac failure
      Occlusive disease:
         Emboli
         Oxalosis (primary hyperoxaluria)
      Thrombocythaemia
      Cryoglobulins
      Cold agglutinins
   Vessel wall disease:
      Arteriosclerosis
      Arteritis:
         Polyarteritis nodosa
         Systemic lupus erythematosus
         Antiphospholipid syndrome
         Rheumatoid arthritis
         Dermatomyositis
         Lymphoma
      Infections:
         Tuberculosis
         Syphilis
         Hepatitis C
Metabolic disease
   Hyperparathyroidism and hypercalcaemia
   Calcific uraemic arteriolopathy

---

limbs leg elevation decreases the appearances of livedo reticularis. Clinically there is a lattice or tracery of thin dusky lines forming a network. It is best appreciated over the shins and on the medial aspects of the knees.

Acquired idiopathic livedo reticularis occurs predominantly in adult women; mild degrees are harmless but severe cases are associated with ulceration, usually in the winter.

Cutis marmorata is a physiological livedo occurring in infants as a response to cold. *Cutis marmorata telangiectatica congenita* is a rare, congenital livedo characterised by a red-purple vascular network which is enhanced by cold and crying.

Livedo racemosa is a livedo in which the network is incomplete; also referred to as a broken livedo. It occurs in cutaneous polyarteritis nodosa.

Differential diagnosis

Erythema ab igne.

Investigations

Laboratory studies should be directed by an underlying disorder (see Box 67.3).

Management

Treatment is directed to the underlying condition, if one is identified.

Raynaud phenomenon

The Raynaud phenomenon (RP) is an episodic digital ischaemia occurring in response to cold or emotional stimuli.

Epidemiology

Primary RP affects 5–20% of women and 3–10% of men. F:M 5:1. Age of onset <40 years.

Pathophysiology

In primary RP the vascular changes are functional resulting in vasoconstriction. In secondary RP (e.g. systemic sclerosis) structural vascular changes include intimal hyperplasia with intravascular thrombi. Primary RP (also called Raynaud disease) is idiopathic and occurs as an isolated innocuous disorder; secondary RP occurs in association with underlying diseases or is caused by physical factors or drugs (Box 67.4).

Clinical features

RP affects the hands and, less often, the feet. It is characterised by sequential colour changes: white (pallor), blue (cyanosis) and red (erythema). A typical attack consists of sudden pallor of one or more digits, followed, after a few

Box 67.4 Causes of Raynaud phenomenon

- Primary Raynaud phenomenon (Raynaud disease)
- Secondary Raynaud phenomenon
  - Trauma or vibration:
    - Reflex sympathetic dystrophy
    - Vibration exposure
    - Arteriovenous fistula
    - Hypothenar hammer syndrome (ulnar artery thrombosis)
    - Intra-arterial drug administration
  - Connective tissue disease and vasculitis:
    - Systemic sclerosis
    - Systemic lupus erythematosus
    - Rheumatoid arthritis
    - Sjögren syndrome
    - Mixed connective tissue disease
    - Dermatomyositis
    - Temporal arteritis
    - Hepatitis B antigen vasculitis
  - Obstructive arterial disease:
    - Atherosclerosis
    - Thromboangiitis obliterans (Buerger disease)
  - Neurological disease:
    - Thoracic outlet syndrome (cervical rib)
    - Carpal tunnel syndrome
  - Haematological disease:
    - Cryoglobulinaemia
    - Cold agglutinins
    - Paroxysmal haemoglobinuria
    - Waldenström macroglobulinaemia
  - Drugs and toxins:
    - Ergot
    - β-blockers
    - Methysergide
    - Bleomycin
    - Amphetamines
    - Bromocriptine
    - Clonidine
    - Ciclosporin
    - Oral contraceptives
  - Miscellaneous:
    - Paraneoplastic syndrome
    - Chronic renal failure
    - Primary pulmonary hypertension
    - Hypothyroidism
    - Anorexia nervosa

minutes, by cyanosis or sometimes by erythema. In primary RP the condition is usually symmetrical and involves several digits; in secondary RP one or a few digits are affected and asymmetry is not unusual. Attacks are usually precipitated by cold or psychological stimuli. In recalcitrant RP attacks of long duration may occur in which the initial pallor is short lived and succeeded by prolonged cyanosis.

Investigations

Investigations are directed towards detecting an underlying cause (Box 67.4).

Management

First line: Keep the hands and feet warm and reduce cold exposure, calcium-channel antagonists (e.g. nifedipine). Long-acting preparations improve compliance and reduce side effects.

Second line: Phosphodiesterase inhibitor (e.g. sildenafil).

Third line: Intravenous infusion of vasodilatory prostaglandins (e.g. iloprost, a prostacyclin analogue), endothelin receptor antagonist (e.g. bosentan), angiotensin II receptor antagonist (e.g. losartan).

Cryoglobulinaemia

See Chapter 54.

In cryoglobulinaemia immunoglobulin complexes precipitate in the small vessels of the skin when cooled below body temperature to produce a variety of signs, including purpura on the lower legs, livedo reticularis, Raynaud phenomenon, atypical ulceration of the legs, digital skin necrosis and cold urticaria.

Cold agglutinins

Cold agglutinin disease is a disorder of autoimmune haemolysis in which cold-sensitive immunoglobulins react against erythrocyte surface antigens. Primary cold agglutinin disease is associated with monoclonal CD20+ κ+ B-lymphocyte population or lymphoplasmacytic lymphoma. Cases may be secondary to *Mycoplasma* and Epstein–Barr virus infections. Cutaneous features include Raynaud phenomenon, acrocyanosis and skin necrosis.

Cryofibrinogenemia

Cryofibrinogenemia is a fibrinogen disorder in which the cooling of an individual's blood plasma to 4°C causes the reversible precipitation of a complex containing fibrinogen and fibrin. Returning the plasma to 37°C resolubilises the precipitate. Clinically the condition is characterised by pathological blood clots in small and medium size arteries and veins. Secondary cryofibrinogenemia occurs in association with another disorder, including infections, lymphoproliferative disorders, myeloproliferative disorders, vasculitis and connective tissue disease. Primary cryofibrinogenemia occurs in the absence of a systemic association.

DERMATOSES CAUSED BY HEAT

Erythema ab igne

A pigmented reticulated dermatosis induced by heat damage.

Pathophysiology

Skin changes result from repeated or prolonged exposure to infrared (IR) radiation, insufficient to produce a burn. Following a single exposure to subthreshold IR radiation, a mild and transient reticular erythema occurs. Repeated exposure causes epidermal atrophy, dermal pigmentation and vasodilatation. Eventually there is keratinocyte atypia and connective tissue degeneration.

Clinical features

Occurs in people who sit close to heaters or habitually use hot water bottles, laptop computers or heated pads. Any surface of the body is susceptible, but it is seen most commonly on the shins. Initially there is reticular pigmentation. Occasionally blisters may be seen (Figure 67.2). With persistent heat trauma poikiloderma and diffuse hyperkeratosis occurs. In severe cases there is confluent pigmentation. There is an increased risk of keratinocyte cancer in affected skin.

Investigations

The diagnosis is made clinically.

Management

Remove the heat source from the skin.

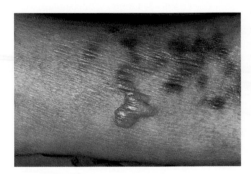

Figure 67.2 Erythema ab igne with subepidermal bulla formation.

Photodermatoses

68

Cutaneous erythema is a normal response following exposure to sunlight [or other ultraviolet radiation (UVR) source] and is termed photosensitivity. Abnormal photosensitivity reactions are called the photodermatoses: idiopathic (immunological) photodermatoses are the commonest; genophotodermatoses are rare (see Chapters 37). Chemical photosensitivity may be caused by an excess of endogenous photoactive chemicals, as in porphyria (see Chapter 39), or by photosensitisation due to a drug.

Patients sometimes undergo specialised tests for the investigation of a suspected photodermatosis: in monochromator phototesting the patient's skin is irradiated with single wavelengths of light, while solar simulator phototesting uses a broad range of wavelengths to mimic sunlight. Both types of test investigate the response of a patient's skin to UVR.

Polymorphic light eruption

(Syn. Polymorphous light eruption)
Polymorphic light eruption (PLE) is a recurrent, delayed-onset, abnormal reaction to sunlight (or artificial UVR source) that resolves without scarring. There are several morphological variants, hence the term 'polymorphic'.

Epidemiology

In Northern Europe and North America the point prevalence is 10–20%. PLE occurs with a lower prevalence in countries near the equator. F > M. It usually starts before 30 years.

Pathophysiology

PLE is believed to be a delayed-type hypersensitivity response to UV-induced allergens (photoallergen). This is supported by (i) the nature of the lymphocytic infiltrate, which comprises T-helper cells early on and T-suppressor cells at 72 h, and (ii) the pattern of adhesion molecule expression, which also resembles that of contact dermatitis. There is disease concordance in 15% of monozygotic twin pairs compared with 5% of dizygotic twin pairs.

Clinical features

A period of sunlight exposure lasting between 10 min and several hours produces, after a delay, an exposed site eruption that is usually intensely itchy. Papules and vesicles are most frequent (Figure 68.1a); other morphologies include plaques, purpura and erythema multiforme-like variants (Figure 68.1b,c). Some patients describe a 'priming phenomenon': the need for 2 or 3 days of initial exposure before PLE occurs. The rash occurs at least 6 h after sun exposure, often noted in the evening after a day in the sun. With subsequent sunlight avoidance, the eruption usually resolves within a few days.

PLE affects sunlight-exposed sites but UV transmission through clothing can provoke the eruption. Sparing of the face and of the dorsal hands is quite common, and is due to tolerance from repeated, perennial UVR exposure. Facial involvement is more commonly seen in children with PLE. There is a tendency for PLE to be less troublesome towards the end of summer; 'hardening' seems to occur with repeated sunlight exposure during the summer months. For many patients marked improvement of PLE occurs over several years.

Rook's Dermatology Handbook, First Edition. Edited by Christopher E. M. Griffiths, Tanya O. Bleiker, Daniel Creamer, John R. Ingram and Rosalind C. Simpson.
© 2022 John Wiley & Sons Ltd. Published 2022 by John Wiley & Sons Ltd.

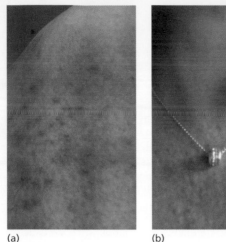

(a)

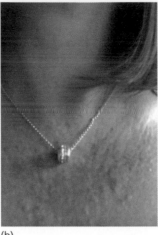

(b)

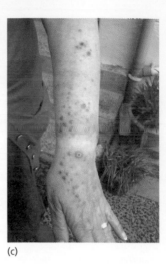

(c)

Figure 68.1 PLE subtypes: (a) papulo-vesicules, (b) urticated papules merging to form a plaque and (c) erythema multiforme-like lesions (note sparing under the watch strap).

Juvenile springtime eruption is a form of PLE in which recurrent papulo-vesicules develop on the upper pinnae of boys following sunlight exposure during spring (Figure 68.2). Male preponderance may be explained by differences in hairstyles: the ears of boys are more often uncovered.

Differential diagnosis

Solar urticaria, drug and chemical-induced photosensitivity, subacute cutaneous lupus erythematosus.

Investigations

In almost all cases the diagnosis is made from the history. Sometimes the patient will produce a photograph of the eruption. If there are atypical features antinuclear antibody (ANA), anti-Ro and anti-La should be performed to exclude lupus erythematosus.

Monochromator phototesting is sometimes undertaken: one-third of patients have a moderately reduced minimal erythema dose (MED) threshold to UVA and/or UVB. PLE can occasionally be provoked by the solar simulator.

Management

First line: Photoprotection measures: patients should avoid sun in the middle of the day (from 11am to 3pm) and wear appropriate clothing (tightly woven fabrics, hat and sunglasses);

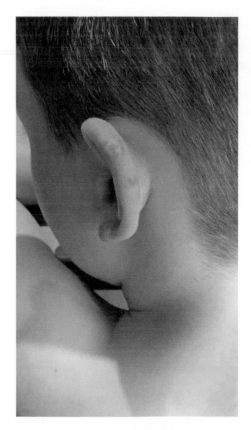

Figure 68.2 Juvenile springtime eruption: papules on the upper pinna of a boy following sunlight exposure during spring.

broad-spectrum high SPF sunscreens should be used and applied correctly (thickly, evenly and frequently). Potent topical corticosteroid is helpful to reduce the inflammation and itching.

Second line: Phototherapy courses of prophylactic narrow-band UVB or psoralen and UVA (PUVA) can be given in the spring to 'harden' the skin. Prednisolone tablets taken at the first onset of PLE in patients affected by holiday-type exposure shortens the duration of the eruption.

Actinic prurigo

Actinic prurigo (AP) is an itchy photodermatosis that is present perennially but tends to worsen during the summer.

Epidemiology
AP is rare in Europe but is common amongst some populations in the Americas. It most commonly starts in childhood. F > M.

Pathophysiology
The action spectrum for abnormal photosensitivity is usually in the UVB and UVA wavelengths (rarely UVA only). AP may represent a persistent form of PLE in genetically susceptible individuals. The majority of AP patients have the HLA-DR4 tissue type, which is common in most populations; more than two-thirds of AP patients express the DRB1*0407 subtype.

Clinical features
AP is usually perennial but most patients are aware of flares related to sunlight exposure. The face, especially the nose, the neck and the chest, are typically affected (Figure 68.3). The distal limbs are also commonly involved. Lesions may also occur on covered skin, such as the buttocks. The eruption is very itchy, and starts with pink papules and vesicles, or small nodules and plaques. The lesions become excoriated, crusted, scabbed and, not infrequently, eczematised and scarred. Cheilitis and conjunctivitis may occur. The condition usually improves by teenage years or early adulthood, but persistence of disease into adult life can also occur.

Differential diagnosis
PLE, atopic prurigo, drug and chemical-induced photosensitivity, discoid lupus erythematosus, subacute cutaneous lupus erythematosus, chronic actinic dermatitis (typically affects older people).

Investigations
Diagnosis is based largely on history and clinical findings. Monochromator phototesting shows severe abnormal photosensitivity in most cases. UVA provocation testing can usually provoke an abnormal papular response. Absence of HLA-DR4 makes AP unlikely, whereas presence of the DRB1*0407 subtype supports the diagnosis of AP.

Management
First line: Photoprotection measures: see PLE. Potent topical corticosteroid is helpful to reduce the inflammation and itching.

Second line: Phototherapy courses of prophylactic narrow-band UVB or PUVA given in the spring serve to 'harden' the skin. Application of a potent topical steroid to the treated areas immediately after each exposure to phototherapy reduces the risk of iatrogenic disease flares.

Third line: Thalidomide may be effective, but its use is restricted by teratogenicity and the risk of irreversible peripheral neuropathy.

Chronic actinic dermatitis

(Syn. **Photosensitivity dermatitis/actinic reticuloid**)
Chronic actinic dermatitis (CAD) is a persistent or recurring dermatitis predominantly affecting photo-exposed sites. CAD is associated with contact and/or photocontact allergy in most patients.

Epidemiology
CAD occurs worldwide, although it is commoner in temperate climates. M > F. It typically occurs in elderly males (mean age at diagnosis is 60 years), although onset in younger life is reported in association with atopic eczema. Patients of skin phototypes IV to VI are over-represented. An association with HIV is reported.

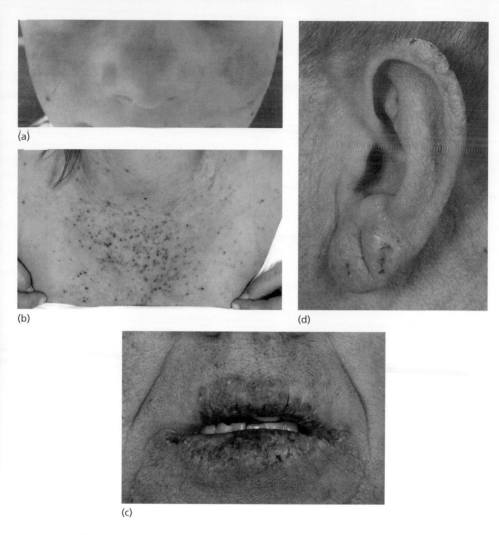

Figure 68.3 Papules and plaques of AP on (a) the cheeks and nose, (b) the chest, (c) AP cheilitis and (d) chronic lesions on the pinna.

Pathophysiology

The most plausible hypothesis is a delayed, cell-mediated hypersensitivity reaction to unknown endogenous photo-induced antigen(s), similar to the mechanisms in allergic contact dermatitis.

Clinical features

Acutely CAD is characterised by an erythematous, exudative, vesicular dermatitis on photo-exposed sites. In chronic disease there is lichenification and sometimes pseudo-lymphomatous infiltrated plaques (actinic reticuloid). Examination reveals prominent and confluent involvement of photo-exposed sites of the head, neck and limbs with a sharp cut-off at the collar and sleeves (Figure 68.4). Alopecia, ectropion and hyper-/hypopigmentation can occur, while in patients of skin phototypes IV to VI there can be a nodular prurigo-like morphology. Some patients are not aware of the association with sunlight exposure.

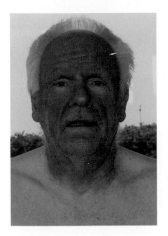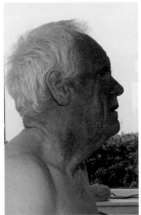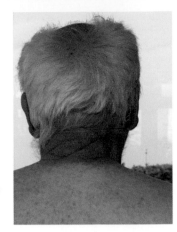

Figure 68.4 CAD with confluent involvement of the face and neck, and demonstrating a sharp cut-off at the collar.

CAD usually develops in the presence of a pre-existing dermatitis: 80% of patients have a preceding history of allergic contact dermatitis, seborrhoeic eczema or endogenous hand eczema.

Differential diagnosis

Allergic contact dermatitis, AP, drug and chemical-induced photosensitivity, photoaggravated atopic and seborrhoeic eczema.

Investigations

Abnormal erythemal responses will be apparent 24 h after phototesting and will become dermatitic. Most patients with CAD will have predominantly UVB sensitivity, although many will also have UVA and visible wavelengths involved. Solar simulator phototesting will induce eczema. Positive patch and/or photo-patch tests are seen in the majority of CAD patients: allergens are often multiple and include fragrances, rubber, nickel, colophony, medicaments, sunscreens and plants, notably to Asteracea (Compositae), lichens and oleoresins.

Management

First line: Photoprotection measures: see PLE. Advice on UVR avoidance may also include the use of UV-excluding window film. For patients who are abnormally sensitive to visible light, the addition of a large-particle, pigmentary-grade,

reflectant sunscreen can provide additional protection. Allergens and photoallergens must be identified and avoided indefinitely. Patients should also be aware of the need to optimise dietary vitamin D intake and if necessary to take supplements.

Treatment of established disease involves the use of potent or super-potent topical corticosteroids. Topical tacrolimus or pimecrolimus can be effective.

Second line: Systemic glucocorticoids may be used in acute flares. Azathioprine, ciclosporin or mycophenolate mofetil can be used as a steroid-sparing agent.

Solar urticaria

Solar urticaria (SU) can be primary (idiopathic) or secondary to drugs, chemicals, porphyria or lupus erythematosus. It is characterised by the immediate development of urticaria following exposure to sunlight.

Epidemiology

Idiopathic SU is uncommon. It can occur at any age, with a peak incidence between the third and fifth decades. It is slightly more common in females.

Pathophysiology

Idiopathic SU is an immunological photo-dermatosis based on a type 1 immediate hypersensitivity reaction to poorly defined photo-induced antigen(s). The proposed pathway is a photochemical alteration of an endogenous chromophore by UVR and/or visible light, resulting in antigen. This is then recognised by specific IgE on mast cells with subsequent mast cell degranulation and histamine release, causing increased vascular permeability and dermal oedema. It is usually cause by wavelengths in the UVA and visible range.

Clinical features

Onset is usually sudden and clearly recalled. Most patients have perennial symptoms due to UVA and/or visible light photosensitivity. The rash can be triggered by light transmitted through window glass. Itch, burning, erythema, and weals occur within seconds to minutes of exposure. Any photo-exposed site can be affected (Figure 68.5), along with lightly clothed sites since loose-weave fabric will not protect against UVA and visible light transmission. If assessed during an acute episode, erythema and urticaria will be evident on involved skin. In most patients urticarial lesions resolve within 2 h. If large areas are involved, systemic symptoms of malaise, headache, wheeze, nausea, dizziness and rarely hypotension and anaphylaxis may occur. For most affected individuals idiopathic SU is a chronic disease.

Differential diagnosis

PLE, cold urticaria (and other physical urticarias), drug and chemical-induced photosensitivity, porphyria (especially erythropoietic protoporphyria).

Investigations

Monochromator phototesting is the investigation of choice: erythema, oedema, weal and flare will occur within minutes at phototest sites (Figure 68.6) and will resolve over an hour or so, often with associated delayed abnormal erythema at 24 h. The immediate minimal urticarial dose and the MED at 24 h should be ascertained at each waveband. Most patients have a fairly broad action spectrum for immediate photosensitivity, with the longer UVA and shorter visible wavelengths being most commonly involved. Secondary causes of SU are uncommon but must be considered: a detailed

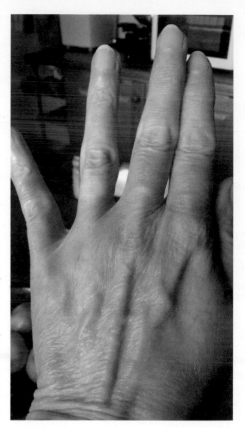

Figure 68.5 Solar urticaria. (a) Acute erythema on the back of the hand after 2 min of wintertime daylight exposure. Note sparing of the distal phalanges and under the wedding ring.

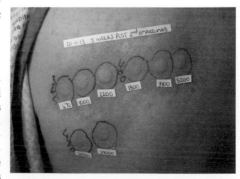

Figure 68.6 Abnormal immediate photosensitivity to UVA (365 nm) and visible (400 and 430 nm) wavelengths in a patient with solar urticaria. Note the erythema, oedema, weal and flare, which developed within 5 min of phototesting.

PART 9: SKIN DISORDERS CAUSED BY EXTERNAL AGENTS

drug history is important, exclude porphyria and lupus erythematosus.

Management

First line: Photoprotection measures: see PLE. Non-sedating H_1 antihistamines: one-third of patients respond completely, one-third respond partially, one-third have no response. Antihistamines are most effective at reducing weal and flare, but not erythema. The addition of an H_2 antagonist may provide additional benefit. Doxepin, ketotifen, chromoglycate and montelukast may also be beneficial in individual patients.

Second line: It may be possible to undertake desensitisation using natural or artificial light, determined by the wavelength dependency and severity of photosensitivity. Desensitisation should only be delivered in a centre with specialist phototherapy expertise.

Third line: Ciclosporin, systemic glucocorticoids, intravenous immunoglobulins and other immunomodulators may be considered. Omalizumab has been shown to be effective.

Hydroa vacciniforme

(Syn. Hydroa aestivale)

Hydroa vacciniforme (HV) is a rare photodermatosis of children and has a characteristic clinical presentation of vesicles, crusts and varioliform scars.

Epidemiology

HV typically occurs in children. There is a bimodal age distribution with onset either between 1 and 7 years, or 12 to 16 years.

Pathophysiology

UVA wavelengths are implicated in the provocation of lesions. A role for Epstein–Barr virus infection has been proposed since the virus has been found in the dermal inflammatory infiltrate of HV patients.

Clinical features

Patients typically present with seasonal symptoms in spring/summer. The commonest sites affected are the cheeks, nose, ears and back of hands (Figure 68.7). Following light exposure

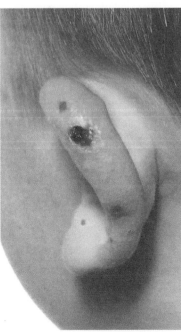

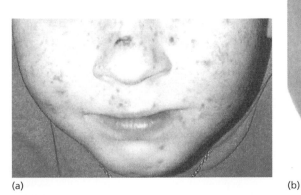

(a)   (b)

Figure 68.7 Hydroa vacciniforme. (a) Papules, vesiculation and haemorrhagic crusting on the cheeks. (b) Papules on the ears.

(from 15 min to a few hours) intensely pruritic crops of papules and vesicles develop on uncovered sites on a background of erythema and oedema. A burning sensation may occur. Haemorrhagic crusts develop as the vesicles resolve. When the crusts detach, varioliform scars remain. There may be systemic malaise and fever during acute episodes. Cartilage destruction of the ears and nose can occur. The eyes can also be affected, with photophobia, conjunctivitis and keratitis. Anterior uveitis may occur acutely and corneal scarring chronically. Usually the condition improves and resolves in later teenage years.

Differential diagnosis

Juvenile spring eruption, PLE, AP, porphyria, atopic eczema.

Investigations

Monochromator phototesting may show predominantly UVA sensitivity. Repeated UVA provocation will usually induce lesions.

Management

First line: Photoprotection measures: see PLE.

Second line: Springtime desensitisation with narrow-band UVB phototherapy can be helpful.

Drug and chemical-induced photosensitivity

(Inc. Phototoxicity, photoallergy)

Drug and chemical-induced photosensitivity is an abnormal cutaneous reaction to UVR and visible radiation induced by photosensitising drugs or chemicals. The reactions are subdivided according to whether the drug/chemical is administered systemically or topically.

Epidemiology

Older patients, whose polypharmacy often includes photoactive drugs, are more at risk of developing drug-induced photosensitivity.

Pathophysiology

Idiosyncratic factors exist which means that not all those exposed to photoactive drugs become photosensitive. Box 68.1 lists the most common culprits in the UK and Europe. Most systemic

and topical drug photosensitivity is phototoxic. Other less common mechanisms include pseudoporphyria, drug-induced lupus, lichenoid reactions and photoallergy. Photoallergy is most frequently seen with topical sunscreens, non-steroidal anti-inflammatory drugs and, less commonly, certain fragrances.

Box 68.1 Exogenous photosenitisers

Systemic

Antibiotics: fluoroquinolones, tetracyclines, sulphonamides
Antifungals: voriconazole, itraconazole, ketoconazole
Antihepatitis C drugs
Antipsychotics: phenothiazines (chlorpromazine)
Azathioprine
BRAF inhibitors
Cardiology: amiodarone, calcium antagonists, angiotensin converting enzyme inhibitors, statins
Celecoxib
Diuretics: thiazides, furosemide, nalidixic acid
Escitalopram
Exogenous porphyrins for photodynamic therapy
Fibrates
Hydroxychloroquine
Hypoglycaemics: sulphonylureas
Imatinib
Leflunomide
Non-steroidal anti-inflammatory drugs
Pirfenidone
Psoralens
Pyridoxine B6
Quinine
Retinoids
Venlafaxine

Topical

Dyes (phototoxic)
Fragrances (phototoxic and photoallergic)
Halogenated salicylanilides (mainly photoallergic)
Non-steroidal anti-inflammatory drugs (phototoxic and photoallergic)
Phenothiazines (chlorproethazine) (phototoxic and photoallergic)
Polycyclic aromatic hydrocarbons (phototoxic)
Psoralens (phototoxic)
Sunscreens (phototoxic and photoallergic)

Clinical features

The commonest presentation is with phototoxicity characterised by an immediate burning sensation on sun-exposed sites, often with erythema, oedema ('exaggerated sunburn') and sometimes urticaria. There may be a delayed erythema and sometimes blistering. Depending on the drug this may follow the same time course as sunburn, peaking at 24 h. Other patterns of presentation are outlined in Table 68.1.

Skin contact with the psoralen-containing sap of Umbelliferae plants (e.g. giant hogweed, cow parsley) or from the juice of Rutaceae fruits (citrus, e.g. lime) and subsequent UVA exposure from sunlight will result in a phototoxic reaction, called phytophotodermatitis. This causes an eruption of linear red streaks and blistering which become apparent 48–72 h post-exposure at the sites of contact (Figure 68.8). Prolonged pigmentation can occur after all forms of drug-induced phototoxicity, but is particularly prominent with phytophotodermatitis.

Differential diagnosis

PLE, SU, CAD, allergic contact dermatitis.

Investigations

Usually a clinical diagnosis, but abnormal photosensitivity can be demonstrated with monochromator phototesting. Testing should be performed whilst the patient is taking the drug, and then repeated when they are off the drug. Most photoactive drugs have maximal absorption in the UVA waveband and therefore photosensitivity is either restricted to UVA wavelengths or disproportionately involves the UVA region. Photopatch testing is the investigation of choice for suspected topical photocontact allergy.

Management

Recognition of the diagnosis and cessation of the suspected drug or chemical is essential. Photoprotection, including broad-spectrum and reflectant sunscreens, is important until photosensitivity has resolved. Topical corticosteroid for a restricted period can be used to control symptoms.

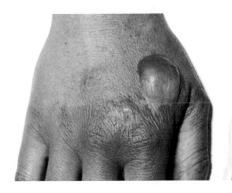

Figure 68.8 Phytophotodermatitis. Erythema and blistering on the back of the hand following contact with lime juice and subsequent exposure to sunlight. Erythema and blistering will be maximal 72–96 h after exposure.

Table 68.1 Patterns of drug- and chemical-induced photosensitivity

Pattern of presentation	Drug and chemical examples
Immediate burning, prickling and subsequent pigmentation	Amiodarone, chlorpromazine, Photofrin, Foscan, topical tar
Exaggerated sunburn	Thiazides, fluoroquinolones, quinine, tetracyclines, amiodarone, chlorpromazine
Delayed erythema and pigmentation	Psoralens
Pseudoporphyria	Non-steroidal anti-inflammatory drugs (particularly naproxen, diclofenac and piroxicam), frusemide, nalidixic acid, tetracyclines, fluoroquinolones, retinoids
Photo-exposed site telangiectasis	Calcium antagonists, venlafaxine
Lupus erythematosus	See Chapter 23
Lichenoid	See Chapter 12

69

Contact dermatitis

Allergic contact dermatitis

(Syn. Contact allergy, allergic contact eczema)

Allergic contact dermatitis (ACD) is an eczematous reaction that occurs as an immunological response following exposure to a substance to which the immune system has previously been sensitised. It is a delayed-type hypersensitivity reaction (type IV).

Epidemiology

In North America and Western Europe the median prevalence of contact allergy to at least one allergen is 21.2% (range 12.5–40.6%). F > M. All ages are affected: children are sensitised as easily as adults. The number of positive patch test reactions tends to increase with age due to an accumulation of allergies acquired over a lifetime.

Pathophysiology

Some compounds react directly with the immune system (e.g. nickel), while others require activation via haptens. Sensitisation is the afferent limb of ACD and elicitation is the effector limb. In sensitisation the hapten interacts with major histocompatibility complex class II molecules on epidermal dendritic cells and Langerhans cells. IL-1β, tumour necrosis factor-α and granulocyte-macrophage colony-stimulating factor mediate activation, maturation and migration of Langerhans cells, which travel via the afferent lymphatics to the regional lymph nodes where they prime naive T lymphocytes. Cytokine release in the lymph node causes proliferation of antigen-specific cytotoxic CD8+ (Tc1) and CD4+ (Th1) lymphocytes. In elicitation these T cells disseminate via the efferent lymphatics and interact with antigen in the skin. On first exposure to a strong sensitiser, such as dinitrochlorobenzene, most subjects develop a local reaction after 5–25 days. During this period, elicitation and sensitisation have been accomplished. If a sensitised person is re-exposed to a specific allergen in sufficient concentration, the clinical reaction subsequently develops much more quickly, usually within 24–48 h.

The dermatopathology of ACD is that of an acute or subacute dermatitis with spongiosis, vesiculation, acanthosis and exocytosis of lymphocytes.

Clinical features

Contact dermatitis can mimic any type of eczema but certain patterns are suggestive of ACD. The history is essential to identify contact with allergens. Although sensitisation and contact dermatitis may result from a single exposure usually several exposures are necessary. A search for possible sources of ACD should include a review of the patient's occupation, home environment, hobbies, clothing, cosmetics and topical medicaments.

An assessment of the primary site of eczema is important. Contact dermatitis begins at a site where contact has taken place with the responsible agent: the site of origin is an important clue to the cause. Table 69.1 highlights the typical patterns of contact eczema and indicates the common sources of allergens in ACD. The

Rook's Dermatology Handbook, First Edition. Edited by Christopher E. M. Griffiths, Tanya O. Bleiker, Daniel Creamer, John R. Ingram and Rosalind C. Simpson.
© 2022 John Wiley & Sons Ltd. Published 2022 by John Wiley & Sons Ltd.

Table 69.1 Common sources of allergens in ACD and their associated patterns of eczema

Body site	Pattern of eczema
Hands and arms	
Rubber gloves	Dorsal aspect of the hands with a sharp line of demarcation at the wrists
Cement	Palms (vesicular dermatitis)
Plants	Streaky involvement of the fingers, dorsal hands and forearms
Garlic and tulip bulbs	Fingertips
Face, lips and ears	
Cosmetics, face creams	Generalised facial involvement (Figure 69.1)
Airborne allergens	Widespread facial involvement with sparing under the chin and behind the ears
Permanent hair dye	Ears, periorbital swelling
Nail varnish	Localised patches of dermatitis on face, eyelids and neck
Eyelid cosmetics, eye drops, contact lens solutions	Upper and lower eyelids
Toothpaste, lip cosmetics	Lips (cheilitis) and perioral skin
Spectacle frames	Skin above and behind ears
Earrings	Ear lobes
Scalp	
Mousses, gels, waxes, shampoos, minoxidil lotion	Generalised scalp involvement
Permanent hair dye	Scalp margins
Neck	
Necklaces	Site of nickel clasp
Nail varnish	Streaky involvement of sides of neck
Collar	Collar-like distribution around neck (textile dye or finishes)
Perfume	Sides of neck (Figure 69.2)
Axillae	
Deodorants	Axillary vault
Clothing	Periaxillary involvement (spares the vault) (Figure 69.3)
Trunk	
Clothing	Sites of contact with clothing, especially when accompanied by friction and sweating, e.g. flexures. Contact with nickel buttons, jeans studs (Figure 69.4) and zip fasteners. Chromate sensitivity from leather and rubber allergy from elastic can all cause ACD on torso, buttocks and proximal limbs (Figure 69.5)
Anogenital	
Medicated creams	Perianal involvement from medicaments used for pruritus and haemorrhoids (Figure 69.6)

(Continued)

Table 69.1 (Continued)

Body site	Pattern of eczema
Moist tissues/wet wipes	Perianal and vulval involvement
Clothing dye in hosiery	Groins
Legs and feet	
Pocket material or contents of pockets	Anterior or lateral thighs from finishes in the material of the pockets or objects kept in the pockets, e.g. nickel coins (Figure 69.7)
Medicated creams/ dressings	Lower leg involvement from ACD to medicaments and dressings, especially in those with varicose eczema and ulcers (Figure 69.8)
Shoes	Dermatitis from shoes: ACD to a component of the shoe upper starts on the dorsal surface of the toes and feet (leather, adhesives) Involvement of the weight-bearing areas of the plantar skin indicates allergy to rubber in the shoes' soles (Figure 69.9)
Exposed skin (face, neck, hands)	
Airborne allergens: sprays, pollens, dust or volatile chemicals	Dermatitis from contact with airborne allergens is confined to the exposed surfaces of the face, neck, hands and arms

behaviour of the dermatitis will help implicate the trigger: relapse at the weekend points to a hobby or the home environment, relapse during the working week indicates an occupational origin. When occupational dermatitis is suspected a knowledge of the materials handled at work will be necessary. A workplace visit may be required to become familiar with the process described.

The primary signs in acute ACD are erythema, swelling, papules and papulo-vesicles. In severe cases there may be blistering and

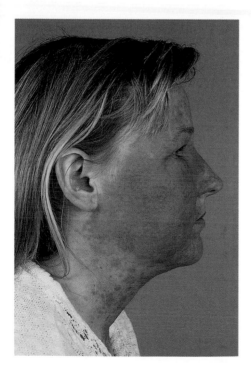

Figure 69.1 Facial ACD, often due to fragrance, preservatives or other ingredients of cosmetics. (Source: Courtesy of Dr J.D. Wilkinson, Amersham General Hospital, Amersham, UK.)

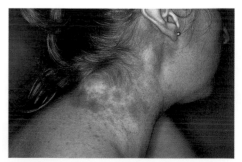

Figure 69.2 An urticated contact dermatitis in a patient allergic to fragrance. (Source: Courtesy of Dr J.D. Wilkinson, Amersham General Hospital, Amersham, UK.)

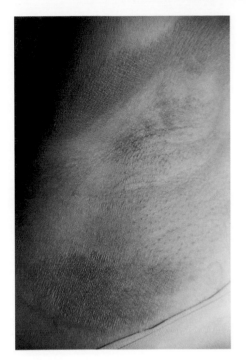

Figure 69.3 Axillary dermatitis (sparing the axillary vault). The characteristic pattern of eczema seen in patients allergic to textile dyes and finishes. (Source: Courtesy of Dr J. D. Wilkinson, Amersham General Hospital, Amersham, UK.)

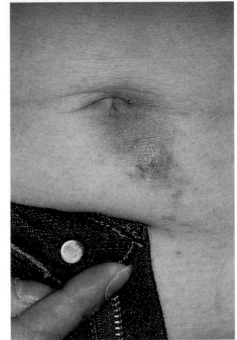

Figure 69.4 ACD to nickel in metal studs on jeans. (Source: Courtesy of Dr J.D. Wilkinson, Amersham General Hospital, Amersham, UK.)

weeping. The dominant symptom is itching. With continued or repeated exposure to the allergen the skin becomes dry, scaly and thickened (lichenification). Sometimes the dermatitis is sharply limited to the site of contact but frequently there is spread of the eczema,

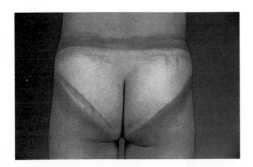

Figure 69.5 ACD to elastic in clothing. (Source: Courtesy of Dr J.D. Wilkinson, Amersham General Hospital, Amersham, UK.)

obscuring the original pattern. Dissemination to distant regions in the absence of allergen spread can also occur, a complication known as systematisation, or an 'id-like' reaction. Contact dermatitis of the hands commonly spreads to the arms and face, dermatitis of the feet tends to spread to the legs and hands. The clinical features of chronic ACD cannot always be distinguished from constitutional or irritant contact dermatitis, indeed the aetiology is often mixed.

Other reaction patterns to allergic contact skin disease are sometimes seen. The major non-eczematous patterns are listed in Table 69.2.

Investigations

The diagnosis of ACD is made by patch testing. The basis of patch testing is to elicit an immune response by challenging an already sensitised person to a defined amount of allergen and assessing the degree of response. Patch testing has a sensitivity and specificity of between 70% and 80%.

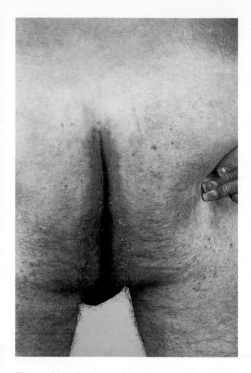

Figure 69.6 Pruritus ani is often complicated by secondary contact dermatitis to local anaesthetics or other medicaments. (Source: Courtesy of Dr J.D. Wilkinson, Amersham General Hospital, Amersham, UK.)

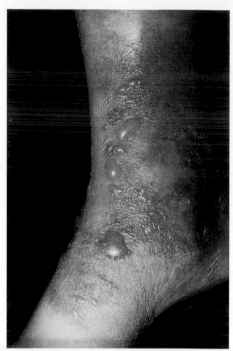

Figure 69.8 Medicament ACD superimposed on stasis eczema. Topical antibiotics/antibacterials, preservatives, lanolin and other constituents of the medicament base are often to blame. (Source: Courtesy of Dr J.D. Wilkinson, Amersham General Hospital, Amersham, UK.)

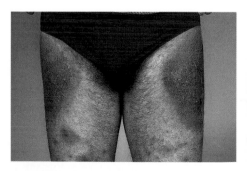

Figure 69.7 ACD due to items kept in trouser pockets. (Source: Courtesy of Dr J.D. Wilkinson, Amersham General Hospital, Amersham, UK.)

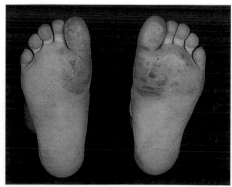

Figure 69.9 Forefoot dermatitis from shoe allergy.

Table 69.2 Non-eczematous responses in allergic contact skin disease

Response	Example
Erythema multiforme-like reaction	Seen in spreading eruption from primary ACD site
Purpuric reaction	Textile dyes, textile resins, rubber chemical accelerators
Lichenoid reactions	On buccal mucosae from metals, cinnamal, spearmint
Lympho-matoid reaction	Contact allergy to gold and nickel can produce lymphoma-like plaques
Pigmented dermatitis	Post-inflammatory hyperpigmentation Also recorded from contact allergy to certain pigments and textile dyes
Depig-mentation	Post-inflammatory hypo-pigmentation or koebnerisation of vitiligo by ACD
Granul-omatous reaction	On buccal mucosae from gold crowns, mercury fillings Also in food additives in oro-facial granulomatosis
Onycholysis	ACD to acrylates (false nails), nail varnish, hairdressing chemicals

Patch tests must be delayed until the acute eczematous eruption has settled. Systemic immunosuppressive drugs should be stopped prior to patch testing. The same applies for systemic corticosteroids, but expert consensus suggests that if the daily dose is no higher than 10 mg prednisolone suppression of positive patch tests is unlikely. If a patient is using potent topical corticosteroids to the back in the 2 days prior to the patches being applied there is a risk of false-negative results. Patch tests should be deferred for 6 weeks after UV exposure (phototherapy and sunbathing) to minimise the chance of false-negative reactions.

Patch testing has a standardised methodology and most patients are tested to a standard series of allergens. These series vary from country to country and should be revised on a regular basis. The British Society for Cutaneous Allergy (BSCA) standard baseline series is shown in Table 69.3. Supplemental series are also recommended; these are important where the baseline series fails to pick up less common allergens such as fragrances or rubber chemicals.

The test site is usually the back, which should be free of eczema. Aluminium discs or chambers (Finn chambers) are used to ensure occluded contact with the skin. The investigator preloads individual allergens onto test discs which are mounted on adhesive tape and stuck onto the back (Figures 69.10 and 69.11). The patches are left in place for 48 h before being removed. A recording of the result is made when the patches are removed (day 2) and then again at day 4. Occasionally a third reading at day 7 is undertaken to pick up positive reactions which were negative at days 2 and 4.

Recording of patch test reactions uses the following scoring scheme:

-     Negative
- ?+   Faint erythema: doubtful reaction
- +   Palpable erythema: weak positive
- ++   Erythema, infiltration, papulo-vesicles: strong positive reaction
- +++   Intense, infiltrated erythema, coalescing vesicles: extreme positive reaction
- IR   Irritant reaction

A positive reaction confirms the person has an allergic contact sensitivity (Figure 69.12), although this does not necessarily mean that the substance is the cause of the dermatitis. An assessment should be made of the relevance of each positive reaction to the patient's presenting dermatitis: (i) current relevance, (ii) past relevance and (iii) relevance not known. Some patch test substances are more likely than others to cause an irritant reaction, leading to a false attribution of allergy.

Table 69.3 Allergens tested in the BSCA standard series and their contact sources

Allergen	Source
Potassium dichromate	Cement, leather
Neomycin sulphate (fradiomycin)	Antibiotic in topical preparations
Thiuram mix	Rubber products (e.g. shoes, gloves, elastic)
p-Phenylenediamine base	Permanent hair dye, 'black' henna
Cobalt chloride ($CoCl_2 \cdot 6H_2O$)	Jewellery, buttons, prosthetic joints, pottery. Added to other metals to increase hardness
Caine mix III	Anaesthetics in topical preparations
Formaldehyde	Preservative: cosmetics, textile resin (wrinkle-free clothing), paint, disinfectants
Colophony (colophonium)	Paper, cosmetics, paint, adhesives, waxes
Quinolone mix	Antimicrobials in medicated creams and ointments
Balsam of Peru (*Myroxylon pereirae*)	Fragrance-containing products, topical medications
N-isopropyl-N'-phenyl-p-phenylenediamine	Rubber products
Lanolin alcohol	Cosmetics, topical creams
Mercapto mix	Rubber products (e.g. shoes, rubber gloves, elastic)
Epoxy resin	Plastics, glues, paint
Parabens mix	Topical medications, cosmetics, antiperspirants
p-Tertiary-butylphenol formaldehyde resin	Resin in adhesives (e.g. shoes, watch straps)
Fragrance mix I	Perfume, fragrance, scented products
Quaternium-15	Preservative in cosmetics, personal care products
Nickel sulphate ($NiSO_4 \cdot 6H_2O$)	Costume jewellery, buckles, zips
Methylchloroisothiazolinone/methylisothiazolinone	Preservative (e.g. shampoo, cosmetics)
Mercaptobenzothiazole	Rubber products (e.g. shoes, rubber gloves, elastic)
Amerchol L101	Products containing lanolin, including cosmetics, topical pharmaceuticals, household products
Sesquiterpene lactone mix	Chrysanthemum family
p-Chloro-m-cresol	Antiseptic and preservative in disinfectants
2-Bromo-2-nitropropane-1,3-diol (Bronopol)	Formaldehyde-releasing antimicrobial preservative
Cetearyl alcohol	Emulsion stabiliser in hair conditioner and other products
Sodium fusidate	Antibiotic in topical medicaments

(Continued)

Table 69.3 (Continued)

Allergen	Source
Tixocortol-21-pivalate	Topical corticosteroids (including hydrocortisone)
Budesonide	Topical corticosteroids (including triamcinolone)
Imidazolidinyl urea (Germal 115)	Formaldehyde-releasing antimicrobial preservative
Diazolidinyl urea (Germal 11)	Formaldehyde-releasing antimicrobial preservative
Methyldibromoglutaronitrile	Preservative in skincare products (e.g. lotions, wet wipes, shampoo)
Ethylenediamine dihydrochloride	Preservative in topical medicaments
4-Chloro-3,5-xylenol	Preservative and antimicrobial in cleansers and cosmetics
Carba mix	Rubber products (e.g. shoes, gloves, elastic)
Disperse Blue mix 106/124	Textile dyes
Fragrance mix II	Perfume, fragrance, scented products
Hydroxyisohexyl 3-cyclohexene carboxaldehyde (Lyral)	Perfume, fragrance, scented products
Compositae mix	Plants of compositae family (e.g. arnica, feverfew, tansy)
Methylisothiazolinone	Preservative in personal care and industrial products
Sodium metabisulphite	Antiseptic and preservative in disinfectants

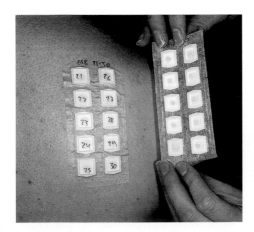

Figure 69.10 Patch tests. Application of patch tests to patient's back. (Source: Courtesy of King's College Hospital, London, UK.)

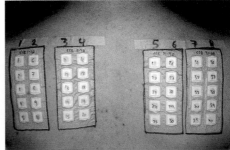

Figure 69.11 Patch tests. Standard baseline series applied to patient's back at the beginning of patch testing. (Source: Courtesy of King's College Hospital, London, UK.)

PART 9: SKIN DISORDERS CAUSED BY EXTERNAL AGENTS

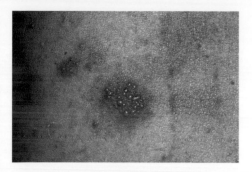

Figure 69.12 A positive allergic (++) patch test response in a patient sensitive to neomycin. (Source: Courtesy of Dr J.D. Wilkinson, Amersham General Hospital, Amersham, UK.)

Irritant contact dermatitis

(Syn. 'Wear-and-tear' dermatitis)

Irritant contact dermatitis (ICD) is the cutaneous response to the physical and/or toxic effects of a wide range of environmental substances. The commonest site of ICD is the hands.

Epidemiology

The prevalence of ICD on the hands in the general population is 1.8%. F:M 2:1.

Pathophysiology

An irritant is any agent, physical or chemical, which is capable of producing cellular perturbation if applied for sufficient time and in sufficient concentration. Strong irritants (e.g. soap) will induce a clinical reaction in all individuals, whereas less potent irritants depend on patient susceptibility and repeated contact. Dermatitis arises when the defence or repair capacity of the skin is exhausted, or when the penetration of chemicals excites an inflammatory response. Skin barrier dysfunction is the major reason for irritation. External factors which enhance the induction of ICD are ambient temperature, air flow (chapping), low humidity and occlusion. Histologically ICD reactions show greater dermatopathological pleomorphism than ACD.

A large number of common substances and products are able to induce an irritant reaction (see Box 69.1). Many occupations are associated with a risk of developing an ICD (see Box 69.2).

> **Box 69.1 Common irritants causing ICD**
>
> Water and wet work: sweating under occlusion
> Household cleaners: detergent, soap, shampoo, disinfectant
> Industrial cleaning agents: including solvents and abrasives
> Alkalis, including cement
> Acids
> Cutting oils
> Organic solvents
> Oxidising agents, including sodium hypochlorite
> Reducing agents, including phenols, hydrazine, aldehydes, thiophosphates
> Certain plants, e.g. spurge, Boracinaceae, Ranunculaceae
> Pesticides
> Raw food, animal enzymes and secretions
> Desiccant powders
> Dust, soil

> **Box 69.2 Occupations associated with ICD**
>
> Hairdressing
> Medical, dental, veterinary
> Cleaning
> Agriculture, horticulture, forestry
> Food preparation and catering
> Printing and painting
> Metal work
> Mechanical engineering
> Construction
> Fishing

Clinical features

ICD has a spectrum of clinical features ranging from dryness, redness and chapping, through various types of eczematous dermatitis to an acute caustic burn.

Hands

Typically there is patchy eczema affecting the dorsal surfaces and sides of the hands (Figure 69.13) and the webs of the fingers (Figure 69.14). Eczema under rings is also associated with wet work and exposure to detergent. The dermatitis starts as dryness and develops

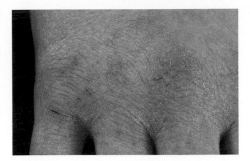

Figure 69.13 Fissuring on the dorsum occurs most commonly as a result of frequent hand washing and outdoor exposure. (Source: Courtesy of St John's Institute of Dermatology, London, UK.)

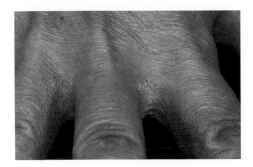

Figure 69.14 Interdigital ICD is frequently caused by inadequate drying of the hands after washing. It is commonly seen in hairdressers on the non-dominant hand. (Source: Courtesy of St John's Institute of Dermatology, London, UK.)

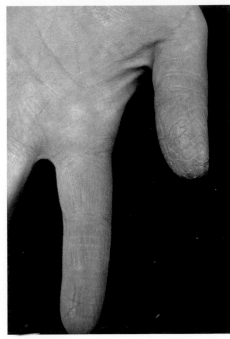

Figure 69.15 Pulpitis (ICD of the finger pulps) is usually caused by wet work. (Source: Courtesy of St John's Institute of Dermatology, London, UK.)

into erythema, scaling and fissuring. The 'apron' pattern is characterised by eczema affecting the palmar aspects of the fingers and distal palm. This pattern of dermatitis commonly occurs in those who frequently hold wet cloths containing detergent or household chemicals. Involvement of the tips of the fingers and thumbs (pulpitis) is another manifestation of wet work (Figure 69.15).

Face

Often caused by an irritant reaction to cosmetics, toiletries and skincare products. The eyelids are particularly susceptible. Those using many products are at risk of 'cosmetic exhaustion', a form of cumulative cosmetic ICD.

Anogenital skin

Can develop in situations of prolonged contact with urine or faeces, thus seen in the very young or elderly in situations of urinary or faecal incontinence (napkin dermatitis). Similar problems can arise on the skin around a stoma. Occlusion, irritant cleansers and secondary infection are all additional complicating factors.

Investigations

ICD is a clinical diagnosis based on knowledge of the chemicals involved and exposure factors. Some chemicals may have both irritant and allergic potential, or the patient may be exposed to several chemicals with irritant or allergic potential. Patch testing should therefore be undertaken to exclude an allergic component. In hand eczema constitutional factors (e.g. atopy) may coexist with irritant and allergic factors. The concept of persistent post-occupational dermatitis, despite avoidance of the original cause(s), may occur following both irritant and ACD.

Management of contact dermatitis (ACD and ICD)

Avoidance

Avoidance of allergens and irritants is central to the management of contact dermatitis. The patient must be educated about the relevance of the causative allergen/irritant. The source of the implicated substance(s) should be identified and avoidance advice given.

Protection

In the context of hand dermatitis protection of the skin against contact with an allergen or irritant most commonly involves the use of gloves. The hands need to be protected at home as well as in the workplace: rubber or polyvinyl-chloride gloves with a cotton lining are recommended for general household tasks. For hand eczema the patient must be given advice about hand care (see Box 69.3).

Workplace visit

If occupational exposure to allergen/irritant is suspected then a workplace visit can help identify which allergens/irritants need to be considered and which procedures in the work environment are leading to exposure. A visit should be organised in conjunction with on-site nursing/medical/safety personnel.

Substitution

Replacement of soap and detergent with an emollient soap substitute is essential in ACD and ICD.

Active intervention

The use of a topical corticosteroid ointment of appropriate potency is usually necessary for a limited period. A short course of oral corticosteroids is sometimes needed. In recalcitrant ACD systemic therapy may be necessary, e.g. alitretinoin, azathioprine, ciclosporin or phototherapy. When ACD fails to improve consider concomitant irritant or constitutional eczema, or the possibility of non-compliance with avoidance advice.

Job change

If a worker is unable to eliminate exposure to the culprit allergen/irritant then the patient occasionally needs to consider a change of career.

Box 69.3 Advice to patients with hand eczema

To speed recovery and prevent your dermatitis from returning, you must take great care of your hands and allow your skin to heal fully. This may take many months, even though the skin may look normal before then.

1. Use a hand cream (moisturiser/emollient) many times per day so that the skin does not become dry.
2. Use the steroid ointment (or cream) prescribed by the doctor.
3. Wash hands using lukewarm water and soap substitute (e.g. aqueous cream). After washing dry thoroughly.
4. If wet work cannot be avoided wear gloves. Plastic gloves are preferable to rubber. Cotton-lined gloves are best.
5. Avoid contact with detergents, shampoo, cleaning agents, solvents (e.g. white spirit).
6. Wear gloves when outdoors in cold weather.
7. If the skin becomes inflamed and throbs, it is likely to be infected. Visit your doctor, who may take a skin swab and prescribe an antibiotic.

Part 10
Neoplastic, Proliferative, and Infiltrative Disorders Affecting the Skin

Benign melanocytic proliferations and melanocytic naevi

70

Benign cutaneous melanocytic proliferations are the most common neoplasms occurring in humans. This chapter describes the spectrum of benign melanocytic lesions, their divergent clinical varieties, pathophysiology and treatment. See Table 70.1 for the basic terminology and definitions.

FRECKLE OR EPHELIS

A small reddish or pale to dark brown macule with a poorly defined border, on sun-exposed areas of the skin.

Epidemiology
Common during childhood. More frequently seen in individuals with fair skin, red hair and blue eyes. Freckles are considered a risk factor for melanoma.

Pathophysiology
Exposure to UV radiation leads to overproduction of melanin by melanocytes, which is subsequently transferred to neighbouring keratinocytes.

Table 70.1 Basic terminology and definitions used in benign melanocytic neoplasms.

Term	Description
Freckle (ephelis)	A pigmented macule on sun-exposed areas consisting of increased melanin pigmentation
Lentigo	A poorly demarcated area of uniform pigmentation consisting of increased melanin pigmentation, epidermal proliferation and replacement of basal cell keratinocytes by melanocytes
Café-au-lait macule	A well-circumscribed, uniformly light to dark brown macule or patch that spares mucous membranes and consists of increased melanin content in the basal cell layer
Junctional naevus	A pigmented melanocytic naevus in which the main histological feature is the presence of nests of melanocytes at the dermal–epidermal junction
Compound naevus	A pigmented melanocytic naevus in which the histological features include both junctional nests and the presence of naevus cells in the dermis
Intradermal/dermal naevus	A melanocytic lesion with naevus cells in the dermis Melanin pigmentation is often absent and there is little or no abnormality of melanocytes in the epidermis The deepest dermal cells tend to neural or fibroblastic differentiation

Rook's Dermatology Handbook, First Edition. Edited by Christopher E. M. Griffiths, Tanya O. Bleiker, Daniel Creamer, John R. Ingram and Rosalind C. Simpson.
© 2022 John Wiley & Sons Ltd. Published 2022 by John Wiley & Sons Ltd.

The basal cell layer appears hyperpigmented, without alteration of the epidermal architecture. In contrast to lentigines, the number of melanocytes is normal.

The melanocortin 1 receptor gene (*MCR1*) has been characterised as the major freckle gene.

Clinical features

Freckles typically appear after excessive sun exposure (either chronic or intermittent) in light-skinned red- or fair-haired individuals. Macular hyperpigmentations with a round or oval shape and ill-defined borders (Figure 70.1a). In winter months freckles tend to lighten or disappear.

Differential diagnosis

Solar lentigines persist even without UV exposure and appear in older ages. Freckling can occur in neurofibromatosis type 1, in which it is more commonly located in non-exposed areas (trunk and axilla) with other manifestations of neurofibromatosis.

Investigations

Under dermoscopy freckles present with a uniform pigmentation and a moth-eaten edge (Figure 70.1b).

Management

No treatment is required other than photoprotection. Chemical peels, lasers, topical depigmenting drugs and dermocosmetic products can be used for cosmetic reasons.

LENTIGINES

UVR-induced hyperperpigmented macules that do not fade in the absence of UV exposure. On microscopy they show increased melanin on the basal cell layer and increased numbers of singly arranged melanocytes, compared with the adjacent non-involved skin.

The subtypes include simple lentigo, actinic (or solar) lentigo, psoralen and UVA (PUVA) lentigo and ink-spot lentigo (Table 70.2). Rarely, lentigines arise as a manifestation of hereditary syndromes (Table 70.3).

MUCOSAL MELANOTIC LESIONS

Mucosal melanotic macules (or mucosal melanosis/genital lentiginosis) are benign pigmented patches of the oral and genital mucosa (see Chapters 59 and 61).

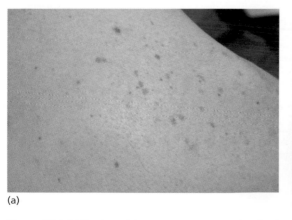

(a)

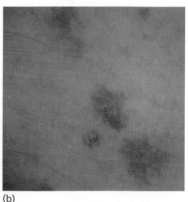

(b)

Figure 70.1 (a) Freckles. (b) Dermoscopic image showing hyperpigmented lesions with reticular pattern and moth-eaten edges.

Table 70.2 Subtypes of lentigenes

	Simple lentigo	Solar/actinic lentigo	Photochemotherapy (PUVA) lentigo	Ink-spot lentigo
Synonym	Lentigo simplex	Senile freckle, Lentigo senilis		
Epidemiology	Common Red hair, fair skin Appears in childhood and increase until 40 years Remains unchanged in adult life	Increases with ageing	Patients who have received a high cumulative dose of PUVA treatment Fair skinned patients	Sunburn in fair-skinned individuals
Pathophysiology	UVR-induced increased melanocytes at the dermal–epidermal junction with melanin hyperpigmentation Multiple lentigines in early life on exposed and non-exposed skin may be manifestation of inherited syndrome (Figure 70.2)	Intermittent, chronic UVR Lesions on back associated with sunburns <20 years Histology as for simple lentigo Clinical and pathological overlap with flat seborrhoeic keratoses	Histology resembles ephelides or lentigines Melanocytes increased in number and may have nuclear atypia	Lentiginous hyperplasia of the epidermis, prominent hyperpigmentation of the basal cells, with 'skip' areas involving the rete ridges, minimal increase in melanocyte number
Clinical features	Up to 5 mm, poorly circumscribed, round or oval, uniformly pigmented macules on photoexposed areas (Figure 70.3) Lesions may coalesce	Sun-exposed sites; face in both sexes, shoulders in males, backs of hands and face in older patients Tan coloured macules which may be large with an irregular border	Relatively large, pigmented macules (Figure 70.4) Increased risk of keratinocyte cancers	Irregular, sharply demarcated, jet-black macules Sun-exposed areas, often shoulders Often solitary (Figure 70.5)
Differential diagnosis	Freckles, junctional naevi, flat seborrhoeic keratoses, lentigo maligna	Simple lentigo, seborrhoeic keratosis, lentigo maligna, melanoma in situ	As for solar lentigo	Lentigo maligna, melanoma in situ
Dermoscopy	Scalloped borders, a faint irregular network or pseudo-network and structureless areas (Figure 70.3b)	Scalloped borders, a faint irregular network or pseudo-network and structureless areas (Figure 70.3b)	Scalloped borders, a faint irregular network or pseudo-network and structureless areas (Figure 70.3b)	Prominent black network with thin and/or thick lines (Figure 70.5b)
Management	Photoprotection Cosmetic treatments, e.g. depigmenting preparations, chemical peels, lasers and PDT	Photoprotection Cryotherapy, topical retinoids, intense pulsed light, pigment-specific (Q-switched) laser	Photoprotection Skin cancer surveillance	Photoprotection

PUVA, psoralen and UVA; UVR, UV radiation; PDT, photodynamic therapy.

Table 70.3 Familial lentiginosis syndromes

Disorder	Clinical manifestations	Inheritance-related gene (chromosomal locus)
Peutz–Jeghers syndrome	Lentigines (lips, oral and bowel mucosa, palms, soles, eyes, nares, perianal region), hamartomatous GI polyps, neoplasms (GI tract, pancreas, breast, ovary, uterus, testis)	Autosomal dominant *LKB1/STK11* (19p13.3)
PTEN hamartomatous syndromes, e.g. Cowden	Macrocephaly, lipomatosis, pigmentation of the glans penis, mental retardation, multiple hamartomas, neoplasms (breast cancer, follicular thyroid cancer, endometrial carcinoma)	Autosomal dominant *PTEN* (10q23.31)
Carney complex	Lentigines (lips, conjunctiva, inner or outer canthi, genital mucosa), PPNAD, cardiac and skin myxomas, schwannomas, acromegaly, breast and testicular tumours Subsets NAME and LAMB syndromes	Autosomal dominant *PRKAR1A* (17q22–24)
Lentiginoses	Lentigines (centrofacial, palmoplantar, trunk) Lentigines (centrofacial, palmoplantar, trunk) plus mental retardation	Autosomal dominant Autosomal dominant/ sporadic
LEOPARD syndrome	Lentigines (mainly on face and upper trunk; rarely on oral mucosa, extremities, genitalia, conjunctiva), cardiac conduction abnormalities, aneurysms, pulmonic stenosis, cephalofacial dysmorphism, short stature, sensorineural deafness, mental retardation, skeletal abnormalities	Autosomal dominant *PTPN11* (12q24.1) – same as in Noonan syndrome Autosomal dominant *RAF1* (3p25)

GI, gastrointestinal; PTEN, phosphate and tensin homologue; PPNAD, pigmented nodular adrenal cortical disease; NAME, naevi, atrial myxoma, myxoid neurofibroma and ephelides; LAMB, lentigines, atrial myxomas, mucocutaneous myxomas and blue naevi; LEOPARD, lentigines, electrocardiogram anomalies, ocular anomalies, pulmonary stenosis, abnormal genitalia, retardation of growth and deafness. Adapted from Guerrero D. Dermocosmetic management of hyperpigmentations. Ann Dermatol Vénéréol 2012;139(Suppl. 4):S166–9.

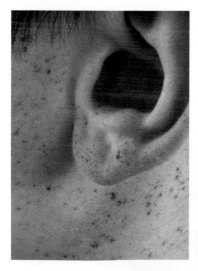

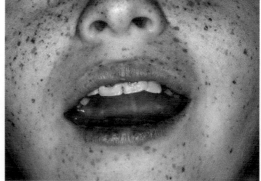

Figure 70.2 Multiple lentigines in a patient with the Carney complex and a PRKAR1A mutation. Only about a third of patients with the complex have this classic pigmentation. (Source: Courtesy of Dr Constantine A. Stratakis, National Institutes of Health, Bethesda, MD, USA.)

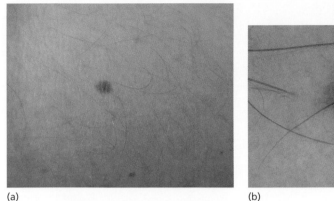
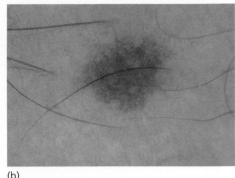

(a)
(b)

Figure 70.3 (a) Simple lentigo. (b) Dermoscopic image of simple lentigo.

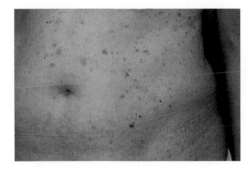

Figure 70.4 PUVA-induced lentigines in a patient with psoriasis.

DERMAL MELANOCYTIC LESIONS

During fetal life, melanocytes migrate from the neural crest to the dermal–epidermal junction. Occasionally they remain entrapped in the dermis, not reaching their destination in the epidermis, and give rise to dermal melanocytic lesions. These lesions have a bluish colour owing to the Tyndall effect (Table 70.4).

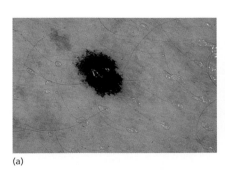
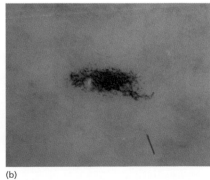

(a)
(b)

Figure 70.5 (a) Ink-spot lentigo. (b) Dermoscopic image of an ink-spot lentigo showing a bizarre-looking black pigment network, which is typical. (Source: Courtesy of Dr S. Puig, Hospital Clinic Barcelona, IDIBAPS, Barcelona, Spain.)

PART 10: NEOPLASTIC, PROLIFERATIVE AND INFILTRATIVE DISORDERS AFFECTING THE SKIN

Table 70.4 Dermal melanocytic lesions

	Lumbosacral dermal melanocytosis (formerly Mongolian spot)	Naevus of Ota	Naevus of Ito
Epidemiology	Present at birth, resolves with time Asian/African descent	Present at birth or develop during first year Occasionally develop around puberty Increase in size and number with age Asian/African descent More common in females	Present at birth Predominantly Chinese and Japanese descent
Pathophysiology	Dermal dendritic melanocytes No dermal fibrosis or melanophages	Dermal dendritic melanocytes No dermal fibrosis or melanophages	Dermal dendritic melanocytes No dermal fibrosis or melanophages
Clinical features	Predominantly lumbosacral, normally single, diffuse blue-grey macule upto 10 cm in size (Figure 70.6)	Normally unilateral, often speckled, blue and brown patch Near/involving the eye (conjunctiva) in distribution of trigeminal nerve (ophthalmic/maxillary) (Figure 70.7) Rarely, melanoma of meninges, choroid, iris or orbit occurs	Normally unilateral, blue-greyish macular discoloration Side of neck and shoulder in distribution of the posterior supraclavicular and lateral cutaneous brachial nerves (Figure 70.8)
Differential diagnosis	Blue naevus	Hori naevus (bilateral Ota-like macules with no mucous membrane involvement)	Becker naevus
Management	No treatment required Q-switched lasers Cosmetic camouflage Close ophthalmological monitoring in naevus of Ito when eye involved, in view of rare malignant transformation	No treatment required Q-switched lasers Cosmetic camouflage Close ophthalmological monitoring in naevus of Ito when eye involved, in view of rare malignant transformation	No treatment required Q-switched lasers Cosmetic camouflage Close ophthalmological monitoring in naevus of Ito when eye involved, in view of rare malignant transformation

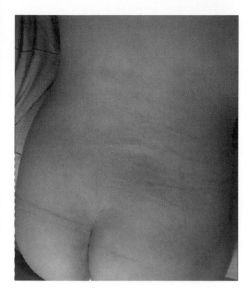

Figure 70.6 Dermal melanocytosis in the lumbosacral area. (Source: Courtesy of Professor A. Katsarou-Katsari, Pediatric Dermatology Unit, Andreas Sygros Hospital, Athens, Greece.)

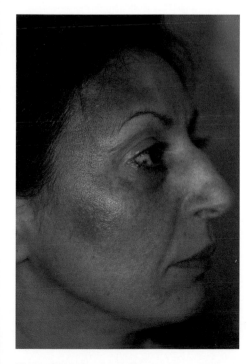

Figure 70.7 Naevus of Ota.

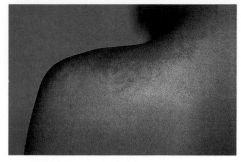

Figure 70.8 Naevus of Ito, showing a typical distribution over the shoulder area.

COMMON ACQUIRED NAEVI

Acquired melanocytic naevi are benign neoplasms of melanocytic neavus cells that begin to proliferate at the dermal–epidermal junction (junctional naevus) and over time tend to migrate into the dermis while a component remains in contact with the basal layer (compound naevus) (Table 70.5). At the end stage of this process all the naevus cells are completely detached from the overlying epidermis (intradermal naevus). Somatic *BRAF* mutations are present in the majority (*c.* 80%) of acquired melanocytic naevi.

NAEVI IN UNUSUAL SITES

See Table 70.6. Although not broadly accepted as a unique entity, these lesions have a different morphological pattern from banal melanocytic naevi. Partially due to anatomical factors, hormonal influences, trauma and epidermal thickness. They are clinically more atypical, presenting with a larger size and colour variegation and exhibit distinct histological patterns such as pagetoid spreading (acral naevi), enlarged junctional nests with discohesion of melanocytes (flexural and genital naevi) or large nests with bizarre shapes that extend down to the follicular epithelium (scalp). Their course is benign and, just as in naevi on other sites, they should be monitored clinically.

Table 70.5 Common acquired naevi

Subtype	Epidemiology	Pathological characteristics	Clinical features	Dermoscopy (Chapter 82)
Junctional naevus (Figure 70.9)	Common, more so in white skin Usually multiple The number increases from childhood to midlife and then decreases	Proliferation of melanocytes in the dermal–epidermal junction	Uniformly pigmented brown macule, with a diameter of 2–10 mm Trunk and extremities more common	Globular, reticular structureless brown and mixed patterns
Compound naevus (Figure 70.10)	A new mole in a patient >60 years should raise concern Patients with >100 naevi have a 7-fold increase in melanoma risk	Proliferation of melanocytes in the dermal–epidermal junction and dermis in the epidermis, showing evidence of migration of cells into the dermis and 'maturation' of those cells within the deeper dermis	Symmetrical slightly raised, oval or round; pigmented with variable shades of brown	Globular, reticular, structureless, brown, multicomponent and mixed patterns
Intradermal naevus (Syn. Dermal naevus) (Figure 70.11)		Proliferation of melanocytes in the dermis Melanocytes tend to lose ability to produce pigment as they progress from epidermis to dermis	Flesh-coloured, dome-shaped, exophytic papule or nodule	Symmetrical homogeneous pattern; may have a slight pigmented globular pattern or black dots Comedo-like openings, crypts and comma vessels may be present

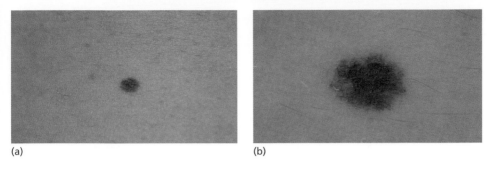

(a)　　　　　　　　　　　　　　　　(b)

Figure 70.9 (a) Junctional naevus. (b) Dermoscopic image of a junctional naevus showing a reticular pattern with a smooth ending at the periphery.

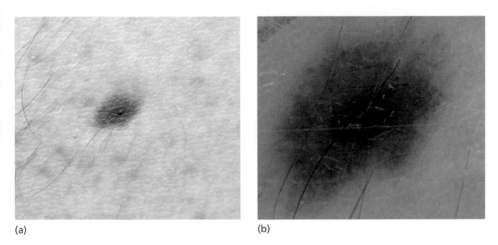

(a)　　　　　　　　　　　　　　　　(b)

Figure 70.10 Compound naevus. (a) Hyperpigmented papule surrounded by symmetrical, lighter brown, macular area. (b) Dermoscopic image showing a structureless brown center with reticulated periphery.

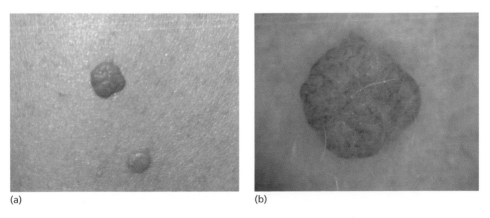

(a)　　　　　　　　　　　　　　　　(b)

Figure 70.11 (a) Intradermal naevi. (b) Dermoscopic image showing a symmetrical, flesh-coloured, homogeneous pattern with coma-shaped vessels.

Table 70.6 Naevi in unusual sites

Subtype	Epidemiology	Pathological characteristics	Clinical features	Dermoscopy
Naevus of the genital area	2.3% of patients undergoing gynaecological examination	Most are compound naevi with florid junctional melanocytic proliferation, cellular discohesion and atypical cytology	Vulva but also perineum, mons pubis, penis and scrotum Usually hyperpigmented and larger than common acquired naevi	Asymmetrical in colour and structure, often with irregular dots/globules or grayish-black blotches
Acral naevus (Figure 70.12)		Junctional, compound or intraepidermal Lentiginous melanocytic proliferation and some degree of upward migration of naevus cells are seen (transepidermal elimination effect from frequent trauma and friction on these sites)	Macular or slightly elevated, uniformly pigmented lesion with irregular and sharp borders Often with a striated appearance, distributed along the parallel furrows of acral skin	Parallel furrow, lattice-like or fibrillar pattern
Conjunctival naevus (Figure 70.13)	Acquired or congenital Melanoma transformation in <1% of naevi	The presence of intralesional cysts is characteristic	Bulbar conjunctiva, often amelanotic (30%), flat or slightly raised macules or papules; often acquire pigmentation after puberty	
Nail-associated naevus (Figure 70.14)	Children and young adults	Junctional or compound naevus with prominent hyperpigmentation and nuclear hyperchromasia	Fingernails more common than toenails Longitudinal parallel and homogeneous light to dark brown to black pigmentation of the nail plate	Brown, longitudinal parallel lines with regular spacing and thickness

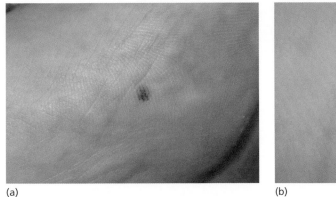
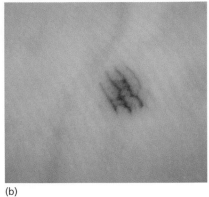

(a)   (b)

Figure 70.12 (a) Naevus on the sole of a foot. (b) Dermoscopic image of acral naevus showing a parallel furrow pattern.

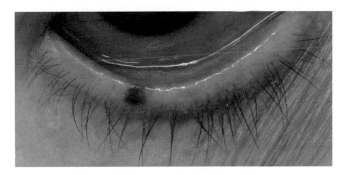

Figure 70.13 Conjunctival naevus. A well-circumscribed papule of various shades of brown (Source: Courtesy of Dr D. Sgouros, Andreas Sygros Hospital, Athens, Greece.)

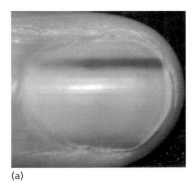
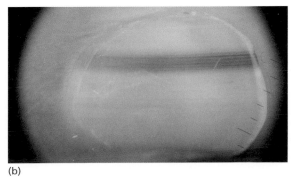

(a)   (b)

Figure 70.14 Nail matrix naevus. (a) A longitudinal pigmented band. (b) Dermoscopic image showing brown, longitudinal parallel lines with regular spacing and thickness.

CONGENITAL MELANOCYTIC NAEVI

See Chapter 36.

NAEVI WITH UNUSUAL MORPHOLOGY

See Table 70.7. A distinct group of naevi that exhibit unusual clinicopathological and dermoscopic features. These naevi, designated as 'special' naevi, include those with clinically atypical presentation that simulate melanoma (e.g. combined and recurrent naevi) and those with targetoid morphology (e.g. halo, Mayerson, cockade and targetoid haemosiderotic naevi).

OTHER NAEVI

Spitz naevus

Spitz naevi remain a subject of controversy due to their clinical and histological variability, their overlapping histological characteristics with melanoma and the uncertainty of their biological behaviour in certain cases (Table 70.8). At one end of the spectrum is the common or classic Spitz naevus, a benign proliferation frequently occurring in children; at the other end

are lesions with extensive pleomorphic features sufficient for the diagnosis of melanoma ('spitzoid melanoma'). In between lies a heterogeneous group of lesions with varying features and unknown malignant potential.

Management

There is a lack of consensus regarding management. Due to the low probability of melanoma in children with typical or classic Spitz naevi, clinical monitoring may be appropriate, provided that a close clinical and dermoscopic follow-up is performed. Exceptions include atypical, large (>1 cm), nodular, ulcerated or rapidly growing lesions. Excision with 1–3 mm margin and histological examination is then advised. The histological diagnosis of an atypical Spitz tumour should be approached more aggressively and treated with a wide margin resection following the guidelines of melanoma resection. Patients can be reassured that the lesion may in fact be benign.

Blue naevus and variants

This is a relatively common blue, blue-grey or blue-black benign melanocytic naevus composed of dermal melanocytes, with several clinical and histological variants (Table 70.9). The blue colour is caused by the 'Tyndall effect': dermal pigment absorbs the longer wavelengths of light and scatters blue light.

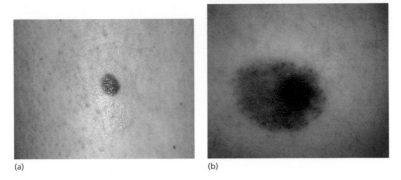

Figure 70.15 (a) Combined naevus. (b) Combined naevus with eccentric, structureless, bluish area, and peripheral, brown, globular pattern. (Source: Courtesy of Dr D. Sgouros, Andreas Sygros Hospital, Athens, Greece.)

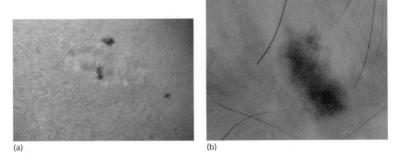

Figure 70.16 Recurrent naevus. (a) Macule developing within the scar of a previously excised melanocytic naevus. (b) Dermoscopic image showing a slightly asymmetrical macule consisting of a smooth reticular network of fine lines and brownish colour on a whitish scar. (Source: Courtesy of Dr D. Sgouros, Andreas Sygros Hospital, Athens, Greece.)

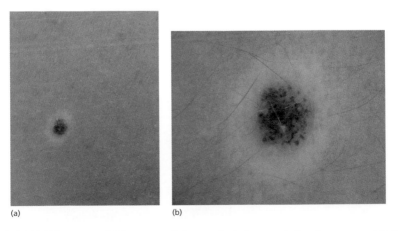

Figure 70.17 (a) Halo naevus. (b) Dermoscopic image of a halo naevus showing a symmetrical compound naevus (globular pattern) surrounded by a whitish halo.

PART 10: NEOPLASTIC, PROLIFERATIVE AND INFILTRATIVE DISORDERS AFFECTING THE SKIN

Table 70.7 Naevi with unusual morphology

Subtype	Epidemiology	Pathological characteristics	Clinical features	Dermoscopy
Combined melanocytic naevus (Figure 70.15)	1% of excised naevi	Blue naevus in combination with a congenital, acquired or spitz neavi	Bluish macule or papule surrounded by a macular brown area often on back	Usually a brownish reticular and/or globular pattern with central or eccentric structureless blue pigmentation
Recurrent melanocytic naevus (Figure 70.16)	Recurrence after incomplete excis on or trauma More frequent in women 20–30 years old	Intraepidermal presence of melanocytes above the level of a scar The atypical appearance has given the term 'pseudo-melanoma'	Back commonest site followed by face and extremities Macular area with hyper- or hypopigmentation, linear streaks and mottled pigmentation arising within a scar	Irregular prominent network, globules and heterogeneous pigmentation, usually within the borders of the scar
Halo naevus (Syn. Sutton naevus) (Figure 70.17)	1% of population Children and young adults Associated with autoimmune disease, e.g. vitiligo, Hashimoto thyroiditis, alopecia areata, atopic eczema	Autoimmune response against naevus cells Dense lymphocytic infiltrate in the early phase and subsequent elimination of naevus cells Triggers include stress and puberty	Predominantly on the back A melanocytic naevus surrounded by a depigmented halo The naevus gradually shrinks and may disappear, leaving a white macule Multiple lesions may occur	Central naevus exhibits globular and/or homogeneous patterns, surrounded by a white rim
Meyerson naevus (Figure 70.18)	Young age May be assoc ated with atopic eczema	Benign naevus with overlying spongiosis of the epidermis	A melanocytic naevus that develops an eczematous-like inflammatory reaction Responds to topical steroid treatment	Pattern of the involved naevus is often blurred by an overlying yellowish superficial crust

Cockade naevus (Syn. Naevus en cocarde) (Figure 70.19)	Children and adolescents	Central junctional or compound component, while the periphery consists of junctional nests	A naevus with a target-like appearance	Darker central globular or homogeneous pattern, surrounded by a structureless inner ring and a more peripheral darker reticular ring
Targetoid haemosiderotic naevus (Figure 70.20)	Children and young and adults Mechanical trauma/ irritation	Naevus cells mingled with extravasated blood vessels	Commonly upper chest Tender, itchy or painful lesion Sudden change of pigmentation in a pre-existing naevus following trauma Brown or red-brown or violaceous papule surrounded by a thin pale area and a peripheral ecchymotic ring	Red to purple colour haemorrhage surrounding a naevus

PART 10: NEOPLASTIC, PROLIFERATIVE AND INFILTRATIVE DISORDERS AFFECTING THE SKIN

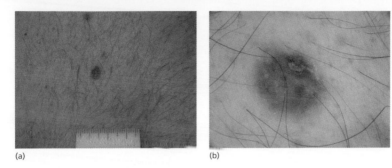

(a)   (b)

Figure 70.18 Meyerson naevus. (a) A small-sized naevus with an eczematous component. (b) Dermoscopic image showing yellowish crusts covering a naevus with a faint brownish network. (Source: Courtesy of Dr I. Zalaudek, Skin Cancer Unit Arcispedale Santa Maria Nuova – IRCCS Reggio Emilia, Italy.)

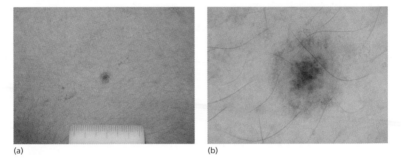

(a)   (b)

Figure 70.19 (a) Cockade naevus. (b) Dermoscropic image of a cockade naevus showing a darker, central homogeneous pattern, a lighter inner ring, and a peripheral brown reticular ring. (Source: Courtesy of Dr I. Zalaudek, Skin Cancer Unit Arcispedale Santa Maria Nuova – IRCCS Reggio Emilia, Italy.)

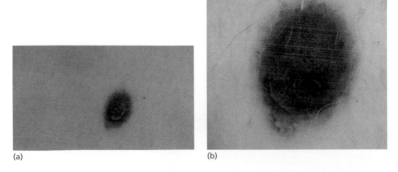

(a)   (b)

Figure 70.20 Targetoid haemosiderotic naevus. (a) Naevus acutely presenting with a haemorrhagic halo. (b) Dermoscopic image showing a peripheral, structureless, purple rim around a central pre-existing compound naevus.

Table 70.8 Spitz naevi

Subtype	Epidemiology	Pathological characteristics	Clinical features	Dermoscopy
Classic Spitz naevus (Figures 70.21 and 70.22)	1% of excised naevi in children <10 years Predominantly white populations	Symmetrical and well-defined compound naevus; epithelio'd/spindle cells arranged in nests showing zonation and maturation at the depth of lesion; intact epidermis, Kamino bodies, few superficial mitoses <2 mm^2	Usually rapidly develop over 3–6 months on the head, neck, and thighs Solitary, firm, symmetrical well defined, round or dome-shaped pink to red or brown nodule (≤5–6 mm in diameter)	Predominantly dotted vascular pattern with reticular depigmentation
Atypical Spitz tumours (Figure 70.23)	>10 years old	Asymmetrical, poorly demarcated, infiltrating, irregular spacing and disorderly arrangement of nests and cells Ulcerated epidermis Absent or few Kamino bodies and >2–6 mm^2 mitoses	Trunk (back in men) >10 mm size, ulcerated, asymmetrical and irregular pigmentation	Often exhibit an asymmetrical peripheral distribution of pigmented streaks, and a heterogeneous pigmentation with bluish-black and whitish hue
Reed naevus (Syn. Spindle cell naevus of Reed) (Figure 70.24)	Young females	Similar to classic Spitz naevi; junctional melanocytic activity with large quantities of melanin pigment	Located on the thighs Solitary, censely pigmented, irregularly shaped, dark-brown or black papule or nodule	'Starburst' pattern (diffuse blue-black pigmentation with radial streaks in the periphery)

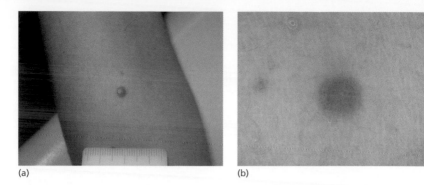

(a)   (b)

Figure 70.21 Classic Spitz naevus. (a) A well-circumscribed pink nodule. (b) A round, symmetrical lesion with dotted vessels and lack of pigmentation. (Source: Courtesy of Dr I. Zalaudek, Skin Cancer Unit Arcispedale Santa Maria Nuova – IRCCS Reggio Emilia, Italy.)

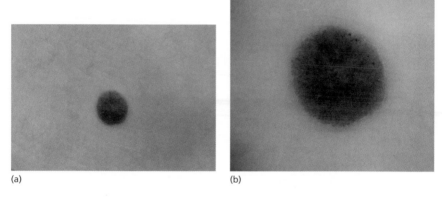

(a)   (b)

Figure 70.22 (a) Pigmented Spitz naevus. (b) Dermoscopic image of a pigmented Spitz naevus showing a well-circumscribed symmetrical nodule with a papillomatous surface and various shades of brown pigmentation. Also seen are locally distributed brownish dots and globules and white perpendicular lines in the centre of the lesion.

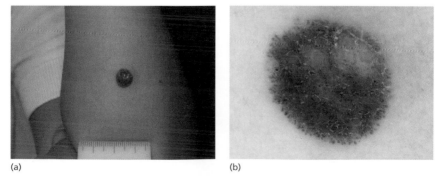

(a)   (b)

Figure 70.23 Atypical Spitz tumour. (a) Asymmetrical nodule with heterogeneous pigmentation. (b) Dermoscopic image of the symmetrical, peripheral distribution of pigmented streaks and heterogeneous pigmentation with bluish/black and whitish hue. (Source: Courtesy of Dr I. Zalaudek, Skin Cancer Unit Arcispedale Santa Maria Nuova – IRCCS Reggio Emilia, Italy.)

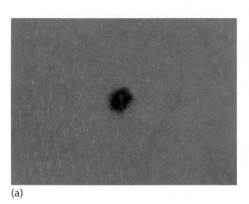
(a)

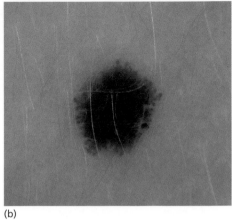
(b)

Figure 70.24 Reed naevus. (a) Darkly pigmented symmetrical macule. (b) Dermoscopic image showing a 'starburst' pattern with diffuse blue-black pigmentation and symmetrically distributed radial streaks in the periphery.

Clinically atypical naevi

(Syn. Dysplastic naevus, Clark naevus, familial atypical multiple mole melanoma syndrome (FAMMM), dysplastic naevus syndrome (DNS), atypical naevus syndrome (ANS))

Clinically atypical naevi are currently considered a distinct subgroup of naevi. Although they are benign lesions, they exhibit clinicopathological characteristics that may resemble early radial growth phase melanomas and are a risk factor of melanoma. For the purposes of this chapter, the term 'atypical naevus' is used as a clinical description, while 'dysplastic naevus' is used as a histological one.

Epidemiology

Typically appear during childhood and become more prominent in puberty. They are more prevalent under 30–40 years of age, probably as a portion of them regress later in life.

The frequency among melanoma patients is higher, ranging from 34% to 59%. Melanoma risk seems to depend on the number of atypical naevi, and on personal and family history of melanoma. Ten or more atypical moles is reported to confer a 12-fold risk of melanoma.

In the setting of melanoma kindreds with increased numbers of atypical naevi and multiple common naevi (FAMMM, DNS, ANS), the relative risk for melanoma is even greater, reaching 85-fold in melanoma-prone family members with dysplastic naevi (Figure 70.28).

Pathophysiology

Family history, sunburn <20 years old. Dysplastic naevi retain their ability to proliferate for an extended period before their maturation, resulting in a larger size and irregular shape and pigmentation compared with common naevi. According to the World Health Organization, a histological diagnosis of dysplastic naevus requires the presence of both major and at least two minor criteria. The major criteria are (i) the basilar proliferation of atypical naevomelanocytes (extending in at least three rete ridges or 'pegs' beyond any dermal naevocellular component) and (ii) the organisation of this proliferation in a lentiginous or epithelioid cell pattern. The minor criteria include (i) the presence of lamellar fibrosis or concentric eosinophilic fibrosis, (ii) neovascularisation, (iii) an inflammatory response and (iv) the fusion of rete ridges.

PART 10: NEOPLASTIC, PROLIFERATIVE AND INFILTRATIVE DISORDERS AFFECTING THE SKIN

PART 10: NEOPLASTIC, PROLIFERATIVE AND INFILTRATIVE DISORDERS AFFECTING THE SKIN

Table 70.9 Blue naevi

Subtype	Epidemiology	Pathological characteristics	Clinical features	Dermoscopy
Common blue naevus (Figure 70.25)	0.5–4% prevalence in white populations Children and young adults, but can occur at any age	Spindle or dendritic melanocytes within the dermis, containing pigment even deeply in the dermis	Blue-black or deep blue dome-shaped papule, with a diameter <1–2 cm Face, scalp, dorsal extremities, buttocks	Structureless, homogeneous, diffuse blue, blue-grey to steel blue pattern
Cellular blue naevus (Figure 70.26)	F > M Multiple epitheliod blue naevi associated with LAMB syndrome	Dermal naevus cells are more numerous and extend into the deep reticular dermis or to subcutaneous fat	Same as common blue naevus; usually larger diameter	Similar to blue naevus; may have pale or yellowish periphery
Deep penetrating naevus		Extension of naevus cells deep into the dermis with a wedge shape	Larger than common blue naevus, may show diffuse and irregular lateral margin Head and neck	Negative globular pattern with blue-brown homogeneous pigmentation
Malignant blue naevus (Figure 70.27) (management as for melanoma, Chapter 81)	Very rare Fourth decade M > F No difference in prognosis to other types of melanoma	A melanoma that arises in association with a blue naevus (usually cellular)	Deep-blue or black ulcerating nodule or plaque Scalp commonest site	

LAMB, lentigines, atrial myxomas, mucocutaneous myxomas and blue naevi.

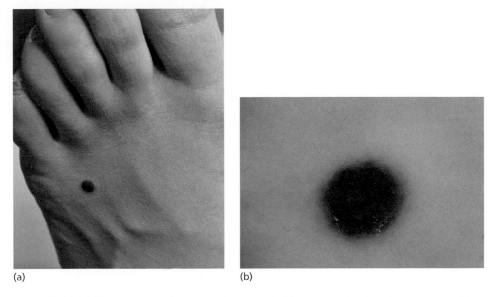

(a)   (b)

Figure 70.25 (a) Blue naevus. (b) Dermoscopic image of a blue naevus showing a homogeneous blue pattern.

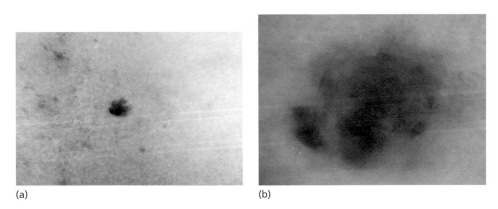

(a)   (b)

Figure 70.26 (a) Cellular blue naevus. (b) Dermoscopic image of a cellular blue naevus showing a well-circumscribed, protuberant nodule with homogeneous dark blue pigmentation and randomly distributed whitish zones corresponding histopathologically to fibrosis.

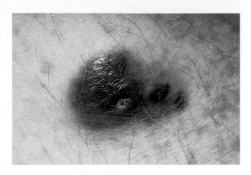

Figure 70.27 Malignant blue naevus that has arisen in a previous cellular blue naevus. This lesion subsequently metastasised to the lymph nodes.

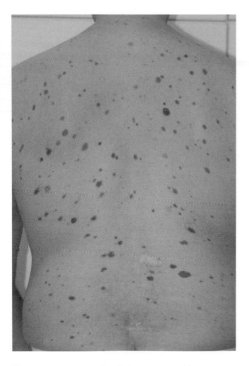

Figure 70.28 Dysplastic naevus syndrome: multiple clinically atypical naevi on the back. The lower surgical scar on the sacral area corresponds to a previously removed superficial spreading melanoma. The patient also had a second primary melanoma on the scalp.

Although a clinically atypical naevus usually exhibits histological dysplasia, and vice versa, this is not always the case.

Clinical features

Atypical naevi are larger than 5 mm with irregular borders and pigmentation (Figure 70.29). They sometimes present with a reddish hue that corresponds to a degree of inflammation. A central papular component is often surrounded by a macular periphery, so that the naevus has a 'fried egg' appearance.

Differential diagnosis

Benign melanocytic naevi, *in situ* or early radial growth phase melanoma.

Investigations

Dermoscopic features that can be seen in atypical naevi vary. It is usual to note an atypical or irregular pigmentation network, irregularly distributed and shaped brown globules and dots, as well as areas of regression (Figure 70.29, right-hand images).

Management

There are currently no data to support the notion that atypical naevi are more likely to progress to melanomas than common naevi; atypical naevi are viewed as risk markers for melanomas rather than true precursor lesions.

There is no need to excise for prophylactic reasons. Patients with atypical naevi, especially those with high numbers of atypical and common naevi and/or a personal or family history of melanoma, are at high risk for melanoma development. These patients should be taught to self-examine and be counselled on sun protection. Skin surveillance including a full skin examination, dermoscopy and photographic recording (either by digital dermoscopic imaging or by total body photography) should be performed. There is no consensus on the frequency of follow-up visits or on the overall time period of surveillance for individual lesions. In the case of particularly atypical lesions, complete surgical excision with a 2–3 mm clinical margin and subsequent histological examination to rule out melanoma *in situ* or early melanoma should be performed.

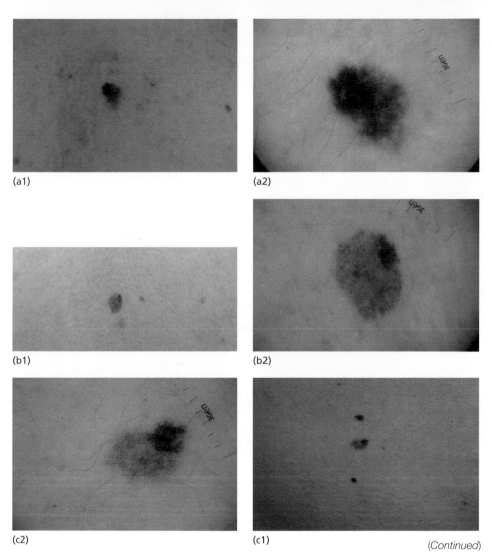

(a1) (a2)

(b1) (b2)

(c2) (c1)

(Continued)

Figure 70.29 (a)–(e) Clinically atypical naevi of variable shapes, sizes and pigmentary patterns (on the left) and their corresponding dermoscopic images (on the right). (Source: (c) and (e) courtesy of Dr D. Sgouros, Andreas Sygros Hospital, Athens, Greece.)

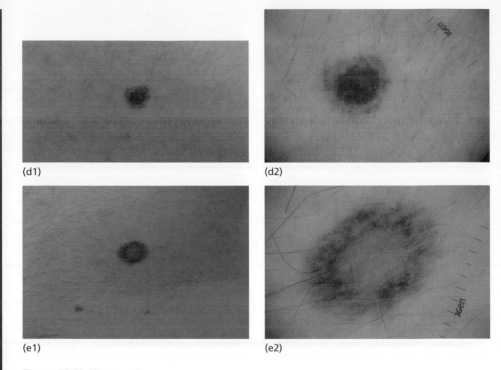

(d1)

(d2)

(e1)

(e2)

Figure 70.29 (Continued)

Benign keratinocytic acanthomas and proliferations

71

BENIGN KERATINOCYTIC ACANTHOMAS

Benign keratinocytic keratoses and acanthomas are a group of benign discrete epidermal proliferative disorders.

Seborrhoeic keratosis

(Syn. Seborrhoeic wart, senile wart, basal cell papilloma)
Seborrhoeic keratoses (SK) are usually asymptomatic with pleomorphic features and are more common in the elderly.

Epidemiology
In Australia, SKs were identified in 30% of subjects under the age of 30 years increasing to 100% of subjects older than 50 years. In UK they were found in 75% of subjects over the age of 70 years. Equal sex incidence.

Pathophysiology
Sunlight has been implicated in the causation. *FGFR3* mutations are present in flat SKs.

The three pathological variants are solid, hyperkeratotic and reticular. The solid SK is the most common and displays a mass of immature keratinocytes seen mainly above the level of the surrounding epidermis. The hyperkeratotic variety is rare and may be clinically mistaken for an actinic keratosis. The reticular form is composed of strands of keratinocytes; this type is frequently seen as a flat lesion on the face.

Clinical features
Usually asymptomatic but may be pruritic. Any body site but most frequently on the face and upper trunk. SKs can be pedunculated or acanthotic, smooth surfaced, domed or heavily pigmented, size varies from 1 mm to several centimetres. The surface has numerous plugged follicular orifices, giving an almost cerebriform appearance (Figure 71.1). The superficial verrucous plaques vary from dirty yellow to black in colour and may have a typical 'stuck-on' appearance with loosely adherent greasy keratin on the surface. Irritation or infection causes bleeding, oozing and crusting, and a deepening of the colour due to inflammation, signs that may indicate subsequent spontaneous resolution.

The rapid development of large numbers of SKs can occur in patients with an inflammatory dermatosis, e.g. eczema, or in association with underlying malignancies where it is known as the sign of Leser–Trélat (gastric and colon cancer). It may be associated with the development of acanthosis nigricans.

Rook's Dermatology Handbook, First Edition. Edited by Christopher E. M. Griffiths, Tanya O. Bleiker, Daniel Creamer, John R. Ingram and Rosalind C. Simpson.
© 2022 John Wiley & Sons Ltd. Published 2022 by John Wiley & Sons Ltd.

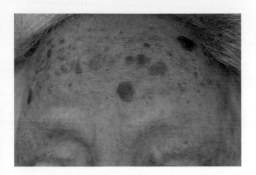

Figure 71.1 Cerebriform appearance of SK.

Clinical variants
Dermatosis papulosa nigra: More common in females and among African Americans and South-East Asians. Clinically, black or dark brown, flat or cupuliform papules (Figure 71.2) 1–5 mm in diameter on the cheeks and forehead. Lesions steadily increase in frequency, number and size after the first decade.

Inverted follicular keratosis (endophytic seborrheic keratosis): Clinically a solitary papule on the head and neck area. Occurring in middle aged and elderly with male predominance. A number arise as a result of infection of the infundibulum of the hair follicle by human papillomavirus (HPV). It may reach a considerable size, and be inflamed and pruritic. Local surgical excision is generally needed, for both diagnostic and therapeutic purposes.

Stucco keratosis: Small, scaly, white or greyish keratotic plaques with a stuck-on appearance predominantly on the lower legs.

Differential diagnosis
Lentigo maligna, actinic keratosis, melanocytic naevi, malignant melanoma, pigmented basal cell carcinomas.

Investigations
The main dermoscopic features of an SK are cerebriform pattern, comedo-like openings, milia-like cysts, moth-eaten border, finger-print structure and hairpin vessels (Figure 71.3). Diagnostic biopsy may be required.

Management
Treatment for symptoms or cosmetic reasons: curettage or cryotherapy.

Warty dyskeratoma

A rare benign skin tumour usually presenting as a solitary papule or nodule.

Pathophysiology
Viral infection, smoking, autoimmunity and UV light have been associated.

Distinct histopathological features include dyskeratotic cells, suprabasal clefting, acantholysis and an overlying keratinous plug.

Clinical features
A pruritic solitary lesion with a central keratotic plug on the head or neck of middle-aged or elderly persons. Other symptoms include recurrent foul-smelling cheesy discharge or bleeding on trauma.

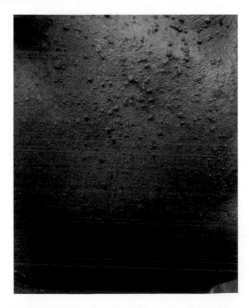

Figure 71.2 Cupuliform papules of dermatosis papulosa nigra.

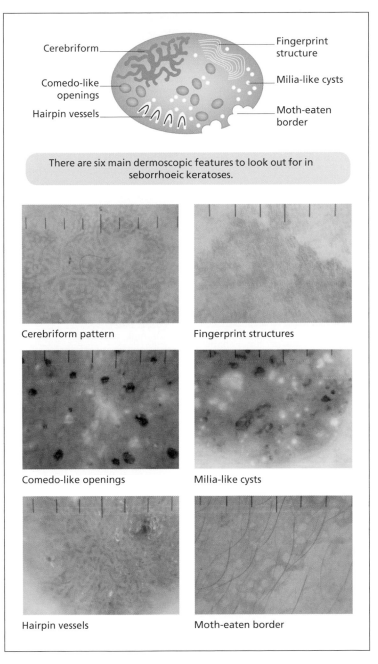

Figure 71.3 There are six main dermoscopic features of SK: (a) cerebriform pattern, (b) fingerprint structures, (c) comedo-like openings, (d) milia-like cysts, (e) hairpin vessels and (f) moth-eaten border. (Source: Reproduced from Jonathan Bowling, Diagnostic Dermoscopy: The Illustrated Guide, 2012. © Jonathan Bowling, John Wiley & Sons, with permission from the copyright holder Dr Jonathan Bowling, Department of Dermatology, Oxford University Hospitals NHS Trust, Oxford, UK.)

PART 10: NEOPLASTIC, PROLIFERATIVE AND INFILTRATIVE DISORDERS AFFECTING THE SKIN

Differential diagnosis

Squamous cell carcinoma, actinic keratosis, basal cell carcinoma and Darier disease.

Management

Excision or curettage.

Clear cell acanthoma

An asymptomatic benign lesion of unknown aetiology.

Epidemiology

Middle-aged to elderly adults.

Pathophysiology

Characteristic histology shows psoriasiform acanthosis with pale periodic acid–Schiff (PAS) positive glycogen-rich keratinocytes (clear cells).

Clinical features

An asymptomatic, red-brown, dome-shaped, solitary papule or nodule on the lower leg, often covered by a thin collarette of scale. Slow-growing, 3–20 mm in size. Giant, pedunculated, atypical, cystic and pigmented patterns may be seen (Figure 71.4).

Differential diagnosis

Actinic or SK, viral warts, pyogenic granulomas, dermatofibromas, eccrine poromas, clear cell hidradenoma, non-melanoma skin cancers and metastatic cancer.

Investigations

Classical dermoscopy is of prominently dilated pinpoint capillary loops ('bunch of grapes' appearance) and reticular or linear patterns.

Management

Excision is only done to exclude more sinister pathology otherwise benign and no treatment required.

Lichenoid keratosis

A common benign solitary asymptomatic lesion on the trunk or distal upper extremities.

Pathophysiology

Epidermal acanthosis, parakeratosis and a band-like lichenoid lymphocyte infiltrate.

Clinical features

Pink to violaceous to hyperpigmented scaly patch on the head and neck, trunk or distal upper extremities.

Differential diagnosis

Basal cell carcinoma, Bowen disease, lentigo simplex, SK, actinic keratosis and melanoma.

Management

Excision for small lesions, curettage or cryotherapy.

OTHER BENIGN PROLIFERATIONS

Skin tags

(Syn. Soft warts, achrochordon, fibroepithelial polyp)
A common benign lesion composed of loose fibrous tissue and occurring mainly on the neck and major flexures as a small soft pedunculated protrusion.

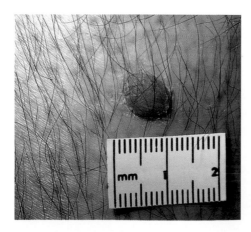

Figure 71.4 Clear cell acanthoma on lower leg.

Epidemiology

Associated with abnormal lipid profile, type 2 diabetes, cardiovascular disease and obesity.

Pathophysiology

Attenuated epidermis, the basal cell layer is flat and often hyperpigmented. The protruding mass is composed of loose fibrous tissue. This is connected to the skin by a narrow pedicle.

Clinical features

Pedunculated, soft, skin-coloured or hyperpigmented. The most common sites are the sides of the neck, axillae and groins.

Differential diagnosis

Melanocytic naevi and neurofibromas are larger.

Management

Snip excision, cautery and cryotherapy.

Epidermoid cyst

(Syn. Epithelial cyst)
Cyst containing keratin and its breakdown products surrounded by an epidermoid wall.

Epidemiology

The commonest cutaneous cyst, most frequently seen in young and middle-aged adults.

Pathophysiology

Due to squamous metaplasia in a damaged sebaceous gland. The result of inflammation around a pilosebaceous follicle. Multiple cysts can be seen in acne vulgaris. May result from deep implantation of a fragment of epidermis by a blunt penetrating injury (inclusion cysts). Those that occur as a part of Gardner and Gorlin syndromes are probably caused by a developmental defect.

Clinical features

Commonly seen on the face and upper trunk (Figure 72.1). Yellowish, white or skin-coloured, firm, smooth, mobile lesions, ranging from a few millimetres to >5 cm. They are tethered to the epidermis and may have a central punctum. Solitary but occasionally multiple. They enlarge slowly and may become inflamed and tender.

Traumatic inclusion cysts usually occur on the palmar or plantar surfaces, buttock or knee. There may be a history of penetrating injury. Suppuration may occur, which leads to an offensive smelling discharge. Rupture of the cyst wall causes intense inflammation.

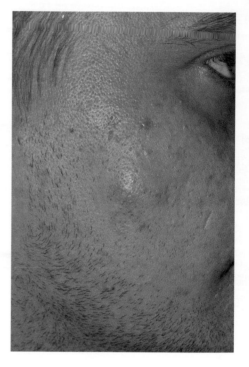

Figure 72.1 An epidermoid cyst on the cheek.

Differential diagnosis

Trichilemmal cysts are usually situated on the scalp and do not have a punctum. Lipomas are soft in their consistency.

Management

Uncomplicated cysts may not require treatment. Non-inflamed cysts can be dissected out, the cyst capsule must be completely removed to ensure that the cyst does not recur.

Rook's Dermatology Handbook, First Edition. Edited by Christopher E. M. Griffiths, Tanya O. Bleiker, Daniel Creamer, John R. Ingram and Rosalind C. Simpson.
© 2022 John Wiley & Sons Ltd. Published 2022 by John Wiley & Sons Ltd.

An inflamed cyst is better incised and drained. Oral antibiotics may be required if signs of infection are present. Inflamed acne cysts may respond to intralesional triamcinolone.

Trichilemmal cyst

(Syn. Pilar cyst)
Trichilemmal cysts contain keratin and its breakdown products. They are usually situated on the scalp.

Epidemiology
5–10% of keratinous cysts. More common in middle age. F > M.

Pathophysiology
Occasionally autosomal dominant. Trichilemmal cysts are lined by stratified squamous epithelium.

Clinical features
These are usually multiple, occur on the scalp and present as smooth, mobile, firm and rounded nodules. Unlike epidermoid cysts, there is usually no punctum.

Inflamed cysts may become tender and the cyst wall can rupture following an infection. The cyst wall may fuse with the epidermis to form a crypt (marsupialised cyst), which can occasionally terminate by discharging its contents and healing spontaneously or form a soft cutaneous horn.

Proliferating trichilemmal tumours are uncommon solitary, multilobular, large, exophytic masses with a predilection for the scalp in elderly females.

Differential diagnosis
Epidermoid cyst.

Management
Excision if treatment wanted.

Steatocystoma multiplex

An uncommon autosomal dominant condition presenting as multiple dermal cysts.

Epidemiology
Presentation is usually in adulthood with lesions appearing around puberty.

Pathophysiology
Most likely to be a genetically determined failure of canalisation between the sebaceous lobules and the follicular pore. Keratin 17 mutations have been implicated. The cyst is situated in the mid-dermis with a thin wall composed of keratinising epithelium without a granular layer. The contents are composed of the unsplit esters (precursors) of sebum.

Clinical features
Multiple, smooth, skin-coloured to yellowish, compressible dermal papules and nodules. Size varies from a few millimetres to 20 mm or more (Figure 72.2). The trunk and proximal limbs are most commonly involved, particularly the presternal area. Lesions may also appear on the face and acral sites. No punctum is usually present, but there may be widespread comedones; differentiation from acne can be difficult. If pricked, an oily fluid can be expressed. Association is with eruptive villous hair cysts and pachyonychia congenita type 2.

Differential diagnosis
Acne, vellous hair cysts.

Management
In most cases treatment is not needed.

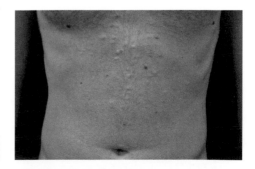

Figure 72.2 Multiple skin-coloured cysts of steatocystoma multiplex.

PART 10: NEOPLASTIC, PROLIFERATIVE AND INFILTRATIVE DISORDERS AFFECTING THE SKIN

First line: Excision. Puncturing and content evacuation can be helpful if cosmetically an issue.
Second line: Isotretinoin. Carbon dioxide laser.

Milium

Milia are isolated or grouped small uniform spherical white papules with a smooth non-umbilicated top.

Epidemiology
Common at all ages. 40–50% of newborns.

Pathophysiology
Small subepidermal keratin cysts. Lesions may be idiopathic or secondary to second-degree burns, epidermolysis bullosa, porphyria cutanea tarda, bullous lichen planus, dermabrasion, topical corticosteroid-induced atrophy and radiotherapy.

The milial cyst has a stratified squamous epithelial lining with a granular layer. The white milium body is composed of lamellated keratin.

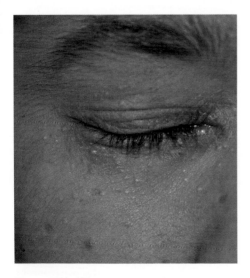

Figure 72.3 Milia on the periorbital area.

Clinical features
Firm, white or yellowish, rarely more than 1–2 mm, usually on the cheeks and eyelids (Figure 72.3).
Milia en plaque appear as a cluster of milia on an erythematous, oedematous base. These are most commonly seen in the post-auricular area.

Management
First line: Incision of the overlying epidermis and expressing the contents is curative. Spontaneous resolution occurs in many milia in infants.
Second line: Laser ablation. Electrodessication. Topical tretinoin.

Eruptive vellus hair cyst

(Syn. Vellus hair cyst)
Occlusion and cystic dilatation of vellus hair follicles.

Epidemiology
Relatively rare, benign lesions. More frequent in pachonychia congenita. Mainly seen in the second decade. In familial cases, lesions present at birth or early infancy.

Pathophysiology
Cysts are located in the mid-dermis and are lined by squamous epithelium. They contain vellus hair and keratin debris. Biopsies from some lesions show features indistinguishable from steatocystoma, with absence of vellus hairs.

Clinical features
Small red or brown papules on the chest. They are usually multiple. Dermoscopy displays an erythematous maroon halo with occasional irregular radiating capillaries at the periphery, vellus hairs can be identified opening onto the epidermis.

Management
Treatments include topical retinoids, curettage and laser therapy. Spontaneous resolution has been reported in 25% of lesions.

Lymphocytic infiltrates

73

Pseudolymphoma

(Syn. Cutaneous lymphoid hyperplasia)
Benign T- or B-cell lymphoid proliferations in the dermis; may be difficult to distinguish from a low-grade malignant lymphoma and rarely transform to lymphoma. B-cell pseudolymphoma is also called lymphocytoma cutis.

Epidemiology
More common <40 years. Lymphocytoma cutis F:M 2:1.

Pathophysiology
Both B- and T-cell pseudolymphomas may occur in tattoos as a reaction to certain pigments or after vaccination, trauma, or acupuncture.

B-cell pseudolymphoma may be associated with infections, e.g. *Borrelia burgdorferi*, *Leishmania*, molluscum contagiosum and herpes zoster.

T-cell pseudolymphomas may be caused by scabies or arthropod bites, as an adverse drug reaction (e.g. anticonvulsants, angiotensin-converting enzyme inhibitors, β-blockers, cytotoxics and antidepressants) or by persistent contact dermatitis.

A lymphoid proliferation is present; usually nodular in B-cell and nodular or band-like in T-cell proliferations with minimal atypical cytology. In B-cell proliferations germinal centres may or may not be present. T-cell pseudolymphomas do not usually show significant epidermotropism. T-cell receptor (TCR) and immunoglobulin gene analysis are usually polyclonal. In B cell the epidermis is usually unaffected and often separated by a relatively acellular grenz zone from the dermis

Clinical features
T-cell pseudolymphomas: Solitary or scattered papules, nodules and plaques (Figure 73.1), but can also present as persistent erythema, which may develop into exfoliative erythroderma, particularly when caused by drug reactions or contact dermatitis; there may be lymphadenopathy, low-grade fever, headache, malaise and arthralgia.

B-cell pseudolymphomas: Solitary or grouped, 3–5 cm asymptomatic, erythematous or plum-coloured papules, nodules or plaques, most common on the face, chest and upper extremities (Figure 73.2). Usually asymptomatic, occasionally itchy or tender. Occasionally photosensitive. Cases due to *Borrelia* infection most frequently seen at sites with low skin temperature such as the earlobes, nipples, nose and scrotum.

Differential diagnosis
Cutaneous B- and T-cell lymphoma.

B-cell pseudolymphoma: sarcoidosis, granuloma faciale, rosacea, Jessner's benign lymphocytic infiltrate, discoid lupus erythematosus (LE), polymorphic light eruption and insect bite reactions.

Investigations
Skin biopsy for histology and TCR/immunoglobulin gene rearrangement analysis.

Rook's Dermatology Handbook, First Edition. Edited by Christopher E. M. Griffiths, Tanya O. Bleiker, Daniel Creamer, John R. Ingram and Rosalind C. Simpson.
© 2022 John Wiley & Sons Ltd. Published 2022 by John Wiley & Sons Ltd.

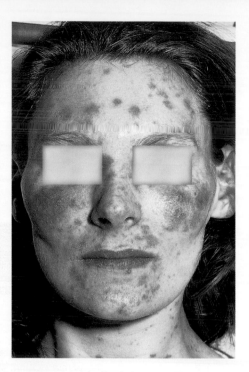

Figure 73.1 Multiple nodules and plaques of T-cell pseudolymphoma affecting the face due to a drug eruption induced by co-trimoxazole.

Borrelia serology and patch test when relevant. Severe drug-induced cases may have eosinophilia and hepatitis.

Management

Remove suspected cause. May take weeks or months to resolve. Drug-induced pseudolymphomas may present months or years after the therapy has been started. Patients with extensive involvement and systemic symptoms may require admission.

Localised disease

First line: Topical steroids for itch, intralesional steroids for solitary small nodules, excision, oral antibiotics if positive borrelia serology.

Second line: Topical 0.1% tacrolius ointment, intralesional interferon-α, intralesional rituximab (B-cell pseudolymphoma), topical photodynamic therapy.

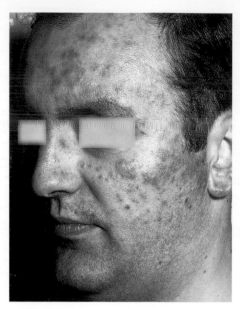

Figure 73.2 Extensive dermal nodules of B-cell pseudolymphoma on the face.

Generalised disease

First line: Hydroxychloroquine.

Second line: Subcutaneous interferon-α, thalidomide.

Pityriasis lichenoides

Pityriasis lichenoides is divided into pityriasis lichenoides chronica (PLC) and pityriasis lichenoides et varioliformis acuta (PLEVA or Mucha–Habermann disease). The distinction between these is based on clinical morphology and histology rather than disease course. Febrile ulceronecrotic Mucha–Habermann disease (FUMHD) is a rare and aggressive form.

Epidemiology

PLC is the most common type. Both PLEVA and PLC last on average 18 months with an episodic course. Seasonal peaks in autumn and winter. More frequent in children and young adults. FUMHD occurs in the second or third decade with male predominance. In PLC M > F in children, M = F in adults.

Pathophysiology

Reported triggers include chemotherapeutic agents, oral contraceptives and astemizole. Infective triggers include toxoplasmosis, cytomegalovirus, Epstein–Barr virus (EBV), varicella-zoster virus, herpes simplex virus, measles and MMR vaccines, streptococci, staphylococci and *Mycoplasma*.

Histology varies with the stage, intensity and extent of the reaction; changes are more severe in PLEVA. In early lesions, an infiltrate of pre-dominantly small lymphocytes surrounds and involves the walls of dilated dermal capillaries. In PLEVA, the infiltrate may be deep, dense and wedge-shaped. The epidermis is oedematous, with an interface dermatitis. Later a parakera-totic scale forms, containing lymphocytic pseudo-Munro abscesses. Mild cytological atypia can be present. If the reaction is more intense, as in FUMHD, frank necrosis is seen.

Clinical features

PLEVA: The eruption develops in crops and so appears polymorphic. Preceding or accompanying constitutional symptoms such as fever, headache, malaise and arthralgia may occur. May cause irritation or burning, but often asymptomatic. An initial oedematous pink papule undergoes central vesiculation and haemorrhagic necrosis. Vesicles may be small or bullous. The trunk, thighs and upper arms, especially the flexor aspects, are chiefly affected, but may be generalised. Lesions of the palms and soles less common; face and scalp often spared. Mucous membranes may be involved. Lesions heal with scarring. Lesions may become infected.

FUHM: In the acute ulceronecrotic form there is high fever and large necrotic lesions (Figure 73.3); new crops may continue to develop over many months. Can be fatal.

PLC: The characteristic lesion is a small, firm, lichenoid papule 3–10 mm in diameter and reddish-brown in colour (Figure 73.4). An adherent 'mica-like' scale can be detached to reveal a shining brown surface, a distinctive diagnostic feature. Over 3–4 weeks, the papule flattens and the scale separates spontaneously to leave a pigmented macule, which gradually fades. Post-inflammatory hypopigmentation may occur,

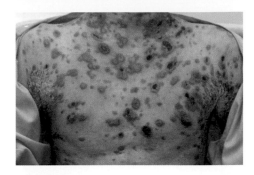

Figure 73.3 Crusted necrotic and ulcerative plaques in a young man with FUMH.

scarring is unusual. Distribution as for PLEVA but an acral and segmental form can occur.

Differential diagnosis

PLEVA: Varicella, vasculitis or pyoderma gangrenosum. Lymphomatoid papulosis is less vesicular with more necrotic papulonodular lesions.

PLC: Guttate psoriasis and lichen planus.

Investigations

Skin biopsy for histology, immunohistochemistry and TCR. FUMH, consider antistreptolysin titre, throat swab, hepatitis, EBV and HIV serology and investigations for *Toxoplasma* infection.

Management

Disease course is variable. Prognosis generally better when onset acute.

PLC

First line: Topical steroids/calcineurin inhibiters.

Second line: In adults UVB, psoralen and ultra-violet A (PUVA), tetracycline, erythromycin. In children erythromycin.

Third line: In adults acitretin (± PUVA), metho-trexate, ciclosporin, dapsone or UVA-1. In children methotrexate, ciclosporin or dapsone.

PLEVA

First line: Erythromycin.

Second line: In adults UVB, PUVA or acitretin plus PUVA. In children UVB.

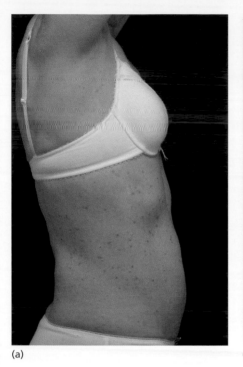

(a)

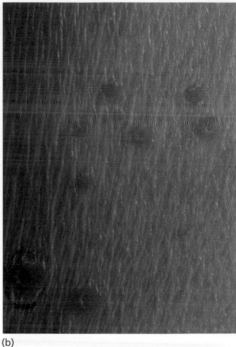

(b)

Figure 73.4 (a) Scattered scaly papules on the trunk in a patient with PLC. (b) Close up of individual lesions of PLC showing the mica-like scale.

Third line: In adults oral steroids, methotrexate, ciclosporin, dapsone or UVA-1. In children oral steroids, methotrexate, ciclosporin or dapsone.

Parapsoriasis

Divided into small and large plaque variants, the term has caused confusion and the synonyms are often preferred. The majority of small plaque parapsoriasis are chronic, benign conditions. In contrast, 11% of patients with large plaque parapsoriasis have been reported to develop mycosis fungoides (MF); whether these cases were MF from the outset remains unclear. Long-term follow-up of these cases is required.

Small Plaque Parapsoriasis
(Syn. Chronic superficial scaly dermatitis, digitate dermatosis)

Epidemiology
Peaks in the fifth decade. M:F 3:1.

Pathophysiology
Histology is non-specific with small focal areas of hyperkeratosis and parakeratosis, with morphologically normal CD4+ T cells in the dermis, mainly around the vasculature. There is no epidermotropism and no Pautrier microabscesses.

Clinical features
Persistent, monomorphic 2.5–5 cm scaly asymptomatic round/oval erythematous plaques, mainly on the trunk. Digitate dermatosis consists of finger-like projections on the lateral aspects of the chest and abdomen (Figure 73.5). Can persist for years and subsequently resolve spontaneously. May be more obvious during the winter. There is sparing of the pelvic girdle area and it lacks the striking polymorphic appearance of individual patches classically seen in MF.

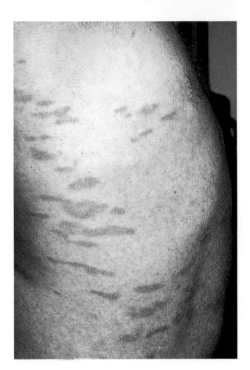

Figure 73.5 Typical pattern of chronic, superficial, scaly dermatosis showing finger-like projections on the sides of the torso.

Differential diagnosis

Discoid eczema, guttate psoriasis, pityriasis versicolor, pityriasis rosea, allergic contact dermatitis, MF.

Investigations

The diagnosis is clinical. A skin biopsy may be required if suspicion of MF.

Management

Often little treatment is needed. Emollients may help scale. PUVA and narrowband UVB phototherapy may result in temporary clearance.

Large Plaque Parapsoriasis

Epidemiology

Slight male predominance.

Pathophysiology

Epidermal atrophy, with a lichenoid or interface reaction at the dermal–epidermal junction and a band-like lymphocytic infiltrate in the papillary dermis. Immunophenotypic studies reveal a normal T-cell phenotype.

Clinical features

Asymptomatic, fixed, large, atrophic, erythematous plaques, usually on trunk and occasionally limbs.

Investigations

Skin biopsy for histology, immunohistochemistry and TCR.

Management

Topical emollients, UVB and PUVA for symptomatic relief. Topical steroids used with caution because of atrophic nature. Monitor in view of the risk of MF.

Jessner's lymphocytic infiltrate

A chronic, benign, inflammatory condition, usually affecting photo-exposed skin.

Epidemiology

Adults < 0 years. Familial cases reported.

Pathophysiology

Not well understood. Controversial as to whether a variant of LE.

The epidermis is usually normal with superficial and deep perivascular dermal mixed polyclonal lymphocytic infiltrate. Direct immunofluorescence (IMF) is negative. Molecular analysis of T and B cells is polyclonal.

Clinical features

Asymptomatic, non-scaly, erythematous papules and plaques, mainly on the face, neck and upper chest. One or more lesions often with central clearing, giving an annular appearance (Figure 73.6). Lesions may last months or years; often resolve spontaneously but can recur, either at the same or a different site.

Differential diagnosis

Polymorphic light eruption, LE and B-cell pseudolymphoma.

Investigations

Skin biopsy for histology, direct IMF and TCR. Consider antinuclear antibody, ESR, anti-Ro and anti-La antibodies, FBC and urinalysis. Phototesting if photosensitive.

Management

Treatment often unsatisfactory.
First line: Topical or intralesional steroids, hydroxychloroquine, cosmetic camouflage and photoprotection.
Second line: Systemic steroids, cryotherapy or excision of smaller lesions.

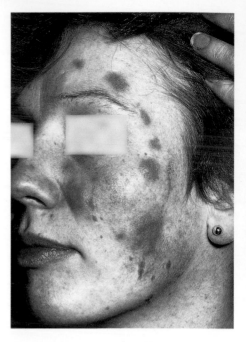

Figure 73.6 Non-scaly erythematous plaques on the face of young woman with Jessner's lymphocytic infiltrate.

Cutaneous histiocytoses 74

Histiocytoses are disorders characterised by abnormal proliferation of dendritic cells and macrophages.

LANGERHANS CELL HISTIOCYTOSIS

Langerhans cell histiocytosis (LCH) is a proliferative disease characterised by excess accumulation of Langerhans cells in various sites, leading to tissue damage. Patients may present with skin, bone, lymph node, pituitary, lung or liver disease.

Epidemiology

A rare disease with an estimated prevalence of 1:50 000 in children under 15 years; most common in 0-4 years. Single system (SS) disease constitutes 70% of paediatric LCH, with bone being the most commonly affected organ and skin in around 10% of SS cases. Multisystem (MS) LCH usually occurs in children less than 2 years old.

In adults, the mean age at diagnosis is 35 years, with 10% being older than 55 years. 69% of adults with LCH have MS disease, with skin and lung involvement in 51% and 62%, respectively.

There is a slight male to female predominance.

Pathophysiology

The clinical heterogeneity of LCH is unified by the histopathology of one abnormal population of LCH cells. LCH cells are round to oval in shape, most commonly found in aggregates and lacking the 'dendritic' morphology. Their nucleus is lobulated, coffee bean or boat shaped, but the most typical LCH nuclei have complex angular and elaborate folds. The cytoplasm is generous and homogeneously pink. CD1a and S100 immunostaining is positive.

Clinical features

The classification of LCH is based on the number of organs involved with an initial subdivision into SS and MS disease.

The appearance of skin lesions in both adults and children is variable with macules, papules, plaques, scales, vesicles, pustules, crusts, bullae and ulcerative lesions (Figure 74.1). The most characteristic cutaneous lesion of LCH in children consists of papulosquamous lesions with greasy scales, affecting the scalp, resembling seborrhoeic dermatitis (Figure 74.2). Other sites include skin folds such as the gluteal cleft and midline of the trunk, but any area can be involved, including the nails. Persistent eruption on the scalp and in skin flexures outside of infancy should raise the suspicion of

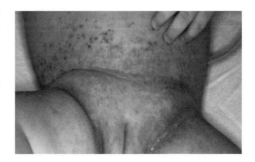

Figure 74.1 LCH showing a polymorphic eruption of papules, vesicles crusts, and telangiectasias affecting the nappy area, including the folds, in an infant.

Rook's Dermatology Handbook, First Edition. Edited by Christopher E. M. Griffiths, Tanya O. Bleiker, Daniel Creamer, John R. Ingram and Rosalind C. Simpson.
© 2022 John Wiley & Sons Ltd. Published 2022 by John Wiley & Sons Ltd.

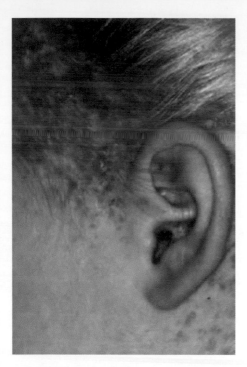

Figure 74.2 LCH showing yellow crusted papules in a seborrhoeic dermatitis distribution in an older child.

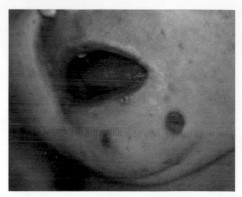

Figure 74.3 Congential self-healing reticulohistiocytosis (Hashimoto–Pritzker disease) showing ulcerated nodules in an infant.

LCH even in the absence of other signs and symptoms. However, unusual persistence of 'cradle cap' or 'nappy rash' even in infancy should suggest the possibility of LCH and warrants a biopsy.

The natural history of paediatric LCH varies from spontaneous regression to a low-grade chronic disease with multiple reactivations and the possibility of significant long-term consequences, to a 'high-risk' disease that can be fatal. In infants from birth to 4 weeks old, skin-only LCH that spontaneously resolves with no other organ involvement is sometimes called Hashimoto–Pritzker disease or congenital self-healing reticulohistiocytosis (Figure 74.3). This form cannot be distinguished from other forms of LCH and all young children with skin-only disease should be carefully observed and the diagnosis of spontaneously regressing disease should only be made retrospectively.

The natural history of LCH in adults is less clear but it is thought that spontaneous regression, even in SS disease, is less likely to occur.

In adult LCH, survival rates of patients with SS disease approach 100%. The survival of adult patients with MS disease, including skin, is better than that seen in children due to the lower number of organs involved.

Skin LCH as part of low-risk multisystem disease, is formerly known as Hand–Schüller–Christian syndrome, a chronic, multifocal form of LCH characterised by lytic bone lesions, exophthalmos, diabetes insipidus and skin lesions. There is a later age of onset between 2 and 6 years.

Skin involvement as part of disseminated disease previously known as Letterer–Siwe disease, is the most extensive and severe form of LCH. Less than 15% of paediatric cases; usually seen under the age of 2 years, often in the neonatal period. The skin is involved in 75–100% of cases, manifesting as a typical seborrhoea-like pattern in the scalp and nappy area, but any part of the body may be affected. Multiple organs are involved including the bones, liver, spleen, lungs, central nervous system (CNS) and bone marrow. This form carries the worst prognosis, is the least likely to resolve spontaneously and always requires systemic therapy.

Differential diagnosis

Dermatophytoses, mastocytosis and scabies. Herpes simplex and herpes zoster for vesicular lesions. The nappy area and retroauricular involvement are often confused with seborrhoeic dermatitis. In adults differentials include hidradenitis suppurativa, extra-mammary Paget disease and Darier disease.

Investigations

Box 74.1 details the investigations that should be conducted on all suspected cases and the indication for more specialised investigations in some patients.

Box 74.1 Investigating patients with LCH

Investigations on all patients

- Full blood count
- U&E, LFT, CRP, ESR, coagulation studies
- Skeletal survey (Figure 74.4)
- Chest X-ray
- Biopsy of site(s) of involvement

Tests indicated in some patients

- MRI of the brain if lytic skull lesions, diabetes insipidus, symptoms suggestive of CNS involvement
- Water deprivation test if polyuria, polydipsia
- High-resolution CT of chest if adult smoker, respiratory symptoms
- Lung function tests if lung involvement
- Abdominal ultrasound, liver biopsy if abnormal liver function tests

---

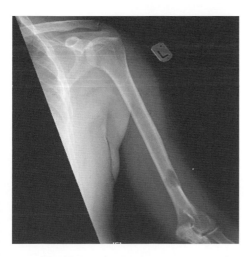

Figure 74.4 Radiograph of a humerus showing a typical punched-out lytic lesion of bone LCH.

Management

Treatment is based on the extent and severity of disease. Management guidelines are updated regularly by the Histiocyte Society.

Paediatrics: With skin-only LCH, patients can be observed and therapy given only if there is pain, bleeding and/or ulceration. If treatment is required, topical corticosteroids are first line; other options include topical pimecrolimus or tacrolimus, narrow-band UVB and PUVA.

Systemic chemotherapy is usually indicated for skin involvement as part of MS LCH. The most commonly used protocol is a combination of vinblastine and prednisolone. Progression of disease after 6 weeks of therapy is a very poor prognostic sign and mandates a change to a salvage protocol and possibly even a reduced intensity conditioning haematopoietic stem cell transplant.

Adults: Possible therapies for skin LCH in adults include surgery for limited disease, topical, e.g. high potency or intralesional corticosteroids, ultraviolet light (UVB or PUVA), radiation or systemic therapy (e.g. methotrexate, vinblastine/steroid combination). Relapse of skin LCH following discontinuation of therapy is common, but the disease often responds again to reintroduction; prolonged therapy and a slow taper may be required.

NON-LANGERHANS CELL HISTIOCYTOSES

The non-Langerhans cell histiocytoses (non-LCHs) are a diverse group of disorders defined by the accumulation of histiocytes that do not meet the phenotypical criteria for the diagnosis of LCH. The non-LCHs are generally benign proliferative disorders, which can be classified according to their dendritic or non-dendritic cell origin (Table 74.1).

Table 74.1 Non-Langerhans cell histiocytoses

Dendritic cell origin

Disorders with mainly skin involvement with/
without a systemic component
Juvenile xanthogranuloma
Benign cephalic histiocytosis
Generalised eruptive histiocytosis
Papular xanthoma
Progressive nodular histiocytosis
Xanthoma disseminatum
Diffuse plane xanthomatosis
Disorders in which skin may be involved but
the systemic component predominates
Erdheim–Chester disease

Non dendritic cell origin

Disorders with mainly skin involvement with/
without a systemic component
Reticulohistiocytoma
Familial sea-blue histiocytosis
Hereditary progressive mucinous
histiocytosis
Malakoplakia
Necrobiotic xanthogranuloma
Disorders in which skin may be involved but
the systemic component predominates
Multicentric reticulohistiocytosis
Sinus histiocytosis with massive
lymphadenopathy

Juvenile xanthogranuloma

A benign proliferative disorder of histiocytes occurring in early infancy and childhood that spontaneously regresses.

Epidemiology

Normally presents during first year of life. There is a male preponderance (M:F 12:1) in children with multiple skin lesions. Ten times more common in white than in black children.

Juvenile xanthogranuloma (JXG) has been associated with neurofibromatosis type 1 (NF1) and juvenile myelomonocytic leukaemia. Patients with JXG and NF1 have a significantly higher risk of developing myeloid leukaemia than normal.

Pathophysiology

Characterised histologically by a dense infiltrate of small histiocytes in the dermis, which stain positively for factor XIIIa, CD68, CD163, CD14 and fascin. Stains for S100 and CD1a are negative. Touton giant cells, seen in 85% of JXG cases, can be distinguished by the characteristic wreath of nuclei around a homogenous eosinophilic centre and prominent xanthomatisation in the periphery.

Clinical features

Cutaneous lesions are the most common presentation of JXG. It presents with single to multiple firm, reddish-yellow papules or nodules (Figure 74.5), with a predilection for the face, head and neck, followed by the upper torso and upper and lower extremities. Single lesions are the most common, but multiple lesions, ranging from a few to hundreds, may occur, particularly in male infants. Systemic involvement occurs in 4% of children, mostly during infancy. Almost half of the patients have no skin lesions. The most common site is a solitary mass in the deep soft tissues (deep JXG) followed by the liver, spleen, lung and CNS. Most systemic lesions undergo spontaneous resolution, but ocular and CNS involvement lead to significant complications. Recognition of eye JXG is important for the prevention of vision loss.

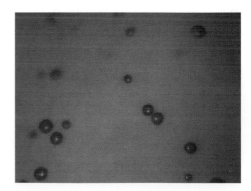

Figure 74.5 JXG showing multiple, disseminated, yellow papules.

JXG, either cutaneous or systemic, usually follows a benign course with spontaneous resolution of lesions within 1 to 5 years. Long-term sequelae are rarely reported. However, CNS involvement may result in significant morbidity with seizures, ataxia, increased intracranial pressure, subdural effusions, developmental delay, diabetes insipidus and other neurological deficits.

Investigations

The diagnosis of JXG is made on immunohistochemistry. Extensive work-up should be reserved for those with clinical suspicion of systemic involvement.

Management

The management of JXG depends upon the site(s) of involvement. Most childhood lesions will resolve spontaneously and do not require treatment; occasionally resolution may result in a scar. Surgical excision may be indicated in some. Ophthalmological surveillance is recommended for high-risk patients less than 2 years of age, who should undergo screening at diagnosis and every 3–6 months until aged 2. For systemic JXG, most incorporate LCH-based agents such as vinblastine, prednisolone and/or methotrexate, but response to chemotherapy is unpredictable.

Benign cephalic histiocytosis

A rare, self-limiting histiocytic disorder. Many consider benign cephalic histiocytosis (BCH) as a clinical variant or a milder form of JXG without systemic involvement. Mean age of onset of 15 months; patients present with asymptomatic, erythematous, brown macules/papules/nodules on the cheeks that spread to the forehead, earlobes and neck (Figure 74.6). Extension onto the trunk, upper limbs and rarely buttocks may be seen. No treatment is required.

Generalised eruptive histiocytosis

A rare cutaneous histiocytosis that mainly affects adults. The disease presents as asymptomatic, multiple, symmetrical, small,

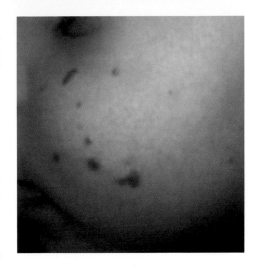

Figure 74.6 BCH showing multiple, asymptomatic, reddish brown papules on the face of a toddler.

red-brown papules on the face, trunk and arms, usually sparing the flexures (Figure 74.7). The characteristic feature of generalised eruptive histiocytosis (GEH) is the rapid appearance of a crop of lesions, which resolve spontaneously or leave a macular area of hyperpigmentation. GEH must be distinguished from the eruptive histiocytomas associated with hyperlipidaemia. The

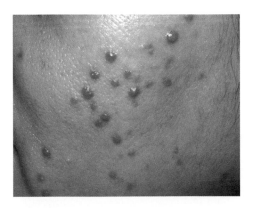

Figure 74.7 GEH showing multiple, small, symmetrical, red-brown papules in an adult. (Source: Courtesy of Dr S. Walsh, Sunnybrook Hospital, Toronto, Canada.)

disease is generally self-limiting and often does not require treatment. The evolution of GEH to other non-LCHs has been reported; if lesions become xanthomatoid or flexural or if systemic symptoms develop then patients should be re-biopsied.

Papular xanthoma

A rare histiocytic disorder. Characterised by 2–15 mm yellow or reddish yellow papules/plaques affecting both the skin and mucous membranes. The back and head are the most common locations. Mucosal involvement and risk for disease progression are features of adult presentation. In contrast, spontaneous resolution is the norm in children, with involution starting after weeks or months and being complete in 1–5 years, often leaving anetoderma-like scarring. No effective treatment.

Progressive nodular histiocytosis

A rare variant of non-LCH disorders that affects skin and mucosa. Predominantly seen in adults. Characterised by the progressive appearance of asymptomatic cutaneous lesions, which can result in severe disfigure-

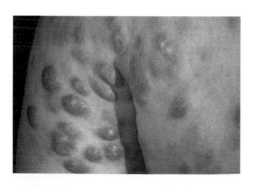

Figure 74.8 Progressive nodular histiocytosis in a 48-year-old man with nodular lesions in the posterior axillary fold. (Source; Courtesy of Professor J.M. Naeyaert, University Hospital, Gent, Belgium.)

ment (Figure 74.8). Superficial papules are 2–10 mm in diameter and yellow-orange, while deep subcutaneous nodules are 1–5 cm in diameter and may be skin coloured or reddish orange due to overlying telangiectasia. Both types of lesions can reach hundreds in numbers. Distribution is random and may also occur in the oral cavity, larynx and conjunctival mucosa. Progressive nodular histiocytosis is not generally associated with systemic involvement or other disorders. There is no effective treatment; large or painful lesions are usually excised.

Xanthoma disseminatum

A rare non-familial disease, characterised by proliferation of histiocytic cells in which lipid deposition is a secondary event, with involvement of the skin, mucous membranes of eyes, upper respiratory tract and meninges.

Epidemiology
Predominantly affects male children and young adults.

Pathophysiology
Thought to be a reactive rather than a neoplastic process, with a pathological immune response triggered by unknown inflammatory triggers. The lesional cell appears to be an inflammatory lipid-laden macrophage with a characteristic foamy appearance.

Clinical features
Patients present with erythematous, yellow brown papules and nodules, symmetrically distributed on the trunk, scalp, face and proximal extremities. The lesions become confluent, especially in flexures, to form xanthomatous plaques, which may become verrucous (Figure 74.9). In 39–60% of patients, the mucous membranes are affected, with particular involvement of the lips, pharynx, larynx, conjunctivae and bronchus. It is a self-limiting disease but may be locally destructive and persist for years. Three clinical patterns have been identified: a rare self-healing form, a chronic, often progressive form and a progressive multiorgan form, which may be fatal.

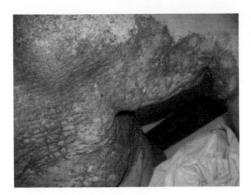

Figure 74.9 Xanthoma disseminatum showing large, yellow-brown plaques affecting the axilla. (Source: Courtesy of Dr S. Walsh, Sunnybrook Hospital, Toronto, Canada.)

Management

Skin lesions are disfiguring and patients often request treatment. Carbon dioxide laser, surgical removal, excision, dermabrasion and electrocoagulation have been used with reported effect. Systemic involvement of lung, liver or CNS requires active treatment but the response to therapy is not predictable and may not be long lasting. Glucocorticoids, chlorambucil, azathioprine and cyclophosphamide have been effective.

Diffuse plane xanthomatosis

A rare, non-lipaemic disease of adults in which xanthomatous lesions develop in the skin in association with paraproteinaemia or an underlying systemic disorder, usually of the haematological or lymphoproliferative type. The condition arises as a result of perivascular deposition of lipoprotein–immunoglobulin complexes.

Patients present with large, flat, plaque-like xanthomatous skin lesions involving the eyelids, neck, upper trunk, buttocks and flexures (Figure 74.10). Serum lipids are usually normal. Multiple myeloma and monoclonal gammopathy are the two most frequently associated diseases and treatment is of the underlying condition.

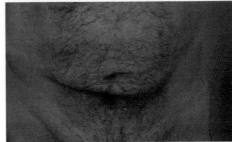

Figure 74.10 Diffuse plane xanthomatosis of 7 years' duration in a 73-year-old man with associated IgG-κ paraprotein.

Necrobiotic xanthogranuloma

A rare, multisystem histiocytic disease strongly associated with haematological malignancy.

Pathophysiology

80–90% of patients have an underlying monoclonal gammopathy of which half are monoclonal gammopathy of uncertain significance and the other half are myeloma, which can manifest years after the skin lesions.

Histologically, confluent granulomatous masses are present as either sheets or nodules, replacing much of the dermis and extending into the subcutaneous tissue. Numerous giant cells are present, with Touton cells and bizarre, angulated giant cells. Less common, but characteristic when present, are palisading cholesterol cleft granulomas and xanthogranulomatous panniculitis.

Clinical features

Slowly progressive, reddish yellow, xanthomatous plaques/nodules that are infiltrative and destructive (Figure 74.11). Over 80% of the lesions are periorbital but may occur on the trunk and limbs where subcutaneous nodules and xanthomatous plaques are present with atrophy and ulceration. The eyes are often affected with conjunctivitis, keratitis, uveitis, iritis and proptosis.

PART 10: NEOPLASTIC, PROLIFERATIVE AND INFILTRATIVE DISORDERS AFFECTING THE SKIN

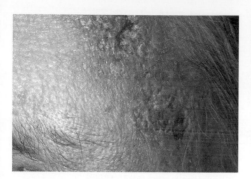

Figure 74.11 Necrobiotic xanthogranuloma showing a reddish yellow, infiltrative plaque with evidence of necrosis. (Source: Courtesy of Dr S. Walsh, Sunnybrook Hospital, Toronto, Canada.)

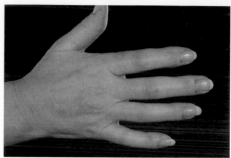

Figure 74.12 Multicentric reticulohistiocytosis. Characteristic 'coral-bead' like lesions along the nail folds. (Source: Courtesy of Dr. T Bleiker.)

Management

Treatment is of the underlying condition.

Multicentric reticulohistiocytosis

Multicentric reticulohistiocytosis is a rare non-LCH disorder characterised by the association of specific nodular skin lesions and destructive arthritis.

Epidemiology

Middle-aged adults, F: M 3:1. 85% of reported adults are white.

Pathophysiology

The characteristic pathological picture is infiltration of mono- and multinucleated giant cells with voluminous ground-glass cytoplasm.

Clinical features

The classic skin lesions are firm brown or yellow papules and plaques, which predominantly affect extensor surfaces, particularly on the hands and forearms. Coral bead-like lesions may occur around the nail folds (Figure 74.12), which may result in nail dystrophy. More than 50% of patients have mucosal involvement, characteristically of the lips and tongue, but it can also affect the mouth, gingiva, pharynx, larynx and sclera.

Two-thirds of patients present with symmetrical polyarthritis of predominantly the hands, followed by the appearance of skin lesions. 15–50% of cases progress to mutilating osteoarthropathy with disabling deformities. Up to 30% of cases may herald an underlying malignancy. 15% of patients have an associated autoimmune disease such as systemic lupus erythematosus, diabetes or Sjogren syndrome.

Disease remission occurs after an average of 7–8 years if there is no underlying malignancy.

Investigation

Screen for underlying malignancy.

Management

The patient is normally managed by both a dermatologist and rheumatologist; any underlying disease should also be treated. There is no consistently effective treatment but there has been success with a variety of agents, including a combination of corticosteroid plus low-dose methotrexate, or other drugs such as cyclophosphamide, ciclosporin, azathioprine, bisphosphonates and anti-TNF agents.

Sinus histiocytosis with massive lymphadenopathy (Rosai–Dorfman disease)

Sinus histiocytosis with massive lymphadenopathy (SHML) is a rare, non-neoplastic disorder of unknown aetiology that is usually self-limiting.

Epidemiology
Most patients are young adults. The disease is slightly more common in males and in black people.

Pathophysiology
Involved lymph nodes show massive sinus infiltration of large histiocytes admixed with lymphocytes and plasma cells. A hallmark of SHML is the presence of emperipolesis (phagocytosis of intact leukocytes, particularly lymphocytes) in histiocytes that express S100, less prominent in the skin than in the nodes.

Clinical features
80% of patients present with bilateral, painless, often cervical lymphadenopathy, which may be associated with fever, malaise, night sweats, weight loss, leukocytosis and hypergammaglobulinaemia. Extranodal involvement is

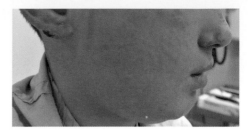

Figure 74.13 Rosai–Dorfman disease showing multiple nodules/tumours with superficial crusting and old scars on the nose.

described in 43% of patients, the skin being the most common (Figure 74.13). Skin lesions are usually yellow but may be violaceous or purple. Macular erythema, papules, nodules or infiltrated plaques have been reported. Other extranodal sites include the lung, urogenital tract, breast, gastrointestinal tract, liver and pancreas.

Management
The outcome is usually good and the disease is often self-limiting. Treatment is only necessary when a vital organ is being compromised or nodal enlargement leads to significant problems such as airway obstruction. Systemic corticosteroids are useful but regrowth often occurs after discontinuation. Up to 10% mortality has been reported.

75

Soft-tissue tumours and tumour-like conditions

FIBROUS AND MYOFIBROBLASTIC TUMOURS

Fibrous papule of the face/nose

A small facial papule with a distinctive fibrovascular component on histological examination.

Epidemiology
Very common. Middle-aged adults.

Pathophysiology
Normal epidermis. In the dermis, there is increased collagen with a hyalinised appearance and scattered, somewhat dilated, vascular channels.

Clinical features
Usually single lesion on the nose. Occasionally occur on the forehead, cheeks, chin or neck and rarely multiple. A dome-shaped, skin-coloured, slightly red or pigmented papule; usually sessile. Mostly asymptomatic, but one-third bleed on minor trauma.

Differential diagnosis
Intradermal melanocytic naevus, basal cell carcinoma.

Management
Shave excision if diagnostic doubt or symptomatic.

Acquired digital fibrokeratoma

A benign lesion on fingers and toes, possibly a reaction to trauma (Figure 75.1).

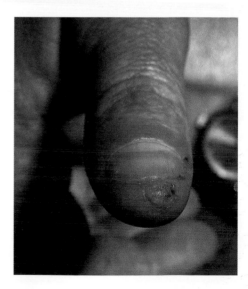

Figure 75.1 Acquired digital fibrokeratoma.

Rook's Dermatology Handbook, First Edition. Edited by Christopher E. M. Griffiths, Tanya O. Bleiker, Daniel Creamer, John R. Ingram and Rosalind C. Simpson.
© 2022 John Wiley & Sons Ltd. Published 2022 by John Wiley & Sons Ltd.

Epidemiology
The incidence is low.

Pathophysiology
The histology shows thick collagen bundles, thin elastic fibres and increased vascularity.

Clinical features
A solitary dome-shaped lesion, with a collarette of slightly raised skin at its base.

Differential diagnosis
Dermatofibroma, viral wart, supernumerary digit and cutaneous horn.

Management
Excision.

Pseudosarcomatous fibromatosis

(Syn. Nodular fasciitis, pseudosarcomatous fasciitis)
A rapidly enlarging subcutaneous neoplasm that histologically resembles a sarcoma.

Epidemiology
Relatively common, more so in young adults but can occur at any age.

Pathophysiology
Histologically may look extremely worrying in view of the high mitotic rate and rapid growth. Composed of bundles of fairly uniform fibroblasts and myofibroblasts with pink cytoplasm, vesicular nuclei and a single small nucleolus.

Clinical features
Tender rapidly growing masses beneath the skin, particularly on the upper extremeties; average size 1–3 cm. Head and neck lesions often present in children.

Management
Simple excision is adequate treatment.

Desmoplastic fibroblastoma

A distinctive subcutaneous fibroblastic tumour consisting of a prominent collagenous stroma.

Epidemiology
Tumours are relatively common. Middle-aged to old adults. M:F 2:1.

Pathophysiology
A well-circumscribed tumour composed of bland elongated or stellate cells, with a background collagenous stroma and focal myxoid change. Mitotic figures rare. Translocation t(2;11)(q31;q12) characteristically found.

Clinical features
Asymptomatic nodule <4 cm, with a predilection for the back and limbs.

Management
Excision.

Palmar and plantar fascial fibromatosis (superficial fibromatoses)

(Syn. Ledderhose disease (plantar), Dupuytren contracture (palmar))
Superficial neoplastic proliferations of fibroblasts and myofibroblasts that have a tendency for local recurrence, but do not metastasise.

Epidemiology
Palmar fibromatosis is more common than plantar fibromatosis.

Middle-aged to elderly patients. M > F. Associations with diabetes, alcoholic liver disease and epilepsy described.

Pathophysiology
Genetic predisposition and trauma thought to play an important role.

Early lesions are fairly cellular and consist of bundles of bland fibroblasts with some collagen deposition. The latter increases in older lesions.

Clinical features
Palmar fibromatosis presents as indurated nodules or as an ill-defined area of thickening, bilateral in about 50% of cases and may result in contracture. Plantar fibromatosis usually consists of a single nodule.

Management
Consider referral to relevant surgical team if symptomatic.

Dermatofibrosarcoma protuberans

Dermatofibrosarcoma protuberans (DFSP) is a locally invasive tumour arising in the dermis and showing fibroblastic differentiation.

Epidemiology

Uncommon but one of the most common dermal sarcomas. Incidence in USA estimated as 4.2 cases per million. More commonly develop during the third and fifth decades. Slight female predilection; more common in black than white patients.

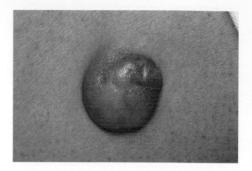

Figure 75.2 Dermatofibrosarcoma protuberans. (Source: Reproduced with permission of Cardiff and Vale University Health Board, Cardiff, UK.)

Pathophysiology

Some cases develop at the site of previous trauma.

Usually a solitary multinodular mass. The dermis and subcutaneous tissue are replaced by bundles of uniform spindle-shaped cells with little cytoplasm and elongated hyperchromatic, but not pleomorphic, nuclei. There is little mitotic activity. Tumour cells infiltrate between collagen bundles of the deeper dermis and blend into the normal dermis, forming a storiform pattern. The subcutaneous tissue is extensively infiltrated and replaced in a typical lace-like pattern. Majority of lesions are CD34 positive. Fibrosarcomatous DFSP is a variant with metastatic potential.

Clinical features

Up to 50% present on the trunk, particularly flexural areas. Involvement of the limbs is usually proximal.

The tumour starts as a plaque, which may occasionally be atrophic. Slow growth over years to become nodules which coalesce and extend, becoming redder or bluish as they enlarge into irregular protuberant swellings (Figure 75.2). The base of the lesion is a hard, indurated plaque of irregular outline. In the later stages, a proportion of lesions become painful and there may be rapid growth, ulceration and discharge.

Differential diagnosis

Histiocytoma, keloid scar, morphoea profunda.

Management

Surgical excision with a margin of between 2 and 4 cm has been recommended. Mohs surgery can reduce the rate of local recurrence and is the preferred treatment in many large centres where there is an experienced pathologist using formalin-fixed paraffin-embedded sections rather than frozen sections.

Local recurrence varies from 15% to 60%. Metastasis is extremely rare but occurs in up to 13% of cases with fibrosarcomatous transformation.

FIBROHISTIOCYTIC TUMOURS

Dermatofibroma

(Syn. Fibrous histiocytoma)
Dermatofibroma (DF) is a benign dermal and often superficial subcutaneous tumour.

Epidemiology

The most common cutaneous soft-tissue tumour often attributed to insect bites.

Young to middle-aged adults; more common in females except cellular and atypical variants, which are more common in males.

Pathophysiology

The overlying epidermis shows a degree of epidermal hyperplasia. In the dermis, there is a localised proliferation of histiocyte-like cells and fibroblast-like cells associated with variable numbers of mononuclear inflammatory cells. A focal storiform pattern is often seen. The tumour blends with the surrounding dermis. Collagen bundles at the periphery of the lesion are surrounded by scattered tumour cells and appear somewhat hyalinised. Older lesions show focal proliferation of small blood vessels in association with haemosiderin deposition and fibrosis.

Variants include cellular, aneurysmal, atypical and epithelioid.

Clinical features

Commonest on the limbs; a firm papule which is frequently reddish-brown in colour and slightly scaly (Figure 75.3). If the overlying epidermis is squeezed, the 'dimple sign' is seen, indicating tethering of the overlying epidermis to the underlying lesion. Giant lesions (>5 cm in diameter) are occasionally seen. Multiple lesions may develop. Eruptive variants may be familial or associated with immunosuppression (e.g. HIV), autoimmune diseases, neoplasia (particularly haematological) and highly active antiretroviral therapy.

Cellular DF, like ordinary DF, has predilection for the limbs. The size is larger than ordinary DF but normally less than 2 cm. Recognition of this variant is important, as it has a local recurrence rate of 25%.

Aneurysmal DF is usually rapidly growing and may be very large. They clinically mimic a vascular tumour. Local recurrence is 19%.

Atypical DF presents as a papule, nodule or plaque, usually less than 1.5 cm in diameter. The rate of local recurrence is around 14%.

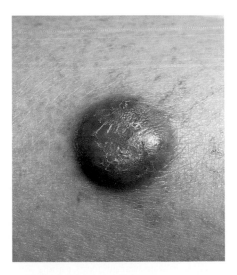

Figure 75.3 Clinical appearance of a dermatofibroma.

Epithelioid DF usually occurs on the limbs of young females. The typical clinical appearance is that of a polypoid, often vascular, lesion resembling a non-ulcerated pyogenic granuloma.

Management

Majority are a cosmetic nuisance and no treatment is necessary. However, cellular, atypical and aneurysmal variants should be completely removed conservatively, in view of recurrence risk.

Atypical fibroxanthoma

Atypical fibroxanthoma (AFX) is a tumour which arises in the sun-damaged skin of elderly people. A paradoxical tumour with histological features of a highly malignant neoplasm and low-grade clinical behaviour.

Epidemiology

Usually occurs in the seventh to eight decades. M > F. Predominantly in white skin.

Pathophysiology

UV radiation-induced *p53* mutations have been observed in these lesions, confirming the association with sun-damaged skin. The diagnosis of AFX is a diagnosis of exclusion.

Exophytic, fairly well circumscribed tumours which are surrounded by an epidermal collarette. The paradoxical feature of AFX is its histological resemblance to a highly malignant soft-tissue sarcoma. It arises in the dermis and may extend very focally into the fat, but the edge is pushing rather than infiltrative. Composed of large spindle-shaped and histiocyte-like pleomorphic cells, many of which appear multinucleated with frequent mitotic figures and atypical forms. Tumours with an infiltrative growth pattern, involvement of deeper tissues, tumour necrosis, lymphovascular invasion and perineural invasion should be classified as dermal pleomorphic sarcomas as they have a more aggressive behaviour than conventional AFXs (see later).

Clinical features

They occur most frequently on the ears (Figure 75.4), bald scalp and cheeks, with less than 6-month duration. Often ulcerated and

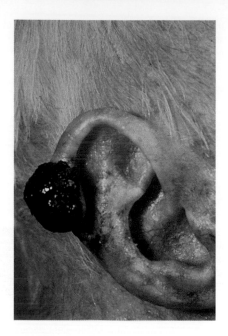

Figure 75.4 Typical clinical appearance of an atypical fibroxanthoma with a polypoid architecture.

have a red fleshy appearance; rarely exceed 30 mm in size.

Management

The benign clinical behaviour of the tumour enables limited local removal. Local recurrence may be seen in about 10% of cases and metastases to lymph nodes and internal organs are rare.

VASCULAR TUMOURS

REACTIVE VASCULAR LESIONS

Intravascular papillary endothelial hyperplasia

A primary phenomenon within a thrombosed blood vessel, usually a vein. The secondary variant is seen as an incidental finding within other vascular tumours.

Epidemiology

A relatively common lesion with a wide age range. Slightly more common in females.

Pathophysiology

All forms of the condition are the result of reactive proliferation of endothelial cells as a result of an organising thrombus most often but not always secondary to trauma.

It is distinguished from angiosarcoma as the latter is only exceptionally purely intravascular; it also displays cytological atypia, multilayering and mitotic figures.

Clinical features

The primary form presents as a slowly growing solitary asymptomatic or slightly painful bluish nodule less than 20 mm in diameter; predominantly on the head and neck, followed by the hand (particularly the fingers).

Differential diagnosis

Vascular tumour.

Management

Simple excision is usually curative.

Glomeruloid haemangioma

This is a rare distinctive multifocal vascular proliferation that occurs in association with POEMS syndrome (*p*olyneuropathy, *o*rganomegaly, *e*ndocrinopathy, *M* protein and *s*kin changes) or with multicentric Castleman disease.

Histologically there is a multifocal dermal proliferation of clusters of closely packed dilated capillaries with a striking similarity to renal glomeruli.

Clinically there are multiple vascular papules on the trunk and limbs. The lesions do not regress spontaneously.

BENIGN VASCULAR TUMOURS

Lobular capillary haemangioma (pyogenic granuloma)

A vascular nodule that develops rapidly, often at the site of a recent injury.

Epidemiology

Common, with a peak in the second decade. M > F.

Pathophysiology

In a minority of cases, a minor injury, usually of a penetrating kind, has occurred a few weeks before the nodule appears. Granuloma gravidarum is a variant that presents in the oral cavity during pregnancy.

Histologically there is a lobular proliferation of small blood vessels, which erupt through a breach in the epidermis to produce a globular pedunculated tumour. Older lesions tend to organise and partly fibrose, and may show focal bone formation.

Clinical features

The common sites are the hands, especially the fingers (Figure 75.5), the feet, lips, head and upper trunk and the mucosal surfaces of the mouth and perianal area. The tumour is vascular, bright red to brownish-red or blue-black in colour. It is partially compressible but cannot be completely blanched and does not show pulsation. Older, darker lesions are frequently eroded and crusted, and may bleed easily. Occasionally, the surface is raspberry-like or verrucous. Between 5 and 10 mm in size, but may reach 50 mm. The initial evolution is rapid, but growth ceases after a few weeks. Spontaneous disappearance is rare. Lesions are not painful; patients mainly complain of the appearance or of recurrent bleeding.

Differential diagnosis

Keratoacanthoma and other epithelial neoplasms, inflamed seborrhoeic keratoses, melanocytic naevi, melanoma and Spitz nevi, viral warts, molluscum contagiosum, angioma, glomus tumour, eccrine poroma, Kaposi sarcoma and metastatic carcinoma.

Management

Curettage and cautery or narrow excision.

Epithelioid hemangioma

(Syn. Angiolymphoid hyperplasia with eosinophilia)
A benign locally proliferating lesion composed of vascular channels lined by endothelial cells with abundant pink cytoplasm and vesicular nuclei.

Epidemiology

The cause is unknown. More common in young adults.

Pathophysiology

A poorly circumscribed lobular lesion composed of clusters of proliferating capillaries and often thicker blood vessels lined by plump epithelioid endothelial with little cytological atypia and rare mitotic figures.

Clinical features

Cluster of small pink nodules on the head and neck, particularly around the ear or hairline (Figure 75.6). The lesions may also involve the oral mucosa and less frequently the trunk and extremities. They rarely exceed 2–3 cm in diameter, but occasionally deeper extension and larger subcutaneous lesions occur. Peripheral blood eosinophilia may be present but only in less than 10% of patients.

Management

Spontaneous regression is seen in some cases. Both surgery and radiotherapy are effective, but local recurrences are common.

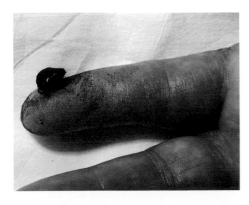

Figure 75.5 Clinical appearance of a pyogenic granuloma on a typical site at the tip of the finger.

PART 10: NEOPLASTIC, PROLIFERATIVE AND INFILTRATIVE DISORDERS AFFECTING THE SKIN

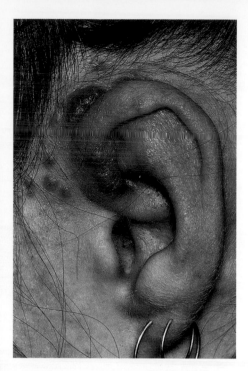

Figure 75.6 Epithelioid haemangioma. (Source: Courtesy of and copyright of Dr R.H. Champion, Addenbrooke's Hospital, Cambridge, UK.)

Hobnail haemangioma

A benign vascular dermal proliferation.

Epidemiology

Relatively uncommon with a predilection for young to middle-aged adults and a slight male predilection.

Pathophysiology

Trauma may play a part in its pathogenesis.

Histology is characterised by small channels lined by endothelial cells with little cytoplasm and a prominent dark nucleus (hobnail cells).

Clinical features

Presents as a rapidly developing asymptomatic solitary red or brown lesion, which in some cases has a central raised violaceous papule and is surrounded by a paler brown halo (targetoid appearance). Any body site may be affected, but it has a predilection for the lower limbs and trunk. The oral mucosa may also be affected.

Management

Simple surgical excision is the treatment of choice; there is no tendency for recurrence.

VASCULAR TUMOURS OF INTERMEDIATE MALIGNANCY

Kaposiform haemangioendothelioma

A locally aggressive vascular neoplasm, often associated with Kasabach–Merritt phenomenon (KMP).

Epidemiology

Rare; predominantly occurs in children under 2 years.

Pathophysiology

The growth pattern is lobular and infiltrative comprising of multiple nodules with haemorrhage and surrounding fibrosis. Tumour lobules are composed of bland spindle-shaped cells with poorly defined pink cytoplasm. Cleft-like spaces are often seen between spindle-shaped cells resembling Kaposi sarcoma.

Clinical features

In 20% of cases there is an association with lymphangiomatosis. Involvement of neighbouring organs and the association with KMP may lead to death.

Management

Complete excision is desirable as local recurrence is frequent, but this may be difficult to achieve when involvement is extensive. Spontaneous regression does not occur. In cases with large and deep-seated lesions and/or KMP, where surgery is not an option, alternative treatments include embolisation, chemotherapy with vincristine, corticosteroids, sirolimus, propranolol, interferon-α and low-dose radiotherapy.

MALIGNANT VASCULAR TUMOURS

Angiosarcoma

This is a malignant vascular tumour arising from both vascular and lymphatic endothelium.

Epidemiology
Angiosarcoma of the scalp and face of the elderly is very rare with male predominance.

Angiosarcoma associated with chronic lymphoedema (Stewart–Treves syndrome) occurs in 0.5% of female patients who survive mastectomy for more than 5 years and the mean interval between mastectomy and the appearance of the tumour is 10.5 years

Post-irradiation angiosarcoma is rare and most cases arise in the skin after radiotherapy for breast or, less commonly, internal cancer.

Pathophysiology
In the well-differentiated tumour, vascular channels infiltrate the normal structures in a disorganised fashion. The collagen is characteristically lined by tumour cells in a pattern that has been described as 'dissection of collagen'. Tumour cells may be plumper than normal, double-layered in places and form solid intravascular buds.

Clinical features
The first sign may be an area of bruising, often thought by the patient to be traumatic. Dusky blue or red nodules develop and grow rapidly, and fresh discrete nodules appear. Haemorrhagic blisters may be a prominent feature. As the tumours grow, the oedema may increase and older lesions may ulcerate (Figure 75.7). Multifocality is frequent, making surgical excision very difficult, particularly in those cases occurring on the face and scalp. Dissemination occurs early, predominantly to the lung and pleural cavity.

Management
In idiopathic angiosarcoma of the head and neck, a very small percentage of patients with smaller lesions (<5–10 cm at presentation) can be successfully treated with radical wide-field radiotherapy and surgery.

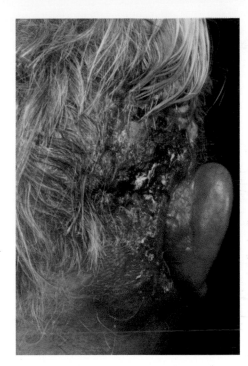

Figure 75.7 Typical haemorrhagic appearance of an angiosarcoma.

All angiosarcomas have a bad prognosis. Idiopathic angiosarcoma of the face, neck and scalp. The reported 5-year survival is low, at between 12% and 33%. Angiosarcomas arising in the setting of chronic lymphoedema and after radiotherapy appear to be equally aggressive.

TUMOURS OF PERIVASCULAR CELLS

Infantile myofibromatosis and adult myofibroma

Infantile myofibromatosis and adult myofibroma/myofibromatosis are best regarded as part of the spectrum of lesions described more recently as myopericytomas.

Epidemiology
Solitary lesions both in children and adults are relatively rare. Multiple lesions are uncommon.

Most cases of infantile myofibromatosis, present before the age of 2 years, with slight male predominance. Congenital tumours occur in up to a third of cases.

Pathophysiology

Rare myopericytomas but not classic myofibromas are associated with Epstein–Barr virus.

Tumours have a distinctive biphasic growth pattern. Areas composed of bundles of mature spindle-shaped myofibroblasts with pink cytoplasm and vesicular nuclei. Areas composed of immature round cells, with scanty cytoplasm arranged around small blood vessels, often displaying a haemangiopericytoma-like pattern ('staghorn-like').

Clinical features

A single nodule that may be skin coloured or blue/red. Multiple lesions are present in 25% of patients. The preferred sites are the head and neck, followed by the trunk. Involvement of other organs, including the gastrointestinal tract, lungs and bone, is seen in some cases.

Lesions tend to regress spontaneously. Visceral tumours may be associated with increased mortality.

Management

Simple excision.

Glomus tumour

A tumour of the myoarterial glomus, composed of vascular channels surrounded by proliferating glomus cells.

Epidemiology

Glomus tumours are uncommon. The incidence increases gradually from 7 years onwards. Multiple tumours are 10 times more frequent in children than in adults. Tumours in adults present during the third or fourth decades.

Pathophysiology

A lobulated, well-circumscribed dermal tumour. The glomus cell is cuboidal, with a well-marked cell membrane and a round central nucleus. The cells align themselves in rows around the single layer of endothelial cells of the vascular spaces and in a somewhat less orderly fashion peripherally. The tumours have variable quantities of glomus cells, blood vessels and smooth muscle. According to this finding, they are classified as solid glomus tumour, glomangioma or glomangiomyoma. More than 50% of tumours can be classified as glomangiomas and a minority (less than 15%) are classified as glomangiomyomas.

The *glomulin* gene is associated with multiple inherited glomangiomas.

Clinical features

A solitary glomus tumour is a pink or purple nodule 1–20 mm in size; it is conspicuously painful (Figure 75.8). Pain provoked by pressure, temperature change or spontaneous. Commonest site hands, particularly fingers, followed by other extremities, including head, neck and penis. Tumours beneath the nail are particularly painful; patients present for

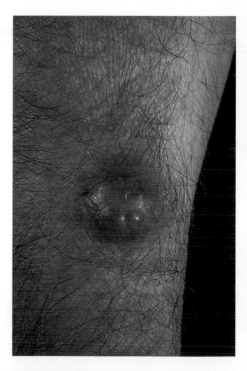

Figure 75.8 Clinical appearance of a glomus tumour.

treatment while the lesions are still very small. The affected nail has a bluish-red flush. Glomus tumours may also involve internal organs.

Multiple glomus tumours are larger, usually dark blue and deep dermal. Less restricted to the extremities, may be widely scattered and not usually painful.

Differential diagnosis
Leiomyoma, eccrine spiradenoma, cavernous haemangioma, 'blue rubber bleb' naevus.

Management
Surgical excision.

PERIPHERAL NEUROECTODERMAL TUMOURS

Multiple mucosal neuromas

In Sipple syndrome, multiple neuromas of the oral mucosa may be associated with phaeochromocytoma, parafollicular thyroid cysts secreting calcitonin, medullary thyroid carcinoma and opaque nerve fibres on the cornea.

Solitary circumscribed neuroma

A distinctive variant of cutaneous neuroma composed of variable proportions of the normal components of nerve tissue.

Epidemiology
Relatively common; mostly in adults.

Pathophysiology
A benign well-circumscribed, partially encapsulated, dermal nodule often associated with a nerve. S100 positive.

Clinical features
Small asymptomatic papule on the face; may resemble a naevus.

Management
Simple excision.

Schwannoma

(Syn. Neurilemmoma)
A tumour of nerve sheaths that arise in the Schwann cells of the myelin sheath surrounding the axons of peripheral nerves.

Epidemiology
The tumour is relatively rare. Most common in the fourth and fifth decades with female predilection.

Pathophysiology
An encapsulated spindle cell tumour in the course of a nerve, usually in the subcutaneous fat. Diagnostic features include fibrous capsule, hypercellular and hypocellular areas, Verocay bodies (palisading arrangement of nuclei) and hyaline vessels. S100 positive.

Clinical features
Arises most frequently from the acoustic nerve. Bilateral acoustic schwannomas are characteristic of neurofibromatosis type 2 (Chapter 38) along with the occurrence of multiple cutaneous plexiform schwannomas. There is no association with neurofibromatosis type 1 (NF1). In the peripheral nervous system, it is found in association with one of the main nerves of the limbs, usually on the flexor aspect near the elbow, wrist or knee, the hands or the head and neck. Other sites include the tongue, wall of the gastrointestinal tract and the posterior mediastinum. Rounded circumscribed pink-grey or yellowish nodules up to 5 cm in size, usually firm (but sometimes soft and cystic) and sometimes painful. Small lesions may be intradermal, but larger ones are subcutaneous. They usually grow slowly.

Management
Simple excision.

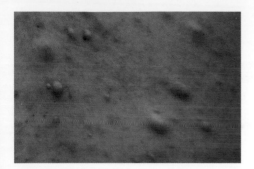

Figure 75.9 Multiple soft papules, typical of neurofibroma in a patient with NF1.

Solitary neurofibroma

An isolated benign nerve sheath tumour. Not specific to NF1.

Epidemiology
Common tumour arising in the second and third decades.

Pathophysiology
Probably arises from the endoneurium made up of a mixture of Schwann cells, fibroblasts and perineurial fibroblasts.

A non-encapsulated tumour composed of bland spindle-shaped cells with wavy nuclei in a myxoid or collagenous stroma.

Clinical features
Any body site may be affected. Slow-growing skin coloured or pink, smooth, soft or rubbery 2–20 mm polypoid lesion. Typical buttonhole effect with finger pressure. Multiple neurofibromas are rare outside the setting of NF1 (Figure 75.9).

Management
Simple excision.

Diffuse neurofibroma

A diffuse poorly defined indurated or plaque-like lesion of the skin and subcutaneous tissue in children or young adults, with a predilection for the trunk and head and neck area, associated with NF1. The histological features are identical to those of a solitary neurofibroma except there is diffuse replacement of involved tissue by the tumour. Local recurrence is frequent unless the lesion is widely excised.

Plexiform neurofibroma

Pathognomonic of NF1 seen in around 30% of patients (see Chapter 38). Single lesions may occur without definitive evidence of NF1.

Epidemiology
Children and young adults of either sex, with a predilection for the lower limbs, head and neck.

Pathophysiology
Tumours are large and located in the dermis, subcutis and even deeper soft tissues. Careful histological examination is necessary as the presence of mitotic activity usually indicates malignant transformation.

Clinical features
The overlying skin is folded and hyperpigmented, and the lesion is described as having an appearance like a 'bag of worms', reflecting the typical histological appearance of nerve trunks of different sizes randomly distributed throughout the involved tissues.

Management
Surgical removal is very difficult because of the extensive involvement.

Granular cell tumour

A tumour composed of cells with characteristic granular cytoplasm, believed to be of neural or nerve sheath origin.

Epidemiology
Tumours are rare and usually seen between the fourth and sixth decades.

Pathophysiology

The tumour is composed of large polyhedral cells arranged in sheets, which infiltrate the dermal connective tissue and subcutaneous fat. The cytoplasm is pale and contains brightly acidophilic granules.

Clinical features

A solitary tumour of the skin or mucosa most commonly found on the head and neck (especially the tongue). It is occasionally found in internal organs (mainly the gastrointestinal tract). The tumour is a firm, slowly growing, 5–20 mm, pink or greyish-brown nodule with smooth or warty surface. Occasionally they are painful. Multiple tumours may occur. Malignant tumours are very rare.

Management

Excision.

TUMOURS OF MUSCLE

Leiomyoma

A benign smooth muscle tumour. Cutaneous leiomyomas classified into three types: pilar leiomyoma (from arrector pili muscle), angioleiomyoma (from media of blood vessels), or genital leiomyoma (from smooth muscle of the scrotum, labia majora or nipples).

Epidemiology

Relatively uncommon. Pilar leiomyoma is the most common.

Pilar leiomyoma occurs generally in early adult life; genital leiomyoma any age. Angioleiomyoma mainly occurs in middle-aged adults. Angioleiomyoma F > M.

Pathophysiology

The smooth muscle cells proliferate to produce interweaving bundles of spindle-shaped cells, which are strongly eosinophilic.

The gene that predisposes to multiple pilar leiomyomas also predisposes to uterine leiomyomas (multiple cutaneous and uterine leiomyomatosis, Reed syndrome) and to renal cancer (mainly papillary renal cell carcinoma,

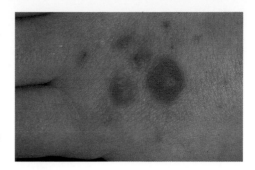

Figure 75.10 Clinical appearance of multiple leiomyomas.

hereditary leiomyomatosis and renal cancer syndrome). This is as a result of mutations in the gene encoding the enzyme fumarate hydratase.

Clinical features

Pilar leiomyoma are pink, red or dusky brown, firm dermal nodules of varying size but usually less than 15 mm in diameter (Figure 75.10). The nodules are often painful. The pain may be provoked by touch, cold temperature or emotion. Some lesions contract and become paler when painful. Adjacent tumours may coalesce to form a plaque. The areas most commonly affected are the extremities, predominantly the proximal and extensor aspects.

Genital leiomyoma is a solitary dermal nodule occurring most commonly in the scrotum, but also appearing on the penis, labia majora and nipple. Pain is less frequent than with pilar leiomyoma. Contraction in response to stimulation by touch or cold can occur.

Angioleiomyoma is usually a solitary, flesh-coloured, rounded, subcutaneous or deep dermal tumour up to 40 mm in diameter more frequent on the lower limb. 50% are painful, triggered by changes in temperature, pregnancy or menses.

Differential diagnosis

The solitary painful lesion may be mistaken for a glomus tumour or an eccrine spiradenoma; a history of contraction is helpful.

Management

Treatment for pain includes surgical excision, calcium-channel blockers and gabapentin.

TUMOURS OF FAT CELLS

Angiolipoma

A benign tumour of mature fat and blood vessels.

Epidemiology
It is a relatively common tumour predominantly in 20–30-year-olds. M > F.

Pathophysiology
An encapsulated tumour composed of mature white adipose tissue admixed with a variable number of thin-walled vessels that contain fibrin microthrombi. Cases with a prominent vascular component have been termed 'cellular angiolipomas'.

Clinical features
Single or multiple variably painful subcutaneous nodules. Usually <2 cm and well circumscribed. A predilection for the upper limbs is observed, particularly the forearm, followed by the trunk and lower limbs.

Familial incidence in 5–10% of cases. Familial angiolipomatosis is autosomal recessive.

Management
Excision.

Lipoma

A benign tumour composed of variable amounts of mature white adipose tissue.

Epidemiology
The most common human mesenchymal neoplasm. Tends to occur in adults (40–60 years old). More frequent in the obese and females. Congenital lesions reported.

Pathophysiology
Tumours are usually encapsulated and consist of lobules of mature adipose tissue divided by delicate fibrous septa. Adipocytes are uniform in size and shape. Nuclear atypia is not a feature. There is no mitotic activity. Degenerative changes frequently occur, usually in the form of fat necrosis.

Clinical features
A slowly growing and painless subcutaneous mass. Predominantly on the trunk, abdomen and neck. Other sites, such as the proximal extremities, face, scalp and less commonly the hands and feet, may be affected. Usually solitary but multiple lesions have been described. Dercum disease is a rare condition characterised by multiple, painful lipomas (Chapter 52)

Size is variable and large lesions may occur. They are most often well-circumscribed but deep-seated variants, such as intramuscular lipomas, may be ill-defined. Progression to liposarcoma is exceptional.

Management
Excision.

TUMOURS OF UNCERTAIN HISTOGENESIS

Acral fibromyxoma

A distinctive benign dermal and/or subcutaneous, fibroblastic tumour with a strong predilection for digits of both the hands and feet.

Epidemiology
Most patients are middle aged. M > F.

Pathophysiology
Lesions are circumscribed and consist of bland stellate and spindle-shaped cells in a variably prominent myxoid and collagenous stroma with small blood vessels in the background.

Clinical features
Most cases present as a longstanding, solitary mass measuring between 1 and 2 cm, with a predilection for the subungual or periungual region of the hands and feet.

Management
Excision.

Tumours of skin appendages

76

The appendageal tumours either differentiate towards or arise from the pilosebaceous apparatus (including the apocrine gland) and eccrine sweat gland.

The pilosebaceous apparatus is concentrated in the head and neck area, with the pilar element predominant on the scalp and the sebaceous element on the face, chest and upper back. Thus, tumours arising from these structures are found predominantly at these anatomical sites. The eccrine sweat glands are, in contrast, found on all body sites.

The great majority of these appendage-derived tumours are relatively benign, with behaviour and prognosis similar to that seen in basal cell carcinoma. Thus, although local recurrence is well recorded, metastases are rare, with the exception of the malignant eccrine and apocrine gland-derived tumours and ocular sebaceous carcinoma.

Only a selection are discussed.

HAIR FOLLICLE TUMOURS

A large number of tumours are theoretically capable of arising from the hair follicle and matrix, depending on the exact type of cell and its situation within the dermis.

Comedo naevus

A rare benign abnormality of the follicular infundibulum presenting as a group of comedo-like lesions. It is part of the naevus comedonicus syndrome.

Epidemiology

Estimated prevalence 1 in 45 000 to 1 in 100 000. They may be present at birth or develop throughout adult life.

Pathophysiology

A rudimentary pilosebaceous follicle is present, with a large overlying keratin-filled crater. The surface of the keratinous material oxidises to give the comedone-like appearance.

Clinical features

Lesions are seen mainly on the head and neck but can also occur at other sites, including the palm and wrist. They appear as a cluster of comedones or as a single giant lesion.

Management

Treatment options, for cosmetic reasons or in complicated cases, include topical therapy, laser and surgery.

EXTERNAL ROOT SHEATH TUMOURS

Trichilemmal cyst

See Chapter 72.

Trichilemmoma

(Syn. Tricholemmoma)
This lesion is classically considered to be a proliferation of the external root sheath of the hair follicle.

Rook's Dermatology Handbook, First Edition. Edited by Christopher E. M. Griffiths, Tanya O. Bleiker, Daniel Creamer, John R. Ingram and Rosalind C. Simpson.
© 2022 John Wiley & Sons Ltd. Published 2022 by John Wiley & Sons Ltd.

Epidemiology

Solitary trichilemmoma is a relatively common lesion presenting in young and middle-aged adults.

Patients with Cowden syndrome (Table 76.1) or multiple hamartoma and neoplasia syndrome, have large numbers of trichilemmomas. Incidence estimated as 1:200 000 with a slight female preponderance.

Pathophysiology

Lesions are well-circumscribed lobular tumours extending down from the epidermis and often connected to a hair follicle. Tumour cells display prominent clear cytoplasm secondary to the deposition of glycogen. A viral aetiology has been confirmed by demonstration of HPV DNA by polymerase chain reaction in some cases. Trichilemmomas are often found within a naevus sebaceous.

Table 76.1 Syndromes associated with multiple adnexal tumours

Syndrome	Gene/locus	Adnexal tumours	Other features
Birt Hogg Dube	FLCN (folliculin) Ch17p12q11 Autosomal dominant	Fibrofolliculomas Trichodiscomas Perifollicular fibromas Acrochordon-like lesions	Lung cysts Spontaneous pneumothorax Renal neoplasms (chromophobe renal carcinoma, oncocytoma)
Brooke–Spiegler	Cylindromatosis (CYLD) gene Ch16q12-13 Autosomal dominant	Trichoepithelioma Cylindroma Spiradenoma	Basal cell carcinoma Salivary and parotid gland tumours
Cowden (multiple hamartoma and neoplasia syndrome)	PTEN, Ch10q23	Trichilemmoma	Cobblestone oral epithelium Skin tags Squamous papillomas Sclerotic fibromas Gastrointestinal, breast and thyroid malignancy
Muir–Torre (hereditary non-polyposis colorectal cancer, Lynch II syndrome) (Chapter 37)	MSH2 gene Ch2p and MLH1 gene Ch 3p Autosomal dominant	Sebaceous adenoma, sebaceous epithelioma, sebaceous carcinoma	Keratoacanthomas, squamous cell carcinoma Colorectal carcinoma Other internal malignancies, predominantly gastrointestinal and genitourinary
Schöpf–Schulz–Passarge syndrome (a form of ectodermal dysplasia syndrome)	Autosomal recessive	Periocular apocrine hidrocystomas	Hypotrichosis Hypodontia Nail dystrophy Palmoplantar keratoderma

Mutations of the *PTEN* tumour suppressor gene on chromosome 10q23 are found in Cowden syndrome.

Clinical features

Lesions are small non-specific papules on facial skin; the diagnosis of multiple trichilemmomas should stimulate a search for other evidence of Cowden syndrome.

Management

Few treatment options are available, ranging from simple surgical excision to carbon dioxide laser tissue ablation for multiple cases.

HAMARTOMAS AND HAIR GERM TUMOURS AND CYSTS

Eruptive vellus hair cyst

See Chapter 72.

Trichofolliculoma

A benign hamartoma of the pilosebaceous follicle.

Epidemiology

Rare, young adults with a slight male predilection.

Pathophysiology

The pathological appearance is that of a dilated and abnormally large pilosebaceous canal containing numerous poorly formed hairs, with several pilosebaceous-like structures opening into the canal.

Clinical features

Predilection for the head and neck, particularly the face. Presenting as small raised nodules with two or three hairs protruding together in a small tuft (Figure 76.1).

Management

Surgical excision.

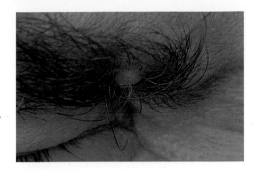

Figure 76.1 Typical example of a trichofolliculoma with a small tuft of hair in the centre.

Trichoepithelioma

A hamartoma of the hair germ. Trichoepithelioma is regarded as part of the spectrum of trichoblastoma.

Epidemiology

Young adults, with a female predilection.

Pathophysiology

The pathology consists of lobules of small dark basaloid cells, often with a degree of peripheral palisading surrounding a central area of eosinophilic amorphous material. There is frequently a strong resemblance to basal cell carcinoma, and differentiating between the two can be very difficult. However, the stroma in trichoepithelioma is distinctive in that it contains clefts, with an absence of retraction artefact between tumour cells and the surrounding stroma.

Multiple lesions are inherited by autosomal dominant transmission.

The Brooke–Spiegler syndrome inherited by autosomal dominant transmission consists of multiple trichoepitheliomas, cylindromas and spiradenomas due to mutations in *CYLD* and *PTCH* tumour suppressor genes (Table 76.1).

Clinical features

A solitary smooth nodule, usually on the face, which clinically resembles a non-ulcerated basal cell carcinoma. Multiple lesions are seen

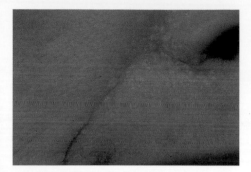

Figure 76.2 Multiple trichoepitheliomas on the central face.

as small pearly lesions, mainly on centrofacial skin (Figure 76.2). Lesions are benign; malignant transformation extremely rare.

Management
Surgical excision, curettage, cryotherapy and dermabrasion. High-energy pulsed carbon dioxide laser is also an option.

HAIR MATRIX TUMOURS

Pilomatricoma

(Syn. Benign calcifying epithelioma of Malherbe, pilomatrixoma)
A benign tumour considered to be a hamartoma of the hair matrix.

Epidemiology
20% of all hair follicle-related tumours. Familial cases can occur. Association with myotonic dystrophy, Turner syndrome, Rubinstein–Taybi syndrome and MYH-associated polyposis. The majority of patients are under 20 years. F > M.

Pathophysiology
A well-circumscribed dermal tumour. The outer cells are small, and their rounded nuclei crowded together make this region deeply basophilic. The cytoplasm is scanty and the cell margins indistinct, but intercellular connections can be seen. Towards the centre of the

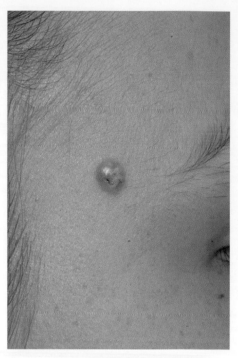

Figure 76.3 Pilomatricoma. Right temple of a child.

mass the cytoplasm becomes more abundant and eosinophilic. The nuclear outline persists, but the chromatin is sparse and clumped in dark granules; when all basophilic material disappears, a mummified 'ghost cell' remains.

Clinical features
The lesion is usually a solitary, deep dermal or subcutaneous tumour 3–30 mm in diameter situated on the head, neck or upper extremities (Figure 76.3). The skin over the tumour is normal and the lesion has a firm to stone-hard consistency and a lobular shape on palpation. In adults, there may be quite a short history and there is usually no evidence of a preceding cyst. It may be subject to periodic inflammation and can present as a granulomatous swelling. Malignant change is very rare.

Management
Surgical excision.

LESIONS OF HAIR FOLLICLE MESENCHYME

According to the World Health Organization trichodiscoma and fibrofolliculoma are now considered to represent the late and early stage, respectively, of the same appendageal tumour which differentiates towards the mantle of the hair follicle.

Trichodiscoma and fibrofolliculoma

Epidemiology
Rare benign lesions. Occur in young to middle-aged individuals (third to fourth decade).

Pathophysiology
Trichodiscoma is a discrete but non-encapsulated area of myxoid, poorly cellular stroma with focal collagen depositionin the dermis, associated with a proliferation of blood vessels, some of which are thick-walled. Trichodiscomas and trichofolliculomas usually show histological overlap.

Fibrofolliculoma shows multiple small poorly formed pilosebaceous follicles set in a striking fibrous stroma.

Multipe trichodiscomas, trichofolliculomas and acrochordon-like lesions as well as perifollicular fibromas and fibrofolliculomas have been described as part of Birt–Hogg–Dubé syndrome (Table 76.1).

Clinical features
Trichodiscomas present as multiple discrete flat-topped papules 2–3 mm in diameter, mainly on the central area of the face.

Fibrofolliculomas are more often multiple either isolated or as a part of Birt–Hogg–Dubé syndrome. They tend to affect the upper part of the body. They can also be associated with other conditions such as thyroid carcinoma and tuberous sclerosis (see Chapter 38).

Management
Excision for cosmetic reasons. In Birt–Hogg–Dubé syndrome skin lesions may be the first manifestation of the disease, therefore screening and follow-up are advisable as the risk for developing renal tumours increases with age.

SEBACEOUS GLAND TUMOURS

Sebaceous adenomas and sebaceomas

Benign tumours composed of incompletely differentiated sebaceous cells of varying degrees of maturity.

Epidemiology
These are relatively rare tumours. Most cases of solitary type occur in the elderly.

Pathophysiology
The tumours are multilobular and usually connected to the epidermis. The lobules are well defined, composed of variable numbers of small basophilic sebaceous matrix cells peripherally and larger cells – mature sebaceous cells – containing cytoplasmic fat globules.

Patients with multiple benign sebaceous tumours (other than sebaceous hyperplasia) should be suspected of having the Muir–Torre syndrome (see Chapter 37).

Clinical features
Tumours are usually rounded, raised and either sessile or pedunculated (Figure 76.4). Normally <10 mm, but older lesions may form plaques or

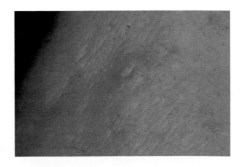

Figure 76.4 Sebaceous adenoma. Small yellowish papule.

ulcerate. Fleshy or waxy yellow colour, and the surface may be papilliferous. Commonly on the face or scalp, may occur on the eyelid. They usually grow slowly, but a sudden increase in growth rate can occur.

Management
Surgical excision.

Sebaceous carcinoma

A malignant tumour composed of cells showing differentiation toward sebaceous epithelium.

Epidemiology
Rare, <1% of all skin malignancies. Lesions may rarely occur in naevus sebaceous.

Most lesions occur in middle-aged and elderly. There is a slight predilection for males.

Pathophysiology
The essential feature is cytological evidence of sebaceous differentiation.

Sebaceous carcinoma may rarely be associated with Muir–Torre syndrome (see Chapter 37).

Clinical features
The tumour is solitary, firm, sometimes translucent and covered with normal or slightly verrucose epidermis. The colour may be yellow or orange. The face and scalp are the commonest sites, especially the eyelid (Figure 76.5). The evolution may be very slow, and a size of 5 cm or more may be reached after many years without metastasis. Some tumours grow rapidly and invade early, but metastasis is uncommon.

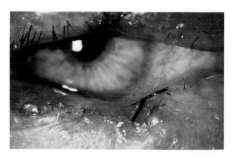

Figure 76.5 Sebaceous carcinoma. Ulcerated yellowish lesion of the lower eyelid.

Management
Complete surgical excision is required.

APOCRINE GLAND TUMOURS

Apocrine hidrocystoma

(Syn. Apocrine cystadenoma)
A benign lesion produced by cystic dilatation of apocrine secretory glands.

Epidemiology
Not uncommon but is most often seen in ophthalmological or surgical clinics. Occurs in adults.

Pathophysiology
Large cystic cavities are found in the dermis if the lesion has been carefully dissected out. The cavities are lined by cuboidal or high-columnar apocrine secretory cells with decapitation secretion and a peripheral layer of myoepithelial cells.

Clinical features
The lesions are solitary or occasionally multiple, asymptomatic, well-defined, dome-shaped, translucent nodules. The surface is smooth and the colour varies from skin colour to greyish or blue-black; pigmentation may affect only part of the cyst. The commonest site is around the eye, particularly lateral to the outer canthus (Figure 76.6). The cyst increases slowly in size and may become >10 mm in diameter. Multiple

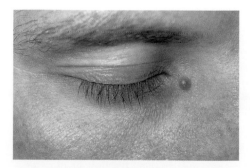

Figure 76.6 Apocrine hidrocystoma. Cystic translucent papule on the right inner canthus.

lesions may be seen in Schöpf–Schulz–Passarge syndrome (Table 76.1).

Management
Surgical excision. Multiple lesions have been treated successfully with trichloroacetic acid.

Syringocystadenoma papilliferum

An exuberant proliferating lesion, commonly seen on the scalp in association with naevus sebaceous.

Epidemiology
May be present at birth or in childhood; the majority are in young adults.

Pathophysiology
The epidermal surface shows papillomatous expansion, and from these areas cystic invaginations are seen. The cystic structures are lined by papillae that have a lining of a double layer of columnar epithelium, which shows an apocrine pattern of secretion.

Clinical features
Papillomatous expansion of a small pre-existing lesion around puberty. The lesion is composed of multiple warty papules, some of which are translucent and pigmented (Figure 76.7).

The lesion is benign. Occasionally, basal cell carcinoma, squamous cell carcinoma (including verrucous carcinoma) or a ductal carcinoma can develop within it.

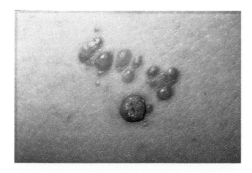

Figure 76.7 Syringocystadenoma papilliferum. Papular lesion with superficial erosion.

Management
Surgical excision is recommended.

ECCRINE GLAND HAMARTOMAS AND TUMOURS

Eccrine hidrocystoma

A benign tumour produced by mature, deformed eccrine sweat units.

Epidemiology
This is a rare tumour. It was formerly reported as being more common in those who had to work exposed to heat, such as cooks.

It typically occurs in middle-aged women.

Pathophysiology
A dermal cystic lesion uni- or multilocular lined by two layers of cells. The inner layer of cells is columnar and the outer layer consists of elongated myoepithelial cells.

Clinical features
Usually solitary but rarely multiple. The lesions are largely confined to the cheeks and eyelids. They are cystic, often blue in colour, and there is frequently a history of enlargement when the skin is exposed to heat and flattening of the lesion when the skin is exposed to cold.

Management
Surgery, electrodesiccation, carbon dioxide laser and pulse dye laser have been used with good results.

Eccrine poroma

A tumour derived from the intraepidermal eccrine duct (acrosyringium).

Epidemiology
Tumours are relatively common. Most patients are adults.

Pathophysiology
There is a clear margin between adjacent normal epidermal keratinocytes and a population

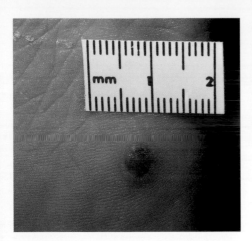

Figure 76.8 Poroma. Note the red shiny surface, which often leads to misdiagnosis of a pyogenic granuloma.

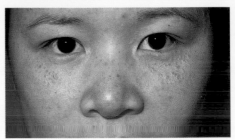

Figure 76.9 Multiple syringomas on the upper cheek area.

of smaller cuboidal cells, usually with darker nuclei protruding down into the underlying dermis.

Clinical features
Predominantly found on the palms and soles (Figure 76.8), in contrast to other skin append-age tumours which tend to be concentrated around the head and neck area. They are moist exophytic lesions, pink or red in colour, and may reach 1–2 cm in diameter. Characteristically have a surrounding moat when the skin is stretched. Occasional lesions are pigmented and look similar to pigmented basal cell carci-noma under dermoscopy.

Disease course and prognosis
The lesion is benign. Malignant change has been recorded in up to 18% of cases (see under porocarcinoma).

Management
Surgical excision.

Syringoma

A benign skin tumour composed of sweat ducts that is usually multiple.

Epidemiology
It is a relatively common benign lesion normally appearing in adolescence. Female predilection.

Pathophysiology
Characteristic architectural pattern. Collections of convoluted and cystic ducts are seen in the upper half of the dermis. Most are lined by a double layer of cells similar to, but flatter than, those that line normal eccrine ducts. The lumina contain amorphous debris. A character-istic feature is the tail-like strand of cells pro-jecting from one side of the duct into the stroma, giving a resemblance to a tadpole or comma.

Clinical features
The individual small dermal papules are skin coloured, yellowish or mauve, but sometimes appear translucent and cystic. The surface may be rounded or flat-topped and the outline sometimes angular. Size varies, most are <3 mm. Usually multiple and symmetrical. Commonest sites are face and neck (Figure 76.9), also found on the chest. Eruptive syrin-gomas have a predilection for the neck, chest, abdomen, pubic area and more rarely the but-tocks. Syringomas are seen more commonly in Down syndrome and may erupt dramatically. Familial cases rarely occur. Syringoma is most likely to be confused with trichoepithelioma on the face, but the latter favour the naso-labial folds.

Management
Careful destruction with diathermy can pro-duce good cosmetic results.

ECCRINE OR APOCRINE/ FOLLICULAR TUMOURS

Hidradenoma

(Syn. Clear-cell hidradenoma)
A relatively rare benign tumour of sweat gland origin.

Epidemiology
Found mainly in adults.

Pathophysiology
The tumour may connect with the epidermis. It forms lobulated circumscribed masses and is composed of two cell types: polygonal cells, whose glycogen content may give the cytoplasm a clear appearance and elongated, darker and smaller cells, which may occur at the periphery.

Clinical features
Firm dermal nodules, 5–30 mm in size and may be attached to the overlying epidermis, which can be either thickened or ulcerated (Figure 76.10). Growth is slow and there may be a history of serous discharge. The lesions are usually solitary on the scalp, face, anterior trunk and proximal limbs.

Management
Surgical excision. Rarely, hidradenocarcinoma, a malignant tumour, arises from a pre-existing hidradenoma. Wide local excision, staging and follow up are required for this poor prognostic tumour.

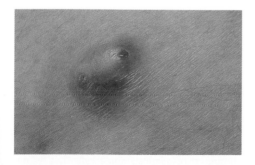

Figure 76.10 Hidradenoma. Red-brown irregular papule.

Cylindroma

(Syn. Turban tumour, Spiegler tumour)
An uncommon benign tumour of the scalp.

Epidemiology
The onset is usually in early adult life but may be in childhood or adolescence. Female predilection.

Pathophysiology
The lesions may be familial (autosomal dominant); a suppressor gene (cylindromatosis gene, *CYLD*) has been identified on chromosome 16q12–13, loss of which is associated with cylindroma development.

Pathologically the tumours have a rounded outline and are composed of closely set mosaic-like masses ('jigsaw-puzzle' appearance) and columns of cells that are invested by a hyaline basal membrane of variable thickness. Thin bands of stroma separate tumour lobules. The cells are of two types: one large, with a moderate amount of cytoplasm and a vesicular nucleus, and the other small, with little cytoplasm and a compact nucleus. Malignant transformation is very rare.

Clinical features
The tumours are frequently multiple, smooth, firm, pink to red in colour and often pedunculated (Figure 76.11). The rate of growth is slow, some tumours become 5 cm or more in diameter, but most are smaller. Pain is an occasional symptom. The commonest site is the scalp and adjacent skin. Tumours on the scalp may be almost hairless when pedunculated, but the smaller lesions form dermal nodules with little loss of overlying hair.

Management
Surgery is the treatment of choice. Extensive involvement of the scalp may require wide excision and skin graft.

Spiradenoma

(Syn. Eccrine spiradenoma)
An uncommon benign solitary tumour of sweat gland origin.

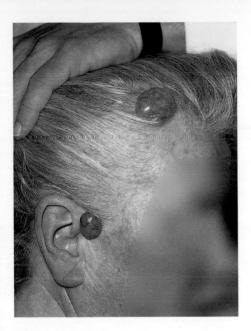

Figure 76.11 Cylindroma. Two large tumours on the head of an elderly woman.

Epidemiology

Rarely familial. It appears mainly in young adults.

Pathophysiology

Multiple lesions may be part of Brooke–Spiegler syndrome (Table 76.1). The tumour is lobular, with two cell types in the islands. Larger paler cells may be grouped around lumina and smaller darker cells form the periphery. Small tubular structures or cystic spaces may occur, and large thin-walled dilated vascular channels are also present. The lobules are surrounded by condensed connective tissue, which may encroach on the islands as hyaline droplets. Malignant transformation may occur and usually presents in longstanding tumours.

Clinical features

The lesion is usually solitary and painful, and consists of a firm rounded bluish dermal nodule 3–50 mm in diameter. The usual site is on the front of the trunk and proximal limbs.

Management

Surgical excision.

SWEAT GLAND CARCINOMAS, INCLUDING DUCTAL APOCRINE/FOLLICULAR CARCINOMAS

These lesions can be divided into two broad groups. The first group represents the situation in which malignant change develops in a pre-existing, apparently benign, lesion such as hidradenoma, mixed tumour, spiradenoma, cylindroma and eccrine poroma. The latter is the most commonly recorded example of such malignant progression. Even when there is unmistakable cytological evidence of malignancy, the biological behaviour of malignant tumours of skin appendages is generally benign, with local recurrence being much more common than cutaneous metastases.

The second group of carcinomas consists of lesions that develop as carcinomas *de novo*. The primary eccrine carcinomas include microcystic adnexal carcinoma, eccrine epithelioma, aggressive digital papillary adenocarcinoma, mucinous carcinoma and adenoid cystic carcinoma.

Malignant eccrine poroma

(Syn. Porocarcinoma)

A malignant tumour arising from intraepidermal eccrine ducts. In up to 18% of cases, tumours arise from a pre-existing benign eccrine poroma

Epidemiology

0.01–0.005% of all cutaneous tumours. Average age at presentation 73 years. F > M.

Pathophysiology

Tumours show multiple connections to the epidermis, and a pre-existing benign eccrine poroma may be present. The tumour infiltrates the dermis and the subcutaneous tissue in nests and lobules composed of relatively small cells that do not have a basaloid appearance. Ductal differentiation is necessary for the diagnosis to be made.

Poor prognostic factors are a large number of mitotic figures, lymphovascular invasion, tumour depth greater than 7 mm and an infiltrating rather than a pushing border.

Clinical features

A papillomatous, often ulcerated tumour, usually on the lower limbs. Tumours may become large and are frequently longstanding.

Management

Wide excision and follow-up are required. Mohs micrographic surgery is useful in those cases with a prominent infiltrative growth. Local recurrence is seen in 17% of cases. Regional lymph node metastases and systemic metastases occur in 19% and 11% of patients, respectively. Mortality rate of 67% in patients with lymph node metastases. Distant metastases are rare.

Microcystic adnexal carcinoma

(Syn. Malignant syringoma)

Epidemiology

Relatively rare. Young and middle-aged patients more frequently affected.

Pathophysiology

Cases have been reported with gneralised immunosuppression and in sites of previous radiotherapy. Histologically there are cords of cytologically banal epithelial cells with focal, variable ductal differentiation set in a sclerotic desmoplastic stroma.

Clinical features

Predilection for the central area of the face, often as an inconspicuous, elevated or depressed sclerotic plaque or nodule in the upper lip area. There may be pain or a burning sensation due to perineural spread. Extensive local recurrence can be a major problem but metastatic spread is very rare. Up to 40% local recurrence rate.

Management

Perineural permeation is common; Mohs micrographic surgery is therefore recommended.

MISCELLANEOUS TUMOURS

Paget disease of the nipple

A progressive, marginated, scaling or crusting of the nipple and areola due to invasion of the epidermis by malignant cells, which usually but not always originate from an intraductal carcinoma of the breast. Extramammary Paget disease is discussed in Chapter 61.

Epidemiology

Paget disease of the nipple is uncommon In one series, it occurred in fewer than 3% of breast cancers.

It is rare before the fourth decade and is most frequent in the fifth and sixth. Predominantly women.

Pathophysiology

The current view is that the majority of cases arise from either invasive or *in situ* ductal carcinoma in the deeper breast tissue. In a minority of cases no underlying *in situ* or invasive carcinoma is found.

The epidermis is thickened, with papillomatosis, enlargement of the interpapillary ridges and hyperkeratosis or parakeratosis on the surface. Characteristic Paget cells are found in the epidermis. The Paget cells are round with clear abundant cytoplasm and hyperchromatic nuclei with a high nuclear/cytoplasmic ratio. An underlying intraductal carcinoma, if present, is not always seen on biopsy, as it may be deeply set.

The main pathological challenge is to distinguish Paget disease from malignant melanoma. Paget disease cells will be carcinoembryonic antigen, epithelial membrane antigen and Cam 5.2 positive, while those of melanoma will be positive for melanocytic markers. S100 protein is not useful, as although it is positive in the great majority of melanomas, it is also positive in a proportion of Paget disease.

Clinical features

The early changes may be minimal, with a small, crusted and intermittently moist area

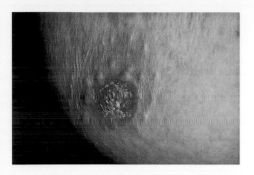

Figure 76.12 Paget disease of the nipple. Close-up view showing erythema and well-marked lateral edge of the lesion.

on the nipple giving a brownish stain on clothing, or producing itching, pricking or burning sensations. Less often, there is a serous or blood-stained discharge from the nipple, or a lump may be noticed in the breast. The surface changes persist and gradually spread to produce an eczematous appearance. The nipple, areola and, at a later stage, skin of the breast are erythematous and moist or crusted (Figure 76.12). Itching may be a prominent symptom and excoriations may be found in the established lesion. Some areas may be ulcerated. The regional glands should be examined. Rarely it is bilateral. The rate of spread of the skin changes is slow and presentation is often delayed.

Differential diagnosis
The main differential diagnosis is eczema of the nipple. This is frequently bilateral and runs a more fluctuating course, improving in response to local treatment and spreading rapidly when irritated. Eczema lacks the sharp, raised and rounded margin and the superficial induration of Paget disease.

Management
Mammogram or ultrasound is essential. Refer to breast team; surgery as per breast carcinoma.

Kaposi sarcoma

77

Kaposi sarcoma (KS) is a multifocal, endothelial proliferation caused by human herpesvirus 8 (HHV-8), most often with cutaneous involvement with or without visceral extension. There are four clinicopathological subtypes: classic, endemic, iatrogenic and AIDS associated, Table 77.1.

Epidemiology

See Table 77.1.

Pathophysiology

Although HHV-8 is considered the causative agent, it is insufficient to cause KS alone. The most powerful co-factor is HIV co-infection, which elevates the risk up to 20 000-fold. The genetic basis for the ethnogeographic predisposition of KS in the classic and endemic subtypes is unclear.

Histopathology is essentially the same in the different epidemiologic types. Patch-stage KS manifests as a mild increase in the number of vessels, which are classically arranged in a horizontal fashion, dissecting through collagen bundles, around adnexae and surrounding pre-existing vessels (promontory sign). The plaque stage has more obvious and extensive vessel expansion, lined by single-layered, plump endothelial cells. In tumour-stage or nodular KS, there is a circumscribed mass of spindled cells with unlined slit-like spaces with extravasated erythrocytes. KS cells stain positively with the endothelial markers (CD31, CD34 and factor VIII-related antigen), several lymphatic specific markers such as D2-40, and with the latent nuclear antigen-1 of HHV-8.

Clinical features

Cutaneous lesions commonly present on the extremities, most often on the feet (Figure 77.1), occasionally on hands, ears or nose. Lesions are typically dark blue or purple and may partially blanche when tumid. They are most often multifocal, fusing to eventually form plaques and tumours to a size of several centimetres (Figure 77.2) often with accompanying lymphoedema. Lesions can ulcerate, fungate or leave pigmented scars. Lymph nodes, mucosae and viscera may be involved as the disease progresses. In the context of immunosuppression lesions may resemble bruises.

Staging of KS was originally developed in the context of AIDS by the AIDS Clinical Trial Group (ACTG) (Table 77.2). Disease outcome depends on tumour extent and systemic involvement. The ACTG T1S1 group has a 3-year survival of 53% versus over 80% for all other groups. Visceral involvement is particularly common in AIDS-associated KS, with lungs, gastrointestinal tract and lymph nodes the most common sites.

Differential diagnosis

Other vascular lesions, particularly haemangiomas, and melanocytic proliferations.

Investigations

Skin biopsy and HIV status.

Management

KS is highly radiosensitive, with complete responses in up to 93% of patients. In localised

Rook's Dermatology Handbook, First Edition. Edited by Christopher E. M. Griffiths, Tanya O. Bleiker, Daniel Creamer, John R. Ingram and Rosalind C. Simpson.
© 2022 John Wiley & Sons Ltd. Published 2022 by John Wiley & Sons Ltd.

Table 77.1 The four clinicopathological subtypes of KS

Subtype	Classic	Endemic	Iatrogenic	AIDS associated
Incidence and prevalence	0.47–8.8 per 100 000 per year in areas of Italy and Greece; more common in Ashkenazi Jews	Up to 10% of cancers in central Africa	0.3–1.6% among transplant recipients in the USA and Europe	30 per 1000 patient-years (pre-HAART) to 0.3 per 1000 patient-years (post-HAART); up to 40% of homosexual men with AIDS (pre-HAART)
Age	Elderly, fifth to seventh decades	Children, adults	Adults, usually younger than classic or adult endemic	Young men, 20–40 years
Sex	M: F > 10:1 ratio	Near unity in childhood; by puberty M:F = 15:1	Male predominance	Male predominance (particularly MSM), up to 7:1
Associated conditions		EBV	Organ transplantation, post-treatment lymphoma, corticosteroid and ciclosporin use	Drug abuse, HIV
Clinical features	Starts in the skin of the lower extremities and progresses very slowly.	In adults, locally aggressive in the skin, but rarely so systemically In children, lymphadenopathic with or without cutaneous involvement; often fatal <2 years	Resembles classic KS in presentation with a more varied site of presentation and more subtle lesions	Rapidly progressive; fulminant disease with widespread nodal and visceral involvement particularly in the absence of HAART

AIDS, acquired immune deficiency syndrome; HAART, highly active antiretroviral therapy; HIV, human immunodefiency virus; EBV, Epstein–Barr virus; MSM, men who have sex with men.

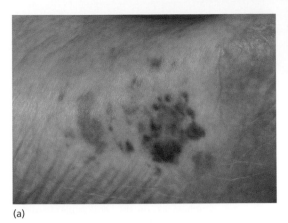

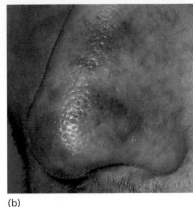

(a)   (b)

Figure 77.1 Patch-stage KS. Clinical lesions consist of violaceous to brown erythematous patches and plaques, most often involving the feet in classic KS (a) and often involving the face in AIDS-associated KS (b).

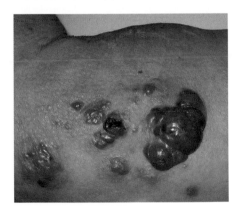

disease, excision and cryotherapy can be used. Intralesional vinblastine, interferon-α2b and imiquimod are effective although recurrence is common. For AIDS-associated KS, HAART often results in regression of KS, but up to 50% never achieve total remission. Reduction of immunosuppression in iatrogenic KS can lead to regression. Liposomal doxorubicin and paclitaxel as first-line and second-line treatments, respectively, for advanced KS.

Figure 77.2 Nodular KS.

Table 77.2 AIDS Clinical Trial Group staging system for KS

	0	1
Tumour (T)	Cutaneous or lymph node-only involvement with few oral macules	Oedema, ulceration, extensive oral KS with papules, extracutaneous and extranodal involvement
Immune (I)	CD4 T-cell count >150/mm^3	CD4 T-cell count <150/mm^3
Systemic (S)	No history of opportunistic infections or thrush; no B symptoms (unexplained fever, night sweats, unintentional weight loss of >10%, diarrhoea) *Karnofsky performance status >70	History of opportunistic infections or oral candidosis; one or more B symptoms Karnofsky performance status <70 Other HIV-related illness such as neurological involvement or lymphoma

*An assessment of functional impairment.

78 Cutaneous lymphomas

The current World Health Organization/European Organisation of Research and Treatment of Cancer (WHO–EORTC) classification is based on clinical, pathological, immunopathological, molecular and cytogenetic findings. It recognises that the site of origin of extranodal lymphomas rather than just tumour morphology determines clinical behaviour, which in turn has a critical influence on prognosis and therapeutic approach (Table 78.1).

PRIMARY CUTANEOUS T-CELL LYMPHOMAS

Mycosis fungoides

This is the most common variant of primary cutaneous T-cell lymphoma (CTCL), generally associated with an indolent clinical course and characterised by well-defined clinicopathological features.

Epidemiology

The incidence of mycosis fungoides (MF) (0.64/100 000) is increasing. Median age at diagnosis is mid-50s.

Pathophysiology

The aetiology of MF is not yet established.

Histological features vary according to the clinical stage. The earliest pathological features are the presence of a moderate lymphocytic infiltrate in the papillary dermis. As the disease progresses with the development of thicker plaques, prominent epidermotropism develops, with selective colonisation of the epidermis by atypical T cells either by single-cell colonisation often along the basal layer, or by clusters of atypical lymphocytes in the epidermis (Pautrier microabscesses). In more advanced stages of disease (IIB–III), the epidermotropic infiltrate may be lost, with scattered larger tumour cells showing marked cellular atypia. Large-cell transformation may occur and is a poor prognostic feature. The tumour cells are CD3+, CD4+, CD45RO+ and usually CD7− T cells. T-cell receptor (TCR) gene analysis in MF is a standard approach that has diagnostic, prognostic and therapeutic implications. Histological involvement of the central lymph nodes and other organs is a very poor prognostic sign.

Clinical features

Polymorphic patches and plaques predominantly affect limb/girdle sites, the breast and buttocks. 34% of patients progress to extensive plaques, tumours or erythroderma.

Patches are subtle, erythematous, fine, scaly and slightly atrophic (wrinkled) (Figure 78.1) and may be pruritic or asymptomatic.

Plaques are more obvious, persistent, polymorphic, erythematous lesions with a similar distribution (Figure 78.2). Individual plaques may become very large, with some degree of regression, giving rise to unusual arcuate lesions that can show considerable variation in colour, degree of scaling and border definition.

Rook's Dermatology Handbook, First Edition. Edited by Christopher E. M. Griffiths, Tanya O. Bleiker, Daniel Creamer, John R. Ingram and Rosalind C. Simpson.
© 2022 John Wiley & Sons Ltd. Published 2022 by John Wiley & Sons Ltd.

Table 78.1 WHO–EORTC classification of primary cutaneous lymphomas

WHO–EORTC classification	Frequency (%)	Disease-specific 5-year survival (%)
Primary cutaneous T-cell lymphoma		
Indolent clinical behaviour		
Mycosis fungoides	44	88
Folliculotropic mycosis fungoides	4	80
Pagetoid reticulosis	<1	100
Granulomatous slack skin disease	<1	100
Primary cutaneous anaplastic large cell lymphoma	8	96
Lymphomatoid papulosis	12	100
Subcutaneous panniculitis-like T-cell lymphoma	1	82
Primary cutaneous CD4+ small medium pleomorphic T-cell lymphoma	2	75
Aggressive clinical behaviour		
Sézary syndrome	3	24
Primary cutaneous NK/T-cell lymphoma, nasal type	<1	NR
Primary cutaneous aggressive CD8+ T-cell lymphoma	<1	18
Primary cutaneous γδ T-cell lymphoma	<1	NR
Primary cutaneous peripheral T-cell lymphoma, unspecified	2	16
Cutaneous B-cell lymphoma		
Indolent clinical behaviour		
Primary cutaneous marginal zone B-cell lymphoma	7	99
Primary cutaneous follicle centre lymphoma	11	95
Intermediate clinical behaviour		
Primary cutaneous diffuse large B-cell lymphoma, leg type	4	55
Primary cutaneous diffuse large B-cell lymphoma, other	<1	50
Primary cutaneous intravascular large B-cell lymphoma	<1	65

Source: Willemze, R. (2005). WHO-EORTC classification for cutaneous lymphomas. *Blood* 2005, 105(10), 3768–3785. doi: https://doi.org/10.1182/blood-2004-09-3502 © 2005 The American Society of Hematology. (Data are based on 1905 patients with a primary cutaneous lymphoma registered at the Dutch and Austrian cutaneous lymphoma database). EORTC, European Organisation of Research and Treatment of Cancer; NK, natural killer; NR, not reached; WHO, World Health Organization.

PART 10: NEOPLASTIC, PROLIFERATIVE AND INFILTRATIVE DISORDERS AFFECTING THE SKIN

Tumours can show considerable variation in size (Figure 78.3). Patients may rarely present with erythrodermic stages of disease and the differential diagnosis for these patients includes inflammatory dermatoses and Sézary syndrome.

The development of peripheral lymphadenopathy in MF may be associated with 'B' symptoms of fever and weight loss. The most common visceral sites involved include the pulmonary, skeletal, naso-pharyngeal and central nevous system (CNS).

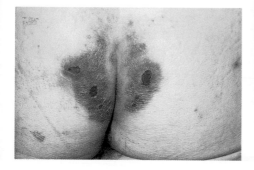

Figure 78.1 MF showing patches in the buttock area.

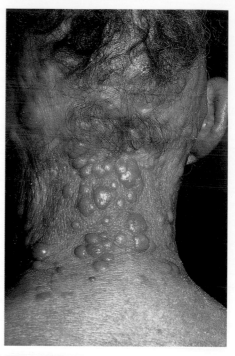

Figure 78.3 Nodular MF showing striking nodules on the back of the neck. Similar lesions were present on all four limbs.

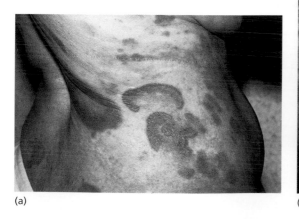

(a)

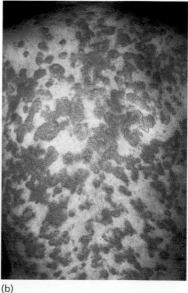

(b)

Figure 78.2 Mycosis fungoides. (a) Typical polycyclic plaques. (b) Plaques involving more than 10% of the body surface.

There is a large number of clinical variants of MF (Box 78.1 and Figure 78.4). Non-white, younger adult patients may present with a hypopigmented variant of MF, often involving the trunk and especially the pelvic girdle area rather than the limbs. In poikilodermatous MF the trunk is usually involved; the breasts and pelvic girdle area may also be affected. The poikiloderma is typically characterised by atrophy, pigmentation and telangiectasia and must be distinguished from poikiloderma resulting from other disorders by appropriate histology. A subset of patients have MF that appears to involve pilosebaceous follicles, giving rise to a follicular clinical pattern often with alopecia (pilotropic or folliculotropic MF); these patients may be resistant to treatment and have a poorer prognosis independent of their stage of disease. The other variants do not have any prognostic significance.

> **Box 78.1 Clinical variants of mycosis fungoides**
>
> - Folliculotropic/pilotropic
> - Poikiloderma
> - Hypopigmented
> - Capillaritis-like
> - Verrucous/hyperkeratotic
> - Psoriasiform
> - Icthyosiform
> - Bullous

Differential diagnosis

In the early stages the clinical differential diagnoses include allergic contact dermatitis, atopic

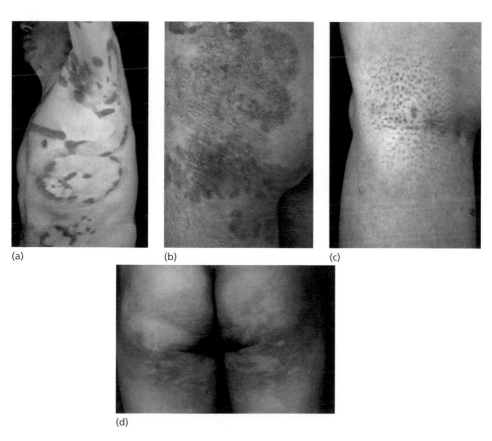

(a) (b) (c)

(d)

Figure 78.4 Clinical variants of MF: (a) annular/polycyclic, (b) poikilodermatous, (c) folliculotropic and (d) hypopigmented.

eczema, pityriasis rosea, psoriasis and fungal infections. Any patient with persistent polymorphic plaques, particularly involving the pelvic girdle area, should have a skin biopsy and histological confirmation.

In early MF, histological differential diagnosis includes a dermatitis reaction, arthropod bites and lymphomatous drug eruptions; clinicopathological correlation is essential.

Investigations

All patients should have a full clinical examination and adequate diagnostic biopsies for histology as well as immunophenotypic and molecular studies (Box 78.2).

An algorithm for establishing an early clinical and histological diagnosis of MF has been proposed by the International Society for Cutaneous Lymphoma (ISCL) (Table 78.2).

Box 78.2 Investigations for mycosis fungoides/Sézary syndrome

- Skin biopsies from representative patches/plaques/tumours (often multiple required every 3–6 months)
- Haematology, LDH, β_2 microglobulin, lymphocyte subsets (flow cytometry), Sézary cell count, HTLV-1 serology
- TCR gene analysis of skin, peripheral blood lymphocytes and any nodal tissue
- PET/CT scans for stages IIB–IV, lymph node excision/core biopsies for palpable peripheral nodes or those nodes >1.5 cm in short axis
- Bone marrow trephine biopsy if unexplained haematological findings

CT, computed tomography; HTLV, human T-cell leukaemia virus; LDH, lactate dehydrogenase; PET, positron emission tomography; TCR, T-cell receptor.

Table 78.2 International Society for Cutaneous Lymphoma diagnostic criteria for early mycosis fungoides (a total of 4 points is required for the diagnosis of MF)

Criteria	Major (2 points each)	Minor (1 point each)
Clinical		
Persistent and/or progressive patches and plaques **plus**	Any 2	Any 1
1 Non-sun-exposed location		
2 Size/shape variation		
3 Poikiloderma		
Histopathological		
Superficial lymphoid infiltrate **plus**	Both	Either
1 Epidermotropism		
2 Atypia		
Molecular/biological		
Clonal TCR rearrangement		Present
Immunopathological		Any 1
1 CD2, 3, 5 <50%		
2 CD7 <10%		
3 Epidermal discordance		

TCR, T-cell receptor.

Table 78.3 Clinical staging system for mycosis fungoides and Sézary syndrome related to the TNM classification

Stage	T (tumour)	N (node)	M (metastasis)	B (blood)
IA	T1: <10% skin surface patches, papules and plaques T1a (patch only) versus T1b (plaque ± patch)	N0 *N0 No palpable nodes or histological evidence of MF*	M0	B0–1 *B0 ≤ 5% Sézary cells* *B1 > 5% Sézary cells but does not meet criteria of B2*
IB	T2: ≥10% skin surface patches, papules and plaques	N0	M0	B0–1
IIA	T1–2	N1 *N1 Palpable node, no histological evidence of MF*	M0	B0–1
IIB	T3: one or more tumours (≥1 cm diameter)	N0–2 *N2 No palpable nodes but histological evidence of MF*	M0	B0–1
IIIA	T4: erythroderma ≥80% body surface area	N0–2	M0	B0
IIIB		N0–2	M0	B1
IVA1	T1–4	N0-2	M0	B2 *B2 ≥ 1000/μL Sézary cells*
IVA2	T1–4	N3 *N3 Palpable nodes and histological evidence of MF*	M0	B0–2
IVB	T1–4	N0–3	M1 *Visceral involvement, histological*	B0–2

Source: Adapted from Olsen, E., Vonderheid, E., Pimpinelli, N., Willemze, R., Kim, Y., ... Knobler, R. (2007). Revisions to the staging and classification of mycosis fungoides and Sezary syndrome: a proposal of the International Society for Cutaneous Lymphomas (ISCL) and the cutaneous lymphoma task force of the European Organization of Research and Treatment of Cancer (EORTC). *Blood*, 110(6), 1713–1722. doi:10.1182/blood-2007-03-055749.

Management

Staging is with the revised ISCL and EORTC system for MF and Sézary syndrome (SS) (see Table 78.3).

The choice of initial treatment for the MF patient will depend on the stage of the disease as well as the patient's performance status. Treatments range from skin-directed therapy consisting of topical agents, phototherapy and radiotherapy, to systemic treatment with biologics, chemotherapy and stem cell transplantation (Table 78.4).

A cutaneous lymphoma prognostic index (CLIPi) has been proposed based on independent multivariate prognostic factors (Table 78.5).

Table 78.4 Treatment algorithm for mycosis fungoides/Sézary syndrome

Prognostic group (stage)	First line	Second line
Mycosis fungoides		
IA–IIA	Expectant SDT	SDT Bexarotene TSEB IFN-α
IIB	SDT TSEB Bexarotene IFN-α	Brentuximab vedotin Clinical trials
III	SDT Methotrexate ECP IFN-α Bexarotene	Brentuximab vedotin Alemtuzumab Clinical trials
IVA2	SDT Chemotherapy Radiotherapy to specific LN basins	Brentuximab vedotin Bexarotene RIC-allo-SCT Clinical trials
IVB	SDT Radiotherapy to LN basins Chemotherapy	Brentuximab Bexarotene Clinical trials
Sezary syndrome		
IVA1–2	ECP Bexarotene IFN-α	Chemotherpay Alemtuzumab Brentuximab RIC-allo-SCT Clinical trials
IVB	Chemotherapy Radiotherapy	Chemotherapy Brentuximab Bexarotene Clinical trials

ECP, extracorporeal photopheresis; IFN-α, interferon α; PUVA, psoralen and ultraviolet A; SDT, skin-directed therapy (emollients with or without moderate potency topical steroids), topical chemotherapy (nitrogen mustard and carmustine), topical rexinoids [targretin 1% (bexarotene) gel], phototherapy (TLO1/PUVA 2–3 times per week until clearance or best partial response) or radiotherapy; TSEB, total skin electron beam therapy; RIC-allo-SCT, reduced-intensity allogeneic stem cell transplantation. Source: British Association of Dermatologists and UK Cutaneous Lymphoma Group guidelines for the management of primary cutaneous lymphomas 2018. Gilson D, et al. *Br J Dermatol* 2019, 180, 496–526).

Follicular mucinosis

(Syn. Alopecia mucinosa)

Boggy cutaneous plaques showing follicular prominence and histological evidence of mucinous degeneration of the hair follicles. There appear to be two distinct forms of follicular mucinosis, one associated with MF and a separate, benign, inflammatory form, although both conditions may represent points on a spectrum.

Table 78.5 Independent prognostic factors (CLIPi) for mycosis fungoides/Sézary syndrome patients

Stage	Adverse factors
Early IA–IIA	Male
	>60 years
	Plaques
	Folliculotropic
	N1/Nx
Late IIB–IVB	Male
	>60 years
	B1/B2
	N2/N3
	Visceral (M1)

Source: Benton et al. (2013). A cutaneous lymphoma international prognostic index (CLIPi) for mycosis fungoides and Sezary syndrome. *European Journal of Cancer*, 49(13), 2859–2868. doi:10.1016/j.ejca.2013.04.018. Reproduced with permission of Elsevier.

Pathophysiology

Degeneration of involved hair follicles, associated in MF with a prominent pilotropic, atypical T-cell infiltrate and interfollicular epidermotropism. Mucin stains such as Alcian blue show the presence of large quantities of mucin. The inflammatory form of follicular mucinosis does not show a prominent atypical pilotropic T-cell infiltrate, although repeated biopsies may be required to fully exclude MF. It may be impossible to distinguish these two forms with confidence and there is an emerging consensus that most, if not all, patients with follicular mucinosis have a form of CTCL (pilotropic MF).

Clonal TCR gene rearrangements can be detected in both MF-associated follicular mucinosis and so-called benign forms of inflammatory follicular mucinosis, consistent with suggestions that both may represent MF variants.

Clinical features

The clinical features of the two types of follicular mucinosis are identical: follicular papules and plaques often associated with severe pruritus and a predilection for the face and scalp, although the trunk and limbs can be affected and classic patches and plaques of MF may also be present. A younger age group is affected by inflammatory forms but there are no satisfactory criteria for distinguishing this from MF-associated follicular mucinosis. Prominent giant comedones are often a feature with acneiform lesions (Figure 78.5) and significant

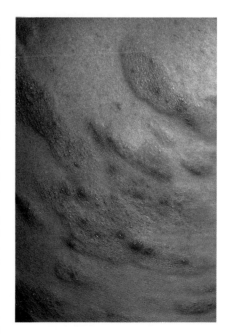

Figure 78.5 Clinical appearance of follicular mucinosis showing boggy mucin-secreting plaques on the trunk.

alopecia may be present. If hair follicles are destroyed, scarring alopecia will be present.

Management

MF associated with follicular mucinosis is treated with skin-directed therapy as for the early stages of MF (Table 78.4); patients may also require systemic treatment with interferon α (IFN-α) or retinoids (bexarotene). Radiotherapy is ideal for isolated plaques of folliculotropic MF. Total skin electron beam therapy may be appropriate for resistant cases. Dapsone can be effective for inflammatory forms of follicular mucinosis. Follicular variants of MF have a worse prognosis, with disease-specific survival rates of 81% at 5 years and 36% at 10 years.

Pagetoid reticulosis

(Syn. Woringer–Kolopp disease)
This is a localised solitary variant of CTCL, which histologically shows intense epidermotropism.

Epidemiology
Rare, affecting younger adults.

Pathophysiology
This entity may either represent a localised epidermotropic variant of MF or be closely related to the more recently described CD8+ epidermotropic CTCL.

Biopsies show an acanthotic epidermis with atypical, large, pale, mononuclear cells, which usually either fail to express lymphoid markers or express an aberrant T-cell phenotype.

Clinical features
Characterised by an isolated, persistent, scaly plaque, commonly involving an acral site (Figure 78.6). The lesion may be asymptomatic and slowly expands, but no further plaques develop on other body sites.

Management
Successful remission and probable cure have been reported with both surgical excision and low-dose superficial radiotherapy. The natural history of this lesion is of very slow local extension with an excellent prognosis.

Granulomatous slack skin disease

A rare disease characterised by the slow development of pendulous folds of lax erythematous skin.

Epidemiology
Middle aged adults.

Pathophysiology
There is a dense granulomatous dermal infiltrate with the destruction of dermal elastic tissue (elastolysis).

Clinical features
The lesions develop slowly and progress over several years. Typically, flexures and consist of thickened, pendulous folds (Figure 78.7). The condition must be distinguished from other forms of cutis laxa.

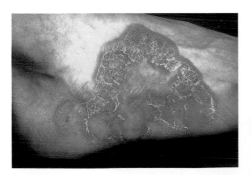

Figure 78.6 Pagetoid reticulosis showing a striking solitary scaling lesion on the side of the foot of a young man.

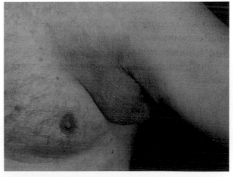

Figure 78.7 Granulomatous slack skin showing prominent, lax folds of markedly indurated axillary skin with superficial scaling and wrinkling.

Management

Radiotherapy, α-interferon, retinoids and surgery can be effective. The prognosis is excellent.

Sézary syndrome

A clinical triad of erythroderma, peripheral lymphadenopathy and atypical mononuclear cells (Sézary cells) comprising more than 20% of total lymphocyte count or a total Sézary count of more than 1000 × 10⁹/L (peripheral blood stage B2).

Epidemiology

The majority are elderly males; may develop the syndrome either *ab initio* or rarely as progression from classic MF.

Pathophysiology

Skin biopsies show large numbers of atypical mononuclear cells in the dermis with epidermotropism. Sézary cells are usually CD3+, CD4+, CD7– and CD26– T cells. Diagnostic

criteria should include the clinical triad of features plus a peripheral blood T-cell clone as indicated by a CD4:CD8 ratio greater than 10, an aberrant expression of pan T-cell antigens, cytogenetics or TCR gene.

Clinical features

Often a prolonged history of 'dermatitis'; rarely patients may have a history of MF.

Patients present with a generalised exfoliative erythroderma, sometimes associated with ectropion, scalp alopecia, palmoplantar hyperkeratosis and fissuring and subungual hyperkeratosis (Figure 78.8). Peripheral lymphadenopathy is often present and there may be systemic features due to the erythroderma.

Differential diagnosis

Includes other causes of erythroderma (Chapter 86).

Management

See Table 78.3 for staging and Table 78.4 for treatment.

The prognosis in SS is poor, with an 11% 5-year overall survival and median survival of 32 months from diagnosis. Most patients die of opportunistic infection.

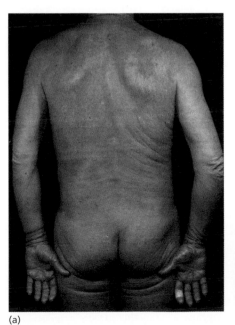
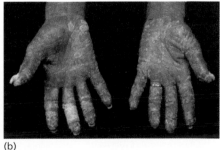

(a) (b)

Figure 78.8 Sézary syndrome showing (a) erythroderma on the back with (b) palmoplantar hyperkeratosis and prominent nail dystrophy.

PRIMARY CUTANEOUS CD30+ LYMPHOPROLIFERATIVE DISORDERS

Primary cutaneous CD30+ lymphoproliferative disorders consist of a spectrum of conditions and represents 30% of all primary cutaneous lymphomas. Lymphomatoid papulosis and CD30+ anaplastic large-cell lymphomas are defined on the basis of clinical and pathological features. Where a distinction cannot be made, patients are designated as 'borderline cases'.

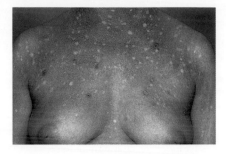

Figure 78.9 Lymphomatoid papulosis. Note multiple scars on the upper chest area of this patient, with a small number of fresh papular lesions.

Lymphomatoid papulosis

A chronic, recurrent, self-healing papulonecrotic or papulonodular eruption with the histological features of a CD30+ cutaneous lymphoma.

Pathophysiology

Clonal TCR gene rearrangements can be identified and are identical in different lesions from the same patient.

There is a mixed dermal infiltrate composed of atypical lymphocytes with large nuclei and frequent abnormal mitoses, eosinophils, neutrophils, extravasated red cells and large histiocytic cells with a relative lack of epidermotropism and Pautrier microabscesses.

Clinical features

Recurrent crops of papular, papulonecrotic or nodular lesions predominantly affecting the trunk, although any body site can be involved and regional localised patterns may occur (Figure 78.9). Lesions grow rapidly over a few days and develop ulcerated necrotic centres. Healing occurs slowly with fine atrophic circular or varioliform scars, but the cycle recurs every few months, with no obvious initiating factor. The lesions generally occur first in adult life and may recur in crops for up to 40 years. Over time, skin lesions will resolve and there may be a persistent remission.

The original description of lymphomatoid papulosis suggested a benign and non-progressive chronic pattern of the disease, but patients may develop primary cutaneous or nodal CD30+ large-cell anaplastic T-cell lymphoma, and Hodgkin disease.

Management

There is no current treatment that alters the natural history of the disease but some therapies may accelerate healing and reduce or prevent the frequency and severity of new lesions. The EORTC, ISCL and US Cutaneous Lymphoma Consortium consensus guidelines for the treatment of primary cutaneous CD30+ lymphoproliferative disorders have been published (Table 78.6).

Long-term follow-up is necessary because of the risk of progression to a more aggressive lymphoma such as a primary cutaneous CD30+ anaplastic lymphoma, MF or Hodgkin disease in less than 5% of cases. The prognosis in patients with both MF and lymphomatoid papulosis appears to be excellent. There are no proven prognostic indicators to identify those patients who are more likely to develop associated lymphomas.

Primary cutaneous anaplastic (CD30+) large-cell lymphoma

A primary cutaneous CD30+ anaplastic large-cell lymphoma (ALCL) in which the CD30+ tumour cells comprise the majority of the infiltrate. Clinical features of MF are absent.

Table 78.6 Treatment algorithm for cutaneous CD30+ lymphoproliferative disorders

Disease	First line	Second line
Lymphomatoid papulosis	Expectant	MTX
	SDT	IFN-α
	Radiotherapy	
Anaplastic large-cell lymphoma	Surgical excision (solitary lesions)	CHOP
	Radiotherapy	Brentuximab vedotin
	MTX	

CHOP, cyclophosphamide, doxorubicin, vincristine, prednisolone; IFN-α, interferon α; MTX, methotrexate; SDT, skin-directed therapy (topical therapy, phototherapy (TLO1/PUVA) or radiotherapy).

Epidemiology
Adults.

Pathophysiology
Biopsies show a dense lymphocytic infiltrate consisting of sheets of large atypical cells with an anaplastic morphology and mitoses; usually no epidermotropism. The vast majority of tumour cells are CD30+. Clonal TCR gene rearrangements are usually detected consistent with a T-cell origin.

'Borderline cases' are closely related to both lymphomatoid papulosis and primary cutaneous CD30+ large-cell lymphoma with the detection of a T-cell phenotype and clonal rearrangements of the TCR gene confirming a T-cell origin.

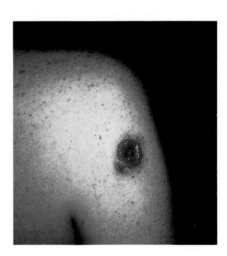

Figure 78.10 CD30+ cutaneous lymphoma showing typical ulcerated lesion on the shoulder.

Clinical features
Presents with large solitary or multiple (often ulcerated) nodules, most often on the trunk (Figure 78.10). Some individuals develop disease localised to a limb. There may be a clinical spectrum with large persistent nodules of ALCL and coexistent lesions of lymphomatoid papulosis. Progression to extracutaneous sites is rare but recorded in ~10%; patients with extensive regional disease may be at risk of disease progression.

Investigation
Careful staging consisting of bone marrow and CT scans are required to exclude systemic CD30+ ALCL in which there is secondary cutaneous involvement.

Management
Both excision and localised radiotherapy are methods of treating isolated lesions (see Table 78.6). Spontaneous clearance of even quite large lesions is recorded and therefore a short period of observation is acceptable.

Disease-related 5-year survival rates of 90% have been reported but they may be as low as 50% for those patients presenting with generalised tumours.

Subcutaneous panniculitis-like T-cell lymphoma

This is a rare, cytotoxic T-cell lymphoma, representing less than 1% of all non-Hodgkin lymphomas.

Epidemiology
Younger adults with an equal sex incidence.

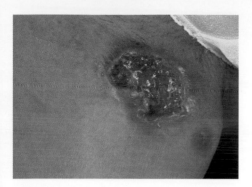

Figure 78.11 Subcutaneous panniculitis-like T-cell lymphoma: indurated and eroded deep plaque on the thigh.

Pathophysiology

There is a diffuse infiltrate restricted to and extending throughout the subcutis without epidermotropism. Lymphocyte atypia combined with adipocyte rimming of CD8+ T cells is also seen.

Clinical features

Patients present with indolent, slowly expanding, subcutaneous nodules usually involving the limbs, which may initially be misdiagnosed as panniculitis (Figure 78.11). Occasionally, patients present with more diffuse erythematous induration mimicking cellulitis. Ulceration is rare. Lymphadenopathy is usually absent at presentation.

Differential diagnosis

Lupus panniculitis, other causes of panniculitis.

Management

Systemic steroids. Superficial radiotherapy can be used for individual lesions. Combination chemotherapy is usually restricted to those with extracutaneous disease. Autologous/allogeneic stem cell transplantation has been successful in patients with refractory disease.

5-year survival is 80%.

PRIMARY CUTANEOUS PERIPHERAL T-CELL LYMPHOMA (UNSPECIFIED)

These are a heterogeneous group of T-cell malignancies, which are not defined by any of the recognised clinicopathological subsets. These include primary cutaneous aggressive epidermotropic CD8+ T-cell lymphoma, primary cutaneous γδ T-cell lymphoma, extranodal NK/T-cell lymphoma (nasal type) and adult T-cell leukaemia–lymphoma (HTLV-1 associated). Only the latter is described here. Primary cutaneous CD4+ small/medium-sized pleomorphic T-cell lymphoma has been downgraded to a lymphoproliferation due to benign behaviour and excellent outcome.

Adult T-cell leukaemia–lymphoma (HTLV-1 associated)

A peripheral T-cell leukaemia–lymphoma caused by the human retrovirus HTLV-1.

Epidemiology

HTLV-1 infection is prevalent in certain parts of the world including Japan, central Africa, the Caribbean, and the south-eastern states of the USA, and consequently adult T-cell leukaemia–lymphoma (ATLL) is endemic in these regions. Sporadic cases are also found. The disease has a long latency period (15–20 years) and the incidence of ATLL among HTLV-1 carriers has been estimated to be 2.5%. There is a slight male predominance and the median age of onset is 55 years.

Pathophysiology

HTLV-1 is randomly integrated into the host genome and induces expression of numerous host genes with additional molecular abnormalities producing a malignant phenotype.

In the skin, a prominent epidermotropic infiltrate consisting of medium to large cells with a pleomorphic nuclear morphology.

Tumour cells are CD2+, CD3+, CD5+ and CD7–. Most tumour cells are CD4+. TCR genes analysis shows clonal TCR gene rearrangements.

Clinical features

Patients with ATLL often have extensive lymph node and peripheral blood involvement but the skin is the most common extranodal site of disease (50% of patients) and primary cutaneous disease can occur. Other extranodal sites of disease include bone, lung, liver, the gastrointesti-

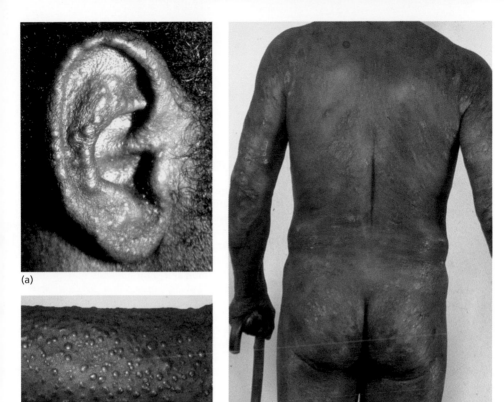

(a)

(b)

(c)

Figure 78.12 Three clinical presentations of cutaneous adult T-cell leukaemia–lymphoma: (a) a pruritic papular eruption confined to the auricle, (b) an extensive nodular eruption on the forearm and (c) superficial patches and plaques involving the limb–girdle area similar to MF.

nal tract and the CNS. Cutaneous involvement is characterised by widespread or solitary papules, nodules, tumours or erythroderma, often associated with intense pruritus (Figure 78.12). Clinically may be indistinguishable from MF.

Opportunistic infections are common including superficial fungal, *Staphylococcus aureus*, scabies, *Strongyloides stercoralis* and tuberculosis.

Investigations

Full staging investigations including PET/CT scans and bone marrow trephine biopsies as well as viral load assays of peripheral blood. HTLV-1 serology is positive. Hypercalcaemia is a common and characteristic finding of acute variants.

Management

Cutaneous disease can respond to skin-directed therapy but patients with the acute and lymphomatous variants have a poor prognosis and require combination chemotherapy. Combination azacytidine and interferon therapy is a standard of care for those with chronic and smouldering variants of ATLL.

Acute and lymphomatous variants have a poor prognosis with less than 10% 5-year survival. In contrast, patients with the chronic (30% 5-year survival) and smouldering (65% 5-year survival) variants can have a prolonged course, although disease transformation eventually occurs for most patients.

PRIMARY CUTANEOUS B-CELL LYMPHOMAS

Primary cutaneous B-cell lymphomas constitute approximately one-quarter of all primary cutaneous lymphomas. The WHO–EORTC classification defines three specific subtypes: marginal zone lymphoma (MZL), follicle centre cell lymphoma (FCL) and diffuse large B-cell lymphoma (LBCL). Full staging investigations are essential for patients with a cutaneous B-cell lymphoma to exclude secondary cutaneous involvement with a nodal lymphoma. Most primary cutaneous B-cell lymphomas are indolent with an excellent long-term prognosis, with the exception of primary cutaneous LBCL. Patients should be managed jointly with a haemato-oncologist.

Marginal zone lymphoma

An indolent primary cutaneous lymphoma derived from post-germinal centre cells.

Epidemiology
There is a slight male predominance and younger adults are more commonly affected.

Pathophysiology
Primary cutaneous MZL is considered to be part of the spectrum of extranodal marginal zone B-cell lymphomas that were first described in the stomach, the so-called mucosa-associated lymphoid tissue lymphoma. Some have been associated with *Borrelia burgdorferi* infection.

Histology is characterised by nodular or diffuse dermal infiltrates of small to medium-sized lymphocytes, marginal B cells (centrocyte-like), lymphoplasmacytoid cells and plasma cells, often with a reactive T-cell infiltrate. There is no epidermotropism.

Clinical features
These lymphomas present as asymptomatic solitary or multiple dermal papules, plaques or nodules on any body site, although the trunk is most often involved (Figure 78.13). Spontaneous resolution can occur.

Investigations
Full staging investigations are indicated and a benign monoclonal paraproteinaemia may be present.

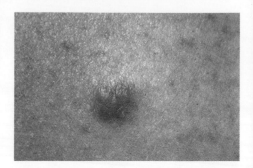

Figure 78.13 Primary cutaneous MZL: typical urticated dermal erythematous papules and plaques predominantly situated on the trunk.

Management
Radiotherapy (low dose) is the standard treatment option but some patients may be managed simply by observation in view of the excellent long-term prognosis. Surgical excision may be used for isolated small lesions. In cases associated with *Borrelia burgdorferi* relevant antibiotic therapy can be appropriate, although evidence is lacking. In patients with multifocal disease chlorambucil may be appropriate.

The estimated 5-year survival is 98–100%.

Follicle centre cell lymphoma

An indolent primary cutaneous B-cell lymphoma derived from follicle centre cells.

Pathophysiology
The histology is variable but the infiltrate shows no epidermotropism and there is a clear Grenz zone in the papillary dermis. In the reticular dermis and subcutaneous fat there is a 'bottom heavy' nodular or diffuse infiltrate composed of a mixture of centrocytes (small/large cleaved cells), centroblasts (large non-cleaved cells with prominent nucleoli), and a prominent infiltrate of reactive T cells with the remnants of poorly formed germinal centres.

Clinical features
Patients present with clinically non-specific solitary or grouped papules, nodules or tumours, most commonly on the head and neck or trunk, although any body site may be involved (Figure 78.14).

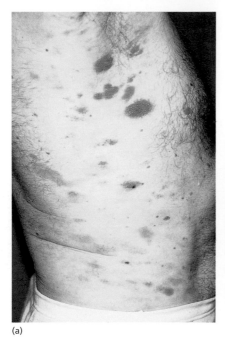
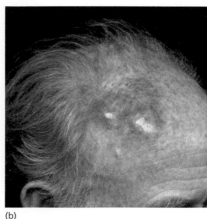

(a)

(b)

Figure 78.14 Primary cutaneous follicle centre cell lymphoma. (a) Extensive erythematous plaque and nodular lesions on the trunk. (b) Typical clinical presentation on the scalp.

Investigations

Full staging investigations are indicated.

Management

Superficial radiotherapy is the treatment of choice for solitary, recurrent and multifocal cutaneous disease. Solitary lesions may be excised, although subsequent radiotherapy is probably advisable to reduce the risk of local recurrence. Recurrences occur in ~30% of cases, are usually confined to the skin, and do not signify a worse prognosis.

The estimated 5-year survival of FCL is 94–97%.

Diffuse large B-cell lymphoma

Primary cutaneous diffuse large B-cell lymphoma (DLBCL) is a rare primary cutaneous lymphoma characterised by a diffuse proliferation of large B cells consisting of centroblasts and immunoblasts, occurring most commonly on the leg.

Epidemiology

Primary cutaneous DLBCL affects an elderly population with a female predominance.

Pathophysiology

There is a diffuse non-epidermotropic infiltrate of large cells with morphological similarity to centroblasts and immunoblasts which may extend to involve the subcutis.

Clinical features

These lymphomas tend to develop on the lower limbs, predominantly as large dermal nodules or tumours, which are either solitary or multifocal and rapidly enlarging (Figure 78.15).

Investigations

Full staging investigations are indicated.

Management

In elderly patients with solitary tumours, radiotherapy may be appropriate but multiagent chemotherapy is usually required, especially for multifocal disease.

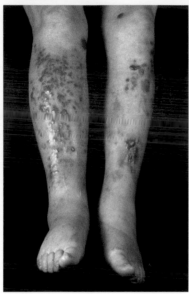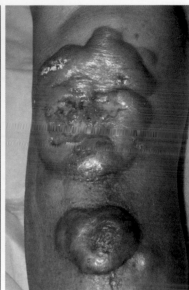

Figure 78.15 Clinical presentation of diffuse large B-cell lymphoma on the legs.

The prognosis of primary cutaneous DLBCL is poor, with a 5-year survival of 41–58%.

OTHER DISORDERS

Leukaemia cutis

Leukaemia cutis is characterised by solitary or multiple dermal skin lesions due to cutaneous infiltration by leukaemic cells (Box 78.3).

Pathophysiology

Skin infiltration favours the lower dermis and subcutaneous fat, with prominent involvement of the adnexal structures, nerves and vessels of the superficial and deep plexus. Cellular atypia may be prominent and mitotic figures are variable.

Clinical features

Generally asymptomatic small, reddish or violaceous/grey-blue macules, papules or nodules (Figure 78.16), which may be fleeting or persistent. Leukaemia cutis occurs in about 20% of patients with acute monocytic leukaemia and extramedullary involvement is often a poor prognostic feature. Gum involvement occurs in 25–50% of patients. Cutaneous involvement

> **Box 78.3 Types of leukaemia causing leukaemia cutis**
>
> - Chronic lymphocytic leukaemia
> - Myelomonocytic leukaemia
> - Hairy cell leukaemia
> - T-cell prolymphocytic leukaemia
> - T-cell acute lymphoblastic leukaemia

usually occurs after the diagnosis of the underlying haematological malignancy but rarely can occur as the presenting feature.

Non-specific lesions are common, but rarely reported by dermatologists. Generalised pruritus may be a presenting symptom and prurigo-like papules develop in some cases.

Differential diagnosis

Sweet syndrome, sarcoidosis, panniculitis, or cutaneous B-cell lymphoma.

Management

The treatment for leukaemia cutis is management of the underlying disease, with symptomatic measures for the skin lesions when required. Superficial radiotherapy can provide useful palliation for symptomatic skin lesions. Some cutaneous lesions may spontaneously regress.

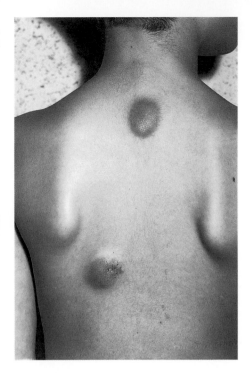

Figure 78.16 Leukaemia cutis in a child with leukaemia.

Cutaneous manifestations of Hodgkin disease

Hodgkin disease does not originate in the skin but rarely can spread in a contiguous manner to the skin as a direct extension from an underlying involved regional lymph node. Cutaneous lesions consist of solitary plaques or tumours that may be ulcerated. Appropriate staging investigations, including CT scans and lymph node biopsies, should be performed. In view of the cytological similarity between primary cutaneous CD30+ lymphoproliferative disorders and Hodgkin disease, this differential diagnosis must be excluded on the basis of clinical and pathological assessment, including immunophenotyping of the infiltrate (only Hodgkin cells are CD15 positive).

Non-specific cutaneous signs associated with Hodgkin disease are very common and occur in 3–50% of cases. These include pigmentation, pruritus, prurigo, atrophy, alopecia, exfoliative dermatitis and herpes zoster.

Pigmentation
This is melanin pigmentation and is very common. It resembles the pigmentation of Addison disease, being most marked in areas that normally show some darkening, such as the axillae, groins and around the nipples. Less often it is more widespread and occasionally a bizarre pigmentation occurs. The mucous membranes are usually spared.

Pruritus
This often occurs together with pigmentation. It is often the presenting feature of the disease and may precede the presence of palpable nodes by months or years. It tends to start on the legs. It is especially severe in patients who show other general symptoms such as fever and weight loss.

Prurigo
This is a sequelae of pruritus. In addition to the widespread irritation, there are excessively itchy papules, predominantly on the trunk, which are scratched until the skin surface is removed and is replaced by a blood crust. When present in association with enlarged superficial glands, it is often called Hodgkin prurigo.

Ichthyosiform atrophy
Hodgkin disease is probably the most common condition to be associated with this acquired icthyosis. It usually starts on the legs and resembles ichthyosis vulgaris, with thin, dry and rather firmly attached scales.

Alopecia
Hair loss is common in Hodgkin disease. It can be caused by rubbing or scratching to relieve itching. It may also be part of the ichthyosiform atrophy or be caused by endocrine dysfunction, when specific infiltration occurs in organs such as the pituitary or adrenal.

Exfoliative dermatitis
Erythroderma and exfoliative dermatitis can occur in Hodgkin disease.

Herpes zoster
Herpes zoster is common in the course of Hodgkin disease, but disseminated zoster is much less likely to occur in Hodgkin disease than in leukaemias.

PART 10: NEOPLASTIC, PROLIFERATIVE AND INFILTRATIVE DISORDERS AFFECTING THE SKIN

79

Basal cell carcinoma

(Syn. Rodent ulcer)

Basal cell carcinoma (BCC) is the most common human cancer. BCC and squamous cell carcinoma (SCC) (Chapter 80), are often grouped together as keratinocyte carcinomas (KCs) and previously as non-melanoma skin cancer, to distinguish them from melanoma. BCC represents approximately 74% of KCs whilst SCC is less common at 23%.

Epidemiology

UV radiation is the most important risk factor for KC. The geographical variability of KC incidence correlates with the amount of ambient sun irradiance and skin type. Unlike SCC, for which cumulative lifetime sun-exposure shows a strong dose–response relationship, for BCC intermittent sun-exposure and exposure during childhood appears more important.

The incidence of BCC varies widely with the highest rates in Australia (>1000/100 000 person-years) and the lowest rates in parts of Africa (<1/100 000 person-years). In England, the incidence of BCC is 76.21/100 000 person-years. Despite underreporting of BCC there is a clear 10% per year rise in incidence worldwide.

80% of cases occur in people aged 60 years and over. The largest annual increase in the numbers of BCCs has been observed among those aged 30–49 years. M > F.

40–50% of patients with a primary BCC will develop at least one or more BCC within 5 years. This risk is highest in the first 6 months after first BCC diagnosis.

Pathophysiology

Risk factors for the development of BCC are listed in Box 79.1. The primary risk factors are ultraviolet (UV) light exposure and genetic predisposition. Both UVB and UVA radiation are mutagenic. UVB radiation causes direct DNA and RNA damage by generation of mutagenic photoproducts. UVA induces indirect DNA damage via formation of reactive oxygen species.

A number of spontaneous and inherited gene defects predispose to the development of BCC. These include mutations in the hedgehog signalling pathway genes, primarily genes encoding patched homologue 1 (*PTCH1*) and smoothened homologue (*SMO*). Hedgehog is a key regulator of cell proliferation and growth; mutations in the pathway leads to proliferation of basal cells in the skin. Other genes of importance include the melanocortin-1 receptor (*MC1R*) genes (associated with fair skin, red hair and melanoma risk) and the p53 tumour suppressor.

Histologically the tumour cells resemble those of the basal layer of the epidermis. Nuclei are compact, darkly staining and closely set. Cytoplasm stains poorly and the cell margins are rather indistinct. The interaction with the dermis produces the characteristic marginal palisade of tumour cells and the well-organised stroma that surrounds it. The cells within the palisade usually show little evidence of organisation or differentiation. Mitotic figures may be frequent.

Histopathological patterns of BCC include superficial, nodular, infiltrative, micronodular and pigmented types.

Superficial BCC: Proliferating atypical basaloid cells form an axis parallel to the epidermal surface.

Rook's Dermatology Handbook, First Edition. Edited by Christopher E. M. Griffiths, Tanya O. Bleiker, Daniel Creamer, John R. Ingram and Rosalind C. Simpson.
© 2022 John Wiley & Sons Ltd. Published 2022 by John Wiley & Sons Ltd.

Nodular BCC: Nests of basaloid cells in either the papillary or reticular dermis where solar elastosis may be evident. The nests are separated from the stroma by a slit-like retraction.

Micronodular BCC: The tumour nests are smaller than those in nodular BCC and more widely and asymmetrically dispersed in the dermis and/or subcutis.

Morphoeic BCC, also known as sclerosing BCC: Displays one- to two-cell thick columns of basaloid cells enmeshed in a dense collagenous stroma. Stromal fibroplasia and fibrosis of the tumour cords is commonly seen with invasion of the deep dermis and subcutis.

Infiltrative BCC: Shows elongated tumour cell strands, five to eight cells in thickness which present as irregularly sized and shaped nests which are poorly circumscribed and may show invasion of the subcutis and adjacent muscular and other structures.

Pigmented BCC: Benign melanocytes produce increased melanin.

Basosquamous or metatypical BCC: Has features of both BCC and SCC and is associated with a significantly higher incidence of metastatic spread.

Table 79.1 Genetic syndromes with BCC as a prominent feature.

Naevoid basal cell carcinoma syndrome (see below)   Bazex–Dupré–Christol syndrome   Rombo syndrome   Xeroderma pigmentosum (see Chapter 37)   Generalised follicular basaloid hamartoma syndrome   Happle–Tinschert syndrome

Source: Adapted from Castori et al. 2012.

Table 79.2 Genetic syndromes with BCC as an ancillary feature.

Genomic instability syndromes
    Muir–Torre syndrome (see Chapter 37)
    Bloom syndrome
    Werner syndrome
    Rothmund–Thomson syndrome
 Disorders of the folliculosebaceous unit
    (see Chapter 76)
    Cowden syndrome
    Brooke Spiegler syndrome
    Schöpf–Schulz–Passarge syndrome
 Syndromes with immunodeficiency
    Epidermodysplasia verruciformis
    Cartilage–hair hypoplasia
 Disorders of melanin biosynthesis
    Oculocutaneous albinism
    Hermansky–Pudlak syndrome

Source: Adapted from Castori et al. 2012.

Box 79.1 Risk factors for BCC

- Solar UV radiation
- Fitzpatrick skin type I and II
- Human papillomavirus
- Iatrogenic immunosuppression
- Acquired immunodeficiency syndrome and non-Hodgkin lymphoma
- Psoralen and UVA therapy
- Photosensitising drugs
- UVB phototherapy
- Ionising radiation
- Occupational factors
- Arsenic exposure
- Previous history of BCC
- >10 actinic keratoses (five-fold increase risk)
- Genetic, e.g. xeroderma pigmentosum, naevoid basal cell carcinoma syndrome (see Tables 79.1 and 79.2)

Clinical features

BCCs typically run a slow progressive course. Approximately 80% occur on the head and neck. Early lesions are usually small, translucent or pearly, with raised telangiectatic edges. More advanced lesions can present as a classical 'rodent ulcer' with an indurated edge and an ulcerated centre. Other common subtypes are nodular or cystic, superficial, morphoeic and pigmented. Between 10% and 40% of BCCs contain a mixed pattern of two or more subtypes. Certain features will divide BCC into high and low risk of recurrence, which may influence the choice of management (see Table 79.3).

Nodular BCC (Figure 79.1): The commonest subtype and usually on the head and neck. There

Table 79.3 Features of high-risk BCCs

Features	High–risk BCC
Clinical subtype	Morphoeic
Tumour size	>5 cm giant BCC
Tumour site	Centrofacial, including periocular and ears
Histological subtype	Infiltrative and micronodular
Histological features of aggression	Perineural and/or perivascular involvement
Host characteristic	Immunosuppression
Lesion type	Recurrent
Lymph node status/other organ involvement	Lymph node involvement or distant metastasis

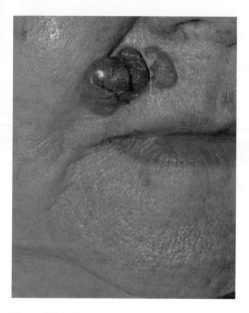

Figure 79.1 Nodular BCC.

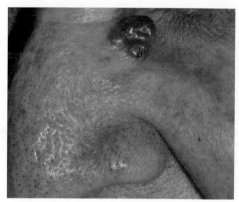

Figure 79.2 Pigmented nodular BCC.

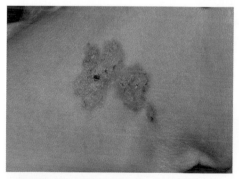

Figure 79.3 Superficial BCC.

may be surface telangiectasia over a pink, red or flesh-coloured mass (Figure 79.2).

Superficial BCC (Figure 79.3): Less common and predominantly on the trunk. Bounded by a slightly raised thread-like margin or a 'whipcord' edge, which is irregular in outline and may be deficient at part of the circumference. The epidermis covering the central zone is usually atrophic and may be scaly. Patients with initially truncal BCC of superficial histology demonstrate the highest rate of increasing BCC numbers.

Morphoeic BCC (Figure 79.4): Also known as sclerodermiform, so named because dense fibrosis of the stroma produces a thickened plaque rather than a tumour. They account for

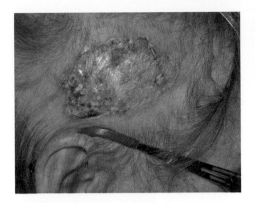

Figure 79.4 Morphoeic BCC.

5% of all BCC, have ill-defined borders, can be difficult to diagnose clinically and often present late. The exact margin of the lesion is impossible to define, but palpation reveals a firm skin texture that extends irregularly beyond the visible changes.

Ulcerated BCC (Figure 79.5): May start as a small macule or papule but with expansion of the thread-like margins, the attenuated surface ulcerates. If left, the tumour and its following ulcer may spread deeply and cause great destruction, especially around the eye, nose or ear. There may be wide extension in the periorbital tissues, the bones of the face, the skull and even the meninges.

Pigmented BCC: A pigmented variant which must be distinguished from a melanoma.

Fibroepithelial BCC (fibroepithelioma of Pinkus): A benign-appearing pedunculated pink tumour that may resemble an acrochordon or skin tag; now classed as a BCC variant. Commonly on the trunk, especially the lower back and extremities. F > M.

Advanced and metastatic BCC (Figure 79.6): A manifestation of prolonged neglect and account for 1–2% of all BCCs. Mutilation of the face or scalp, with destruction of the nose or eye and exposure of the paranasal sinuses or the skull, dura or brain may eventually result in death. Progression of advanced BCC to a

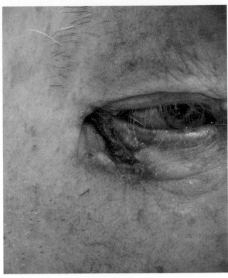

Figure 79.5 Ulcerated BCC.

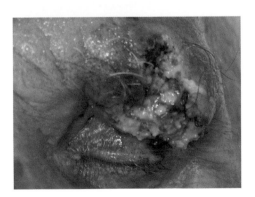

Figure 79.6 Advanced BCC.

metastatic form is extremely rare (0.0028–0.55% of BCCs) and usually have a basosquamous histological subtype.

Differential diagnosis
See Table 79.4.

Investigations
The diagnosis is primarily clinical. A biopsy may be required for diagnosis or to aid management decisions. In nodular BCC this may be a

Table 79.4 Differential diagnosis of BCC

Diagnosis	Distinguishing clinical features	Image
Naevus	Lack of rolled telangiectatic edge May be hairy	
Sebaceous hyperplasia	Central depression, usually multiple on a background of sebaceous quality skin	
Molluscum contagiosum	Central punctum is characteristic	
Keratoacanthoma	A central keratin plug is typical, history of evolution followed by involution	
SCC	Shorter history and indurated base (better felt on palpation)	
Bowen disease	Scaly edge, lack of thread-like margin	

(Continued)

Table 79.4 (Continued)

Diagnosis	Distinguishing clinical features	Image
Psoriasis	Silvery scales and response to topical antipsoriatic therapy	
Eczema	History of eczema and response to topical eczema therapy	
Melanoma	Grey-black discoloration and pigment spill. Shorter history	
Chondrodermatitis nodularis helicis	Usually tender	
Viral warts	Keratotic 'warty' surface	

shave biopsy; a punch biopsy may be more appropriate in morphoeic lesions.

Dermoscopy is a useful clinical adjunct as identification of features such as white and grey-brown structureless areas, blue-grey ovoid nests, blue-grey globules, maple-leaf like areas, spoke-wheel areas, concentric structures, ulcerations and blue-grey dots may help differentiate BCC from Bowen disease and melanomas and also help in subtyping the tumour (Figure 79.7). The most frequently observed vasculature include atypical red vessels, arborising, comma and telangiectactic vessels, short fine telangiectasias and vascular blush.

Management

Both tumour (clinical and histological nature, size and site) and patient factors determine the choice of treatment of BCC. An approach to the treatment of a patient with a BCC is illustrated in Figure 79.8.

The primary aim of treatment is complete removal of the BCC. Achieving a good and acceptable cosmetic outcome is an important secondary goal. For low-risk superficial and small nodular BCC, non-destructive therapies such as topical treatments and photodynamic therapy have a high success rate, usually with an excellent cosmetic outcome. Conversely, high-risk and recurrent BCC require histological examination of the excision margins.

Surgical treatments

Excision with predetermined margins: Surgical excision is one of the most effective treatments for well-defined BCCs. Complete clearance can be achieved in 95% of the well-defined small BCC with a 4–5 mm surgical margin. Recurrence rates are low (<2% in 5 years) following histologically complete excision and cosmetic outcomes are good.

Mohs micrographic surgery: Certain high-risk lesions should be considered for Mohs micrographic surgery. Criteria include:

- Size (especially larger (>2 cm) lesions).
- Site (especially the perioral, periorbital, perinasal and periauricular areas where a combination of a high cure rate and maximal preservation of normal tissues and structures is vital).

- Lesions with very poorly defined clinical borders (where it is difficult to accurately identify appropriate surgical resection margins).
- Failure of previous treatment (recurrent disease).
- Histologically incompletely excised lesions.
- High-risk histological features (Table 79.3).

Curettage and electrodesiccation (Syn. Curettage and cautery): Can be considered for low-risk non-facial lesions.

Cryosurgery: Liquid nitrogen cryosurgery can be used for low-risk primary BCC. A single 30-s freeze–thaw cycle for superficial truncal BCC is recommended. Compared to surgical excision, for low-risk primary BCC cryosurgery may achieve a similar recurrence rate but pain and subsequent hypopigmentation are common.

Medical treatments

Imiquimod: Topical 5% imiquimod cream is an immune response modifier. Applied five times per week for 6 weeks. Licensed for use in superficial BCC in immunocompetent adults, with a maximum tumour diameter of 2.0 cm. Erythema, pruritus, erosion, ulceration, dyspigmentation and scabbing are commonly observed side effects of topical imiquimod therapy (Figure 79.9). Patients may also experience flu-like symptoms, which may be severe enough to stop treatment.

5-Fluorouracil (5-FU): An antimetabolite. Despite high histological cure rates and good cosmesis with topical 5-FU treatment of small and superficial BCC, it is rarely used for this indication.

Photodynamic therapy (PDT): MAL PDT using red light LED irradiation at 37.5 J/cm² is licensed for superficial BCC with two treatments 1 week apart, repeated at 3 months if there is only partial response. Clearance rates of 92–97% are reported at 3 months follow-up.

Vismodegib: A hedgehog pathway inhibitor used in the treatment of metastatic and locally advanced BCCs.

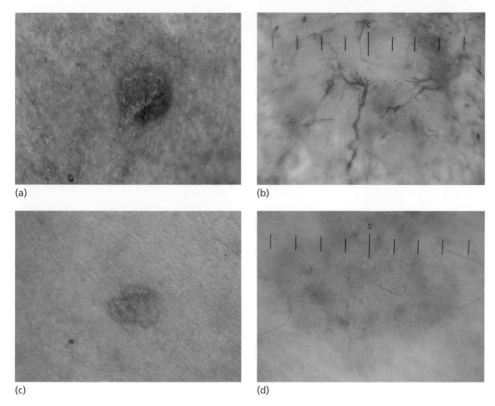

(a)

(b)

(c)

(d)

Figure 79.7 Dermoscopic images of BCC. (a) Nodular BCC. (b) Corresponding dermoscopic image showing white and grey-brown structureless areas, blue-grey globules and telangiectactic vessels. (c) Superficial BCC. (d) Corresponding dermoscopic image: spoke-wheel areas, concentric structures, arborising, comma and telangiectactic vessels.

Radiotherapy

Superficial and electron beam radiotherapy or brachytherapy are effective therapeutic strategies in primary or surgically recurrent BCC as well as high-risk BCC in patients who are unwilling or unable to tolerate surgery. Palliative radiotherapy may be used in patients with advanced and/or incurable disease. Incomplete clearance of BCC and recurrences after radiotherapy are higher and cosmesis poor when compared with surgical excision. Frequent out-patient attendances need to be taken into account.

Radiotherapy should be avoided for radiotherapy-treated recurrent BCC or for patients with naevoid basal cell carcinoma syndrome (NBCCS). It should be used cautiously in young patients (<65 years) in view of the risk of latent tumours in radiotherapy-treated sites. Other situations where radiotherapy is best avoided include BCC on the lower limbs, ear and eyelid, recurrent tumours, lesions previously treated with radiotherapy and tumours with poorly defined clinical margins.

Lasers

The tissue-heating properties of the carbon dioxide laser can be used to ensure precise ablation of BCC. Whilst high clinical cure rates have been reported, the lack of histological confirmation of cure restricts use to low-risk BCC.

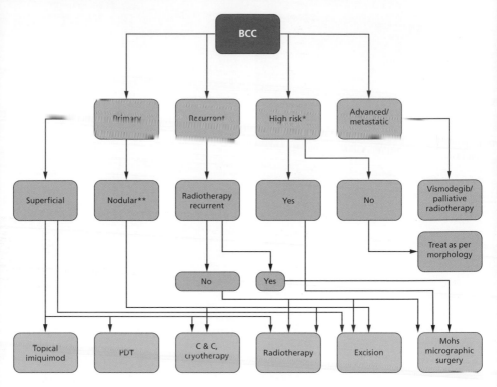

Figure 79.8 An algorithm for the treatment of BCCs. *High-risk BCCs include morphoeic lesions/ infiltrative and micronodular growth pattern/greater than 5 cm in size/centrofacial and ear location/ perineural and perivascular invasion on histology/host immunosuppression. **Only small nodular BCCs can be treated with photodynamic therapy (PDT). C&C, curettage and cautery.

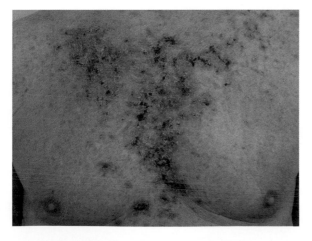

Figure 79.9 Skin reaction to topical imiquimod therapy for superficial BCC.

Naevoid basal cell carcinoma syndrome

(Syn. Gorlin syndrome, Gorlin-Goltz syndrome)
NBCCS is an autosomal dominant familial cancer syndrome in which affected individuals are predisposed to the development of multiple BCCs at an early age.

Epidemiology
UK prevalence approximately 1 in 56 000 of the population. Skin lesions, including BCCs, may develop in infancy but more frequently develop between puberty and 35 years with an average age of onset at 25 years.

Pathophysiology
NBCCS is caused by mutations in the *PATCHED* (*PTCH1*) gene.

Clinical features
Skin manifestations include BCCs, skin tags, palmoplantar pits (Figure 79.10), milia, epidermoid cysts and lesions that clinically resemble dermal naevi. BCCs are often smaller and much more numerous (from a few to thousands) than sporadic BCC. They can present on both sunexposed and non-exposed areas, and are most common on face, back and chest.

Other features include jaw cysts (multiple odontogenic keratocysts), highly characteristic facies (broad nasal root, hypertelorism, frontal bossing), dysgenesis of the corpus callosum, calcification of the falx cerebri (Figure 79.11) and macrocephaly. Skeletal abnormalities include spina bifida occulta, bifid or splayed ribs, scoliosis or kyphosis.

In addition to BCCs, the syndrome is associated with an increased susceptibility to other neoplasms, including rhabdomyosarcoma, ovarian and cardiac fibromas and, in particular, medulloblastoma. Less common associations are not listed here.

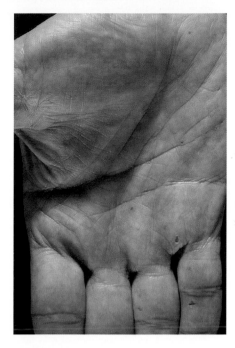

Figure 79.10 Palmar pits in a patient with Gorlin syndrome.

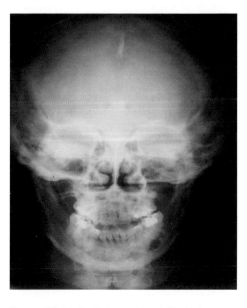

Figure 79.11 Skull X-ray with calcified falx cerebri and jaw cyst.

Investigations

See Box 79.2.

Management

NBCCS is a complex multisystemic disease and a multidisciplinary approach is crucial in the management of these patients. Such multidisciplinary teams should include input from dental teams, maxillo-facial surgeons, oncologists, radiation oncologists, prosthodontist, dermatologists, geneticists and psychiatrists.

The large number of lesions in patients with NBCCS means that primary excision of all lesions is not always practicable. Radiotherapy is contraindicated as many patients show an accelerated rate of development of new BCCs within an irradiated field. Surveillance of NBCCS patients who have developed BCCs for the early detection and treatment of new lesions. Other treatment options as per BCC above.

Box 79.2 Assessment of a patient with NBCCS

- Detailed medical and dental history
- Multisystem clinical examination
  - Dental
  - Skin examination: annual from puberty and every 2–3 months for adult patients, who should also receive training for self-skin examination[a]
  - Neurological evaluation: MRI brain 6 monthly until age 3 years and annually from ages 3 to 8 years[a]
  - Head circumference measurement
  - Ophthalmological[a]
  - Cardiological[a]
  - Orthopaedic[a]
  - Gynaecological and urological[a]
- Genetic tests: *PTCHH* (patched), *SMO* (smoothened), *SHH* (sonic hedgehog)
- Radiological examinations
- Annual panoramic radiographs from age 8 to 40 years: chest, skull, cervical and thoracic spine, hands and pelvis in female patients[a]
- CT scans of the facial bones[a]
- Ultrasonography of the abdominal cavity and pelvis minor (focused on finding ovarian and mesentery fibromas and cysts)[a]
- Echocardiograms and electrocardiogram[a]

[a]Once diagnosis confirmed.
Source: Based on Kiwilsza, Małgorzata, and Katarzyna Sporniak-Tutak (2012) Gorlin–Goltz syndrome – a medical condition requiring a multidisciplinary approach. Medical Science Monitor. International Medical Journal of Experimental and Clinical Research, 18 (9), RA145-53. doi:10.12659/msm.883341.

Squamous cell carcinoma, its precursors and skin cancer in the immuno-compromised patient

80

LESIONS WITH UNCERTAIN OR UNPREDICTABLE MALIGNANT POTENTIAL

Actinic keratosis

(Syn. Solar keratosis)
Actinic keratoses (AK) are hyperkeratotic lesions on chronically light-exposed adult skin, which are focal areas of abnormal proliferation and differentiation that carry a low risk of progression to invasive squamous cell carcinoma (SCC). Patients with AK may have coexisting keratinocyte cancers [KC; SCC and basal cell carcinoma (BCC)] or melanoma.

Epidemiology

Increased incidence in older age (>50 years), males, white population and areas of high sunlight exposure.

In the UK and Ireland there is a reported prevalence of 19–24% of at least one AK in individuals >60 years. In Japan a lower prevalence rate at 0.4% (diagnosed histologically), whilst in Australia up to 60%.

Pathophysiology

The most important factor in the development of AK is excessive ultraviolet radiation (UVR).

Risk factors include:

- *Patient characteristics*: Fair skin, blue eyes, red hair, freckling, Fitzpatrick type I and II skin (burns doesn't tan).
- *Occupation*: Outdoor worker, cumulative sun exposure.
- *UV exposure*: Chronic cumulative exposure, history of sunburn, iatrogenic phototherapy, ionising radiation, sunbed use.
- *Immunosuppression*: Organ transplant recipients (OTR), immunosuppression.
- *Genetic*: Xeroderma pigmentosum, albinism.

UVR results in DNA damage, causing keratinocyte mutations and eventually development of AK. The tumour suppressor gene, tumour protein 53 (*TP53*), located on chromosome 17p13.1, helps to repair DNA damage; mutations of this gene are frequently seen in AK. Human papillomavirus (HPV) may also play a role.

Histologically there is solar elastosis and disordered epidermal keratinocyte maturation with cytological atypia. The typical lesion shows hyperkeratosis, parakeratosis and hypogranu- losis. Histological variants of AK include atrophic, hypertrophic, lichenoid, acantholytic, pigmented and bowenoid.

Clinical features

1 mm to >2 cm scaly macules, papules or plaques, which are usually multiple and asymptomatic. Located on sun-exposed sites, such as the face, scalp and dorsa of the hands (Figure 80.1). The sides of the neck are involved in both sexes; ears predominate in men. The vermilion of the lower lip is involved more so in men than women.

The adherent scale can be picked off with dif- ficulty, revealing a hyperaemic base with punc- tate bleeding points. Scaling may be prominent and become thick and horny. There is often associated 'field change', with areas of photoda- mage, skin atrophy, telangiectasias and pig- mentary change which surrounds and extends beyond clinical AKs. Many patients give a his- tory of relapsing and/or remitting lesions, which often disappear either spontaneously or after sun avoidance and use of sunscreens.

The rate of progression of an individual AK to invasive SCC has been estimated to be low (less than 1 in 1000/year); an individual with an average of 7.7 AKs has a probability of around 10% of one AK transforming to a SCC over a 10-year period.

Reported high-risk features of AK are listed in Box 80.1 (Figure 80.2).

Differential diagnosis
see Table 80.1.

Investigations
Diagnosis is clinical unless diagnostic doubt, when a biopsy is indicated.

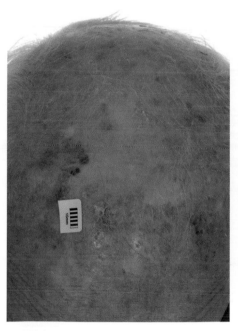

Figure 80.2 'High-risk' disease characterised by multiple thick AKs in an immunosuppressed patient.

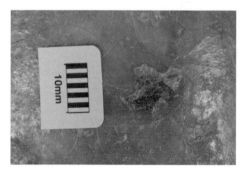

Figure 80.1 Actinic keratosis.

Box 80.1 High-risk clinical features of AK

The presence of one or more of these features may increase the risk of progression to SCC, but evidence for some individual factors, such as extensive actinic damage, although reasonable, is lacking.

- Multiple thick AKs
- Past history of KC
- Extensive actinic damage
- Patient immunosuppressed
- Tender enlarging lesion(s)

Table 80.1 Common clinical differential diagnoses of AK

Diagnosis	Differentiating features	Image
Seborrheoic keratosis	May mimic pigmented AK Usually larger, darker and multiple Raised 'greasy' warty surface	
Squamous cell carcinoma	Enlarging lesion Induration raised shoulder or nodule Tenderness	
Bowen disease	Usually larger and solitary Irregular erythematous base Mainly occur on lower legs in females	
Keratoacanthoma	Enlarging lesion Generally larger and solitary Usually more hyperkeratotic than AK	
Basal cell carcinoma	Often solitary Usually less hyperkeratotic than AK Irregular erythematous base	

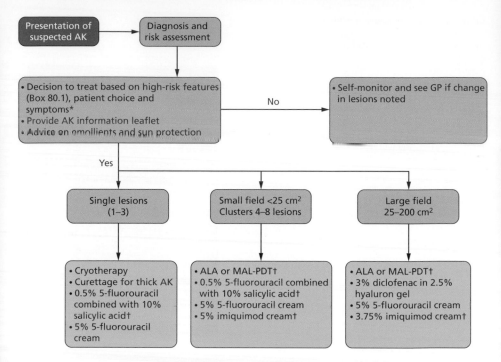

Figure 80.3 AK management algorithm. *Treatment should be decided following discussion with the patient, assessment of treatment availability and of local expertise with the aim of optimising patient concordance. †Topical therapy without specific licence for the treatment of AK on the trunk and extremities. ALA, aminolaevulinic acid; MAL-PDT, methyl aminolevulinate photodynamic therapy.

Management

AKs are an important biomarker of excessive UV exposure and increased skin cancer risk; patients should be educated in the recognition of skin malignancy. Regular sunscreen reduces the rate of development of new lesions.

A number of therapeutic options are available, with the aim to control and reduce the number of AKs and to reduce the rate of progression of AK to SCC (Figure 80.3). Treatment protocols, precautions and field use for all the topical treatments, including PDT, currently available in the UK are documented in Table 80.2.

Cutaneous horn

Hard conical projections from the skin, made of compact keratin. They arise from benign, premalignant or malignant skin lesions.

Epidemiology

Peak incidence 60–70 years and Fitzpatrick skin types I and II. There is an increased chance of pre-malignant or malignant change in the base with increasing age.

Pathophysiology

UVR exposure and possible association with HPV-2 subtype. Histologically, usually no atypicality or loss of polarity of the epidermal cells, but the granular layer may be deficient or absent. Many have benign pathology at the base, such as seborrhoeic keratosis, viral wart or trichilemmal cysts. Just under 40% have pre-malignant (AK, intraepidermal carcinoma) or malignant change, usually an SCC.

Clinical features

Defined as a keratotic lesion with a height of at least half the widest diameter of its base

(Figure 80.4). Often solitary and asymptomatic on exposed areas, particularly the upper part of the face and the ears. A curved hard, yellow to brown keratotic outgrowth with circumferential ridges, with surrounding normal-looking epidermis or an acanthotic collarette. Recurrent injury may cause the base to be inflamed. Malignant change is suggested by pain and erythema, induration at the base, increase in size and a wide base or low height-to-base ratio (Figure 80.5).

Management
Surgical excision is usually advised to obtain pathology and rule out malignancy.

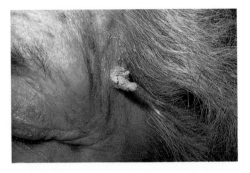

Figure 80.4 Typical cutaneous horn. Underlying this lesion, a carcinoma *in situ* was identified after biopsy.

Disseminated superficial actinic porokeratosis

A disorder characterised by hyperkeratotic papules surrounded by a thread-like elevated border. It appears on sun-exposed areas, becoming more prominent in summer and may improve in winter. It is the commonest porokeratosis (see Chapter 43).

Epidemiology
Uncommon, average age of onset 40 years, F > M.

Pathophysiology
An autosomal dominant disorder. Risk factors include genetic factors, UVR exposure and immunosuppression.

The distinctive pathological feature of porokeratosis is the cornoid lamella at the margin, a narrow column of altered or parakeratotic keratin, seated in a slight depression in the epidermis. The granular layer of the indented epidermis is usually missing and there may be dyskeratotic cells.

Mutations in the mevalonate kinase gene (*MVKK*) have recently been reported in Chinese patients with familial and sporadic disseminated superficial actinic porokeratosis.

Clinical features
Usually affects light-exposed sites mainly on the distal extremities. Tend to be asymptomatic but may be mildly pruritic, particularly after sun exposure, and are often unsightly. 1–3 mm conical, brownish red or brown papule usually around a follicle containing a keratotic plug. It expands and a sharp slightly raised keratotic ring develops and spreads out to a diameter of 10 mm or more. The skin within the ring is atrophic and mildly reddened or hyperpigmented (Figure 80.6).

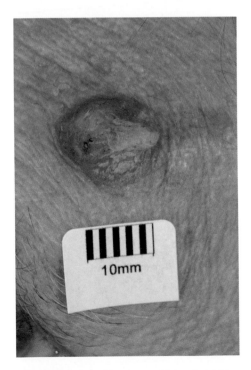

10mm

Figure 80.5 Cutaneous horn with low height-to-base ratio. Pathology showed SCC at the base.

PART 10: NEOPLASTIC, PROLIFERATIVE AND INFILTRATIVE DISORDERS AFFECTING THE SKIN

Table 80.2 Topical therapies for AK

Therapy	Protocol	Precautions
Diclofenac 3% gel	Twice daily for 60–90 days Max 4 g/application (as 0.5 g maximum area 200 cm²)	Usually well tolerated, occasionally causes a rash
5% fluorouracil	Once or twice daily for 3–4 weeks Facial lesions usually respond quicker than those on trunk/legs Lesions on hands/forearms respond more slowly Maximum area of skin treated at any one time 500 cm²	Normal response is an early and severe inflammatory phase then necrotic phase, followed by healing
0.5% 5-fluorouracil combined with 10% salicylic acid	Once daily to slightly palpable and/or moderately thick hyperkeratotic AK Response can be seen from 6 weeks Optimal effect may not be evident for up to 8 weeks after cessation Maximum area of skin treated at any one time 25 cm²	Peel off existing coating before reapplication Apply with brush applicator
Imiquimod 5%	Apply three times a week to AK on face or scalp for 4 weeks. Assess after a 4-week interval, repeat cycle if required Maximum recommended is 1 sachet, limit to ~25 cm²	Apply prior to normal sleeping hours, wash off after 8 h Local inflammatory reactions are common Advise rest period of several days if inflammation severe Flu-like symptoms uncommon
Imiquimod 3.75%	Apply once daily before bedtime for two treatment cycles of 2 weeks, each separated by a 2-week interval Up to 2 sachets, approximately 200 cm² (whole face or scalp)	Local inflammatory reaction common Rest period if required Flu-like symptoms are uncommon

| PDT | Ameluz is new nanoemulsion of 5-ALA, Metvix is methylester of 5-ALA
Apply to lesions and 5–10 mm of surrounding skin | Single treatment, repeat at 3 months if required, to AK on face/scalp (applied under occlusion for 3 h before illumination with red light)
Pain/burning sensation is common during PDT
Erythema common after treatment and scab formation |

5-ALA, 5-aminolaevulinic acid; PDT, photodynamic therapy.

Source: Adapted from Morton C, Mowbray M, Clark C, Gupta G, Herd R, Fleming C. Update on the treatment of actinic keratosis. Dermatology in Practice 2013, 19, 14–17. © Hayward Medical Communications.

PART 10: NEOPLASTIC, PROLIFERATIVE AND INFILTRATIVE DISORDERS AFFECTING THE SKIN

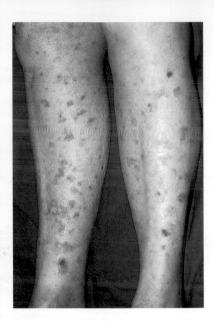

Figure 80.6 Disseminated superficial actinic porokeratosis on the lower legs.

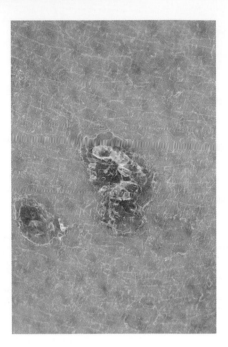

Figure 80.7 Bowen disease.

The number of lesions tends to increase over time but the risk of malignant change remains very low.

Differential diagnosis
AK, Bowen disease, superficial BCC.

Investigations
The diagnosis is clinical in most cases, biopsy if doubt.

Management
First line: Reassurance, emollients and high-factor broad-spectrum sunscreen.
Second line: Cryotherapy, topical diclofenac gel, vitamin D$_3$ analogues, 5% 5-fluorouracil cream, 5% imiquimod cream and PDT.

IN SITU CARCINOMA OF THE SKIN

Bowen disease

(Syn. **Intraepithelial carcinoma, SCC *in situ***)
A form of intraepidermal (*in situ*) SCC.

Epidemiology
Rare <30 years, more common >60 years. F > M. 30–50% of cases have a history of previous or subsequent skin cancers, mainly BCC.

Pathophysiology
Risk factors include chronic UVR exposure, immunosuppression (OTR, haematological malignancy, HIV), arsenic, chronic skin injury or inflammation (e.g. lupus vulgaris or chronic lupus erythematosus).

Charaterised by full-thickness epidermal dysplasia and disordered differentiation with loss of epithelial polarity. The dermal–epidermal junction remains distinct.

Clinical features
Usually a solitary plaque but multiple in 10–20% of cases. Typically found on the lower legs of elderly women, but can be found on any body site with an increased incidence on the head and neck. A gradually enlarging red, scaly, slightly raised, well-demarcated plaque with a flat surface that may become hyperkeratotic or crusted (Figure 80.7). Ulceration is usually a sign of the development of invasive carcinoma.

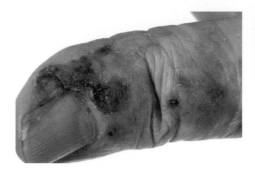

Figure 80.8 Periungual Bowen disease.

The lifetime risk of malignant transformation to invasive SCC is low, around 3–5%.

Bowen disease of the nail unit (subungual, periungual) affects younger women and is associated with high-risk HPV types such as HPV16 with a higher risk of invasion and recurrence (Figure 80.8).

Bowen disease arising in mucosal genital skin (anal intraepithelial neoplasia, penile intraepithelial neoplasia and vulval intraepithelial neoplasia) is described separately (see Chapter 61).

Differential diagnosis
See Table 80.3.

Investigations
If the diagnosis is uncertain, the lack of improvement with topical steroids is suggestive of

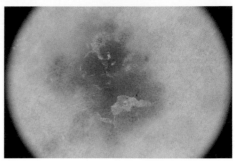

Figure 80.9 Dermoscopy of Bowen disease showing irregular erythematous base, mild hyperkeratosis with vascular structures throughout the lesion.

Bowen disease. Where diagnosis remains in doubt, a diagnostic biopsy is necessary. Coiled glomerular vessels are a characteristic dermatoscopic feature which clears with treatment (Figure 80.9).

Management
Advice on high-factor broad-spectrum sunscreen and emollients. There is a wide range of therapeutic options available for the treatment of Bowen disease (Figure 80.10). The preferred treatment option is based on the size of the lesion, site, previous treatment and number of lesions.

For cryotherapy a single freeze–thaw cycle (FTC) of 30 s, or two FTCs of 20 s with a thaw

Table 80.3 Common clinical differential diagnoses of Bowen disease

Diagnosis	Differentiating features
Seborrhoeic keratosis	Usually larger, darker and multiple Raised 'greasy' warty surface
Basal cell carcinoma	Superficial variant may mimic Bowen disease Usually less hyperkeratotic Often solitary
Squamous cell carcinoma	Enlarging lesion Induration Raised shoulder or nodule Tenderness
Nummular eczema	Often large multiple plaques Pruritus is main symptom
Psoriasis	Thickened plaque with marked scale Often multiple, large and on other body sites

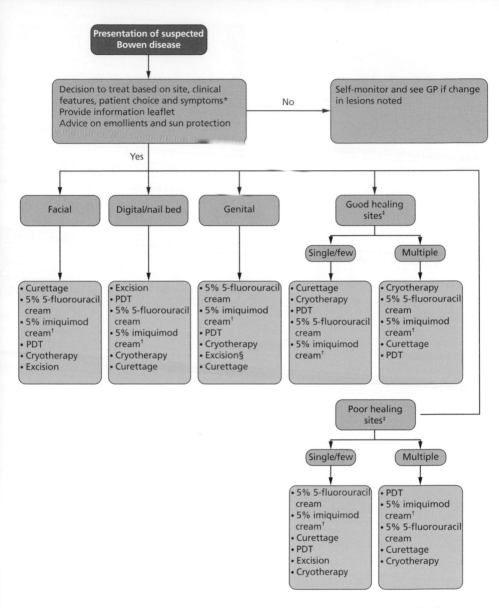

Figure 80.10 Bowen disease management algorithm. *Treatment should be decided following discussion with patient, treatment availability and local expertise with the aim of optimising patient concordance. †Topical therapy without specific licence for treatment of Bowen disease. ‡Clinician's perceived potential for good or poor healing at affected sites. §Consider surgery or Mohs micrographic surgery (MMS) for mucosal genital Bowen disease. PDT, photodynamic therapy.

period, yields better results, but such doses can cause significant discomfort and ulceration.

In some patients with slowly progressive thin lesions, especially on the lower leg of elderly patients where healing is poor, observation may be preferred.

Due to the recurrent nature of perianal and subungual Bowen disease, surgery with wide excision for perianal disease and digital amputation or Mohs micrographic surgery for nail unit disease may be necessary.

SQUAMOUS CELL CARCINOMA OF THE SKIN

A keratinocyte cancer arising from epidermal keratinocytes or its appendages. Patients are more susceptible to developing other UVR-induced skin cancers.

Epidemiology

The second commonest skin cancer after BCC, the ratio of BCC:SCC in an immunocompetent population is 3–4:1. Worldwide incidence is increasing but accurate figures are not available. Pooled data from England suggest an average annual incidence of 22.65/100 000 person-years. In the USA and Australia rates are 290 and 387/100 000 person-years, respectively.

In non-white populations SCC is still the most common skin cancer due to trauma, albinism, burn scars, ionising radiation, chronic inflammation and chronic discoid lupus erythematosus

The SCC risk in OTRs is discussed below.

Pathophysiology

The most important factor of SCC development is excessive UVR.

Risk factors include:

- *Patient characteristics*: Male, increasing age, fair skin, blue eyes, red hair, freckling, Fitzpatrick type I and II skin.
- *Occupation*: Outdoor workers.
- *UV exposure*: Chronic cumulative exposure, history of sunburn, iatrogenic phototherapy, ionising radiation, sunbed use.
- *Immunosuppression*: OTR, immunosuppression due to disease (e.g. chronic lymphocytic leukaemia, HIV) and drugs (e.g. azathioprine, ciclosporin).
- *Genetic*: Xeroderma pigmentosum, albinism.
- *Other conditions*: Long-standing chronic ulceration/post irradiation and other diseases, e.g hidradenitis suppurativa, morphoea, lymphoedema, Hailey–Hailey disease, cutaneous lupus and dystrophic epidermolysis bullosa. Verrucous carcinoma can develop

in areas of chronic inflammation and in association with HPV (types 11 and 16).

A number of DNA mutations are associated with SCC. Mutations of *TP53* caused by UVR, leading to pyrimidine dimers, are seen in 90% of SCCs. UVR can also cause mutations in the CDKN2A gene, which encodes p16, a tumour suppressor protein, leading to continuous cell cycling and thought to advance AK to SCC.

Invasive SCC begins when atypical keratinocytes breach the epidermal basement membrane and invade the dermis. Differentiation from precursor lesions is thus architectural rather than cytological.

Histological variants of SCC have been described: classic/no special type, acantholytic, spindle cell, desmoplastic, basaloid, verrucous, pseudovascular and follicular. The cells of SCC vary from large, polygonal cells with vesicular nuclei, prominent nucleoli and an abundant cytoplasm, overt evidence of keratinization and well-developed intercellular bridges (well-differentiated lesions) to pleomorphic cells which provide no clear cytological evidence of their origin (poorly differentiated lesions). The possibility of metastatic SCC (not necessarily cutaneous) should be considered when an *in situ* component is not identified.

The histopathological report of excision specimens for SCC should include tumour type, grade of differentiation, tumour thickness, level of invasion, perineural invasion, lymphovascular invasion, excision margins and pathological stage.

Clinical features

See Figures 80.11–80.13.

Sun-exposed sites, backs of the hands and forearms, the upper part of the face and, especially in males, on the lower lip and pinna. The evolution of SCC is usually faster than that of BCC, but slower than that of KA. The first clinical evidence of malignancy is induration. The area may be plaque-like, verrucous, tumid or ulcerated, but in all cases the lesion feels firm. The limits of the induration are not sharp and usually extend beyond the visible margin of the lesion.

The better-differentiated tumours are usually papillomatous with a keratotic crust, this may then become ulcerated or eroded with an indurated margin and a purulent exuding surface that bleeds easily.

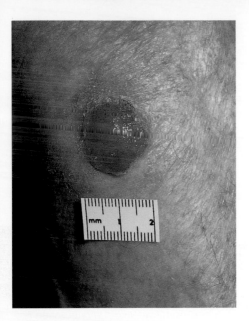

Figure 80.11 Raised friable nodule. Poorly differentiated SCC.

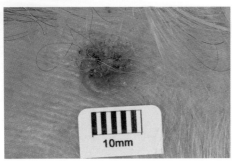

Figure 80.12 Well-differentiated SCC on the forehead with even circumscribed edge and central crusting.

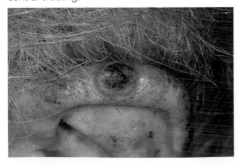

Figure 80.13 Well-differentiated SCC on the helix of the ear (high-risk site).

In OTRs, lesions are frequently multiple and often deceptively banal resembling either KA or AK. All such lesions should be regarded with suspicion.

Verrucous carcinoma of the foot is a slow-growing, well-differentiated SCC which rarely metastasises, characterised by an exophytic verruciform appearance.

SCC has a low rate of metastasis of 5%. Low-grade tumours carry an excellent prognosis but the risk of developing metastasis increases significantly in SCCs displaying high-risk features A Table has been omitted, my error, on High-risk features. This is Table 142.6 from Parent Book. Staging systems stratify patients according to their risk of developing local and/or disseminated disease (Table 80.4).

Differential diagnosis

AKs tend to be multiple and lack a dermal component on palpation. Warty lesions such as viral warts or seborrhoeic keratoses are not indurated and often multiple. BCC, amelanotic melanoma and skin metastases from internal malignancy may resemble SCCs.

Investigations

Biopsy if diagnostic doubt.

There are no clear indications for when radiological imaging is warranted to search for nodal metastases. Conventional CT and MRI scans add little to the clinical examination of a node-negative region. Ultrasound with a guided fine-needle aspiration or core biopsy should be performed if lymph node or parotid gland involvement suspected.

Management

Patients should be given information on diagnosis, sun-avoidance and self-examination of the skin and lymph nodes.

First line: The tumour should be completely excised taking a peripheral and deep margin of normal skin. In low-risk SCCs a 4-mm margin is recommended; in high-risk tumours a 6-mm margin or Mohs micrographic surgery may be desirable. In certain clinical situations curettage and cautery may be acceptable for low-risk SCCs.

Adjuvant radiotherapy: May be an effective therapeutic option in decreasing the risk of

Table 80.4 Union for International Cancer Control (UICC) tumour, node and metastasis (TNM8) staging of primary cutaneous SCC

Primary tumour (pT)	Definition
pTX	Primary tumour cannot be assessed
pT0	No evidence of primary tumour
pTis	Carcinoma in situ
pT1	Tumour ≤20 mm in maximum dimension[a]
pT2	Tumour >20 mm to ≤40 mm in maximum dimension[a]
pT3	Tumour >40 mm in maximum dimension[a] OR pT1 or pT2 can be upstaged to pT3 by one or more high-risk clinical/pathological features[b]
pT4a	Tumour with gross cortical/marrow invasion
pT4b	Tumour with axial skeleton/skull base/foraminal invasion

Source: Brierley JD, Gospodarowicz MK, Wittekind CH (2017) Union for International Cancer Control. TNM Classification of Malignant Tumours Eighth Edition. Wiley Blackwell, Oxford. (UICC TNM8 adopted by Public Health England and Royal College of Pathologists UK for skin cancer staging excluding eyelid, vulval, penile and perianal skin).
[a] Clinical dimension but macroscopic pathological dimension can be used if the clinical is not available.
[b] High-risk features include deep invasion defined as tumour thickness >6 mm and/or invasion beyond the subcutaneous fat OR perineural invasion of named nerve (≥0.1 mm and/or located beyond the dermis), which may be detected clinically or by imaging OR minor bone erosion.

tumour progression when an SCC has been excised with close or involved margins, or where there are specific high-risk features such as perineural invasion.

In the absence of high-risk features, SCCs carry an excellent prognosis and following definitive treatment patients may be discharged after one visit. SCCs with high-risk features have a greater potential for local invasion and to develop metastases and a 2-year follow up is recommended, longer for those on immunosuppression or those with multiple tumours.

KERATOACANTHOMAS AND ASSOCIATED SYNDROMES

Keratoacanthoma

(Syn. Well-differentiated SCC [keratoacanthoma type])
Keratoacanthoma (KA) behaves differently to invasive SCC clinically and there is considerable debate whether KA is a separate entity or a variant of SCC.

It has been reclassified as a well-differentiated SCC (keratoacanthoma type) in the World Health Organization and Royal College of Pathologists UK classifications.

Epidemiology
A relatively common tumour in the white population, M:F = 3:1. The incidence is higher in immunosuppressed patients and increases with higher levels of UVR. Most frequent in middle life.

Pathophysiology
Risk factors are as for SCC. In addition, the solid tumour multikinase inhibitor (e.g. sorafenib), *BRAF* inhibitors (e.g. vemurafenib and dabrafenib) and the hedgehog signalling pathway inhibitor (vismodegib) may lead to the development of KA, which resolve or stop developing when therapy is discontinued.

Multiple KAs are found in patients with Muir Torre syndrome (Chapter 37), multiple self-healing squamous epithelioma (MSSE, see below), and generalised eruptive KA of Grzybowski.

The diagnosis of KA requires close clinico-pathological correlation. Examination of the whole/intact lesion is needed to assess architecture. Early-stage KA is characterised by an exoendophytic growth pattern that evolves into a symmetrical central structure that contains keratin. Frank dermal invasion or solid growths of atypical cells are not KA features.

Clinical features

The most frequently affected area is the central part of the face: the nose, cheeks, eyelids and lips, followed by the dorsum of the hand, wrist and forearm. In most cases, the tumour presents as a solitary lesion. Multiple or recurrent tumours are more likely to be present in patients who are immunosuppressed, have associated syndromes or who have been exposed to pitch or tar.

There is no precursor lesion and they evolve in three clinical phases: proliferative, maturing, and resolving. The first evidence of KA is a firm, rounded, flesh-coloured or reddish papule, which may resemble molluscum contagiosum or, if keratotic, a viral wart. There follows a rapid growth phase and in a few weeks it may become 10–20 mm across. There is no infiltration at the base. The nodule is smooth and shiny, skin-coloured to red with telangiectasia. The centre contains a horny plug or is covered by a crust which conceals a keratin-filled crater (see Figure 80.14). The keratin may project like a horn or it may soften and break down. Spontaneous healing usually takes about 3 months to leave a pitted scar.

Differential diagnosis

Molluscum contagiosum, viral warts, hypertrophic AK and SCC.

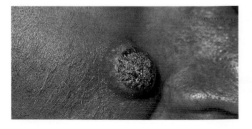

Figure 80.14 Keratoacanthoma, which is often larger and more hyperkeratotic than actinic keratosis.

Investigations

Investigations are generally not necessary.

Management

First line: Solitary lesions that are not resolving should be removed by surgical excision or curettage and cautery. Despite it being reclassified as a well-differentiated SCC (keratoacanthoma type), small lesions possess a low risk of invasion and so could be treated with curettage and cautery particularly if they are less than 2 cm in diameter. For larger lesions over 2 cm in diameter, subungual lesions, and where diagnosis is not clear then surgical excision is recommended.

Second line: Radiotherapy.

Multiple self-healing squamous epithelioma

(Syn. Ferguson–Smith disease)

MSSE is an autosomal dominant condition characterised by the intermittent development of spontaneously regressing skin tumours, predominantly on sun-exposed sites, which are histologically identical to well-differentiated SCCs. Susceptibility to MSSE is conferred by heterozygous loss-of-function mutations in the *TGFBR1* gene. Most tumours regress spontaneously leaving a scar, solitary lesions may be excised or curetted; radiotherapy should be avoided. Advice on sun protection should be given.

SKIN CANCER IN THE IMMUNOCOMPROMISED PATIENT

Certain primary immunodeficiencies predispose to skin cancer but the greatest burden of disease is associated with acquired immunodeficiency, including immunosuppressive drug therapy (e.g. following solid-organ and haematopoietic transplantation and for immune-mediated inflammatory disorders), non-Hodgkin lymphoma/chronic lymphocytic leukaemia (NHL/CLL) and HIV infection (Chapter 6) (Table 80.1).

Non-Hodgkin lymphoma/chronic lymphocytic leukaemia

A 5- to 8-fold increase risk of skin cancer has been documented with higher risk in CLL compared with non-CLL NHL. In CLL the cumulative incidence by 20 years was 43.2% for SCC and 30.6% for BCC in the USA.

Solid-organ transplantation

Overall risk for any cancer in OTRs is 2- to 6-fold greater than that of the general population with a disproportionate increase in four tumour types: keratinocyte cancers (SCC, BCC), post-transplant lymphoproliferative disorders, ano-genital malignancy and Kaposi sarcoma (KS), with smaller but significant increases in hepatocellular and renal cancers and some sarcomas.

Epidemiology

Spectrum of skin cancers post-transplant: KC account for >95% of all post-transplant skin cancer; SCCs are more than 150-fold more common, BCC are 5- to 10-fold increased, with reversal in the 3–4:1 BCC:SCC ratio usually seen in the general population. Melanoma incidence is increased 2- to 8-fold, KS 40- to 200-fold, appendageal tumours 20- to 100-fold and Merkel cell carcinoma (MCC) up to 60-fold.

Tumour burden and accrual: The incidence of skin cancers in OTRs increases with time post-transplantation. In a UK cohort, 10% of OTRs at 5 years had developed a skin cancer rising to almost 75% at 30 years. After the first KC more than 30% will develop a further KC by 1 year and almost 75% by 5 years compared with 14.5% and 40.7%, respectively, in the general population.

Type of solid-organ transplant: SCC risk appears to be greatest after cardiac and/or lung transplantation, followed by renal transplantation with risk lowest in liver transplant recipients. The reasons for this are not clear but may relate in part to intensity of immunosuppression.

Pathophysiology

Pathogenesis of skin cancers in immunosuppressed patients is multifactorial, including UVR, altered immune surveillance, drugs and oncogenic viruses, with likely additional roles for host genetic susceptibility factors, chronic inflammation and donor-derived cells.

The degree of risk of individual non-biological immunosuppressive drugs is difficult: azathioprine may pose an increased risk over ciclosporin and corticosteroids, and mammalian target of rapamycin inhibitors (rapamycin/sirolimus, everolimus) confer reduced skin cancer risk compared to the other immunosuppressants.

The most common immunosuppression-associated skin malignancies due to known or suspected oncogenic viruses include KS (HHV-8) (see Chapter 77), post-transplant lymphoproliferative disorders (EBV) and MCC (Merkel cell polyomavirus, MCPyV) (see Chapter 83). An oncogenic role for HPV in SCC in OTRs remains unproven.

Clinical features

Skin tumours in the setting of immunosuppression may have atypical presentations and altered clinical courses.

Clinical features predicting OTRs at greatest risk for developing skin cancer:

- *Duration of immunosuppression:* 50% of OTRs will have developed a skin cancer by 20 years post-transplant in the UK, whereas it is greater than 80% in Australia.
- *Age at transplant:* Risk increased 12-fold if transplanted >55 years compared with <34 years.
- *Skin phototype* and sunburn pre-transplant (particularly in childhood) are associated with time to first skin cancer; these factors together with male sex and chronic UV exposure are associated with cumulative skin cancer burden.
- *Presence of AKs in OTR:* Increases SCC risk >30-fold.

Squamous cell carcinomas are predominantly located on UV-exposed sites but are more common on sites other than non-head and neck sites in immunocompromised compared with immunocompetent individuals. Appearances may be atypical, and pain is a useful symptom of invasive malignancy. The metastatic risk is up to 7%, more than twice that in the general population; prognosis for metastatic disease is worse in immunocompromised individuals with an overall 5-year survival of 14–39%.

Field cancerization is a common problem in OTRs and other immunocompromised individuals (Figure 80.15) with areas of confluent AK and Bowen disease, and increased SCC development. AK may be contiguous with multiple plane warts in areas such as the dorsum of the hand and forehead and it may be difficult to distinguish viral, and dysplastic lesions from each other without diagnostic biopsy.

Management

A multidisciplinary approach with dermatologists, transplant clinicians, oncologists, surgeons

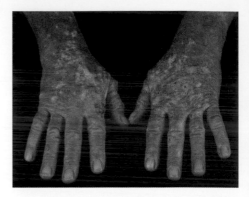

Figure 80.15 Field cancerization in a patient with Crohn disease who was taking azathioprine for many years. Confluent AK and Bowen disease (field cancerization/field change) are present and an SCC has developed on the dorsum of the right hand.

and other relevant healthcare professionals is important. All OTRs and other at-risk patients should be monitored in a dedicated skin cancer surveillance clinic.

Melanoma

81

A malignant tumour arising from melanocytes.

Epidemiology

Melanoma represents 4% of skin cancers and 80% of skin cancer deaths; currently it is the fifth leading cancer in males and seventh in females. Incidence rates are doubling every10–20 years. Global incidence is about 160 000 new cases per year and 48 000 deaths per year, with the highest rate in sunnier climates and in white skin. Mortality rates have remained relatively stable since the 1980s.

Median age at diagnosis is around 60 in the USA; 7% of patients are >85 years. Men more affected in high-incidence countries and in central, eastern and southern Europe, whereas females are more affected in western and northern Europe. Recent trends show an increase in young females and of thicker melanomas in >60-year-old males.

Pathophysiology

75–80% of cutaneous melanomas arise *de novo*. 20–25% arise from pre-existing naevi. There are a number of risk factors (Box 81.1).

Major melanoma susceptibility genes (high penetrance genes): These include CDKN2A, CDK4, *MC1R*, *ASIP* and *TYR*. They are rare and account for a minority of melanomas. Genetic

---

Box 81.1 Melanoma risk factors

- Increasing age
- Naevi characteristics:
  - Naevus count (100–120 naevi 7× increased risk compared to <15 naevi)
  - Congenital melanocytic naevi: large (>20 cm) 5–15% lifetime risk; small (<4.5 cm) lifetime risk 2.6–4.9% (probably similar to common naevi)
  - >5 atypical/dysplastic naevi
  - Dysplastic/atypical naevus syndrome (familial atypical multiple mole melanoma)
- Fitzpatrick's skin type 1, fair skin, blue eyes, freckles and red hair
- Ultraviolet (UV) light exposure:
  - Intermittent exposure with sunburn history particularly in childhood; melanoma on the trunk more common
  - Chronic sun exposure; head and neck melanoma more common, e.g. lentigo maligna
  - Artificial UV, e.g. sunbeds (particularly if first used <35 years), therapeutic psoralen and UVA (risk more than doubled when >200 treatments)
  - No increased risk with narrow-band UVB
- Family history (×2 increased risk)
- Personal history of melanoma, squamous cell carcinoma, basal cell carcinoma or actinic damage
- Immunosuppression (drugs or HIV)
- Genetic
  - Melanoma susceptibility genes: CDKN2A, CDK4, *MC1R*, *ASIP* and *TYR*
  - Xeroderma pigmentosum

Rook's Dermatology Handbook, First Edition. Edited by Christopher E. M. Griffiths, Tanya O. Bleiker, Daniel Creamer, John R. Ingram and Rosalind C. Simpson.
© 2022 John Wiley & Sons Ltd. Published 2022 by John Wiley & Sons Ltd.

Table 81.1 Candidacy for consideration of genetic testing

Low melanoma incidence area/population	Moderate to high melanoma incidence area/population
• Two (synchronous or metachronous) primary melanomas in an individual and/or	• Three (synchronous or metachronous) primary melanomas in an individual and/or
• Families with at least one invasive melanoma and one or more other diagnoses of melanoma and/or pancreatic cancers among first- or second-degree relatives on the same side of the family	• Families with at least one invasive melanoma and two or more other diagnoses of invasive melanoma and/or pancreatic cancer among first- or second-degree relatives on the same side of the family

Source: Leachman, Sancy A. et al. (2009) Selection Criteria for Genetic Assessment of Patients with Familial Melanoma. Journal of the American Academy of Dermatology, 61, 4. © 2009 Elsevier.

testing is not routine but should be offered in certain situations (Table 81.1).

Classification of melanoma: Four main histo-clinical subtypes: nodular melanoma (NM), superficial spreading melanoma (SSM), lentigo maligna melanoma (LMM) and acral lentiginous melanoma (ALM). Melanoma first grows along the basal membrane (radial growth phase) before penetrating into the dermis (vertical growth phase), which gives rise to the potential metastatic process. NM, SSM, LMM and ALM are four points within a spectrum of tumours. At one end of the spectrum there are melanoma with a long horizontal phase (LMM and ALM), with plenty of time to detect them before they turn into an aggressive vertical phase. At the other end of the spectrum, the NM have virtually no horizontal phase and turn immediately into a vertical progression. For histopathology see investigations below.

Distinct mutations in proteins along the RAS-RAF-MEK-ERK pathway resulting in the aberrant activation of the mitogen-activated protein kinase pathway are present in over 80% of primary melanomas. The three most frequently activated oncogenes in melanoma are *B-RAF* (around 40%), *N-Ras* (15–18%) and *c-KIT* (7% in cutaneous melanoma but up to 20% in mucosal melanoma).

Clinical features
Early diagnosis is key. Four general principles are applied:

1. **Analytical examination**
   ABCDE algorithm:
   • Asymmetry
   • Border irregularity
   • Colour variegation
   • Diameter >6 mm
   • Evolution
2. **Pattern recognition**
   When an individual sees a new object, a cognitive pattern for this object is built unconsciously, which will then be used to recognise it when faced with the object again.
3. **Intraindividual comparative analysis ('ugly duckling' sign)**
   A naevus which does not fit the dominant pattern of naevi in an individual, the ugly duckling sign, should raise suspicion of melanoma.
4. **Dynamic analysis (evolution)**
   Changes in size, colour or shape of pre-existing pigmented lesions, or of any new growing skin lesion. Whole-body photographs or 'mole mapping' are important in people with multiple atypical naevi.

Superficial spreading melanoma: 60–70% of melanomas present as a flat pigmented macule (Figure 81.1) which progressively becomes more irregular in shape and colour (Figure 81.2a) with shades of brown, black, grey and red as well as depigmented areas (regression) over several months or more rarely years. As growth continues, the diagnosis will become obvious; the lesion will become palpable with the development of a nodule, reflecting the vertical growth phase (Figure 81.2b).

Nodular melanoma: 10–20% of- melanomas present as regular, symmetrical, elevated, dome-shaped or more rarely polypoid or pedunculated lesions (Figure 81.3). Colour ranges from black or dark brown to red. They tend to be fast-growing and are usually thick tumours at diagnosis. Ulceration and bleeding are common.

Lentigo maligna melanoma: Flat, brown or black, irregularly shaped lesion which grows slowly over months and years on chronically sun-exposed areas of the skin (e.g. the face, neck, forearms) in the elderly (Figure 81.4). The early intraepidermal (*in situ*) phase known as a lentigo maligna (LM/Hutchinson's melanotic freckle) can be mistaken for a solar lentigo, a pigmented actinic keratosis or a flat seborrhoeic keratosis. In time, a nodule may develop.

Acral lentiginous melanoma: Initially a discrete light brown or black macule, with indistinct borders on the soles of patients usually >60 years (Figure 81.5). The frequency differs by race ranging from 2–10% of melanoma in white to 60–72% in black populations because

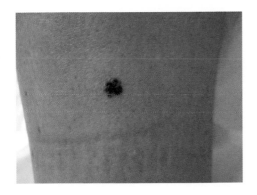

Figure 81.1 Superficial spreading melanoma (early presentation).

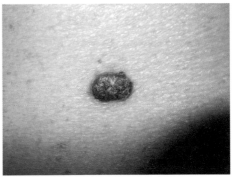

Figure 81.3 Nodular melanoma.

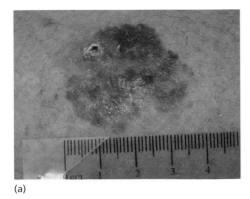

(a)

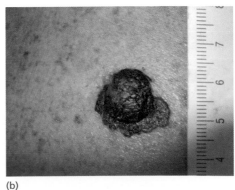

(b)

Figure 81.2 Superficial spreading melanoma (late presentation).

PART 10: NEOPLASTIC, PROLIFERATIVE AND INFILTRATIVE DISORDERS AFFECTING THE SKIN

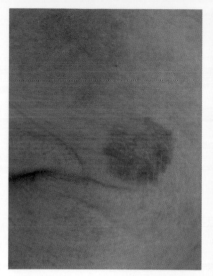
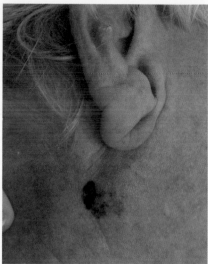
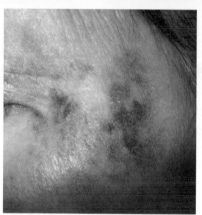

Figure 81.4 Lentigo maligna melanoma.

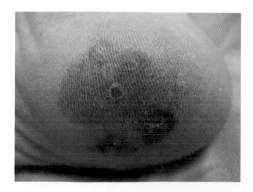

Figure 81.5 Acral lentiginous melanoma.

of the position the diagnosis is often delayed by years. At later stages, a nodule or ulceration can develop (Figure 81.6).

Subungual melanoma: Approximately 2–3% of the melanomas in white-skinned but a higher proportion in dark-skinned populations. The first sign is a brown to black linear discoloration in the nail bed hard to differentiate from benign melanonychia, which is quite common (Figure 81.7). Changes in the width and colour of the nail band should raise suspicion of melanoma. Later, symptoms become prominent with the Hutchinson's sign

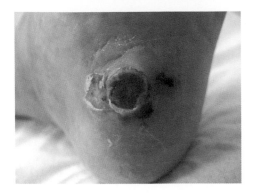

Figure 81.6 ALM of the sole (late presentation).

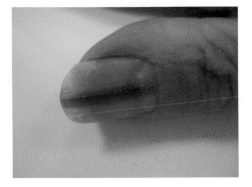

Figure 81.7 ALM in the nail area. Early presentation as a longitudinal melanonychia.

(pigmentation in the adjacent skin) and inflammatory or pigmented paronychia (Figure 81.8). Differential diagnoses: onychomycosis, paronychia, naevus and pyogenic granuloma.

Mucosal melanoma: Primary melanoma arising from the mucosal epithelia lining the respiratory, alimentary and genito-urinary tracts are rare (<5%). Melanoma of the mouth and vulva are the most frequent. They present as an irregular macular pigmentation (Figure 81.9). Ulceration and bleeding are common at later stages. Prognosis is poor due to late diagnosis.

Ocular melanoma: Arising from melanocytes situated in the conjunctival membrane and uveal tract of the eye. Uveal melanoma can affect any part of the uveal tract, but choroidal melanoma is predominant (86.3%).

Amelanotic melanoma: As diagnosis of melanoma is often suggested by pigmentation, amelanotic melanoma can be easily missed (Figures 81.10 and 81.11). They may mimic inflammatory lesions, angiomas, sarcoma, squamous cell carcinoma, basal cell carcinomas or others.

Regressive melanoma: Inflammation can lead to focal regression of a melanoma, which is usually visible as an irregular focus of

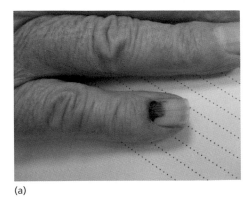

(a)

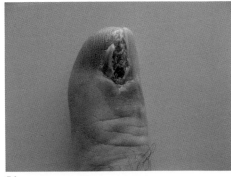

(b)

Figure 81.8 ALM in the nail area. Late presentation.

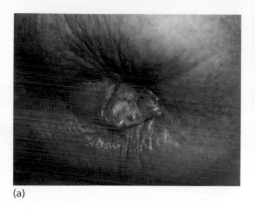

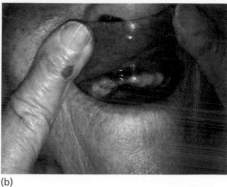

(a) (b)

Figure 81.9 Mucosal melanoma: (a) anal and (b) oral.

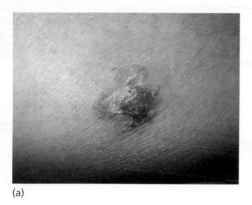

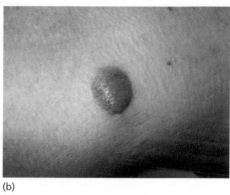

(a) (b)

Figure 81.10 Amelanotic melanoma: (a) amelanotic superficial spreading melanoma and (b) amelanotic nodular.

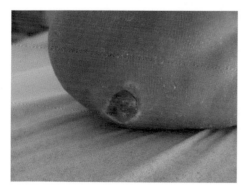

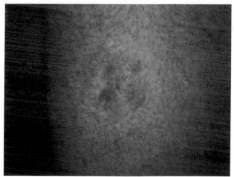

Figure 81.11 Amelanotic acral lentiginous melanoma.

Figure 81.12 Regressive melanoma.

hypopigmentation (Figure 81.12). However, when the regression is more severe, the melanoma may no longer be visible. Up to 8% of melanomas present as metastatic disease from an unknown primary.

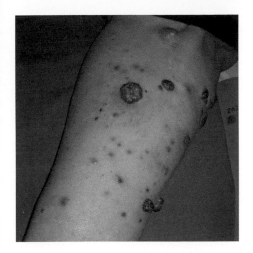

Figure 81.13 Melanoma skin metastasis.

Metastatic melanoma: The initial site of metastasis is most commonly the skin or subcutaneous tissue but 18–27% of the initial recurrences involve a distant organ: lung, brain, liver and bones are the commonest sites (Figure 81.13).

Investigations

Dermoscopy (see Chapter 82).
Reflectance confocal microscopy uses a near infrared laser to obtain *in vivo* imaging of the top layers of the skin. Specific morphological patterns are observed, allowing for differentiating benign and malignant, but also melanocytic from non-melanocytic lesions.

Histopathology
Pathological criteria of malignancy

- *Architecture*: Asymmetry, loss of architecture and heterogeneity in the size, shape and placement of nests, with confluence or fusion of the nests. Lack of top-down morphological maturation.
- *Pagetoid spread*: Upward individual migration of atypical melanocytes (pagetoid spread) within the epidermis; unusual in benign naevi.
- *Cytology*: Nuclear pleomorphism, enlargement and hyperchromatism, prominent nucleoli, and mitotic activity.
- *Brisk and asymmetrical host inflammatory response*: Regression figures with focal disappearance of melanocytes replaced by pigment, dermal fibrosis, verticalisation of the blood vessels and lymphocytic inflammation; interpreted as an immune reaction against melanoma.

Main pathological patterns

- *Nodular melanoma*: A predominantly dermal proliferation raising the epidermis with little or no junctional/pagetoid spread.
- *ALM and LMM*: Typical lentiginous pattern of melanocytes along the dermo–epidermal junction. LM is intraepidermal/*in situ*; LMM has dermal invasion. LM/LMM are associated with elastosis and epidermal atrophy often with extension of melanocytes down the appendages.
- *SSM*: Intraepidermal melanocytic proliferation made of nests with pagetoid spread and a dermal component of predominantly epithelioid cells. SSM has a prolonged radial-growth phase, where the lesion remains thin, with no potential for metastasis, followed by a vertical growth phase with an expanding tumour nodule and metastatic potential.

Immunohistochemistry
S100 protein is expressed by 99% of melanomas and melanocytic naevi but also by tumours with cartilaginous, nervous or myoepithelial differentiation. HMB-45 is most specific but does not stain desmoplastic melanoma and may not stain spindle cell melanoma. Other markers include Melan-A (MART-1) and MITF.

Prognostic factors (Box 81.2)
The best prognostic factor is the tumour thickness, the Breslow index (Figure 81.14) corresponding to the measurement (in millimetres) of the distance between the overlying epidermal granular layer and the deepest level of invasion of the primary lesion. Thicker tumours have a higher metastatic potential.

Management
Surgical

Primary excision: Suspected melanoma should be excised with a narrow ~2 mm margin for determination of diagnosis, key melanoma parameters and accurate microstaging. The biopsy should be oriented with definitive wide excision in mind. A wide local excision (WLE) or flap closure as the initial biopsy may prevent the option of subsequent sentinel lymph node biopsy

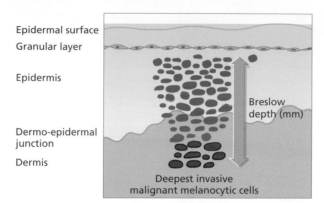

Figure 81.14 Breslow depth.

Box 81.2 Main prognostic factors for primary melanoma

- Thickness (Breslow index)***
- Sentinel node status***
- Ulceration**
- Mitotic rate** (negative value especially in thin tumours)
- Regression* (underestimation of Breslow)
- Age* (negative for older age)
- Sex* (negative for males)
- Location* (negative for head and neck)

Predictive value from *** high to * low.

(SLNB) or overtreat a benign lesion so should be avoided. In some situations, due to size or location, a biopsy through the thickest darkest portion is performed; this does not increase risk of metastasis.

Subclinical extension and local recurrence are characteristic features of LM/LMM, increasing the risk of incomplete excision margins. Margins of 0.5 cm for *in situ* LM are often inadequate. Techniques to consider, particularly on the head and neck, include standard excision with delayed reconstruction to allow for permanent section margin analysis, Mohs surgery with immunostaining and Johnson's square technique (a staged surgical procedure involving removal of the peripheral margin followed by paraffin wax embedded histopathological analysis to achieve total peripheral margin control prior to removal of the primary lesion).

Wide local excision: Prior to WLE regional draining lymph node basins must be clinically examined; any lymphadenopathy should be investigated with ultrasound and fine-needle aspirate. WLE aims to prevent local recurrence from persistent microscopic disease. Recommended margins are listed in Table 81.2. Depth of excision is to the deep adipose tissue for thin melanoma and melanoma *in situ*, and the plane of the muscular fascia for intermediate and thick melanoma. WLE on sites such as the face, hands and feet may require amendment of the recommended margin due to anatomical considerations.

Sentinel lymph node biopsy: SLNB is a staging test to identify patients with occult nodal disease providing useful prognostic information. Accurate identification of patients with stage III disease allows for better surveillance, consideration of adjuvant treatment, counselling and entrance into clinical trials. The benefits, risks and limitations of the procedure must be discussed with patients.

Table 81.2 Recommended clinical margin for WLE of melanoma

Melanoma tumour thickness	Recommended clinical margin*
Melanoma *in situ*	0.5–1 cm
Breslow depth ≤1.00 mm	1 cm
Breslow depth 1.01–2.00 mm	1–2 cm
Breslow depth >2.00 mm	2 cm

* For LMM pattern melanoma, especially on the head and neck, wider margins may be required for histological tumour clearance.
Sources: Adapted from Coit DG, Andtbacka R, Anker CJ, *et al*. (2012) Melanoma. J Natl Comp Cancer Network, Mar, 10(3), 366–400, Coit DG, Andtbacka R, Anker CJ, *et al*. (2013) Melanoma, version 2. 2013: featured updates to the NCCN guidelines. J Natl Comp Cancer Network, Apr 1, 11(4), 395–407, Bichakjian CK, Halpern AC, Johnson TM, *et al*. (2011) Guidelines of care for the management of primary cutaneous melanoma. American Academy of Dermatology. J Am Acad Dermatol, Nov, 65(5), 1032–1047.

Lymph node dissection: Total lymph node dissection of metastases to regional lymph nodes (either occult or palpable), without distant disease, is potentially curative. Adjuvant radiation to the nodal basin following surgery can be considered in the presence of nodal metastasis with extracapsular extension or high nodal disease burden.

Staging primary melanoma
The eight edition of the American Joint Committee on Cancer (AJCC) melanoma staging system was published in 2017 (Tables 81.3–81.5).

Systemic treatment
Systemic treatment options have evolved rapidly over the last decade and are still in a dynamic state of change (Figure 81.15). Treatment decisions are based on basic prognostic parameters such as tumour thickness, involvement of the regional lymph nodes, extent of internal organ involvement with special attention to brain metastases, growth dynamics and molecular assessment of the tumour.

In patients with metastatic melanoma there are three main systemic treatment options (see Figure 81.15): immunotherapy, targeted therapy and conventional chemotherapy.

Table 81.3 TNM staging categories for cutaneous melanoma

Classification	Breslow thickness (mm)*	Ulceration status/mitoses
T		
TX	Primary tumour thickness cannot be assessed (e.g. diagnosis by curettage)	N/A
T0	No evidence of primary tumour (e.g. unknown primary or completely regressed melanoma)	N/A
Tis	N/A	N/A
T1	≤1.00	Unknown or unspecified
T1a	<0.8	Without ulceration
T2b	<0.8 0.8–1.0	With ulceration With or without ulceration
T2	>1.0–2.0	Unknown or unspecified
T2a T2b	>1.0–2.0	Without ulceration With ulceration

(Continued)

Table 81.3 (Continued)

Classification	Breslow thickness (mm)*	Ulceration status/mitoses
T3	>2.0–4.0	Unknown or unspecified
T3a T3b	>2.0–4.0	Without ulceration With ulceration
T4	>4.0	Unknown or unspecified
T4a T4b	>4.0	Without ulceration With ulceration
N	Number of tumours involved regional lymph nodes	Nodal metastatic burden
NX	Regional nodes not assessed (e.g. SLN biopsy not performed, no regional nodes previously removed for another reason)	
N0	0	N/A
N1	0–1	a: One clinically occult (i.e. detected by SLN biopsy) b: One clinically detected c: No nodes with any number of in-transit, satellite and/or microsatellite metastases
N2	1–3	a: 2–3 clinically occult (i.e. detected by SLN biopsy) b: 2–3, at least one of which was clinically detected c: One node (occult or detected) with any number of in-transit, satellite and/or microsatellite metastases
N3	≥2	a: >4 clinically occult (i.e. detected by SLN biopsy) b: ≥ 4, at least one of which was clinically detected, or the presence of any number of matted nodes c: ≥2 nodes clinical or occult and/or presence of any number of matted nodes with any number of in-transit, satellite and/or microsatellite metastases
M	Anatomic site	Serum LDH
M0	No distant metastases	N/A
M1a	Distant skin, subcutaneous or nodal metastases	1a(0) normal, 1a(1) elevated
M1b	Lung metastases	1b(0) normal, 1b(1) elevated
M1c	Distant metastasis to non-CNS visceral sites	1c(0) normal, 1c(1) elevated
M1d	Distant metastasis to CNS	

* Tumour thickness measurements are recorded to the nearest 0.1 mm.
CNS, central nervous system; LDH, lactate dehydrogenase; N/A, not applicable; SLN, sentinel lymph node.
Source: Adapted from AJCC Cancer Staging Manual, 8th edition (2017) published by Springer International Publishing (Gershenwald JE, Scolyer RA, Hess KR, et al. Melanoma of the skin. In: Amin MB, Edge SB, Greene FL, et al, eds. AJCC Cancer Staging Manual. 8th ed. New York: Springer International Publishing, 2017, 563–585).

Table 81.4 Anatomical stage groupings for cutaneous melanoma.

Clinical staging*				Pathological staging**			
	T	**N**	**M**		**T**	**N**	**M**
0	Tis	N0	M0	0	Tis	N0	M0
IA	T1a	N0	M0	IA	T1a & b	N0	M0
IB	T1b	N0	M0	IB	T2a	N0	M0
	T2a	N0	M0				
IIA	T2b	N0	M0	IIA	T2b	N0	M0
	T3a	N0	M0		T3a	N0	M0
IIB	T3b	N0	M0	IIB	T3b	N0	M0
	T4a	N0	M0		T4a	N0	M0
IIC	T4b	N0	M0	IIC	T4b	N0	M0
III	Any T	N > N0	M0	IIIA	T1a/b-T2a	N1a or N2a	M0
				IIIB	T0	N1b, N1c	M0
					T1a/b-T2a	N1b/c or N2b	M0
					T2b/T3a	N1a-N2b	M0
				IIIC	T0	N2b, N2c, N3b or N3c	M0
					T1a-T3a	N2c or N3a/b/c	M0
					T3b/T4a	Any N	M0
					T4b	N1a-N2c	M0
				IIID	T4b	N3a-c	M0
IV	Any T	Any N	M1	IV	Any T	Any N	M1

* Clinical staging should be used after biopsy of the primary melanoma, with clinical assessment for regional or distant metastases (including radiological assessment if indicated).
** Pathological staging is completed after additional information is gathered from pathological assessment of the primary site from the wide-excision specimen, and pathological assessment of the regional lymph nodes after sentinel lymph node biopsy or therapeutic lymph node dissection.
Source: Adapted from AJCC Cancer Staging Manual, 8th edition (2017) published by Springer International Publishing (Gershenwald JE, Scolyer RA, Hess KR, et al. Melanoma of the skin. In: Amin MB, Edge SB, Greene FL, et al, eds. AJCC Cancer Staging Manual. 8th ed. New York: Springer International Publishing, 2017, 563–585.)

Immunotherapy: Anti-programmed-death 1 (anti-PD-1) antibodies nivolumab and pembrolizumab can be used alone or, preferably, if the patient is fit enough, a combination of nivolumab with the cytotoxic T-lymphocyte associated protein 4 (anti-CTLA-4) antibody ipilimumab.

Targeted therapy: *BRAF* inhibitors (vemurafenib, dabrafenib, encorafenib) and MEK (mitogen-activated protein kinase kinase) inhibitors (trametinib, cobimetinib) can only be used in *BRAF* and *NRAS* mutated melanoma. These selective kinase inhibitors are able to block tumour proliferation within a few days and are therefore the recommended first-line treatment in patients with aggressive disease characterised by high tumour burden, elevated lactate dehydrogenase, fast growth and significant visceral involvement, including metastases in the liver and brain. Imatinib and nilotinib can be used in melanoma with *KIT* mutations (more common in acral and mucosal melanomas) and selumetinib has been used

Table 81.5 Estimated 5- and 10-year survival rates according to AJCC staging (8th edition)

Pathological staging subgroups	5-year survival (%)	10-year survival (%)
Stage IA	99	96
Stage 1B	97	94
Stage IIA	94	88
Stage IIB	87	82
Stage IIC	82	75
Stage IIIA	93	88
Stage IIIB	83	77
Stage IIIC	69	60
Stage IIID	32	24

Source: Data from Gershenwald JE, Scolyer RA, Hess KR, et al. Melanoma staging: evidence-based changes in the American Joint Committee on Cancer, 8th edition, Cancer Staging Manual. CA Cancer J Clin 2017, 67(6), 472–492.

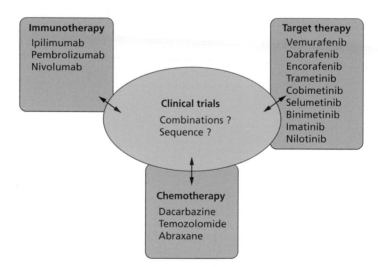

Figure 81.15 At present there are three main systemic treatment options for advanced melanoma: immunotherapy, kinase inhibitors and conventional chemotherapy.

for metastatic uveal melanoma, but effectiveness is varied and immunotherapy would generally be first line in these rarer melanoma types.

Chemotherapy: In the absence of other treatments, cytotoxic drugs such as dacarbazine, temozolamide and taxanes may be used.

Other: Imlygic (talimogene laherparepvec, or T-VEC) is an oncolytic virus therapy locally administered by injection to metastases in the skin and lymph nodes. It has also been used in combination with immmunotherapy. Limb perfusion or infusion as well as electro-chemotherapy can be useful for localised metastases in carefully selected patients.

Adjuvant therapy: Immunotherapy and targeted therapy are now offered to patients with stage III and stage IV no evidence of disease (NED) melanoma, depending on stage, age, comorbidity, BRAF mutation status and patient choice. Careful counseling by the oncology team for eligible patients is required.

Follow-up

The main purposes of follow-up are to detect any local recurrence around the scar of the excised melanoma, to palpate the draining lymph nodes for any clinically detectable evidence of nodal spread and to examine the rest of the skin for second primary melanomas. Second primary melanomas develop in 1.0–4.4% of patients diagnosed with a first melanoma. All patients should be taught self-examination to detect early recurrence, how to palpate lymph nodes and how to detect a second primary melanoma. Patients should have a point of contact to enable early review in case recurrence is suspected.

Guidance on follow-up varies between countries. Medical surveillance is usually every 3–6 months for the first 3–5 years after diagnosis and then with a lower frequency.

In view of the development of treatments in advanced disease, periodic radiological examination in asymptomatic patients is now performed for stage 3 melanoma at variable intervals.

For melanoma *in situ* some individuals can be discharged after appropriate surgery and education on self-examination and sun protection. Those with atypical moles should receive surveillance for additional melanomas. For LM, follow-up is required in view of the risk of another focus of melanocytic dysplasia at the excision margins.

82

Dermoscopy of melanoma and naevi

BENIGN DERMOSCOPIC PATTERNS IN NAEVI

One of the main objectives of dermoscopy is to differentiate benign naevi from melanoma. There are 10 well-defined benign patterns commonly seen in naevi (Figure 82.1) exhibiting symmetry in the distribution of colours and structures:

1. *Reticular diffuse*: Lines homogeneous in colour, thickness and size; network fades toward periphery. Seen in melanocytic naevi with a prominent junctional component (Figure 82.2a).
2. *Reticular patchy*: Focal patches distributed symmetrically separated by homogeneous structureless areas (same colour or slightly darker than the surrounding skin) (Figure 82.2b).
3. *Peripheral reticular with central hypopigmentation*: Uniform network at the periphery with central homogeneous and hypopigmented structureless area (same colour or slightly darker than the surrounding skin). Seen in acquired melanocytic naevi, fair skin (Figure 82.2c).
4. *Peripheral reticular with central hyperpigmentation*: Uniform typical network at the periphery with central homogeneous and hyperpigmented structureless area or blotch. Seen in acquired melanocytic naevi, especially darker skin (Figure 82.2d).
5. *Homogeneous*: Diffuse homogeneous structureless pattern. May appear grey-blue as seen in blue naevi (this pattern can also be seen in epidermotropic metastatic melanoma), brown as seen in congenital naevi, or tan-pink as seen in acquired naevi in fair skin (Figure 82.3).
6. *Peripheral globules with central network or homogeneous area, including the starburst pattern*: Correlates with the active radial growth phase of some naevi. Central component consists of a reticular or homogeneous pattern. The peripheral component can be (i) a single row of globules as seen in some actively growing dysplastic naevi, (ii) multiple rows of globules (i.e. tiered globules) creating a starburst pattern as commonly seen in Spitz naevi or in dysplastic naevi with spitzoid features, or (iii) streaks (classic starburst pattern) as seen in Spitz/Reed naevi (Figure 82.4).
7. *Peripheral reticular with central globules*: A uniform typical network at the periphery with central globules. Seen in naevi with a congenital pattern on histology (Figure 82.2e).
8. *Globular*: Globules of similar shape, size and colour distributed throughout the lesion. Globules may be large and angulated, creating a cobblestone pattern as seen in some congenital naevi (Figure 82.2f).
9. *Two-component*: Combination of two patterns with one half manifesting one pattern and the other half another pattern. The most common two-component pattern is the reticular–globular pattern (Figure 82.2g).

Rook's Dermatology Handbook, First Edition. Edited by Christopher E. M. Griffiths, Tanya O. Bleiker, Daniel Creamer, John R. Ingram and Rosalind C. Simpson.
© 2022 John Wiley & Sons Ltd. Published 2022 by John Wiley & Sons Ltd.

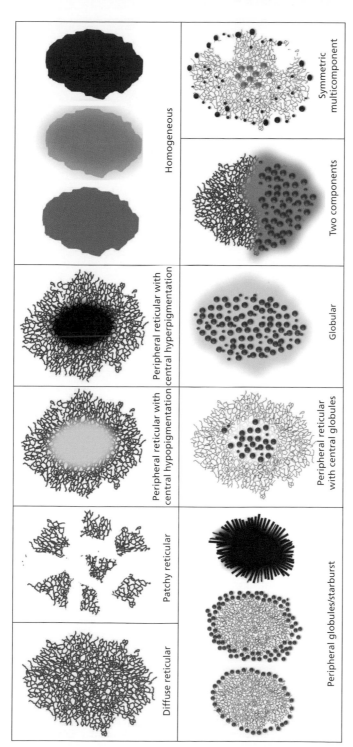

Figure 82.1 Dermoscopic naevi patterns.

PART 10: NEOPLASTIC, PROLIFERATIVE AND INFILTRATIVE DISORDERS AFFECTING THE SKIN

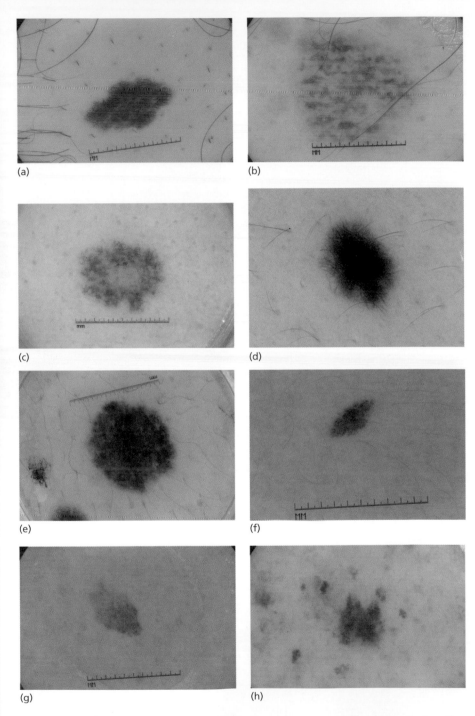

Figure 82.2 (a) Reticular diffuse naevus. (b) Reticular patchy naevus. (c) Peripheral reticular with central hypopigmentation naevus. (d) Peripheral reticular with central hyperpigmentation naevus. (e) Peripheral reticular naevus with central globules. (f) Naevus with globular pattern. (g) Two-component pattern naevus. (h) Multicomponent pattern naevus.

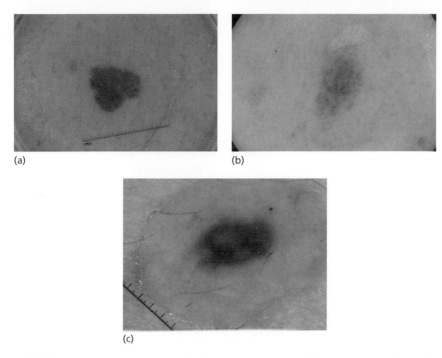

Figure 82.3 Homogeneous pattern naevi: (a) homogeneous brown, (b) homogeneous pink and (c) homogeneous grey-blue.

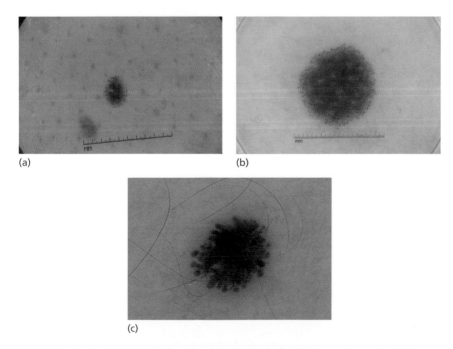

Figure 82.4 Naevi with peripheral globules: (a) growing naevus with a single row of globules, (b) Spitz naevus with multiple rows of globules and (c) Spitz naevus with streaks giving the appearance of an exploding star.

PART 10: NEOPLASTIC, PROLIFERATIVE AND INFILTRATIVE DISORDERS AFFECTING THE SKIN

10. *Multicomponent*: Combination of three or more patterns and/or structures distributed symmetrically in at least one axis (Figure 82.2h).

Most patients have a predominant naevus pattern with one or two of the above; a lesion that has a different dermoscopic pattern deserves closer scrutiny and perhaps biopsy. Lesions with the same pattern as the predominant naevus pattern can be safely monitored.

DERMOSCOPY OF MELANOMA

Melanoma-specific structures are dermoscopic structures with a heightened odds ratio for melanoma. Most melanomas developing on non-glabrous skin are of the superficial spreading subtype, and tend to reveal three or more colours (i.e. brown, black, red, white and/or blue-grey) and at least one of the 10 melanoma-specific structures listed in Table 82.1 (Figure 82.5).

Table 82.1 Melanoma-specific structures

Dermoscopic structure	Definition	Schematic illustration
Atypical pigment network	Increased variability in the width of the network lines, their colour and distribution. The hole sizes also have increased variability. The network can appear broken up (non-contiguous), appearing as branched streaks, and may end abruptly at the periphery	
Angulated lines	Angulated lines creating a zig-zag pattern or coalescing to create polygonal structures such as rhomboids	
Negative pigment network	Serpiginous interconnecting hypopigmented lines, which surround irregularly shaped pigmented structures that resemble elongated curvilinear globules. Diffuse or focally and asymmetrically located within the lesion	
Streaks	Radial projections located at the periphery of the lesion, which extend from the tumour toward the surrounding normal skin. *Pseudopods* are finger-like projections with small knobs at their tips, whereas *radial streaming* are the same structures without the knobs	
Crystalline structures	Shiny white, linear streaks that are often orientated parallel or orthogonal to each other. Also known as shiny white streaks or lines	

(Continued)

Table 82.1 (Continued)

Dermoscopic structure	Definition	Schematic illustration
Atypical dots or globules	*Dots* are small, round structures, which may be black, brown and/or blue-grey In melanoma dots vary in size, colour and distribution, tending to be located towards the periphery of the lesion and not associated with the pigmented network lines *Globules* consist of well-demarcated, round to oval structures that may be brown, black, blue and/or white in colour Larger than dots. In melanoma usually multiple and of differing sizes, shapes and colours Often asymmetrically and/or focally distributed within the lesion	
Off-centre blotch or multiple asymmetrically located blotches	Dark-brown to black, usually homogenous areas with varying hues of pigment that obscure visualisation of any other structures In melanoma, blotches are asymmetrically and/or focally located towards the periphery of the lesion or can present as multiple blotches Eccentric peripheral hyperpigmentation is often found in melanoma	
Regression structures (white scar-like depigmentation and/or blue-grey granularity or peppering overlying macular areas and not associated with vessels)	Regression structures consist of *granularity* (also known as peppering) and *scar-like areas* When both are present together, it gives the appearance of a blue-white veil over a macular area Tend to be asymmetrically located and often involve more than 50% of the lesion's surface area	
Blue-white veil overlying raised areas	Confluent blue pigmentation of varying hues with an overlying white 'ground glass' haze, asymmetrically located or diffusely present throughout the lesion	

(Continued)

Table 82.1 (Continued)

Dermoscopic structure	Definition	Schematic illustration
Atypical vascular structures	*Dotted vessels* over milky-red background *Serpentine vessels:* linear and irregular vessels *Polymorphous vessels:* two or more vessel morphologies within the same lesion *Corkscrew vessels:* usually seen in nodular melanoma, desmoplastic melanoma, or melanoma metastases	
Peripheral tan structureless areas	Structureless light brown area/s located at the periphery of the lesion and encompassing more than 10% of a lesion's surface area	

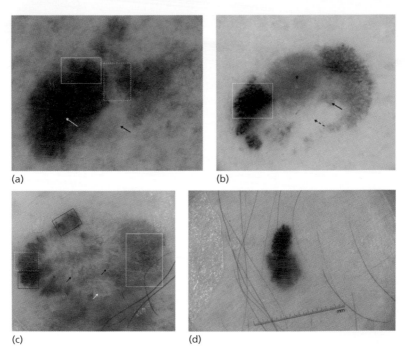

Figure 82.5 Melanoma dermoscopic images. (a) Atypical network (solid box), regression structures including granularity and scar-like depigmentation (dashed box), peripheral tan structureless area (black arrow) and atypical blotch area (white arrow). (b) Atypical network (solid box) and regression structures (arrows), with the solid arrow pointing to granularity/peppering and the dashed arrow pointing to scar-like depigmentation. The lesion also has a peripheral tan structureless area (asterisk). (c) Atypical network (black solid boxes), atypical globules (white dashed box), negative network (white solid box), scar-like areas (white arrow) and atypical vessels, including serpentine, dotted and irregular hairpin vessels (black arrows). (d) Atypical peripheral streaks (i.e. radial streaming).

Table 82.2 Melanoma structures seen on facial or on sun-damaged skin

Dermoscopic structure	Definition	Schematic illustration
Perifollicular granularity	Dots aggregated around adnexal openings	
Asymmetrical grey perifollicular openings	Dots or grey pigment aggregated around hair follicles in an asymmetrical fashion This asymmetrical distribution often creates a crescent shape around the hair follicles	
Angulated lines	Brown to bluish grey dots and/or lines arranged in an angulated linear pattern creating a zig-zag pattern or coalescing to create polygonal structures such as rhomboids	
Rhomboidal structures	Hyperpigmented brown and grey lines surrounding hair follicles and creating shapes like rhomboids	
Follicle obliteration	Rhomboidal structures become broader, obliterating hair follicles	
Circle within a circle (isobar pattern)	Concentric pigmented rings encircling each other	

Lentigo maligna melanoma is the most common melanoma subtype on facial and chronic sun-damaged skin. They more frequently display a different set of dermoscopic structures, as shown in Table 82.2 and Figure 82.6.

Some melanomas manifest a non-specific pattern, including lesions that are structureless or featureless. These dermoscopically non-diagnostic lesions should raise suspicion for melanoma.

MELANOMAS IN SPECIAL LOCATIONS

Acral melanoma

Most do not display melanoma-specific structures but show features listed in Table 82.3. The *acrolentiginous type* is the commonest subtype. It is imperative to identify the furrows and ridges of the dermatoglyphics, since pigment on the ridges (parallel ridge pattern) is highly suggestive of melanoma (Table 82.3 and Figure 82.7a,b). Most benign naevi reveal patterns with pigment predominantly in the furrows.

Clues to assist in recognising the ridges:

- Ducts of the eccrine glands; row of tiny white dots overlying ridges.
- Ridges wider than the furrows.
- Ink applied to the skin highlights the furrows, ridges and eccrine openings.

Melanoma involving the nail unit

Evaluating melanonychia striata requires inspection of the nail plate, cuticle, paronychium and hyponychium. Dermoscopy findings are listed in Table 82.4.

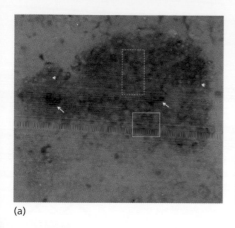
(a)

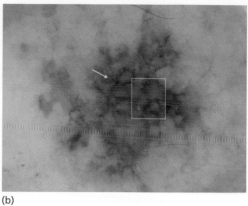
(b)

Figure 82.6 (a) Dermoscopic image of a lentigo maligna on the nose with perifollciular granularity and asymmetrical grey perifollicular openings (solid box), polygonal structures (dashed box), rhomboidal structures (solid arrows) and circle within a circle (arrowheads). (b) Dermoscopic image of a melanoma on chronic sun-damaged skin on the shoulder, revealing perifollicular granularity and asymmetrical grey perifollicular openings (solid box) and polygonal structures (white arrow).

Table 82.3 Melanoma structures in acral melanoma (melanomas on volar skin)

Dermoscopic structure	Definition	Schematic illustration
Parallel ridge pattern	Pigmentation located on the ridges of palms and soles	
Irregular diffuse pigmentation	Irregular, diffuse pigmentation with different shades of tan, brown, black and/or grey	
Irregular fibrillar pattern	Any fibrillar pattern on the palms, or fibrillar pattern on the soles that reveals an increased variability in the thickness or colours of the lines Line colour other than brown is also considered atypical	
Large-diameter lesion	Newly acquired lesion greater than 7–10 mm in diameter, especially in individuals over the age of 50 years	

Mucosal melanoma

Mucosal melanomas often reveal a multi-component pattern composed of irregular brown-black dots, blue-white veil, atypical vessels and/or a negative network. Other dermoscopic structures include focal areas of pigment network, globules, parallel structures or ring-like structures. The combination of one of three colours (blue, grey or white) and structureless areas is highly predictive of melanoma.

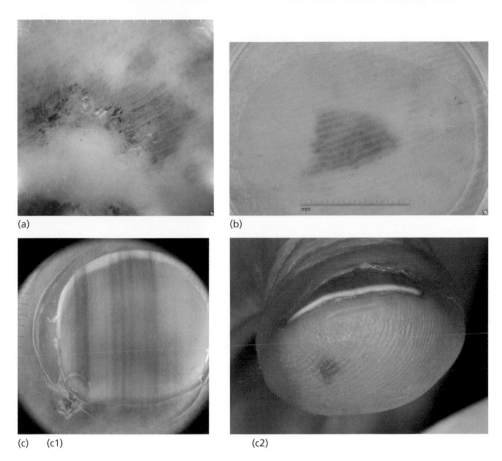

(a)   (b)

(c)   (c1)   (c2)

Figure 82.7 (a) and (b) Dermoscopic images of melanomas on the soles with a parallel ridge pattern. (c) Dermoscopic image (c1) of a melanoma involving the nail unit with multiple, longitudinal, irregular, brown bands with irregular spacing and thickness and the micro-Hutchinson sign. Also present is irregular pigmentation the hyponychium, c2.

OTHER MELANOMA VARIANTS

Amelanotic melanoma

Vascular structures are the main dermoscopic features, in particular serpentine or linear irregular vessels, milky-red areas and dotted vessels (Figure 82.8a).

Nodular melanoma

Nodular melanomas (NMs) do not have any pigment network, pseudo-network or regression structures (Figure 82.8b). Pigmented NMs tend to reveal areas of homogeneous blue pigmentation, blue-white veil, crystalline structures, pink or black colours and irregular blotches. Other features include atypical dots or globules, in particular black ones at the periphery and atypical vascular structures, including milky-red areas and atypical vessels with large diameters (most frequently linear irregular/serpentine vessels and hairpin vessels in a pink background). Some may present with pseudo-lagoons, characterised by red lacunae-like structures not separated by septae, as is the norm for haemangiomas. Some of these lacunae-like structures have small vessels within them (Figure 82.8b).

Table 82.4 Melanoma-specific structures of the nail unit

Dermoscopic structure	Definition	Schematic illustration
Hyponychial pigment with any features described in Table 82.3	Irregular pigmentation on the distal periungual skin, with any of the features associated with melanomas on acral skin	
Hutchinson or micro-Hutchinson sign	Pigmentation of the proximal nail fold that can be seen with the naked eye (Hutchinson) or only with dermoscopy (micro-Hutchinson)	
Triangular shape	Width of the melanonychia striata is wider at the proximal end of the nail plate	
Irregular band pattern	Multiple, longitudinal, irregular bands of different colours (i.e. black, brown, grey) with irregular spacing, thickness and disruption of parallelism	
Nail dystrophy	Complete or partial nail destruction and/or absence of the nail plate	

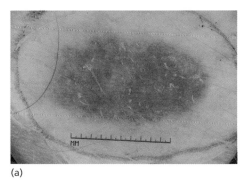

(a)

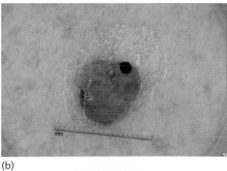

(b)

Figure 82.8 Dermoscopic images of amelanotic melanomas. (a) Serpentine vessels, dotted vessels and vascular blush. (b) Serpentine and hairpin vessels within pseudo-lagoons.

Merkel cell carcinoma

83

(Syn. Neuroendocrine carcinoma of the skin)
Merkel cell carcinoma (MCC) is a highly aggressive neuroendocrine skin cancer characterised by early and frequent metastasis, resulting in a 5-year disease-associated mortality rate of more than 40%.

Epidemiology

Although rare, the incidence is rapidly increasing. Most recent studies have reported an age-adjusted annual incidence rate of 0.18–0.41 per 100 000 persons in the USA and Europe, and almost one per 100 000 persons in Australia.

Mean age mid-70s with a 5- to 10 fold increase in incidence after the age of 65. M > F.

In organ transplant patients, MCCs develop 7–8 years post-transplantation and affect the head and neck areas.

Patients with MCC have an increased risk of a second primary cancer compared with the general population, including basal cell carcinoma (BCC) and chronic lymphocytic leukaemia.

Pathophysiology

Predisposing factors include immune suppression (e.g. organ transplant, AIDS and haematolymphoid disorders), sun exposure and advanced age.

Most MCCs are characterised by a clonal integration of the Merkel cell polyomavirus (MCPyV) into the host genome, and virally encoded proteins appear necessary to maintain tumour cell growth.

MCCs tend to occur in the mid-dermis with either a solid, sheet-like or nodular growth pattern or a diffuse growth pattern. Mitotic and apoptotic features are usually numerous and can easily be identified. Most MCCs have lymphatic and vascular invasion at diagnosis. Features associated with poor outcome include tumour size (≥5 mm), extension into the subcutaneous tissue, diffuse growth pattern, absence of an intratumoral T-cell infiltrate and high mitotic rate.

Immunohistochemistry is necessary for diagnosis and to distinguish from other conditions such as BCC, melanoma, lymphoma and metastases of small cell carcinomas of the lung. Staining for chromogranin A, synaptophysin or CD56 may be used to assess neuroendocrine differentiation. The perinuclear 'dot-like' reactivity of antibodies to low-molecular-weight keratins such as CK20 is typical although not pathognomonic of MCC.

Clinical features

A rapidly growing reddish nodule with a smooth shiny surface and firm consistency occurring on chronically sun-damaged skin (Figure 83.1). Predominant sites are the head and neck (over half of cases) and extremities (one-third of cases); the trunk and the oral and genital mucosa are involved in less than 10% of cases. Plaque-like variants occur rarely, especially on the trunk. Satellite metastases are frequently observed (Figure 83.2). Distant metastases are often present at diagnosis. Common sites include the skin, the lymphatics and the liver.

A mnemonic to remember the common clinical characteristics is AEIOU: *a*symptomatic, *e*xpanding rapidly, *i*mmune suppressed, *o*lder than 50 years, *u*ltraviolet-exposed site on fair skin.

Staging MCC is divided into stages based on the primary tumour size and extent of disease using the 8th edition of the American Joint

Rook's Dermatology Handbook, First Edition. Edited by Christopher E. M. Griffiths, Tanya O. Bleiker, Daniel Creamer, John R. Ingram and Rosalind C. Simpson.
© 2022 John Wiley & Sons Ltd. Published 2022 by John Wiley & Sons Ltd.

PART 10: NEOPLASTIC, PROLIFERATIVE AND INFILTRATIVE DISORDERS AFFECTING THE SKIN

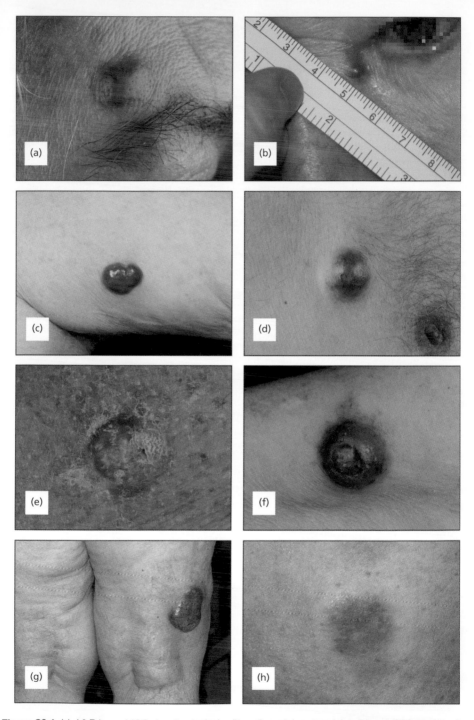

Figure 83.1 (a)–(d) Primary MCC showing typical solitary, firm, pink-red nodules. (e) and (f) Ulceration of MCC primaries is rarely observed and is mostly seen in advanced tumours. (g) and (h) Besides the more frequent nodular type of MCC, plaque-like variants occur, especially on the trunk and the lower extremities.

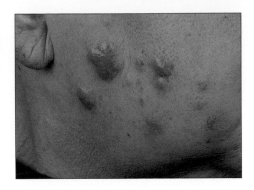

Figure 83.2 Metastatic MCC with satellite lesions.

Committee on Cancer (AJCC) staging system for MCC (Amin MB et al. (eds.) Springer International Publishing, 2017).

Investigation

Skin biopsy, including immunohistochemistry for diagnosis. Further investigations can be helpful including ultrasound scan, CT scan, and positron emission tomography/computed tomography (PET/CT). Sentinel lymph node biopsy (SLNB) is increasingly undertaken as at least half of patients with MCC will develop lymph node metastases. When distant metastases are expected, the appropriate organ imaging should be performed.

Management

General principles include wide local excision of 1–2 cm of primary tumour. Consideration of SLNB and adjuvant radiation should be discussed. Management of systemic disease is challenging; while the tumour shows high response rates to chemotherapy, these responses are mostly short lived, and no therapy regimen has proven survival benefit. Avelumab, an anti-programmed death ligand 1 inhibitor (PD-L1) is recommended for the treatment of adult patients with metastatic MCC.

A multidisciplinary approach to the treatment of MCC is essential to optimise outcomes. Clinical follow-up at 3-month intervals is performed given the high risk of local recurrences or regional lymph node metastases in the first 2 years. In high-risk patients 6-weekly clinical follow-ups may be considered. After 2 years, follow-up is recommended at 6-month intervals and generally restricted to 5 years given that the majority of recurrences occur during this time.

84 Cutaneous markers of internal malignancy

The following categories embrace most associations and interactions between skin and internal malignancy:

1. Multisystem and haematopoietic tumours that involve the skin.
2. Tumour spread from adjacent and distant tissues.
3. Genetically determined syndromes with cutaneous manifestations.
4. Paraneoplastic disorders.
5. Dermatoses associated with internal malignancy.

MULTISYSTEM AND HAEMATOPOIETIC TUMOURS THAT INVOLVE THE SKIN

See Chapters 78 and 85.

Tumour spread from adjacent and distant tissues

Cutaneous involvement by direct invasion, local metastasis or from cutaneous metastases from an internal tumour.

Direct invasion of the skin from a deeper tumour usually causes nodular infiltration, ulceration or inflammation, but may present in less obvious ways (Figure 84.1).

Peau d'orange (orange peel appearance)

Commonly occurs in the vicinity of the primary tumour, usually breast cancer.

Carcinoma en cuirasse

May have an early inflammatory stage and include some nodularity, but at a later stage is sclerodermoid in appearance. It may also occur with lung, gastrointestinal, renal and other malignancies.

Carcinoma erysipeloides

Resembles erysipelas, presenting as an extensive, warm, oedematous, tender plaque but without pyrexia or toxaemia; accounts for nearly a third of cases of cutaneous metastases from breast cancer. Similar presentations have been reported in melanoma, mesothelioma, cutaneous squamous cell carcinoma and carcinomas of the lung, prostate, oesophagus, bladder, colon, larynx, rectum, stomach, cutaneous squamous and pancreas. The clinical picture is due to plugging of dermal lymphatics by tumour cell emboli.

Rook's Dermatology Handbook, First Edition. Edited by Christopher E. M. Griffiths, Tanya O. Bleiker, Daniel Creamer, John R. Ingram and Rosalind C. Simpson.
© 2022 John Wiley & Sons Ltd. Published 2022 by John Wiley & Sons Ltd.

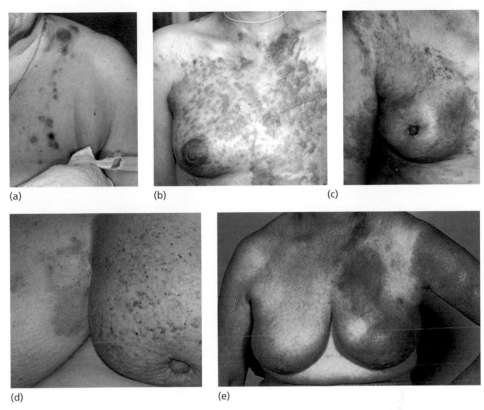

(a) (b) (c)

(d) (e)

Figure 84.1 Patterns of skin infiltration by carcinoma of the breast. (a) Limited and (b) extensive nodular infiltration. (c) Sclerotic infiltration (carcinoma en cuirasse) of breast skin and telangiectatic infiltration (carcinoma telangiectodes) extending beyond the breast. (d) Peau d'orange appearance due to infiltrative carcinoma skin of left breast. (d) and (e) Erysipelas-like changes (carcinoma erysipeloides) involving the right breast at an early stage (d) and at an advanced stage involving the left upper extremity as well as the breast (e). Note also nipple retraction in (c) and (d). Source: (a)–(c) Courtesy of Dr Olga Mikheeva, Moscow Region Oncological Dispensary, Russia; (d) Courtesy of Dr Ken Tsai; (e) Courtesy of Dr R. Emmerson, Royal Berkshire Hospital, Reading, UK.)

Telangiectatic metastatic carcinoma

Typically associated with breast cancer and may be difficult to diagnose as tumour cells may be scanty and the telangiectasia subtle. The vascular changes may be florid and resemble angiosarcoma.

Cutaneous metastasis

Metastasis to the skin is not as common as metastasis to liver, lung or bone; 10% of all metastases are cutaneous. The most common sources, in order of frequency, are breast, lung, colon, stomach, upper aerodigestive tract, uterus, kidney and melanoma from any source (Figures 84.1 and 84.2). The most common skin metastases from a previously unknown primary tumour originate from kidney, lung, thyroid or ovary.

Cutaneous metastases generally present as painless, firm to hard nodules, which may be skin-coloured, blue-brown or reddish-purple. The commonest pattern presents with a nodule that is solitary (Figure 84.3), which is twice as frequent as multiple nodules (Figure 84.4). Dermal or subcutaneous nodules may be more readily detected by palpation as they may not initially be apparent or symptomatic

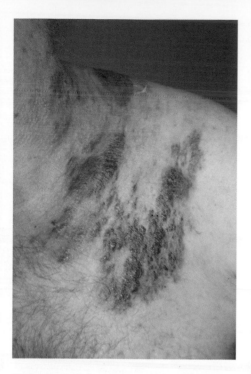

Figure 84.2 Metastatic bronchial carcinoma resembling cutaneous angiosarcoma (Source: Courtesy of Dr Olga Mikheeva, Moscow Region Oncological Dispensary, Russia.)

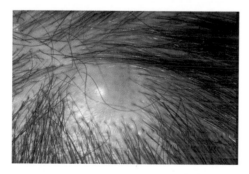

Figure 84.3 Solitary metastasis of squamous carcinoma to the scalp from an unknown primary.

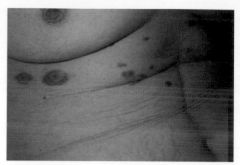

Figure 84.4 Metastatic pancreatic carcinoma manifesting as haemorrhagic nodules in the skin. (Source: courtesy of Dr Olga Mikheeva, Moscow Region Oncological Dispensary, Russia.)

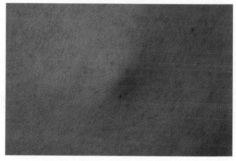

Figure 84.5 Subcutaneous metastasis from lung carcinoma; such metastases are typically multiple and many more firm nodules can usually be palpated if the patient is carefully examined.

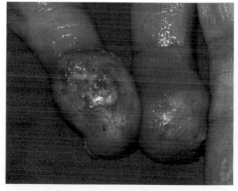

Figure 84.6 Embolic metastasis to the little finger of each hand from carcinoma of oesophagus.

(Figure 84.5). Other patterns include morphoea-like sclerotic plaques, scar infiltration, erysipelas-like diffuse skin infiltration, infiltrated areas of alopecia (alopecia neoplastica) and embolic metastasis to digits (Figure 84.6).

75% of cutaneous metastases occur on the head, neck and upper trunk. Metastases to

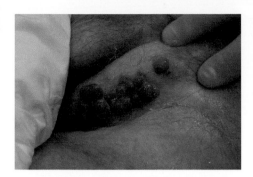

Figure 84.7 Metastasis to the groin in a patient with extensive pelvic prostatic carcinoma.

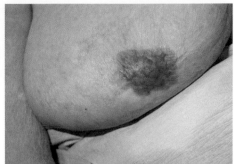

Figure 84.8 Paget disease of the breast causing destruction of the right nipple.

extremities suggest intra-arterial embolic spread, widespread skin metastases suggest that tumour cells are present in the general circulation, whilst metastases to the skin in the vicinity of the affected organ is more suggestive of dissemination by lymphatic vessels or by veins (Figure 84.7). Other than the scalp, notable sites for skin metastasis include umbilicus (Sister Mary Joseph nodule, related most commonly to bowel tumours) and recent operative scars.

Metastases to the scalp, usually from carcinomas of the breast, lung or kidney, may give rise to focal alopecia. Alopecia over a scalp 'cyst' should alert the physician to the possibility of malignancy (Figure 84.3).

Biopsy of a suspected skin metastasis will usually confirm or exclude malignancy. It is not always useful in determining the organ of origin if the tumour cells are poorly differentiated. Lymphatic spread of tumour cells may lead to an 'Indian filing' appearance in some cases.

PAGET DISEASE

Paget disease occurs in mammary and extramammary forms (see Chapter 61).

Mammary Paget disease

Presents with scaling and erythema, sometimes with oozing and crusting, on or around the nipple (Figure 84.8). It is a direct epidermal extension of an underlying ductal adenocarcinoma. Useful histopathological markers for mammary

Paget disease include epithelial membrane antigen, carcinoembryonic antigen, cytokeratins CK7 and CK8/18, as well as mucins such as MUC1. Differential diagnosis includes eczema, psoriasis, hyperkeratosis and erosive adenomatosis.

Clinical features include itch, burning, oedema, bleeding and reddish-brown plaques, often with a prominent margin. The margin maybe obscured by secondary infection and difficult to define in vaginal mucosa. Differential diagnosis: eczematous process, psoriasis or tinea. Histological and immunohistochemical features are similar to those of mammary Paget disease.

GENETICALLY DETERMINED SYNDROMES WITH CUTANEOUS MANIFESTATIONS

Many genodermatoses are associated with an increased risk of internal malignancy (Table 84.1).

PARANEOPLASTIC DISORDERS

There is a broad range of dermatoses which can present as markers of internal malignancy. The likelihood of finding a neoplasm in some of the better known paraneoplastic disorders may be graded as high, intermediate or low (Table 84.2).

Table 84.1 Examples of genodermatoses associated with internal malignancies

Main organ affected or usual mode of presentation (many are multisystem disorders)	Genodermatosis	Main neoplasms (may be limited to some families in some of the disorders listed)
Gastrointestinal tract	Gardner syndrome	Gastrointestinal polyposis and carcinomas, central nervous system tumours
	Bannayan–Riley–Ruvalcaba syndrome	
	Turcot syndrome (mismatch repair cancer syndrome)	
	Peutz–Jeghers syndrome	Gastrointestinal polyposis and carcinomas, pancreatic carcinoma, genital tumours (especially Sertoli cell, sex cord and cervix), breast cancers, lung cancers
Neurological	Ataxia–telangiectasia	Lymphomas, leukaemias
	Neurofibromatosis	Neurological tumours, sarcomas, phaeochromocytoma
Skin	Xeroderma pigmentosum	Skin cancers, sarcomas, central nervous system tumours, leukaemia, various solid organ tumours
	Naevoid basal cell carcinoma syndrome (Gorlin)	Basal cell carcinomas of skin, medulloblastoma
	Bazex–Dupré–Christol syndrome	Basal cell carcinomas of skin, possible leukaemia
	Porphyria cutanea tarda	Hepatocellular carcinoma
	Tylosis (Howel Evans syndrome)	Oesophageal carcinoma
	Sclerotylosis (Huriez syndrome)	Squamous cell carcinoma of skin; oral and bowel cancers also reported
	Muir–Torre syndrome	Colorectal tumours, sebaceous carcinoma
	Birt–Hogg–Dubé syndrome and Hornstein–Knickenberg syndrome	Medullary carcinoma of thyroid, renal cell carcinoma
	Familial leiomyomas (also uterine)	Renal cell carcinoma
	Incontinentia pigmenti	Wilms tumour, rhabdomyosarcomas (renal, paratesticular), retinoblastoma, leukaemias
	Familial atypical naevi and melanoma	Pancreatic carcinoma, cutaneous and ocular melanoma
	Melanoma–astrocytoma syndrome	Melanomas, astrocytomas and other central nervous system tumours

(Continued)

Table 84.1 (Continued)

Main organ affected or usual mode of presentation (many are multisystem disorders)	Genodermatosis	Main neoplasms (may be limited to some families in some of the disorders listed)
	Supernumerary nipples	Genito-urinary tumours: renal cell carcinoma, Wilms tumour, bladder, testicular, prostate
	Ichthyoses (autosomal dominant and X-linked)	Testicular carcinoma
Endocrine	Multiple endocrine neoplasia syndromes	Medullary carcinoma of thyroid, phaeochromocytoma
Growth/skeletal	Werner syndrome	Many, especially sarcomas
	Rothmund–Thomson syndrome	Skin, osteosarcoma
	Bloom syndrome	As general population but early onset
	Maffucci syndrome	Chondrosarcomas, gliomas, ovarian cancers
	Goltz syndrome	Chondrosarcomas, giant cell tumour of bone
	Fanconi anaemia (usually presents due to congenital malformations)	Myolodysplastic syndrome, acute myelogenous leukaemia, hepatic carcinoma
Haematopoietic	Dyskeratosis congenita	Mucosal squamous cell carcinoma, haematopoietic malignancy and others
Immunological	Wiskott–Aldrich syndrome	Lymphoreticular malignancies
	Chediak–Higashi syndrome	Lymphoreticular malignancies
Multisystem	Cowden's (multiple hamartoma and neoplasia) syndrome	Breast, thyroid, gastrointestinal, cerebellum, endometrial and renal carcinomas
	Carney complex	Myxomas, schwannomas, testicular Sertoli cell tumour, pituitary adenomas, thyroid cancer
	Von Hippel–Lindau disease	Phaeochromocytoma, renal carcinoma, haemangioblastoma, pancreatic carcinoma
	Beckwith–Wiedemann syndrome (exomphalos–macroglossia–gigantism syndrome)	Wilms tumour, adrenal carcinoma, hepatoblastoma, pancreatoblastoma, others (especially in patients with hemihypertrophy)

Acrokeratosis paraneoplastica

(Syn. Bazex syndrome)

A rare paraneoplastic condition. M > F. Particularly associated with squamous cell carcinoma of the upper respiratory or gastrointestinal tracts.

Cutaneous changes develop gradually, often in several phases, initially with violaceous erythema and scaling on the peripheries, especially the helices of the ears, tip of the nose, hands and feet (particularly the distal portion of digits). The eruption then becomes more hyperkeratotic, with a palmar-plantar keratoderma. Subsequently the eruption may become

Table 84.2 Strength of correlation of some potentially paraneoplastic dermatoses with internal malignancy

Strength of correlation	Type of reaction pattern	Examples
Strong	Papulosquamous and figurate eruptions	Bazex syndrome
		Erythema gyratum repens
		Necrolytic migratory erythema
	Epidermal conditions	Acanthosis palmaris (tripe palms)
		Florid cutaneous papillomatosis
	Deposition disorders	Primary amyloidosis
		Scleromyxoedema
		Necrobiotic xanthogranuloma
		POEMS syndrome
	Others	Acquired hypertrichosis lanuginosa
		Paraneoplastic pemphigus
		Carcinoid syndrome
		Trousseau syndrome
Moderate	Papulosquamous and neutrophilic eruptions	Sweet syndrome
		Pyoderma gangrenosum
		Dermatomyositis
	Others	Multicentric reticulohistiocytosis
		Pityriasis rotunda Mastocytosis (see Chapter 18)
Weak	Epidermal conditions	Acanthosis nigricans in isolation
		Acquired ichthyosis (unless widespread, deeply fissured, truncal pattern)
		Eruptive seborrhoeic keratoses (sign of Leser–Trélat)
	Deposition disorders	Scleredema
		Calcinosis cutis
	Others	Vasculitis, Raynaud phenomenon, digital ischaemia
		Erythromelalgia
		Relapsing polychondritis
		Erythroderma/exfoliative dermatitis
		Digital clubbing (unless with hypertrophic osteoarthropathy)
		Pruritus
		Erythema annulare centrifugum
		Cushing syndrome

POEMS, *polyneuropathy, organomegaly, endocrinopathy, M-protein, skin changes.*

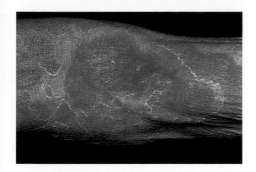

Figure 84.9 Erythema gyratum repens of the arm secondary to carcinoma of the bronchus. (Source: Courtesy of Dr Kristian Thomsen, Finsen Institute, Copenhagen, Denmark.)

generalised. Differential diagnosis: seborrheic dermatitis, contact dermatitis, acral psoriasis or reactive arthritis. Histological changes are non-diagnostic.

Erythema gyratum repens

A rare, bizarre, cutaneous eruption consisting of mobile, concentric, often palpable, erythematous, wave-like bands, which give a 'woodgrain' appearance to the skin (Figure 84.9). A peripheral scale or collarette may be present. The whole torso is frequently affected. There is often severe pruritus. Lesions migrate, usually changing position by about 1 cm daily. It has a strong association with internal malignancy (over 80% of cases), particularly lung cancer, which is present in about a third of cases.

Necrolytic migratory erythema

Strongly associated with a glucagon-secreting α-cell tumour of the pancreas. It presents as a widespread painful migratory rash with repeated eruptions of irregular polycyclic, intensely inflammatory erythematous patches with expanding scaling margins; these blister and break down with superficial epidermal necrolysis and crusting. It has a predilection for the anogenital region and trunk. Necrolytic migratory erythema is strongly associated with the presence of an underlying glucagon-secreting pancreatic islet cell adenoma. It is one of the components of

glucagonoma syndrome along with weight loss, diabetes, stomatitis and diarrhoea.

Deposition disorders

Can be associated with internal malignancy and include amyloidosis (myeloma), mucinoses, e.g. scleromyxedema (paraproteinaemia), lipids, e.g. necrobiotic xanthogranuloma (paraproteinaemia), calcium, e.g. metastatic and dystrophic calcification (lung and pancreatic carcinomas).

Paraneoplastic pigmentation

Can be associated with internal malignancy (Table 84.3).

DERMATOSES ASSOCIATED WITH INTERNAL MALIGNANCIES

Several dermatoses have a significant association with internal malignancy.

Raynaud phenomenon and digital ischaemia

Persistent, painful digital ischaemia, with an unusual Raynaud syndrome-type appearance but often progressing to gangrene, has been linked to a variety of solid tumours and reticuloendothelial neoplasms. The process may have a vasculitic element.

Hyperviscosity syndromes such as polycythaemia vera, leukaemias or myeloma-linked cryoglobulinaemia may give rise to cutaneous ischaemia and phlebitis by microvascular occlusion. Cancer-associated coagulopathy may also cause vascular occlusion.

Erythromelalgia

Linked with myeloproliferative disorders, most commonly polycythaemia vera or essential thrombocythaemia in over a third of adult

Table 84.3 Pigmentary abnormalities associated with internal malignancy

Pigmentary change	Pattern	Examples
Hyperpigmentation	Diffuse, or diffuse with localised accentuation (Addisonian pattern of pigmentation)	Melanoma (rarely causes diffuse slate grey pigmentation)
		Phaeochromocytoma (Addisonian pattern)
		Ectopic ACTH syndrome (Addisonian pattern; occurs with bronchial adenocarcinoma)
		POEMS syndrome (diffuse or semiconfluent speckled pattern)
		Hyperpigmentation with scleromyxoedema and gammopathy
		Diffuse mastocytosis
		Lymphomas (uncommon)
		Ependymoma (mild increase in pigmentation)
		Werner syndrome (localised or diffuse pigmentation)
		Cachexia due to neoplasia
	Patchy or reticulated	Fanconi anaemia (various pigmentary changes)
		Dyskeratosis congenita (reticulate pigmentation)
	Other distributions	Carcinoid syndrome (photodistributed)
		Pancreatic, gastric and renal tumours (erythema ab igne due to local application of heat)
	Lentigines and freckles	Peutz–Jeghers syndrome (lentigines)
		Carney complex (lentiginosis is characteristic, freckles also occur)
		Xeroderma pigmentosum (freckles)
		Neurofibromatosis (flexural freckle-like macules)
		Cowden's disease and Bannayan–Riley–Ruvalcaba syndrome (genital lentigines)
		Gardner syndrome (freckles)
		Paraneoplastic acral lentiginosis
	Café-au-lait macules	Neurofibromatosis
		Bloom syndrome
		Multiple endocrine neoplasia types 1 and 2B
		Fanconi anaemia
		Von Hippel–Lindau disease

(Continued)

Table 84.3 (Continued)

Pigmentary change	Pattern	Examples	
	With epidermal hyperplasia	Acanthosis nigricans	
	Melanocytic naevi and melanoma	Associated with pancreatic neoplasia, astrocytomas and other cerebral neoplasms in some families	
		Blue naevi and ordinary naevi occur in Carney complex	
Mixed hyper- and hypopigmentation	Poikiloderma	Dermatomyositis (speckled pigmentation on hypopigmented background)	
		Rothmund–Thomson syndrome (photodistributed poikiloderma)	
Hypopigmentation	Generalised	Chediak–Higashi syndrome	
	Localised, multiple	Tuberous sclerosis complex (ash leaf macules)	
		Mycosis fungoides (hypopigmented variant)	
		Halo depigmentation around primary tumour or metastases	
	Melanoma-associated (other than regression within the primary lesion)	Distant leukoderma, usually with centrifugal spread starting on the trunk	
	Dystrophic calcification	Pancreatic carcinoma	Calcification of fat

POEMS, *polyneuropathy, organomegaly, endocrinopathy, M-protein, skin changes.*

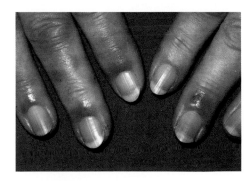

Figure 84.10 Chilblain-like lesions in acute myeloid leukaemia.

cases. The feet are most commonly affected, with severe burning pain and erythema; symptoms may occur 2 years or more before the haematological disorder presents. The mechanism involves microvascular occlusion (typically with platelet aggregates, termed 'white thrombi'); Raynaud phenomenon may occur.

Vasculitis

There is an association of cutaneous vasculitis with neoplasia, particularly in myeloproliferative disorders and myeloma. Hairy cell leukaemia appears to be especially associated with vasculitis, which may be of leukocytoclastic or polyarteritis nodosa pattern.

When linked with a haematological malignancy, vasculitis often antedates bone marrow involvement, as opposed to the more predictable purpura due to thrombocytopenia, which reflects bone marrow infiltration by myeloproliferative disease or carcinoma. It is difficult in some reports to distinguish between microvascular occlusion (e.g. by a monoclonal type I cryoglobulin) versus primary vasculitis or therapy-related vessel injury.

Chilblain-like lesions

Lesions resembling perniosis may be a manifestation of leukaemias and myeloproliferative disorders (Figure 84.10). They are persistent rather than episodic, tend to be refractory to treatment with drugs (such as calcium-channel blockers) and on biopsy may show blast cells as well as vascular changes.

Flushing

May be a feature of carcinoid syndrome, mastocytosis, phaeochromocytoma, medullary carcinoma of thyroid, hypogonadism in males, pancreatic tumours producing vasoactive intestinal peptide (VIPomas), basophilic leukaemia, horseshoe kidney (Rovsing syndrome) and renal cell carcinoma. It is also a feature of POEMS (*p*olyneuropathy, *o*rganomegaly, *e*ndocrinopathy, *M* protein, *s*kin changes) syndrome, which is associated with myeloma. Plethora, but not flushing, may be apparent in polycythaemia vera.

Hyperhidrosis

Generalised hyperhidrosis may rarely be associated with malignant disease. It is an almost consistent finding in phaeochromocytoma.

Nocturnal hyperhidrosis ('night sweats') may also occur in lymphoma and carcinoid syndrome. Localised hyperhidrosis may occur in POEMS syndrome.

Paroxysmal unilateral hyperhidrosis of the face and neck, usually severe and unrelated to stimuli such as eating, may be due to an ipsilateral thoracic tumour (adenocarcinoma, squamous cell carcinoma or mesothelioma) compressing or infiltrating the sympathetic trunk. Associated features may include Horner syndrome, facial weakness, sensory disturbance and other features of the primary tumour.

Cancer-associated thrombosis

Includes migratory thrombophlebitis, deep vein thrombosis and Mondor disease. Mondor disease is a rare condition in which a cord-like lesion is palpable in the subcutaneous tissue of the anterior or lateral thorax; the underlying lesion is a thrombophlebitis. Up to 15% of patients may have an associated breast carcinoma.

Paraneoplastic pruritus

Internal carcinoma is a non-specific, rare, but important cause of pruritus (see Chapter 40).

Part 11
Systemic Disease and the Skin

The skin and systemic diseases

85

The skin is involved in the clinical expression of many systemic disorders. Tables 85.1–85.10 provide a summary of the main skin associations encountered in the diseases of each organ system.

Table 85.1 Skin manifestations of rheumatological diseases

Rheumatological disease	Skin disorder *Systemic features*
Dermatomyositis (see Chapter 24)	Nail fold erythema, ragged cuticles, Gottren's papules, extensor surface erythema, 'shawl' sign, upper chest erythema, heliotrope eyelid erythema, scalp erythema, photosensitivity, poikiloderma, panniculitis, erosions and ulcers, calcinosis *Proximal limb myositis, dysphagia, interstitial lung disease*
Fibroblastic rheumatism	Skin nodules *Symmetrical polyarthropathy, flexion contractures (especially fingers)*
Gout	Tophi (tophus = singular) on pinna, elbow, Achilles tendon and fingertip (Figure 85.1) *Inflammatory monoarthritis*
Multicentric reticulohistiocytosis	Papulonodular skin lesions *Symmetrical polyarthritis, arthritis mutilans, fever, weight loss, malaise*
Osteoarthritis	Heberden nodes at distal interphalangeal joints of fingers; Bouchard nodes at proximal interphalangeal joints *Degenerative arthritis of hands, feet, spine and large weight-bearing joints*
Psoriatic arthritis (see Chapter 10)	Chronic plaque psoriasis, generalised pustular psoriasis, palmo-plantar pustulosis *Seronegative spondyloarthropathy*
Reactive arthritis	Palmo-plantar pustulosis, geographic tongue, circinate balanitis (Figure 85.2) *Genito-urinary or gastrointestinal infection inducing inflammatory arthritis of large joints, conjunctivitis, uveitis*
Relapsing polychondritis	Chondritis of cartilage in pinnae and nose (Figure 85.3) *Chondritis of respiratory tract cartilage*

(Continued)

Rook's Dermatology Handbook, First Edition. Edited by Christopher E. M. Griffiths, Tanya O. Bleiker, Daniel Creamer, John R. Ingram and Rosalind C. Simpson.
© 2022 John Wiley & Sons Ltd. Published 2022 by John Wiley & Sons Ltd.

Table 85.1 (Continued)

Rheumatological disease	Skin disorder *Systemic features*
Rheumatoid arthritis	Rheumatoid nodules, pyoderma gangrenosum, rheumatoid neutrophilic dermatitis, vasculitis, interstitial granulomatous dermatitis, leg ulcers *Seropositive inflammatory polyarthritis, anaemia, interstitial lung disease, accelerated atherosclerosis*
Systemic lupus erythematosus (see Chapter 23)	Photosensitivity, malar erythema, discoid lupus, nail fold erythema, livedo reticularis, Raynaud phenomenon, mouth ulcers, alopecia, panniculitis, acute cutaneous LE, bullous LE, subacute cutaneous LE, TEN-like LE *Non-erosive arthritis, blood disorders, renal disorders, neurological disorders, serositis, fatigue*
Systemic sclerosis (see Chapter 25)	Nail fold erythema, sclerodactyly, Raynaud phenomenon, digital ulcers, scleroderma, microstomia, calcinosis, leg ulcers *Symmetrical polyarthritis, pulmonary hypertension, right-sided heart failure, reflux oesophagitis, renal disease*

LE, lupus erythematosus; TEN, toxic epidermal necrolysis.

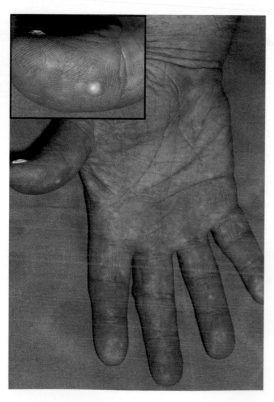

Figure 85.1 Gout with multiple cream-coloured tophi on the palmar surfaces of the digits.

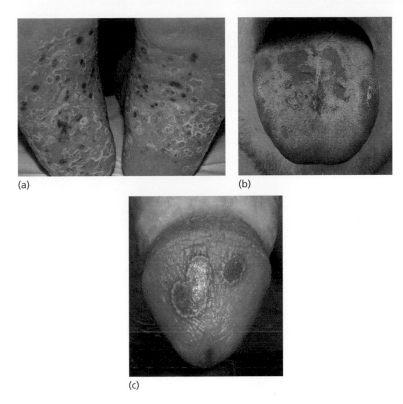

Figure 85.2 Reactive arthritis with (a) plantar pustulosis, (b) geographic tongue and (c) circinate balanitis.

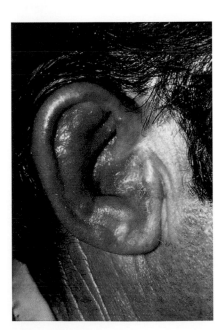

Figure 85.3 Relapsing polychondritis, showing inflammation of the pinna.

Table 85.2 Skin manifestations of respiratory diseases

Respiratory disease	Skin disorder *Systemic features*
Eosinophilic granulomatosis with polyangiitis (see Chapter 54)	Vasculitis with purpura, nodules, ulcers *Rhinitis, asthma, pneumonitis, eosinophilia, neuropathy, renal involvement*
Granulomatosis with polyangiitis (see Chapter 54)	Vasculitis with purpura, nodules, ulcers *Upper airway disease, pulmonary infiltrates, pulmonary nodules/cavities, alveolar haemorrhage, renal involvement*
Microscopic polyangiitis (see Chapter 54)	Vasculitis with purpura *Pulmonary infiltrates, pulmonary nodules/cavities, alveolar haemorrhage, renal involvement*
Mycoplasma infection	Erythema multiforme, often mucosal *Pneumonia*
Tuberculosis (see Chapter 5)	Erythema nodosum, lupus vulgaris, scrofuloderma, other forms of cutaneous tuberculosis, erythema induratum *Pneumonia, disseminated mycobacterial infection*
Yellow nail syndrome (see Chapter 48)	Thickened yellow finger- and toenails (Figure 85.4) *Dyspnoea, cough, bronchiectasis, pleural effusions, chronic sinusitis, lung infections*

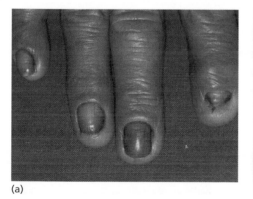
(a)

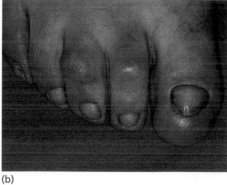
(b)

Figure 85.4 Yellow nail syndrome affecting the nails of (a) the fingers and (b) the toes.

Table 85.3 Skin manifestations of haematological diseases

Haematological disease	Skin disorder *Systemic features*
Acute myeloid leukaemia	Leukaemia cutis (Figure 85.5), cutaneous small vessel vasculitis, neutrophilic eccrine hidradenitis, Sweet syndrome, pyoderma gangrenosum *Anaemia, thrombocytopenia, frequent infections, fatigue*
Adult T-cell leukaemia/lymphoma	Leukaemia cutis *Anaemia, thrombocytopenia, frequent infections, fatigue, hypercalcemia, lytic bone lesions.*
Chronic lymphocytic leukaemia	Leukaemia cutis (Figure 85.6), cutaneous small vessel vasculitis, exaggerated insect bite-like reactions (Figure 85.7) *Fever, weight loss, fatigue, lymphadenopathy*
Myelodysplastic syndrome	Leukaemia cutis, Sweet syndrome, pyoderma gangrenosum, malignant extramedullary haematopoiesis *Anaemia, thrombocytopenia, frequent infections, fatigue*
Hodgkin lymphoma	Pruritus, lymphomatous infiltrates *Fever, night sweats, weight loss, fatigue, lymphadenopathy*
non-Hodgkin lymphoma	Pruritus, lymphomatous infiltrates, paraneoplastic pemphigus *Fever, night sweats, weight loss, fatigue, lymphadenopathy, bone pain*
Multiple myeloma	Pyoderma gangrenosum (Figure 85.8), type I cryoglobulinaemia, plasma cell infiltrates, macroglobulinaemia cutis, scleredema, scleromyxoedema, necrobiotic xanthogranuloma, POEMS syndrome, AL amyloidosis *Bone pain, anaemia, hypercalcaemia, renal impairment, hyperviscosity syndrome, frequent infections, fatigue*
Plasmacytoma	POEMS syndrome, cutaneous deposits (macroglobulinaemia cutis) (Figure 85.9) *Bone pain*
Monoclonal gammopathy of unknown significance	Scleredema (Figure 85.10), scleromyxoedema (Figure 85.11), necrobiotic xanthogranuloma, AL amyloidosis *Usually no systemic features*
Waldenström macroglobulinaemia	Plasma cell infiltrates, cutaneous small vessel vasculitis, type I cryoglobulinaemia, macroglobulinaemia cutis, Schnitzler syndrome *Fatigue, weight loss, bleeding from the nose and gums*

POEMS, polyneuropathy, organomegaly, endocrinopathy, monoclonal gammopathy, skin changes (hyperpigmentation, hypertrichosis, haemangiomas, acrocyanosis, scleroderma, leuchonychia); AL, amyloid light chains.

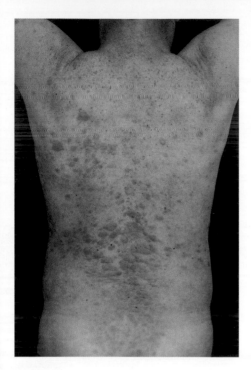

Figure 85.5 Leukaemia cutis in acute myeloid leukaemia: extensive infiltrative, papulonodular lesions over the back. (Source: Courtesy of Professor Lorenzo Cerroni, University of Graz, Austria.)

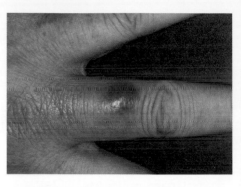

Figure 85.7 Exaggerated insect bite-like reaction in chronic lymphocytic leukaemia. (Source: Courtesy of Professor Lorenzo Cerroni, University of Graz, Austria.)

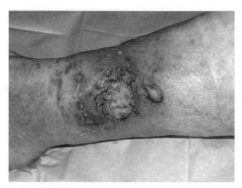

Figure 85.8 Pyoderma gangrenosum in patient with IgA paraproteinaemia. (Source: Courtesy of Dr Ian Coulson, Burnley General Hospital, UK.)

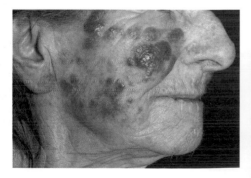

Figure 85.6 Leukaemia cutis in chronic lymphocytic leukaemia: infiltrated nodules and plaques on the cheek. (Source: Courtesy of Professor Lorenzo Cerroni, University of Graz, Austria.)

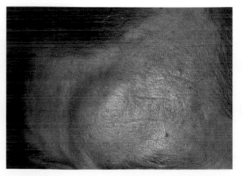

Figure 85.9 Plasmacytoma cutis. (Source: Courtesy of Professor Lorenzo Cerroni, University of Graz, Austria.)

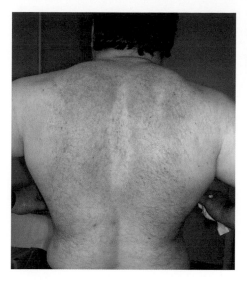

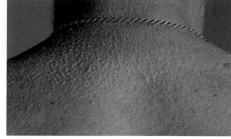

Figure 85.11 Scleromyxoedema in patient with monoclonal gammopathy of undetermined significance.

Figure 85.10 Scleredema in a patient with monoclonal gammopathy of undetermined significance. (Source: Courtesy of Dr Ian Coulson, Burnley General Hospital, UK.)

Table 85.4 Skin manifestations of primary immunodeficiency syndromes

Immunodeficiency syndrome	Skin disorder *Systemic features*
Chediak–Higashi syndrome	Hypopigmented skin, silvery hair (partial albinism), pyogenic and fungal skin infections *Neuropathy, neutropenia*
Hermansky–Pudlak syndrome	Oculocutaneous albinism *Platelet coagulopathy, bleeding tendency, pulmonary fibrosis, granulomatous colitis*
Griscelli syndrome	Albinism, pyogenic skin infections *Hepatosplenomegaly, neutropenia, thrombocytopenia*
Wiskott–Aldrich syndrome	Eczema, recurrent staphylococcal skin infections *Coagulopathy due to thrombocytopenia, leukaemia, lymphoma, reduced IgM levels*
Omenn syndrome	Graft-versus-host-like disorder, hyperkeratotic eczema, desquamation, erythroderma, persistent bacterial skin infections *Diarrhoea, hepatosplenomegaly, leucocytosis, lymphadenopathy, elevated IgE*
DiGeorge syndrome	Mucocutaneous candidosis, cutaneous calcification *Thymic hypoplasia, absence of T cells, congenital heart disease, seizures, hypocalcaemic tetany, characteristic facial features (short philtrum, low-set ears, hypertelorism)*

(Continued)

Table 85.4 (Continued)

Immunodeficiency syndrome	Skin disorder *Systemic features*
Hyper-IgE syndrome	Eczema, staphylococcal folliculitis and abscesses, mucocutaneous candidosis *Increased IgE, eosinophilia, scoliosis, retained primary teeth, characteristic facial features (prominent forehead, deep-set eyes, broad nasal bridge)*
Chronic granulomatous disease	Pyogenic and fungal skin infections, perioral dermatitis, granulomatous cheilitis *Lymphadenopathy*
Congenital CD4 deficiency	Multiple, large viral warts (Figure 85.12) *Increased risk of lymphoma, including MALT lymphoma, Burkitt lymphoma, diffuse large cell lymphoma*
WHIM (warts, hypoimmunoglobulinaemia, infections, myelokathexis)	Multiple, large viral warts, recurrent skin bacterial infections *B-cell dysfunction, neutropenia*
Common variable immunodeficiency	Recurrent pyogenic skin infections, eczema *Recurring infections in different organs, bronchiectasis, asthma, viral infections, enlarged lymph nodes and spleen, hypogammaglobulinaemia: low levels of IgG, IgA, IgM*
X-linked agammaglobulinaemia	Recurrent pyogenic skin infections *Recurring infections in different organs, as in common variable immunodeficiency*

MALT, mucosa-associated lymphoid tissue.

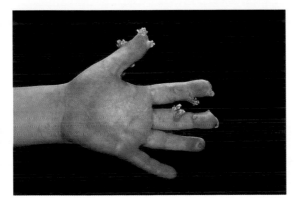

Figure 85.12 Multiple large viral warts in a child with congenital CD4 deficiency.

Table 85.5 Skin manifestations of endocrine diseases

Endocrine disease	Skin disorder *Systemic features*
Acromegaly	Cutis verticis gyrata (Figure 85.13), acne and sebaceous gland hyperplasia (Figure 85.14), hypertrichosis, hyperhidrosis, soft tissue swelling of hands, feet, nose, lips and ears, macroglossia (Figure 85.15) *Pituitary adenoma, visual field deficit (bitemporal hemianopia), headache, facial bone changes, arthritis, cardiomegaly and heart failure, diabetes mellitus*
Addison disease	Generalised hyperpigmentation (Figure 85.16), oral hyperpigmentation *Fatigue, postural hypotension, muscle weakness, weight loss, anxiety, Addisonian crisis*
Cushing syndrome/disease	Acne, easy bruising, telangiectasiae, striae, hypertrichosis *Moon face, central obesity, buffalo hump, weight gain, hypertension, muscle weakness, fatigue, menstrual irregularities, osteopenia*
HAIR-AN syndrome (hyperandrogenism, insulin resistance, acanthosis nigricans)	Acne, hirsutism, acanthosis nigricans *Polycystic ovarian syndrome, menstrual irregularities, obesity, insulin resistance*
Hyperprolactinaemia	Seborrhoea *Pituitary adenoma, amenorrhoea, galactorrhoea, hypogonadism, gynaecomastia, erectile dysfunction, bitemporal hemianopia*
Thyroid disease (autoimmune)	Alopecia areata, finger clubbing (thyroid acropathy), urticaria, vitiligo, pretibial myxoedema (notably in Grave disease) (Figure 85.17), palmar erythema (hyperthyroidism) *Hyperthyroidism: irritability, weakness, tachycardia, heat intolerance, diarrhoea, weight loss* *Hypothyroidism: depression, weakness, bradycardia, cold intolerance, constipation, weight gain*

PART 11: SYSTEMIC DISEASE AND THE SKIN

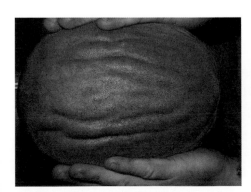

Figure 85.13 Cutis verticis gyrata in acromegaly.

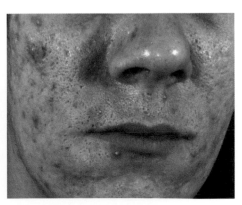

Figure 85.14 Acromegaly: note the coarse features, severe acne and seborrhoea.

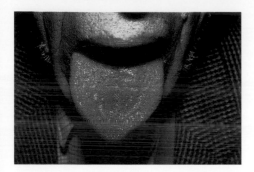

Figure 85.15 Acromegalic macroglossia.

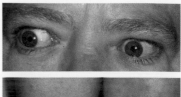

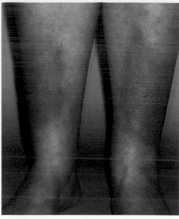

Figure 85.17 A patient with Graves disease with pretibial myxoedema and exophthalmos.

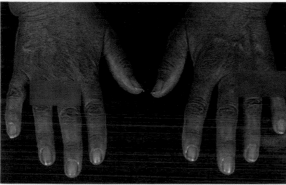

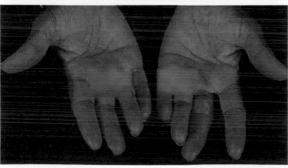

Figure 85.16 Addisonian pigmentation of the dorsal hands and palmar creases.

Table 85.6 Endocrine tumours associated with dermatological features

	Carcinoid tumour	Glucagonoma	Phaeochromocytoma
Epidemiology	Rare	Rare	Rare
Pathophysiology	Tumour generally develops in small intestine Main secretory products of carcinoid tumours are serotonin, histamine, tachykinins and prostaglandins	Tumour of pancreas (alpha cells) Secretory product is glucagon, which causes increase in blood glucose and hypoaminoacidaemia	Tumour of adrenal medulla Main secretory products are catecholamines (adrenaline and noradrenaline) and other vasomediators
Clinical features	Flushing is the most prominent symptom lasting from 30 s to 30 min (Figure 85.18) Other symptoms include diarrhoea, hypotension, tachycardia, abdominal cramping, sweating, bronchospasm	Necrolytic migratory erythema is characterised by oedema, erythema and blistering with an active spreading margin (Figure 85.19) Occurs on low abdomen, genitalia, groins, perineum and buttocks Other symptoms include diabetes, weight loss	Paroxysmal flushing of face, neck and chest Attacks last 15 min to hours Other symptoms include hypertension, tachycardia, palpitations, anxiety, headaches, chest/abdominal pain
Investigations	24-h urinary excretion of 5-hydroxyindoleacetic acid Appropriate imaging	Serum glucagon levels Appropriate imaging	24-h urinary excretion of catecholamines and metanephrines Appropriate imaging
Management	Surgical resection of tumour Octreotide or other somatostatin analogues may decrease secretory activity of the carcinoid	Surgical resection of tumour Glucagon secretion can be reduced by octreotide	Surgical resection of tumour

PART 11: SYSTEMIC DISEASE AND THE SKIN

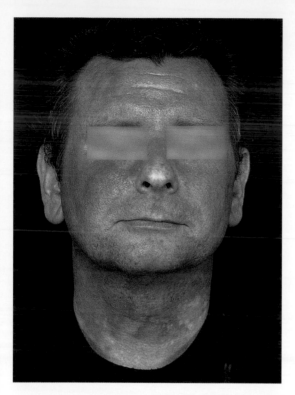

Figure 85.18 Histamine-evoked 'geographical' pattern of flushing due to foregut carcinoid tumour. (Source: Courtesy of Professor M. Greaves, London, UK.)

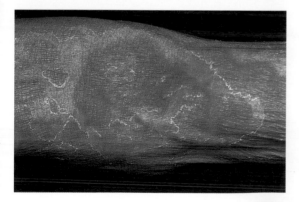

Figure 85.19 Necrolytic migratory erythema due to glucagonoma. (Source: Courtesy of Dr Kristian Thomsen, Finsen Institute, Copenhagen, Denmark.)

Table 85.7 Skin manifestations of diabetes

	Acanthosis nigricans	Diabetic dermopathy	Necrobiosis lipoidica	Scleredema of Buschke
Epidemiology	Common	Common	Rare	Rare
Pathophysiology	Mostly associated with obesity and insulin resistance Overexpression of EGFR and IGF-1 receptors stimulates keratinocyte proliferation	Caused by diabetic microvasculopathy Thickened arteriolar walls, haemosiderin and melanin deposition in dermis	Inflammatory disorder of dermal collagen Perivascular and interstitial mixed inflammatory infiltrate with extensive areas of collagen necrobiosis	Occurs mostly in middle-aged men with poorly controlled insulin-dependent diabetes Increased synthesis of collagen and mucin by dysfunctional fibroblasts
Clinical features	Symmetrical velvety dark patches in axillae, groins and neck	Red papules evolving into round, hyperpigmented atrophic lesions Occurs on shins	Indurated plaque(s) on shins with raised red margins and sunken yellow centre with visible telangiectasiae Can ulcerate	Indurated thickening of skin on posterior neck spreading to shoulders and upper back Erythema and peau d'orange appearance of lesional skin
Investigations	Clinical diagnosis	Clinical diagnosis	Often a clinical diagnosis Biopsy sometimes needed	Biopsy needed to exclude other sclerotic conditions
Management	Maximise diabetic control Topical retinoid may reduce hyperkeratosis	Maximise diabetic control, moderately potent topical steroid, compression hosiery	Maximising diabetic control does not appear to help resolution	Maximise diabetic control Phototherapy (narrow band UVB, PUVA, UVA-1)

EGFR, epidermal growth factor receptor; IGF-1, insulin-derived growth factor; PUVA, psoralen and UVA photochemotherapy.

PART 10: SYSTEMIC DISEASE AND THE SKIN

Table 85.8 Skin manifestations of gastrointestinal and liver diseases

Gastrointestinal/liver disease	Skin disorder *Systemic features*
Chronic liver disease	Hyperpigmentation, jaundice, pruritus, spider naevi, palmar erythema, loss of secondary sexual hair in males, easy bruising, porphyria cutanea tarda, Terry's nails *Fatigue, cirrhosis, ascites, portal hypertension, liver failure*
Coeliac disease	Dermatitis herpetiformis, aphthous ulcers, cutaneous small vessel vasculitis, erythema nodosum, erythema elevatum diutinum *Fatigue, anaemia, malabsorption, weight loss, failure to grow (in children)*
Crohn disease	Anal tags, perineal abscesses, fissures and fistulae, lip swelling, cobblestoning of gingivae, oral ulceration (Figure 85.20), extra-gastrointestinal cutaneous Crohn disease Other skin associations: psoriasis, erythema nodosum, pyoderma gangrenosum (Figure 85.21), Sweet syndrome, bowel-associated dermatosis-arthritis syndrome, cutaneous PAN *Fatigue, anaemia, fever, diarrhoea (may be bloody), malabsorption, weight loss, bowel obstruction*
Hepatitis C	Jaundice, cryoglobulinaemia, cutaneous small vessel vasculitis, lichen planus *Fatigue, cirrhosis, ascites, portal hypertension, liver failure*
Multiple hamartoma and neoplasia syndrome (Cowden syndrome) (see Chapter 38)	Tricholemmomas, palmar keratosis, oral papillomas, epidermal naevi, café-au-lait macules, lipomas *Gastrointestinal polyposis, thyroid follicular adenoma, multinodular goitre, thyroid cancer, macrocephaly, breast cancer*
Primary biliary cholangitis, sclerosing cholangitis	Jaundice, pruritus *Fatigue, cirrhosis, ascites, portal hypertension, liver failure*
Ulcerative colitis	Erythema nodosum, pyoderma gangrenosum, Sweet syndrome, pyodermatitis-pyostomatitis vegetans, cutaneous small vessel vasculitis, epidermolysis bullosa acquisita, bowel-associated dermatosis-arthritis syndrome *Fatigue, anaemia, fever, diarrhoea (may be bloody), malabsorption, weight loss*

PAN, polyarteritis nodosa.

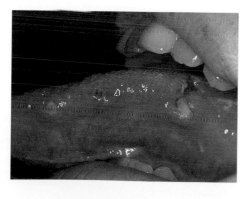

Figure 85.20 Recurrent major aphthae in 26-year-old man with longstanding severe Crohn disease.

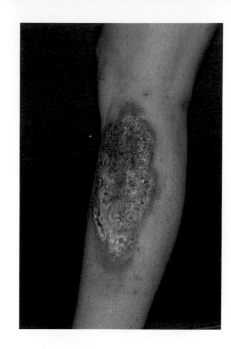

Figure 85.21 Pyoderma gangrenosum in a patient with Crohn disease.

Table 85.9 Skin manifestations of renal diseases

Renal disease	Skin disorder *Systemic features*
Acquired partial lipodystrophy (Barraquer–Simons syndrome) (see Chapter 52)	Progressive lipoatrophy of face, arms and torso *Mesangiocapillary glomerulonephritis*
Birt–Hogg–Dube syndrome (see Chapter 84)	Fibrofolliculomas, tichodiscomas, perifollicular fibromas *Renal tumours (chromophobe renal carcinoma and renal oncocytoma), renal cysts, subpleural lung cysts, pneumothorax, thyroid nodules*
End-stage renal disease (chronic renal failure)	Pruritus, xerosis, pigmentation, half-and-half nails (Figure 85.22), perforating dermatoses (Figure 85.23), calcific uraemic arteriolopathy (calciphylaxis) (Figure 85.24), pseudoporphyria (Figure 85.25) *Nausea, anorexia, fatigue, oedema, hypertension, hyperparathyroidism*
Fabry disease	Angiokeratomas, anhidrosis, red hands and feet (secondary to neuropathy) *Chronic kidney disease, restrictive cardiomyopathy, generalised pain, painful extremities (acroparasthesia), abdominal pain*
Hereditary leiomyomatosis and renal cell carcinoma syndrome (see Chapter 75)	Multiple cutaneous leiomyomas *Uterine leiomyomas, uterine leiomyosarcomas, renal cell cancer*
Nail-patella syndrome (see Chapter 48)	Poorly developed finger- and toenails *Proteinuria, nephritis, hypoplastic patellae, arthrodysplasia of elbows, hypothyroidism*

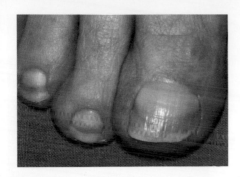

Figure 85.22 'Half-and-half' toenails in a patient with uraemia.

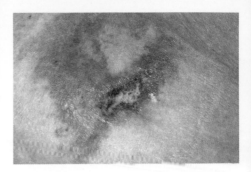

Figure 85.24 Early calcific uraemic arteriolopathy (calciphylaxis) resulting from diabetic nephropathy.

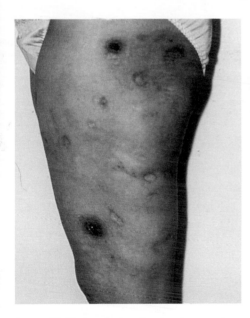

Figure 85.23 Acquired perforating dermatosis on the thigh of a woman with diabetic nephropathy.

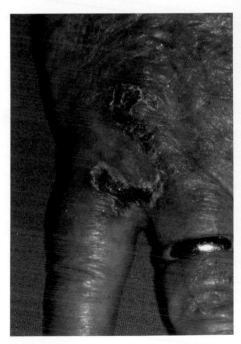

Figure 85.25 Pseudoporphyria on the backs of the hands of a man with end-stage chronic kidney disease.

Table 85.10 Skin manifestations of neurological disorders

Neurological disease	Skin disorder *Neurological features*
Complex regional pain syndrome	Erythema, oedema, cyanosis and dyshidrosis of affected limb *Pain and progressive tissue damage in affected limb*
Gustatory hyperhidrosis (Frey syndrome)	Unilateral scalp and facial sweating immediately after eating hot/spicy food *Facial nerve damage from parotid gland surgery or parotid gland tumour*
Hereditary sensory and autonomic neuropathies types I–V	Dyshidrosis *Severe sensory dysfunction, other symptoms and features vary according to the subtype*
Horner syndrome	Unilateral facial anhidrosis *Ipsilateral ptosis and small pupil*
Parkinson disease	Seborrhoea, seborrhoeic dermatitis, xerosis, hyperhidrosis *Tremor, bradykinesia, rigidity, postural instability* *Non-motor features: autonomic dysfunction, neuropsychiatric problems*
Peripheral neuropathy with neuropathic ulcer	Painless ulcer on weight-bearing surfaces of foot, especially over the metatarsal heads (Figure 85.26) *Distal polyneuropathy with motor, sensory and autonomic components: vast majority of neuropathic ulcers occur in type II diabetes*
Spinal dysraphism	Lumbo-sacral skin abnormalities, e.g. hypertrichosis ('faun tail') (Figure 85.27), lipoma, pit, dimple, haemangioma *Cauda equina syndrome, walking difficulties, lower sacral sensory problems, cyanosis of feet, trophic changes to toes*
Sympathetic nerve injury	Vasodilatation and anhidrosis *Peripheral nerve injury with loss of somatic sensation*
Syringomyelia	Loss of pain and temperature sensation in hands and arms, with retention of touch and position sense (dissociated sensory loss) *Chronic pain, abnormal sensations in the hands, paralysis or paresis, neuropathic arthropathy (Charcot joint)*
Tuberous sclerosis	Ashleaf macules, facial angiofibromas, periungual fibromas, shagreen patches, dental enamel pits, intraoral fibromas *Brain tumours, epilepsy, autism spectrum disorder, other neuropsychiatric disorders, renal angiomyolipomas, polycystic kidney disease, cardiac rhabdomyomas*

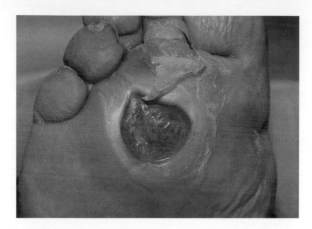

Figure 85.26 Neuropathic ulcer over metatarsal heads.

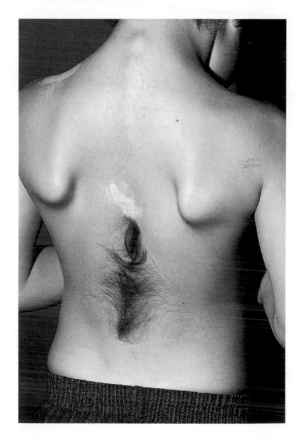

Figure 85.27 Tuft of hair in association with spina bifida.

Acute dermatoses

Rook's Dermatology Handbook, First Edition. Edited by Christopher E. M. Griffiths, Tanya O. Bleiker, Daniel Creamer, John R. Ingram and Rosalind C. Simpson.
© 2022 John Wiley & Sons Ltd. Published 2022 by John Wiley & Sons Ltd.

PART 11: SYSTEMIC DISEASE AND THE SKIN

Acute Painful Ulcer in adults

Causes

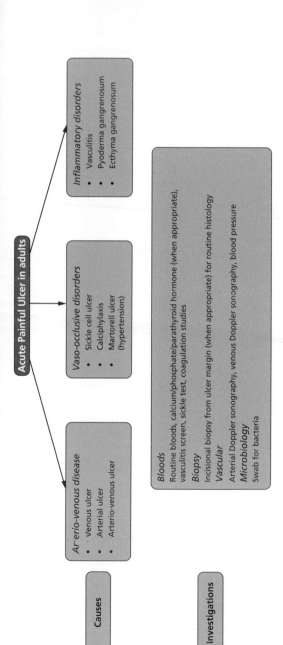

Arterio-venous disease
- Venous ulcer
- Arterial ulcer
- Arterio-venous ulcer

Vaso-occlusive disorders
- Sickle cell ulcer
- Calciphylaxis
- Martorell ulcer (hypertension)

Inflammatory disorders
- Vasculitis
- Pyoderma gangrenosum
- Ecthyma gangrenosum

Investigations

Bloods
Routine bloods, calcium/phosphate/parathyroid hormone (when appropriate), vasculitis screen, sickle test, coagulation studies
Biopsy
Incisional biopsy from ulcer margin (when appropriate) for routine histology
Vascular
Arterial Doppler sonography, venous Doppler sonography, blood pressure
Microbiology
Swab for bacteria

Management

Arterio-venous disease
- Venous ulcer: See Chapter 56
- Arterial ulcer: See Chapter 56
- Arterio-venous ulcer: See Chapter 56

Vaso-occlusive disorders
- Sickle cell ulcer: Treatment directed by haematologists
- Calciphylaxis: Treatment directed by internal physicians
- Martorell ulcer: Treat hypertension

Inflammatory disorders
- Vasculitis: see Chapter 54
- Pyoderma gangrenosum: see Chapter 21
- Ecthyma gangrenosum: see Chapter 4

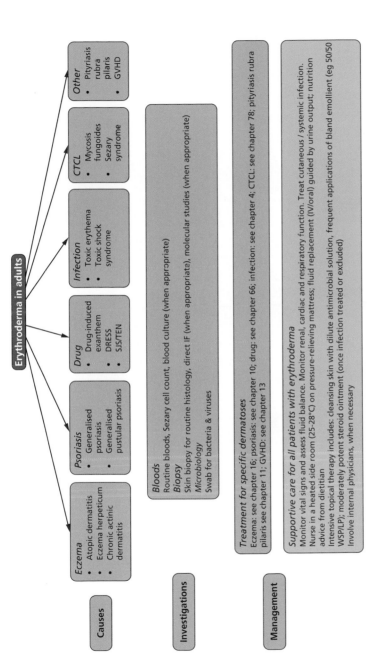

Erythroderma in adults

Causes

Eczema
- Atopic dermatitis
- Eczema herpeticum
- Chronic actinic dermatitis

Psoriasis
- Generalised psoriasis
- Generalised pustular psoriasis

Drug
- Drug-induced exanthem
- DRESS
- SJS/TEN

Infection
- Toxic erythema
- Toxic shock syndrome

CTCL
- Mycosis fungoides
- Sezary syndrome

Other
- Pityriasis rubra pilaris
- GVHD

Investigations

Bloods
Routine bloods, Sezary cell count, blood culture (when appropriate)

Biopsy
Skin biopsy for routine histology, direct IF (when appropriate), molecular studies (when appropriate)

Microbiology
Swab for bacteria & viruses

Management

Treatment for specific dermatoses
Eczema: see chapter 16; psoriasis: see chapter 10; drug: see chapter 66; infection: see chapter 4; CTCL: see chapter 78; pityriasis rubra pilaris see chapter 11; GVHD: see chapter 13

Supportive care for all patients with erythroderma
Monitor vital signs and assess fluid balance. Monitor renal, cardiac and respiratory function. Treat cutaneous / systemic infection. Nurse in a heated side room (25-28°C) on pressure-relieving mattress; fluid replacement (IV/oral) guided by urine output; nutrition advice from dietitian
Intensive topical therapy includes: cleansing skin with dilute antimicrobial solution, frequent applications of bland emollient (eg 50/50 WSP/LP); moderately potent steroid ointment (once infection treated or exuded)
Involve internal physicians, when necessary

CTCL, cutaneous T-cell lymphoma; DRESS, drug reaction with eosinophilia and systemic symptoms; GVHD, graft-versus-host disease; SJS/TEN, Stevens–Johnson syndrome/toxic epidermal necrolysis; 50/50 WSP/LP, 50% white soft paraffin/50% liquid paraffin.

PART 11: SYSTEMIC DISEASE AND THE SKIN

PART 11: SYSTEMIC DISEASE AND THE SKIN

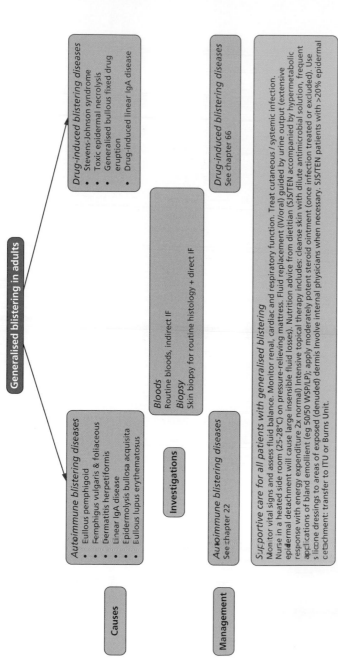

Generalised blistering in adults

Causes

Autoimmune blistering diseases
- Bullous pemphigoid
- Pemphigus vulgaris & foliaceous
- Dermatitis herpetiformis
- Linear IgA disease
- Epidermolysis bullosa acquisita
- Bullous lupus erythematosus

Drug-induced blistering diseases
- Stevens–Johnson syndrome
- Toxic epidermal necrolysis
- Generalised bullous fixed drug eruption
- Drug-induced linear IgA disease

Investigations

Bloods
Routine bloods, indirect IF

Biopsy
Skin biopsy for routine histology + direct IF

Management

Autoimmune blistering diseases
See chapter 22

Drug-induced blistering diseases
See chapter 66

Supportive care for all patients with generalised blistering
Monitor vital signs and assess fluid balance. Monitor renal, cardiac and respiratory function. Treat cutaneous / systemic infection. Nurse in a heated side room (25–28°C) on pressure-relieving mattress. Fluid replacement (IV/oral) guided by urine output (extensive epidermal detachment will cause large insensible fluid losses). Nutrition advice from dietitian (SJS/TEN accompanied by hypermetabolic response with energy expenditure 2x normal) Intensive topical therapy includes: cleanse skin with dilute antimicrobial solution, frequent applications of bland emollient (eg 50/50 WSP/LP); apply moderately potent steroid ointment (once infection treated or excluded). Use silicone dressings to areas of exposed (denuded) dermis when necessary. SJS/TEN patients with >20% epidermal detachment: transfer to ITU or Burns Unit.

SJS/TEN, Stevens–Johnson syndrome/toxic epidermal necrolysis; 50/50 WSP/LP, 50% white soft paraffin/50% liquid paraffin.

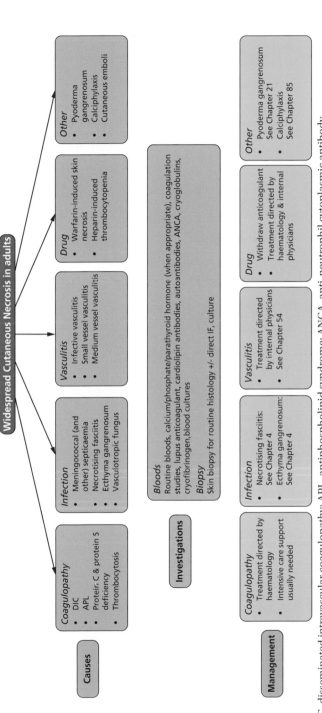

Widespread Cutaneous Necrosis in adults

Causes

Coagulopathy
- DIC
- APL
- Protein C & protein S deficiency
- Thrombocytosis

Infection
- Meningococcal (and other) septicaemia
- Necrotising fasciitis
- Ecthyma gangrenosum
- Vasculotropic fungus

Vasculitis
- Infective vasculitis
- Small vessel vasculitis
- Medium vessel vasculitis

Drug
- Warfarin-induced skin necrosis
- Heparin-induced thrombocytopenia

Other
- Pyoderma gangrenosum
- Calciphylaxis
- Cutaneous emboli

Investigations

Bloods
Routine bloods, calcium/phosphate/parathyroid hormone (when appropriate), coagulation studies, lupus anticoagulant, cardiolipin antibodies, autoantibodies, ANCA, cryoglobulins, cryofibrinogen, blood cultures

Biopsy
Skin biopsy for routine histology +/- direct IF, culture

Management

Coagulopathy
- Treatment directed by haematology
- Intensive care support usually needed

Infection
- Necrotising fasciitis: See Chapter 4
- Ecthyma gangrenosum: See Chapter 4

Vasculitis
- Treatment directed by internal physicians
- See Chapter 54

Drug
- Withdraw anticoagulant
- Treatment directed by haematology & internal physicians

Other
- Pyoderma gangrenosum See Chapter 21
- Calciphylaxis See Chapter 85

DIC, disseminated intravascular coagulopathy; APL, antiphospholipid syndrome; ANCA, anti-neutrophil cytoplasmic antibody.

PART 11: SYSTEMIC DISEASE AND THE SKIN

Widespread Pustules in adults

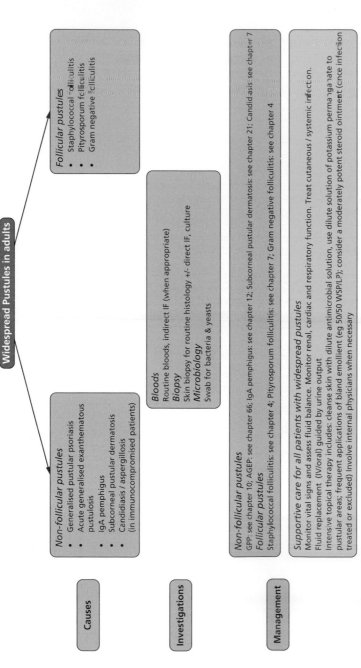

Causes

Non-follicular pustules
- Generalised pustular psoriasis
- Acute generalised exanthematous pustulosis
- IgA pemphigus
- Subcorneal pustular dermatosis
- Candidiasis / aspergillosis (in immunocompromised patients)

Follicular pustules
- Staphylococcal folliculitis
- Pityrosporum folliculitis
- Gram negative folliculitis

Investigations

Bloods
Routine bloods, indirect IF (when appropriate)
Biopsy
Skin biopsy for routine histology +/- direct IF, culture
Microbiology
Swab for bacteria & yeasts

Management

Non-follicular pustules
GPP: see chapter 10; AGEP: see chapter 66; IgA pemphigus: see chapter 12; Subcorneal pustular dermatosis: see chapter 21; Candidiasis: see chapter 7
Follicular pustules
Staphylococcal folliculitis: see chapter 4; Pityrosporum folliculitis: see chapter 7; Gram negative folliculitis: see chapter 4

Supportive care for all patients with widespread pustules
Monitor vital signs and assess fluid balance. Monitor renal, cardiac and respiratory function. Treat cutaneous / systemic infection.
Fluid replacement (IV/oral) guided by urine output
Intensive topical therapy includes: cleanse skin with dilute antimicrobial solution, use dilute solution of potassium permanganate to pustular areas; frequent applications of bland emollient (eg 50/50 WSP/LP); consider a moderately potent steroid ointment (once infection treated or excluded) Involve internal physicians when necessary

GPP, generalised pustular psoriasis; AGEP, acute generalised exanthematous pustulosis; 50/50 WSP/LP, 50% white soft paraffin/50% liquid paraffin.

Differential diagnosis

In this chapter, commonly occurring dermatological presentations are used as the starting point for a framework to aid the thought process involved in distinguishing between potential diagnoses. The purpose is to aid diagnosis in the clinical setting, providing a quick reference guide, and the flow diagrams are not intended to be exhaustive. The reader is encouraged to refer back to the relevant Handbook chapter for more information and representative clinical images.

Rook's Dermatology Handbook, First Edition. Edited by Christopher E. M. Griffiths, Tanya O. Bleiker, Daniel Creamer, John R. Ingram and Rosalind C. Simpson.
© 2022 John Wiley & Sons Ltd. Published 2022 by John Wiley & Sons Ltd.

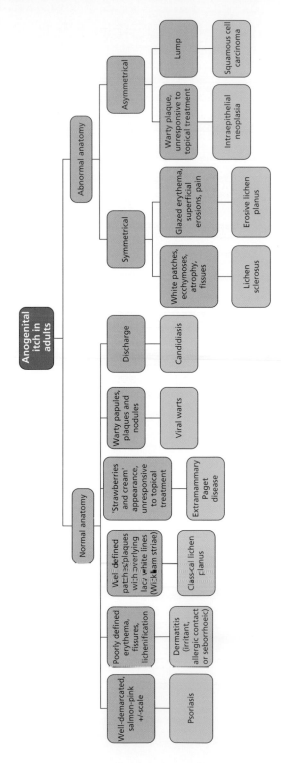

Figure 87.1 Differential diagnosis of anogenital itch in adults.

NB: Candidiasis may occur on its own or in conjunction with an inflammatory dermatosis.

NB: Intraepithelial neoplasia or squamous cell carcinoma may occur with normal anatomy if they do not arise from a background of an inflammatory dermatosis

See Chapter 61 for management of anogenital conditions.

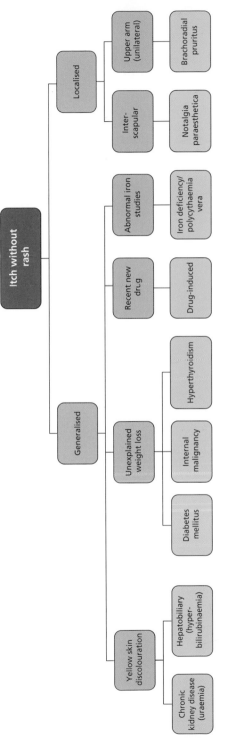

Figure 87.2 Differential diagnosis of itch without rash.

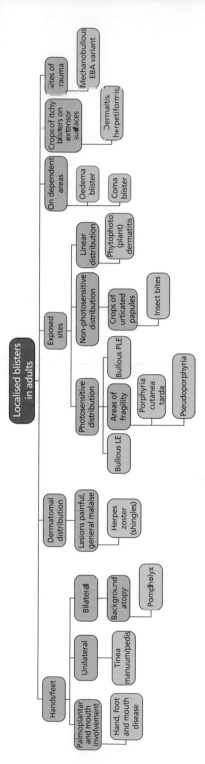

Figure 87.3 Differential diagnosis of localised blisters in adults. EBA, epidermolysis bullosa acquisita; LE lupus erythematosus.

Box 87.1 Other causes of localised blisters without specific site distribution

- Episodic recurring in same site
  - Crops of vesicles, painful: Herpes simplex virus
  - Single or few lesions, central blister: Fixed drug eruption
- Due to external agents
  - Drug-induced bullous dermatoses
  - Friction blisters
  - PUVA-induced acrobullous dermatosis
  - Bullous lichen planus
  - Bullous morphea
  - Burns, e.g. thermal, caustic
  - Dermatitis artefacta
- Metabolic disorders
  - Diabetic bullae (bullous diabeticorum)
  - Bullous amyloidosis (rare)
- Occurs in area of cellulitis
  - Bullous cellulitis
- Urticated itchy lesions that develop blisters
  - Localised bullous pemphigoid
  - Linear IgA bullous dermatosis
  - Flaccid blisters, spread rapidly
  - Bullous impetigo

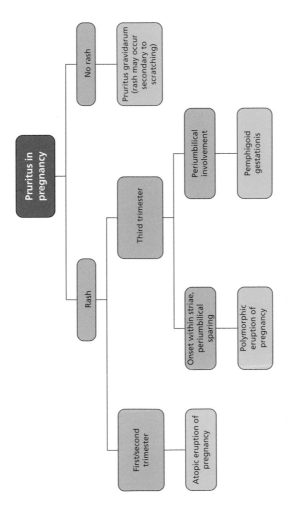

Figure 87.4 Differential diagnosis of pruritus in pregnancy. See Chapter 62 for management of pruritus in pregnancy.

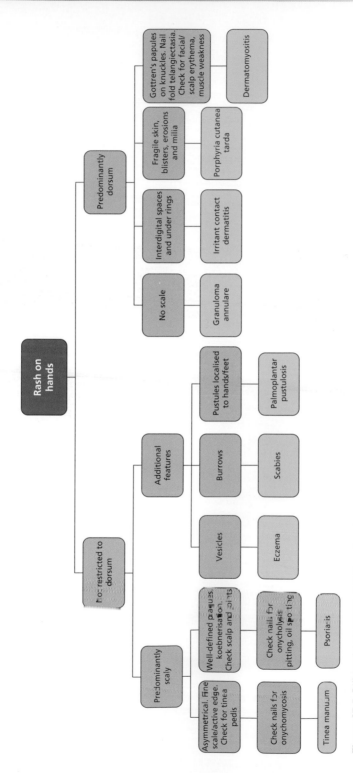

Figure 87.5 Differential diagnosis of rash on hands.

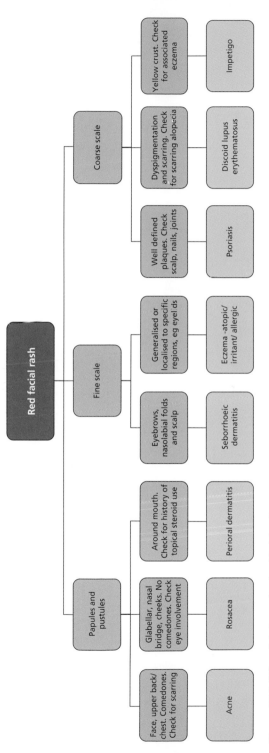

Figure 87.6 Differential diagnosis of red facial rash.

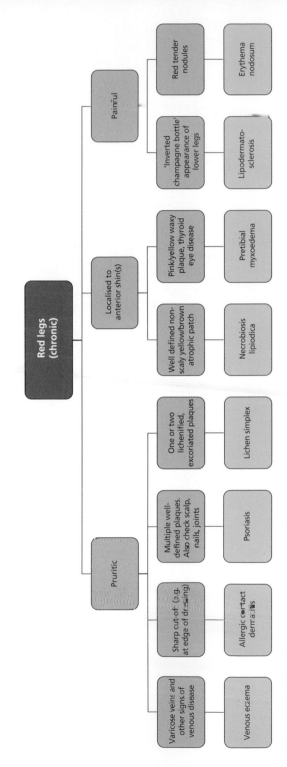

Figure 87.7 Differential diagnosis of chronic red legs.

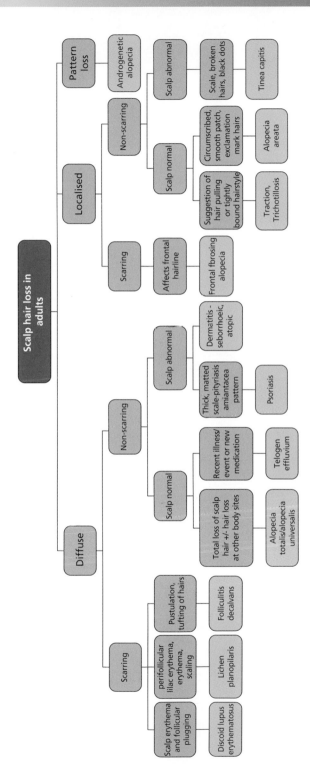

Figure 87.8 Differential diagnosis of scalp hair loss in adults.
See Chapter 31 for management of hair loss in adults.

88 Drugs in dermatology

Many systemic drugs are used off-licence within dermatological practice. Due to potential international differences we have not specified the licensed indications within this chapter. Local guidelines should be followed with regard to vaccination (e.g. varicella) and prophylaxis (e.g. influenza, COVID-19) where relevant.

The authors gratefully acknowledge the local systemic treatment guidelines shared by Dr Sarah Cockayne and team at Sheffield Teaching Hospitals, which have been adapted for this chapter.

Acitretin

Dose	Oral medication, up to 1 mg/day in a single dose, ideally taken with fatty foods
Mode of action	Retinoid (vitamin A-related), major metabolite of etretinate, inhibiting excessive keratinocyte proliferation via retinoid receptors
Indications	Psoriasis, palmoplantar pustulosis, ichthyosis, Darier disease Also considered for lichen planus, lichen sclerosus, lupus erythematous, palmoplantar keratoderma, extensive warts, cutaneous SCC prevention in immunosuppressed
Most important things to counsel patient about	Women must avoid pregnancy and breast-feeding during treatment and for 3 years afterwards due to teratogenicity Photosensitivity and need for increased sun protection Skin dryness and fragility likely to occur – avoid physical hair removal methods Avoid blood donation during treatment and for 3 years afterwards
Contraindications	Inability to attend for monitoring Pregnancy/breast-feeding Hyperlipidaemia, hepatic and renal impairment
Interactions	Tetracyclines (increases risk of benign intracranial hypertension) Drugs for diabetes (increased risk hypoglycaemia) Vitamin A (potential for vitamin A overdose) Warfarin/nicoumalone (reduced anticoagulant effect) Excessive alcohol, carbamazepine, keratolytics, methotrexate, phenytoin, progestogen-only contraceptives
Adverse effects	Hyperlipidaemia (especially hypertriglyceridaemia), dry skin, dryness of lip and conjunctival mucous membranes, epistaxis, paronychia, hair dryness and thinning or alopecia, myalgia, arthralgia and bone pain, premature epiphyseal fusion in children, headache, hepatitis, decreased night vision
Baseline investigations	Pregnancy test and written consent for women of child-bearing potential (acitretin usually avoided in this patient group), U+E, LFT, fasting lipids, HbA1c
Monitoring requirements	U&E, LFT, fasting lipids: at 4 weeks, 12 weeks and 3–4 monthly thereafter; monthly pregnancy test for women of child-bearing potential; frequent blood glucose monitoring in those with diabetes
Actions in the event of abnormal monitoring/ adverse effects	Severe headache (especially early morning), vomiting or visual disturbance: discontinue, may need neurology referral ?raised intracranial pressure Persistently elevated LFTs: increased frequency of monitoring; stop acitretin if ALT or AST >3× upper limit and consider hepatology referral Persistently elevated fasting lipids: dietary advice and GP to consider statin; stop acitretin if triglycerides >6 Pregnancy: stop drug immediately; confirm with pregnancy test; refer to specialist teratogenicity obstetric services

Rook's Dermatology Handbook, First Edition. Edited by Christopher E. M. Griffiths, Tanya O. Bleiker, Daniel Creamer, John R. Ingram and Rosalind C. Simpson.
© 2022 John Wiley & Sons Ltd. Published 2022 by John Wiley & Sons Ltd.

Apremilast

Dose	Oral medication, 30 mg twice daily At onset, gradual dose increments over 7-day period, starting with 10 mg once daily, supplied as induction pack
Mode of action	Inhibitor of phosphodiesterase 4 enzyme
Indications	Moderate to severe chronic plaque psoriasis (also licensed for active psoriatic arthritis unresponsive to first-line systemic therapy)
Most important things to counsel patient about	Gastrointestinal adverse effects are common, particularly during treatment initiation Apremilast increases the risk of depression and, uncommonly, suicidal ideation Ensure women of child-bearing potential are using effective contraception
Contraindications	Inability to attend for monitoring Pregnancy/breast-feeding: teratogenic in animal studies
Interactions	Avoid concomitant use with the following due to reduced apremilast plasma concentrations: carbamazepine, phenobarbital, phenytoin, rifampicin, St John's wort
Adverse effects	Common: gastrointestinal (nausea, vomiting, decreased appetite, dyspepsia, diarrhoea, gastroesophageal reflux, upper abdominal pain) Uncommon: weight loss, depression, suicidal ideation
Baseline investigations	Psychiatric history must be taken from all patients Pregnancy test if appropriate
Monitoring requirements	Monitor weight, mood and response to treatment, check ongoing effective contraception in women if relevant
Actions in the event of abnormal monitoring/ adverse effects	Depression: link with patient's GP and consider dose reduction/discontinuation Suicidal ideation: stop apremilast; immediate referral to psychiatry Severe weight loss: stop apremilast

ROOK'S DERMATOLOGY HANDBOOK

Azathioprine

Dose	Oral medication, 1–3 mg/kg daily for normal TPMT enzyme levels Dose for intermediate TPMT level 0.5–1 mg/kg; this lower dose is also used in the elderly and if renal/hepatic impairment Avoid azathioprine in those with low TPMT level
Mode of action	Inhibits purine metabolism, limiting synthesis of DNA and RNA Suppresses both T-cell and B-cell production, impacting cellular and humoral immunity
Indications	Atopic dermatitis, bullous pemphigoid, chronic actinic dermatitis, dermatomyositis, pemphigus, pityriasis rubra pilaris, pyoderma gangrenosum, SLE, vasculitis, granulomatosis with polyangiitis
Most important things to counsel patient about	Hypersensitivity reaction causing acute flu-like illness involving dizziness, malaise, vomiting, diarrhoea and arthralgia possible during initiation and requires treatment to be stopped immediately Excessive bone marrow suppression may be indicated by easy bruising or sudden-onset mouth ulcers: seek medical advice and check FBC Avoid live vaccines Flu vaccination encouraged Azathioprine may be prescribed in pregnancy and breast-feeding if the severity of the dermatosis/disorder warrants continuation of its use
Contraindications	Inability to attend for monitoring Hypersensitivity Severe infection/recent live vaccines Severe liver impairment/bone marrow suppression Very low or absent TPMT activity
Interactions	Allopurinol (relatively contraindicated), ACE inhibitors, aminosalicylates, clozapine, co-trimoxazole, febuxostat, live vaccines, phenytoin, ribavirin, trimethoprim, warfarin
Adverse effects	Hypersensitivity reaction, bone marrow suppression, hepatitis and cholestatic jaundice, gastrointestinal disturbances-nausea/vomiting, increased susceptibility to infections in combination with prednisolone, acute pancreatitis (extremely rare), increased risks of lymphoma and skin cancers in other patient groups but not currently documented in inflammatory dermatoses
Baseline investigations	FBC, U&E, LFT, TPMT level, virology screen (hepatitis B, C, HIV, varicella), pregnancy test if appropriate Consider varicella vaccination if not immune (but will delay treatment because live vaccine)
Monitoring requirements	FBC, U&E, LFTs weekly for first month, then monthly thereafter and 3-monthly when stable If dose increased, repeat bloods after 2 weeks Initial monitoring more frequent if TPMT level intermediate
Actions in the event of abnormal monitoring/adverse effects	Hypersensitivity reaction: stop drug Falling FBC parameters (even if still out of normal range); temporary treatment cessation and discuss with haematology Gastrointestinal disturbance: if early in treatment may be helped by gradual dose escalation Increased mean cell volume: check B12, folate and TFTs and discuss with haematology if continues to rise Elevated LFTs: moderate derangement: dose reduction; AST/ALT ×2 normal: stop drug Severe infection: stop drug, at least temporarily Contact with chickenpox or shingles in those non-immune: consider varicella immunoglobulin Acute abdominal pain/vomiting: check serum amylase

Anti-IL-17 biologics

Dose	Variable and dependent on biologic All SC Secukinumab 300 mg weekly to 4 weeks, then 4-weekly Ixekizumab 160 mg week 0, 80 mg week 2 to week 12, then 80 mg 4-weekly Brodalumab 210 mg at 0, 1 and 2 weeks, then 210 mg 2-weekly
Mode of action	Secukinumab and ixekizumab bind and inhibit the action of IL-17A Brodalumab binds the IL-17 receptor and inhibits IL-17 in general
Indications	Psoriasis
Most important things to counsel patient about	Increased risk of infection Avoid live vaccines Recommend pneumococcal and annual flu vaccine Keep up to date with screening tests, e.g. cervical smear test, mammograms Injection site reactions Candidiasis Exacerbation or induction of inflammatory bowel disease
Contraindications	Active infection and latent TB until treated Pregnancy/breast-feeding
Interactions	No drug interactions but caution if used in combination with other immunomodulators
Adverse effects	Infection, increased risk of malignancy Atopic eczema, asthma Candidiasis Neutropenia Inflammatory bowel disease
Baseline investigations	FBC, U&E, LFT, CXR, ANA, virology screen (hepatitis B, C, HIV, varicella), IGRA Physical examination Discussion about family history of inflammatory bowel disease
Monitoring	FBC, U&E, LFT: every 3 months Annual review with repeat IGRA If pregnant: individual advice but low risk for first and second trimesters
Actions in the event of abnormal monitoring/ adverse effects	Rising LFTs: no action unless 2× upper limit of normal Infection: stop drug until resolved Neutropenia: stop drug Positive IGRA: TB treatment according to local guidelines

Anti-IL-23 biologics

Dose	Variable and dependent on biologic All SC Guselkumab 100 mg at weeks 0 and 4, then 8-weekly Risankizumab 150 mg at weeks 0 and 4, then 12-weekly Tildrakizumab 100 mg at weeks 0 and 4, then 12-weekly; consider 200mg dose if bodyweight ≥ 90 Kg
Mode of action	Inhibit IL-23 by binding to p19 subunit
Indications	Psoriasis
Most important things to counsel patient about	Increased risk of infection, including TB Avoid live vaccines Recommend pneumococcal vaccine and annual flu vaccine Keep up to date with screening tests, e.g., cervical smear test, mammograms Injection site reactions
Contraindications	Active infection and latent TB until treated Pregnancy/breast-feeding
Interactions	No drug interactions but caution if used in combination with other immunomodulators
Adverse effects	Infection, possible increased risk of malignancy Atopic eczema, asthma Cutaneous adverse drug reactions
Baseline investigations	FBC, U&E, LFT, CXR, ANA, virology screen (hepatitis B, C, HIV, varicella), IGRA Physical examination
Monitoring	FBC, U&E, LFT: every 3 months Annual review with repeat IGRA If pregnant: individual advice but low risk for first and second trimesters
Actions in the event of abnormal monitoring/ adverse effects	Rise in LFTs: no action unless 2× upper limit Infection: stop drug until resolved Positive IGRA: TB treatment according to local guidelines

Anti-TNF biologics

Dose	Variable depending on drug and disease
	Adalimumab SC:
	  Psoriasis: 80 mg week 0, 40 mg week 1, 40 mg 2-weekly
	  Hidradenitis suppurativa: 160 mg week 0, 80 mg week 2, 40 mg weekly
	Etanercept SC: 50 mg once weekly
	Infliximab IV: 5 mg/kg week 0, week 4 then 8-weekly

Mode of action	Inhibition of TNF Adalimumab and infliximab are neutralising antibodies for TNF Etanercept is a soluble receptor for TNF
Indications	Etanercept: psoriasis Adalimumab: psoriasis, hidradenitis suppurativa, pyoderma gangrenosum Infliximab: psoriasis, hidradenitis suppurativa, pyoderma gangrenosum, generalised pustulosis
Most important things to counsel patient about	Increased risk of infection, especially TB Risk of demyelination Exacerbation of cardiac failure Avoid live vaccines and soft cheeses Recommend pneumococcal vaccine and annual flu vaccine Keep up to date with screening tests, e.g. cervical smear test, mammograms Infliximab: anaphylaxis, infusion reactions Adalimumab and etanercept: injection site reactions
Contraindications	Active infection and latent TB until treated Personal or family history of demyelination Pregnancy/breast-feeding Cardiac failure New York Heart Association grade III/IV
Interactions	No drug interactions but caution if used with other immunomudulators
Adverse effects	Infection, exacerbation of pre-existing cardiac failure, increased risk of malignancy, demyelination Atopic eczema, asthma Agranulocytosis
Baseline investigations	FBC, U&E, LFT, CXR, ANA, virology screen (hepatitis B, C, HIV, varicella), IGRA Physical examination
Monitoring	FBC, U&E, LFT: every 3 months Annual review with repeat IGRA If pregnant: individual advice but low risk for first and second trimesters
Actions in the event of abnormal monitoring/ adverse effects	Rise in LFTs: no action unless 2× upper limit of normal Infection: stop drug until resolved Positive IGRA: TB treatment according to local guidelines

Ustekinumab

Dose	SC 45 mg (<100 kg) or 90 mg (≥100 kg) at weeks 0 and 4, then 12-weekly
Mode of action	Inhibits IL-12 and IL-23 by binding to common p40 subunit
Indications	Psoriasis Pityriasis rubra pilaris
Most important things to counsel patient about	Increased risk of infection, including TB Avoid live vaccines Recommend pneumococcal vaccine and annual flu vaccine Keep up to date with screening tests, e.g. cervical smear test, mammograms Injection site reactions
Contraindications	Active infection and latent TB until treated Pregnancy/breast-feeding
Interactions	No drug interactions but caution if used in combination with other immunomodulators
Adverse effects	Infection, possible increased risk of malignancy Atopic eczema, asthma Cutaneous adverse drug reactions
Baseline investigations	FBC, U&E, LFT, CXR, ANA, virology screen (hepatitis B, C, HIV, varicella), IGRA Physical examination
Monitoring	FBC, U&E, LFT: every 3 months Annual review with repeat IGRA If pregnant: individual advice but low risk for first and second trimesters
Actions in the event of abnormal monitoring/ adverse effects	Rise in LFTs: no action unless 2× upper limit Infection: stop drug until resolved Positive IGRA: TB treatment according to local guidelines

Ciclosporin

Dose	Oral 2.5–5 mg/kg daily in two divided doses Short term: 6 months
Mode of action	Calcineurin inhibition: inhibits T-cell activation
Indications	Psoriasis, atopic eczema, urticaria, alopecia areata, lichen planus, pyoderma gangrenosum, Behcet disease, prurigo nodularis, palmo-plantar pustulosis
Most important things to counsel patient about	Do not take with grapefruit juice (impairs absorption) Avoid live vaccines Be aware of potential drug interactions Headache
Contraindications	Hypertension (uncontrolled) Breast-feeding, malignancy, lymphoproliferative disease Active infection Impaired renal function Severely impaired hepatic function Concomitant phototherapy
Interactions	Many drug interactions, mainly on account of shared cytochrome P450 metabolism, including carbamazepine, phenytoin, St John's Wort, macrolide antibiotics, erythromycin, clarithromycin, azole antifungals, calcium antagonists, metoclopramide, oral contraceptives, danazol, allopurinol, statins, amiodarone, NSAIDs, digoxin, potassium sparing diuretics, potassium supplements, ACE inhibitors
Adverse effects	Hypertension, nephrotoxicity, hyperlipidaemia, hyperuricemia, hypomagnesaemia, gastrointestinal upset, gingival hypertrophy, hepatic dysfunction, myalgia, fatigue, muscle cramps, tremor, headache, paraesthesia Rarely: haemolytic anaemia, gynaecomastia, pancreatitis, lymphoproliferative disease, acceleration or reactivation of malignancy
Baseline investigations	FBC, U&E (creatinine two separate occasions), LFT, urate, lipids and HbA1C Blood pressure (two separate occasions), local guidelines for breast, prostate and cervical cancer screening if indicated Pre-immunosuppression virology screen (hepatitis B and C, HIV and varicella)
Monitoring requirements	Serum creatinine, U&Es, eGFR and blood pressure every 2 weeks for first 2 months FBC and blood lipids 3-monthly
Actions in the event of abnormal monitoring/ adverse effects	Maintain blood pressure below 140/90 If creatinine rises by 25% above baseline reduce dose by 1 mg/kg/day (even if still within normal range)

Dapsone

Dose	Start at 50 mg od and increase by 50 mg increments according to response Maximum dose is 300 mg/day
Mode of action	Dapsone has anti-inflammatory activity via the suppression of neutrophil recruitment and neutrophil function It is also an antimicrobial agent, being structurally related to the sulphonamide antibiotics
Indications	In dermatology dapsone is used primarily in the treatment of dermatitis herpetiformis Also used in linear IgA disease, chronic bullous disease of childhood, erythema elevatum diutinum, granuloma faciale, Sweet syndrome, Behcet disease, subcorneal pustular dermatosis, cutaneous small vessel vasculitis, pyoderma gangrenosum, acne conglobata and pyoderma faciale Dapsone is licensed for the treatment of leprosy
Most important things to counsel patient about	The rash of dermatitis herpetiformis is gluten sensitive; adherence to a gluten-free diet can reduce dapsone requirements Patients must report any medical condition which might reflect bone marrow suppression
Contraindications	Severe G6PD deficiency, anaemia, severe ischaemic heart disease, chronic respiratory problems, adverse reactions to sulphonamides, acute porphyria
Interactions	Trimethoprim: raised dapsone levels Cimetidine: raised dapsone levels Probenecid: raised dapsone levels Rifampicin: reduced dapsone levels
Adverse effects	Haemolytic anaemia, sometimes catastrophic (increased risk with G6PD deficiency) Also methaemoglobinaemia, agranulocytosis, severe hypersensitivity reactions (including SJS/TEN and DRESS)
Baseline investigations	FBC, reticulocyte count, renal function, liver function tests, G6PD levels
Monitoring requirements	FBC, reticulocyte count, renal function, liver function tests: weekly for first month, then monthly for 2 months, then 3-monthly Methaemoglobin levels if patient is developing breathlessness, headache, lethargy, cyanosis
Actions in the event of abnormal monitoring/ adverse effects	Adverse effects of dapsone can be life threatening At any sign of haemolytic anaemia, hypersensitivity reaction, or significant methaemoglobinaemia: stop dapsone If methaemoglobinaemia is severe, administer oxygen and IV 1% methylene blue solution (which will restore iron in haemoglobin to the reduced state, its oxygen carrying state)

Dupilumab

Dose	SC administration Weight >60 kg: 600 mg week 0, 300 mg 2-weekly Weight <60 kg: 400 mg week 0, 200 mg 2-weekly
Mode of action	Inhibits IL-4 and IL-13
Indications	Atopic dermatitis
Most important things to counsel patient about	Increased risk of infection Avoid live vaccines Recommend pneumococcal vaccine and annual flu vaccine Keep up to date with screening tests, e.g. cervical smear test, mammograms Injection site reactions
Contraindications	Active infection Pregnancy/breast-feeding
Interactions	No drug interactions but caution if used in combination with other immunomodulators
Adverse effects	Ophthalmic inflammation Ocular pruritus Conjunctivitis and allergic conjunctivitis Oral herpes simplex infection Eosinophilia Serum sickness
Baseline investigations	FBC, U&E, LFT, virology screen (hepatitis B, C, HIV, varicella)
Monitoring	FBC, U&E, LFT: every 3 months Annual review If pregnant: individual advice
Actions in the event of abnormal monitoring/ adverse effects	Infection or conjunctivitis: stop dupilumab until resolved

Fumaric acid esters/dimethyl fumarate

Dose	Start at 30 mg od in week 1, increasing to 30 mg bd in week 2 and 30 mg tds in week 3 In week 4 increase dose to 120 mg od, increasing to 120 mg bd in week 5, 120 mg tds in week 6 In week 7 240 mg, 120 mg, 120 mg (am, midday, nocte), week 8 240 mg, 120 mg, 240 mg, week 9 240 mg, 240 mg, 240 mg and maintain at this dose
Mode of action	The immunomodulation of FAEs is effected by release of IL-10 from cutaneous dendritic cells instead of IL-12 and IL-23 This leads to Th2 cell activation and production of Il 4
Indications	FAEs are used to treat moderate-to-severe psoriasis FAEs have also been used in the treatment of sarcoidosis, disseminated granuloma annulare and necrobiosis lipoidica
Most important things to counsel patient about	A slow onset of therapeutic action is usual with FAEs (6 weeks to several months)
Contraindications	Pregnancy and breast-feeding, severe liver or renal impairment, active symptomatic gastrointestinal disease (e.g. peptic ulceration)
Interactions	None known
Adverse effects	Abdominal pain and diarrhoea are common dose-dependent adverse effects Patients may experience flushing and headaches Lymphopenia may occur Liver tests need to monitored for hepatic dysfunction Progressive multifocal leukoencephalopathy has been reported with FAEs
Baseline investigations	FBC, renal function, liver function tests, urinalysis
Monitoring requirements	FBC, renal function, liver function tests: 2-weekly for first 3 months, then monthly
Actions in the event of abnormal monitoring / adverse effects	Gastrointestinal adverse effects will diminish with dose reduction and when taking FAEs with milk Lymphopenia and liver enzyme abnormalities reverse with dose reduction or drug cessation

Hydroxychloroquine

Dose	Start at 200 mg od or 400 mg od Maintenance dose is 200 mg od, or 400 mg od, or 200 and 400 mg on alternate days Maximum dose of HCQ is 6.5 mg/kg/day ideal body weight
Mode of action	Anti-inflammatory action via inhibition of TLR9 and TLR7, which in turn down-regulate expression of TNF-α and type 1 interferons
Indications	Used in the treatment of the skin features of DLE, subacute LE and systemic LE HCQ also has efficacy in the management of fatigue and arthralgia in SLE Other indications for HCQ are sarcoidosis, Jessner's lymphocytic infiltrate, reticulate erythematous mucinosis syndrome, urticarial vasculitis, lichen planus
Most important things to counsel patient about	An annual ophthalmic examination at an optician (including a retinal assessment) is recommended Report any change in vision
Contraindications	Pre-existing maculopathy Severe liver or renal impairment
Interactions	Amiodarone: increased risk of ventricular arrhythmias Digoxin: raised digoxin levels Ciclosporin: raised ciclosporin levels Antacids: reduced HCQ absorption
Adverse effects	Irreversible retinopathy (bulls-eye maculopathy) Risk is related to long-term exposure to HCQ (>5 years) Causes central scotoma, decreased visual acuity and loss of peripheral visual fields Other HCQ adverse effects include gastrointestinal disturbance, skin pigmentation, headache, psychosis
Baseline investigations	FBC, renal function, liver function tests, visual acuity: if there are acuity problems refer to ophthalmology
Monitoring requirements	Monitor visual acuity annually; refer to ophthalmology if there is decreased acuity or blurred vision The American Academy of Ophthalmology recommends annual ophthalmology screening after 5 years of HCQ treatment
Actions in the event of abnormal monitoring / adverse effects	Stop HCQ with any new visual disturbance Only restart HCQ following a satisfactory ophthalmological review Many patients receive HCQ only during the spring and summer months to reduce cumulative drug exposure

Isotretinoin

Dose	Oral medication, up to 1.0 mg/kg per day in a single dose taken with fatty foods for 4–6 months Duration adjusted to give at least 90% clearance of acne followed by 4–8 weeks of consolidation
Mode of action	Reduces sebum production, influences comedogenesis, lowers surface and ductal *Propionibacterium acnes* and has anti-inflammatory properties
Indications	Severe acne that has failed to respond to antibiotic therapies Resistant rosacea
Most important things to counsel patient about	Women of childbearing potential must be counselled about teratogenicity; must not become pregnant during or for 1 month after treatment Mental health issues: psychiatric referral if significant depression Do not donate blood during and for at least 1 month after treatment Avoid waxing/dermabrasion during and for 6 months after treatment Long-term risks on night vision with patients who drive for a living Some brands contain peanut and soya oil Sun protection (more likely to burn) Intolerance of contact lenses
Contraindications	Inability to attend for monitoring, pregnancy/breast-feeding, hepatic impairment, uncontrolled hyperlipidaemia, hypervitaminosis A, airline pilots Allergy to soya bean
Interactions	Tetracyclines (increases risk of benign intracranial hypertension), vitamin A Refer to Drug Formulary for full list
Adverse effects	Dryness of nasal, buccal, lip or conjunctival mucous membranes/epistaxis Nail fragility and paronychia Teratogenic Psychiatric disorders, very rarely suicide reported Arthralgia, myalgia Photophobia, impaired night vision Headaches Raised lipids, hepatitis, anaemia, neutropenia
Baseline investigations	Pregnancy prevention programme as per local guidelines Liver enzymes and lipids
Monitoring requirements	Liver enzymes and lipids repeated at 1 month and 3-monthly during treatment Monthly pregnancy test and 5 weeks post treatment in women of childbearing potential Mood assessed each visit
Actions in the event of abnormal monitoring / adverse effects	Intracranial hypertension: discontinue if severe headache If AST/ALT >3 times upper limit, discontinue isotretinoin Triglyceride above or approaching 6, stop treatment Pregnancy: stop drug immediately; refer to teratology/obstetric services Mood change: drug may need reducing or discontinuing

Methotrexate

Dose	Oral/subcutaneous 2.5–25 mg once weekly Test dose of 2.5 mg as first dose may be given Dose adjusted according to response Folic acid 5 mg once weekly not on the same day as methotrexate; 6 days per week if nausea
Mode of action	Inhibits the enzyme dihydrofolate reductase, essential for purine and pyrimidine synthesis
Indications	Psoriasis, eczema, pemphigus/pemphigoid, sarcoidosis, scleroderma, CTCL stage ≥IIB, lymphomatoid papulosis, SLE/cutaneous lupus
Most important things to counsel patient about	Once weekly medication Report immediately: blood disorders (sore throat, bruising, mouth ulcers), liver toxicity (nausea, vomiting, dark urine, abdominal pain), respiratory effects (cough, shortness of breath), gastrointestinal toxicity (stomatitis) If have coincidental diarrhoea and vomiting:omit treatment until symptoms subside No live vaccines Other members of house cannot have polio vaccine
Contraindications	Dialysis (greater risk of fatal pancytopenia), severe renal impairment (eGFR less than 20 ml/min), active hepatitis (B/C) or TB, alcohol excess, severe hepatic dysfunction/ cirrhosis, pregnancy/breast-feeding/wishing to conceive (avoid conception for 6 months after cessation in both genders), bone marrow failure, pulmonary fibrosis
Interactions	Alcohol <4–6 units per week or abstention Sulphonamides, trimethoprim and phenytoin increase toxicity Azathioprine, statins, tetracyclines, aspirin, NSAIDs, penicillin, probenecid and ciclosporin Check drug formulary for full list
Adverse effects	Gastrointestinal (e.g. nausea, mouth ulceration, anorexia, dyspepsia), bone marrow suppression, hepatitis/liver fibrosis, pulmonary fibrosis
Baseline investigations	FBC, U&E, LFTs, B12, folate Procollagen III/PIIINP if treating psoriasis (without psoriatic arthritis) CXR if >40 years old and smoker or symptoms present Pre-immunosuppression virology screen (includes hepatitis B, C, HIV and varicella) TB testing if suspected Methotrexate patient information and monitoring booklet
Monitoring requirements	LFTs, FBC and U&E at 1, 2, 4, 6, 10 and 14 weeks, 3-monthly thereafter, 2-monthly if renal impairment, comorbidity, advanced age, concomitant NSAIDs Procollagen III/PIIINP 3-monthly if psoriasis
Actions in the event of abnormal monitoring / adverse effects	FBC: Hb drop of more than 10 g/L, WCC $< 3 \times 10^{-9}$/L, neutrophils $<1.0 \times 10^{-9}$/L or platelets <100, withhold/decrease treatment If acute toxicity urgent folinic acid rescue Elevated LFTs: AST and ALT less than twice normal, repeat in 2–4 weeks ALT and AST more than twice normal may require reduction or cessation of methotrexate Albumin: stop drug if unexplained fall PIIINP: If pre-treatment >8 µg/mL, three samples >4.2 µg/mL in a 12-month period, two samples >8 µg/mL or one sample >10 µg/mL consider referral to hepatology for fibroscan Severe renal impairment: withhold methotrexate and give folinic acid rescue

Mycophenolate mofetil

Dose	Oral medication, 1–3 g/day in divided doses
Mode of action	Reversible inhibitor of inosine guanosine nucleotide synthesis leading to cytostatic effects on T and B lymphocytes
Indications	Atopic dermatitis, bullous pemphigoid, dermatomyositis/polymyositis, pemphigus vulgaris, psoriasis, pyoderma gangrenosum, SLE
Most important things to counsel patient about	Bone marrow suppression: seek medical advice for inexplicable bleeding or bruising, fever, sore throat, rash, mouth ulcers or purpura Teratogenic: advise against pregnancy, must not become pregnant for 6 weeks after stopping the drug Increased risk of skin cancer/need for sun protection Avoid live vaccines but recommended pneumococcal and annual flu vaccine Keep up to date with screening tests, e.g. cervical smear test
Contraindications	Inability to attend for monitoring Pregnancy/breast-feeding Infection Avoid live vaccines 2 weeks before and 6 months after treatment
Interactions	Antacids Antibiotics: metronidazole, norfloxacin, rifampicin Antivirals: aciclovir, ganciclovir Cholestyramine Clozapine Iron Phenytoin Probencid Sevelamer
Adverse effects	Anaemia/red cell aplasia, thrombocytopenia, leucopenia, gastrointestinal disturbances, increased risk malignancy
Baseline investigations	FBC, U&E, LFT, CXR, virology screen (hepatitis B, C, HIV, varicella)
Monitoring requirements	FBC, U&E, LFT: every week for 4 weeks, every 2 weeks for 2 months, monthly for 12 months and then every 3 months once dose is stabilised
Actions in the event of abnormal monitoring/ adverse effects	Hb drop of more than 1 g/100 mL, WCC or platelets below normal range suggests bone marrow suppression Discontinue if neutropenia develops (absolute neutrophil count $<1.3 \times 10^9$) Nausea, vomiting, diarrhoea: divide or reduce the daily dose Change from tablet to syrup formulation Rising LFTs: reduce dose or stop drug Severe infection: may need to stop drug Chickenpox, shingles or measles: if contact with these and patient not had in past, consider giving varicella immunoglobulin

Prednisolone

Dose	Oral medication, usually 0.5 mg/kg on tapering regimen Can use up to 1 mg/kg lean body weight (NB: Can be used as an IM depot injection)
Mode of action	A highly potent glucocorticoid steroid which has an anti-inflammatory effect
Indications	Short-term: inflammatory dermatoses, e.g. atopic eczema, lichen planus (use short course with tapering regimen) Long-term: SLE, blistering disorders, sarcoidosis, vasculitis, dermatomyositis (use lowest possible maintenance dose and consider steroid as early as possible)
Most important things to counsel patient about	Do not stop long-term steroids abruptly (risk of adrenal failure) Need for gastroprotection and bone density protection if using long term Avoid live vaccines
Contraindications	Inability to attend for monitoring Systemic infection Relative contraindications: pregnancy, breast-feeding, history of TB, hypertension, diabetes, thromboembolic disorders, recent myocardial infarction, congestive cardiac failure, osteoporosis, glaucoma, peptic ulcers, hypothyroidism, renal and hepatic impairment
Interactions	Multiple, e.g. many drugs in combination with prednisolone increase risk of hypokalaemia; many increase risk of gastrointestinal bleeding
Adverse effects	Acute pancreatitis, adrenal suppression, behavioural disorders and psychiatric disturbance, bruising, cataracts, congestive cardiac failure, diabetes mellitus, exacerbation of peptic ulcers, fluid and sodium retention, glaucoma, headaches, hirsuitism, hyperhidrosis, hypertension, increased susceptibility to infection, indigestion, joint pain (hip or knee avascular necrosis possible and serious), leucocytosis, malaise, mood change, muscle weakness, myocardial rupture following recent MI, nausea, osteoporosis, papilloedema, potassium and calcium loss, skin thinning, sleep disturbance, striae, vertigo, weight gain
Baseline investigations	Recommend FBC, U&E, LFT, glucose, blood pressure
Monitoring requirements	Blood pressure at each visit (if on higher doses) Repeat bone densitometry 2-yearly (or as per local protocol), FBC, U&E, glucose every 6 months if used long term
Actions in the event of abnormal monitoring/ adverse effects	Diastolic BP >95 mmHg on two occasions: arrange antihypertensive treatment Low Hb and reduced MCV suggestive of iron deficiency and gastrointestinal bleeding: arrange gastrointestinal review Raised plasma glucose: request diabetic advice Infection, acute illness or surgery: if on long-term steroids will need to increase dose

Index

Note: Page numbers with f denotes figure, t denotes table and b denotes box

Rook's Dermatology Handbook, First Edition. Edited by Christopher E. M. Griffiths, Tanya O. Bleiker, Daniel Creamer,
John R. Ingram and Rosalind C. Simpson.
© 2022 John Wiley & Sons Ltd. Published 2022 by John Wiley & Sons Ltd.